HISTOLOGY

SEVENTH EDITION

HISTOLOGY

Arthur W. Ham, M.B., F.R.S.C., D.Sc.

Professor Emeritus, Department of Anatomy,
Faculty of Medicine, University of Toronto

SEVENTH EDITION

J. B. Lippincott Company

Philadelphia and Toronto

Library of Congress Cataloging in Publication Data

Ham, Arthur Worth
 Histology.

  1. Histology. I. Title.
QM551.H147 1974   611'.018   74-7262
ISBN 0-397-52062-X

Preface

For those who are not familiar with any previous edition of this book it should be explained that this, like former ones, has been written not only for students in general but in particular for students who may not have had any previous acquaintance with the subject. This has required that it be written so as to permit a student of the latter type, or one who because of choice or necessity depends on self instruction, to begin reading on page 1 and read through the remainder of the book without encountering concepts or terms which are not explained as simply as possible when they are encountered. It is therefore hoped it will permit such a student to begin reading on page 1 with his vocabulary of terms and concepts being built up progressively as he continues to read.

Writing a textbook designed primarily for undergraduate students permits an author to more or less express his philosophy about teaching the subject with which the book deals. In this connection, my chief impression from teaching has been that perhaps the most important goal to achieve is to have students develop an interest in the subject. So in writing each edition of this book, I have tried to present the subject matter of histology in as interesting a way as possible. As a student, I found the course in histology that I took, which dealt exclusively with microscopic structure, extremely dull and I remembered almost nothing from it. I think furthermore that it is still not unusual for students, after their initial interest in looking down a microscope has waned, to find a course that confines itself to microscopic structure somewhat uninspiring. From teaching histology, I soon learned that students were much more interested in microscopic structure if it was learned about in relation to its function. Teaching structure in relation to function probably takes advantage of the inherent curiosity in all of us that led us as children to take our toys apart to see how they worked. In any event, the dual approach of describing microscopic structure in relation to function is used a good deal in this book, not only because it makes the subject more interesting but also because it makes it easier to learn. Microscopic structure is so admirably adapted to its function that with a knowledge of the tissues, a student who knows about the function of say, an organ, can almost anticipate the kind of structure it will be found to possess.

There are other helpful ways to teach or write about histology that makes the subject more interesting. If a student knows why he is studying a particular subject he is much more inclined to become interested enough in it to learn it well. In the instance of medical and paramedical students, it is comparatively easy to show them that knowing the histology of almost anything in the body is essential to their later understanding the disease processes that may affect it. This means that it arouses interest when, in describing the histology of polymorphonuclear leukocytes, one tells enough about inflammation for students to understand why they must learn about these particular cells. Likewise, the importance of learning about red blood cells is easily demonstrated if it is accompanied by a brief discussion of the anemias. Learning about the microscopic structure of bone can be made to seem worthwhile if a student realizes he must know about how new bone is formed and dead bone resorbed if he is to understand how a fracture heals or why there is such a condition as osteoporosis. Because this is so useful a way to stimulate the interest of students in learning histology, there are many examples of its application to the understanding of various disease conditions throughout the book.

From the foregoing it should be apparent that the author believes that, so far as is practicable, a discipline should be taught in a medical school so that its subject matter is easily integrated with what will be taught in more detail in other disciplines encountered later in the medical course.

Two other aims that I have had in this and previous editions might also be mentioned. First, structure at the microscopic and submicroscopic level presents an ever changing scene because so many processes are proceeding constantly in it. These have to be explained. If explanations are to be understood, they usually require the use of a good many words and if words seem to be required I do not think one should be stingy with them in the interest of brevity. Second, many research-minded students are interested not only in the impressive discoveries that have been made in biological science as, for example, that the physical basis of genes exists in DNA, but also in how knowledge developed in so many of the areas dealt with in histology, and, for this reason, in discussing various topics I often include sections headed "Development of Knowledge." These of course have a second advantage in that they provide a background for understanding the present state of knowledge that exists about these various topics.

Since this preface is supposed to describe not only the character of this book but also how this present (7th) edition differs from the previous one, brief comment will now be made on this matter.

First, some changes have been made in the order in which material is presented. In previous editions, most of the technics employed in histology were described in the first few chapters. However, by the time the last edition was written, these had become so numerous that to describe almost all of them at the beginning of the book made the first chapters somewhat dull, and I am grateful to Dr. Arthur Axelrad for suggesting that students would find different technics more interesting to read about if they were each placed in connection with the descriptions of the new information their use had elicited. So in this edition the various technics by which cells and other components of tissue are investigated are presented throughout the book with reference to the particular topic the study of which they facilitate.

This change permitted the book to be divided into 3 parts instead of 4 parts as formerly. The first 5 chapters now deal with the cell. The first chapter is relatively elementary and provides suitable instruction for a beginner to obtain a fairly well-rounded concept of the general structure of cells and how they are studied. The next 3 chapters (2, 3 and 4) deal with the nucleus. Chapter 2 contains a much more extensive account of mitosis than that of previous editions. It also deals in more detail with chromosome structure and with some of the more common chromosome anomalies and how they arise. My colleagues Drs. Axelrad and Kalnins were both most helpful in preparing this chapter. Chapter 3 is concerned chiefly with what happens in the S phase of the cell cycle and how it can be studied by radioautography and how the latter method can be used to study cell lineages. How the times required for the various stages of the cell cycle can be determined is also described. In Chapter 4 the interphase nucleus is considered in more detail and distinctions are made between the functions of extended and condensed chromatin. An account of protein synthesis as directed by genes is included and the formation of ribosomal RNA is described in connection with the nucleolus, which structure is dealt with in some detail. Chapter 5 presents a very extensive description of the organelles of cytoplasm, beginning with the cell membrane and ending with cell junctions. This chapter is much enlarged over previous editions and suitably illustrated by electron micrographs; many of the new ones were provided by my colleague Dr. V. I. Kalnins.

The theme then shifts from cells to the study of tissues; hence, Chapter 6 is appropriately entitled "From Cells to Tissues." It deals with the origin and development of the 4 basic tissues and explores the problem of cell differentiation to some extent, in particular the conditions essential for cell environment to influence cell differentiation. The problem of how genes are turned on or off is considered again here in addition to what was described about this in Chapter 4. The possible control of cell populations by chalones is also considered.

Chapter 7 deals with epithelial tissue and 8 and 9 with loose ordinary connective tissue. In the latter the concept and nature of intercellular substances and their formation are considered in some detail. The origin and nature of tissue fluid are described and why it accumulates so as to sometimes cause edema is also discussed.

In Chapter 9, after describing fibroblasts and the synthesis of collagen, and the structure and function of fat cells, a new theme is introduced by dealing with plasma cells. This theme, which is carried from here through to the end of Chapter 13, relates to the cellular basis for immunological reactions. As indicated above, it begins with the description of plasma cells and is carried along further in this chapter in relation to mast cells, macrophages and leukocytes which immigrate into loose connective tissue. This leads to the next chapter (10) which deals exclusively with leukocytes. Inflammation is described here and the role of polymorphonuclear leukocytes in this process is described. Lymphocytes are considered in detail and the respective roles of T and B types are dealt with extensively. The theme relating to immunology is briefly suspended in the next chapter which is concerned with red blood cells and platelets but it is resumed again in the two succeeding chapters (12 and 13) which deal with the hemopoietic tissues.

Perhaps there is no area in histology in which there have been more revolutionary changes in thinking than in connection with the formation of blood cells and in which more difficulties have arisen in connection with associating what was known or believed in the past with what is now apparent. Hence a great deal of time was spent on writing the chapter on myeloid tissue (12) and in explaining at least in part the developments that were concerned in providing for the new concepts. As might be expected, the nature of the stem cell that accounts for the formation of blood cells receives a good deal of consideration. Chapter 12 thus provides an excellent background for understanding how the cell populations of the various lymphatic organs—the thymus, lymph nodes and spleen, dealt with in Chapter 13 —are developed and maintained and the particular functions these different structures perform in the body.

The next chapter (14) deals with cartilage and the following one with bone. In this chapter the subject matter was rearranged to provide for better sequence and new material and illustrations were added. As usual, this chapter was written with many practical applications in mind. Chapter 16 is concerned with joints, and through the courtesy of Dr. R. B. Salter of the Department of Surgery, University of Toronto, I was able to include a description of some new and as yet unpublished research which shows that articular cartilage can be regenerated at sites of experimentally induced injuries.

At this point it might be mentioned that, in order to provide proper continuity from one chapter to the next and to ensure that what is discussed in any given chapter provides a proper background for the next, my way of revising the book is begin with chapter 1 and revise each successive chapter in turn. By the time I had finished Chapter 16 I realized that if I were to attempt to revise all the remaining chapters this edition would not see the light of day this summer as was planned. I therefore asked my good friend Dr. C. P. Leblond if he would assume responsibility for revising Chapters 18 (muscle tissue) and 22 (digestive system), a proposal to which he agreed, for which I am deeply grateful. Accordingly, credit for the revision of Chapter 18 is entirely due to Dr. Edward Schultz and Dr. C. P. Leblond of the Department of Anatomy, McGill University, and credit for the revision of Chapter 21 is due to Dr. Hershey Warshawsky, who revised the section on teeth, and to Dr. C. P. Leblond, who revised the part of the chapter dealing with the intestinal tract. Although there is more information in these chapters than I could have provided, I do not think the reader will notice any particular difference in the way it is presented, perhaps because Dr. Leblond had already read so many of the previous chapters in manuscript and provided me with comment on them, that he did not find it difficult to present the new material in these chapters in much the same manner.

Continuing with the chapters that I revised, that on nervous tissue (17) was changed a good deal, with much new material being added particularly with regard to the central nervous system. The systems were dealt with in the same order as in the previous edition. Changes were made when indicated in each of these, and in particular the chapter on the male reproductive system (27) was extensively altered. Because the descriptions of technics have been included in later chapters and certain chapters in the first half of the book have been combined, there are only 28 chapters in this edition instead of the 31 that were in the previous edition.

Arthur W. Ham

Acknowledgments

Three friends in particular helped to make this edition much better than it otherwise would have been: they are Dr. C. P. Leblond of McGill University and my colleagues, Dr. Arthur Axelrad and Dr. Vic Kalnins of the Department of Anatomy, University of Toronto.

As described in the preface, when time began to run out, I asked Dr. Leblond if he would assume responsibility for revising Chapters 18 and 21 for me which he most kindly did with the collaboration of Drs. E. Schultz and H. Warshawsky for the two chapters respectively. Furthermore, Dr. Leblond read the manuscript of most of the chapters in the first half of this edition and made many helpful suggestions about improving them and other chapters not yet begun. Dr. Axelrad assumed much responsibility not only in connection with the material in Chapter 2 that deals with chromosomes and chromosome anomalies but also with much of the extensive subject matter that deals with lymphocytes, the formation of blood cells and the immunological reactions that occur in the body; this material is to be found in Chapters 10 to 13 in this edition. I am most grateful for this help. I am greatly indebted also to Dr. Vic Kalnins who was of the greatest assistance in preparing both the account of mitosis in Chapter 2 and that dealing with the organelles of cytoplasm in Chapter 5; the number of his illustrations that appear in this chapter is indicative of the breadth of his assistance. I am also grateful to him for allowing me to encroach on his time in preparing this edition whenever any topic arose about which some consultation would be helpful. In a similar connection I thank Dr. David McLeod for much constructive comment on the book as it applies to a student's needs.

I received much help and new illustrations from Dr. G. T. Simon and Dr. S. C. Luk in connection with the hemopoietic tissues. Furthermore, Dr. Luk helped in many other areas as well with the greatest goodwill. Dr. Carl Grant read the manuscript of the chapter on bone and made most helpful suggestions. I thank Dr. R. B. Salter for providing me with information and illustrations about his, and his colleagues', studies on the repair of articular cartilage. I am grateful to Dr. Ian Robertson and Dr. Phil Seeman for providing me with micrographs for the chapter on nervous tissue and most helpful comments. I am also obliged to Dr. Arthur Hand for his micrographs and informative comments on nerve terminations in glands.

I continue to be impressed with the almost universal graciousness of those histologists and biologists whose research lies in special fields when help is requested by the author of a teaching textbook for information and illustrations. In this connection I thank Dr. L. A. Chouinard of Laval University for a great deal of information and splendid micrographs relating to the nucleolus. I am particularly indebted to Dr. Marilyn Farquhar for allowing me to use her beautiful micrographs of the cells of the adenohypophysis and the information relating to them and to Dr. Dorothy Bainton for information and micrographs, particularly the one of the cell that would seem to be the stem cell of myeloid tissue. Such help and illustrations were also received from Dr. Peter Moens in connection with the preparation of the section on spermatogenesis, and with regard to this chapter I am grateful to Andy Wrybeck for extensive assistance. Dr. Richard W. Young was most helpful in supplying me both with information and illustrative material in connection with the retina. Dr. Ken Money provided me not only with further information about the ear but also with some new illustrations. Dr. M. Weinstock supplied me with several new micrographs dealing with different topics. I am grateful to Dr. Roger Daoust for some special photomicrographs about whose preparation he went to considerable trouble. I thank also my friend of many years, Harry Whittaker, for the same reason. Several new illustrations from other individuals were also requested and used; these are acknowledged in the text and I am grateful to all who supplied them.

I thank June Pitter for typing the thousands of pages of manuscript, not easy to interpret, that were required before final copy was achieved and also managing to do this with the utmost encouraging cheerfulness.

It has always been a pleasure to deal with the staff of J. B. Lippincott Co. and in connection with this edition it has been a pleasure to deal with Mr. George Stickley of that company. I am grateful that the editing of the manuscript was assigned to Miss Naomi Coplin with whom it was a pleasure to work and who, in changing any sentences, always made things clearer.

A.W.H.

Contents

PART ONE: CELLS

PART TWO: TISSUES

16 JOINTS **448**

17 NERVOUS TISSUE **466**

18 MUSCLE TISSUE **526**

PART THREE: THE SYSTEMS OF THE BODY

PART ONE

Cells

1 Microscopy and Biology of Cells

Introduction

The word *cell* was first used in biology by Robert Hooke, a brilliant physicist and biologist of the 17th century. Having built a compound microscope, he did something that any student can now easily repeat by cutting a slice of cork thin enough to transmit light and then examining it with his microscope. What is seen if this is done is shown in Figure 1-1. Since cork is dead, dried out plant tissue, it appears under the microscope to be composed of innumerable tiny, empty chambers separated from each other by thin walls which are now known to consist of cellulose. Since in Hooke's time the word *cell* was in common use to describe small chambers such as those in monasteries, he appropriately gave the name *cells* to the chambers in cork.

Over the next two centuries, however, further microscopy showed that freshly obtained living plant tissue was different from cork. Although it contained similar compartments, each was filled in living plant tissue with a little jellylike body. Furthermore, many animal tissues were found to consist of similar little jellylike bodies seemingly packed together without any compartment walls between them. As a result, the word *cell* began to be used for the little jellylike bodies as well as for the compartments and, of course, its use with two meanings caused some confusion. It even seems that, when the general notion of the cell doctrine—that cells are the ultimate units out of which plants and animals are constructed—was enunciated independently by Schleidin and Schwann in 1832, there was still some uncertainty about what a cell was; but before long the term *cell*, so far as animal tissue was concerned, came to be used exclusively for little jellylike bodies. Then in due course it was noticed that each jellylike body contained a generally rounded structure of a somewhat different refractive index than the rest of the cell; this was termed its *nucleus* (nut) and still later this was found to contain a still smaller relatively dense body which was called the nucleolus (little nut). The remainder of the cell came to be called cytoplasm. This led to the common practice of

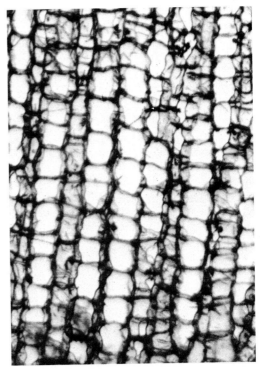

FIG. 1-1. A freehand section of cork. Under the microscope it can be seen that it is composed of many tiny empty chambers separated from each other by thin walls.

depicting a cell graphically (on, say, a blackboard in the classroom) as is shown in Figure 1-2.

Eucaryotic and Procaryotic Cells. Although the kinds of cells with which this book deals all contain nuclei, it should be pointed out here that in the general field of cell biology two kinds of cells, in due course, came to be recognized—those with, and those without nuclei. Those with nuclei are termed *eucaryotic* cells, which term from its origin (*eu*, good; *karyon*, nucleus) indicates that this kind of cell possesses nuclear material that is enclosed by a nuclear membrane or envelope (the inner ring in Fig. 1-2). Eucaryotic cells are the kind of which all animals, plants and micro-

3

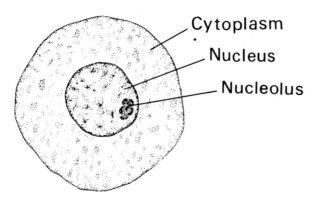

Fig. 1-2. Diagram of a eucaryotic cell.

organisms, excepting bacteria and blue-green algae, are composed. The latter contain nuclear material but it is not enclosed by a nuclear membrane or envelope. Cells of this type are termed *procaryotic,* which term infers they evolved before cells of the eucaryotic type.

Eucaryotic cells differ from procaryotic in another respect in that their cytoplasm is much more highly organized, containing, as we shall see in Chapter 5, a vast number of specialized structural arrangements that perform specifically different functions for the cell.

Although, as mentioned above, the kind of cells with which this book deals are the eucaryotic type, it should be said that much of what has been learned about how they work at the level of molecular biology has come from the study of procaryotic cells. But unless otherwise mentioned, all of the following accounts of cells refer to those of the eucaryotic type.

The Advent and Decline of the Use of the Term Protoplasm. With the increasing interest in cells it was inevitable that scientists would begin to inquire into the basis for life that was manifested by these tiny objects and this led to attempts to define the properties of living cells. At this point some confusion was introduced by the term *protoplasm.* This word was coined to denote the substance from which cells were made and which provided the physical basis for life, but this concept unfortunately led easily to another—that protoplasm was itself a living substance that possessed certain properties (soon to be mentioned) that were supposed to characterize living things.

Although the term protoplasm is still sometimes used as a general synonym for cell substance, the concept of its being a special substance of unknown composition that possesses the properties of life was gradually eroded as more was found out about cells.

It is now known that a cell contains a host of specialized macromolecular structures that are arranged in special ways so that they function in an integrated manner to bring about the chemical reactions required for the cell to exhibit the properties of life. Life emerges from the integrated activity of a vast number of different subcellular components which we shall soon study, one by one; it is not the property of any single given substance.

Why Cells To Live Must Be in a Certain Size Range. Although cells of different kinds vary somewhat in size, there are limits to how small or how large they can be; the mean is probably around 0.015 mm. First, they have to be large enough to house the great number of different subcellular macromolecular components that are essential for the integrated reactions on which life depends. However, since the reactions between these subcellular components must be fueled with nutrients and oxygen, and since these substances have to be absorbed by cells from their surfaces, cells could not exist if they became too large because their innermost parts would be too far removed from their exterior to be adequately serviced.

The Physiological Properties of Cells. In seeking to compile a list of properties manifested by animal cells, a list that could distinguish them from the non-living objects, much study was made of animals consisting of only one cell, such as amebae. A unicellular animal is in a sense a jack-of-all-trades. It exhibits physiological properties that enable it to do a lot of things but not all of them exceedingly well. For cells or people to become expert at anything requires that they become specialized, and this, of course, occurs in the multicellular animal such as man, for, as a body consisting of billions of cells develops, some cells become specialized to perform one kind of function and other cells to perform other functions. As we shall see later, a high development of one function in the multicellular animal is often associated with the loss of some other property that in turn becomes highly developed in some other type of specialized cell. The time-honored list of the physiological properties of cells is given below, for much reference will be made to them later.

1. *Irritability.* This term refers to a cell's being sensitive to a stimulus of some kind—for example, mechanical prodding, exposure to light, a chemical of some sort or an electric current. However, the only way it can be shown that a cell is sensitive to a stimulus is by observing that it reacts to it by manifesting one of the responses listed below. It should be noted

that some kinds of cells, like some kinds of people, are more sensitive to stimuli than others. Irritability is brought to its highest state of development in nerve cells.

2. *Conductivity.* This particular response to a stimulus is manifested by a wave of excitation beginning at the point of the stimulus and passing along the surface of the cell to reach its other parts. A wave of excitation passing along a cell is associated with a changing electric potential along its course, and this can be measured. Both irritability and conductivity are the chief physiological properties exhibited by nerve cells which are often long drawn-out structures that can conduct waves of excitation over long distances, some for over a few feet. The two properties of irritability and conductivity will be discussed in detail in Chapter 17, which deals with nerve cells and nervous tissue.

3. *Contractility.* This is manifested by a cell shortening in some direction in response to a stimulus. It is brought to a high state of development in muscle cells. The structural components within muscle cells that provide for this property will be dealt with in detail in connection with muscle in Chapter 18.

4. *Absorption and Assimilation.* All cells can take in food and other substances from their surface and utilize or otherwise deal with the substances. Comment on these two properties will begin when we deal with cytoplasm in Chapter 5.

5. *Secretion.* In the multicellular animal, certain cells, from substances they absorb, can synthesize new substances and deliver these through their surrounding membranes to serve as useful secretions which exert specific functions elsewhere. The cell components involved in secretion are described in detail in Chapter 5 and the cellular structures called glands, which are specialized organs for secretion, are described in Chapter 7.

6. *Excretion.* All cells can rid themselves of waste products resulting from their utilizing food and oxygen. The way this is done is described in Chapter 5.

7. *Respiration.* Cells absorb oxygen which is used to bring about the oxidation of food substances within them, which provides energy. This is called cell respiration; the cell components involved in the process will be discussed in connection with mitochondria in Chapter 5.

8. *Growth and Reproduction.* Growth requires the synthesis of more cell substance. As already mentioned, cells become inefficient if they exceed a certain size, so growth is almost always attained by cells staying at about the same size and multiplying in numbers instead of becoming larger. How this is done will be the main topic described in the next chapter.

Cells As Structural and Physiological Units

A cell is the smallest unit of structure that can manifest the physiological properties described above while surviving independently by utilizing nonliving materials. It should be noted that while it is true that unicellular animals can reproduce their own kind in a nonliving environment, many of the more specialized cells of the multicellular animals cannot reproduce so this ability is not essential for them to be true cells. Furthermore, the ability to reproduce one's own kind does not necessarily imply life, because viruses can reproduce their own kind if they are in a living environment, i.e., inside a suitable kind of cell; but to multiply and so manifest this property of life, they require much help from the living cell they parasitize. Viruses, unlike bacteria (which are unicellular organisms), cannot reproduce in nutritive solutions of nonliving materials. Viruses are not cells.

For the microscopist, one very important consequence of the specialization of cells in the multicellular animal is that cells that become specialized with regard to exploiting some particular property come to have a different appearance from those that particularly exploit some other property. As a consequence, a cell specialized for contractility has a very different appearance under the microscope from a cell that is specialized to secrete. As a result, we can recognize different kinds of specialized cells with the microscope. In subsequent chapters we shall discuss other consequences of the specialization of the structure and function of cells.

The Chemical Composition of Cells

Biochemistry is the discipline that deals with the chemistry of cells. However, it is necessary to discuss some aspects of this subject here for three reasons. First, in most curricula, instruction in the microscopy and function of cells precedes formal instruction in biochemistry and hence it cannot be assumed in a book such as this that the reader will be familiar with either those terms or those concepts of biochemistry that are essential for the intelligent study of cell structure and function. Second, electron microscopy has disclosed a new world of organized macromolecular structures within the cell, the individual structures being termed *organelles,* and the study of the function of these and the roles they play in the chemical reactions that proceed in the cell has become more or less a common ground for both microscopy and biochemistry, which of course has had the desirable effect of helping relate structure, function and chemistry at the microscopic level. Finally, there are certain aspects of the chemistry of cells that should receive special emphasis in relation to their microscopy because they are essential for understanding ordinary staining reactions and special histochemical tests which are commonly employed to demonstrate certain chemical features of cells with the microscope.

Four main types of substances (aside from water, mineral salts, and some special substances in very low concentrations) enter into the composition of cells; these are: proteins, nucleic acids, carbohydrates and lipids (fats).

Proteins

Of the four main substances, proteins by themselves or conjugated with other chemical entities, such as nucleic acid so as to form nucleoproteins, or carbohydrate to form glycoproteins, or lipid to form lipoproteins, are the essential component of cells. As Mulder wrote in 1838, "without protein, life would be impossible on our planet."

Proteins exist in the form of huge molecules (called macromolecules) which are assembled in linear fashion from building blocks called amino acids. There are 20 or so of these acids and they are characterized by each containing an amino group, NH_2, and a carboxyl group (COOH). Thus proteins contain nitrogen. Plants can synthesize amino acids (and hence proteins) from simple components—water, carbon dioxide and inorganic nitrogen. Animals, however, cannot synthesize amino acids from these simple components so they must acquire these or their special building blocks by eating plants (or other animals). In the digestive system of an animal, proteins are broken down to amino acids and from the intestine these are absorbed into the blood which carries them to body cells in various parts of the body and in these various body cells amino acids are variously linked together to form different kinds of proteins.

Apart from such carbohydrate and lipid that becomes conjugated with protein, carbohydrate and lipid taken in by cells are generally used as fuel for energy. In some instances, as we shall see, either carbohydrate or lipid can be stored as such in cells as a reserve of fuel.

Protein also can be used as a fuel for the production of energy, but its main function is to comprise the metabolic machinery responsible for the chemical reactions on which life depends. To discuss the latter we must introduce the word *metabolism.*

The Role of Proteins in Metabolism

The sum total of all the chemical reactions that proceed in a cell, and confer on it the properties of life, constitute its *metabolism (metabolē,* change). Some metabolic reactions are concerned with the breakdown of protoplasm; these are termed catabolic (*kata,* down; *ballein,* to throw). Others are concerned with the synthesis of protoplasm; these are termed anabolic (*anabolē,* a rising up). In some cells anabolic and catabolic activity remain in balance; such cells are said to be in a *steady state.* Growth is dependent on the anabolic reactions exceeding the catabolic reactions.

Almost all of the important chemical reactions involved in metabolism are catalyzed by *enzymes,* all of which are proteins. But not all proteins are enzymes. Another important function of proteins in cells is to provide the structural material out of which the various little organelles that exist in the cell are composed. Most organelles (as will be explained in detail in Chapter 5) are composed of *membranes* which are made of protein associated with lipid. Membranes permit different substances to be separated from one another in the cell, as we shall learn in detail later. However, the membranes may have enzymatic protein associated with them, so that reactions catalyzed by enzymes may occur on the surfaces of membranes. Enzymatic proteins are also present both inside organelles and in that part of the cell which permeates everywhere between the organelles and is sometimes called cell sap or matrix. Protein enzymes are required to bring about the reactions by which carbohydrate and lipid are metabolized in cells to provide energy.

Both the protein-containing organelles and the enzymes in cells are not permanent fixtures; they are to different extents always being catabolized or otherwise lost, while new ones are always being synthesized to take their place. Life, then, depends on the continuous occurrence of protein synthesis in cells—it is necessary both for the continuous renewal of their enzymes and organelles and also for the performance of their functions.

The Colloidal Properties of Proteins

The fact that proteins exist in colloidal solution is of almost incalculable importance in understanding many of the features of cell and fluid behavior in the body. It is also important with regard to understanding the methods that are used in preparing stained thin slices of tissue for examination with the microscope (soon to be described) so we shall deal briefly with colloids here.

From its derivation the word *colloid* means gluelike. The term was coined to refer to certain soluble substances, including many proteins that on evaporation of their solutions—e.g., the white of an egg—leave a residue that is amorphous and sticky (rather than crystalline, as occurs when a solution of a crystalloid such as common salt is evaporated). Solutions of colloids differ from solutions of crystalloids in another respect: they will not pass through membranes easily permeable to solutions of crystalloids, because in general the particles or molecules in a colloidal solution are too large to pass through the infinitesimally tiny pores in this type of membrane. As already mentioned, protein molecules are so large they are termed macromolecules. It might be wondered why such large molecules do not settle from solution because of gravity; an important reason for this not happening is that they all bear similar electrical charges so that in solution they constantly repel each other, which of course helps to keep them well apart. Another factor is that proteins are *lyophilic* (*lyo*, solution; *philein*, to love) colloids, which means that protein macromolecules like the state of solution; indeed, they attract water to them, which helps further in keeping them in solution and accounts for their being termed *hydrophilic* colloids.

Sols and Gels. The colloidal state in which proteins normally exist can be that of either a sol or a gel. Sols are fluids that are generally more or less viscous; gels are at least semisolid. At least some sols may become gels under certain circumstances and vice versa. A common animal-derived protein that is easily shown to undergo sol-gel transformations is gelatin. Gelatin is an important component of consommé (beef broth). However, if you order consommé, a waiter does not ask if you wish it as a sol or a gel, but if you wish it hot or cold. If it comes hot from the stove it is in the form of a sol but if the same soup has been kept in the refrigerator it will come to you as a jellied consommé. If you order the latter but do not immediately eat it, it will begin to change back again to a sol. Gelatin thus provides an example of a colloid that undergoes sol-gel transformations because of temperature changes. Sol-gel transformations can occur for other reasons—for example, changes in pH.

It might be asked where the water goes when a sol becomes a gel. It becomes bound in the brush-heap arrangements into which the macromolecules become arranged when the gel forms. Since there is just as much water in the gel as was present in the sol, a gel provides a material through which diffusion of ions can occur, as is shown by the fact that, if a dye is painted on the surface of a gel, it can be seen to diffuse into the substance of the gel. This is of vast importance in the body because, as we shall learn, certain cells of *connective tissue* surround themselves with a material called *intercellular substance* which in many sites is in the form of a gel and hence nutrients have to diffuse through this gel to nourish the cells. For example, this is the way the cells that are buried in the cartilage of joints receive their nourishment; it diffuses to them from the fluid in the joint (as will be described in due course).

As we shall see in later chapters, the fact that protein colloids exert a certain amount of osmotic pressure, so that they tend to draw water to them, and yet can be kept behind membranes, such as the membrane that surrounds the cell, is also of the greatest importance in understanding the factors that affect the movement of fluids and inorganic ions—for example, between the interior of the cell and its environment.

The proteins of a cell are partly gels and partly sols. The membranes of the organelles inside the cell and the membrane that surrounds the cell all have their structural basis in gels. Between the organelles and other little structures within cells (that will be described later), much of the protein is in the form of a sol; this constitutes much of the cell sap or cytoplasmic matrix. This fact creates a problem with regard to cutting groups of cells into thin slices for microscopic study because, if cells are cut, the part of the protein that is a sol runs away. To prevent this, and for other reasons soon to be described, small pieces of body parts that are to be prepared for microscopic study must be *fixed*, a procedure which coagulates the sols and holds them, and the structures they surround, in place. Fixation is usually accomplished by immersing small pieces of some body part into certain chemical solutions—a 4 percent solution of buffered formaldehyde is a common one. Fixation can even be accomplished by boiling. For example, egg white is a protein sol but if an egg is boiled, the white is irreversibly converted to a firm gel which is hard enough to slice for sandwiches. The same kind of thing happens to the sols of cells if they are boiled.

With this discussion of proteins, we are now in a position to discuss the microscopy of cells, in which account the other main components of cells—nucleic acids, carbohydrates and fats—will be described briefly.

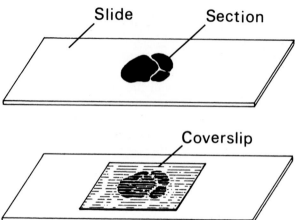

Slide   Section

Coverslip

FIG. 1-3. (*Top*) A stained section on a glass slide. (*Bottom*) The same section with a coverslip on top.

How Cells Are Studied With the Microscope

Although cells from the body may be isolated by special methods and examined in various ways as will be described later, the easiest and commonest way to study cells is by examining them in their normal position in the body where they are in association with one another. This method has the advantage of showing how cells of different types are fitted together in different parts of the body and it depends on preparing and studying what are termed "sections" of various body parts.

What Are Sections? A section is an extremely thin, transparent shaving cut from a little piece of body substance, laid flat on, and caused to adhere to, a glass slide and stained (Fig. 1-3, *top*). It is then covered first with a small amount of mounting fluid of the proper refractive index and finally with a thin glass coverslip, which is pressed down firmly on the flat shaving of stained tissue (Fig. 1-3, *bottom*). In the laboratory the student will have access to, and study, sections mounted on glass slides that have been prepared from all important parts of the body. The term *section* is sometimes also used to distinguish the complete preparation (glass slide, stained shaving, mounting medium and coverslip). We shall use the term indiscriminately.

How Sections Are Prepared

In order to study sections intelligently it is helpful to know something about how they are prepared; hence, successive steps in the technic of preparing a section from some body part, for example, the liver, will now be described briefly. Since the first step in the process is termed "Obtaining the Tissue," we must explain here that although the word *tissue* has a special meaning as will be described in Part 2 of this book, the word is also commonly used in a nonspecific way to denote any body substance. For example, if a surgeon cuts away a little piece of body substance at an operation, he is said to have removed a piece of tissue, or if anyone hits his thumb with a hammer, he is said to have caused tissue damage.

1. **Obtaining the Tissue.** A little piece of tissue for sectioning should be obtained with the greatest care. Pinching it with forceps or squeezing it with dull scissors or cutting it with a dull knife can profoundly change the appearance of its cells. Tissue should be removed with a very sharp knife and with the use of very little pressure. As soon as possible, the little piece that is taken, and thereafter referred to as a *block*, should be immersed in fixative. Fixatives, in hardening the sols in the tissue, inactivate certain of the enzymes in cells that would otherwise begin to digest the cells and thus cause what is termed *postmortem degeneration* which spoils cells for subsequent microscopy. To allow for rapid permeation of fixative, any block of tissue taken from a body should not be more than a few mm. thick.

2. **Fixation.** Besides coagulating the protein sols of cells, hardening the gels, and inactivating enzymes, fixatives have several further actions. The general coagulation of protein sols imprisons to some extent certain carbohydrates and even some fatty materials that would otherwise escape. Most fixatives, moreover, are good antiseptics and so kill bacteria and other disease agents which might be in infected tissue and present a health hazard to those subsequently handling the tissue. Fixatives also can affect tissue so that it reacts better to certain stains. Some special fixatives (listed in books on histologic technic) are better than others for preserving certain cell and tissue components.

3. **Sectioning.** This refers to cutting slices from a block that are thin enough to study with the microscope. For routine light microscopy the slices should not be *more than 5 to 8 microns (micrometers) thick*. A micron, or micrometer, is $\frac{1}{1000}$ mm. (10^{-6} *meter*). Microns, or micrometers, are depicted by the symbols μ or μm.

In order to cut such thin slices there are three requirements:

(1) A slicing machine that has an advance that can be adjusted so as to cut successive sections this thin; such a machine is called a microtome (Fig. 1-4).

(2) A heavy and very sharp knife for the microtome.

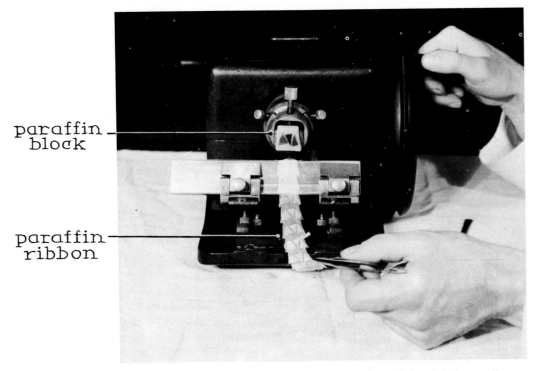

paraffin block

paraffin ribbon

Fig. 1-4. A microtome being used to cut a ribbon of paraffin sections. Notice that the paraffin block has 3 pieces of tissue embedded in it. The outline of these may be seen in each of the sections whose edges are adhering to one another to form the ribbon.

(3) The block of tissue must be so treated as to make it uniformly hard enough to slice very thin. This is done in two usual ways, either by freezing the block of tissue (the frozen section technic) or impregnating the block with paraffin wax (the paraffin technic) or some plastic material.

The Frozen Section Technic

The freezing method is the faster and hence is commonly used when a surgeon, during an operation, wants a microscopic examination made, for example, on a lump or mass of tissue which might possibly be cancer. A block of tissue is removed from the lump and a section is prepared immediately by a histopathologist who, on examining the stained slice with a microscope, can, within a few minutes, tell the surgeon the nature of the diseased tissue. This enables the surgeon to finish the operation in a way to most effectively treat the disease that is present.

One procedure is to place a block of fresh, but preferably fixed, tissue on the stage of a microtome that has an outlet below the stage through which carbon dioxide gas (under pressure) can be released to cool the stage sufficiently to freeze the tissue. Fairly thin slices can then be cut from its surface by the microtome knife, which in this type of microtome is arranged so that it sweeps over the surface of the frozen block of tissue horizontally. However, nowadays frozen sections are commonly cut in a *cryostat,* an apparatus that permits the microtome knife as well as the block of tissue to be kept below freezing so that the whole operation of preparing the section is conducted at the same low temperature, and this gives better results.

Aside from the speed with which they can be prepared, frozen sections have certain other advantages as well as certain disadvantages, as will be mentioned later.

Preparing Sections by the Paraffin Technic

Dehydration. Possibly in the past some ingenious person, having noticed how easy it was to whittle thin shavings from a candle, conceived the idea of infiltrating tissue with wax, so that it, like a candle, could be cut in thin slices. However, about 65 percent of tissue is water, which is not miscible with wax, particularly the paraffin wax which is routinely used. In order to introduce wax into tissue, one of the procedures used is to take the block through a substance which is miscible with both water and melted paraffin. A frequently used substance is dioxane. The block is first placed in several baths of dioxane, which mixes with tissue water and eventually replaces it. The block is then placed in warmed paraffin that mixes with the dioxane of the block and in turn replaces it. In this manner the block becomes infiltrated with paraffin.

Another procedure is to use two different solvents to obtain paraffin infiltration. First, the water in the block of tissue is removed by immersing it in alcohols of graded strength until it contains no water but only absolute alcohol; this step is called *dehydration*. Then another step called "clearing" is employed. Clearing agents—for example, xylol—are soluble in both wax and alcohol. From absolute alcohol the block of tissue is immersed in xylol until all alcohol is displaced by xylol and then it is placed in warm melted paraffin and allowed to remain there until all the xylol is replaced by melted paraffin; this step is called *embedding*.

Sectioning. When a block of tissue is embedded in paraffin by either method described above the paraffin is allowed to harden, and excess wax is cut away from it. The paraffin-embedded block is then mounted on a microtome and shavings are cut from it. The last step is called *sectioning*. As is shown in Figure 1-4, as sections come off the knife, the edge of one adheres to the edge of the next so that a paraffin ribbon of sections is obtained, from which individual sections are easily separated.

Staining and Mounting. To stain sections cut by the paraffin technic there is a further problem because most stains act only in aqueous solution. So, before the section can be stained, the paraffin that permeates each shaving of tissue has to be removed and replaced by water. To do this, each shaving is laid flat on a

glass slide to which it is made to adhere by first making the slide a little sticky with some material that will not interfere with the staining. The slide, with its adhering slice of tissue, is then dipped in xylol to remove the paraffin, then in absolute alcohol to remove the xylol, then in alcohols of decreasing strength and finally into water. It can then be dried, and the tissue slice which still remains on the slide can be stained with dyes that are in aqueous solution. After staining, the section is passed through alcohols of increasing strength to absolute, and then into xylol. Now it can be *mounted* in a mounting medium that is soluble in xylol and of the correct refractive index. Last of all, a coverslip is pressed down firmly on the section, and generally this makes a fairly permanent type of preparation (Fig. 1-3, *bottom*).

STAINS AND STAINING

Why Sections Are Stained. With the light microscope little detail can be seen in cells in (1) a slice of unstained tissue, (2) whole mounts of unstained cells, or (3) living cells that are immersed in suitable fluids, because cell components are of much the same optical density. It is the optical density of anything through which light passes that reduces the amplitude of the light that passes through it (Fig. 1-5). The optical densities of the various little structures within an unstained cell are similar, so that they all affect the amplitude of the light that passes through them similarly and, thus, these structures do not appear lighter or darker than one another and cannot be individually distinguished. The common way to overcome this difficulty is to treat sections of dead fixed tissue with stains, as will be described shortly. These combine with different cell and tissue components to different extents and so bring about relative changes in both

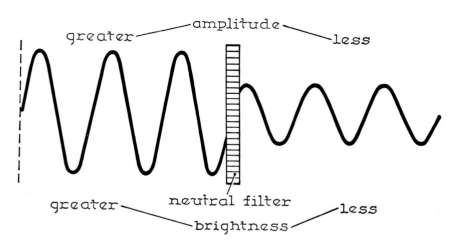

Fig. 1-5. Diagram showing how the amplitude of light waves is decreased by the waves' passing through a neutral filter.

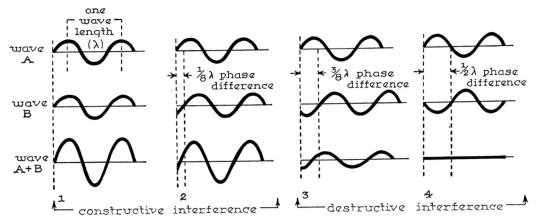

Fig. 1-6. Diagrams showing how light waves can interfere with one another to increase or decrease the amplitude of the resultant waves.

their optical densities and their color so that they may be distinguished from one another. However, in research studies it is often very important to be able to study fresh living cells that are in nutritive solutions and even record their movements and behavior by means of cinematography as is shown in Figure 5-11. This can be done by use of what is termed the *phase microscope*, which we shall now describe briefly because a full explanation of how it works is a matter for physics.

The Phase Microscope. As already noted, the components of cells are of such a similar optical density that different cell components do not affect the amplitude of the light that passes through them differently enough to allow them to be distinguished from one another with the ordinary light microscope. Different cell components do alter the *phase* of the light waves that pass through them to different extents, but phase differences in light reaching the eye cannot of course be distinguished. It is well known that light waves, like water waves, can interfere with one another so as to increase or decrease the amplitude of the resultant waves, as shown in Figure 1-6. Hence, if phase differences could be converted into differences of amplitude, different cell components could be distinguished from one another in the microscope. This is accomplished in both the *phase microscope* and the *interference microscope*. In both types it is necessary to use two sets of waves and these are combined with one another to create differences in amplitude in the light that reaches the eye from different cell components. This is done in the phase microscope, the more commonly used instrument, by using two sets of waves, those of the light incident to the object and those diffracted by the object. These two sets are recombined

in the objective where the two sets from different cell components interfere with each other to different extents so that the amplitude of the light from waves from different cell components is different and hence they are seen by the eye as objects that are darker or lighter than one another as is shown in Figure 5-1.

The Use of Dyes to Provide Color and Contrast in Sections

What Is an H and E Section? Although treating a section with a single dye increases contrast between cell and tissue components because they take up a single dye to different extents, it was found that using two dyes, first one of one color and then a second of a different color, would produce even more contrast because one dye would combine with some cell and tissue components and the other dye with others and so the two-dye method became usual. The two most commonly used in the histology laboratory for students' sections are *hematoxylin* and *eosin*. A section stained by this method is called an *H and E section*. The reason for each of these dyes staining different cell and tissue components will be explained, because understanding why some components take up one dye, and others the other, can be informative about the chemical nature of the material that takes up the particular dye.

But first we should mention a matter of particular interest to medical students: As more and more dyes were produced, it was found that some seemed to have extraordinarily specific effects, and this led to the dream that it might be possible to find a dye that would combine with and kill organisms causing disease in the body without the dye harming body cells. It was through exploring this possibility that two great medical discoveries were made and the modern science of chemotherapy initiated, as will now be described briefly.

When Paul Ehrlich (1854-1915) was a medical student, he devised a method by which sections prepared from the diseased tissue of people who died of tuberculosis could be stained so as to specifically color the bacteria that were present in the tissue and responsible for the disease. He was so fascinated by the fact that a dye could be so specific in its action that he spent many years of his life testing one dye after another by injecting it into animals suffering from infections caused by different disease-causing organisms to see if he could find one that would kill the organisms and leave the body cells unharmed. After years of work he had found only one (trypan red) and this had an effect only on a type of animal trypanosomiasis. However, he read in a journal about a new form in which arsenic could be prepared as a drug, and so he turned to experiments with arsenicals and eventually found one that he called compound 606; this later became known as the magic bullet because it seemed to have a profound and selective effect on the spirochete that caused syphilis and became the universal drug by which this disease was treated until it was superseded by penicillin. In 1932 Gerhard Domagk took up the same kind of search with dyes. Among others, he tested the effects of a red dye called Prontosil on some mice that had been infected with a virulent strain of streptococci (bacteria) and found that the mice recovered. This dye was then tested on people with streptococcus and certain other bacterial infections and was found to have what seemed to be a truly wonderful curative effect. It was soon found, however, that the effect of Prontosil was due not to the dye's being taken up selectively by bacteria, but to its being converted in the body to another substance called sulfanilamide, which is not a dye but a compound that does selectively interfere with bacterial metabolism. Actually, sulfanilamide had been synthesized several decades before and had been sitting on a shelf, as it were, all that time, while countless people died without anyone knowing that it would be a wonderfully effective chemotherapeutic agent against streptococcus and certain other bacterial infections and that it would become known as the first of the "wonder" drugs of the 20th century.

We shall now return to our discussion of staining.

Acid and Basic Stains. Most dyes used in histology are classed as acid or basic stains. However, they are not frank acids or bases but neutral salts that dissolve in water where they dissociate into anions and cations. Whether a stain is termed acid or basic depends on whether the component that imparts color is in the anion or the cation of the dissociated salt. If it is in the anion (the acid radical), the stain is termed an acid or anionic stain whereas if the dye is associated with the cation, the stain is termed a basic or cationic stain. The first stain used in preparing an H and E section is hematoxylin and this as it is used acts as a basic stain. This is followed by eosin which is an acid stain.

Basophilic and Acidophilic Substances. We can now understand the meaning of the two common histological terms, *basophilia* and *acidophilia*. Any substance seen in a section is termed basophilic (*philein*, to love) if it has an affinity for a basic stain; likewise, a substance is said to be acidophilic if it takes up an acid stain. (The terms acidophilic and eosinophilic are commonly used as synonyms.) Since hematoxylin used with a mordant is a blue to purple dye, it imparts this color to substances that have an affinity for it; hence, basophilic substances are blue-purple in an H and E section. Since eosin imparts a pink to red color to substances that have an affinity for it, acidophilic substances are pink to red in an H and E section. A glance at the upper left illustration in Figure 1-14 will show that some things in a cell are blue (basophilic) and some are pink to red (acidophilic). What these things are will be described shortly.

How To Identify Cells in H and E Sections

The student who as yet has had no lengthy experience in examining stained sections of animal tissues with the LM but has seen lots of diagrams of isolated cells (such as in Fig. 1-2), may think that identifying cells in stained sections would be easy. But it is not as simple as might be thought. There are a few problems, and we shall try to solve these as we proceed.

Choosing a Suitable Section. The first problem for a beginner is that of choosing a section in which it is easy to follow an oral or written description of how to recognize cells. Sections from many parts of the body contain a variety of cells of different shapes and sizes and arranged in various groupings, and it is very difficult to describe to a beginner how to locate cells in such a section. It is much easier to identify cells in a section from a description if a section is chosen in which most of the cells are of the same kind and in the same kind of arrangement. This desirable state of affairs is realized in a section of the liver, for in this organ, 60 percent of the cells are of the same kind and they are all arranged in a similar manner.

Comparing What You See With Illustrations. In order to learn to recognize cells readily in sections it is of the greatest assistance to be able to compare what you see with your microscope with a labeled illustration of sections of the same tissue that you are studying. Since liver cells are our first topic, several illustrations of how they appear in sections will soon follow. But we should first comment on two matters: (1) Why black and white pictures are so commonly used to illustrate what you will see with the LM in H and E sections, and (2) how large a cell should be in relation to the field of the section that you see with different objectives and eyepieces.

WHY BLACK AND WHITE ILLUSTRATIONS?

Although there are stains that are extremely selective for certain particular cell components and for which color illustrations are desirable, about all that H and E staining accomplishes is for hematoxylin to color basophilic substances blue-purple and for eosin to color acidophilic substances pink to red. In black and white *prints* made from negatives obtained by photographing H and E sections with the LM, the degree of darkness observed generally coincides with the depth of staining by hematoxylin, whereas the grays are due either to staining with eosin or to lighter staining with hematoxylin. Since color illustrations are extremely expensive, they will be used here only for special purposes; this is a practice that is followed in the various journals you will read. Furthermore, there are no colors in sections photographed with the electron microscope so electron micrographs are always in black and white. Since the latter are widely used in this book, there is another reason for developing familiarity with black and white photomicrographs of H and E sections,—it helps in interpreting the electron micrographs that will come later; why it does so will be explained in the next chapter.

SOME GENERAL ADVICE ABOUT HOW TO STUDY SECTIONS IN THE LABORATORY AND ABOUT COPING WITH COMMON PROBLEMS THAT MAY ARISE

Before placing a section on the stage of the microscope, hold it to the light and examine it with the naked eye. There are two reasons for doing this: First, the coverslip may be covered with dust, dirt or hardened immersion oil; if so it can be cleaned with xylol and soft tissue. Second, as you learn more and more histology you can often tell, from the naked eye appearance of the little stained slice of tissue, the organ from which it was taken.

Next, although we shall move quickly to the use of the higher power objective in order to study cells, in later work studying tissues and organs the temptation to use the greatest magnification as quickly as possible should be resisted in the study of both normal histology and histopathology. A famous histopathologist is said to have removed all the high-power objectives from the microscopes of the graduate students who came to study with him so that they would appreciate the great value of the low-power objective in diagnosing pathological conditions. One reason for this is that it discloses a larger area of the section than the high-power objectives so by moving the section around, it is possible with it (or easier still with a scanning objective) to examine every part of the section. Often the important clue about the part of the body that the section was taken from (which is of importance in practical examinations in normal histology), or the nature of the disease process that is present (which is important in diagnostic histopathology) may be present at only one little site in the section which could be easily missed if the whole section was not investigated with a low-power objective. Furthermore, inspection with the low-power objective should reveal the best area to center for subsequent examination with the higher power objectives.

The High-Power Objective. There should be no problem to swinging this objective in place to examine the area centered with the low-power objective. But if the high-power objective cannot be focused, the chances are that the slide is upside down—that is, the coverslip and slice of tissue are below instead of above the slide and hence the slice of tissue is too far away to be focused with the high-power. The chief reason for this occurring is that someone has attached the label on the wrong side of the slide; it should, of course, be on the same side as the coverslip.

The Oil-Immersion Objective. This must approach the coverslip so close there is danger of lowering it onto the coverslip and breaking the latter or the objective in trying to get it into focus.

Probably the best way to bring the oil-immersion objective into focus safely is this: After centering the particular area to be examined with the high-power objective, the tube of the microscope should be raised with the coarse adjustment. Then the oil-immersion objective is switched into place. A drop of oil is then put on the part of the slide that lies directly over the center of the condenser. Watching the bottom of the oil-immersion objective from the side, the microscope tube is then lowered until the objective is seen from the side with the naked eye to just enter the drop of oil. At this point the oil-immersion lens is still *above* the point of focus. The eye is then applied to the eyepiece and the microscope tube is slowly lowered with the fine adjustment until the field comes into focus. If it does not come into focus with 1 or 2 turns of the fine adjustment, it is best to stop and question whether or not something has gone wrong. Two possibilities should be considered: (1) there may be no stained part of the section under the very small area of the section seen with the oil-immersion objective, or (2) the objective is *below* the level at which it is in focus. If color can be seen on looking down the microscope, the first possibility can be ruled out, and if color has become better defined with focusing downward, the chances are that the objective is still above the point of focus and can be safely lowered somewhat farther. But if there is reason to doubt, the tube should be raised, the oil wiped off the objective and the slide, the area centered again with the high-power objective, and the rest of the procedure repeated. It is always best to proceed very cautiously until considerable experience has been gained.

Poor Illumination. If the section is not properly illuminated when the condenser seems to be raised to its usual position, it may be the result of the part of the condenser that contains the lens having slipped down the sleeve that is attached to the mechanism by which the condenser is raised.

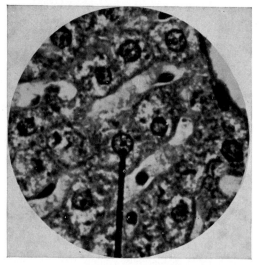

FIG. 1-7. This shows how a pointer in the eyepiece can be used to indicate a particular structure in the section under view. In this section of liver, the end of the pointer reaches and extends slightly over the edge of the nucleus of a liver cell. The nucleolus is seen just off the end of the pointer.

Dirty Eyepieces or Objectives. If a field under view seems irregularly clouded or covered with specks, (1) the coverslip of the section may be dirty, (2) the objective lens may have become smeared with oil or, (3) the eyepiece may be dirty. If the cloudy appearance or specks move when the eyepiece is turned, the trouble is a dirty eyepiece. To clean it, a common procedure is to breathe on the lenses and then rub them with lens paper or some soft tissue until they are clear and bright. However, loose specks generally remain after this procedure, and they must be blown off, not with the breath (which is moist air), but with a blast of dry air from a rubber syringe that is kept for this purpose. Any small syringe, such as an ear syringe, that can be purchased very cheaply from any medical supply house, serves this purpose well, and every student should have one. The coverslip of the section or oil on the bottom of the objective lens can be cleaned off with soft tissue and xylol.

Desirability of Having a Pointer in an Eyepiece. A student, on seeing something in a section which he cannot identify, can waste an enormous amount of his and his instructor's time by trying to describe it and where it is in the field under view so that the instructor can tell him what it is. Such are the difficulties of attempting to identify appearances by descriptions that the student and the instructor may end by looking at different things in the section. The quickest and most certain way of having an instructor identify something for the student, or of making it possible for the instructor to show something easily to a student, is to have a pointer in the eyepiece so that the object to be identified or demonstrated can be indicated clearly and definitely by the pointer as in Figure 1-7. In the type of eyepiece commonly used a few years ago, there was a diaphragm which formed a shelf as is illustrated in Figure 1-8, and a short hair could be attached to the shelf with a drop of balsam. However, there is no shelf in the eyepieces of some of the microscopes made today; if yours is of this type, it would help to get an eyepiece of the older type and fit it with a pointer, or borrow one, when it is necessary to point to something in a section.

HOW LARGE IN RELATION TO THE FIELD UNDER VIEW SHOULD CELLS APPEAR WITH DIFFERENT OBJECTIVES AND EYEPIECES?

A liver cell has a polyhedral shape and so it is about as deep or long as it is wide. A rough estimate of its average diameter would be around 20 microns. Next, the size of the circular area of the section that is seen with the microscope varies in relation to the magnifica-

Microscope Eyepiece Pointer

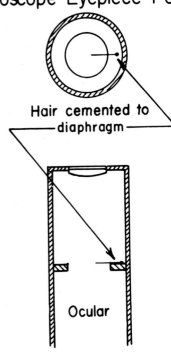

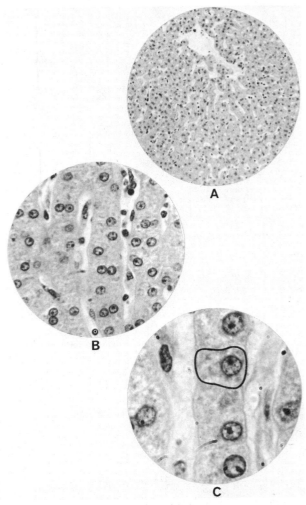

FIG. 1-8. If the top lens is unscrewed from the eye-piece, it will appear as in the upper picture, and a hair can be cemented to the diaphragm with a small drop of Canada balsam. The lower diagram shows the position of the hair in a longitudinal section of the eyepiece.

tion being employed, *becoming decreased as the higher power objectives are used.* The data are given in Figure 1-9 along with illustrations to indicate the width of the area of the section that is under view at different magnifications. Since a liver cell is around 20 μ in either length or width and since the area under view with the low-power objective is around 1,500 μ wide, it takes about 75 liver cells in a row to stretch from one side of the field to the other. But with the oil-immersion objective the area of the section under view is only around 105 microns wide so it takes only around 5 liver cells to cross the field from one side to the other and individual cells of course appear much larger. In order to help you identify an individual liver cell, one is outlined in black in Figure 1-9, C.

In the black and white drawing (Fig. 1-10) which was made at a magnification of around 200 ×, it is easy to see that the main component of the liver, which is represented as gray material (reddish in the section), is arranged in what appear to be irregular branching cords separated by lighter spaces. The cords

FIG. 1-9. Photomicrographs showing how the size of the circular area of a section of liver that is seen with the microscope varies in relation to the magnification being employed. One cell is outlined in black in C.

	Eye-piece	*Objec-tive*	*Magni-fica-tion*	*Width of area under view*
A. Low Power	× 10	× 10	× 100	1500 μ
B. High Power	× 10	× 43	× 430	970 μ
C. Oil Immer-sion	× 10	× 98	× 980	105 μ

of reddish material contain more or less circular blue bodies along their course. The reddish material is the *cytoplasm* of liver cells and the blue bodies contained within the reddish material are the *nuclei* (labeled in

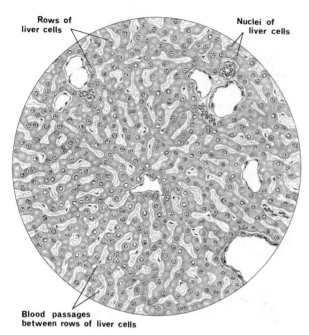

Rows of
liver cells

Nuclei of
liver cells

Blood passages
between rows of liver cells

FIG. 1-10. If an H and E section of liver is examined
with the low-power objective, a field similar to the one
shown above should be easy to find. The important
thing to see here is that there are rows of liver cells that
are separated from one another by blood passages. Next,
it should be noted that there are rounded blue-staining
nuclei within the substance of the rows of liver cells,
which is colored pink to red. The pink-to-red material
is the cytoplasm of liver cells.

Fig. 1-10) of the liver cells. The spaces between the
rows of liver cells are passages for blood (labeled in
Fig. 1-10), and they may be disregarded temporarily.

The next problem is that of deciding how much of
the length of a cord is occupied by one liver cell. It is
very easy to make a mistake at this point because the
boundaries between individual liver cells in a cord
seen in an H and E section are generally not very
obvious, and, indeed, sometimes they cannot be seen
at all (as in Figs. 1-10 and 1-11, "cell boundary not
apparent here"). Hence those students who have seen
many pictures of cells as individual rounded bodies
are tempted to assume that the blue bodies seen in
the cords are whole cells and that the smaller blue
bodies seen within the larger blue bodies are the nuclei
of these rounded cells. To avoid this mistake keep in
mind that the cytoplasm of the cell is reddish, not blue,
and that the blue rounded bodies within the nuclei are
nucleoli (labeled as such in Fig. 1-11) which will be
described in detail in a subsequent chapter.

Since it is easy enough to see the width of a liver
cell because a cord of liver cells is so often only one

cell wide (Fig. 1-10), it can be assumed that each cell
of a cord is about as long as it is wide.

Although our purpose at this time is to study only
liver cells, and not the liver as an organ, it should be
mentioned that the spaces between the branching rows
of liver cells are blood passageways called sinusoids
that are lined with more or less elongated flattened
cells that have dark ovoid nuclei (labeled as nucleus
with condensed chromatin in Fig. 1-11) and are only
loosely attached to the cords, from which they frequently shrink away when tissue is fixed (Fig. 1-11).
The nature and content of these blood passages will
both be described in detail when we investigate this
organ thoroughly in Chapter 22.

**Interpretation of Three-Dimensional Structures
From Sections Cut Through Them.** Even though we
are at this time only using sections to study a representative type of cell (liver cell), it is not too soon to
begin a practice which can be of inestimable help in
interpreting the structure of organs which, of course,
will come later. Even here it will explain why cells of
the same size may appear in sections to be of different
sizes and why some cells may seem to have no nuclei
or why the size of nuclei seems to vary. The practice
we refer to is that of always being conscious that (1)
what you see in a section is a slice that has been cut
through some object, and (2) different slices cut
through the same object may present different appearances. For example, if slices were cut through
different parts of a hard-boiled egg and laid flat on
pieces of glass and examined from above, it would be
readily apparent that some of the slices would not
indicate that the egg had a yolk (see Fig. 1-12).
Furthermore, if only one slice was examined and it
was a slice that had been cut through the yolk it
might be concluded that the yolk extended from one
end of an egg to the other. Different sections, moreover, would suggest different sizes for an egg (Fig.
1-12).

From the above it is easy to realize that if slices
about 5 μ in thickness are cut through a group of
irregularly arranged cells that are each 15 μ in diameter, those cells that are sliced close to their sides
would seem small and would reveal either no nucleus
(Fig. 1-13) or the edge of one which would appear
as a small nucleus (Fig. 1-13), while slices that
passed through the centers of the cells in the group
would show them to be 15 μ or so wide and to have
a nice large rounded nucleus, as is shown in Figure
1-13.

Finally, we have spoken of branching cords of liver
cells. As we shall learn when we study the structure
of this organ later, the cords are not composed of a

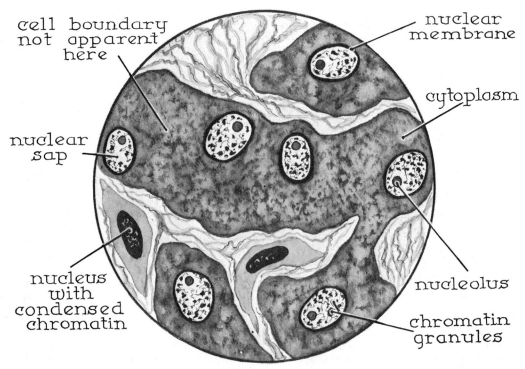

cell boundary not apparent here

nuclear membrane

nuclear sap

cytoplasm

nucleus with condensed chromatin

nucleolus

chromatin granules

FIG. 1-11. Drawing of cords of liver cells from an H and E section as seen with the oil-immersion objective and a 15 × eyepiece. The circular area of the section that can be seen with this magnification is less than 100 μ wide, and it takes only about 4 large liver cells to bridge the area from side to side. Notice that cell borders are not apparent.

single row of cells; instead, what appears as a cord of cells, one or two cells thick in a section, could, of course, have more cells above the ones that you see in the slice and more cells below the ones you see in the slice. Actually, what appears as a cord in the liver is just what is seen in a slice cut through uneven perforated plates of cells with the perforations being occupied by the blood sinusoids (labeled "blood passages" in Fig. 1-10). The arrangement of cells in the liver will be explained in more detail when we study the liver as an organ.

THE CHEMICAL BASIS FOR THE COLORS OF, AND OTHER APPEARANCES SEEN IN, LIVER CELLS IN AN H AND E SECTION

The chief chemical entities involved in the structure and metabolism of cells are proteins, nucleic acids, carbohydrates and lipids. We shall now comment briefly as to how the presence of these can be identified by their color or by other means in an H and E section of liver.

Why the Cytoplasm Is Colored Red. The cytoplasm of cells, aside from the water it contains, consists chiefly of proteins. To understand how proteins react with dyes, it helps to know that proteins act as one of the buffers of the body; that is, if any condition arises whereby extra acid or alkali is produced or ingested, the proteins of the body can assist other buffer systems to prevent the extra acid or alkali from materially altering the pH of body fluids. Proteins act this way because they are *amphoteric* (*ampho*, both): they can act either as acids or as bases. If body fluids tend to become acid, proteins act as bases, and vice versa. Proteins are able to act either way because the amino acids of which they are composed have side chains, some of which donate H^+ when the pH goes up and others that can combine with H^+ when the pH goes down. Many proteins of the body, including those of the cytoplasm of liver cells, have enough (positively charged) basic groups in their side chains at the usual pH at which staining is done to combine with acid dyes, such as eosin, which of course have their color in their (negatively charged) anions;

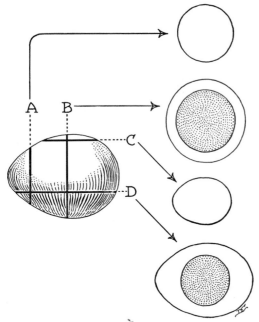

FIG. 1-12. Diagram showing how sections cut through an object in different planes or at different levels may give different impressions about its structure. A hard-boiled egg is shown at the left side of this illustration. Notice how cross sections cut at A and B would be different from one another and in turn different from longitudinal sections cut at C and D.

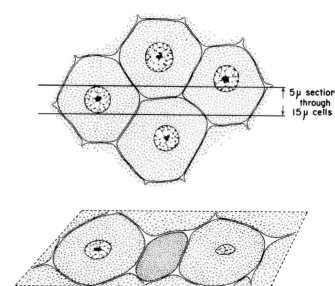

FIG. 1-13. If on looking through the microscope the student saw some cells as they appear in the bottom picture, he might conclude that the cells of the material were of different sizes, that some had no nuclei, and that in those that had nuclei, the nuclei were of different sizes. The top picture shows that a slice of a given thickness cut through a group of cells of the same size could on being examined with the microscope present the appearance seen in the bottom illustration.

hence the protein of the cytoplasm is colored pink to red with eosin (Fig. 1-14, *upper left*). The protein of red blood cells (hemoglobin) and that of muscle cells also bind eosin and so they too, like the cytoplasm of liver cells, are pink to red in an H and E section.

Why Nuclear Components Are Colored Blue. A basic stain has its color in its cations. Hematoxylin in itself is not a basic stain but it is used with what are called mordants which have positive charges, and these attach both to hematoxylin and to sites which would be colored with a basic stain so that hematoxylin acts like one.

There are two kinds of nucleic acid in the nucleus; these are termed deoxyribose nucleic acid (DNA) and ribonucleic acid (RNA) respectively. Their chemistry will be described in more detail in the next three chapters as will the fact that the units of heredity, namely genes, have their chemical basis in DNA; in fact, a gene is a short segment or group of segments in an enormously long DNA molecule. Furthermore, different types of RNA are instrumental in cells in picking up chemical information that is coded in DNA

molecules and conveying this information to sites in the cytoplasm where other forms of RNA assist in permitting the information to be translated into the synthesis of specific proteins, as will be explained in sufficient detail with proper illustrations in Chapter 4. Here, however, we have to stress the fact that both DNA and RNA possess acidic phosphate radicals which combine with the positively charged combination of mordant and hematoxylin and this explains why so much of the nucleus is blue in an H and E section (Fig. 1-14, *upper left*).

Some Basophilic Material Can Usually Be Detected in the Generally Acidophilic Cytoplasm of Liver Cells. As indicated in the color illustration (Fig. 1-14, *top left,* labeled "cytoplasmic RNA") and in the black and white illustration (dark mottling in Fig. 1-11), liver cell cytoplasm is irregularly mottled with little irregular clumps of blue material scattered about in the pink to red cytoplasm. This blue material is RNA. Its significance will be discussed in Chapters 4 and 5.

Why the Cytoplasm of Liver Cells Seen in Some H and E Sections Seems To Have Empty Spaces in It. Liver cells play a very important role in regulating

Figure 1-14

Fig. 1-14. This plate is designed to help the student interpret the colors he sees in stained sections.

At upper left a single liver cell is shown as it appears in an H and E section. The nucleus has a blue rim; this is due to a concentration of the nucelic acid, DNA, around the inner surface of the nuclear membrane. Within the nucleus there are granules of blue material; these are little aggregations of DNA, and there is also a larger rounded body within the nucleus called the nucleolus. This is blue because of its content of another nucleic acid, RNA. The cytoplasm reveals some pink material; this is protein, and this stains with eosin. There are also little aggregations of blue material in the cytoplasm; these are due to little aggregations of RNA in this position. Empty ragged-appearing spaces are also seen in the cytoplasm; these are due to deposits of glycogen. These appear as empty spaces because glycogen is not stained by either H or E.

At upper right a similar cell stained by both the PA-Schiff technic (which colors certain carbohydrate macromolecules a magenta color) and hematoxylin is seen. The chief difference between its appearance and that of the cell at the left is that the protein of the cytoplasm is not stained red (because no eosin was used), but the glycogen is colored specifically (magenta) by the PA-Schiff technic.

The middle illustration shows a row of epithelial cells that lie on loose connective tissue. The staining here is PA-Schiff plus hematoxylin. Two of the epithelial cells in the row are goblet cells, and these secrete a glycoprotein called mucus. The secretion within these cells, which they are pouring onto the free surface, is stained magenta by the PA-Schiff technic. The nuclei of the epithelial cells are stained blue with hematoxylin because of nucleic acids. In the loose connective tissue below the epithelial membrane there are some strands of intercellular substance; these would stain better if eosin could have been used here. A capillary is also shown with some red cells which are not as red as they would be if eosin could have been used. There are seemingly empty spaces in the loose connective tissue; these contain certain mucopolysaccharides, but these do not stain sufficiently by the technic used here to be colored. Part of the seemingly empty areas in the loose connective tissue results from the former presence of tissue fluid, which is washed out in preparing a section.

The lower two pictures illustrate fat cells. The left picture shows fat cells in an H and E section prepared by the usual paraffin technic; by this technic the fat is dissolved away and leaves a rounded empty space in its place. At the right, fat cells are shown as they appear in a section prepared by the freezing technic; by this technic the fat is retained in the cell so that it can be stained with a special stain for fat, which colors it red.

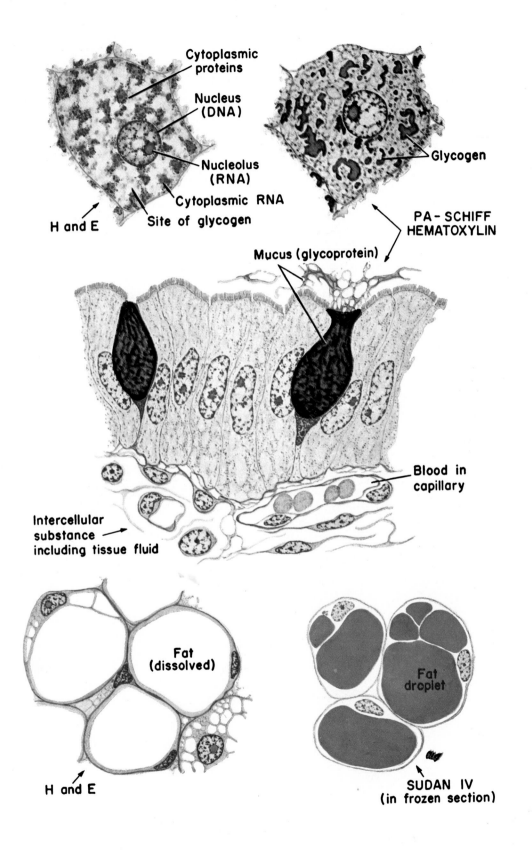

Cytoplasmic proteins

Nucleus (DNA)

Nucleolus (RNA)

Cytoplasmic RNA

Site of glycogen

H and E

Glycogen

PA - SCHIFF
HEMATOXYLIN

Mucus (glycoprotein)

Blood in capillary

Intercellular substance including tissue fluid

Fat (dissolved)

H and E

Fat droplet

SUDAN IV
(in frozen section)

the level of sugar in the blood. Monosaccharides are absorbed from the intestine, not at a constant rate but in relation to meals, and so it might be thought that the level of the blood sugar would go up after meals and down between meals. However, the liver cells regulate the level of the sugar in the blood by removing it from the blood and storing it in their cytoplasm whenever the level begins to rise. On taking sugar from the blood, liver cells convert it to a polysaccharide called *glycogen* which, like starch, is composed of a large number of interconnected glucose residues. Glycogen is not stained with either hematoxylin or eosin and so translucent deposits of it in the cytoplasm of a cell appear as irregularly shaped, ragged, seemingly empty spaces in the reddish cytoplasm (Fig. 1-14, *upper left*) and as ragged empty spaces in the black and white illustration (G, in Fig. 1-15, *left*).

Spaces indicating the presence of glycogen are seen only in sections of some livers. The reason for this is that if the human liver tissue used for preparing the section was taken from a person (as often happens) who died after a lengthy illness in which his appetite had failed, his liver cells would not have been storing glycogen. However, if liver tissue is obtained from a healthy normal person who, for example, is killed in a motor accident shortly after eating a hearty meal, the cells of his liver may be so riddled with seemingly empty spaces that a student hospital pathologist, who is accustomed to seeing the liver cells of people who have died after lengthy illnesses, can scarcely recognize it as liver. The liver cells shown in Figures 1-14 and 1-15 were taken from a healthy, well-fed laboratory animal.

The Staining of Glycogen in Sections by the PA-Schiff Technic. Since glycogen is a polymer, it is not very soluble in water; hence it is not readily dissolved in the preparation of a stained section. However, if fixation is not prompt, hydrolytic enzymes begin to operate in cells soon after death occurs, and these convert glycogen to glucose, which, of course, is soluble and washed out as the section is prepared. If fixation is less than perfect, the fixative, in penetrating cells slowly from one side to the other, coagulates protein progressively from one side of the cell to the other, and in doing so pushes the glycogen ahead of it to some extent; as a result, the glycogen is displaced toward one side of each cell which position for it is, of course, an artifact.

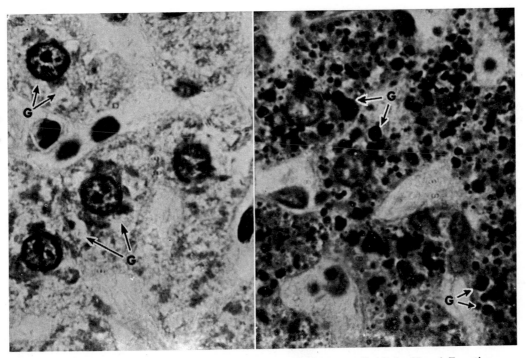

FIG. 1-15. Photomicrographs of sections of liver of well-fed rat. (*Left*) An H and E section, and the sites of glycogen in the cytoplasm are indicated by irregular ragged clear areas (G). (*Right*) A smilar section stained by the PA-Schiff technic, which colors the glycogen magenta; this appears black in the photograph (G).

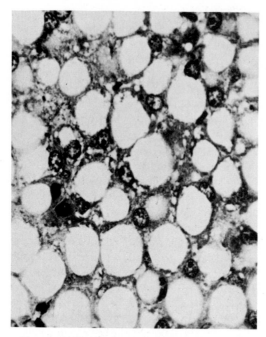

Fig. 1-16. Photomicrograph of a section of liver from a rat which had experienced a choline deficiency for 12 days. (McGregor stain, × 600.) The liver cells that are distended with fat are almost twice as wide as normal cells. The black structures seen are capillaries that have been injected with India ink. (Hartroft, W. S.: Anat. Rec., *106*:61)

The PA-Schiff technic is a 2-step procedure based on the application to histology of 2 reactions well known to chemists. Periodic acid reacts with certain 1,2 glycol groups (–CHOH–CHOH–), which occur in the glucose residues making up the glycogen chain. On treating sections containing glycogen with periodic acid, both members of each glycol group yield an aldehyde group (–CHO), so that the polysaccharidic chain of glycogen becomes a polyaldehyde chain. The second step is to treat the sections with a well-known reagent for aldehydes; this is a dye known as basic fuchsin, which can be bleached with sulfurous acid, when it is then known as the Schiff reagent. Aldehydes combine with the bleached dye to produce a *magenta-* or *purple*-colored complex (Fig. 1-14, *upper right*) which is readily seen in the microscope. In the case of glycogen, a bright purple reaction product is seen (Fig. 1-14, *upper right*). In black and white illustrations it is black (Fig. 1-15, *right*). Accordingly, it is said that glycogen is a PA-Schiff-positive substance.

Glycogen is readily broken down by alpha amylase, the enzyme present in saliva, and after treatment with this enzyme, it can be washed out of sections. Hence

when a PA-Schiff-positive substance is found in a cell, it is customary to incubate a section in a solution of purified alpha amylase (or in saliva, which is rich in amylase) to extract glycogen and stain again by the PA-Schiff method. Disappearance of the purple material proves that the material was glycogen.

Fat in Liver Cells. Another kind of seemingly empty space can be seen in the cytoplasm of the cells of some livers. These differ from those of glycogen by being round and having sharp edges (Fig. 1-16) instead of having irregular shapes and fuzzy edges. Round empty spaces are left by stored droplets of fat which dissolved away in the reagents employed in making a paraffin section. If the cells of a liver contain a great many of these round holes, the person who died is said to have had a *fatty liver*. Commonly this condition is seen in individuals who have, for a lengthy period, replaced nourishing food in their diets in favor of the steady heavy consumption of alcohol.

Since fat in liver cells dissolves away in preparing a paraffin section, frozen sections are commonly used to demonstrate it with special fat stains such as Scharlach R or Sudan III (see bottom row of illustrations in Fig. 1-14).

With this preliminary study of cells, we should now be able to consider their two parts, nucleus and cytoplasm, in detail, which will be done in the next four chapters. However, since this will entail the study of further sections, you should now be made aware of the fact that sections are not always as perfect as might be hoped for and one class of imperfections known as artifacts may puzzle you unless you know what they are. So, before beginning on the detailed study of the nucleus, we shall now comment briefly on some of the common artifacts so that you will not be puzzled if you encounter them.

ARTIFACTS

To understand artifacts it should be realized that each of the steps involved in preparing a section provides an opportunity for something to happen that will make the final product less than perfect. Artifacts are not the result of anything that occurred in the tissue during life but only to alterations made in it subsequently because of its manipulation by man as he prepares sections from it.

Some common ones are listed below and illustrated in Figure 1-17.

Shrinkage. The different chemicals with which tissue is treated, or the heat of the melted paraffin, may cause *shrinkage*. As a result, portions of tissue which were adjacent in life may be pulled away from

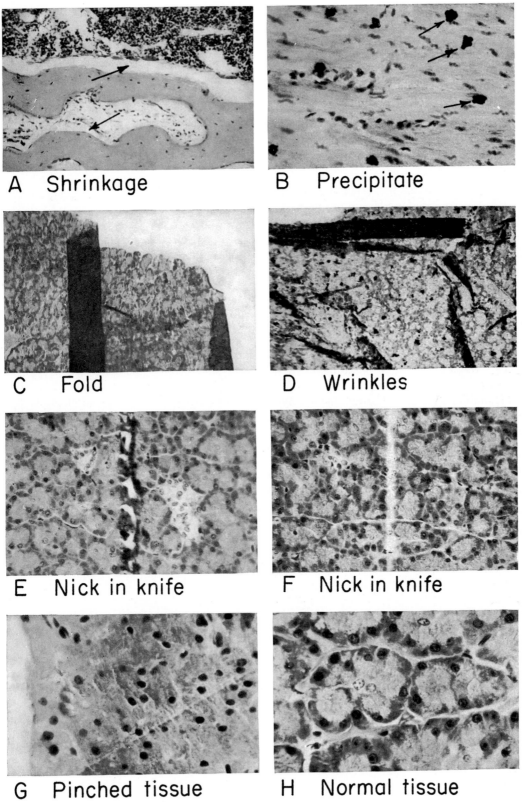

FIG. 1-17. Photomicrographs showing various kinds of artifacts.

one another, as has occurred at the sites indicated by arrows in Figure 1-17, A.

Imperfect Removal of Fixative. Sometimes the fixative is imperfectly removed from tissue, and crystals of it precipitate and remain behind. The appearance of any other foreign material (dust or dirt in the air) added during the preparation of the section is somewhat similar, but it depends, of course, on the nature of the material. See Figure 1-17, B.

Folds and Wrinkles. Paraffin sections are so thin that it is not unusual for them to become somewhat wrinkled or folded as they are cut, and sometimes these little *wrinkles* or *folds* cannot be entirely smoothed out when the section is being mounted on a slide. These then appear in a section, as shown in Figure 1-17, C and D.

Nicks in the Knife. Microscopic nicks in the microtome knife cause a characteristic defect. As the knife sweeps across a paraffin block in a straight plane, any nick in it creates a defect in the section and appears as a straight line across it. Figure 1-17, E and F, show examples of defects caused in this way. The picture in E shows one caused by a large nick, and the one in F by a small nick. Any defect that is seen as a straight line passing across the section is most likely to be an artifact of this type.

Rough Handling of Fresh Tissue. Another type of artifact often seen in sections, which may lead to the incorrect surmise that the tissue under view has been the seat of pathological change, is produced by rough handling of tissue as it is being cut from the animal body. Commonly, in obtaining tissue, forceps are used to hold a piece that is being cut away; sometimes the cutting is done by scissors (instead of a very sharp knife), and dull ones at that. The pinching caused by holding living tissue firmly with forceps and cutting it with dull scissors profoundly affects the appearance it presents in stained sections. This appearance is illustrated in Figure 1-17, G. Figure 1-17, H shows how the tissue would have appeared if it had not been mistreated.

Postmortem Degeneration. This, although it is a very important cause of sections of poor quality is, strictly speaking, not an artifact. It and its cause will be described and illustrated in connection with lysosomes in Chapter 5.

References and Other Reading

Since this chapter is of a general nature no specific references to any particular topic need be given. However, since several technics are mentioned, it should be pointed out to any student who wishes more detailed information about any of these that the library of the college or university that he is attending would have a variety of books dealing with light microscopy, photomicrography, phase microscopy, histologic technics, stains and staining and histochemistry. So far as attempting to visualize three dimensional structure from the study of single sections is concerned, anyone who has difficulty in this matter will find more extensive treatment of this subject in earlier editions of this book which are also probably to be found on library shelves.

2 The Nucleus

Division of Function Between Nucleus and Cytoplasm. The cytoplasm performs the particular work for which any given cell is specialized. For example, the contractile mechanism of a muscle cell is a cytoplasmic component. Likewise the production lines along which secretions are assembled in various gland cells are located in their cytoplasm. We might, therefore, ask what responsibilities are delegated to the nucleus. There are two.

The first is that the nucleus, since it contains the genes, is chiefly responsible for ensuring that when a cell divides into two daughter cells, each daughter cell inherits the same genes as those possessed by the mother cell.

The second is also dependent on the nucleus containing the genes; however, its function in carrying out this responsibility is performed, not while a cell is dividing but when it is performing its specialized work. In the latter phase the genes from their nuclear position direct the synthesis of the proper proteins in the cytoplasm for the cell to have the proper enzymes and organelles to perform the particular functions for which that particular type of cell is specialized.

The Conflict Involved in the Nucleus Having Two Functions. A professor is generally interested in performing research as well as in teaching. He obviously cannot engage in both of these activities at the same time and so he has to alternate his time between them. Nuclei are in much the same position, for when a nucleus is engaged in the process of duplicating its genes and going through all the other events concerned in cell division, the genes have to temporarily stop their work of directing the usual type of protein synthesis they direct when the cell is performing its specialized work.

A Conflict Between Specialized Function and the Ability to Divide. There is a second conflict between the two functions of the nucleus. This appears seemingly when the task of its genes in directing protein synthesis in the cytoplasm becomes so specialized and exacting that the nucleus loses its ability to undergo division. The fact that there are many kinds of highly specialized body cells that can no longer divide poses a problem in connection with maintaining cell populations in various parts of the body, as will next be described.

How Cell Populations Are Maintained (or Not Maintained) in Three Categories of Body Cells

When a body stops growing in stature, cells must continue to divide, because in many parts of the body cells wear out and die or are lost from some surface; hence, to maintain a normal cell population in these parts of the body, more cells must be produced at the same rate as that at which cells are lost. Cell division is, therefore, required all through life to provide for the *maintenance* of the body. Furthermore, as a result of injury or disease, parts of the body may be destroyed, and effective *repair* in these instances is brought about because cells that remain undergo division to provide daughter cells to take the place of those that have been destroyed. Thus, the normal growth, maintenance and repair of body tissues hinges on the ability of at least certain cells of the body to be able to undergo cell division. However, as noted, most kinds of highly specialized cells cannot divide, and this brings up the problem of how cell populations are maintained under these circumstances. This problem is most easily dealt with at an introductory level by classifying body cells according to the way their populations are affected, into 3 categories, as was suggested by Leblond.

Category 1. By the time of birth or at most after a very few years of postnatal life, there are some cells in the body in which a highly specialized state has been attained only at the expense of a complete loss of reproductive capacity. Moreover, no provision is made for the replacement of these specialized cells if they wear out or are destroyed. Nerve cells are the classic and almost the only example of cells in this category. After we are a few years old we have all the nerve cells that we shall ever possess. As they wear out and die there is throughout life a continuous diminution of their number. To compensate for this discouraging thought there is a comforting one: there is perhaps some advantage in their not being able to divide, for, if they did, it would probably upset our memories and reflexes.

23

Category 2. Many kinds of body cells (all of which we shall study in due course) that become highly specialized to perform some particular function either wear out or are lost from body surfaces, often at a rapid rate. Furthermore, like nerve cells, the highly specialized cells of this second category are unable to reproduce. However, there is provision for the replacement of the specialized cells of this category. This is accomplished by division of cells of the same lineage (family type) that have not yet become sufficiently specialized to have lost their ability to reproduce. These cells are termed the *stem cells* * or *germinative cells* of the lineage to which they belong, and by reproducing themselves they keep up a supply of stem cells of the particular family type to which they belong. As a result, new cells that can specialize are always available to take the place of those specialized cells that are lost. This means that in many parts of the body (all of which will be described in detail later) there is a continuous, often rapid *turnover of the cell population,* with young cells dividing and yielding daughter cells that mature to take the place of those that are lost. There exists a balance between cell production and cell loss in the adult, so that the total number of cells remains the same although its individual members change. It is said that the cell population of these parts of the body is in a *steady state.*

Category 3. Still other kinds of cells in the body appear to represent an exception to the rule that specialized function interferes with reproductive capacity, for there are several examples of highly specialized cells that under certain circumstances can reproduce themselves. However, the highly specialized cells in this category are generally not called upon very often to use their reproductive capacity after the growth of the organ in which they live is completed. Cells of this category are found mostly in organs in which the cells have a long life-span, and in which cell division seldom occurs after full growth of the organ has been attained. The cells of the liver are examples of this category. However, if two thirds of the liver of

* Whereas it is usual to use the term *stem cell* for the mother cell of a given particular family of cells of a certain type in the body, a particular family may embrace more than one related but different subsidiary cell line, and the stem cell in this instance has the capability of becoming specialized along any of these sublines—as occurs, for example, in the formation of blood cells. There may, furthermore, be intermediate steps between the stem cell and the end product in any of the cell lines of a family, with cells of the intermediate types being somewhat more restricted than the stem cell both with regard to their reproductive capabilities and the breadth of the number of sub-lines of cells along which it can specialize. The problem will be explored in more detail later in relation to the various cell families which we shall encounter.

an experimental animal is removed at an operation, the cells of the remaining third undergo division and reproduce themselves so rapidly that the liver is restored to its former size in less than two weeks. The cells of many glands that make hormones are highly specialized. Under normal conditions they seldom reproduce themselves, for they, like liver cells, live a long time; but under altered conditions they, too, can undergo division and so demonstrate that, even though they are specialized, they have not lost the ability to reproduce themselves.

Why some cells that are highly specialized, such as those in Category 3, are still able to undergo cell division while the highly specialized cells of both Categories 1 and 2 are not is not understood. However, the highly specialized cells of Categories 1 and 2 demonstrate that the specialization of a cell for a particular function is only obtained at the cost of the loss of reproductive capacity.

Technics Required To Study the Nucleus

Our next task, therefore, is to describe the microscopic appearance of both the interphase and the dividing nucleus and relate what is seen in them to what is happening and, so far as is reasonable at the level of this book, to changes that occur at the molecular level. In order to achieve this end we must, however, take into account what has been learned from electron microscopy and radioautography and so, before describing and interpreting the appearance of the interphase nucleus at the level of the LM, we shall describe the electron microscope (EM) so that we shall be able to correlate, in our description of the nucleus, its appearance in the LM with that in the EM. Later on it will become necessary to deal with radioautography.

The Search for Greater Effective Magnification. The resolving power of the light microscope is irrevocably limited by the wave length of visible light. No two objects separated by less than 0.2 micron can be resolved clearly as distinct entities by the ordinary LM. One attempt made to obtain greater effective magnification was to build microscopes that would take advantage of the shorter wavelength of ultraviolet light. This required that lenses be made out of quartz or some other material that transmits UV. Since ultraviolet light is invisible, the image has to be focused on a fluorescent screen which acts to transform light of shorter wavelengths into visible light. However, ultraviolet light affects photographic emulsions directly so, after the image is focused with the screen, a film can be substituted for the screen and a photomicrograph can be taken at an effective magnification approximately twice that possible with the ordinary microscope. But the revolutionary advance in microscopy came in the 1920's when it was discovered that suitably shaped magnetic or electrostatic fields could be used as lenses for an electron beam, and that the wave length of electrons is such that this factor would be almost negligible in resolving objects with them. This knowledge led to building a microscope that would use electrons instead of light.

The Electron Microscope

Development. The first electron microscope was built in 1931 by Knoll and Ruska in Germany, and by 1933 they had made one that had a resolving power greater than the LM. The first EM built in North America (1932) was constructed in the Department of Physics at the University of Toronto by Prebus, Hillier and Burton. Soon afterward commercial instru-

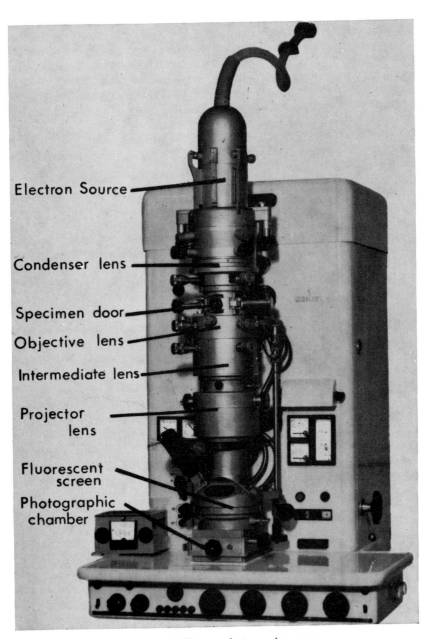

Fig. 2-1. A Siemens electron microscope.

ments of high quality became available and were steadily improved. But many years elapsed before it became possible to study tissue sections with this new instrument. It was not until around 1950 that means were evolved for preparing sections of cells that were thin enough and otherwise suitable to be profitably studied. Since then a stream of information has flowed from EM studies of cells that has opened up a new world of knowledge.

Electron Micrographs. Like ultraviolet light, an electron beam that has passed through a section has to be focused on a fluorescent screen where the image is converted to one of visible light. However, like ultraviolet light, electrons affect photographic emulsions directly, hence photographic film can be substituted for the fluorescent screen and a picture termed an *electron micrograph* taken of the image that was focused on the screen.

Because electron microscopes are very expensive and because their use requires special training, the undergraduate student usually will not use one as he uses his own LM to study sections but instead will learn what is called *fine structure* or *ultrastructure,* which terms designate structure visible at the magnification obtain-

able only with the EM, mostly from the study of electron micrographs. Fortunately, these often reveal more detail than can be seen on the fluorescent screen of an electron microscope. However, in most laboratories the student will have the opportunity of seeing an EM (Fig. 2-1) and perhaps observing a few sections with one. Furthermore, in some laboratories the image projected on the fluorescent screen can be televised and so watched by students as an instructor examines different parts of a section and at different magnifications with the EM.

Since a description of an EM is a subject for physics, and since there are now many books on the instrument and its use in the biological fields, we shall here give only a brief account of the instrument but then make detailed comments on interpreting electron micrographs.

COMPARISON OF OPTICS OF LIGHT AND ELECTRON MICROSCOPES

The optics of the LM are shown on the left side of Figure 2-2 but in order to compare these with those of the EM, the LM is upside down.

In the LM, light from a suitable source is focused with a condenser lens (Fig. 2-2, *left*) and directed as a strong beam through the object—for example, a stained section that is on the stage (Fig. 2-2, *left, "object"*). The light that passes through the object is focused by the objective lens (Fig. 2-2, *left*) to bring an image of the object into focus somewhere between the objective and the projection lens (Fig. 2-2, *left*). The projection lens (the one in the eyepiece of the LM) can further magnify the image up to 10 or 15 times. This lens can be used to bring the enlarged image into focus on either a ground glass or a photographic film placed at the site indicated by the bottom arrow (Fig. 2-2, *left*).

The optics of an EM are illustrated on the right side of Figure 2-2. In the EM, the paths of electrons are influenced by magnetic fields in the same way that light is influenced by glass lenses. The strength of these fields can be varied by changing the amount of current passing through the coils of wire in the electromagnetic lenses of the EM (stippled in Fig. 2-2, *right*). The whole instrument (Fig. 2-1) is, in essence, a cathode-ray tube in which a vacuum must be maintained by continuous pumping because electrons can travel only for very short distances in air. From the electrically heated cathode, which is a V-shaped tungsten filament (Fig. 2-2, *top right*) electrons are emitted and attracted toward the anode (by a potential difference of 50,000 to 100,000 volts). The anode has a hole or an aperture in it so that a stream of electrons passes through it

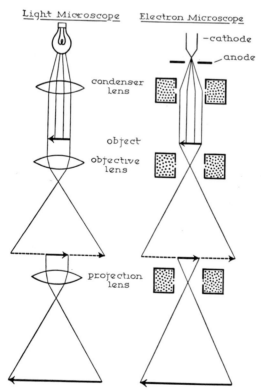

FIG. 2-2. Diagram showing optical paths in light and electron microscopes.

(Fig. 2-2, *right*) and is then focused by the condenser lens (a magnetic field) and directed at the object (Fig. 2-2, *right*), which for our purposes is generally an unbelievably thin slice of tissue prepared as will be described presently. As the electrons pass through the section, more are scattered out of the beam by the denser parts of the section than by the less dense parts.

Those electrons that are scattered by the specimen are removed from the beam by blocking action of a very fine aperture (not shown in the diagram) placed just above the objective lens. The role of this aperture, which is usually about 30 microns in diameter, is to provide more contrast in the final image. The remaining electrons (those not scattered and, hence, not subtracted from the beam) are focused by the objective lens, and an enlarged image is obtained thereby (Fig. 2-2, *right*). This image is enlarged further, first by a lens known as an intermediate lens (not shown in diagram) and then by a projection lens; the latter projects the image onto the fluorescent screen (Fig. 2-1) or a photographic film which can be substituted for it.

How Sections Are Examined in the EM

Thin sections, prepared as will be described later, are placed on the specimen holder of the microscope and inserted into the instrument. A high vacuum must be produced in the instrument before the electron beam can be switched on and the specimen examined. The black round knobs at the bottom of Figure 2-1 are controls for moving the specimen around, for changing the magnification, the brightness of the image, and so on. The magnification can be changed easily by turning a knob that controls the current passing through the intermediate or the projector lens. Focusing of the image is accomplished by altering very slightly the objective lens current. The focal length of the objective lens is altered thereby, to bring the image into sharp focus on the fluorescent screen. Since focusing must be done accurately, it is customary to observe the screen through a low-power binocular microscope while bringing the image into focus.

The Kind of Sections Required for the EM

The electron beam penetrates matter so poorly that it took a long time to evolve methods for cutting sections thin enough (roughly a millionth of an inch thick) for study in the EM.

Fixation. For many years a buffered solution of osmium tetroxide, introduced by Palade, was the only fixative of practical importance to electron microscopists. After its use, however, certain cell components are not preserved and it is impossible to make certain histochemical tests which depend on enzyme reactions. It was then that a procedure using two fixatives was introduced. Fixation in an aldehyde followed by fixation in osmium tetroxide usually produced results better than the best osmic fixation. The buffered aldehydes that give the best results are formalin, acrolein and particularly, glutaraldehyde; these preserve the cell's fine structure and still permit the use of many histochemical technics after the aldehyde and before the osmic acid fixative.

Embedding Media. New embedding media harder than wax were also necessary for cutting the very thin sections required for the EM. At first, a plastic material, butyl methacrylate, was used but it had some disadvantages. Since then new ones have been discovered and among these the epoxy resins, Epon and Araldite, are the most popular.

Microtomes. First, microtomes with special mechanisms capable of advancing the blocks of tissue to be cut roughly from only $\frac{1}{10}$ to $\frac{1}{40}$ micron, each time, the range required for electron microscopy, had to be designed. Next, it was found important to avoid having the block pass back over the knife edge on the return stroke after completion of the cutting stroke. Accordingly, ultramicrotomes are usually designed so that the block takes a circuitous course and bypasses the cutting edge on the return stroke.

Knives. Another improvement resulted from the use of the fractured edge of a piece of plate glass to cut sections. Then specially ground diamond knives became available: the cutting edge of these is no sharper than that of a glass knife, but it is so hard that it can be used for a much longer time and also to cut very hard tissues such as bone and teeth.

Mounting. The problem of obtaining proper support for the very thin sections required for the EM and yet permitting the passage of electrons through them is solved by mounting the sections on little copper grids, each of which is often coated with a very thin supporting film of Formvar (a plastic) or carbon. The copper grid supports the film and the film supports the section. The electron beam can pass through the section and its supporting film in the spaces between the bars of the grid. These spaces are each sufficiently large to allow a relatively extensive part of a section to be examined at a time.

Staining. Because no colors are involved, the term *staining* is used only in the sense that material is treated with solutions of heavy metals to make certain cell components more electron dense than others so as to produce a greater black-and-white contrast in images on the fluorescent screen or on photographic film. It is fortunate that osmium is so commonly used for fixation, because osmium, which scatters electrons strongly, is normally taken up to different extents by different cell components. Other salts of heavy metals commonly used are uranium acetate and lead hydroxide. They act in a similar manner to increase contrast and are usually applied to the thin sections after they have been placed on the copper grids.

Since the production of an image on a fluorescent screen or the taking of an electron micrograph on a film by the electron microscope as has been described above requires that electrons pass through a section (the object), the technic is referred to as transmission electron microscopy. Micrographs prepared by this technic are the common kind used to illustrate a book such as this. However, we should mention here that micrographs also can be taken of objects by a different method that is termed *scanning electron microscopy;* this method does not require that electrons pass through an object. To avoid confusion this type of electron microscopy, which is very useful for providing three-dimensional surface views of objects, will not be described here but in connection with the first micrograph prepared by this method that is used in the text. In the following section we shall therefore deal only with some of the problems associated with interpreting electron micrographs of the transmission type. *Any reference to electron micrographs in the following implies micrographs made by transmission electron microscopy.*

Interpreting Electron Micrographs

The student should, at this stage, acquire some competence in interpreting electron micrographs, for they are widely used as illustrations in lectures, books and journals encountered not only in histology but also in almost all fields of medical and biological science. A few points, now to be described, should help in this matter.

Similiarities Between Black and White Photomicrographs and Electron Micrographs

Familiarity with interpreting black and white photomicrographs can stand the beginner in good stead when he first begins to study electron micrographs because the latter are, of course, always in black and white. Furthermore, one very important component of cells, the nucleic acids that combine strongly with hematoxylin in ordinary sections and so print out black in photomicrographs, combine strongly with the heavy metals used as stains for electron microscopy, and hence print out black in electron micrographs. This

fact in itself helps establish a few landmarks when one first examines electron micrographs of cells: for example, compare a nucleus in the drawing of a liver cell in H and E section made with the LM (Fig. 2-3) with the electron micrograph of a similar nucleus (Fig. 2-4). Proteins in general are not heavily stained in either H and E sections or electron micrographs and so print out lightly in both. Glycogen must be stained if it is to be black in either photomicrographs or electron micrographs, otherwise it appears as clear areas. Fat, however, generally combines with the osmium used in fixing material for electron microscopy and so it is black in electron micrographs whereas in ordinary H and E sections its site is marked by empty spaces. The fact that lipid is stained with the osmium tetroxide used in preparing tissue for electron microscopy probably assists in demarcating lipoprotein membranes—which, as will be described in Chapter 5, abound in cells—from a protein background in cytoplasm.

Some Differences Between Electron Micrographs and Black and White Photomicrographs

1. *Why Electron Micrographs Are Enlarged.* An oil-immersion photomicrograph taken on a good-sized negative reveals all the detail that can be resolved with the light microscope. To enlarge it does not reveal any more detail; it just makes everything larger. However, because of the extremely short wave length of an electron beam an incredible amount of detail can be registered on suitable film, more than can be seen with the eye in a contact print and hence enlargements are necessary to make it apparent. Accordingly, substantial enlargements of micrographs taken with the EM are essential to take full advantage of the resolving power of the instrument.

2. *Different Units of Measurement Are Used.* We are in a period of transition in which the units of measurement that have been in use for both the LM and the EM are being replaced by units that adhere more strictly to the metric system. First, the term micron which gained universal use in connection with light microscopy, and was described in the first chapter as being one thousandth of a millimeter and designated by the symbol, μ, is being displaced by the term micrometer which is designated by the symbol μm and, of course, is one thousandth of a millimeter. The advent of electron microscopy with its much greater effective magnifications made the use of still smaller units of measurements essential. The two units that came into general use for this purpose were first, the term millimicron, characterized by the symbol, mμ, which represented one thousandth of a micron and the term Ang-

strom unit, characterized by the symbol Å, which represented one tenth of a millimicron. The term millimicron, however, is now being displaced by the term nanometer, which is characterized by the symbol nm, and the term Angstrom unit is being replaced by 0.1 nm.

New Terminology	*Old Terminology*
micrometer μm	= micron μ
nanometer nm	= millimicron mμ
0.1 nm	= 1 Å

Since the older units of measurement were used in all the literature up to the time of the introduction of the new units, anyone who wants to know what was learned in the past as well as what will be learned in the future needs to become conversant with both sets of units, and in order to facilitate this, both will be used in this book, often giving the same measurement in both.

3. *The depth of focus* of the oil-immersion objective of the light microscope is so short that it is impossible to have all the thickness of even a very thin paraffin section in focus at the same time. As a result, in inspecting various parts of a section with the oil-immersion objective, the observer has to focus up and down continually. This, however, has an advantage as well as a disadvantage; by focusing up and down, the observer can generally tell whether some minute object is above or below an adjacent object. It is not possible to do this with the EM. In the EM everything within the thickness of a section is in focus at the same time. This makes it impossible to tell whether one small object is above or below any other small object. *For example, a tiny granule below part of a larger thin-walled sac would appear in the EM as if it was inside the sac.*

4. An important difference between photomicrographs and electron micrographs is due to the sections used for the EM being so much thinner than those used for the LM. Whereas only a few paraffin sections would be required to section completely one liver cell for the LM, about 400 such sections would be required to section the same cell for electron microscopy. This explains why, for example, when a certain kind of cell is examined with the LM, it may seem to be very well filled with granules, but when the same cell is examined in the EM, it may seem to contain only an occasional granule. However, if a whole pile of sections were cut at the thickness required for the EM from this cell, and if these were placed one above the other until the thickness of the section used for the LM was attained and then if these piles of sections were viewed with the LM, the cell would, of course, again appear to be heavily granulated. With the LM one has a much greater thickness of a cell to see through and hence one sees many more of the kinds of things that are in it, provided that they are visible in the LM.

Further information on the interpretation of electron micrographs will be given in Chapter 5 in relation to the appearance of cytoplasmic organelles.

We are now in a position to make a detailed study of the nuclei of cells in which we can compare their structure as seen with the LM and the EM.

The Nuclei of Nondividing Cells (Interphase Nuclei)

Terminology. Long ago it was noticed with the LM that when a cell undergoes division, a series of changes occur in the appearance of its nucleus (all of which will be described in detail presently) and, when the process terminates, the original cell has divided into two daughter cells. The whole process which results in one cell thus becoming two was termed *mitosis,* for reasons that will also be described presently. Next, when the method of *tissue culture* was devised whereby living cells could be grown in glass receptacles in suitable fluids, it was found that there were certain kinds of animal cells that multiplied vigorously under these conditions by passing through mitosis at regular and relatively short intervals. The period of time between the end of one mitosis and the beginning of the next was termed the interphase (*inter,* between). The period of time occupied by one mitosis plus one interphase was the time taken for what is termed a *cell cycle.* Soon it became customary to refer to the nucleus of any cell that was not in the process of mitosis as an interphase nucleus. However, this is not a good term because, as was described earlier in this chapter, many body cells seen in sections are of kinds that will never divide again and so they are not *between* two phases of mitosis. It therefore becomes difficult to find a term which properly depicts nuclei that are in body cells that are not dividing at the moment but can divide, as well as those that will never divide again.

Since only a very small percentage of the cells of the body are at any given time in the process of cell division, most of the nuclei that are seen in sections are in cells that are either working or resting. Perhaps the best way to refer to these is by calling them nondividing cells. However, it is more or less common practice to refer to their nuclei as interphase nuclei so we shall follow this practice and use it because it is so common, but with the understanding that it does not refer exclusively to cells that are *between* two mitoses.

APPEARANCE OF THE NONDIVIDING (INTERPHASE)
NUCLEUS IN H AND E SECTIONS

As we study the various tissues and organs of the
body with the LM, we shall find that the interphase
nuclei present a considerable variety of appearances in
different cell types. Some kinds of cells have interphase
nuclei which are small and in which the nuclear contents are tightly packed together. Sinusoid lining cells
(Fig. 2-3) show this type of nuclei. The nuclei of still
other kinds of cells will be found to have unusual
shapes; for example, instead of being round to ovoid
they may be elongated and, in some instances, pinched
along their lengths so that they resemble short strings
of beads, as in the cell called a neutrophil or polymorph
illustrated in Chapter 10. However, generally speaking,
all nuclei have the same components, and the easiest
way to see these with the LM is to study the cells in
which the nuclei are large enough to have their components spread sufficiently apart for them to be identi-

fied, as in nuclei of liver cells in Figure 2-3. There are
many cell types in the body that have nuclei of this
sort but, since we have already learned how to identify
cells in the liver and since liver cell nuclei are almost
always in the interphase and have their components
fairly well spread apart, we shall take them for our
example and describe the appearance of their components. We shall then compare what can be seen in
the LM (Fig. 2-3) with what is seen in the EM (Fig.
2-4).

THE FOUR COMPONENTS OF THE INTERPHASE
NUCLEUS AS SEEN WITH THE LM IN AN
H AND E SECTION

1. With the oil-immersion objective the interphase
nucleus appears to be limited by a dark-blue-staining
line; this is termed the *nuclear envelope* or *nuclear
membrane* (Fig. 2-3).

2. Within each nucleus there are one or more
rounded blue-staining bodies; these are the largest and
roundest of the bodies within the nucleus. These bodies
are termed *nucleoli,* and each one is a nucleolus (Fig.
2-3).

3. Within each nucleus there are also numerous,
often poorly defined particles of blue-staining material
that are of irregular shapes and smaller than the
nucleoli. Sometimes they may appear as if they were
more or less strung together. This material is referred
to as *chromatin* (chrome-color) because it stains
strongly with basic stains (Fig. 2-3). What appear to
be individual particles of chromatin with the LM are
sometimes termed *chromatin granules* although, as
noted, they are not sharply defined.

4. The space in the nucleus not occupied by chromatin and nucleoli is filled with a semifluid material
called *nuclear sap.* In stained sections this material is
represented by very pale-staining or almost clear areas
(Fig. 2-3).

We shall deal first with the nuclear envelope.

The Nuclear Envelope or Membrane

In photomicrographs or drawings of cells in H and E
sections, the nuclear envelope generally appears as a
dark blue-purple line (Fig. 2-3). Hence, before the
days of electron microscopy it was assumed that the
nuclear envelope was thick enough to be resolved with
the LM after it had been stained. However, when it
was studied with the EM, it was found that in sections
that cut across it at right angles the nuclear envelope
appeared as two roughly parallel fine lines, as can be
seen in Figure 2-4 but to better advantage in the lower
picture in Figure 2-6. These two lines represent slices

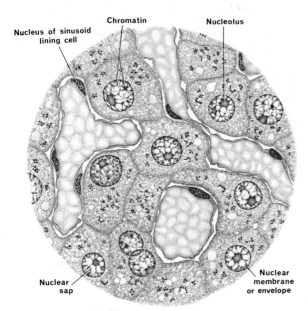

FIG. 2-3. This is what should be seen with oil-immersion
when a section of liver is examined. The detail to note is as
follows: First, each nucleus of the liver cells contains a blue-
staining nucleolus (*upper right*). The remainder of each nucleus
is made up of fine strands or granules of blue material (which
is chromatin, *upper middle*), between which there are seemingly
little empty spaces; the latter contain nuclear sap (*lower left*).
Each nucleus is surrounded by a nuclear membrane or envelope
(*lower right*). Notice also (*upper left*) that the nuclei of the
cells that line the blood spaces are darker, smaller and more
elongated than the nuclei of liver cells; in these the chromatin
is more condensed. Within the blood passages the outlines of
red blood cells can often be seen.

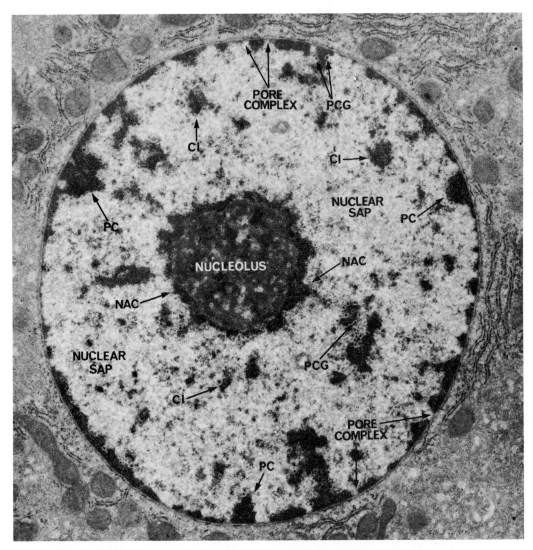

Fig. 2-4. Electron micrograph ($\times$ 14,000) of the interphase nucleus of a rat liver cell. Material was fixed in glutaraldehyde and postfixed in osmium tetroxide. This procedure allows a clear visualization of the condensed parts of chromosomes, forming peripheral chromatin (PC), chromatin islands (CI) and nucleolus-associated chromatin (NAC). The intranuclear channel of a pore complex can be seen as a pale area of nuclear sap between two adjacent masses of peripheral chromatin. Careful inspection shows perichromatin granules (PCG). (Miyai, K., and Steiner, J. W.: The fine structure of interphase liver cell nuclei in subacute ethionine intoxication. Exp. Molec. Path., *4:525*)

cut across two very thin membranes, more or less at right angles to them. The two are separated from each other by a space.

Why It Seems That the Nuclear Envelope Is Visible With the LM in Stained Sections. The nuclear envelope actually consists of two membranes, each about 70 Å thick, which are separated by a space of around 250 Å; thus the total thickness of the en-velope is only around 400 Å. The amount of substance in the two 70-Å-thick membranes is much too thin to be visible as a blue-purple line in an H and E section with the LM. The reason for the dark line seen with the LM and in Figure 2-3 is that there is a good deal of dark granular chromatin scattered along and more or less adherent to, the inner surface of the nuclear en-velope (Fig. 2-4). Chromatin is very basophilic and so

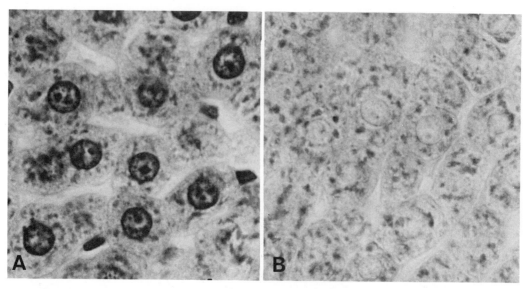

Fig. 2-5. H and E sections of rat liver (*A*) before, and (*B*) after extraction with DNAase. The nuclei stain much less intensely and the nuclear envelope is less prominent after the extraction with DNAase. (Courtesy R. Daoust)

it seems that what has been assumed to be basophilic nuclear envelope in stained sections with the LM is not the envelope itself but the chromatin that adheres to its inner surface. This chromatin has a smooth outer surface in H and E sections because it is limited by the invisible membranous nuclear envelope.

It is easy to verify the above concept with the LM if advantage is taken of the fact that the enzyme DNA-ase dissolves the DNA from chromatin and so destroys its characteristic staining properties. As is shown in Figure 2-5, A, what appears to be nuclear envelopes are seen in an H and E section. But if sections are treated with DNA-ase before they are stained with a basic stain, as is shown in Figure 2-5, B, the structures that appeared to be nuclear envelopes in the control section (Fig. 2-5, A) are not nearly as apparent because the DNA in the peripheral chromatin that ordinarily accounts for this blue staining is removed by the DNA-ase.

Why the Nuclear Envelope Is Not Seen As Two Membranes With the EM in Oblique Sections. A thin section cut through the nuclear envelope more or less at a right angle to it reveals two membranes (Figs. 2-4 and 2-6, *bottom*). But if the plane of the section passes through the membrane so obliquely that it is almost parallel to the membrane, the two membranes of the nuclear envelope cannot be seen as such (Fig. 2-6, *top*). The reason is that the individual membranes have so little density that they scatter enough electrons to become visible as two lines *only if the*

electron beam has to pass through an envelope disposed more or less at right angles to the plane of the section. If envelopes slant through a section or run parallel to it, the electron beam has to pass through their thickness only, and because they are so thin this does not scatter many electrons. (The same principles hold for demonstrating the layers of the cell membrane; see Fig. 5-4.)

The outer membrane of the nuclear envelope, the one next to the cytoplasm, is similar to, and often connects with, a cytoplasmic membrane system called the rough-surfaced endoplasmic reticulum which will be described in detail in the chapter on Cytoplasm.

Nuclear Pores. Knowledge of the biochemical interactions that occur between the nuclear and the cytoplasmic compartments indicates that there must be means by which macromolecules of considerable size can pass between nucleus and cytoplasm. The probable pathway is through little gaps in the nuclear envelope which are disclosed by the EM (Fig. 2-6, *bottom* and Fig. 2-7, large arrows). These gaps are termed *nuclear pores*. They appear circular but it has been shown by Gall that their outline is actually octagonal. In most cells they are numerous, fairly evenly distributed and generally separated from one another by only 1,000 to 2,000 Å (100 to 200 nm). Around the edge of each pore, the outer and the inner membranes of the nuclear envelope are continuous. The diameter of pores found in different types of cells varies somewhat; it can range from about 300 to 1,000 Å (30 to 100 nm). Thin

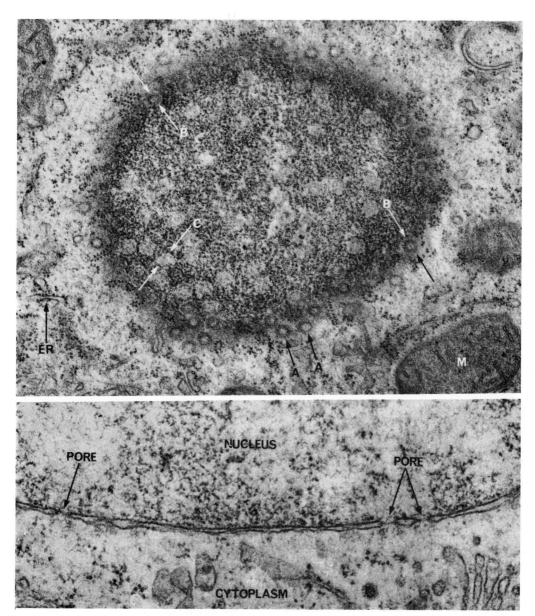

F<small>IG</small>. *2-6.* Electron micrographs of interphase nucleus of rat liver cell. (*Top*) ($\times$ 35,000) Slightly oblique section across part of the nucleus showing nuclear pore complexes. Where pore complexes are sectioned through their cytoplasmic portion (A), they lie within the cytoplasm, some distance from the chromatin of the nucleus. When sectioned through the intranuclear channel (C), the pore complex lies within the peripheral chromatin. Pores designated as (B) are seen in sections between levels A and C (M, mitochondria; ER, endoplasmic reticulum). (*Bottom*) Electron micrograph ($\times$ 56,000) of section cut at right angles to the nuclear envelope, showing nuclear pores. The outer and the inner membranes of the nuclear envelope fuse at the periphery of the nuclear pores. Note the appearance of a diaphragm across the pore opening on the right of the micrograph. (Miyai, K., and Steiner, J. W.: The fine structure of interphase liver cell nuclei in subacute ethionine intoxication. Exp. Molec. Path., *4:525*)

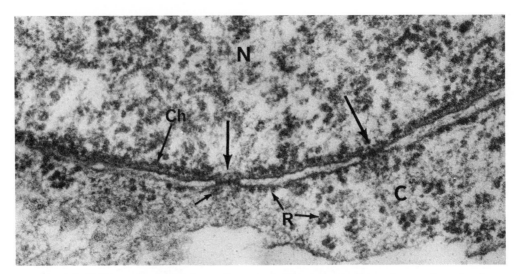

FIG. 2-7. Electron micrograph of a section cut at right angles to the nuclear envelope showing nuclear pore complexes (large arrows). The outer and the inner membranes of the nuclear envelope fuse at the periphery of the nuclear pores. A thin diaphragm extends across the pore openings. A ring of dense material (small arrow) surrounds the pore and extends out into the cytoplasm (C). On the side of the nucleus (N) chromatin (Ch) lines the inner membrane of the nuclear envelope except at the nuclear pores. Granules called ribosomes (R) are found on the cytoplasmic side of the outer membrane and in the cytoplasm. $\times$ 90,000. (From V. I. Kalnins)

sections cut more or less parallel with the surface of nuclei, sections in which the nuclear envelope itself cannot be seen distinctly as composed of two membranes, reveal the pores (Fig. 2-6, *top*). Detailed studies of pores have shown that a channel projects for a short distance from both aspects of the pore into the nucleus on one side and into the cytoplasm on the other. Within the nucleus the channel is bounded by condensed chromatin (Figs. 2-4 and 2-6, *top*, and 2-7, Ch). On the cytoplasmic side of the nuclear pore it is sometimes seen that the channel is surrounded by a ring of material of slightly increased density (Fig. 2-6, *top*). The whole arrangement is sometimes described as the *pore complex.*

There has been some question as to whether a nuclear pore is ever completely open, or whether a very thin diaphragm always extends across it as shown in Figures 2-6, *bottom,* and 2-7. Since pores that are completely closed with thin diaphragms can be found in micrographs of good quality, it has become conceivable that diaphragms control and determine what molecules pass from the nucleus into the cytoplasm and vice versa. The finding that some pores reveal no diaphragms is generally interpreted as indicating not that pores are sometimes open, but that their diaphragms are so thin and so difficult to fix that they may be present but defy demonstration.

Detailed information is available about nuclear pores in many species; those interested should see Further Reading.

Having dealt with the envelope of the interphase nucleus, we shall deal with chromatin as seen with the LM and the EM.

Chromatin

Since the DNA of cells exists as a constituent of chromatin, it could be argued that chromatin is not only the most important component of nuclei but the most important substance in the body. There are so many aspects of chromatin to describe or discuss that chromatin will be directly or indirectly concerned with what is said in the remainder of this chapter and in the following two chapters. In the present chapter we shall describe briefly the appearance of chromatin in interphase nuclei as seen with the LM and the EM and then in more detail describe the changes that occur in the arrangement of chromatin as a cell divides to form two daughter cells.

THE CHROMATIN OF THE INTERPHASE NUCLEUS OF A LIVER CELL

Appearance in H and E Sections. The chromatin as seen with the LM in H and E sections of liver cells is in the form of fine to coarse blue-purple granular material scattered about in the nuclear sap (Fig. 2-3, chromatin, and Fig. 2-8, chromatin granules). Its distribution in the nuclei of liver cells is seen to better advantage in low-power electron micrographs, as will now be described.

Distribution of Chromatin. In thin sections of liver fixed in gluteraldehyde and post-fixed with osmium tetroxide, chromatin appears in a low-power electron micrograph in the form of aggregates of electron-dense (dark) material (Fig. 2-4). These aggregates of chromatin are distributed throughout the nucleus, but there is more chromatin in some parts of the nuclei than in others. First, islands of chromatin are seen scattered about in the nuclear sap (Fig. 2-4, CI); these are the counterparts of the so-called chromatin granules seen with the LM. Secondly, chromatin can be seen with the EM to be distributed along the inner surface of the nuclear envelope; this is what accounts for the deep blue staining of what was supposed to be the nuclear envelope from LM studies. It is called the peripheral chromatin (PC in Fig. 2-4). Thirdly, some chromatin can be seen with the EM on the surface of, and sometimes even inside, the nucleolus; this is called the nucleolus-associated chromatin (NAC in Fig. 2-4). It should be noted here that the bulk of the nucleolus itself is for the most part electron-dense but, as will be explained later, most of this is not due to chromatin.

The Nature of Chromatin. Chromatin is not a chemical compound for which a formula can be written. Chromatin received its name because it was a substance seen in the nucleus that had an avidity for stains. Although it is now known that the characteristic basophilia of chromatin is due to DNA, it is also known that chromatin is not naked DNA because it can be shown that other components in chromatin, mainly basic proteins, provide a large part of its substance. The existence of these other substances can be shown by extracting the DNA from chromatin with DNA-ase. What is left behind can then be stained with stains that have an affinity for basic proteins. Histones (one type of basic protein) are important constituents of chromatin and it has been thought that they may serve very important roles in connection with the blocking or permitting the release of genetic information by DNA. There are other proteins and also a small amount of RNA as well in chromatin. In other words, chromatin is a very complex material and how its components are related to one another is only in part understood.

The Physical Form of Chromatin. It was once believed from the appearance of chromatin in LM sec-

tions that it actually consisted of isolated granules that were scattered about in the nucleus. It is now conceded that chromatin exists in the form of long threads which at various sites along their course may be coiled, folded or crumpled so as to form little masses that are large enough, when stained, to be visible with the LM (with which instrument they appear as granules). It is now also conceded that other parts of a chromatin thread, instead of being coiled, folded or crumpled in some fashion, may be extended and that these extended parts of chromatin threads are not dense enough even when stained to be visible with the LM.

The Terms Condensed and Extended Chromatin. The portions of threads of chromatin which are coiled, folded or aggregated to form visible masses are said to constitute what is termed the *condensed chromatin* of a nucleus and this, of course, is the only kind visible with the LM. The parts of threads of chromatin that are extended and are invisible with the LM in the nuclear sap constitute what is termed the *extended chromatin* of a nucleus. (The appearances of condensed and extended chromatin seen with the EM at high magnifications will be described in Chapter 4).

Proportions of Condensed and Extended Chromatin in Nuclei of Different Cell Types. This varies. For example, in nerve cells the nuclei may be very large and with the LM almost no chromatin can be seen in them; hence, it must almost all be extended and it would be most interesting to know what purpose this serves in nerve cells. On the other hand, in a type of blood cell termed the lymphocyte, the chromatin is almost all of the condensed type and hence the nuclei of lymphocytes are small and appear with the LM as being almost solidly blue. In the nuclei of liver cells there seems to be a mixture of the two types.

The Significance of Extended and Condensed Chromatin in Nuclei. A good deal of evidence will be presented in Chapter 4 which indicates that in interphase nuclei it is only the extended chromatin that is active in directing the synthesis of proteins in the cell. Thus the genes of the condensed chromatin of a nucleus appear to be inactive. Hence the extended chromatin of a nucleus is sometimes referred to as the *euchromatin* (*eu,* good), the good kind, and the condensed chromatin is sometimes referred to as *heterochromatin* (*hetero,* other), the other kind. However, since the term heterochromatin carries with it certain other inferences, it is best to use the terms condensed and extended chromatin.

We shall now consider the changes that occur in the appearance of chromatin as a cell divides into two daughter cells.

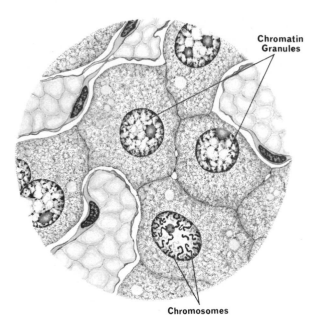

Chromatin
Granules

Chromosomes

FIG. 2-8. This drawing illustrates the difference in the appearance of the nucleus of a cell that is in the interphase and one that has entered the prophase of mitosis. The nuclei of the cells in the middle are typical interphase nuclei, and in them chromatin granules can be seen. When the interphase cell enters the prophase of mitosis, dark blue-staining chromosomes are seen instead of chromatin granules (bottom cell). The nucleolus is still present in this cell, which is in an early stage of prophase. It disappears later, along with the nuclear membrane.

THE REARRANGEMENT OF CHROMATIN SEEN IN THE PROCESS OF CELL DIVISION (MITOSIS)

When an interphase cell begins to divide by the process called *mitosis* (the reasons for this term will be explained below) there is a dramatic change in the appearance of the chromatin of its nucleus. Instead of irregular aggregates and/or fine granules, it becomes visible as blue-staining threads that are called chromosomes (*chrome,* color; *soma,* body) because they are colored bodies. Compare A with B in Figure 2-10. The term *mitosis* (*mitos,* thread; *osis,* a process) was coined because of these threadlike bodies that appear in its first stage. The threadlike chromosomes soon become shorter and thicker to appear as little curved rods. Compare the upper interphase nuclei in Figure 2-8 with the lower nucleus which has begun mitosis and in which chromosomes are labeled.

When chromosomes from cells that are beginning mitosis are spread out on glass slides and stained, each can be seen with the LM to have become a double

structure in that it is split longitudinally into two halves which are attached together at only one site called the *centromere* of the chromosome (Fig. 2-9, *bottom*). Each longitudinal half of a chromosome is called a *chromatid.* Since each chromatid has a full complement of the genes carried by that chromosome, two important events must occur just before mitosis begins.

First, the genes of each chromatin thread that existed in the interphase nucleus must become duplicated just before mitosis begins and chromosomes become

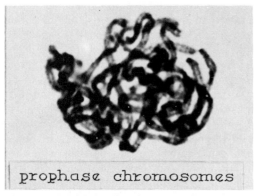

prophase chromosomes

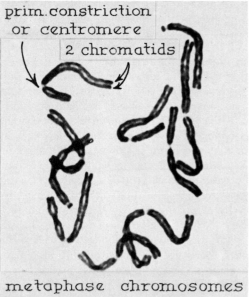

prim. constriction
or centromere

2 chromatids

metaphase chromosomes

FIG. 2-9. Oil-immersion photomicrographs of squash preparations of chromosomes from root tips of *Trillium.* Feulgen stain. These illustrations show that both prophase and metaphase chromosomes each contain 2 chromatids. A careful inspection of the lower picture will enable the student to match the 10 chromosomes shown into 5 pairs. (Preparation by Dr. K. H. Rothfels)

visible. This means that the long DNA molecule of each chromatin thread must give rise to a second identical DNA-containing molecule. Second, each of the two molecules must become housed in separate chromatin threads which become the two chromatids of each chromosome. The way this is done is best left to be described in the next chapter after we have in this one described the stages of mitosis.

How Interphase Chromatin Becomes Mitotic Chromosomes. A few decades ago it was believed that the chromatin of an interphase nucleus was actually in the form of free granules and that these became assembled in some way to become chromosomes when mitosis began. With the development of knowledge about the chemical basis of genes, to be described in the next chapter, it became obvious that this old concept could not be correct and it was concluded that, in the interphase, chromosomes must exist as such even though they could not be seen as threadlike structures. The reasons they cannot be seen in the interphase as chromosomes is that they exist as enormously long fine threads of chromatin that are beyond the limits of resolution with the LM. Hence, in the interphase only parts of the chromosomes can be distinguished—those parts of the long thread that became coiled, folded or crumpled together sufficiently to form a mass large enough to be stained and seen with the LM. The parts of chromosomes that are seen in interphase nuclei are of course the condensed chromatin of the interphase nucleus. What happens at the beginning of mitosis is that the two chromatids of each of the former chromatin threads (which become doubled just before mitosis begins) become coiled, folded or crumpled in some fashion *along their whole lengths* so that the two chromatids of each chromosome as well as the whole chromosome can be seen with the LM.

The Main Events in Mitosis. As mitosis begins there are 46 chromosomes in a human cell. During mitosis the 2 chromatids of each chromosome separate from each other completely and when this occurs each former chromatid is said to have become a chromosome in its own right. The cell at this stage has 92 chromosomes. Half of these (one of the 2 chromatids from each of the original chromosomes) move toward one end of the cell (which in the meantime has usually become elongated) and the other half move toward the opposite end of the cell. In each of these sites the new chromosomes (that were formerly chromatids) organize nuclei which soon become interphase type, so that the cell would now be binucleated, were it not for the fact that in the meantime the cytoplasm has become constricted at the midline to pinch the cell

into two halves, each of which is then a daughter cell complete with a nucleus and a full complement of genes. The various stages in mitosis are illustrated in a diagram in Figure 2-10 and in sectioned material in Figure 2-21, both of which figures will be explained in detail in the following text.

One of the more fascinating events observed in mitosis is the development of a delicate transient structure termed the *spindle* which plays a most important role mechanically in bringing about first an alignment of the chromosomes at the midline of the cell and then the movement of the chromosomes described above toward each end of the elongated cell (Fig. 2-10, B, C and D). Next, although mitosis is thought of chiefly as a nuclear event concerned with chromosomes, the first step in the process depends, as will now be described, on the formation of a spindle from cytoplasmic components. So the first event in the prophase concerns both chromosomes and the spindle which is derived from the cytoplasm.

Mitosis has four consecutive phases—*prophase, metaphase, anaphase* and *telophase*. When mitosis begins, the process is normally continuous, with each stage merging imperceptibly into the next. The whole process takes from 1 to $2\frac{1}{2}$ hours, according to the cell type.

We shall now describe the four phases in detail.

THE PROPHASE

The prophase lasts longer than any other phase, taking as much as $1\frac{1}{2}$ hours until it merges with the beginning of the metaphase.

Growth and Movement of the Centrioles. Each cell of every kind of body cell that can divide has in its cytoplasm two very small structures called *centrioles* because they seemingly try to take up a position in the center of the interphase cell (Fig. 2-10, A). However, they generally cannot attain this position because of the usual shape and position of the nucleus, but they get as close to the cell center as possible, so if the nucleus is indented on one of its sides, the centrioles commonly lie in the indentation (Fig. 2-10, A).

With the LM and specially stained material, it is just barely possible to see the centrioles in the interphase as two little dots. With the EM centrioles are revealed as structures which have a cross section diameter of 0.2 μ (Fig. 2-11). Their walls are composed of 9 longitudinally disposed bundles of what are termed microtubules. Since these are cytoplasmic structures, they will be described in connection with cytoplasm. In the meantime, it is enough to say that microtubules are slender, rodlike structures 240 Å (24 nm) in diameter and, as seen in high-power micrographs, they

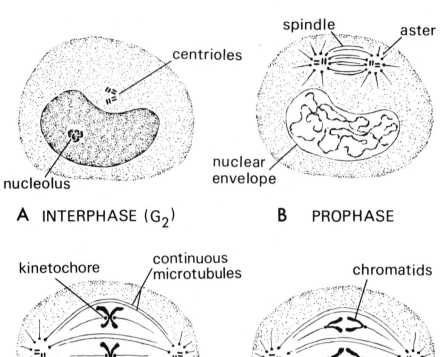

Fɪɢ. 2-10. Diagram illustrating the various stages in mitosis, including the condensation of chromatin into chromosomes, the formation of the mitotic spindle and the separation of chromosomes and centrioles equally into the two daughter cells. (Courtesy of V. I. Kalnins)

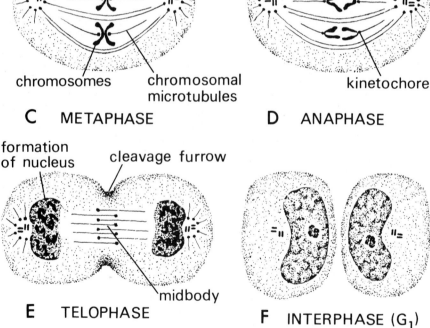

resemble tubules in that their central core is less dense than their periphery, which gives them a somewhat hollow appearance. They materialize in cytoplasm from a precursor protein called tubulin. In the centriole they are arranged as bundles of three which in turn are embedded in a finely fibrillar material (Fig. 2-11).

Following mitosis each daughter interphase cell has two centrioles arranged at right angles to each other (Fig. 2-10, F). However, if such a cell prepares for division again (A, in Fig. 2-10) a small daughter centriole is assembled beside, and at right angles to, each of the original two centrioles (Fig. 2-10, A). This daughter centriole acquires microtubules and grows as is shown in the longitudinal sections of centrioles in Figure 2-12, A and B. As a result there are two pairs of centrioles in a cell (Fig. 2-10, A) just before the prophase begins, and soon one pair begins to move toward one pole of the cell and the other pair toward the other (Fig. 2-10, B).

More or less simultaneously what appear with the LM to be delicate fibrils can sometimes be seen to begin to form and to radiate out from the region of each pair of centrioles (Fig. 2-10, B). When these were first seen in dividing sea-urchin eggs, they seemed so much like rays of light from stars they were called astral *(astron,* stars) rays or asters. However, this starlike appearance around centrioles is not prominent in dividing mammalian cells. What the EM discloses is that as the two pairs of centrioles move to take up positions at opposite ends of the nucleus, a set of microtubules is assembled (from a cytoplasmic pool of previously synthesized protein called tubulin) at microtubule-organizing sites located close to each pair of centrioles (Fig. 2-10, B). The microtubules that assemble near one pair of centrioles grow toward those that are assembling at and growing from the other

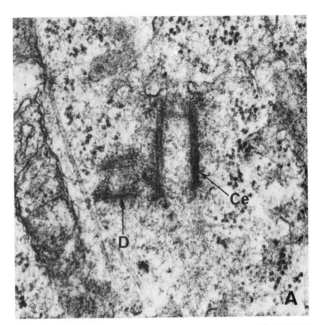

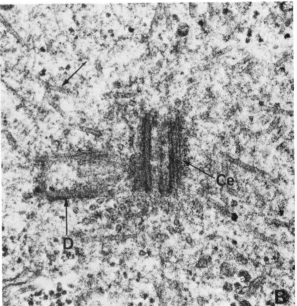

FIG. 2-12. Ependymal cell of rat embryo, in interphase (*A*), and in metaphase (*B*). Two different stages in the assembly of daughter centrioles (D) at right angles to mature parent centrioles (Ce) are shown. In both *A* and *B* the parent centriole and the daughter centrioles are cut in longitudinal sections. The daughter centriole in *A* is much shorter than the adjacent parent centriole. In *B* the daughter centriole has grown to the same length as the parent centriole and remains oriented at right angles to it. Many microtubules (arrow) terminate in the region near the centrioles in *B*. × 50,000. (From J. D. Marshall and V. I. Kalnins)

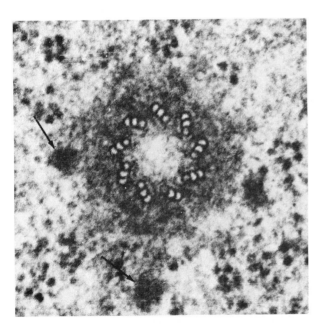

FIG. 2-11. Electron micrograph showing a centriole in cross section. The 9 bundles of microtubules arranged in a specific pattern can be distinguished in the wall of the centriole. Each bundle consists of 3 microtubules and is embedded in a fine fibrillar material. Aggregates of dense material (arrows) called centriolar satellite(s) are often found in the vicinity of centrioles. × 140,000. (From M. Wassman and V. I. Kalnins)

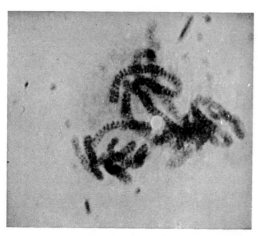

FIG. 2-13. The coiled nature of a mitotic chromosome can be shown in squash preparations of plant cells that are in mitosis if the preparation is treated with sodium cyanide before it is stained; this causes the individual coils of the coiled threads to become slightly separated from each other, as is shown here. This preparation is stained by the Feulgen technic, which is specific for DNA. (Courtesy of Dr. A. R. Gopal-Ayengar and Prof. Lesley Coleman, Department of Botany, University of Toronto)

pair (Fig. 2-10, B). These microtubules elongate further to become what are termed the *continuous microtubules* of the delicate temporary structure called the spindle (Fig. 2-10, B). Reasons for this name will be given presently and a further component of the spindle will also be described.

At the beginning of prophase the nuclear envelope of light microscopy is still partly discernible; this is probably to be accounted for by the chromosomes that are forming from the pre-existing peripheral chromatin tending to lie along the inner aspect of the true nuclear envelope (see Fig. 2-21, B). But as the prophase proceeds, the true nuclear envelope (the one seen with the EM) breaks up and so there is no longer any organized barrier between the chromosomes and the cytoplasm and this permits the spindle to complete its development in the metaphase. Moreover, as the prophase proceeds, the nucleolus, or at least most of it, disappears as an entity (how this happens will be explained in Chapter 4) and, finally, as the prophase continues, the chromatin thread of each chromatid becomes increasingly coiled or folded (more condensed) so that the chromosomes become shorter and thicker. In squash preparations of mitotic chromosomes of dividing plant cells, it can be shown that the chromatin thread of a chromatid is tightly coiled along its length, for, if it is treated with suitable reagents, the coils be-

come sufficiently separated for a histochemical reaction for DNA (which is contained in the coiled thread) to demonstrate with the LM that the thread is coiled (Fig. 2-13). The way in which the chromatin thread in mammalian cells becomes condensed seems to be more complex, as will be described shortly.

THE METAPHASE

The shortening and thickening of the chromosomes which begins in the prophase continues for a time in the metaphase, which makes metaphase chromosomes dense enough objects to be studied profitably with the LM. Spreads of human metaphase chromosomes can be prepared from ruptured cells (Fig. 2-14) and they are much employed clinically for reasons to be described presently. As is seen in Figure 2-14, the chromosomes of man differ from each other considerably in length and with regard to the position of the centromere along their respective lengths. The portions of a chromosome between its centromere and its ends are termed arms and arms are, of course, double structures consisting of two adjacent chromatids, as can be seen if the metaphase chromosomes in Figure 2-14 are inspected carefully. (For a diagram of a chromosome see Fig. 2-23.)

The Fine Structure of Metaphase Chromosomes. The study of these in sections has revealed many things of interest (as will be described presently) but a section of a metaphase chromosome is not very informative about the manner in which a very long chromatin thread of a mammalian mitotic chromatid is condensed. In a section the chromatids or chromosomes of a dividing cell are sliced at various angles and they appear as dark bodies of irregular size and shape. Slices through two chromatids are apparent in Figure 2-15. (See also Chr in Figs. 2-18 and 2-19.) Close inspection shows their substance to be made up of what appear to be closely packed roughly round dark dots and short segments of curving strands (arrow in Fig. 2-15) of dark material of the same diameter as the dots, which is around 100 Å (10 nm). Less dense material is seen between the dots and short curved strands; in some sites it is little more than a film and in other sites it appears as areas much larger than the dark dots or curved structures. The nature of the electron-dense material will be discussed in the next chapter.

Another way of studying the fine structure of mitotic chromosomes with the EM was devised by Du-Praw who by special technics was able to prepare whole mounts of metaphase chromosomes and study

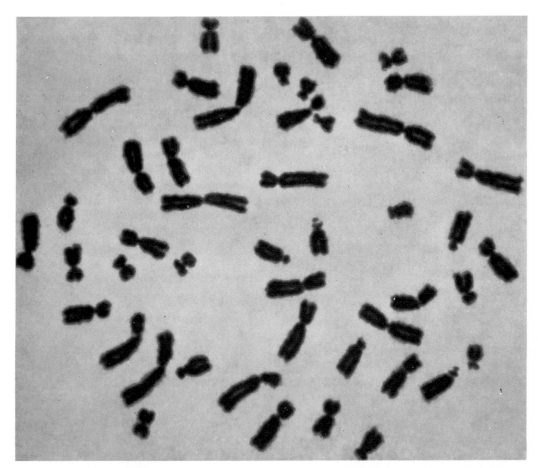

Fɪɢ. 2-14. Photomicrograph of metaphase chromosomes of normal human male. Preparation made from blood cells that were cultured as described in text. (Preparation by Charles E. Ford)

these with the EM. One of his beautiful micrographs of a human mitotic chromosome is shown in Figure 2-16. His observations are consistent with the concept of a chromatid's being composed of a single long thread (which he terms a fiber) of a diameter of from 200 to 500 Å (20 to 50 nm) that is tightly folded in the manner shown in the micrograph to account for its being condensed into a chromatid. This is termed the folded fiber model of chromosome structure. DuPraw points out from many detailed experiments that the continuous DNA molecule that lies within this continuous fiber is enormously longer than the fiber and hence to fit into the fiber it must be tightly coiled along its length. Furthermore, as will be described in the next chapter, the two strands of the DNA molecule itself are in a helical arrangement so there are two orders of coiling within the chromatin fiber which itself is folded on itself (Fig. 2-16). Some other features of DuPraw's model will be described in the next chapter

when DNA and its duplication are considered. Here we must continue with what happens in the metaphase.

The most striking feature seen with the LM in the metaphase is that all its chromosomes become arranged with their centromere regions in the same plane (Figs. 2-10, C, and 2-17). This plane is called the *equatorial plane* because it crosses from one side of the cell to the other at right angles to the longitudinal axis of the spindle. From the centromeres of the chromosomes arranged in this plane, the two chromatids of each arm tend to diverge from one another and stick out to either side of the equatorial plane (Fig. 2-10, C). The two chromatids of each chromosome then separate from each other at the centromere where they were previously joined together and so the two chromatids of each chromosome move apart (Fig. 2-10, D). It is interesting to inquire into possible mechanisms that may operate to cause the centromeres of chromosomes (1) to become arranged in the equatorial plane and

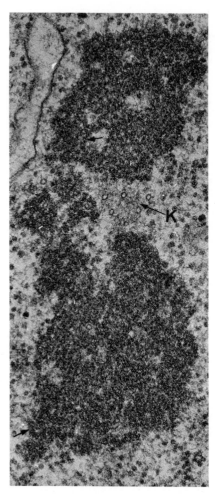

FIG. 2-15. Electron micrograph ($\times$ 100,000) of a section cut through a dividing cell. The two dark masses seen represent cuts through two different parts of a chromatid that has just become a chromosome in its own right because a kinetochore (labeled K, and to be described presently) is seen between the two. The dark masses are granular in appearance and it is assumed that this is due to the DNA-containing chromatin thread of the chromatid being cut innumerable times in cross or oblique section. In a few instances the thread has been cut over a short distance more or less longitudinally and in these instances it appears as a short curving rod (arrows). (From V. I. Kalnins)

ferent sources, as will now be described. The first kind to form grow out in the prophase from the vicinity of each pair of centrioles toward the other pair. When there is no longer any nuclear membrane to impede their progress, the microtubules of the developing spindle push into the area formerly bounded by the nuclear membrane. Hence, in the metaphase the elongating microtubules from one pair of centrioles are able to meet and interdigitate with those from the other pair (Fig. 2-10, B). The effect of this is to push the two pairs of centrioles farther apart and this of course causes the spindle to elongate so that it clearly has a long axis.

In a section cut longitudinally through a dividing cell at the metaphase stage, it is sometimes possible with the LM to see the spindle which, with the LM,

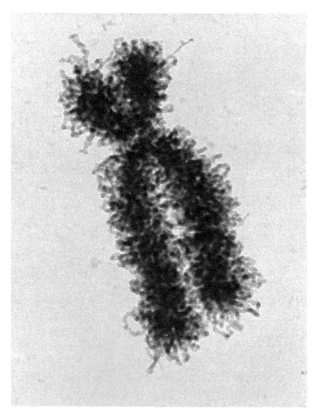

FIG. 2-16. Electron micrograph ($\times$ 60,400) of a wholemount preparation of human chromosome 12. This type of preparation suggests that each chromatid consists of a single long fiber of from 200 to 500 Å (20 to 50 nm) in diameter that is tightly folded on itself; this accounts for the loops that can be seen around the periphery of each chromatid. See text for details. (From DuPraw, E. J.: DNA and Chromosomes. New York, Holt, Rinehart and Winston, 1970)

(2) to separate and move. To discuss these questions we must discuss the spindle in more detail.

The Mitotic Spindle. The mitotic spindle is composed of microtubules. These develop from two difappears as a delicate fibrillar structure extending from one pole of the cell to the other but is expanded in its midsection (Fig. 2-17) so that it has a shape somewhat similar to the spindles once used for weaving, which were rods tapered toward each of their ends. The EM has shown, of course, that the fibrils of light microscopy are actually bundles of microtubules (Fig. 2-18 labeled Mt). The microtubules that grow from the vicinity of each pair of centrioles, as mentioned, are termed the *continuous microtubules,* and early in the metaphase stage the chromosomes have become more or less enmeshed in the spindlelike arrangements of continuous microtubules that have formed between the two pairs of centrioles (Figs. 2-17, 2-18 and 2-10, C).

The Development of Chromosomal Microtubules. As the continuous tubules, originating from the vicinity of one pair of centrioles, are growing toward those from the other pair of centrioles in the metaphase a second set of microtubules begin to develop. The reason for a second set being able to develop, after the nuclear envelope has broken down, is that the microtubule precursor substance (tubulin) which is synthesized in the cytoplasm is now able to enter readily the area previously occupied by the nucleus. With this substance becoming available it is possible for special microtubule-organizing structures called kinetochores (Figs. 2-15, 2-19 and 2-20, labeled K), two of which are present in the centromere region of each chromosome (Fig. 2-10, C), to initiate microtubule formation. The kinetochores are little disklike structures visible only in the EM (Figs. 2-19 and 2-20, labeled K). The microtubules that form from them are termed *chromosomal microtubules* (top arrows in Fig. 2-19). Since each centromere region contains two kinetochores, two sets of microtubules develop from each chromosome, one from each of its two chromatids. One set extends out toward one pole of the spindle and the other set in the opposite direction. Both chromosomal microtubules from a kinetochore of a chromosome and continuous microtubules are shown in Figure 2-20. We can now theorize about how the formation and growth of these chromosomal microtubules could cause the centromeres of the chromosomes to line up across the equatorial plane.

The problem perhaps is somewhat similar to that of a man holding a two-part extension ladder in its middle and trying to open it in a hallway. If he holds the ladder in the middle and then slides the two parts along each other to elongate the ladder, he soon finds that it has become too long to fit into the hallway any way except along its length. Furthermore, if he continues to stand in the middle of the ladder he finds

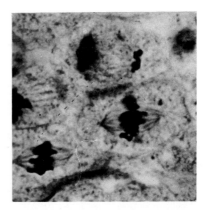

Fig. 2-17. Oil-immersion photomicrograph of cells in the first mitotic metaphase in the rat testis. Spindles appear to advantage because the tissue was fixed in Flemming's solution and stained with iron hematoxylin. (From Y. Clermont and C. P. Leblond)

that, when the ladder is fully opened and reaches from one end of the hall to the other, he is halfway between the two ends of the hall. Hence it might be thought that mechanical factors alone, due to chromosomal microtubules growing out from the kinetochores in opposite directions into a maze of roughly parallel continuous tubules (Fig. 2-10, C) would tend to lead to the centromere regions of the chromosomes all ending up in a position halfway between the two ends of the spindle. It seems likely that chemical energy changes to mechanical energy to achieve this effect.

In order to discuss how the chromosomal microtubules could be involved in the movement of the chromatids from the equatorial plane we must describe the anaphase.

THE ANAPHASE

The anaphase (Figs. 2-10, D and E, and 2-21, D and E) is characterized by two events. First, the centromere region of each of the chromosomes splits so that the two chromatids of each chromosome become completely separated from each other, whereupon, as already mentioned, each former chromatid is considered as a chromosome in its own right. Second, after the centromeres divide, half of the 92 chromosomes begin to move toward one pole of the cell and the other 46 to the other pole. There has been much speculation through the years about how this movement occurs. When it was believed that the microtubules were fibers it was thought that the fibers must contract

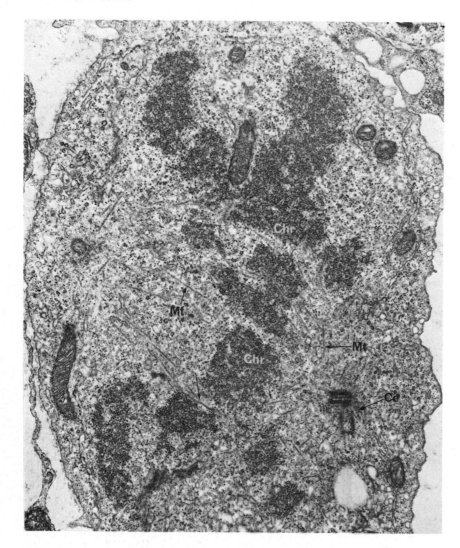

FIG. 2-18. Electron micrograph of a cell in the metaphase stage of mitosis. This section has passed through both poles of the mitotic spindle and shows a pair of centrioles (Ce) in longitudinal section at right angles to each other at one pole, and one of the two centrioles at the other pole. The dense staining masses in the central part of the spindle are sections through chromosomes (Chr). Continuous microtubules of the spindle may be seen running between the chromosomes (arrows). Many of the other microtubules (Mt) in the region between each of the poles and the chromosomes are chromosomal microtubules. Ependymal cells of rat embryo. × 22,000. (From J. D. Marshall and V. I. Kalnins)

so as to pull chromatids toward each pole. More recently, it has been suggested that chemicomechanical interactions between the continuous and the chromosomal microtubules in the spindle may be responsible for the movement of the chromosomes toward the poles of the cell that occurs in the anaphase. Both kinds of microtubules are shown in Figure 2-20. McIntosh, Hepler and Van Wie have suggested that this interaction may be mediated by what are termed *cross bridges,* which represent delicate temporary attachments between adjacent continuous and chromosomal microtubules in the spindle. It is thought that as a result of reactions that utilize energy, the cross bridges operate to cause the two types of microtubules, i.e., continuous and chromosomal, to slide past each other, for example, as the two parts of an extended extension

ladder are moved in relation to one another as the ladder is closed. Since both kinds of microtubules seem to move, there are two results. The first is that as a result of each of the two sets of chromosomal microtubules sliding toward opposite poles of the spindle, the kinetochores and the chromosomes to which they are attached are pulled toward the two poles; this would account for the movement of the chromosomes seen in the anaphase (Fig. 2-10, D). The second result would be that the continuous microtubules would be pulled away from each pole toward the midpart of the cell, where they would be temporarily aggregated to become a significant part of a transient structure termed the *midbody* (see Figs. 2-10, E and 2-22) which is seen in the telophase, the next stage of mitosis to be described.

THE TELOPHASE

Toward the end of the anaphase and at the beginning of the telophase a constriction begins to develop at the midpoint of the elongated cell (Figs. 2-10, E and 2-21, F and G). This constriction encircles the cell as what is known as the *cleavage furrow,* because as it deepens it splits the cell into two daughter cells (Figs. 2-10, F and 2-21, H). The cleavage furrow probably develops because of an accumulation and contraction of fibrillar material in the cytoplasm immediately beneath the cell membrane at this site (Figs. 2-10, E and 2-22), and it is possible that the filaments of this material may individually be contractile, but perhaps it is more likely that individual fibrils, by sliding past each other, tighten and contract and thus make the cleavage furrow deeper and deeper. In order to cover the extra surface there has to be an increase in the amount of cell membrane; extra membrane is probably provided from intracytoplasmic membranous organelles which fuse with the membrane, as can be shown to occur in plant cells.

While the cleavage furrow is deepening, a bundle of the tubules still connects the two cells that are just about to separate; these constitute what is known as the midbody of the dividing cell (Figs. 2-10 E and 2-22).

When cleavage is complete, the remnants of the midbody are indicated by an increased density along the cell membrane of one of the two daughter cells at the point where they are separated; this increased density is occasioned by what is left of the midbody.

Meanwhile, as is shown in Figure 2-10, F, the chromosomes in each daughter cell have become uncoiled to various extents to assume the form of chromatin threads characteristic of chromosomes in interphase nuclei. Nucleoli have re-formed and a new nuclear envelope has developed in each daughter cell to surround the chromatin, the nucleoli and the nuclear sap of the nucleus.

Mitotic Figures

A cell in any phase of mitosis is commonly called a *mitotic figure.* Their presence in a section indicates that cellular growth was occurring in the tissue obtained for sectioning. Mitotic figures are encountered

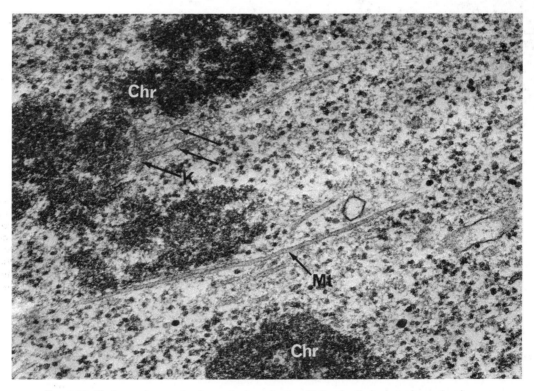

FIG. 2-19. Electron micrograph of a part of a mitotic spindle of cells in metaphase, showing continuous microtubules (Mt) between adjacent chromosomes (Chr) and chromosomal microtubules (arrows) attached to a kinetochore (K) of a chromosome. × 50,000. (From V. I. Kalnins)

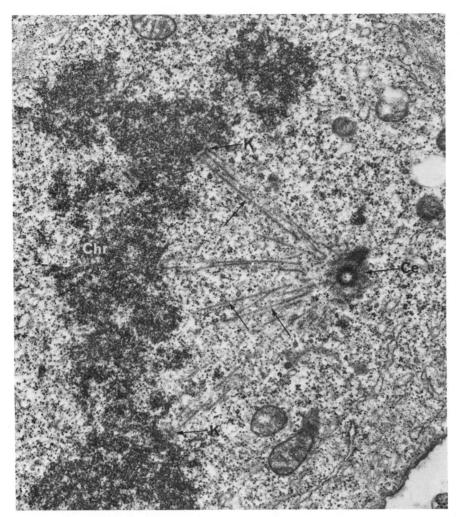

FIG. 2-20. Electron micrograph of a cell in anaphase showing one of the poles of the mitotic spindle. Two centrioles (Ce), one cut in cross section and the other in an oblique grazing section, are present at this pole. Dense material surrounds the two centrioles. Microtubules (arrows) of the spindle radiate out from this region toward the densely staining chromosomes (Chr). The chromosomal microtubules are attached to the chromosomes at kinetochores (K). Rat embryo ependymal cells. × 22,000. (From J. D. Marshall and V. I. Kalnins)

in many normal body tissues until full growth is attained. Afterward they are seen in sites where cells must divide in order to maintain cell populations. In addition, in abnormal conditions they appear in specific sites where repair of damage is in progress and also in abnormal cellular growths such as cancer where their prevalence is an aid to diagnosing the condition with the microscope. The presence of mitotic figures in a section is so significant that learning to recognize them readily is a *must*. The way they appear in the various stages of mitosis in H and E sections is shown in Figure 2-21.

How To Identify Mitotic Figures. First, in an ordinary H and E section, do not look for centrioles or spindle fibers, for they will almost never be seen. The identification of most mitotic figures is made from seeing deeply staining chromosomes lying in the more central part of a cell (which is often pale) without

their being enclosed by a nuclear envelope. (See Fig. 2-21, C, D, E, and F.) Furthermore, in routine sections you cannot count on seeing individual chromosomes clearly in mitotic figures, for they may be clumped together to form an irregular, deeply basophilic conglomerate (Fig. 2-21, C, D, E, and F). Accordingly, in the routine scanning of an H and E section with a low-power objective, what attracts the eye as being a possible mitotic figure is that there is some condensed basophilic material that is of a *deeper blue* than the blue of the usual interphase nucleus in the central part of some cell in the field (provided, of course, that the tissue under examination is not one of the few in which the interphase nuclei are all of the condensed chromatin type).

Metaphases, anaphases and telophases are easiest to identify in tissue in which the cells are all oriented in the same plane and which has been sectioned in the

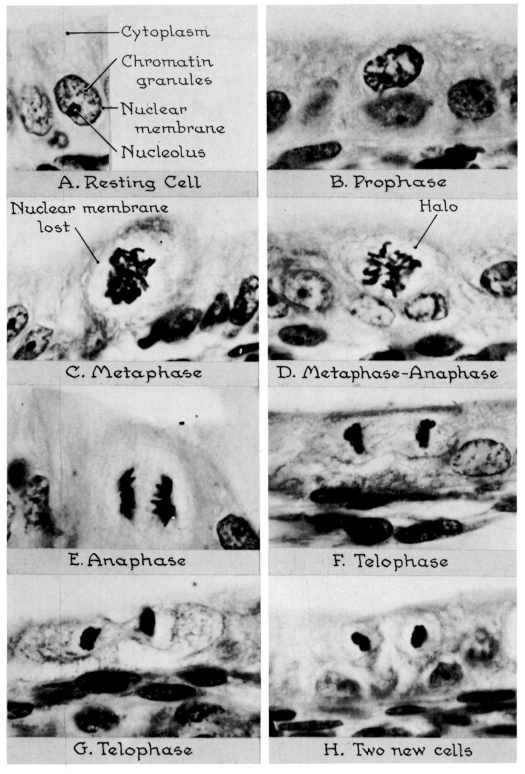

FIG. 2-21. Oil-immersion photomicrographs taken from sections of the lining of the uterus of a rat that was injected 48 hours previously with a large dose of female sex hormone. The illustrations show the different stages of mitosis.

same plane as that in which the cells are oriented. In such sections the appearances seen, as is shown in Figure 2-21, C, D, E, and F, will approximately match those seen in the common diagrams that are used to illustrate mitosis. These conditions can be met more easily in plant than in animal tissues and that is one reason for sections of a growing onion root to be commonly used to study mitosis. But in most sections of human material these two requirements are not met, either because the cells of the tissue being examined are not all disposed in the same plane or, if they are, because the section was not cut in a plane parallel to the long axes of the cells. Accordingly, you have to be able to visualize how metaphases and anaphases would appear if the cell containing them was sectioned in some plane other than its long axis.

To be sure you are seeing mitotic figures it helps to find some clear-cut example of anaphases, for an anaphase is the easiest kind of mitotic figure for the beginner or anyone else to identify, provided that it is sectioned in a plane that is reasonably close to being parallel to that joining the two poles of the dividing cell, as is shown in Figure 2-21, E. But since the chances of mitotic figures sectioned in this plane in most kinds of mammalian cells are not nearly as great as they are of their being sectioned in some other plane, it may take a lot of time and patience and the use of

several suitable sections to find mitotic figures illustrating various stages of mitosis that are sectioned in the plane that shows them to best advantage. However, if a clump of deep-staining material is seen to be lying free in cytoplasm, often with a pale area around it and *not* surrounded by a nuclear membrane, and with a *spiky appearance* (Fig. 2-21, C, D, or E) due to individual chromosomes projecting from it at various angles, the chances are excellent that it is a mitotic figure. It sometimes happens that nuclei die and shrink to form a dark blue mass that may be mistaken for a mitotic figure. To be certain, find mitotic figures with a spiky outline (Fig. 2-21, C and E) that is characteristic of clumps of chromosomes.

A common mistake made by beginners is to think that two interphase nuclei that are close together is a telophase and hence that they have seen a mitotic figure. Without seeing good examples of earlier phases in the same preparation the presence of telophases would be unlikely.

Effects of Colchicine on Mitosis

An alkaloid, cholchicine, extracted from the corm of the plant *Colchicum autumnale* has two remarkable biological properties. The first has meant a lot to those who suffered from gout because colchicine was the first

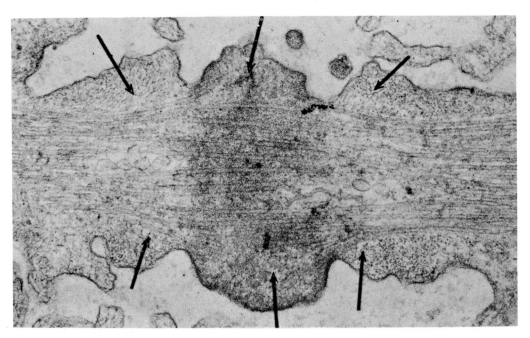

FIG. 2-22. Electron micrograph ($\times$ 60,000) showing cell cleavage in the telophase stage of mitosis. A bundle of continuous tubules still connects the two daughter cells; these constitute the midbody. Bundles of filaments cut in cross section are indicated by arrows. (Preparation by S. Dales)

drug found that effectively relieved the excrutiatingly painful inflammations of joints that occur in this condition. The second effect is of more general interest because colchicine has the remarkable effect of arresting the process of mitosis at the metaphase stage. Under the influence of colchicine, the mitotic spindle is not formed and therefore the chromatids do not separate from one another and so they have a longer time to keep on shortening; hence metaphase chromosomes seen after colchicine treatment are both shorter and thicker than normal.

Information is now available about the way in which colchicine arrests mitosis. It has been shown that it binds to the monomers of microtubule protein (tubulin) and prevents this protein from being assembled into microtubules. As a consequence, in the presence of colchicine, microtubule assembly and hence spindle formation is inhibited and, as a result, the two pairs of centrioles are not pushed apart to the two poles of the cell. In the absence of a spindle, the chromosomes arrange themselves in a sphere around the two pairs of centrioles at the cell center and continue shortening. In sections this arrangement of chromosomes resembles a mitotic figure and has been called a colchicine metaphase or a C-metaphase. When such cells are no longer subjected to the influence of colchicine, a typical spindle forms. A true metaphase follows in which the chromosomes become typically aligned at the equator of the spindle and normal separation of chromatids occurs.

The finding that mitosis can be arrested by the use of colchicine has been put to two very important uses:

Use of Colchicine in Studying Cell Turnover. If colchicine is given to an animal, or added to a culture of cells in which cell multiplication is occurring, any cells that enter mitosis after colchicine has taken effect do not complete it, and as a result, mitotic figures accumulate until such time as the dose wears off. If, however, at some given time (before the dose wears off) the mitotic figures are counted, the number obtained will be, for all practical purposes, the number of cells in that tissue or cell culture that entered the process of mitosis over the period of time allowed for the experiment. In those structures and organs in the body in which cell multiplication is matched by cell loss or death, it is therefore possible to use colchicine to estimate the turnover rate of the cell population by determining the proportion of cells that enter mitosis over a given period of time.

Use of Colchicine in Preparing Karyotypes. Colchicine is used to study the chromosomes of any given individual. The common way this is done in the laboratory is by obtaining some blood from the person and then separating some leukocytes (described in Chap. 10) from it which are then placed in a culture medium to which a substance called phytohemagglutinin is added; this has the extraordinary ability to stimulate certain of the leukocytes to undergo division. After two or three days, colchicine can be added to the culture which causes the dividing cells in the culture to be arrested in the metaphase stage. Such cells are then made to swell in a hypotonic medium, which procedure separates the chromosomes from one another, and the cells are then fixed. Since the fixative contains alcohol, a drop of it containing the cells can be ignited on a glass slide and this makes the cells flatten and spread out on the glass. The preparations may then be stained so that the chromosomes of single cells can be studied and photographed. Figure 2-14 is an illustration of how an excellent spread of a metaphase mitotic figure appears under the microscope.

After the chromosomes of a given cell are counted, photomicrographs of them can be cut up and the chromosomes of that cell arranged, as will soon be described, so as to construct what is called a *karyotype* (*karyon*—a nut, a nucleus) of the particular chromosomes of the individual from which the cells were taken. The karyotype or map so constructed can be studied conveniently to see if any abnormalities exist in the number or the form of the chromosomes of that individual.

The Chromosomes of Man

The development of methods by which the chromosome complement of the body cells of man and other species can be determined has been of vast importance to the study of genetics and the practice of medicine wherein it has become apparent that chromosome *anomalies* (variations in number or structure) are responsible for many recognized clinical conditions, the causes of which were previously obscure. Before discussing normal and abnormal karyotypes, we must first comment briefly on the chromosomes of the body cells of man.

The fertilized ovum from which a human body develops has 46 chromosomes; hence the body, or as they are commonly termed, the *somatic* (*soma*, body) cells that develop from the fertilized ovum have 46 chromosomes each. The chromosomes of the fertilized ovum are derived from germ cells, half from the unfertilized ovum, and half from the male germ cell that fertilizes the ovum. How germ cells come to have only half the number of chromosomes of somatic cells will be explained presently. Of the 23 chromosomes of a normal female germ cell, one is a sex chromosome; the other

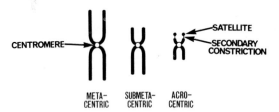

Fig. 2-23. Diagrammatic representation of the three types of human chromosomes. (Adapted from Thompson, J. S., and Thompson, M. W.: Genetics in Medicine. Ed. 2. Philadelphia, W. B. Saunders, 1973)

22 are termed *autosomes* (*auto,* self). The sex chromosome of female germ cells is always of the X type. Male germ cells also each possess 22 autosomes and 1 sex chromosome but the sex chromosome may be either an X chromosome or a Y chromosome (the morphology of these will be described later). Maleness is dependent on the Y chromosome. Consequently, a female germ cell (which always has an X chromosome) that is fertilized by a male germ cell carrying an X chromosome will have an XX combination of sex chromosomes, and so will become a female, with each of its somatic cells afterward possessing 44 autosomes and 2 X chromosomes. If the male germ cell that fertilizes an ovum has a Y chromosome, the fertilized ovum will possess 44 autosomes and an XY combination of sex chromosomes and, because of its having a Y chromosome, it will develop into a male, with all of its somatic cells possessing 44 autosomes plus an X and a Y chromosome.

Why the Chromosomes in a Spread Can Be Arranged in Pairs. The chromosomes in a spread made from a cell of a normal individual differ sufficiently in appearance for them to be arranged into groups and in many instances, to be individually identified—with, however, one important qualification—they always have to be arranged in pairs (Fig. 2-24). There are always two autosomes that have an identical appearance because each of the 22 autosomes derived from one side of the family has the same appearance as its homologue (*homo,* the same; *legein,* to speak) derived from the other side of the family. The same holds true for the 2 sex chromosomes in a spread in the instance of a female because the X chromosome from the female side of the family has an appearance identical with that of the X chromosome derived from the male side of the family. However, if the subject is a male he will, of course, have an XY combination of sex chromosomes in his cells and the Y chromosome will have a different appearance from the X, so in males the sex chromosomes are not paired.

It should be noted that whereas the 22 autosomes

from one side of the family have appearances identical with the 22 from the other side of the family, they do not carry identical genes. Furthermore, even the two X chromosomes in the cells of females which have identical appearances do not carry identical genes.

Terminology Used for Classifying Chromosomes. A chromosome whose centromere (the nonstaining area joining the two chromatids and represented as a circle in each chromosome in Figure 2-23) is approximately at the midpoint of its long axis is said to be *metacentric* (*meta,* between) and its two arms are, therefore, of roughly equal length (Fig. 2-23). A chromosome whose centromere is situated between its midpoint and one of its ends is termed *submetacentric;* it has one shorter and one longer arm (Fig. 2-23). A chromosome whose centromere is very near one end is referred to as *acrocentric* (*acro,* at the end); it has one very short arm and one long arm (Fig. 2-23). The corresponding positions of the centromeres are called median, submedian and subterminal, respectively. No human chromosomes have centromeres situated exactly at the end.

Making a Karyotype. Chromosomes are cut out from a photomicrograph or drawing such as the one in Figure 2-14. They are at first arranged in a descending order according to their total lengths and with their centromeres along a horizontal line (Fig. 2-24). When arm lengths are unequal, each chromosome is oriented with its shorter arm upward and its longer arm downward (Fig. 2-24). The chromosomes are then divided into groups, with the members of a group all having approximately the same ratio between the lengths of their two arms. This criterion of arm-length ratio sometimes can take precedence over the total length of a chromosome in establishing the position of the chromosome in the karyotype, for it will be found, after arranging them into groups according to relative arm lengths, that sometimes the first member of a later group may be somewhat longer than the last member of the preceding group. By arranging the chromosomes according to their lengths and then rearranging them into groups according to the relative lengths of their two arms, it becomes obvious that there are two identical autosomes of each type (but not pairs of identical sex chromosomes if the preparation is from a male). The identical autosomes are, of course, paired in the karyotype (Fig. 2-24).

Satellites are small spherical stained portions of chromosomes that are separated by a narrow thread from the end of the short arms of certain acrocentric chromosomes (see Fig. 2-23, *right*). They are regularly found on chromosomes 13, 14 and 21 and sometimes on other acrocentric chromosomes but never on the Y chromosome. Secondary constrictions are nonstaining areas in a chromatid or chromosome (Fig. 2-23). They resemble primary constrictions (another name for centromeres) but, unlike them, are not sufficiently constant in position to be very useful for identifying chromosomes.

In a karyotype the individual pairs of human chromosomes that are arranged primarily in a descending order of length are numbered serially 1 to 22 (Fig. 2-24). The further criteria described above permit the 22 pairs to be arranged into 7 groups. These 7 groups are referred to as the 1 to 3 or A group, the 4 to 5 or B group, the 6 to 12 or C group, the 13 to 15 or D group, the 16 to 18 or E group, the 19 to 20 or F group and the 21 to 22 or G group. Group A, for example, consists of chromosome pairs 1 to 3, which are the longest metacentric chromosomes, and group G includes pairs 21 and 22, which are the shortest acrocentric chromosomes. In males group G also contains the Y chromosome (Fig. 2-24), which is an acrocentric chromosome like the others but is usually the longest in the group, and its long arms are usually parallel to one another rather than divergent as in the other members of the G group. The X chromosome is very similar to certain members of the 6 to 12 (C) group (Fig. 2-24) and cannot always be distinguished as a separate entity from certain members of that group.

The new techniques of culturing blood cells have been scaled down and improved so that very small quantities of whole blood can be used to initiate cultures from large numbers of individuals. This has made it possible to produce chromosome preparations of excellent quality from the members of a variety of human populations in institutions etc. The preparation of karyotypes is, however, time consuming and tedious work and so it cannot be readily used to obtain numerical information on chromosomes from large numbers of metaphases. This problem is being overcome through the development of automatic systems that are designed to scan stained metaphase plates either on photographic negatives or even directly on slides and to feed the numerical information into a computer programmed to identify chromosomes on the basis of these measurements.

Chromosome Anomalies

The term *anomaly* signifies marked deviation from a standard. The standard used for establishing chromosome anomalies is the number and morphology of the chromosomes in a normal karyotype as seen with the LM. Hence an anomaly exists in the chromosomes of an individual if a karyotype prepared from his or her cells shows more or fewer chromosomes than 46 or if

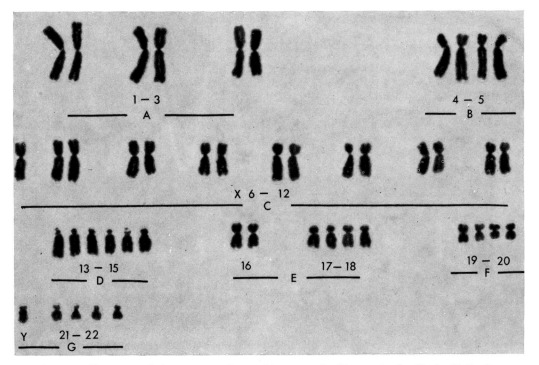

Fig. 2-24. Karyotype of chromosomes of normal human male. (Preparation by Charles E. Ford)

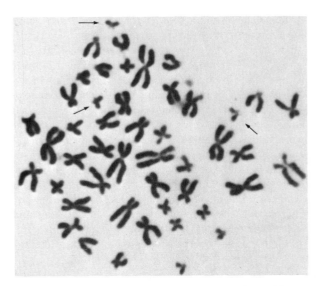

FIG. 2-25. Chromosome preparation of cell obtained by *amniocentesis* (fluid removed from the amniotic cavity surrounding the fetus). The fact that there are three no. 21 chromosomes (arrows) shows that the fetus had the chromosome constitution of *Down's syndrome,* thus allowing a diagnosis to be made prenatally. (Preparation courtesy of Dr. Henry L. Nadler, Children's Memorial Hospital and Northwestern University, Chicago, Ill.)

any chromosome exhibits a morphology different from that of the same chromosome in a normal karyotype.

Chromosome anomalies can originate at either of two levels and it helps in understanding their effects if this is kept in mind. One kind can originate at the level of the germ cells that fuse to constitute a fertilized ovum that in turn gives rise to a whole body. Chromosome anomalies that originate at this level will appear in every cell of the body that develops. A second group of anomalies can originate in somatic cells. Anomalies of this type are seen only in the cell in which they originate or in any somatic cells that descend from that cell and inherit the type of anomaly that developed in it.

Since it is confusing to discuss both of the above types together, we shall first deal with anomalies that originate in germ cells and are transmitted to all of the somatic cells of the individual that develops. Following this, we shall discuss anomalies that originate in somatic cells.

CHROMOSOME ANOMALIES THAT ORIGINATE
AT THE LEVEL OF GERM CELLS

These occur in about three out of every 100 pregnancies. Some are incompatible with the continuance

of pregnancy and cause a spontaneous abortion or miscarriage. It was only in the last decade or so that karyotypes of aborted embryos were studied and found to reveal chromosome anomalies of the embryo or fetus and so permitted this cause of many spontaneous abortions or miscarriages to be determined. However, some anomalies do not cause abortion. Probably about one of every 200 babies that are born have some kind of a chromosome anomaly. The effects of various anomalies differ greatly. Many involve anomalies of the sex chromosomes and others involve anomalies of autosomes. A few examples will be given here; for details see Further Reading.

Example of an Anomaly of an Autosome

It was long known that around one out of 500 babies that were born had a curious but characteristic facial expression, a placid disposition, and short hands and certain other physical features and that such babies would be mentally retarded. When the condition was first described it was, unfortunately, and for no good reason, termed *mongolism* and babies so affected were termed mongoloids. The condition is now referred to as Down's syndrome or trisomy-21 disease. The latter and best term for this condition became possible when it was discovered in 1959 by Lejeune and his co-workers that babies of this kind had 47 chromosomes in their cells instead of the normal 46. It was established that the extra chromosome was a member of the G group and it was agreed to call it an extra 21 (even though 21 and 22 are very much alike). Since there are normally two number 21 chromosomes, the extra one made three and so the condition was termed trisomy-21 which, since *soma* means body, indicates that there are three little chromosome bodies of the 21 type present (Fig. 2-25).

In order to describe how this anomaly originates it is necessary to comment briefly on how germ cells are formed in the body because the anomaly occurs as an accident in the process called meiosis.

MEIOSIS

Difference Between Diploid and Haploid Cells. As already noted, each body (somatic) cell of man contains 46 chromosomes which are constituted of 23 pairs, with one member of each pair being derived from the germ cell of the mother and the other member of each pair from the germ cell of the father. The members of each pair are said to be homologous and are called homologues (*homo,* same) because they have the same form and structure, as is shown in Figure 2-24 (but, as already noted, the genes they carry are not necessarily identical). Since each body cell thus has a double set of chromosomes of the same form and structure (except for the pair of sex chromosomes of the cells of males, which have an XY combination of sex chromosomes), body cells are said to have a diploid (*diplous,* double) number of chromosomes.

Germ cells, however (the egg cell of the female and the spermatozoon of the male), each have only one member of each of the 23 pairs found in diploid cells so they are said to have a haploid (*haplo,* single) number of chromosomes.

Haploid Cells Develop From Diploid Cells. In both the male and the female the germ cells with their haploid number of chromosomes are derived from mother cells that have a diploid number of chromosomes. In each sex this is accomplished by the mother cell of the germ cells undergoing two consecutive divisions of a special kind called *meiosis* (*meio,* to make smaller) which results in each mother cell giving rise to four cells, each of which has only the haploid number of chromosomes. Meiotic divisions are also referred to as reduction divisions. In the male the four daughter cells are all viable germ cells called spermatozoa but in the female only one of the four daughter cells is a viable egg cell; the other three fail to develop and are discarded as what are termed *polar bodies.* Meiosis in the male is described in Chapter 27.

The Formation of Germ Cells in the Female. The mother cell from which haploid germ cells develop is termed a primary oocyte. By the time a female baby is born there are about 2,000,000 of these diploid cells in the baby's ovaries, and they have already duplicated their DNA and entered the counterpart of the prophase of an ordinary mitosis. However, the prophase that begins before birth is arrested and is only resumed in any primary oocyte when it begins to form an ovum that is capable of being fertilized, and this does not occur until puberty. But beginning at puberty it happens in a female roughly every 28 days (unless pregnancy occurs) and it only ceases when a woman reaches the menopause. The last oocytes that develop into germ cells in women who are close to the menopause have therefore been in prophase for over forty years.

The prophase begins in the oocyte as it does in mitosis, with the 46 chromosomes becoming visible; they appear long and threadlike. But before the prophase is arrested, certain changes occur that are different from those seen in mitosis, for each of the 23 threadlike chromosomes of paternal origin seeks out its homologue of maternal origin (or vice versa) and becomes arranged in intimate association with it along its whole length. Each homologous pair so arranged is

called a *bivalent.* There are now 23 bivalents in the nucleus. As the prophase continues the two chromosomes in each bivalent become more tightly coiled and shorter. Since each chromosome consists of two chromatids held together at its centromere, there are four chromatids with 2 centromeres in each bivalent. The two chromosomes of each bivalent then begin to separate from one another except at certain sites where one of the two chromatids of maternal origin adheres to one of the two chromatids of paternal origin. It is at these sites that a phenomenon of the greatest interest with regard to heredity occurs which involves the maternal chromosomes exchanging genetic material with the paternal ones. This is termed *crossing over.* The sites of exchange are visible microscopically and are called *chiasmata.* This is a very important stage for it provides for the reshuffling of genes and this in turn leads to enormous possibilities for variation in the new combinations of genes in the offspring. It is upon these inherited variations that selective forces have acted throughout evolution. The reshuffling of genes occurs as a result of breakages in the chromatids that develop naturally at the time when the paternal and maternal chromatids are lying close to and intertwined with each other; this permits broken pieces of chromatid material to be exchanged between them, and so genetic exchange is effected. After exchanges have occurred the bivalents gradually extend until the nucleus appears as if it were in the interphase. It is now that the oocytes enter their long rest period and are not awakened from it until puberty at the earliest. At puberty or after, in an oocyte that begins to mature, the bivalents rapidly condense so as to once more appear as chromosomes which now enter the metaphase. In the anaphase which follows, the two chromatids of each chromosome *do not separate* from each other as occurs in mitosis. Instead, the two chromosomes of each bivalent, each with a single centromere and two chromatids, separate from one another. Moreover, whether a paternal or a maternal chromosome of a bivalent faces one or the other pole is a matter of chance so that when the homologous chromosomes separate from one another, some of the chromosomes that go to one pole are from the paternal side and some from the maternal. However, one member of each bivalent chromosome pair normally goes to each pole, which leads to each daughter cell's possessing only 23 chromosomes.

It is at the above described stage that trisomy-21 is most likely to occur. The bivalent consisting of the pair of chromosomes 21 probably never forms in this instance. The chromosomes 21 remain as univalents instead. This may result from either a failure of pairing in the first place or a failure in the formation of a chiasma after pairing has occurred. As the chance of forming a chiasma is related to the length of the chromosomes that are paired, the shortness of chromosome 21 would tend to favor failure of chiasma formation but in either case, 2 univalents rather than one bivalent would result.

Univalents have an equal chance of going to either daughter cell and so occasionally both chromosomes 21 would end up in the same daughter cell, giving it 24 chromosomes (Fig. 2-25). The other daughter cell thus has only 22 chromosomes. The failure of two homologous chromosomes to go to two daughter cells separately is termed *nondisjunction* and this is the usual cause of trisomy-21. Nondisjunction is an accident that can happen to any chromosome. The one affecting chromosome 21 leads to Down's syndrome; if nondisjunction affects the X chromosome, it can result in XXX as well as XO females and XXY males.

The second meiotic division resembles an ordinary mitosis except that it is not immediately preceded by a duplication of the DNA of the chromosomes or the formation of more chromatids. The chromosomes in the cell that begin the second meiotic division already each have two chromatids and one centromere. So all that happens is that the chromosomes line up in the equatorial plane and there the centromere divides, each chromosome thus splits into its two chromatids which then become chromosomes in their own right and in due course these become the chromosomes of the two daughter cells that form. But because under normal conditions there were only 23 chromosomes in each daughter cell that resulted from the first meiotic division, the second meiotic division results in each of the two daughter cells that form from it having only the haploid number of chromosomes. However, if one of the two daughter cells that enters the second meiotic division has 24 chromosomes because of an extra chromosome 21 and if either of these should become an ovum and be fertilized, the baby will have cells with 47 chromosomes and suffer from the trisomy-21 syndrome. If either of the daughter cells with only 22 chromosomes should become the ovum and be fertilized it will never form a viable fetus.

Trisomy-21 is the most common of the chromosome anomalies observed in newborn infants, although it is not a particularly common condition. It does not always require an extra complete chromosome 21, for the condition is sometimes caused as a result of only an extra piece of chromosome 21 being present in the cells of the infant; this can be caused by a piece of chromosome 21 being translocated to another chromosome so that the infant has not only its normal pair of chromosomes 21 but an extra piece of a chromosome 21 in another chromosome. The incidence of trisomy-21 increases with the age of the mother. A woman over 40 is over 50 times more likely to give birth to an affected child than a woman of 25. Her chances are, in fact, about one in 60 of doing so. The reason for this has to do with the increasingly longer time an oocyte has remained in an arrested prophase before it completes its meiotic divisions to give rise to a viable ovum. Nondisjunction can occur in the production of male germ cells but it is most unlikely. This is probably related to the fact that they are made freshly all through life and so there is no prophase that is kept in arrest for years as occurs in the female.

Some Examples of Anomalies of Sex Chromosomes

These in general exert their primary effect on the development and function of the reproductive system of the affected individual.

The Y chromosome has a gene whose function seems to be that of directing the development of the testes (the male sex glands) in embryonic life. X chromosomes, in addition to exerting genetic effects which direct development along the female type unless overpowered by a Y, have, in contrast to a Y chromosome, an extensive complement of genes which have nothing specially to do with sex and so X chromosomes in this sense are of more *general* importance to a body than Y chromosomes.

The commonest anomaly of the sex chromosomes is due to an extra X being present in a male who therefore has an XXY combination in all the cells of his body. Males with this anomaly develop small testes and are infertile. For some reason not understood, having a pair of X chromosomes in their cells instead of one may affect the development of their intelligence so that in some it may be somewhat less than that of normal males. The condition is called *Klinefelter's syndrome* and, like trisomy-21, is probably to be explained by nondisjunction during one of the meiotic divisions of the oocyte which gives rise to the ovum, which leads in this instance to the pair of X chromosomes not separating but both going to the ovum which became fertilized by a spermatozoon carrying a Y chromosome. It can also arise, but less frequently, when an XY-bearing sperm (from nondisjunction at meiosis in the father) fertilizes a normal X-bearing ovum. Nondisjunction at both meiotic divisions in one of the parents can give rise to XXXY or XXXXY chromosome constitutions, conditions which clinically are indistinguishable from the regular Klinefelter's syndrome except that *all* of these individuals are mentally retarded.

Another condition, called *Turner's syndrome,* is seen in females that have only one X chromosome instead of a pair. This state of affairs is termed *monosomy* (only one body). Monosomies are nearly always incompatible with life but sometimes full-term babies are born with it. Two X chromosomes are required if an individual is to develop normal ovaries and hence those with an XO (O as used here means *nothing*) instead of an XX combination do not develop normal ovaries or even normal stature. Otherwise their development is essentially female though not normal in certain respects. This anomaly also can be caused by nondisjunction at the germ cell level, for if both X chromosomes of the oocyte go to one daughter cell (which is lost as a polar body), the other daughter cell has no X chromosomes left and so if it is fertilized by a spermatozoon carrying an X chromosome, the somatic cells of the individual that develops have only the one X chromosome that was derived from the male germ cell. The XO condition can probably also arise by loss of an X chromosome during spermatogenesis; if so, a spermatozoon having neither an X nor a Y would have to have fertilized a normal X-bearing ovum.

Another anomaly of interest is the male that has an XYY chromosome complement. Males with this combination tend to be tall and there is some indication that they may be more aggressive than normal males, although there is no firm evidence as yet that it is the extra chromosome that is responsible for the antisocial behavior seen in some of these individuals. Several other anomalies of the sex chromosomes involving numbers are now known; those interested should consult "Further Reading."

Example of an Anomaly Involving the Form of a Chromosome Instead of Total Number. An anomaly of this type occurs as a deletion of part of the short arm of chromosome 5. It results in the infant having facial deformities of various degrees of severity, probably depending on how much of the arm of the chromosome is deleted. Another clinical feature resulting from the defect is that the sound of the cry of the baby with this defect is unusual and characteristic, accounting for the term, the "cri-du-chat" syndrome.

A Note on the Symbols Used To Denote Chromosome Anomalies. For any student pursuing this subject further it may help in reading the literature to be aware that when karyotype findings in man are being described, it is now customary to record first the total number of chromosomes. This is followed by a comma and then the sex chromosome constitution. Autosomes are mentioned only if there is an abnormality. The normal human male karyotype is thus designated as 46,XY. The karyotype of a female who has Down's syndrome with an extra chromosome 21 would be referred to as 47,XX, 21+ and of a male with Klinefelter's syndrome with 2 XX chromosomes, as 47,XXY.

We shall next comment on some chromosome anomalies that originate at the somatic cell level.

ANOMALIES THAT ARISE AT THE SOMATIC CELL LEVEL

Some Further Terminology. It has already been mentioned that normal somatic (body) cells are termed *diploid* cells and that diploid means double. Actually diploid is derived from *di,* twice or double, and *ploos,* folded. The word fold is used here with the meaning it has in twofold which word means twice or multiplied by two. So diploid has reference to something that is multiplied by two and that something is the haploid (*haplod,* single) number of chromosomes in germ cells which is, of course, 23.

Another term is *polyploidy,* which means many times folded or multiplied so polyploid cells are cells which have multiples of the haploid number, for example, a *tetraploid* cell has four times the haploid number (double the diploid number) and so on. Still another term that is much used is *aneuploidy;* since *an* means want or absence, aneuploidy means an absence of the property of being a normal (*eu,* health) multiple, so the number in a cell manifesting aneuploidy is not an exact multiple of the haploid number. Hence a human cell with say 45, 47 or any number that is not an exact multiple of 23 is an aneuploid cell. We can now see that (almost) all the clinical conditions resulting from anomalies involving a change in the number of chromosomes that originate at the germ cell level, and which we have just described, are examples of aneuploidy. Aneuploid numbers of chromosomes can also arise at the level of somatic cells, as will soon be described, but first we shall discuss polyploidy originating at the somatic cell level.

Polyploidy Originating in Somatic Cells

This occurs in certain somatic cell families under normal conditions; indeed there is one kind of cell to be described in a later chapter (the megakaryocyte) that is normally polyploid. Certain other types of cells, for example, liver cells, are occasionally polyploid. Seen in the interphase, a polyploid liver cell has a

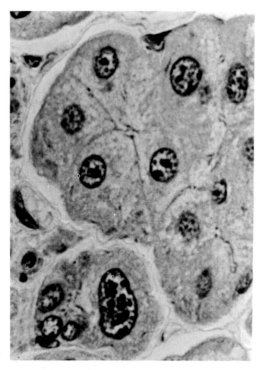

FIG. 2-26. Photomicrograph showing a cell (*lower middle*) that demonstrates polyploidy. The nucleus is much larger and contains more nucleoli than the nuclei of the cells in the group above, which are normal and so have a diploid number of chromosomes.

only two cells, but each would have a tetraploid content of chromosomes because the original nucleus has divided twice. An example of two sets of chromosomes caught in a single spindle is illustrated in Figure 2-27.

Aneuploidy Originating in Somatic Cells

Aneuploidy originates at the somatic cell level under two conditions, as will now be described.

Species of higher animals such as man are perpetuated indefinitely because of their germ cells creating successive new individuals to carry on the species. Since bodies which are composed of somatic cells have a limited life span, the question arises as to whether or not a factor in causing the limited life span is that those somatic cells which must continue to multiply throughout life in order to maintain the structure of the body have some inherent limitation placed on the number of times they can reproduce themselves. It would, of course, be of great interest to know whether, if the kind of somatic cells that can divide were transferred from one individual to another compatible one, they would through succeeding generations demonstrate the same type of immortality as is demonstrated by germ cell lineages. One way by which the question of somatic cell immortality can be investigated is by cultivating somatic cells outside the body in suitable media. Many studies of this kind have shown that somatic cells with proliferative capacity can indeed be propagated outside the body in nutritive media

larger nucleus than its diploid counterpart (Fig. 2-26, *bottom*). So far as is known, polyploid liver cells function normally. The first and probably the most common way polyploidy occurs is by a cell passing through the prophase and the metaphase of mitosis but then, after the chromosomes have each separated into their two chromatids, the two sets do not pull apart to opposite ends of the cell but remain in the region of the equatorial plane until a new nuclear membrane forms to enclose them all in the same nucleus. Another way polyploidy can occur is by means of the nuclear membrane failing to break down even though the chromatids separate, so as a consequence, the nucleus comes to contain a double number of chromosomes. Still another way is more indirect and takes place in two stages; first mitosis occurs and results in 2 nuclei. But the cytoplasm does not divide and, as a result, a binucleated cell is formed. Then both nuclei in the binucleate cell enter mitosis at the same time, and when the nuclear membranes simultaneously disintegrate, the chromosomes of both cells become caught in the same spindle and are pulled together again. Therefore, when division is complete there would be

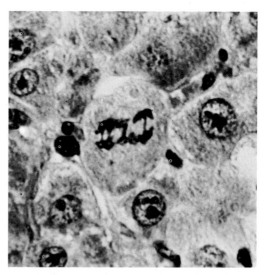

FIG. 2-27. High-power photomicrograph of an H and E section of regenerating rat liver, showing double the usual number of anaphase chromosomes arranged in a common spindle, which is just visible above them.

long enough to suggest that they could go on multiplying forever. However, since methods for chromosome analysis have become available it has also become evident that most of these lines of cells that have been cultured acquire in due course an aneuploid number of chromosomes and so they can no longer be considered to be normal cells.

The suspicion is thus aroused that the long-continued multiplication of somatic cells is associated with the risk of some genetic change occurring in the cell which makes it less responsive to factors that would ordinarily suppress its rate of reproduction or capacity for unlimited reproduction, and which often leads to frank aneuploidy.

Aneuploidy and Cancer Cells. Aneuploidy evolves under conditions of the more or less continuous multiplication of cells also in the disease commonly termed cancer. It is believed that cancer originates because some somatic cell, of a type that has reproductive capacity, undergoes a genetic change of such a nature that the cell is much less susceptible than its neighbors to those factors that control cell populations in the body, and so it multiplies under conditions in which the multiplication of normal cells would be restrained. The constantly enlarging and invading cellular aggregate that thus forms is called a malignant tumor or a cancer. The escape of cancer cells from growth-control mechanisms is associated more or less reciprocally with a loss of their ability to attain the kind of highly specialized structure normal cells of the same type would attain, and hence, they are usually not proficient functionally, or, if they can function at all, their function is unregulated, as if they did not relate to the rest of the organism. Accordingly, cancer cells are commonly said to use energy for growth instead of function. Whereas normal cells stop moving and stop proliferating when they come in contact with other normal cells, cancer cells characteristically lose this quality of contact inhibition of movement and of growth, and they spread over any cells in their vicinity.

Since the change that turns a somatic cell into a cancer cell is a genetic change, cancer cells pass on their asocial characteristics to all their progeny. One result of the alteration at the level of genes (and a most desirable result) may be that the altered genetic nature of the cell may result in the synthesis of protein being sufficiently altered in the cancer cells for them to be considered foreign by the immunological mechanisms of the host (to be described in Chapters 9 and 10), and if this occurs, cells of the beginning cancer may be destroyed by the same type of rejection mechanism that so often operates to reject improperly matched transplants of tissues and organs. However, if this does not occur, the fact that cancer is due to a genetic change means that the cancer cells pass on their asocial and aggressive characteristics to all their progeny and so if a cancer is not all surgically removed, or destroyed in some other fashion before it has grown for too long a period, its cells may be disseminated by way of blood or lymph to parts of the body distant from its origin. In these sites the cells set up new foci of invasive and destructive growth called *metastases,* and by this means cancer cells can overwhelm the body.

By losing their ability to respond to the influences that control the growth of normal cells, cancer cells in a sense achieve the requisites for somatic cell immortality. They do not, of course, demonstrate immortality in the body in which they develop, for if they are left to multiply in that body, they will destroy it. But if they are removed, and thereafter grow in cultures, some kinds at least can be propagated indefinitely. Furthermore, if the cells of a cancer originating in an experimental animal are regularly transferred to other animals of the same strain, they will continue to multiply indefinitely, and, indeed, on continued transplantation they often experience further genetic changes by which they become even more malignant than when they originated. Some cancers have been maintained in mice by this means for decades. Cancer cells, therefore, seem to be able to reproduce themselves indefinitely.

The cells of a cancer commonly exhibit aneuploidy; indeed, the demonstration of aneuploidy in growing cells taken from the body is regarded as a positive test for the cells concerned being cancer cells. The absence of aneuploidy, however, does not rule out the presence of cancer, for some cancer cells may not be aneuploid—at least, not at first, but only as their multiplication continues.

From the behavior both of diploid cells in cultures and of cancer cells in the body, we are left with the impression that aneuploidy, originating at the somatic cell level, is probably more or less the final outcome of some genetic disorganization that in its beginning is responsible for releasing the cells in which it occurs from the influences, both inherent and environmental, which ordinarily place restraints on their proliferative activities and capacities.

An Example of a Chromosome Anomaly Originating at the Somatic Cell Level Which Involves Form Instead of Number

Patients with the disease chronic granulocytic leukemia, in which there is an overproduction of certain white cells of the blood, characteristically have in the chromosome complement of their bone marrow cells a unique minute chromosome, which, because it was discovered in Philadelphia, is referred to as the "Philadelphia chromosome," "Ph¹" or simply "Ph." It is a small acrocentric chromosome (no. 22) with about half of its long arm missing. The individual's chromosomes may be otherwise normal in number and morphology. Since it is present in nearly all cases of this condition and absent in other conditions, the Philadelphia chromosome has been valuable in the diagnosis of chronic granulocytic leukemia. In several instances it has also been found before symptoms of the disease were apparent, and it tends to persist even when the disease is arrested.

Somehow this chromosome anomaly is intimately involved in the process that leads to the leukemia, possibly being a necessary if not sufficient condition for the development of the disease.

The Philadelphia chromosome is not inherited from one generation to another. It is not present in the children of patients with the disease, nor is it found in all the cells of the body when it is present. While nearly all the cells of the bone marrow in patients possess the unusual chromosome, the cells of other tissues in the same individuals have normal appearing chromosomes. It thus arises at the somatic rather than at the germinal cell level, probably early in the development of the disease, in a precursor of the white blood cells, by the accidental loss of part of the long arm of chromosome 22. Once this has happened, the chromosome anomaly is transmitted to all the somatic cells that thereafter develop from this altered cell. It will be mentioned again in Chapter 12.

How Every Human Chromosome Can Be Individually Identified

The identification of each and every one of the individual pairs of human chromosomes is beyond the scope of the methods already described. But recently several methods of staining chromosomes have been developed which bring out chromosomal banding patterns that are invisible in routinely stained preparations. Since the banding patterns are unique for each chromosome pair and the bands of chromosomes belonging to the same pair are identical, it is now possible to identify individual members of each chromosome group.

In the first of these methods, quinacrine, a fluorescent dye, is used to stain the chromosome preparations. The dye molecules are preferentially taken up by certain regions of the chromosomes, rendering these bands

visible with the fluorescence microscope. The distal part of the long arm of the Y chromosome in man is seen to fluoresce especially brightly by this method. Since this is also true in the interphase, it makes it possible to identify male cells readily even when they are not dividing.

The new staining method has revealed some abnormalities of chromosome structure that could not be seen before, such as deletions of chromosome material, inversions and translocations of part of one chromosome to that of another. It has also made it possible to distinguish between chromosomes 21 and 22. As already mentioned, trisomy of chromosome 21 occurs in Down's syndrome, while deletion of part of the long arm of chromosome 22, which results in what is called the "Philadelphia chromosome," is characteristic of the disease chronic myelogenous leukemia. Until recently it was believed that these two conditions were associated with different abnormalities of the same chromosome. Trisomy-22 is now a recognized condition distinct from trisomy-21 (Down's syndrome).

The use of fluorescence under ultraviolet light of chromosome regions stained by quinacrine requires expensive equipment. For routine purposes, other methods have been developed that utilize the old Giesma stain (a much-used stain for blood cells) in new ways. Like quinacrine, the modified Giesma procedure stains certain chromosome regions preferentially and the bands can then be seen with an ordinary light microscope. Figure 2-28 shows a normal human karyotype made from a chromosome preparation that was stained by this procedure.

In most human chromosomes the regions that are stained are situated near the centromere. The mechanism of this differential staining effect is still not clearly understood but it is somehow related to the presence of protein in the chromosomes, for treatment of the chromosomes with proteolytic enzymes has the same effect in unmasking the bands as the heat, alkali, alcohol, etc. that are normally used prior to staining in all these procedures (see Wang and Federoff).

Several modifications of these methods have appeared; one of these permits the banding patterns of human chromosomes to be seen with an ordinary microscope in as little as 10 minutes from the beginning of the staining procedure.

Effect of Radiation on Cells and Chromosomes

The fundamental way that radiation can damage cells is very different from the way that body parts

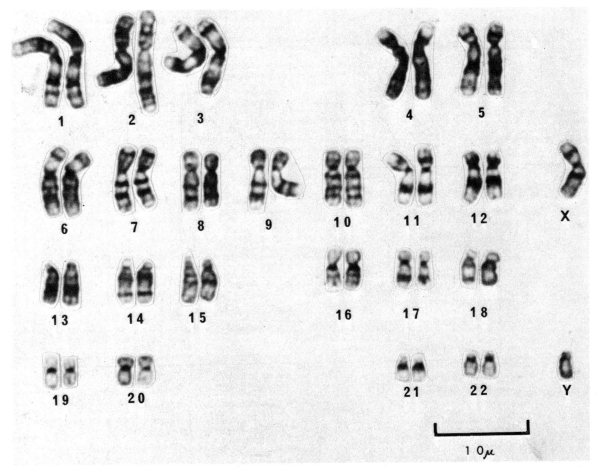

FIG. 2-28. The normal male karyotype, showing the banding pattern seen after staining by Giemsa technic as described in text. The characteristic banding pattern of chromosomes obtained by this technic permits each human chromosome to be identified. (Preparation courtesy of Mrs. M. Seabright, Cytogenetics Unit, Salisbury General Hospital, Salisbury, England)

are injured by other kinds of physical agents. Indeed, a knowledge of the way damage is done by a thermal burn or frostbite may hinder the student rather than help him understand radiation damage. For example, heat, as when a person touches a hot stove, causes localized damage to the skin and underlying tissue which quickly becomes apparent. Furthermore, the damage done by heat applied to the skin is greatest at the surface and diminishes in relation to depth from the surface. The damage done by radiation, on the contrary, may not become apparent for a relatively long time and, furthermore, does not necessarily diminish in relation to depth from the surface; indeed, high-energy radiation may do more damage considerably below than at the skin surface.

The effects of harmful amounts of x- or gamma rays on living cells that are in their path, and through which they may pass, is due to the high-energy photons of the radiation setting energetic electrons in motion in the nucleus and cytoplasm of the cells. The energetic electrons can knock other electrons out of atoms in the cell components, which causes these atoms to become intensely reactive so that they immediately enter into new chemical combinations in their immediate environment, thus causing changes in the chemical composition of the particular cell component with which they react.

We must now ask what effect this would have on the appearance, at the level of the LM, of cells such as those of the liver with whose normal appearance we are now very familiar and which we know seldom undergo mitosis under ordinary circumstances. The

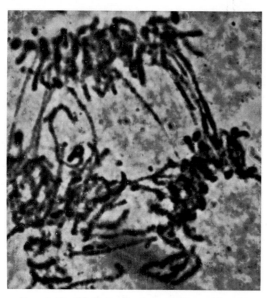

FIG. 2-29. Oil-immersion photomicrograph of a squash preparation of an L cell in mitosis following 5,000 r of x-rays that was given to the culture in which this cell was growing. The radiation has interfered with the normal process of cell division in that (1) the spindle in this cell has 3 poles instead of 2; (2) many of the chromosomes are lagging, and as a result they form *chromosomal bridges;* and (3) many are of an abnormal form. (Till, J. E., and Whitmore, G. F.: Effects of x-rays on mammalian cells in tissue culture. *In* Proc. 3rd Canadian Cancer Res. Conf., New York, Academic Press)

catabolized. So the cell could appear as it did before and could soon probably continue to function much as it did before.

The fact that cells in the interphase may appear normal but may, however, have suffered damage from irradiation becomes apparent when the cells attempt to undergo mitosis, as has been shown experimentally. As previously mentioned, the cells of the liver of a normal adult animal seldom divide. But if a large portion of the liver is removed, the cells of the remaining portion of the liver soon divide so actively that they restore the liver to almost its normal size in a few days. If this type of experiment is performed on an animal whose liver had previously been given sufficient radiation, it has been found that instead of finding normal mitotic figures in the liver cells, many abnormal mitotic figures make their appearance. The same phenomenon is observed if cells that are multiplying in cell cultures are irradiated—the subsequent mitosis of cells is profoundly affected. The mitotic chromosomes may be altered in form or broken up, or joined together in abnormal ways and fragments of them may be completely lost. The spindle may show abnormalities—for example, it may have three poles instead of two, with the result that chromosomes are draw to three points instead of two (Fig. 2-29). The mitotic chromosomes act as if they were sticky and in the anaphase the chromatids do not pull apart from one another evenly. Some may lag and form bridges between the two groups of chromosomes (Fig. 2-29). The chromosomes may divide without the nucleus dividing; this gives rise to large nuclei with more than the normal number of chromosomes. Or the nuclei may divide without the cytoplasm dividing. In the last two instances the cells affected may become much larger than normal and are then called giant cells.

A possible explanation for the radiation damage to cells becoming apparent when cells attempt to undergo mitosis may be that this is the first time that all of the damage done to the chromatin of an interphase cell has the opportunity to manifest itself. As will be described in the next chapter, the genes of cells have to be duplicated before a cell undergoes division, and, to accomplish this, the two strands of every DNA molecule have to separate, with each strand thereupon serving as a template for the synthesis of a second strand so that two complete double-stranded molecules become available to provide for the double number of genes required for the two daughter cells that soon form. To understand why undisclosed injuries to DNA should become apparent at this time it should be reiterated that in its ordinary work in the interphase

answer is, very little, if any. The reason for specialized functioning cells not necessarily evidencing damage from a dose of radiation that has actually done some damage is to be explained, at least in part, as follows:

First, in a normal specialized cell only a small fraction of its genes are required to direct the synthesis of the particular proteins that characterize that particular kind of cell. The chances of any of these genes being injured would be much less than the chances of some of the much larger number of unused genes in that cell being injured. Furthermore, if one or more of the active genes are injured by the radiation, there may be uninjured duplicate genes to take over their work. Third, any chemical alterations that occur because of intensely reactive atoms in the *cytoplasm* entering into new chemical combinations could be of only temporary significance if the genes that direct the synthesis of fresh protein were unaffected because new proteins and conjugated proteins are always being synthesized and the altered material would soon be

of mitosis, a cell uses only a small fraction of its total number of genes—only those required to direct protein synthesis required in that particular kind of cell. The great number of the genes of most cells, for reasons to be given in the next chapter, are not used in a functioning cell. But for a cell to divide normally, *every molecule of the very large amount of previously unused DNA of the cell* in its condensed chromatin, as well as of the much smaller amount used for normal function, has to be duplicated and it is then that the previously hidden injuries done to any of the chromatin of the nucleus becomes apparent, for all the chromosomal material has to be duplicated, with chromatids separating, if mitosis is to be normal. If the damage is severe enough it is manifested in the mitotic figures that are seen in the ways described previously and it can be serious enough for an attempted mitosis being not only unsuccessful but lethal.

The above might explain part of the rationale for radiation being used in the treatment of cancer. The aim is not to kill cancer cells that are in the interphase but to affect them in such a way that they become unable to undergo successful mitosis. The aim is to slow up or stop their further growth. Furthermore, radiation can be delivered in ingenious ways so that the site of a tumor receives more than the tissues in the surrounding or nearby territories, which, of course, is desirable because radiation can cause any cells in the affected area to thereafter have diminished reproductive ability.

Mutagenic Effects. These are the results of small doses that do not do enough damage to make a cell unable to undergo mitosis but just enough to affect the genetic material so that it becomes slightly altered. The gene or genes lost or altered may not affect the duplication of genes as a whole so that mitosis will be normal, but if altered genes duplicate as a prelude to mitosis they duplicate their altered character. Lost genes, of course, are not duplicated. Thus the descendants of the affected cell will not only lack the normal qualities of genes that are lost but may also be affected by the qualities imparted by altered genes that duplicate. This is the way in which radiation, in doses that are not lethal to a cell, can induce cell mutations. A mutation in a body cell caused this way can initiate a cancer, as was shown all too often by those who worked with x-rays before their dangers were fully appreciated. A mutation resulting from the irradiation at the level of the formation of germ cells can result in an anomaly in an offspring.

What Is Meant by "Sensitivity to Radiation." This term is often misunderstood.

First, under different environmental conditions the same kind of cells that receive the same amount of irradiation can have different amounts of damage done to their DNA. A very important factor influencing the amount of damage done to cells by irradiation is oxygen tension. Cells in sites of high tension are more sensitive to irradiation than cells in sites of low oxygen tension.

Second, there has been an old theory to the effect that cells are more sensitive to radiation if it is given when they are actually in mitosis. This theory has been shown to be only partly true, for although its truth has been demonstrated in certain cells of animals of some species, it is not true of the same kinds of cells in other species.

Third, it could be said that cells which remain in the interphase for long periods, or even for life, are less sensitive to irradiation than those kinds of cells which divide frequently, because the former cells do not pass into the stage in which the lethal effects of irradiation become operative. However, granted the same turnover rate, it seems that all kinds of body cells in the same environment are, roughly, equally sensitive to irradiation.

References and Other Reading

The order of the headings follows that in which various matters are dealt with in the text.

THE TURNOVER OF CELL POPULATIONS

Altmann, G. G., and Enesco, M.: Cell number as a measure of distribution and renewal of epithelial cells in the small intestine of growing adult rats. Am. J. Anat., 121:319, 1967.
Bertalanffy, F. D., and Lau, C.: Cell renewal. Int. Rev. Cytol., 9:357, 1962.
Cairnie, A. B., Lamerton, L. F., and Steel, G. G.: Cell proliferation studies in the intestinal epithelium of the rat. Exp. Cell Res., 39:528 and 539, 1965.
Fry, R. J. M., Griem, M. L., and Kirsten, W. H. (eds): Normal and Malignant Cell Growth. New York, Springer-Verlag, 1969.
Goss, R. T.: Turnover in Cells and Tissues. In Prescott, D. M., Goldstein, L., and McConkey, E. (eds.): Advances in Cell Biology. vol. 1, New York, Appleton-Century-Crofts, 1970.
Leblond, C. P., Clermont, Y., and Nadler, N. J.: The pattern of stem cell renewal in three epithelia (esophagus, intestine and testis). Can. Cancer Res. Conf. (Pergamon Press), 7:3, 1967.
Leblond, C. P., and Walker, B. E.: Renewal of cell populations. Physiol. Rev., 30:255, 1956.
Marques-Pereira, J. P., and Leblond, C. P.: Mitosis and differentiation in the stratified squamous epithelium of the rat esophagus. Am. J. Anat., 117:73, 1965.
Stohlman, F., Jr.: The Kinetics of Cellular Proliferation. New York, Grune & Stratton, 1959.

The Electron Microscope and Technics Employed

History

Bradbury, S.: The Evolution of the Microscope. New York, Pergamon Press, 1967.

Burton, E. F., and Kohl, W. H.: The Electron Microscope. ed. 2. New York, Reinhold, 1946.

Freundlich, M. M.: Origin of the electron microscope. Science, *142*:185, 1963.

Technics

Everhart, T. E., and Hayes, T. L.: The scanning electron microscope. Sci. Am., *226*:54, 1972.

Hayat, M. A.: Basic Electron Microscopy Technics. New York, Van Nostrand Reinhold, 1972.

———: Principles and Techniques of Electron Microscopy. New York, Van Nostrand Reinhold, 1972.

Koehlered, J. K.: Advanced Techniques in Biological Electron Microscopy. New York, Springer-Verlag, 1973.

Meek, G. A.: Practical Electron Microscopy for Biologists. p. 498. New York, Wiley-Interscience, 1970.

Pease, D. C.: Histological Techniques for Electron Microscopy. ed. 2. New York, Academic Press, 1964.

Sjostrand, F. S.: Electron Microscopy of Cells and Tissues. New York, Academic Press, 1967.

Wischnitzer, S.: Introduction to Electron Microscopy. ed. 2. New York, Pergamon Press, 1970.

For Atlases and Books on the Fine Structure of Cells, see Chapter 5.

The Nuclear Envelope

Feldherr, C.: Structure and Function of the Nuclear Envelope. Adv. Cell Molecular Biology. vol. 2. DuPraw, E. J. (ed.), New York, Academic Press, 1972.

Franke, W. W.: Isolated nuclear membranes. J. Cell Biol. *31*: 619, 1966.

Gall, J. G.: Octagonal nuclear pores. J. Cell Biol., *32*:391, 1967.

Kessel, R. G.: Structure and Function of the Nuclear Envelope and Related Cytomembranes. *In* Progress in Surface and Membrane Science. vol. 6, p. 243. 1973.

The Interphase Nucleus

Beams, H. W., and Mueller, S.: Effects of ultracentrifugation on the interphase nucleus. Zeit. Zellforsch. *108*:297, 1970.

Bonner, J., Dahmus, M., Fambrough, D., Huang, R. C., Marushinge, K., and Tuan, D.: The biology of isolated chromatin. Science, *159*:47, 1968.

Brown, S. W.: Heterochromatin. Science, *151*:417, 1966.

Dalton, A. J., and Haguenau, F. (eds.): Ultrastructure in Biological Systems. vol. 3. The Nucleus. New York, Academic Press, 1968.

DuPraw, E. J.: DNA and Chromosomes. New York, Holt, Rinehart and Winston, 1970.

Gurndon, J. B.: Transplanted nuclei and cell differentiation. Sci. Am., *219*:24, 1968.

Harris, H.: The reactivation of the red cell nucleus. J. Cell Sci., *2*:23, 1967.

Milner, G. R.: Nuclear morphology and ultrastructural localization of deoxyribonucleic acid synthesis during interphase. J. Cell Sci., *4*:569, 1969.

Mirsky, A. E., and Osawa, S.: The Interphase Nucleus. *In* Mirsky, A. E., and Bracket, J. (eds.): The Cell. vol. 2. New York, Academic Press, 1961.

Mitchell, J. S. (ed.): The Cell Nucleus. New York, Academic Press, 1960.

Ris, H.: Ultrastructure and molecular organization of genetic systems. Canad. J. Genet. Cytol., *3*:95, 1962.

Swift, H. S.: Molecular morphology of the chromosome. In Vitro, *1*:26, 1966.

For further references about the chromatin, including the sex chromatin, of the interphase nucleus, see Chapter 4.

The Chromatin of the Interphase Nucleus—*See* Chapter 4.

Mitosis—Centrioles and Microtubules

Bajer, A., and Mole-Bajer, J.: Architecture and function of the mitotic spindle. Adv. Cell Molec. Biol., *1*:213, 1971.

Brinkley, B. R.: The fine structure of the nucleolus in mitotic divisions of Chinese hamster cells in vitro. J. Cell Biol., *27*: 411, 1965.

Brinkley, B. R., and Stubblefield, E.: Ultrastructure and Interaction of the Kinetochore and Centriole in Mitosis and Meiosis. *In* Prescott, D. M., Goldstein, L., and McConkey, E. (eds.): Advances in Cell Biology. vol. 1. New York, Appleton-Century-Crofts, 1970.

Comings, D. E., and Okada, T. A.: Architecture of meiotic cells and mechanisms of chromosome pairing. *In* DuPraw, E. J. (ed.): Adv. Cell Molec. Biol. vol. 2. New York, Academic Press, 1972.

De Harven, E.: The Centriole and the Mitotic Spindle. *In* Dalton, A. J., and Haguenau, F. (eds.): The Nucleus. New York, Academic Press, 1968.

Forer, A.: Chromosome movements during cell division. *In* Lima-de-Faria A. (ed.): Handbook of Cytology. Amsterdam, North Holland, 1969.

Friedlander, M., and Wahrman, J.: The spindle as a basal body distributor. J. Cell Sci. *7*:65, 1970.

Fulton, C.: Centrioles. *In* Reinert, J., and Ursprung, H. (eds.): Origin and Continuity of Cell Organelles. vol. 2, p. 170. New York, Springer-Verlag, 1971.

Inoue, S.: On the physical properties of the mitotic spindle. Ann. N.Y. Acad. Sci., *90*:529, 1960.

Inoue, S., and Sato, H.: Cell motility by labile association of molecules. The nature of mitotic spindle fibers and their role in chromosome movement. J. Gen. Physiol., *50*:259, 1967.

Jokelainen, P. T.: The ultrastructure and spatial organization of the metaphase kinetochore in mitotic rat cells. J. Ultrastr. Res., *19*:19, 1967.

Kristan, A., and Buck, R. C.: Structure of the mitotic spindle in L. strain fibroblasts. J. Cell Biol., *24*:433, 1965.

Levine, L.: The Cell in Mitosis, New York, Academic Press, 1963.

Mazia, D.: How cells divide. Sci. Am., *205*:101, Sept. 1961.

———: Mitosis and the Physiology of Cell Division. *In* Brachet, J., and Mirsky, A. E. (eds.): The Cell. vol. 3. New York, Academic Press, Inc., 1961.

McIntosh, J. R., Hepler, P. K., and Van Wie, D. G.: Model for mitosis. Nature, *224:*659, 1969.

McIntosh, J. R., and Landis, S.: The distribution of spindle microtubules during mitosis in cultured human cells. J. Cell Biol., *49:*468, 1971.

Murray, R. G., Murray, A. S., and Pizzo, A.: The fine structure of mitosis in rat thymic lymphocytes. J. Cell Biol., *26:*601, 1965.

Nicklas, R. B.: Mitosis. *In* Adv. in Cell Biol. vol. 2, 1971.

Porter, K. R.: Cytoplasmic microtubules and their functions. *In* Wolstenholme, G. E. W., and O'Connor, M. (eds.): Principles of Biomolecular Organization. Ciba Foundation Symposium. London, J. and Churchill, A. Ltd., 1966.

Rhoades, M. M.: Meiosis. *In* Brachet, J., and Mirsky, A. E. (eds.): The Cell. vol. 3. New York, Academic Press, 1961.

Robbins, E., and Gonates, N. K.: The ultrastructure of a mammalian cell during the mitotic cycle. J. Cell Biol., *21:*429, 1964.

Robbins, E., Jentzsch, G., and Micali, A.: The centriole cycle in synchronized HeLa cells. J. Cell Biol., *36:*329, 1968.

Szollosi, D.: Cortical cytoplasmic filaments of cleaving eggs: A structural element corresponding to the contractile ring. J. Cell Biol., *44:*192, 1970.

Tilney, L., and Marsland, D.: A fine structural analysis of cleavage induction and furrowing in the eggs of Arbacia. J. Cell Biol., *42:*170, 1969.

Tucker, J. B.: Microtubules and a contractile ring of microfilaments associated with a cleavage furrow. J. Cell Sci., *8:*557, 1971.

MITOTIC INHIBITORS

Bertalanffy, F. D.: Tritiated thymidine vs. colchicine technique in the study of cell population cytodynamics. Lab. Invest., *13:*871, 1964.

Borisy, G. G., and Taylor, E. W.: The mechanism of action of colchicine. Binding of colchicine-H³ to cellular protein. J. Cell Biol., *34:*525, 1967.

Brinkley, B. R., Stubblefield, E., and Hsu, T. C.: The effects of colcemid inhibition and reversal on the fine structure of the mitotic apparatus of Chinese hamster cells in vitro. J. Ultrastr. Res., *19:*1, 1967.

Inoue, S.: The effect of colchicine on the microscopic and submicroscopic structure of the mitotic spindle. Exp. Cell Res., Suppl. *2:*305, 1952.

Stevens Hooper, C.: Use of colchicine for measurement of mitotic rate in the intestinal epithelium. Am. J. Anat., *108:*231, 1961.

CHROMOSOME STRUCTURE

Comings, D., and Okada, T.: Whole mount electron microscopy of meiotic chromosomes and the synaptonemal complex. Chromosoma, *30:*269, 1970.

Diacumakos, E., Holland, S., and Pecora, P.: Chromosome displacement in and extraction from human cells at different mitotic stages. Nature, *232:*33, 1971.

DuPraw, E. J.: DNA and Chromosomes. New York, Holt, Rinehart and Winston, 1970.

Golomb, H., and Bahr, G. F.: Scanning electron microscopic observations of surface structure of isolated human chromosomes. Science, *171:*1024.

Huberman, J. A., and Attardi, G.: Isolation of metaphase chromosomes from Hela cells. J. Cell Biol., *31:*95, 1966.

Lampert, F.: Coiled supercoiled DNA in critical-point dried and thin sectioned human chromosome fibers. Nature (Biol.), *234:*187, 1971.

Pavan, C.: Modern concept of chromosome structure and function. Triangle, *6:*287, 1964.

Prescott, D. M.: The structure and replication of eukaryotic chromosomes. Adv. Cell Biol., *1:*57, 1970.

Stern, H.: Function and reproduction of chromosomes. Physiol. Rev., *42:*271, 1962.

Taylor, J. H.: Replication and organization of chromosomes. Proc. XIIth Int. Conf. on Genetics, Tokyo. New York, Pergamon Press, 1969.

Valencia, J. I., and Grell (eds.): Genes and chromosomes structure and function. Nat. Cancer Inst., Monogr. 18, 1965.

White, M. J. D.: The Chromosomes ed. 5. London, Methuen & Co., 1961.

Wolff, S.: Strandedness of chromosomes. Int. Rev. Cytol., *25:*279, 1969.

CHROMOSOME IDENTIFICATION AND CHROMOSOME ANOMALIES

Bartalos, M., and Baramki, T. A.: Medical Cytogenetics. Baltimore, Williams and Wilkins, 1967.

Book, J. A., *et al.*: A proposed standard system of nomenclature of human mitotic chromosomes. Lancet, *1:*1063, 1959.

Burdette, W. J. (ed.): Methodology in Human Genetics. San Francisco, Holden Day, 1962.

Casperson, T., Zech, L., Johansson, C., and Modest, E.: Identification of human chromosomes by DNA-binding fluorescent agents. Chromosoma, *30:*215, 1970.

Eggen, R. R.: Chromosome Diagnostics in Clinical Medicine. Springfield, Illinois, Charles C Thomas, 1965.

Friedmann, T.: Prenatal diagnosis of genetic disease. Sci. Am., *225:*34, 1971.

Golomb, H. M., and Bahr, G. F.: Analysis of an isolated metaphase plate by quantitative electron microscopy. Exp. Cell Res., *68:*65, 1971.

Lampert, F.: Chromosome alterations in human carcinogenesis. Adv. Cell Molec. Biol., *1:*185, 1971.

Lewis, K. R., and John, B.: Chromosome Marker. London, J. & A. Churchill, 1963.

———: The chromosomal basis of sex determination. Int. Rev. Cytol., *23:*277, 1968.

Kihlman, B. A.: Molecular mechanisms of chromosome breakage and rejoining. Adv. Cell Molec. Biol., *1:*59, 1971.

McKusick, V.: The mapping of human chromosomes. Sci. Am., *224:*104, April, 1971.

Mendelsohn, M., Hungerford, D., Mayall, B., Perry, B., Conway, T., and Prewitt, J.: Computer oriented analysis of human chromosomes. Ann. N.Y. Acad. Sci., *157:*376, 1969.

Nowell, P. C., and Hungerford, D. A.: A minute chromosome in human chronic granulocytic leukemia. Science, *132:*1197, 1960.

Rudkin, G. T.: Photometric measurements of individual metaphase chromosomes. *In* Yerganian, G. (ed.): The Chromosome: Structural and Functional Aspects. p. 12. Baltimore. Williams & Wilkins, 1967.

Sasaki, M., and Makino, S.: The meiotic chromosomes of man. Chromosoma, *16:*637, 1965.

Seabright, M.: The use of proteolytic enzymes for the mapping of structural rearrangements in the chromosomes of man. Chromosoma, *36:*204, 1972.

Sumner, A. T., Evans, H. J., and Buckland, R. A.: A new technique for distinguishing between human chromosomes. Nature, New Biology, *323:*31, 1971.

Thompson, J. S., and Thompson, M. W.: Genetics in Medicine. ed. 2. Philadelphia. W. B. Saunders, 1973.

Wang, H. C., and Federoff, S.: Banding in human chromosomes treated with trypsin. Nature (New Biol.), *235:*52, 1972.

Yunis, J. J.: Human chromosome methodology. New York, Academic Press, 1965.

For references about Barr bodies *see* Chapter 4.

POLYPLOIDY AND ANEUPLOIDY

Beams, H. W., and King, R. L.: The origin of binucleate and large mononucleate cells in the liver of the rat. Anat. Rec., *82:*281, 1942.

Herman, C. J., and Lapham, L. W.: Neuronal polyploidy and nuclear volumes in the cat central nervous system. Brain Res., *15:*35, 1969.

Thompson, R. Y., and Frazer, S. C.: The desoxyribonucleic acid content of individual rat cell nuclei. Exp. Cell Res., *7:*367, 1954.

Wilson, J. W., and Leduc, E. H.: The occurrence and formation of binucleate and multinucleate cells and polyploid nuclei in the mouse liver. Am. J. Anat., *82:*353, 1948.

EFFECTS OF RADIATION ON CHROMOSOMES AND CELLS

Bender, M. A., and Wolff, S.: X-ray induced chromosome aberration and reproductive death in mammalian cells. Am. Naturalist, *95:*39, 1961.

Cellular Radiation Biology. A collection of papers presented at the 18th Annual Symposium on Fundamental Cancer Research, 1964, U. of Texas, M. D. Anderson Hospital and Tumor Institute. Baltimore, Williams & Wilkins, 1965.

Elkind, M. M., and Whitmore, G. F.: The Radiobiology of Cultured Mammalian Cells. New York, Gordon and Breach, 1967.

Evans, H. J.: Chromosome aberrations induced by ionizing radiations. Int. Rev. Cytol., *13:*221, 1962.

Wolff, S.: Chromosome aberrations. *In* Hollaender, A. (ed.): Radiation Protection and Recovery. pp. 157-174, New York, Pergamon Press, 1960.

3 The Nucleus (Cont'd)

The Steps in Cell Division That Precede Mitosis

In the previous chapter the process of mitosis was described as beginning when threadlike chromosomes can be detected in a nucleus. But when chromosomes appear as such in the prophase, the process of cell division has already been underway, for the genes of the chromosomes have already been duplicated and each chromosome has developed two chromatids, each of which has a full complement of genes. Strictly speaking, the term cell division is therefore not a synonym for mitosis, for it is a lengthier process and includes the preliminary steps mentioned above.

This chapter will deal with these steps in cell division that precede mitosis and in which the genes of the interphase cell are duplicated. Since genes have their basis in DNA (deoxyribonucleic acid) we shall in this chapter have to deal first, to some extent, with (1) the chemistry of nucleic acids so that the way DNA is doubled can be understood. Following this we will show (2) how the doubling of the DNA can be followed by

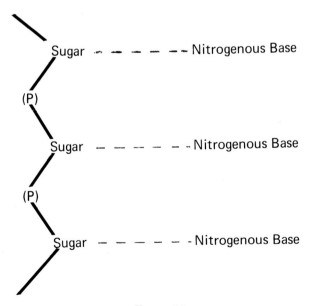

the histological technic of radioautography (which will be described) and (3) how the technic enables newly synthesized DNA to be traced into daughter cells and their progeny.

Nucleic Acids

Their Discovery and the Early Development of Knowledge. Freidrich Miescher (1844–1895) became interested in investigating the chemical composition of cell nuclei. He knew that the pus that exuded from suppurating wounds contained large numbers of white blood cells (which migrate from the bloodstream to sites of infection, as will be described in Chapter 10) and that these blood cells contained nuclei. In his first studies he used white blood cells obtained from the bandages removed from suppurating wounds of hospital patients. He treated the cells with gastric juice which we now know contains the enzyme pepsin, which digests the protein components of cells. The nuclear material that was left was then submitted to analysis. Later he used a better source of material, salmon sperm, and in due course established that there was a component in the nucleus that was a phosphorus-containing poly-acid of high molecular weight. Hence, this substance was not, like other cellular materials discovered to date, a protein, but a new type of biological substance to which he gave the name, nuclein. Shortly afterward it came to be called *nucleic acid*.

Intensive work continued on nucleic acids in the 20th century and it became established that a nucleic acid exists in the form of an enormously long unbranched macromolecule; indeed, nucleic acids were found to be the largest naturally occurring polymers that are known. The long macromolecule (then believed to consist of a single strand) was shown to be made up of alternating units of a sugar and phosphoric acid with side chains consisting of nitrogenous bases attached to the sugars (Fig. 3-1).

Two Kinds of Nucleic Acid. In due course it was shown that there are two kinds of nucleic acid—deoxyribonucleic acid (DNA) and ribonucleic acid (RNA). The two differ with regard to the kind of

FIGURE 3-1

sugar their molecules contain: DNA contains 2-deoxy-D-ribose and RNA, D-ribose. The two nucleic acids differ also in another respect. The nitrogenous bases in DNA are adenine, guanine, thymine and cytosine. In RNA, three (adenine, guanine and cytosine) are the same as in DNA but uracil is present instead of thymine, which fact becomes important, as we shall see, in connection with studying the nucleic acids by means of radioautography.

Identification of Nucleic Acids in Sections

Since both DNA and RNA are acids, they combine avidly with basic stains; hence, the sites where they exist in cells are indicated in an H and E section by deep blue to purple staining (Fig. 1-14, upper left). With other basic stains such as methylene blue, they both take on the color of the stain.

The Feulgen Reaction for DNA. It became of importance to be able, in sections, to distinguish the two nucleic acids from each other and from other possible cellular components that might absorb basic stains. In 1924, a specific test for DNA was devised by Feulgen and Rossenbeck; this is now commonly termed the *Feulgen reaction*. Sections of properly fixed material are subjected to a strong acid to break the bond between the nitrogenous base purine and deoxyribose in any DNA that is present; this releases the aldehyde group of the 2-deoxy-D-ribose and the released aldehyde is then detected by means of the Schiff reaction (described in connection with the PA-Schiff technic in Chapter 1) by which the sites in which DNA is present in a section are colored magenta. Mitotic chromosomes are thus demonstrated by the Feulgen reaction (see Fig. 2-13).

Identification of RNA. In an H and E section both the condensed chromatin and the nucleolus of interphase nuclei are colored purple, and varying amounts of blue material are also seen in the cytoplasm of many kinds of cells.

If sections of the same material are stained by the Feulgen reaction, magenta staining is seen only in the condensed chromatin of the nucleus. The reason for this is that in an H and E section, the purple color of the nucleolus and of the little masses of material in the cytoplasm is due to their content of RNA which, of course, stains as avidly with hematoxylin as DNA. Thus by comparing similar sections stained with a basic stain and with the Feulgen technic, the main sites of RNA in a cell are roughly indicated. Sites of DNA and RNA are more positively identified by using the specific enzymes for digesting DNA and RNA that have become available. These are termed DNA-ase

and RNA-ase. These can be used on sections to remove DNA (Fig. 2-5) or RNA (Fig. 4-7); so that comparison of sections stained with basic stains with or without previous treatment with one or the other of these enzymes shows the sites occupied by DNA and RNA.

Measuring the DNA Content of Cells. This can be done by making a biochemical analysis of known numbers of cells of various kinds from an animal. It was thus shown that the DNA content of all that animal's diploid nuclei is the same. The DNA content of the diploid cells of animals of different species is, of course, different, just as their chromosome numbers are different. Subsequently, a way of measuring the DNA content of individual cells in sections stained by the Feulgen reaction was devised; this depends on how much light is absorbed from the magenta band as it passes through the individual nuclei in a section. This method (called cytophotometry) also shows that diploid nuclei in the cells of a given individual all have the same DNA content. Furthermore, aneuploidy can be detected in individual cells in a section by this method—as, for example, would occur if certain cells in a section were cancer cells.

Relation of DNA to Genes

The Discovery of Transformation. For purposes of perspective it is important to realize that a vast amount of knowledge had accumulated about genes and their effects before their dependence on DNA, or the way they exerted their effects, could be visualized. It was known that genes must reside in chromosomes and as it became increasingly obvious that DNA was localized in chromosomes, the suspicion was, of course, aroused that DNA must have something to do with genes. Two strains of a pneumonia-causing kind of bacteria (pneumococcus) played an important role in showing that DNA was indeed the hereditary material of cells. Briefly, the story began with an early (1928) experiment, in which two strains of pneumococci were used, one type being lethal for mice and the other not lethal. An important difference between the two strains was that those of the first formed a sugar-containing capsule around themselves while those of the second strain lacked the capsule; this difference accounted for the first strain being lethal and the other not, because the capsule protected the bacteria of the lethal strain from the defenses of their hosts so they continued to multiply in them and killed their hosts. Members of the noncapsulated strain were destroyed by their hosts. It was shown, however, that a mixture of bacteria of the nonlethal strain and *heat-killed members* of the lethal strain would also kill mice and when cultures were made from the dead mice, the bacteria recovered were found to be of the lethal type in that they possessed capsules. Somehow something from the dead heat-killed bacteria of the lethal type had changed some nonlethal living bacteria into the lethal variety in the injected mice. At first the results of this experiment did not attract much attention, but later it was repeated by others and it was concluded that some active substance must pass from one type of bacteria to the other to *transform* the second type so that it had certain characteristics of the first type and, furthermore, that these characteristics would be passed on to future generations. The substance that could transform the bacteria of one type into another was sought by chemical methods and finally it was shown to be DNA. Since the bacteria that were transformed by the DNA extracted from those of the lethal strain passed on their new characteristics to subsequent generations, it was apparent that the *DNA in this instance acted as a gene.* From this beginning many further experiments were performed which showed eventually that *genes have their chemical basis in DNA.*

After this was established it was inevitable that certain questions would be asked, and that answers would be sought to these questions. To serve more or less as a guide for the subsequent discussion, we shall list 3 questions that could be asked.

1. How could genetic information be stored in DNA?

2. How could a huge macromolecule of DNA in a chromosome be duplicated in such a way so that when a chromosome splits into two chromatids that separate from each other, they would have precisely the same genetic information?

3. How could information stored in DNA be transmitted in the interphase to the various parts of the cell where the enzymes that determine the functions of the cell are located, and by what means would the transmitted information be implemented?

We shall deal with the first two questions in this chapter and with the third in the next chapter.

How Information Is Stored in DNA

To help understand how information is stored in the DNA molecule, it is helpful to consider briefly how information is contained by words. Words are composed of letters. Words give different information not only because they are composed of different letters but also because the same letters can be used in words in *different sequences.* When we consider the DNA molecule, we shall find that it has an alphabet of only 4 chemical "letters" with which "words" that convey

different information are written and arranged into long sentences. We shall find, moreover, that this 4-letter alphabet is used to write only 3-letter words. Now we know that with 4 letters, for example, a, e, p and r, it is possible to write several different 3-letter words that convey different information, for example, ear, par, are, pea, per, ape and pep. If it were not for the fact that words have to be pronounced, which requires that attention be paid to the placement of vowels and consonants, there would be 64 possible 3-letter code words that could be written with a 4-letter alphabet, and, of course, each 3-letter word could code for a different meaning. As will be explained later, no more than 20 code words need be spelled out by the chemical letters of the DNA molecule, because the only way genes can act is by prescribing the amino acids that are to be assembled into proteins so all that is needed is that there be a different code word for each of the 20 amino acids.

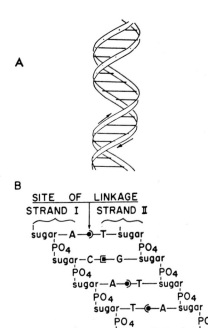

Fig. 3-2. (A) Diagram of a portion of a double-stranded DNA molecule according to the model prepared by Watson and Crick. (B) Portion of a double-stranded DNA molecule showing how deoxyribonucleotides of one strand are joined to those of the other strand through their bases; by adenine being joined to thymine or cytosine being joined to guanine.

The 4 chemical letters in the 4-letter alphabet of the DNA molecule are 4 nitrogenous bases, *adenine, cytosine, guanine* and *thymine*. These will be represented in the illustrations by using A for adenine, C for cytosine, G for guanine and T for thymine. In order to explain how these 4 bases are arranged in DNA molecules to code information, how the words are read and how DNA molecules can be duplicated as a prelude to mitosis, we must comment on the DNA molecule in more detail.

Due to the brilliant research of Watson and Crick, it is now known that the DNA molecules of mammalian chromosomes each consist of two long thin strands that are wound together in the form of a double helix (Fig. 3-2, A). Each strand has a backbone consisting of alternating phosphoric acid and sugar units. A side chain which is one of the four nitrogenous bases already mentioned extends inward into the helix from each sugar along each backbone of the double helix to meet and attach to one of the nitrogenous bases connected to the other backbone (Fig. 3-2, B). The segment of the DNA molecule consisting of one sugar and one phosphoric acid unit plus one nitrogenous base is termed a deoxyribonucleotide residue; in the free form it is a deoxyribonucleotide. There may be as many as 40 million deoxyribonucleotide residues strung along one strand of a single DNA molecule.

WHEN DO DNA MOLECULES IMPART INFORMATION?

DNA molecules impart information under two sets of circumstances. First, when the DNA of a cell is duplicated as a preliminary to mitosis, the molecule must somehow impart information to the agencies that are responsible for synthesizing whatever is required to provide for the pre-existing molecule being duplicated. Second, in the interphase, DNA molecules must impart information to the agencies that control the synthesis of proteins in the cell so that the normal protein constitution of the cell is maintained for its life and function. We shall now comment on how DNA molecules store information and impart it so new molecules with the same information are produced.

Information Storage in DNA Molecules

As already noted, information is stored in DNA molecules in the form of an enormously long string of 3-letter words composed from a 4-letter alphabet (A, C, G, T).

If we seek information that is stored in the words in a book, we have to open the book to see the words printed on its pages. Likewise for the 3-letter words

written along the course of a DNA molecule by various combinations of its 4 nitrogenous bases (A, C, G and T), the molecule, like a book, has to be opened. As long as the nitrogenous bases on each strand of the two-stranded molecule are bonded to one another, the pages of the book, as it were, are closed. This does not mean that for a DNA molecule to impart information its two strands have to come apart along its whole length at the same time, any more than a book, to impart information, has to be opened at all its pages simultaneously. A book is read one page at a time. However, there are enough chemical "eyes" available to read simultaneously different parts of the DNA molecule that are open at one time, which speeds up the reading process.

With this introduction we can now describe how the molecule imparts information required for it to be duplicated as a preliminary to cell division. In this connection it is very important to appreciate that the nitrogenous bases of the two strands are not bonded together in a haphazard way but instead in a very special way termed complementary base pairing which means that *adenine bonds only with thymine* and *cytosine bonds only with guanine,* these bases being complementary to each other. Accordingly, as shown in Figure 3-2, B, whenever there is an A along one strand, there is a T on the other strand and whenever there is a C on one strand, there is a G on the other strand. Furthermore, as the two strands begin to come apart in the first step in the duplication of the two-stranded molecule (Fig. 3-3 shows them apart) each strand has a new strand build beside it. The information that is given off by an exposed A on the old strand leads to the addition of a newly formed deoxyribonucleotide molecule with a T on the new strand; as shown in Figure 3-4 this T then becomes bonded to the A of the original strand (complementary base pairing). Likewise an exposed T of the original strand leads to the addition of a new deoxyribonucleotide molecule with an A on the newly forming strand. This same phenomenon occurs in connection with the C's and G's that become exposed as the process continues at different sites along the length of the original molecule, so that two new double-stranded molecules are formed, with half of each being new and half of each being one half of the original molecule (see Fig. 3-4).

From the above it follows that in the duplication of a DNA molecule neither of the two new strands that are synthesized is an identical copy of the strand beside which it is synthesized. Instead each is *complementary* to the strand beside which it is formed (complementary means something required to complete a whole, which in this case is a double-stranded

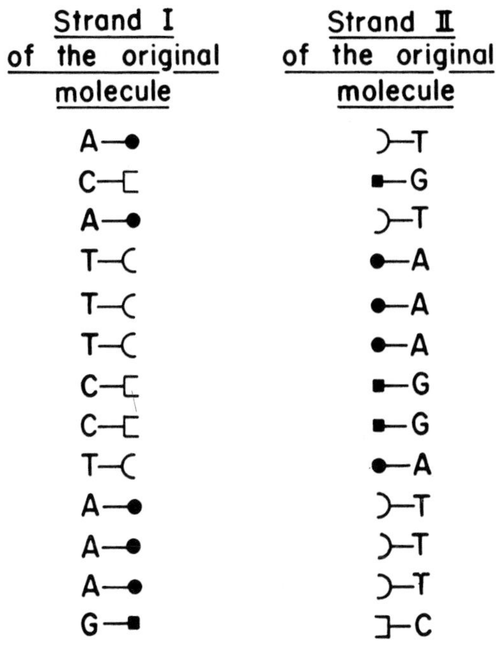

Strand I of the original molecule	Strand II of the original molecule
A—●	)—T
C—⊏	■—G
A—●	)—T
T—⊂	●—A
T—⊂	●—A
T—⊂	●—A
C—⊏	■—G
C—⊏	■—G
T—⊂	●—A
A—●	)—T
A—●	)—T
A—●	)—T
G—■	⊐—C

FIG. 3-3. The first step in the duplication of a DNA molecule is the separation of its two strands.

DNA molecule). Since the two strands of the original double-stranded molecule were not identical (Fig. 3-3) but were complementary (because wherever there was, for example, an A on one, there was a T on the other), the two strands of each of the two daughter molecules are likewise complementary (Fig. 3-4).

Hence the two new double-stranded molecules are identical to one another and to the mother molecule from which one strand of each was derived. (Compare Figs. 3-3 and 3-4.)

We shall next describe how the duplication of DNA can be studied by means of radioautography. To do this we must first describe the technic which in addition to having application here, has a vast number of other applications as will become apparent in subsequent chapters.

Radioautography

INTRODUCTION

Radioautography Provides Information Impossible To Obtain by Older or Other Technics. Neither staining nor histochemical tests provide any direct information on how long it takes for the various cell or tissue components seen in sections to be synthesized, or how long they last. Hence, they give no information about the turnover time of cell and tissue components. Moreover, they give no direct information about the exact site where the synthesis of different substances occurs in cells or from what chemical building blocks they are assembled, or about the nature of their movements from one part of a cell to another or from cells to other sites. The development of the method of radioautography has permitted information to be obtained on all these points because it permits the various substances that are taken in by cells to be traced with a label that can be followed with the LM or the

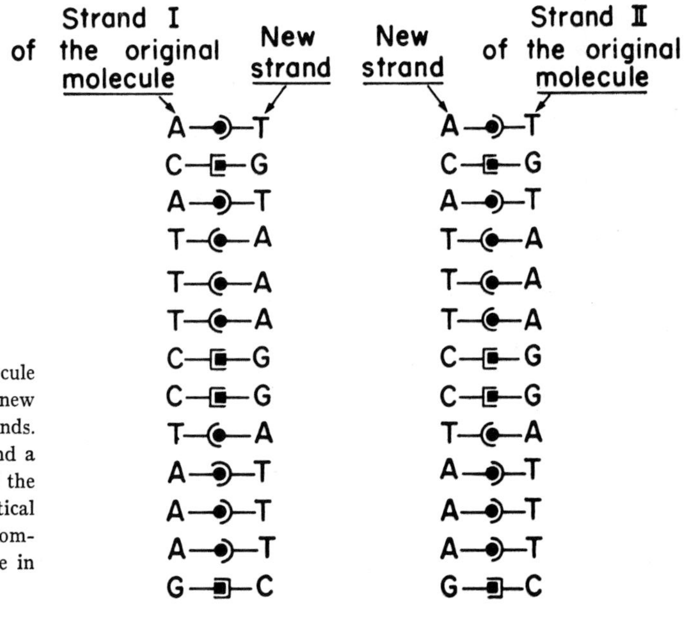

Strand I of the original molecule	New strand		New strand	Strand II of the original molecule
A—◑—T			A—◑—T	
C—◧—G			C—◧—G	
A—◑—T			A—◑—T	
T—◖—A			T—◖—A	
T—◖—A			T—◖—A	
T—◖—A			T—◖—A	
C—◧—G			C—◧—G	
C—◧—G			C—◧—G	
T—◖—A			T—◖—A	
A—◑—T			A—◑—T	
A—◑—T			A—◑—T	
A—◑—T			A—◑—T	
G—◨—C			G—◨—C	

FIG. 3-4. After the two strands of a DNA molecule have separated, as is shown in Figure 3-3, a new strand is synthesized beside each of the two strands. An A always forms beside a T, and vice versa, and a C beside a G, and vice versa. As a result, each of the double-stranded molecules that are formed is identical with the one whose strands become separated. Compare both of these with each other and with one in Figure 3-2 B.

EM in sections obtained from animal tissues at various times after the labeled substance is given. It is also practicable to add labeled material to the medium in which cells are grown in cultures and then follow the label in spreads of cultured cells with the LM.

The label used is a radioactive isotope of some element, hence the development of the method had to await the era of nuclear physics and the production by the cyclotron or atomic pile of the kind of radioactive isotopes that could be injected into animals, or added to cell cultures in a dose small enough to avoid interfering with the metabolism of the cells. At first only a few such isotopes were available—for example, radioactive phosphorus was an important one used in many early studies. Later, a large number became available, most notably tritium (^{3}H), a radioactive isotope of hydrogen. In due course it became possible to incorporate ^{3}H into many different types of chemical compounds which are utilized by cells. For example, it can be used to label the substance thymidine that is incorporated into newly forming DNA, as will be explained shortly.

Precursors and Products. The chemicals labeled with a radioactive isotope which are used to investigate biological problems are called *precursors*. Precursors are usually substances similar to those available from the foods which serve as building blocks for tissue components and they are incorporated into more complex constituents of cells and tissues in the same way that unlabeled building blocks would be incorporated. The tissue constituent into which a labeled precursor is incorporated is called a *product,* and when this event occurs, the product, of course, emits radiation. Precursors are usually soluble, the products usually are not. Hence, in fixing and sectioning tissue taken from an animal during or after a time a labeled precursor was available, such precursors as are still present are washed away because they are soluble, while the insoluble products remain. Any radioactivity detected in a section, therefore, is due to the presence of a label in a *product* that has become insoluble and is thus *locked in position* by fixation.

To detect sites of radioactive products in a section, advantage is taken of the fact that labeled products serve as point sources of radiation, and the emission of

electrons from them will affect photographic emulsion that is placed above the section. There are 2 methods for applying photographic emulsion to sections (or spreads of whole cells) for this purpose.

The Coating Technic. This method, developed by Belanger and Leblond in Leblond's Laboratory in 1946, marked the birth of modern radioautography. Coated radioautographs are prepared as follows:

Tissue from animals given some kind of labeled building block—a precursor—is fixed and sectioned. Indeed, the section may even be stained. (No substance capable of inhibiting the response of the emulsion, such as heavy metallic salts, should be present in the fixative or stain used.) The sections are then taken to the darkroom, where they are coated with photographic emulsion and dried. The coated sections are left in a lightproof box for a suitable length of time, during which each minute amount of isotope in the section of tissue acts as a point source of radiation, bringing about ionization of the silver atoms in each crystal of silver bromide in the emulsion hit by the emitted rays. The preparation is subsequently developed and fixed like an ordinary photographic negative, and a coverslip is added (Fig. 3-5). The crystals of silver bromide that have been hit appear as little dark dots, which are commonly called grains (Fig. 3-5). The sites of grains in the emulsion indicate radioactivity in sites below the grains, and, indeed, as will be described presently, by using beta emitters with short tracks, and very thin sections and thin layers of emulsion, the grains that are seen can be related to the particular cell or tissue component directly or almost directly under them.

The Stripping Film Method. This method, developed in 1947 by Pelc, employs a special kind of film which readily permits the emulsion to be stripped from its backing. This step is, of course, carried out in the darkroom, and the stripped emulsion is placed on the surface of water in a dish. A glass slide with a section mounted on it, but with no coverslip, is then slipped under the floating stripped emulsion and brought up under it, so that the layer of emulsion rests flat on the section. Subsequent steps are much the same as in the previous technic.

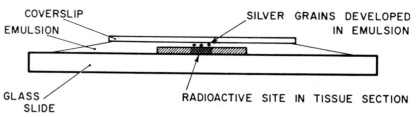

FIG. 3-5. Diagram of a radioautograph prepared by the coating technic.

Some Factors Concerned in Obtaining Precise Localization of Radioactive Emitters in Sections

Since a radioactive label in a tissue section serves as a point source of radiation, it gives off rays in all directions. If the label used is a high-energy emitter such as ^{32}P, an emitter of beta particles (i.e., electrons) endowed with high energy, the localization in the cell spread or section is not very precise, because not only do the electrons emitted at right angles to the section affect the emulsion directly above the label, but the electrons given off by the point source at other angles also reach the emulsion even though they have to travel longer distances to reach it. Hence the emulsion for considerable distances on either side of the emitter is affected, and as a consequence the site of the label cannot be localized with precision. It is therefore desirable to use low-energy beta emitters, since they give off electrons with short tracks, which ideally are only long enough to reach emulsion that is directly above the label and not long enough to reach the emulsion if they extend off at various angles from the point source. This is an important reason for ^{3}H being so commonly used for radioautography: the electrons that it emits have a low average energy (5.7 KeV), which gives them a range in water of about 1 micron. It is therefore obvious that some of the emission from tritium in the deeper part of anything except a very thin section would not reach the emulsion at all; hence, it is desirable to have the emulsion as close as possible to the tissue components in the section, and the sections used for detecting tritium should be so far as possible of a thickness that only the short tracks of the emitted particles that pass at right angles through the section will reach the emulsion. If this ideal is realized, the emitter sites will be directly under the dots seen in the developed emulsion.

The Kinds of Labeled Building Blocks Used for Labeling the Different Chemical Compounds of Tissue

Proteins. The usual precursor used to label newly forming protein is an amino acid, for example, leucine, into which ^{3}H has been incorporated. Since collagen contains much glycine and proline, these two amino acids labeled with ^{3}H are excellent precursors to use to label collagen that is being synthesized.

Carbohydrates. The synthesis of glycogen can be followed by using glucose labeled with ^{3}H. If, after injection of labeled glucose, some radioactivity is present in control radioautographs but absent from sections that are first treated with the enzyme alpha-

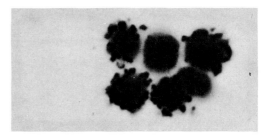

Fig. 3-6. Radioautograph of a smear preparation of some bone marrow cells obtained from an animal that had been given some radioactive iron. Iron is a component of hemoglobin, and so by using radioactive iron and radioautographs the cells that are synthesizing hemoglobin, i.e., the cells which are the precursors of red blood cells, can be identified.

amylase which breaks down glycogen, the radioactivity observed is attributed to this polysaccharide.

Radioactivity remaining in sections after alpha-amylase treatment is usually due to labeled glucose being incorporated into either mucopolysaccharides or glycoproteins, substances to be described in later chapters, and into which glucose may be incorporated as they are synthesized.

Lipids. The synthesis of lipids labeled by radioautography may be examined after injection of labeled acetate or other suitable precursors. Care must be taken to avoid dissolving out the lipids in the course of histological processing.

Inorganic Substances. The calcium phosphates that are being deposited in cartilage or bone can be labeled with radioactive isotopes of either calcium or phosphorus (see Fig. 15-31). The iron that enters into the formation of the hemoglobin of developing red blood cells can be labeled with a radioactive isotope of iron (Fig. 3-6), and this is much used in the study of blood diseases. The hormones of the thyroid gland have iodine as one of their components, and so it is possible to follow their formation by administering a radioactive isotope of iodine, as will be described in the chapter on the Endocrine System.

Nucleic Acids. The study of the synthesis of nucleic acids by means of radioactive labels and radioautography will be dealt with in the following section.

The Study of DNA Synthesis by the Use of a Radioactive Label and Radioautographs

Why Labeled Thymidine Is Used. The two new strands of DNA that are formed when a DNA molecule is duplicated must be synthesized out of simpler

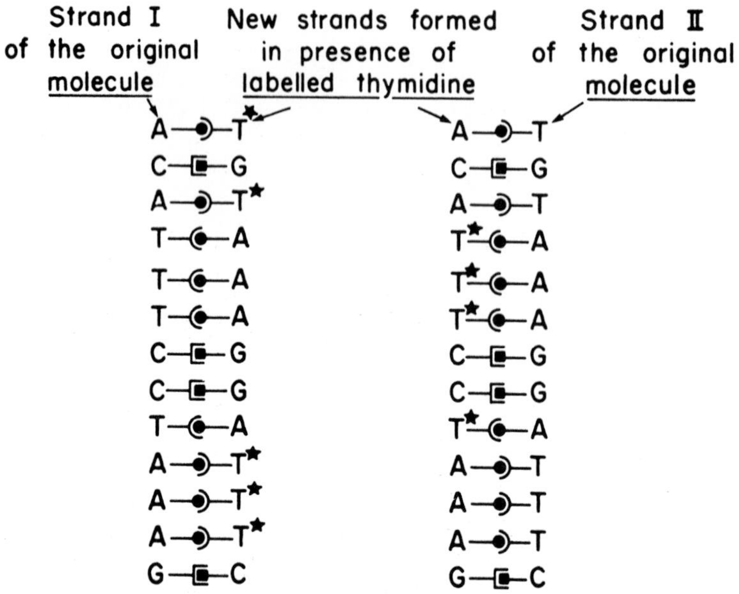

Strand I of the original molecule	New strands formed in presence of labelled thymidine	Strand II of the original molecule
A—●—T		A—●—T
C—■—G		C—■—G
A—●—T*		A—●—T
T—◖—A		T*—◖—A
T—◖—A		T*—◖—A
T—◖—A		T*—◖—A
C—■—G		C—■—G
C—■—G		C—■—G
T—◖—A		T*—◖—A
A—●—T*		A—●—T
A—●—T*		A—●—T
A—●—T*		A—●—T
G—■—C		G—■—C

FIG. 3-7. If labeled thymidine is available as the two new strands are being synthesized (the period of time that elapses between Figs. 3-3 and 3-4), such thymine as is synthesized in the two new strands will be labeled. This is indicated by an asterisk.

ingredients. Obviously, if one of these ingredients could be labeled with a radioactive isotope, the synthesis of new DNA could be studied by the radioautographic method. In choosing a precursor of DNA for labeling purposes, the important consideration is finding a precursor that is not incorporated into any other product synthesized by cells, for if a specific precursor were available, all the labeling seen in cells after such a labeled precursor was used would be in DNA. It so happens that the only product in which thymine is found in the body is DNA, and so thymine would seem to be an ideal product to label for study of DNA synthesis. However, pure thymine is not incorporated into newly forming DNA molecules. Thymine is incorporated into newly forming DNA molecules only when it is attached to sugar, and sugar does not become attached to thymine that is given an animal; sugar must be attached to thymine as thymine is being synthesized by an animal. But if thymine that is already attached to sugar (and this is called thymidine) is labeled and given an animal, the thymidine will be incorporated into such new DNA as is being synthesized, just as thymine that was being synthesized and attached to sugar in the cell would be incorporated into newly forming DNA. So thymidine labeled with tritium is universally used to label specifically the new DNA that is synthesized.

Since both of the original strands of a DNA molecule serve as a template against which a new strand is synthesized (Figs. 3-3 and 3-4), each one of the two double-stranded molecules of DNA that result when DNA synthesis is completed has one old strand and one new strand, as is shown in Figure 3-4. If labeled thymidine is available during the period of DNA synthesis, the thymine that appears in each of the new strands is labeled; this is shown in Figure 3-7 by putting a star beside the T that represents thymine that carries a label. The pre-existing thymine on the old strands would of course *not* be labeled.

An important point to appreciate from the foregoing is that when labeled thymidine is sufficiently abundant, every new two-stranded molecule of DNA that forms when it is available would carry a label. But the label would be present only in the *new strand* of each DNA molecule and not in the strand that was part of the previous DNA molecule. Hence, when a cell enters the process of mitosis, after having doubled its DNA content under conditions in which label is available, *all* the chromosomes of both daughter cells will carry a label, because every molecule of the DNA of which they are composed would carry some label in *one of its two* strands (the recently formed strand that was synthesized in the presence of label). And even though labeled thymidine is incorporated only into newly forming strands of DNA molecules, it labels DNA very satisfactorily for radioautographic studies of DNA synthesis, as is shown in Figure 3-8. Figure 3-8 is a photomicrograph showing the way "silver grains" appear over chromosomes in a radioautograph of a mitotic cell in which DNA synthesis took place in the preceding interphase in the presence of labeled thymidine.

Various Ways in Which Labeling Nuclei With Radioactive Thymidine Has Furthered Knowledge

In Connection With Determining Mitotic Activity. Although the use of colchicine, as described in the previous chapter, often helped, the common way that the extent of cell division occurring in any tissue during its growth, repair or maintenance was estimated before labeled thymidine became available, was by taking sections at different times and trying to count the numbers of mitotic figures present in them. However, as noted, mitotic figures are sometimes difficult to identify, particularly when they are cut in planes other than the long axis of cells that are dividing.

In experimental work it is much easier to obtain a more accurate estimate of the extent to which cell division is occurring in any given tissue by giving the animal a dose of labeled thymidine. This is allowed to act for only a very brief period, after which the tissue that is to be examined is removed and fixed. Radioautographs are then prepared from the tissue that was removed.

Since it takes about 7 hours for a cell to double its DNA, it can be reasoned that, in the radioautographs taken from a tissue which was subjected to labeled thymidine for say an hour, there would be three general categories of cells that would be labeled:

1. Cells that were in the phase of DNA duplication during the *whole* hour.

2. Cells that entered the phase of DNA duplication during the hour and so were exposed to the labeled thymidine for only the latter part of the hour.

3. Cells that were in the last stages of DNA duplication and finished it during the hour so they would take up labeled thymidine for only the first part of the hour.

The period during which the cells are subjected to the labeled thymidine in this type of experiment must be very short (e.g., 1 hour), so that there should not be time for any labeled cells to have passed through mitosis, for, if any labeled cells had time to divide, there would be two labeled cells that could be counted instead of one. If the time is short, every cell that is labeled in the radioautograph marks a cell that is *destined* to undergo mitosis in the next few hours. This gives the same *kind* of information obtained by counting mitotic figures because it provides an index of the extent to which cell division is occurring in a tissue; but, quantitatively, the counts would not be the same, because mitosis takes longer than an hour. (If one observer counted how many automobiles—all

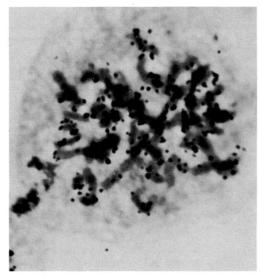

Fig. 3-8. Radioautograph of an air-dried preparation of an L cell from a culture that was given a 16-hour exposure to tritium-labeled thymidine. The labeled thymidine was taken up as the DNA was being duplicated, and enough time elapsed for the cell to enter mitosis; this cell was obtained when it was in the metaphase. The dark grains that are seen over the chromosomes are due to the short tracks of beta particles from the tritium causing ionization in the overlying photographic emulsion. (Stanners, C. P., and Till, J. E.: DNA synthesis in individual L-strain mouse cells. Biochim. Biophys. Acta, *37*:406)

traveling at the same speed—were present on a two-mile stretch of road, he would not get the same figure as another observer who counted those present on a four-mile stretch over the same period.)

Establishing the Kinds of Cells That Are Responsible for Providing New Cells in Growth, Repair, and Maintenance of Cell Populations. It is not as easy as might be thought to determine, in areas where there is a mixture of cell types, which particular kind of cell is the one that responds to the need for more cells by undergoing cell division. It might be thought that the type of cell that responds could be ascertained by examining the cells that are seen to be in mitosis. But once a cell is actually in the process of mitosis the usual characteristics by which it is recognized in the interphase as being of a particular type may mostly disappear and, as a consequence, different kinds of cells, when they are in the process of mitosis, may look very much alike.

Since, as has been described in the preceding section, thymidine labels cells in the interphase *before* they actually enter the process of mitosis, a labeled cell retains most of its usual interphase appearance until it enters mitosis and this makes it possible to ascertain the type of cell that provides the new cells that appear in the repair process.

Using Labeled Thymidine To Trace Cell Lineages. One of the most difficult problems that has beset those who have studied cells in the human body has been encountered in trying to establish which kind of cell gives rise, in growth, maintenance and repair, to the new cells that appear. For example, the development of knowledge about the origin of the various cells of the blood, or of the cells that repair a fracture in a bone, or of the cells that variously participate in the immunological reactions of the body, has been associated with a great amount of controversy which is still not all dispelled. Modern technics have helped a great deal by making it possible in some instances to label a stem cell in some way so that its progeny will all carry the label. If this is done, it becomes possible to trace the label from a stem cell into the various types of cells into which its progeny develop as they become increasingly specialized. One way of achieving this aim is by labeling stem cells with radioactive thymidine and then tracing the label into their progeny by means of radioautography. We shall first give an example of how a cell lineage can be traced by this method and then afterward describe how the method suffers from some limitations.

A very simple example which illustrates that thymidine can be used both (1) to show the kinds of cells that have proliferative capacity and (2) to trace cell lineages is provided by its use in studying how new bone is added to pre-existing bone. As will be explained in detail in the chapter on Bone, there is a layer of cells on the surface of a growing bone that consists of more or less elongated flattened cells mixed with larger and more rounded cells. Then below the surface of the bone there are bone cells buried in intercellular substance. During growth, mitotic figures can be seen in the surface cells but, as already noted, when a cell enters mitosis it becomes difficult to be sure what kind of cell it is; in this case it was sometimes assumed that it was the elongated cells that divided but it was also sometimes assumed that the larger more rounded cells on the surface also divided. However, after animals were given a brief exposure to labeled thymidine, sections taken from the bone immediately afterward showed that label was present in the flattened cells and not in the rounded cells; this then is an example of how thymidine can be used to identify the kind of cells that undergo mitosis in any given situation.

If, from a bone of an animal treated similarly, sections are taken a day or so after treatment, the label is found in the rounded cells on the surface. Since label was not available over this period of time, the only label that will be seen must be that which was taken up by the elongated cells when label was available; therefore, the elongated cells after a day or so have turned into the larger rounded type of cell. Next, if sections are cut from animals similarly treated a week or so afterward, the label will be seen in the bone cells that are buried in intercellular substance just below the surface. Again, this shows that the larger rounded surface cells have, during this time, produced intercellular substance with which they surrounded themselves to become the bone cells of the new layer of bone that was thus formed on its old surface.

From the above type of experiment it can be concluded that the more flattened surface cells are the cells with proliferative capacity and that they can turn into the larger rounded surface cells which produce intercellular substance and become buried in it to become still more mature cells which are called bone cells; this shows how thymidine can be used to trace a cell lineage.

How Label in Cells Becomes Diluted on Continuous Cell Division

While generally most useful, the method of tracing cell lineages by labeling cells with thymidine suffers from one restriction. If the daughter cells of the labeled stem cell are in turn capable of proliferating and continue to divide, the label becomes diluted. Because of this and for other reasons too, it is very important to understand how and why thymidine label does not *all* go to one of the two daughter cells at each subsequent division but is always divided between the two with consequent dilution.

All the DNA molecules that result from the duplication of DNA in the presence of labeled thymidine will be labeled, but only in one of their strands, as is shown in Figure 3-7. It was shown by Taylor and his associates that if a labeled daughter cell subsequently divided in the absence of label, only one of the two chromatids of each chromosome seen at the metaphase will carry label. To explain this phenomenon, it is helpful to study Figure 3-9. The molecule at the top has one strand (indicated by a broken line) that was synthesized in the presence of label, so it is the newer strand of that molecule. The unlabeled strand (indicated by a continuous line) is the older. Then, as a prelude to another mitosis, if the duplication of this two-stranded molecule occurs *in the absence of label,* as is illustrated in the middle diagrams, each strand of the former molecule gains a new unlabeled strand beside it. Both of these *new strands* are unlabeled and are of the same age, being the youngest of all 4. Each of the two DNA molecules now has a new strand and an older strand, but the older strand in the molecule on the right is older than the older (labeled) strand in the molecule on the left because it served originally as the template for the labeled strand. So, the complete molecule on the left can be considered to be as a whole younger than the one on the right. When the chromosomes in which this type of duplication of DNA has occurred divide into chromatids, in preparation for the next mitosis, it seems that the "younger" DNA molecules all go to what might be termed the daughter chromatids, and the "older" molecules all stay in the mother chromatids. As a result of this, all the labeled DNA molecules (the younger ones) end up in the daughter chromatids.

It might be thought from the previous discussion, that the "daughter" chromatids with the newer DNA molecules would, in turn, all go to the same daughter cell and that as a result one daughter cell from that division would contain all the label and that after division all of the label would always be in one daughter cell. But this is not what happens, for at the metaphase, when the chromosomes that have one labeled chromatid and one unlabeled chromatid line up in the region of the equatorial plane, the direction they face is a matter of chance. Accordingly, the labeled chromatid of one chromosome may face one pole of the cell and the labeled chromatid of another chromosome, the other pole of the cell. Hence when the centromeres of the chromosomes separate, half of the labeled chromatids (on the average) are moved toward one pole and become the chromosomes of that daughter cell, and half are moved toward the other pole and become the chromosomes of the other daughter cell. Accordingly, the label in each daughter cell is diluted on the average by 50 percent with each cell division. The same thing happens on subsequent divisions of daughter cells; the label becomes diluted again with each subsequent division of daughter cells by 50 percent, and soon there is so little label left in dividing cells that it can no longer be detected.

INVESTIGATING THE CELL CYCLE

Labeled thymidine has been useful in establishing the times taken by cells to pass through the different stages of the cell cycle.

The term cell cycle came into use primarily from studying cells that continue to divide regularly, such

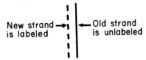

When DNA duplication occurs in the presence of label, the new strand of every DNA molecule of every chromosome is labeled as in the molecule illustrated below

New strand is labeled → ← Old strand is unlabeled

If next duplication of DNA occurs in the absence of label, both the old strand and the new strand act as templates for still newer strands, neither of which is labeled

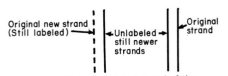

Original new strand (Still labeled) → ← Unlabeled still newer strands → Original strand

Since the original strand of the molecule on the right is older than the labeled strand of the molecule on the left, and since the two new strands are of the same age, the double-stranded molecule on the right is on the whole the older molecule

After DNA duplication is complete, each chromosome separates into two chromatids One of these can be thought of as the mother chromatid and the other as the daughter chromatid. The older DNA molecules all stay in mother chromatids, and the newer molecules all go to the daughter chromatids as shown below.

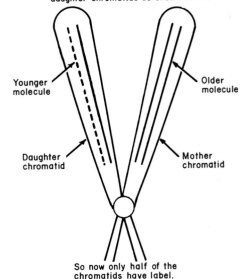

Younger molecule

Older molecule

Daughter chromatid

Mother chromatid

So now only half of the chromatids have label.

FIG. 3-9. Diagrams showing newer DNA molecules going to daughter chromatids.

as those that are growing in the type of cell cultures in which they continue to pass consecutively through interphase, mitosis, interphase, mitosis and so on without any of them becoming specialized for functioning which would require that they cease dividing in a

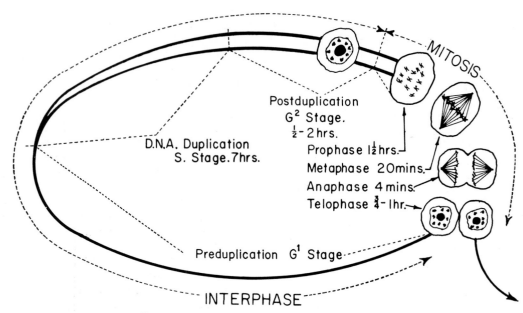

FIG. 3-10. Diagram illustrating stages of cell cycle.

regular cycle. In cell cultures in which cells of the same type do nothing but continuously multiply, one complete passage through the interphase and mitosis is termed a *cell cycle*. The time taken for a cell to complete a full cell cycle is termed its *generation time* (see Fig. 3-10).

As is shown in Figure 3-10, there are 3 stages through which a cell passes as it proceeds through the interphase. After finishing mitosis the cell enters what is termed the G_1 (Gap 1) stage. Where cells of the type we have described are being cultivated in cultures, the length of time the cells remain in this stage can be ascertained fairly readily and is fairly constant for a given type of cell.

After this time has elapsed, a cell enters the DNA duplication stage, also called the S (S = synthesis) stage. It takes about 7 hours for all of the DNA of a cell to be duplicated; this is ascertained by using labeled thymidine, as will be described below.

After finishing the S phase the cell enters the G_2 (Gap 2) phase, which occupies a relatively brief interval before it begins mitosis.

TIMES TAKEN FOR THE STAGES OF THE CELL CYCLE AND HOW THEY ARE DETERMINED

The common way this is done in cell cultures in which different cells of the same kind are in different phases of the cell cycle is to add some labeled thymidine to a culture for a very brief period, after which the culture medium is changed. Thereafter, samples of cells are taken from the culture at regular intervals and examined by making radioautographs of them.

Radioautographs made from cells taken immediately after the momentary exposure to labeled thymidine show label in only some interphase nuclei. Hence at the time of exposure to labeled thymidine only a percentage of the cells in a culture are in the S stage; the unlabeled interphase cells in the sample could have been in a stage either preceding the S phase (the G_1 stage) or following it (the G_2 stage).

Determination of Time Taken For the G_2 Phase. Those cells that take up label on the momentary exposure will range all the way from those that are just beginning the S phase to those that have almost completed it. So, if samples are taken regularly from the culture, a time will come when label will be seen over the chromosomes of a few cells that have entered the prophase of mitosis. Since the cells in which label is *first seen* over prophase chromosomes would be cells that were labeled just as they were finishing the duplication of their DNA, the interval between the time when label was made available and the time when label is *first seen* over prophase chromosomes is the duration of the G_2 stage.

How Time Taken For the S Phase Is Determined. First, the time is noted when 50 percent of metaphase mitotic figures in samples are found to be labeled. After this the percentage increases until 100 percent of metaphase mitotic figures show label. Further samples are taken until the time when the percentage of labeled metaphase mitotic figures has fallen to 50 percent. The time that elapses between the time when 50 percent first become labeled and when 50 percent are last seen to be labeled is the time for the DNA duplication stage of the interphase (averages are used).

Determination of Time Taken For the G_1 Phase. The figure obtained by adding the time taken for the process of mitosis, the time taken for the G_2 stage and the time taken for DNA duplication, is subtracted from the time taken for a complete cell cycle (the generation time); this gives the time for the G_1 stage. The time taken for the G_1 stage, though the same for cells of a given cell line in cultures, varies with different cell lines; it is not nearly as constant as the times taken for mitosis or the other stages of the interphase. In man, cells may stay in this phase as long as they live, as is explained below.

The Cell Cycle Concept in Relation to Body Cells. Although the cell cycle concept is important in general cell biology, it should not be assumed that all body cells can pass through cell cycles or that any of them do so steadily at a constant rate. As was described in Chapter 2, there are three general categories of body cells. Those of category 1 and many of those of category 2 are unable to divide and hence they cannot pass through cell cycles. The reason for the problem being so different in the body cells of man from that of cells in cultures is that body cells must become specialized to perform their various functions and specialization for function is, in general, antagonistic to continuing proliferation. It is possible for

there to be stem cells in the body which are responsible for maintaining the population of certain cell families and in order to maintain their numbers these stem cells must of course pass through cell cycles; the stem cell that probably undergoes the most constant constant cycle is the stem cell responsible for maintaining the cellular lining of the intestine. But in order to maintain a cell family in which the most differentiated members have only a short life span, stem cells from the pool that is being maintained by cell cycles must leave the pool and become specialized to take the place of those specialized cells of the family which wear out or are otherwise lost. Once a stem cell begins to differentiate, it ceases to be in cycle. The point at which it leaves the cycle is in the G_1 phase and hence most body cells that are specialized for function are said to be in the G_1 phase but since most of them have left the cycle and will never enter the S phase again, it is sometimes said they are in the G_0 phase. This is of course different from what happens in the type of cell culture in which all the cells continually proliferate because in this type of cell culture cells never leave the cycle so as to become specialized for function.

The study of the cell cycle in cultures has provided valuable information in demonstrating the duration of the S phase and indicating that once a cell enters the S phase it is irrevocably committed to passing through the G_2 phase and mitosis. How long a cell will remain in the G_1 or G_0 phase in the human body depends on its type and other factors.

For **References and Other Readings** see end of Chapter 4.

4 Microscopy and Biology of Interphase Nuclei of Functioning Specialized Cells

Perspective. In Chapter 2 the four components of the interphase nucleus were listed as (1) the nuclear envelope, (2) chromatin, (3) the nucleolus and (4) nuclear sap and were dealt with to different extents:

(1) The nuclear envelope as seen with both the LM and the EM was described in detail.

(2) The appearance of chromatin in the interphase nucleus was described briefly at the level of both the LM and the EM and it was pointed out that chromatin existed in the form of long single threads and that these could be present in a cell in an extended or condensed form.

The changes that occur in the chromatin of an interphase cell as it enters and passes through mitosis, during which process all the chromatin of each chromosome becomes condensed to form chromosomes, was described. Following this a good deal of attention was paid to the identification of the chromosomes of man and to chromosome anomalies.

In Chapter 3 the changes that occur in chromatin as a prelude to mitosis in the S phase of the cell cycle were described in some detail. This included an explanation of how DNA molecules are duplicated and how this can be followed by radioautography which method was also described. The latter led to a consideration of the many uses of labeled thymidine in connection with the study of cell multiplication and cell lineages.

In the present chapter we shall try to round out our account of the nucleus by considering certain matters that could not be dealt with until the background provided by Chapters 2 and 3 had been laid. These matters are:

1. The functional differences between condensed and extended chromatin and the significance of the existence of each type in any given specialized cell.

2. The ways and means whereby the DNA of the extended chromatin of a cell directs the synthesis of protein in that cell. Comment on this matter involves: (A) Defining a gene (a term coined long before the discovery of DNA to denote a biological unit of heredity) in terms of a segment of a strand of a DNA molecule; (B) the roles played by three types of RNA whereby information stored in DNA results in the synthesis of specific proteins, and (C) some comment on how the regulation of gene activity could be controlled by environmental factors.

3. A detailed account of the nucleolus which, as will be shown, provides one of the types of RNA required for proteins to be synthesized from amino acids in the cell.

4. Brief comment on the nuclear sap in which the extended chromatin of a cell is contained.

We shall deal with these four topics in the order given above.

Functional Differences Between Condensed and Extended Chromatin

Introduction. The only way genes can determine or control the nature and function of an interphase specialized cell is by directing the synthesis of the particular proteins that are required in that cell to enable it to have a particular structure and perform a particular function. Interphase cells that serve different functions in the body must have somewhat different protein constitutions in order to perform these different functions; for example, a muscle cell, in order to be able to contract, must have different amounts of certain proteins than a cell designated to secrete. Furthermore, the protein secretions of secretory cells are of many different varieties. Hence the assortment of proteins produced in different kinds of cells differs greatly and this requires that their enzymes differ. Furthermore, some of the proteins produced in the cells of a given individual of a species that practices random breeding differ from those produced in any other individual of the species except in the instance of identical twins.

It is now generally accepted that the information needed by a given cell to produce any particular protein is stored somewhere along the course of its DNA molecules in the form of a sentence (or sentences) written in specific 3-letter words from the A, C, G and T alphabet.

Because of the exact way DNA molecules are duplicated, there is no reason to believe that the code on the DNA molecules of any given body cell could, except for accidents, ever become different from that of any other body cell. Accordingly, it is thought that the reason for one cell producing one assortment of proteins while another cell produces a different assortment is not that the information inscribed in the DNA of different body cells is different but instead that different parts of DNA molecules are "read" in different kinds of cells and this, of course, results in one kind of cell synthesizing proteins that are different from those that are synthesized in other kinds of cells where other parts of the DNA molecules are "read."

EVIDENCE INDICTING THAT THE DNA OF CONDENSED CHROMATIN DOES NOT DIRECT PROTEIN SYNTHESIS

There is evidence indicating that the parts of the DNA molecules being read in any given specialized cell are located exclusively in the portions of chromatin threads that are extended. In other words, the parts of the DNA molecules that are in the condensed chromatin that is observed in a specialized cell are thought not to be providing any information for protein synthesis in that particular cell. Two kinds of evidence support this concept. One kind was more or less an unexpected sequela of the discovery that the nuclei of cells of males and females could be distinguished from one another (in most mammals) by examining them with the LM in sections or spreads. The other kind of evidence hinges on radioautographic studies. We shall first describe how it was discovered that the cells of females could be distinguished from the cells of males and how this helped to lead to the concept that condensed chromatin is inactive.

BARR BODIES

Their Discovery. By 1949 good light microscopes had been available for around a hundred years and thousands of microscopists had examined probably millions of sections and spreads of mammalian cells and no one had noticed that there was a sufficient difference between the appearance of the interphase nuclei of the cells of males and females of most types of mammals for them to be distinguished from one another. Hence it seemed more or less incredible when Barr and Bertram in 1949 described how they found it was possible to determine the sex of cats by examin-

ing their nerve cells and that the same method was equally effective with regard to human nerve cells. They and their colleagues quickly extended their studies to various species and to different kinds of body cells and soon Moore had described a method for easily making, on ordinary glass slides, spreads (smears) of cells wiped from the oral mucosa of people that enabled a microscopist to quickly determine whether their cells contained what are now termed Barr bodies, which are characteristic of females as will presently be explained. But first it is of interest to research-minded students to tell how this discovery was made.

Barr and Bertram were studying the changes that occur in the cytoplasm of certain nerve cells of cats when the nerve fibers that extended off from the cells were stimulated. Although they were concerned primarily with the cytoplasm, the generally pale large nucleus of the nerve cells (Fig. 4-1) helped in bringing to their attention a little rounded basophilic body that was in the nucleus of the first cats they studied. The fact that it seemed to change its position under different experimental conditions furthered their interest in it. Commonly, however, it was close to the nucleolus (Fig. 4-1, *left, on right side of nucleolus*). As they continued their experiments they, therefore, continued to look for this little rounded body and were surprised when they were unable to see it in some of the cats they studied while in others it was as clear as in the first ones. Puzzled by this, like the good scientists they were, they went over the careful records they had kept and discovered that the tiny body was present only in the nerve cell nuclei of *female* cats.

When other kinds of body cells of female cats and other mammals were studied thoroughly, it became apparent that the common position of the little body in nerve cells (close to the nucleolus) was unusual, for in most kinds of cells it was almost always located on the inner aspect of the nuclear membrane, as is shown in Figure 4-2, *top;* furthermore, in these it appears as a plano-convex body instead of the rounded body seen in nerve cells.

Terminology. By this time it was concluded that the little body must have something to do with the body cells of females each containing two X chromosomes while those of males have only one. Accordingly it came to be referred to as the *sex chromatin* and for a time it was generally assumed that the two X chromosomes of female cells must constitute a large enough body of chromatin in the interphase to be visible with the LM whereas the one X chromosome of male cells did not. But this concept soon changed when it was established that the little body was only one of the

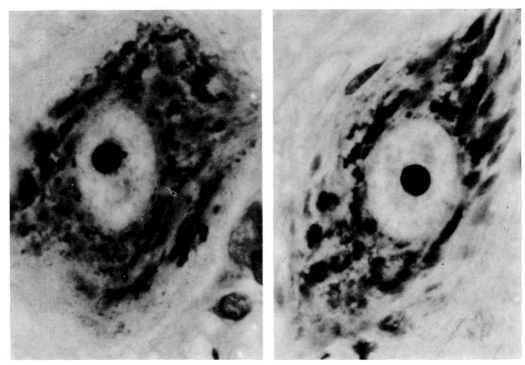

FIG. 4-1. Oil-immersion photomicrographs of two nerve cells from the anterior horn of the spinal cord of two different cats. The nuclei of such cells have almost all their chromatin extended, and hence the nuclei are large and pale. Each nucleus, moreover, has a prominent nucleolus. Barr and Bertram noticed that the nucleus of the female cat (*left*), however, contained a little round body (on the right side of the nucleolus in this illustration). This body was not seen in the nuclei of male cells (*right*). (Barr, M. L., Bertram, L. F., and Lindsay, H. A.: Anat. Rec., *107:*283)

two X chromosomes and that the reason for one X chromosome being visible was that it remained condensed while the other was extended and hence invisible. It is necessary for only one X chromosome to be extended and give off such information as is carried by its genes. So in females one of the X chromosomes remains condensed in the interphase to constitute a small visible body of chromatin. Since male cells have only one X chromosome, it has to be extended (in which state it is invisible with the LM) in order to give off the information its genes contain. (An X chromosome is concerned with much more than sex; it has over 50 genes that have nothing to do with sex and are important in both males and females.) From all this it became apparent that the term *sex chromatin* was not appropriate for a single inactive condensed X chromosome and it was generally agreed to name the little body after its discoverer, so that it is now termed a *Barr body.*

Why only one of the two X chromosomes of a female body cell should become extended in the interphase is not understood. However, what is important

for us to note is that, if one X chromosome remains condensed when the other is extended and functioning, the possibility of the existence of a mechanism for suppressing gene activity is suggested—a mechanism that results in the chromatin, in which the genes to be suppressed are contained, being in a condensed form. Further evidence for the existence of an inactivation mechanism of this sort is provided by the fact that, if some genes belonging to an autosome become translocated to an X chromosome, they become inactivated if the X chromosome becomes a Barr body. That a mechanism for causing chromatin to become condensed operates to cause all but one of the X chromosomes in a cell to become condensed is also shown in anomalies (described in Chapter 2) in which there are an excessive number of X chromosomes in a cell whether it is a female or a male cell. If, for example, there are two X chromosomes in a male cell, one will appear as a Barr body; if there are three X chromosomes in a female cell, two will appear as Barr bodies, i.e., every one but one becomes a Barr body except when polyploidy occurs, for in tetraploid cells of a female one

X chromosome per diploid set unwinds so that there are two Barr bodies in these cells.

Why Human Females Are Mosaics. Barr bodies make their appearance in body cells when a female embryo is about two weeks old, at which time it consists of only a few hundred cells and has become implanted in the lining of the uterus (Fig. 26-23). At this time one of the two X chromosomes of its body cells can be seen to be condensed while the other is extended. Which of the two chromosomes in a cell becomes a Barr body at this time is a matter of chance. Since the genes of the two X chromosomes may be somewhat different because one X chromosome is derived from the father and one from the mother, the cells of an embryo in which the X chromosome from the father's side becomes active will be slightly different from those in which the X chromosome from the mother's side becomes active. After chance has made the original decision about which one will be active in each body cell of the early embryo, the one that becomes active gives rise to the active ones in subsequent generations of cells arising from that cell as the body develops. Hence the different clones of cells that are set up, which in due course populate the adult body, differ slightly. In the cells of some the father-derived X chromosome is always active and in the others, the mother-derived X chromosome is always active. For this reason, normal human females are mosaics composed of two kinds of slightly different cells.

The Significance of Barr Bodies in Somatic Cells. When the technics for the chromosome analysis of mitotic cells became available and various anomalies were studied with these technics, it became apparent that Barr bodies do not always prove an individual to be female. As was described in Chapter 2, sex is not determined by whether or not individuals possess two or more X chromosomes, but by whether or not they possess a Y chromosome, because it is the Y chromosome that is responsible for the development of testes (the sex glands of the male). Through the use of the Barr body test, and the study of chromosome spreads, it was disclosed that there are certain chromosomal anomalies in which individuals who are females do not reveal Barr bodies and some individuals who are males possess them. For example, in the anomaly known as Turner's syndrome (described in Chapter 2) the cells of a female have only one sex chromosome which is an X. Since it would be extended and active there would be no Barr bodies seen in the cells of such a female. In Klinefelder's syndrome (also described in Chapter 2) an individual has a Y chromosome in all his cells and, in addition, he has two X chromosomes.

Since only one X is active and extended, the other appears as a Barr body, yet because of the Y chromosome, the individual is a male. As noted, in anomalies in which there are more than two X chromosomes present in cells, only one is extended, so every additional X appears as a Barr body.

Strictly speaking, a negative sex chromatin test, i.e., the establishment of the absence of Barr bodies in the somatic cells of an individual, although enormously useful for detecting various anomalies, is not conclusive proof that the individual is a male. Likewise, the presence of Barr bodies in the cells of an individual, although equally useful, is not conclusive proof that the individual is a female; it is merely proof that the somatic cells of that individual contain at least two X chromosomes. Final proof of the chromosomal sex of an individual is determined by establishing whether or not the somatic cells have one or more Y chromosomes; this is done by the study of spreads of metaphase chromosomes as outlined in Chapter 2.

How a Simple Test for Barr Bodies Is Made. Moore and Barr showed that instead of having to remove tissue (such as a bit of skin) and cut sections, the test can be performed by lightly scraping cells off the inside of the cheek with a metal spatula, such as the type commonly used for analytical weighing. The cells are smeared onto a glass slide that has been coated with a thin layer of egg albumin. Fixation is accomplished by immersing the slide in 90 percent ethyl alcohol. The slide is then passed through graded alcohols to distilled water and stained with cresyl violet (Fig. 4-2).

Form and Disposition. In most kinds of cells a Barr body appears as a little dark mass, often planoconvex in form, that is pressed against the inner side of the nuclear envelope (Fig. 4-2). Generally it has a diameter of about 1 μ so that it is clearly visible in smears with the LM or in sections if the plane of the section passes through it. But it should not be expected that it will be seen in every female nucleus that is examined, because a section may not cross the nucleus in the right plane. Even in smears, every female nucleus need not show sex chromatin, because it may be on the upper or lower part of the flattened nucleus and not at its side where it shows up best. Also, some nuclei of male cells may show bits of condensed chromatin close to the nuclear membrane which look like Barr bodies.

Accordingly, since a Barr body cannot be seen in every female nucleus and since chromatin masses approximating the appearance and the position of Barr bodies can sometimes be seen in male nuclei, the pres-

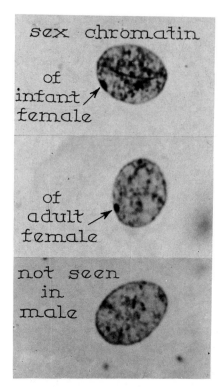

FIG. 4-2. Photomicrographs of epithelial cells from the oral mucosa stained with cresyl-echt violet ($\times$ 2,000). The upper two nuclei have Barr bodies, which are indicated by arrows. (Moore, K. L., and Barr, M. L.: Lancet, *269:57*)

ence or absence of Barr bodies cannot be determined by a hasty examination of a section or a smear but only by examining say, 100 consecutive nuclei and then calculating the percentage of cells in which this appearance was noted. The number of Barr-body-like structures is usually of the order of 90 percent in female cells and only 10 percent in male cells.

Significance With Regard to Functional Activity of Chromatin. The discovery of Barr bodies and the development of knowledge that followed and was due to the devising of technics for making chromosome analysis of mitotic cells not only opened up the very important aspect of modern medicine dealing with chromosome anomalies and their effects but also suggested that chromatin that remains condensed in the interphase of specialized functioning cells is inactive and that only extended chromatin gives off information that directs the synthesis of proteins in the interphase. Thus the condensation of chromatin would seem to be associated with one means for the suppression of gene

function and although the above-described evidence to this effect relates to sex chromosomes, evidence for the condensed chromatin of autosomes also being inactive has received support from radioautographic studies of RNA synthesis in the nuclei of specialized cells. For example, in 1964 Littau et al., using uridine-^{3}H to label newly forming RNA, showed that the grains that appeared over the nuclei of calf thymocytes, in which cells most of the chromatin is that of autosomes and of the condensed type, were almost exclusively located over the small amount of chromatin that was extended. From their study they concluded that the condensed chromatin was virtually inactive as a template for synthesis of RNA.

It therefore seems ironic that although chromatin was both described and named by light microscopy, the only chromatin that is seen with the LM in interphase nuclei is not the chromatin that is directing the particular type of protein synthesis that is occurring in that cell. The parts of the chromatin threads that are active in directing protein synthesis are probably only those that cannot be seen with the LM and are distributed in what was termed the nuclear sap. With the EM, however, while the distinction between dense and extended chromatin is generally clear (as it is, for example, in Fig. 4-3), at high magnifications, more or less of a gradual transition between the two types can sometimes be seen. For example, toward the left side of Figure 4-4, there appears to be a gradual transition between the narrow band of perinuclear (condensed) chromatin above and the extended chromatin that lies below it. Furthermore, short longitudinal segments of chromatin threads (which conceivably could be giving off information) can be seen in the extended chromatin (arrows at left and middle). Part of a thread cut in longitudinal section can also be seen at the edge of condensed chromatin at the right where it is indicated by two arrows. In general, the fine structure of any discrete mass of condensed chromatin in the nuclei of interphase cells is the same as that of the chromatin seen in sections of mitotic chromosomes (compare Fig. 4-3 with Figs. 2-19 and 2-20).

It is also worth noting that whereas some of the genes that are in the extended chromatin of the nuclei of various kinds of specialized cells are the same as those that are active in other kinds of specialized cells, others may differ. Hence some of the genes that are active and hence reside in the extended chromatin in some kinds of cells are inactive and tucked away in the condensed chromatin in other kinds of cells. The condensed chromatin seen in different kinds of inter-

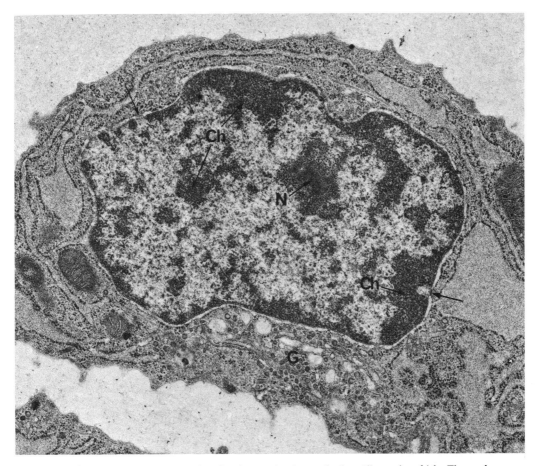

Fɪɢ. 4-3. Electron micrograph of a chondrocyte in the tracheal cartilage of a chick. The nucleus shows regions of both condensed and extended chromatin. Much of the condensed chromatin is distributed along the inner surface of the nuclear membrane but it is also scattered about in the nucleus in the form of islands. Both types are indicated by arrows from Ch. Note that the condensed chromatin is absent at the sites of nuclear pores (shown by arrows, lower right and upper left, which point to pores). A nucleolus (to be described presently) is labeled N. For those who refer to this illustration when reading the chapter on Cartilage note the Golgi apparatus which is indicated by G in the cytoplasm below the nucleus. (From V. I. Kalnins)

phase nuclei therefore differs not only in quantity but also in genetic content. It seems probable that the genes of the extended chromatin of any specialized cell vary in the extent of their activities at different times with regard to directing protein synthesis—that they are turned "on" or "off" in relation to demand (possible mechanisms for this will be described later in this chapter) and hence that a gene that is used sometimes in a cell can be turned "off" while it is still in the extended chromatin without its having to be tucked away in the condensed chromatin. In general it would therefore seem that the condensed chromatin in the nucleus of a

particular kind of cell is more or less superfluous so far as the present functioning of that cell is concerned. But there are examples, as we shall see later, of cells engaging in new functions and it seems most probable that under these conditions chromatin threads from the previously condensed chromatin become extended and active. Lastly, when a cell divides, all of the chromatin of the cell, both the condensed and extended, must of course be duplicated.

We shall next deal with how information stored in the DNA of the extended chromatin of an actively functioning interphase cell directs protein synthesis in

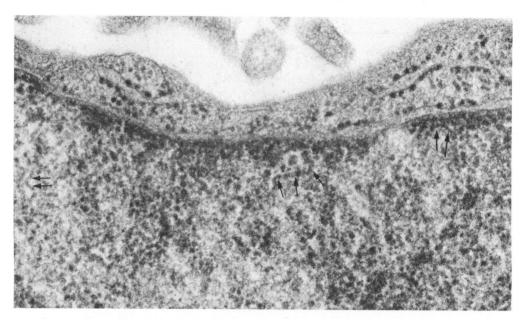

FIG. 4-4. Electron micrograph ($\times$ 80,000) of part of a nucleus of a fibroblast. The nuclear envelope extends across the illustration and there is a relatively narrow layer of condensed (perinuclear) chromatin lying immediately beneath it except at the site of a pore which can be seen to the left of the two arrows which are near the right side of the illustration. The two arrows here indicate a short segment of a curving chromatin thread. The two arrows at the left indicate a site where some chromatin threads have been cut over a short distance in longitudinal section. The arrows in the center also indicate a portion of a longitudinally disposed chromatin thread. In this illustration there appears to be more or less of a gradual transition between the condensed perinuclear chromatin and the extended chromatin that lies below it. (From V. I. Kalnins)

the cytoplasm of that cell. Three types of RNA are required for this to happen, as will now be described.

The Function of Extended Chromatin

How Information Stored in DNA Molecules Directs the Synthesis of Particular Proteins

The Triplet Code. In the preceding chapter it was explained that information is stored in DNA molecules in the form of sentences written in three-letter words from an alphabet of four letters, A, C, G and T, each letter standing for a different base in the DNA molecule, adenine, cytosine, guanine and thymine respectively. Proteins are assembled from only about 20 amino acids. In order to have a separate and distinct code word for each amino acid, the code words would have to be more than two letters long because 20 different two-letter words cannot be written from a 4 letter alphabet. It took a good deal of brilliant research to establish that the code words were each three-letter words (the triplet code) and that the letters used were

from the four-letter alphabet of A, C, G and T. For example, CCT, specifies the amino acid glycine and TTT specifies phenylalanine. There are, however, 64 possible three letter words that could be written. Since there are only 20 or so amino acids, there are a lot of excess words that could be used. Some of these are used as duplicates for coding for a particular amino acid—that is, a particular amino acid is sometimes coded for by more than one code word. For example, on DNA the sequences TTT and TTG both can specify the amino acid phenylalanine.

The order of the three-letter words in sentences written along a DNA molecule prescribe the order in which amino acids should be strung together to form either a whole protein (if it consists of only one long strand of amino acids it is called a polypeptide) or each of the polypeptides involved if several of them are required to form a more complex protein molecule. If the sentence codes for only one polypeptide of a complex protein molecule, other sentences on the same or on some other DNA molecule code for the other polypeptides required to form the protein.

Genes. In the light of the knowledge about the chemical basis for genes, a gene came to be defined as having its chemical basis in a segment of a strand of a DNA molecule that codes for a polypeptide chain which is equivalent to (1) a complete simple protein molecule or (2) a part of a more complex protein molecule composed of several polypeptide chains. However, it soon was realized that there may also be other kinds of genes (soon to be described), so the kind defined above are now called *structural genes*. Other kinds will be described presently.

We shall now consider how the code inscribed on a strand of a DNA molecule can direct the synthesis of particular proteins. The reactions concerned involve three different kinds of RNA.

Types of RNA

Three kinds of RNA are required in order for the information coded in DNA to be translated so as to link the amino acids of the prescribed protein together and in proper sequence; they are (1) Messenger RNA (mRNA), (2) Transfer RNA (tRNA) and (3) Ribosomal RNA (rRNA). Their respective roles will now be described.

How the DNA Code Is Read

Messenger RNA

The code inscribed along a DNA molecule in three-letter words from the A, C, G and T alphabet is read by means of its being transcribed onto a long single-stranded molecule of messenger RNA (mRNA). Transcription is effected by means of long single-stranded molecules of mRNA being synthesized alongside the exposed sentences written on one strand of a DNA molecule. Such a transcription occurs by means of its bases A, C, G and T serving as sites for the synthesis of complementary bases on an RNA molecule. (Complementary base pairing is described in Chapter 3 and illustrated in Figs. 3-3 and 3-4.) However, the bases in RNA differ from those of DNA in one respect, as will now be described.

RNA differs from DNA not only in its sugar but also because one of the four nitrogenous bases of its molecules (uracil) is different from the corresponding base in DNA (thymine). The other three bases, adenine, cytosine and guanine, are the same as those in the DNA molecule. Hence, in transcription, complementary base pairing results in guanine always being synthesized in the mRNA molecule wherever there is cytosine on the DNA molecule and cytosine wherever there is guanine on the DNA molecule. Furthermore,

wherever there is thymine on the DNA molecule, adenine is synthesized in the RNA molecule. But wherever there is adenine in the DNA molecule, uracil is synthesized in the RNA molecule. So the three-letter words of the DNA molecule that are *transcribed* onto a newly forming mRNA molecule are spelled out in three-letter words from an alphabet of four letters that are A, C, G and U respectively.

Messenger RNA reaches the cytoplasm where it appears in the form of long threadlike strands; a portion of one seen in the cytoplasm is shown in Figure 5-20.

The three-letter words inscribed along DNA molecules are called *codons,* and each codes for a particular amino acid. As noted, there may be more than one codon for the same amino acid. Since the codons are transcribed onto mRNA by complementary base pairing, the codon on the DNA molecule for the amino acid glycine, CCT, would be transcribed by complementary base pairing onto mRNA as GGA, as shown below:

$$\text{DNA molecule—CCT}$$
$$\text{mRNA molecule—GGA}$$

The next question is how the three-letter words along molecules of mRNA result in the amino acids for which they code being brought together in proper sequences to form particular polypeptides and proteins.

The linkage of amino acids occurs at the sites of ribosomes next to be described.

Ribosomes and Ribosomal RNA (rRNA)

Ribosomes are electron-dense little *bodies* of nucleoprotein around 150 Å in diameter. Their nucleic acid component is rRNA. They are seen most clearly and abundantly in the cytoplasm at sites of protein synthesis. Since they are a type of cytoplasmic organelle, they will be described in detail in the next chapter, which deals with cytoplasm. A ribosome is assembled from two subunits (Fig. 4-5), both of which are produced in the nucleolus. How these are made involves the synthesis of rRNA in the nucleolus, which will be described later in this chapter. In Figure 4-6, which shows amino acids being linked together on a ribosome, the latter is depicted as a black sphere. (This illustration was made some years ago before it became evident that the shape of a ribosome is actually that shown in Fig. 4-5.)

Ribosomes serve as essential but nonspecific sites on which amino acids are linked together in the order prescribed by the order of the codons along the mRNA molecule which moves along a ribosome or ribosomes in the cytoplasm.

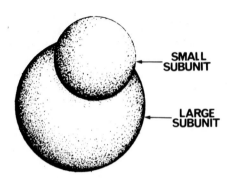

Fig. 4-5. Diagram of a ribosome.

Transfer RNA (tRNA)

Messenger RNA, as has been described above, carries a string of code words that specify different amino acids in a special order so that, when strung together in this order, they will constitute a specific polypeptide or protein. Ribosomes provide sites upon which the amino acids are linked together in the order specified by the code words on mRNA. But how do code words recognize the various amino acids that they specify? How does an amino acid recognize the code word that specified it? Mutual recognition is achieved because there is a go-between, which is transfer RNA (tRNA).

Molecules of tRNA have, as it were, two faces (Fig. 4-6). One face recognizes and becomes attached to a particular amino acid—for example, glycine (Fig. 4-6). The other face of this tRNA molecule possesses a particular three-letter word of the A, C, G, U alphabet that by complementary base pairing will recognize and attach to the suitable three-letter word exposed along the course of the molecule of mRNA. For example, the code word for glycine along the mRNA molecule is GGA (Fig. 4-6) and this pairs with a CCU sequence on a molecule of tRNA (Fig. 4-6) which, as described above, would have glycine attached to its other face.

Protein Synthesis

How Specific Polypeptides Are Assembled

What happens, very roughly, is that a long molecule of mRNA moves to a cytoplasmic site where there are ribosomes (Fig. 4-6). The ribosomes are in the midst of a pool of 20 amino acids. Each of the amino acids is attached to one face of a molecule of tRNA which on its other face exposes a three-letter word of the A, C, G, U alphabet that will pair in a complementary fashion with the three-letter word on the mRNA molecule that specifies this particular amino acid. As the molecule of mRNA moves along the ribosome the vari-

ous amino acids specified by the code words along its course are thus brought together in the proper order and, as they are brought together, they become linked in what will be a polypeptide chain, as is shown in Figure 4-6. The tRNA to which each amino acid was previously attached then becomes detached from it, and more or less simultaneously the tRNA also becomes detached from the codon on the mRNA with which it was paired. The molecule of tRNA is, therefore, available to combine with the same kind of amino acid again and be used again. The mRNA, once it has served its purpose usually becomes degraded but there are some important examples of mRNA persisting and coding for protein synthesis for a long time, as, for example, in certain cells that have lost their nuclei.

By using various amino acids labeled with tritium, the synthesis of different proteins can be studied by radioautography in many parts of the body with both the LM and the EM. Several examples will be mentioned later. The synthesis of mRNA can be investigated by using uridine specially labeled with tritium.

The Regulation of Protein Synthesis

The rate of protein synthesis in cells differs under different circumstances which relate to different needs for growth and function. Since the synthesis of proteins in cells is directed by genes, it would seem that, when protein synthesis in cells increases, the genes that direct the synthesis of the proteins concerned must become either more active than they were before or active for longer stretches of time. Likewise, when protein synthesis decreases in a cell it seems that the genes that direct the synthesis of the proteins concerned become either less active than before or active for shorter periods of time. Accordingly it has become more or less common language to say that there must be a mechanism for turning genes "on" or "off" in cells to meet the different requirements for protein synthesis under different conditions.

Next, since the genes of a cell are confined to the chromatin of the nucleus, they are not in direct touch with the external environment of the cell. Furthermore, it seems logical to think that the demand for more protein synthesis for growth (as in the repair of an injury), or the demand for more secretion by secretory cells that make protein-containing secretions, must arise somewhere in the body outside of the cells that will be called upon to respond to that demand. This demand must somehow be conveyed to the immediate environment of the cell that will respond to it. Then from the immediate environment of the cell the demand must some-

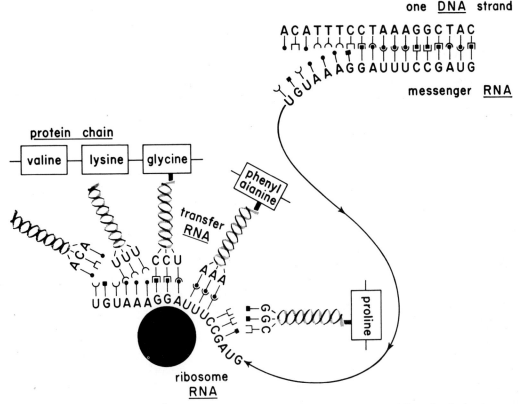

FIG. 4-6. Diagram to show how information coded on one strand of a DNA molecule in the nucleus (*upper right*) is transferred to a strand of messenger RNA which forms beside it (*upper right*), and how the latter peels away from the DNA molecule (*upper right*) and moves (*arrow on right side*) to the cytoplasm to a ribosome (*lower left*). Here the strand of messenger RNA is surrounded by a pool of amino acids, each of which is identified (so far as the messenger RNA is concerned) by a particular 3-letter code word of transfer RNA; thus valine is identified by ACA, lysine by UUU, glycine by CCU, phenylalanine by AAA and proline by GGC. The first 3-letter code word inscribed along the strand of messenger RNA (*bottom, left*) fits ACA so that the amino acid valine is the first selected by the messenger RNA. The next 3-letter code word selects UUU so that lysine is added to valine as the construction of a protein molecule is begun. The next word selects glycine, which is added to the protein chain. The diagram shows that phenylalanine and proline will be added next (*right side*) and that the transfer RNA responsible for identifying valine and lysine (*left side*), having done its work, has become detached both from the messenger RNA and from the amino acids they identified.

how affect the cytoplasm of the cell in some way so that by chemical means the demand is directed into the nucleus to the genes that would be concerned with directing the synthesis of the required protein.

Although still enormously difficult, it is much easier to investigate in bacteria possible ways by which alterations in the external environment of a cell can set up chemical reactions within the cell which are reflected to the genes that control the synthesis of the proteins required so that they are turned "on" or "off" than it is to study this problem in the specialized cells of

mammals. We shall now give an example of how certain genes in a bacterial cell can be turned "on" by a change in the external environment of a cell; this example concerns the *induction of an enzyme.*

If certain strains of *E. coli* (a variety of bacteria) are grown in a medium that contains no galactoside (a galactose-containing glycoside), the bacteria synthesize only traces of the enzyme β-galactosidase (a specific protein that breaks down the galactoside, lactose, to simpler sugars). But if lactose is added to the medium, the bacteria soon produce large quantities of this enzyme. For the synthesis of a particular enzyme to be produced abundantly by the presence in the environment of an abundant substrate for the enzyme proves, first, that the sequences of three-letter words that code for this particular enzyme must have pre-existed somewhere along the course of the DNA of the bacterial cell and, second, that without substrate for the enzyme the gene was inactive. Lactose is therefore said to be an inducer of this enzyme—that is, it somehow causes the gene that codes for this enzyme and was previously inactive to begin transcribing mRNA which, in turn, directs the synthesis of the protein, β-galactosidase. This, then, is an example of a substrate inducing an enzyme. (There are, however, inducers that are not substrates.)

The next question relates to how an inducer causes a gene that is not transcribing to begin transcribing.

An Introduction Only to the Operon Concept

It is now known that three enzymes are synthesized rather than one when lactose, the inducer, is added to the medium, with all three participating in bringing about changes that occur subsequently. Since three enzymes are induced, three genes must be involved. These are arranged one after the other on the DNA molecule. Genes of the sort that code for particular proteins which are either enzymes or proteins that become nonenzymatic parts of the structure of the organelles of a cell, are termed *structural genes*. To explain how structural genes are turned on or off, however, required the postulation of further kinds of genes. In this connection it was found that the three genes that are turned on with lactose are turned on or off together. The control of the three in this respect is believed to be under what is termed an *operator gene*. The operator gene plus the three structural genes constitutes what is termed an *operon*. The operator gene is, in turn, controlled by another kind of a gene called a *regulator gene*. The regulator gene codes for the formation of a protein substance termed *repressor*. The repressor, in the absence of an inducer, combines with and keeps the operator gene from turning on the structural genes that it controls. An inducer, however, has an affinity for the repressor, so when lactose, in this instance, is added to the medium, it combines so strongly with the repressor that the repressor is unable to repress the operator gene which is thereby enabled to turn on the three structural genes so that they begin transcribing and this leads to the production of the three enzymes in quantity. Thus we have an example to show how it is possible for an environmental in-

fluence to exploit a previously undisclosed potentiality of a cell for profound activity of a particular kind, provided that the cell has the code in its genes to direct that activity.

The operon concept evolved from the brilliant research of Jacob and Monod and has been much investigated in recent years. It explains not only how a particular kind of external environmental influence, by affecting a repressor, can lead to the genes responsible for directing the synthesis of particular proteins becoming unmasked, but also how feedback mechanisms from certain metabolic reactions in a cell can affect the repressor so that it binds with the operator gene so as to turn it "off." An example of this is provided by experiments that show that if cells that are synthesizing a particular amino acid have that amino acid added (in sufficient quantity) to the medium in which the cells are living, the production of that amino acid by the cells ceases. In this instance the end product of this particular synthetic process on the part of the cell (the amino acid) acts by combining with the repressor so as to make it actively combine with and hence turn off the operator gene that controls the synthesis of the enzymes concerned with the production of this particular amino acid. This, therefore, is an instance of the end product of an enzyme-controlled reaction making the repressor more active. Substances which act this way are called *co-repressors*.

In an instance such as the one described above, the co-repressor cannot immediately stop the synthesis of the amino acid because the enzymes concerned in the reactions that produce the amino acid would persist and function for a considerable length of time even if the genes that controlled their synthesis were turned off. There is another kind of mechanism, however, that can automatically affect the overproduction of the end product. As the concentration of the end product mounts, the end product itself may act to inhibit the enzyme that controls the first step in the synthetic process.

The operon concept derived from bacterial studies provides a most important clue as to how the genes of mammalian cells that control protein synthesis for maintenance and function could be regulated. It also provides a background for understanding how genes could be turned on or off for the extra protein synthesis required for growth. Finally it has still another application, in that it provides a clue as to how the cells that form from a fertilized ovum as a body develops can be of a great many different varieties because of their having been exposed at critical times in their development to different environments, as will be discussed in more detail in Chapter 6. Also in Chapter 6, there will be some description of the way that hormones can act so as to turn on certain genes in their target cells (the cells on which they more or less specifically act) and how this phenomenon seems to be involved with their affecting the formation of what is termed cyclic AMP in their target cells. Here, however, we must continue our discussion of the various RNA's, so we shall next discuss rRNA and the nucleolus where rRNA is formed.

Nucleoli and rRNA

The general LM appearance of the nucleolus was described in Chapters 1 and 2 and illustrated and labeled in Figure 1-12. This nuclear organelle of great importance is not enclosed by a membrane. It has two main functions: (1) to produce most, if not all, of the ribosomal RNA (rRNA) of the cell, and (2) to serve as the site in which two kinds of ribonucleoprotein particles called preribosomal particles are produced (which later and elsewhere come together to form complete ribosomes). Chemically 80 to 90 percent of the nucleolar mass is protein. Part of this protein is that of the nucleoprotein of the ribosomal subunits and the remainder is either concerned with the enzymatic reactions that occur in this organelle (which is metabolically very active) or is located in its structural components.

Problems Associated With Seeing Nucleoli in Sections or Smears With the LM. Nucleoli are seen to best advantage in nuclei that contain extensive amounts of extended chromatin and very little condensed chromatin, as in the nerve cell shown in Figure 4-1, *right*. In nuclei with much condensed chromatin, the presence of nucleoli is obscured (Fig. 1-11). A small nucleus with much condensed chromatin and little nuclear sap may be wholly contained within the thickness of a routine-type section, and hence to see a nucleolus in it, the observer has to look through condensed chromatin both above it and below it, as well as beside it. Since both condensed chromatin and nucleoli are blue-purple in an H and E section, a nucleolus cannot be distinguished with any assurance in this type of preparation. The same holds true for this type of nucleus seen in a smear or film, as is apparent in Figure 10-3, *upper left*. To see nucleoli in small dense nuclei, sections that are much thinner than nuclei must be used; this procedure gets rid of much of the chromatin that is above or below the nucleolus. Very thin sections examined with the EM usually demonstrate nucleoli in the type of nuclei in which they do not appear to advantage with the LM in ordinary H and E sections.

The Basis for the Basophilia of Nucleoli in H and E Sections. The thickness of an H and E section may allow it to contain a whole nucleus and it follows that, since nucleoli are much smaller than nuclei, most of the nucleoli seen in H and E sections would be whole nucleoli and not slices cut through them. As was mentioned in connection with chromatin in Chapter 2, there is a tendency for chromatin to adhere more or less to the exterior of a nucleolus; this chromatin is termed the nucleolus-associated chromatin and was illustrated in the electron micrograph of a thin section (Fig. 2-4, NAC). In the thicker sections used for the LM, the nucleolus-associated chromatin, which is seen in the thin section in Figure 2-4 to be present only around the periphery of the nucleolus, may be present both above and below the nucleolus. It can be shown that this nucleolus-associated chromatin (which, of course, contains DNA) accounts for much of the basophilia of the nucleolus seen in ordinary H and E sections, because, if sections are treated with RNA-ase, which dissolves the rRNA from the body of the nucleolus, the nucleoli of most cells (as is seen in Fig. 4-7, *top*) still appear as basophilic rounded bodies in the nucleus. Although what seem to be nucleoli can still be seen, all cytoplasmic basophilia—which is due to RNA, chiefly rRNA—has disappeared. In the lower picture, which is a section that was treated with DNA-ase, the cytoplasmic basophilia (which is due to RNA) is present and, although some nucleoli are visible, their staining is not very intense because the nucleolus-associated chromatin has been removed by the DNA-ase.

Size. It is of interest that the total amount of nucleolar substance was shown by Shea, working in Leblond's laboratory on Purkinje cells of the nervous system, to be always the same in that type of cell whether there were one or more nucleoli in a nucleus. Hence, the more nucleoli there are, the smaller they are. However, whereas the total amount of nucleolar substance of cells of the same kind and in approximately the same state of function is probably the same, there is much evidence indicating that nucleoli tend to be larger than normal in cells that are very actively engaged in protein synthesis. The cells of rapidly growing cancers, in which protein synthesis for growth is very active, often reveal very large nucleoli (see Fig. 4-11, *upper left corner*).

Nucleolar Organizers. For rRNA to be constantly formed in the nucleolus there must be one or more threads of extended chromatin within it that possess genes that code for the formation of rRNA. Long ago it was shown that the formation of nucleoli was associated with only certain of the chromosomes, and the parts of these that seemed to be associated with the

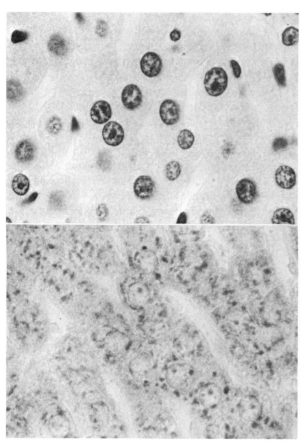

Fig. 4-7. Oil-immersion photomicrographs of two sections of normal liver stained with H and E. The upper section was treated with RNA-ase before staining and the lower section with DNA-ase. Note that nucleoli can still be seen in the nuclei of the upper picture even though the RNA has been removed from them. That the appearance of nucleoli in the upper picture is due to DNA is indicated by the fact that they stain somewhat faintly when the nucleolus-associated chromatin which contains DNA is removed from them as is shown in the lower picture. (Photomicrographs courtesy of Roger Daoust)

formation of nucleoli were termed *nucleolar organizers*. It was next shown that nuclear organizers were limited to chromosomes that in chromosome spreads were shown to possess satellites.

Satellites are found in only five of the pairs of chromosomes of the cells of man, in the members of pairs 13, 14, 15, 21 and 22. The nucleolar organizer of each can be seen in spreads of metaphase chromosomes as the thin poorly stained portions of the chromosomes that are adjacent to the satellites (see Figs. 2-23 and 2-24).

The fact that there are several chromosomes that possess nucleolar organizers could account for there sometimes being several nucleoli in the same nucleus. It is often said that if several nucleoli form they tend to fuse to become a single body. What seems equally likely is that the common single large nucleolus is the result of several nucleolar organizers being close together when they begin to transcribe for the formation of rRNA so that the rRNA that is formed in association with different organizers becomes confluent to form a single large nucleolus.

THE SYNTHESIS OF rRNA IN THE NUCLEOLUS

What is seen with the EM in the different parts of the nucleolus will be easier to interpret if we first describe the synthesis of rRNA in that organelle.

Subunits of Ribosomes and of rRNA. It is known that fully formed ribosomes recovered from cytoplasm can each be readily separated by chemical means into two subunits which are designated by their sedimentation coefficient as determined by centrifugation and expressed as Svedberg units. One is referred to as the 60S or large subunit and the other as the 40S or small subunit. However, each of these subunits of a ribosome consists of both rRNA and protein. So far as the rRNA itself is concerned, the 60S subunit of nucleoprotein contains rRNA with a sedimentation coefficient of 28S while the 40S subunit of nucleoprotein contains 18S rRNA. Since ribosomes are so easily split into two subunits, it is easy to visualize that the subunits are produced first as separate entities in the nucleolus and subsequently joined together. However, the pathway from the synthesis of rRNA to its incorporation into subunits has been found to be somewhat complicated. We shall begin by commenting on nucleolar genes.

Nucleolar Genes. In describing the triplet code, a gene was described as a segment of a DNA molecule that codes for a sequence of amino acids which when linked together constitute a particular polypeptide molecule which would be the equivalent of a simple protein molecule or part of a more complex protein molecule composed of several polypeptide chains. Earlier in this chapter we described how the code of a gene is transcribed onto mRNA and how when it moves to the cytoplasm it directs the linking, in the correct order, of the amino acids specified by the code of the gene that was read by the mRNA. Since different assortments of proteins are produced in different cells, different assortments of mRNA are produced in different cells. However, the RNA of ribosomes (rRNA) is probably of exactly the same composition in all kinds of body cells. Its role in protein synthesis, unlike that of mRNA, is nonspecific. Accordingly, there must be segments of DNA molecules in every body cell that carry exactly the same code which is responsible for rRNA being transcribed beside it. Since these segments of DNA molecules are not concerned with transcribing mRNA that will direct the synthesis of particular polypeptides, they do not fit into the usual concept of a gene; nevertheless, they are termed *nucleolar genes*. They are distributed repetitively along the DNA molecules of the extended chromatin of the portions of those chromosomes that organize the formation of nucleoli.

The Formation of rRNA in the Nucleolus. First, the DNA of a nucleolar organizer in the substance of the nucleolus carries a code for transcribing RNA.

The same code "sentence" is repeated many times along the DNA strand of a nucleolar organizer. The pieces of RNA that are formed along the DNA molecule are, however, not of precisely the same composition as the RNA that later appears in the ribosomes, for it has a sedimentation coefficient of 45S but contains within it 18S and 28S rRNA segments (which later become incorporated into ribosomes) together with some other RNA whose function is, at the moment, unknown.

Studies of the Formation of rRNA With the EM. The extrachromosomal nucleoli of amphibian oocytes possess certain features which make them suitable for studying the synthesis of preribosomal RNA. By using these nucleoli, Miller and Beattie were able to

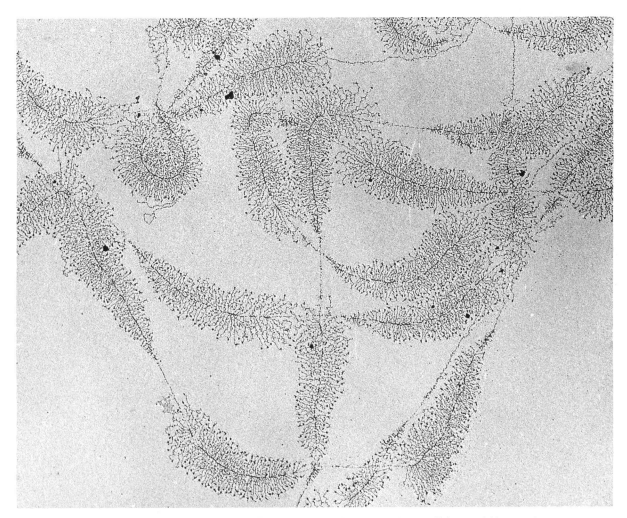

FIG. 4-8. Nucleolar genes isolated from an oocyte of the spotted newt *Triturus viridescens*. ($\times$ 25,000) (O. J. Miller, Jr., and Barbara R. Beatty, Biology Division, Oak Ridge National Laboratory) See text for description.

isolate strands containing the DNA that codes for the synthesis of what is assumed to be the 45S rRNA and to obtain remarkable electron micrographs illustrating the formation of this rRNA beside the "sentences" that code for it and are repeated along the course of the DNA molecule (Fig. 4-8). Along a strand of DNA each "sentence" is separated from the next by a segment of the DNA molecule which appears to be inactive. As their illustration shows, many molecules of what is probably 45S rRNA are being synthesized simultaneously on each of the many "sentences" coding for rRNA written along the DNA strand. The synthesis of rRNA molecules, as seen in the electron micrographs, has almost gone to completion at one end of each "sentence" and is just beginning at the other, which accounts for each having an appearance similar to that of a Christmas tree (Fig. 4-8). Several "sentences" along a strand of DNA, each coding for rRNA, result in an appearance similar to that which would be seen if a series of Christmas trees were arranged end to end, with the branch-free bottom part of the trunk of each touching the tip of the next tree (Fig. 4-8). The branching portion of the trunk of each tree would contain the portion of a DNA strand coding for 45S rRNA while the branches of each tree would consist of different lengths of rRNA that had just been synthesized and in which maturation had begun.

The 45S rRNA that is formed beside the genes along the DNA-containing cores is pushed away from the cores as more is formed beneath it and soon becomes altered. By a series of complicated steps, each molecule of 45S rRNA is cleaved gradually to yield one molecule of 18S rRNA and one of 28S rRNA. Ribosomal proteins become associated with the 45S rRNA shortly after its synthesis and as a result of what is termed maturation, 18S rRNA and 28S rRNA combined with protein come to constitute the two different types of ribonucleoprotein particles that eventually become associated to constitute ribosomes. The particles containing the 28S rRNA tend to accumulate in the nucleoli before moving to the cytoplasm. There is much controversy at this time as to how the nucleoprotein particles reach the cytoplasm, although most workers in this area believe that it is via the nuclear pores. It is believed that in the cytoplasm and, perhaps, already in the nucleus, the 40S particles of ribonucleoprotein which contain the 18S rRNA become attached to mRNA and that this is followed in each instance by a 60S particle which contains the 28S rRNA combining with the 40S particle so as to form a complete ribosome.

Ribosomes will be considered further as cytoplasmic organelles in the next chapter.

The Fine Structure of the Nucleolus

As seen in thin sections with the EM, the nucleoli of the cells of various plants and animals differ in certain respects, and probably many kinds have to be studied to understand the basic structure of this organelle. We shall begin with the appearance of the nucleolus of a mouse oocyte in a thin section as illustrated in Figure 4-9.

The first point to make is that the same structure that is seen with the LM in a routine H and E section as a rounded homogeneous blue body that is surrounded by nuclear sap (Fig. 2-3) appears in a thin section examined with the EM at greater magnification not as a solid dense mass but as a dark network of electron-dense material (Fig. 4-9, a) that lies free (with no surrounding membrane) in the substance of the nucleus (Fig. 4-9). The interstices of this network are filled with a light material (labeled b in Fig. 4-9) which usually appears as islands surrounded on all their sides by dark material.

Is the Dark Material in the Form of a Crumpled Cord or a Sponge? Studies with the LM made before the days of the EM did not all indicate that the nucleolus was a relatively solid structure; some studies made with special technics had suggested that it contained within its substance a convoluted cord which was called the *nucleolonema* (*nema*, thread). Subsequently when thin sections of nucleoli, viewed with the EM, revealed dark material that was arranged in a network, it was often assumed that this was the appearance that a convoluted or crumpled cord of dark material would present in a thin section, and this sometimes led to the conclusion that the EM appearance confirmed the existence of a cordlike nucleolonema. However, if the dark material was in the form of a cord, there would be many examples in a section of its being cut in cross or oblique section where it would be seen to be completely surrounded by light material. Actually the reverse is true, for it is the light material (labeled c in Fig. 4-9) that appears as islands surrounded by the dark material (labeled a in Fig. 4-9). Hence the dark material must exist more or less in the form of a sponge, with the light material filling individual holes or communicating spaces that exist within the substance of the sponge. Accordingly, if there is such a thing as a nucleolonema in the nucleolus, it is not the network of dark material seen in a thin section but something that winds about within the dark material, as will be described later.

FIG. 4-9. Electron micrograph (× 26,000) of a section of a mouse oocyte as it enters the dictyate stage of meiotic prophase. The general appearance of the nucleolus in a section is compatible with what might be expected if a section were cut through a spongelike structure of dark material (a) the interstices of which were filled with light material (b). The nature of (c) and (d) is described in the text. ne, Nuclear envelope; nac, nucleolus-associated chromatin. (Illustration courtesy of L. A. Chouinard, Université Laval)

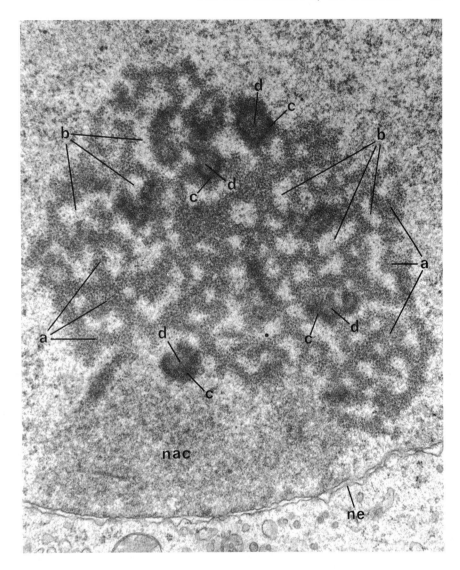

THE TWO COMPONENTS OF THE DARK MATERIAL

The Pars Granulosa. As is apparent in Figure 4-9, much of the material of the dark network (the part labeled a) has a granular appearance; this is often termed the *pars granulosa* of the nucelolus. The granularity is due to accumulated particles of ribonucleoprotein that are for the most part the 60S subunits of future ribosomes. The particles are held in place by a delicate protein matrix (a matrix is a ground substance in which something is embedded) in which they lie until they migrate from the nucleolus. It is to be noted that it is the granular kind of dark material that commonly abuts on the nuclear sap in which the nucleolus lies and, furthermore, it is very often this type of dark substance that borders the islands of light material. It is from the edge of the granular material that faces the nuclear sap that most ribosomal subunits escape into the nucleus and it is probable also that some may leave by way of what appear to be islands of light material in sections but could be cross sections of channels that lead to the exterior of the nucleolus.

The Pars Fibrosa. The second component of the dark material consists of very fine electron-dense filaments that are commonly packed closely together. They too contain much rRNA. Aggregations of these filaments or fibrils are labeled c in Figure 4-9. This figure shows the densely packed filaments that are arranged in thick dark rings around rounded or elongated cores of a less dense material; these cores are termed *fibrillar centers* and are labeled d in Figure 4-9. The dense fibrillar material that constitutes the rings (labeled c) is considered in part to be 45S rRNA that has just been synthesized alongside chromatin threads that lie in the fibrillar centers, as will be described in more detail presently. The peripheral part of the rings that border the granular material is probably the site at which maturation of the first-formed ribonucleoprotein is being completed to give rise to the particles of nucleoprotein that will become the subunits of ribosomes. The border between pars fibrosa and pars granulosa cannot therefore be sharp, because it is a zone of transition where the fibrillar material is changing into granular material.

Fibrillar Centers. A fibrillar center (d, in Fig. 4-9) is the less dense region that is seen to be surrounded by a thick ring of dense fibrillar material (c, in Fig. 4-9) in a thin section. The appearance of rounded cen-

ters in a section is due to a cross or oblique section having been cut through cords that are composed of some material of only moderate electron density (indicated by arrows in Fig. 4-10) which contain electron-dense chromatin threads which run along in their substance, as can be seen in Figure 4-10, where the chromatin in the cores of the cords are as electron dense as the chromatin seen outside of the nucleolus. It has been shown that after treatment with DNA-ase both the chromatin in the fibrillar centers and the chromatin of the nucleus are no longer electron dense in sections. Accordingly, the appearances seen in fibrillar centers substantiates the concept that the organizing region of a nucleolar chromosome, associated with some other material, winds its way through the dark component of the nucleolus, serving along its course to code for the formation of 45S rRNA which appears as a sheath of electron-dense fibrillar material around it.

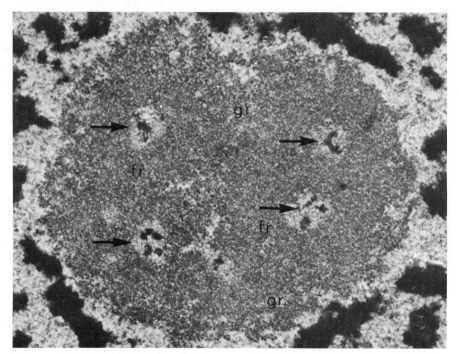

FIG. 4-10. Electron micrograph ($\times$ 22,000) of an interphase nucleus of meristemic cells of *Allium cepa* which shows fibrillar centers to advantage. Four are indicated by arrows. The fibrillar centers are seen to contain several very dark electron dense little bodies which appear to be sections cut through the chromatin thread of the nucleolus-organizing portion of a chromosome. The electron density of these is similar in this section to that of the chromatin of the nucleus which appears as very dark material scattered about around the nucleolus. The organization of the fibrillar and granular material in this type of nucleolus is different from that of the nucleolus shown in Figure 4-9, for the granular material (gr) is located around the edge and toward the center of the structure, with some in between. The fibrillar component (fr) is disposed in patches which are associated with the fibrillar centers. (Illustration courtesy L. A. Chouinard, Université Laval)

In other words it would seem that the chromatin threads that run along in fibrillar centers are the counterparts of the trunks of the "Christmas trees" shown in Figure 4-8, and that the branches of the trees become the dark fibrillar material (c in Fig. 4-8) that surrounds the centers.

If there is such a thing as a nucleolonema in a nucleolus it would probably be a cord containing the chromatin of the nucleolus-organizing segment of a nucleolar chromosome that has become ensheathed with electron-dense fibrillar material.

The Light Component of the Nucleolus: Its Nature and Origin

Light areas scattered about in thin sections of the nucleolus appear mostly as islands but around the periphery of the nucleolus they commonly are seen to be continuous with the nuclear sap (Fig. 4-9). Indeed, there is no reason to think that the light material has a composition that differs from that of the nuclear sap (which will be discussed presently) or that it is not just part of the nuclear sap. Its presence within the nucleolus is to be explained by the fact that, as a nucleolus develops, the dark component is synthesized around the threadlike nucleolar organizing segments of nucleolar chromosomes. Loops of these threads are close enough together for the dark material that forms around them to here and there fuse with that which forms around other portions of the thread or threads (which pursue convoluted courses), and so the dark material thus comes to surround areas of nuclear sap. It is therefore somewhat debatable as to whether the light component of the nucleolus should be considered part of the nucleolus or merely the nuclear sap of the region in which the spongelike nucleolus develops. The way a nucleolus forms can be studied by following through mitosis, as will next be described.

Behavior of the Structural Components of the Nucleolus During Mitosis

Clues to the functional significance of the various structural components of the nucleolus have been obtained in part through studies of the behavior of these components during the process of mitosis. As is well known, the nucleolus, as an organized entity, usually disappears from view at late prophase and is formed anew in the daughter nuclei at late telophase. Also, in the course of both nucleolar dissolution at late prophase and nucleolar reconstitution at late telophase

(in *Allium cepa*), the nucleolar body remains intimately associated with a specific region (usually referred to as the nucleolar organizing region) of a specific chromosome (the so-called nucleolar chromosome). It has been shown that in the undifferentiated embryonic cells of the onion, the interphase nucleolus is seen to be made up of a contorted loop of chromatin material extending from the nucleolar organizing region of the nucleolar chromosome; this chromatin loop (which courses along the fibrillar centers seen in sections) is invested with a coating of dense fibrillar material (pars fibrosa) which in turn is surrounded by a mantle of moderately electron-dense primarily granular material (pars granulosa). The fibrillar centers (arrows) and contained chromatin of the nucleolar organizing region are easily recognized in the section shown in Figure 4-10.

It was also found that during late prophase as an early step in the dissolution of the nucleolus, the intranucleolar chromatin loop retracts, presumably as a result of its becoming coiled (condensed). More or less at the same time there is a gradual and complete dispersion of the fibrillar granular components of the nucleolus into the surrounding nuclear sap. From early to mid telophase, the nucleolus consists of no more than the dense chromatin occupying the nucleolar organizing region of the nucleolar chromosome. Toward the end of mid telophase, this nucleolar chromatin gradually transforms (presumably through uncoiling) into a convoluted loop structure around which a dense fibrillar material (pars fibrosa) becomes deposited. Subsequent growth of the nucleolus during late telophase is accomplished partly by an increase in the amount of dense fibrillar material surrounding the chromatin loop structure and partly through the appearance of more peripherally located granular material (pars granulosa). By very late telophase, the nucleolar mass already exhibits all of the organizational features of the mature interphase nucleolus. The general conclusion that has been drawn from these observations is that the chromatin loop should be considered as the only structural component of the nucleolus showing continuity from one cell generation to the next. It has therefore been surmised that such intranucleolar chromatin contains most, if not all, of the genetic information necessary for the synthesis and aggregation of the nucleolar material.

Nuclear Sap

So far we have considered three of the main components of the nucleus: (1) the nuclear envelope, (2)

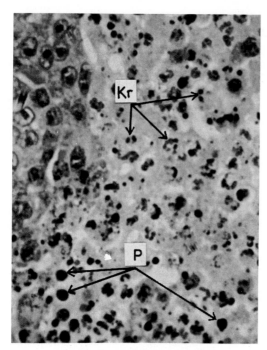

FIG. 4-11. High-power photomicrograph of a section of a malignant tumor. The cells at the left side were still alive and growing (notice their large nucleoli) when the specimen was taken, but those on the right side had died previously and, as a consequence, their nuclei had undergone changes which are indicative of these cells having died. Some nuclei have shrunken into rounded dark-staining bodies (P); this is termed *pyknosis*. Other nuclei have become broken up into fragments (Kr); this is termed *karyorrhexis*. Areas of tissue in which the cells die during life are described as constituting areas of necrosis (*nekros*, corpse). See also karyolysis (Fig. 4-12).

rapid diffusion of metabolites and the movement of ribosomal subunits, mRNA and tRNA, to the pores.

Nuclear Changes Indicative of Cell Death

It is obvious that all the cells in a section cut from fixed materials are dead. When histologists or pathologists speak of seeing "dead cells" in a section, they do not refer to these but to cells that died while the body in which they were contained was still alive.

Dead cells are encountered in a living body for two main reasons. First, in some tissues it is normal for cells to die and be replaced by others; this occurs, for example, in the outer layer of the skin. Likewise, certain of the white cells of the blood have only a short life-span and die within the body. Accordingly, in tissue removed from a healthy body, it is normal to see nuclear changes that are indicative of cell death in sites where it is normal for cells to die. Second, dead cells may be present as a result of disease. For example, an artery supplying some limited area of tissue may, as a result of disease, become plugged, and as a consequence the cells in the area supplied by the artery die from lack of oxygen and food. In such areas the nuclei of the cells at some time variously demonstrate the various changes described below. Rapidly growing cancers are prone to contain areas of dead tissue, probably because the blood supply to the rapidly growing cells is inadequate (Fig. 4-11).

Although the cytoplasm changes greatly in dead cells, the most positive indication that cells are dead is given by their nuclei. The changes here that indicate cell death are of 3 kinds. The commonest change is called *pyknosis* (dense mass). This consists of shrinkage of the nuclear material of a cell into a homogeneous hyperchromatic mass (Fig. 4-11). The student must take care not to confuse a pyknotic nucleus with a normal nucleus of the condensed chromatin type or with a poorly fixed mitotic figure. If difficulty is encountered in any instance, it is advisable to examine the cytoplasm of the cell, for, if the nucleus is dead, the cytoplasm will become altered also in some way so that it no longer has a normal appearance, as may be seen in Figure 4-11. However, in other instances death is indicated by the nucleus breaking up into fragments. This is termed *karyorrhexis*. When many nuclei break up in this fashion, nuclear "dust" may be formed (Fig. 4-11). In still other instances cell death is indicated by dissolving of the nucleus. This is termed *karyolysis* (Fig. 4-12).

chromatin and chromosomes, and (3) the nucleolus. We shall now consider briefly the fourth component of the nucleus, the *nuclear sap*. This term originated from light microscopy to denote the contents of the seemingly empty areas seen in nuclei with the LM. This was long before it was known that chromatin is immersed in the nuclear sap, where it exists in the nucleus of an interphase cell in an extended invisible form—the form in which it gives off information.

The nuclear sap is a semifluid colloidal solution that contains protein but stains poorly and does not have enough density to appear to advantage in the EM. An important function of the sap must be that of serving as a medium through which there can be both the

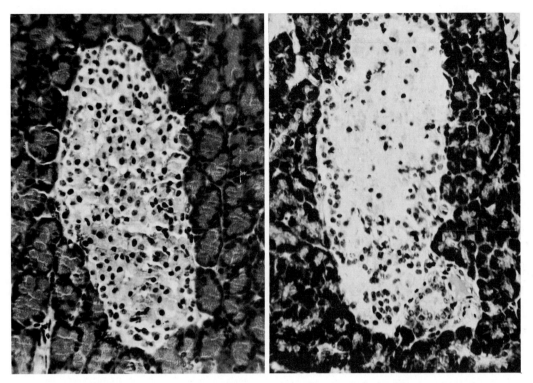

Fig. 4-12. Medium-power photomicrographs of sections of pancreas obtained from rats some hours after they had been given alloxan, a material which destroys many of the cells of the islets of Langerhans. (*Left*) The nuclei of the cells in the oval islet may be seen; there are some examples of pyknosis. (*Right*) The nuclei have mostly dissolved away; this picture illustrates karyolysis.

References and Other Reading for Chapters 3 and 4

DNA, RNA AND PROTEIN SYNTHESIS

Brown, W. V., and Bertke, E. M.: Textbook of Cytology. St. Louis, C. V. Mosby, 1969.

De Robertis, E. D. P., Nowinski, W. W., and Saez, F. A.: Cell Biology. ed. 5. Philadelphia, W. B. Saunders, 1970.

Dowben, R. M.: Cell Biology. New York, Harper & Row, 1971.

DuPraw, E. J.: The Biosciences: Cell and Molecular Biology. Cell and Molecular Biology Council, Stanford, Calif., 1972.

———: Cell and Molecular Biology, New York, Academic Press, 1968.

Lima-de-Faria, A. (ed.): Handbook of Molecular Cytology. Amsterdam, North Holland, 1969.

Loevy, A. G., and Siekevitz: Cell Structure and Function. ed. 2. New York, Holt, Rinehart and Winston, 1970.

Novikoff, A. B., and Holtzman, E.: Cells and Organelles. New York, Holt, Rinehart and Winston, 1970.

Rosenberg, E.: Cell and Molecular Biology, An Appreciation. New York, Holt, Rinehart and Winston, 1971.

Watson, J. D.: Molecular Biology of the Gene. ed. 2. New York, W. A. Benjamin, 1970.

RADIOAUTOGRAPHY

General

Leblond, C. P., and Warren, K. B. (eds.): The Use of Radioautography in Investigating Protein Synthesis, New York, Academic Press, 1965.

Special

Belanger, L. F., and Leblond, C. P.: A method for locating radioactive elements in tissues by covering histological sections with a photographic emulsion. Endocrinology, *39:*8, 1946.

Cranboulan, P.: Comparison to emulsions and techniques in electron microscope radioautography. (Page 43 in general reference given above)

Kopriwa, B. M.: A semiautomatic instrument for the radioautographic coating technique. J. Histochem. Cytochem., *14:* 923, 1966.

———: The influence of development on the number and appearance of silver grains in electron microscope radioautography. J. Histochem. Cytochem., *15:*501, 1967.

Kopriwa, B. M., and Leblond, C. P.: Improvements in the coating technique of radioautography. J. Histochem. Cytochem., *10:*269, 1962.

Pelc, S. R.: The stripping-film technique of autoradiography. Int. J. Appl. Radiat., *1:*172, 1956.

Pelc, S. R., Appleton, T. C., and Weldon, M. E.: State of light radiography. (Page 9 of the general reference given above)

Salpeter, M. M., and Bachmann, L.: Assessment of technical steps in electron microscope radioautography. (Page 23 of the general reference given above)

THE STUDY OF THE CELL CYCLE AND CELL MIGRATION BY LABELING DNA

Mazia, M.: The cell cycle. Sci. Am., *230:*54, 1974.

Messier, B., and Leblond, C. P.: Cell proliferation and migration as revealed by radioautography after the injection of thymidine-H^3 into male rats and mice. Am. J. Anat., *106:*247, 1960.

Prescott, D. M.: Comments on cell life cycle. Nat. Cancer Inst., Monographs, *14:*55, 1964.

Stanners, C. P., and Till, J. E.: DNA synthesis in individual L-strain mouse cells. Biochem. Biophys. Acta, *37:*496, 1960.

Taylor, J. H.: Chromosome reproduction. Int. Rev. Cytol., *13:*39, 1962.

————: The time and mode of duplication of chromosomes. Am. Naturalist, *91:*209, 1957.

RESPECTIVE SIGNIFICANCE OF CONDENSED AND EXTENDED CHROMATIN (INCLUDING BARR BODIES) IN THE INTERPHASE NUCLEUS

Barr, M. L.: The significance of the sex chromatin. Int. Rev. Cytol., *19:*35, 1966.

————: The sex chromosomes in evolution and in medicine. Canad. Med. Assoc. J., *95:*1137, 1966.

————: The significance of nuclear sexing. *In* Howells, J. G. (ed.): Modern Perspectives in World Psychiatry. Chapter 2, pp. 20-49. Edinburgh, Oliver & Boyd, 1968.

Barr, M. L., and Bertram, E. G.: A morphological distinction between neurons of the male and female, and the behaviour of the nucleolar satellite during accelerated nucleoprotein synthesis. Nature, *163:*676, 1949.

Bartalos, M., and Baramki, T. A.: Medical Cytogenetics. Baltimore, Williams & Wilkins, 1967.

Lewis, K. R., and John, B.: The chromosomal basis of sex determination. Int. Rev. Cytol., *23:*277, 1968.

Littau, V. C., Allfrey, V. G., Frenster, J. H., and Mirsky, A. E.: Active and inactive regions of nuclear chromatin as revealed by electron microscope autoradiography. Proc. Nat. Acad. Sci., *52:*93, 1964.

Mittwoch, Ursula: The Sex Chromosomes. New York, Academic Press, 1967.

Moore, K. L. (ed.): The Sex Chromatin. Philadelphia, W. B. Saunders, 1966.

THE NUCLEOLUS

Bernhard, W., and Granboulan, N.: Electron microscopy of the nucleolus in vertebrate cells. *In* Dalton, A. J., and Haguenau, F. (eds.): Ultrastructure in Biological Systems. vol. 3, p. 81. New York, Academic Press, 1968.

Chouinard, L. A.: Localization of intranucleolar DNA in root meristematic cells of *Allium cepa*. J. Cell Sci., *6:*73, 1970.

————: A light- and electron-microscope study of the nucleolus during growth of the oocyte in the prepubertal mouse. J. Cell Sci., *9:*637, 1971.

————: Behaviour of the Structural Components of the Nucleolus During Mitosis in *Allium cepa*. *In* Advances in Cytopharmacology. vol. 1. New York, Raven Press, 1971.

Lafontaine, J. G., and Chouinard, L. A.: A correlated light and electron microscope study of the nuclear material during mitosis in *Vicia faba*. J. Cell Biol., *17:*167, 1963.

Miller, O. L., Jr., and Beatty, B. R.: Visualization of nucleolar genes. Science, *164:*955, 1969.

Miller, O. L., Jr., Beatty, B. R., Hamkalo, B. A., and Thomas, C. A., Jr.: Electron microscopic visualization of transcription. Cold Spring Harbor Symp. Quant. Biol., *35:*505, 1970.

Miller, O. L., Jr.: The visualization of genes in action. Sci. Am., *228:*34, 1973.

Vincent, V. S., and Miller, O. J., Jr. (eds.): The Nucleolus, Its Structure and Function. Nat. Cancer Inst. Monograph No. 23, December 1966.

5 Cytoplasm and Cytoplasmic Organelles

Although the nucleus, through synthesis of specific mRNA molecules directs the kind of work a cell will do, the various kinds of specialized functions performed by interphase cells are performed by their cytoplasm.

The performance of work requires energy. This is obtained through the oxidation of foodstuffs in cytoplasm. For this to occur, both nutrients and oxygen must be absorbed by the cytoplasm of a cell from its environment. The way food and oxygen reach the environment of body cells will therefore be the first matter to be described.

How Food and O_2 Reach Body Cells

There are two steps by which food and oxygen reach the cytoplasm of cells. In the first, food and oxygen travel to the neighborhood of almost all cells by way of the bloodstream (Fig. 5-1). From small blood vessels, termed capillaries, food and oxygen then diffuse outward into the extracellular fluid (called *tissue fluid*) in which most cells live (Fig. 5-1). It is from the latter fluid that food and oxygen are absorbed by cytoplasm (Fig. 5-1).

Tissue Fluid and Intercellular Substance. The tissue fluid that exists between blood capillaries and body cells is seldom in the form of free fluid. As will be explained in detail when we study connective tissue in Chapter 8, the spaces between capillaries and body cells are filled with a combination of jellylike materials and fibers which constitute what is called *intercellular substance* (Fig. 5-1). This material is permeated and kept wet with tissue fluid through which diffusion (indicated by arrows in Fig. 5-1) between capillaries and cells can take place.

How Food and Oxygen Are Supplied to the Bloodstream

The food eaten by a person consists of three main components—proteins, carbohydrates and fats. These basic foodstuffs are digested in the gastrointestinal tract. As a result of digestion, proteins are broken down to amino acids, and these are absorbed through the lining of the intestinal tract into the bloodstream. Carbohydrates are broken down to monosaccharides, and these, too, are absorbed into the bloodstream in the intestine, and from the bloodstream both the amino acids and monosaccharides pass through capillary walls into the tissue fluid from which they are absorbed as such by cells. Fat is also broken down in the intestinal tract, but it is mostly resynthesized after it

FIG. 5-1. Diagram to show the routes by which food and oxygen in blood capillaries reach cells that are not adjacent to capillaries, and how waste products from the metabolism of cells travel in the opposite direction. Both routes depend on substances diffusing through the tissue fluid that permeates the intercellular substances between capillaries and cells. In order to enter the epithelial cells shown above, dissolved substances in the tissue fluid have to pass through the basement membrane of the epithelium, which is shown as a dark line, and then through the surrounding membrane of the epithelial cells themselves (shown as a light line).

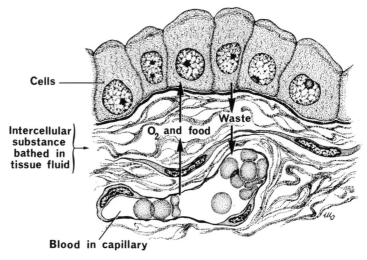

Cells

Intercellular substance bathed in tissue fluid

O_2 and food

Waste

Blood in capillary

99

is absorbed. The resynthesized fat enters the blood-stream, not directly but indirectly through lymphatic vessels (which will be described in due course) and, when it reaches the bloodstream, is in the form of tiny droplets called *chylomicrons*. The subsequent fate of these is described in connection with fat cells in Chapter 9; it is enough to say here that fatty acids become available to be absorbed by cells where they serve as nutrients.

Oxygen is absorbed into the blood in the lungs; in these organs fresh air, drawn in regularly by inspiratory movements, is separated from blood circulating through capillaries by only a thin membrane, through which oxygen diffuses. In the blood the oxygen combines with hemoglobin (which is contained in red cells). The oxygenated blood is then transported through capillaries to the vicinity of body cells (Fig. 5-1). Here the oxygen is released from the hemoglobin of the red cells and diffuses through the capillary walls into the tissue fluid, from which it is absorbed by cells (Fig. 5-1).

Waste products of metabolism that form in cells pass out into the tissue fluid and, from there, back into the bloodstream (Fig. 5-1). They are then eliminated from the blood by the kidney and other organs, as will be described later.

The General Structure of Cytoplasm

Cytoplasm is generally described as consisting physically of two main components. The first is called its *matrix* or ground substance. The word matrix is a very general sort of term which means the basic material or groundwork on or from which anything develops. The term is used with reference to the intercellular substances of cartilage, bone and dentin as well as cytoplasm, so the term refers to substances of different kinds. The matrix of cytoplasm is essentially a colloidal solution of enzymatic and nonenzymatic proteins which varies in viscosity and contains various soluble substances that have been absorbed by the cell and others that are being excreted by the cell. The matrix of cytoplasm serves as the material in which formed structures which are mostly what are termed *organelles* are housed. However, in addition to organelles, there are in some kinds of cells accumulations in the cytoplasmic matrix of materials termed *inclusions,* such as stored glycogen or fat, pigments of various sorts and so on, all of which will be described at the end of this chapter. We shall next describe and discuss the more important structures—the organelles.

The Organelles

An organ is defined as a particular part of the body in which some important special function is segregated. Thus the lung, liver, kidney, thyroid gland, etc. are all regarded as organs, for each has a specialized structure and function to enable it to play a different role in the body. Likewise, the term *organelle* (*little organ*) refers to different structures variously located in the cytoplasmic matrix in or by which various special functions, including those essential to the life and metabolism of the cells, are carried out. As will be explained presently, most of the organelles are membranous structures. Most of the information about them is of relatively recent origin; when the first edition of this book was published in 1950, the cytoplasmic organelles could be described in a few pages, whereas today so much is known about them that an adequate description of an organelle of the cytoplasm may take as much space as a description of the structure and function of some of the organs of the body.

The elucidation of the nature, structure, distribution and function of the various cell organelles became possible only with the development of modern methods. These include (1) electron microscopy; (2) various cell fractionation procedures which allowed biochemists to isolate from disrupted cells, in relatively pure form, the various cell organelles that had been recognized by electron microscopy and, consequently, to study the particular metabolic reactions with which each of the organelles was concerned; and, finally, (3) radioautography, which enabled direct studies to be made on the metabolic reactions that occurred in various organelles. These technics will all be described in due course.

The major membranous cytoplasmic organelles are:

(1) The cell or plasma membrane
(2) Mitochondria
(3) The rough endoplasmic reticulum (rER)
(4) The Golgi apparatus
(5) Lysosomes
(6) Coated vesicles
(7) The smooth endoplasmic reticulum (sER)

The nonmembranous organelles are:

    (1) Free ribosomes
    (2) Microtubules
    (3) Centrioles, cilia and flagella
    (4) Filaments and fibrils

Some of the nonmembranous organelles may be associated with membranes. Thus the cilia and flagella are partially enclosed by the cell membrane and at least some types of filaments and fibrils may be attached to membranes. Centrioles and microtubules have already been considered to some extent in the discussion of mitosis (Chapter 2). Likewise, ribosomes were dealt with extensively in the previous chapter. We shall, however, consider these organelles somewhat further in this one.

Since so many of the organelles are membranous structures, we shall first discuss the importance of membranes.

The Importance of Membranes

If all the enzymes and substances within a cell were allowed to mix freely, the metabolic reactions on which the life and function of cells depend could not occur; indeed, the cytoplasm would soon be liquefied and dead. Life is possible in cells only if various enzymes and substances are kept from mixing freely, and this is done by means of membranes. The membranes that serve this purpose within the cell are the delicate walls of the membranous organelles; thus the contents of a membranous organelle are chemically different from the cytoplasmic matrix in which it lies. The membranous walls of organelles are such that they selectively restrain the passage of certain molecules or inorganic ions through them while permitting the passage of others. Many enzymes are firmly bound to membranes and are disposed in orderly arrays within or along the membranes, an arrangement that permits products of the reactions they catalyze to be segregated to the proper side of the membrane.

The fact that so many fluids of different composition are separated from one another in the body has led to a terminology whereby the different media that are separated from one another are said to be in different *compartments*. Thus the blood, which is confined in blood vessels, is said to comprise one compartment, the tissue (extracellular) fluid, another compartment and the matrix of the cytoplasm still another. All these compartments are separated from one another by membranes of one kind or another. Within the cytoplasm are still further compartments, because the contents of various membranous organelles are separated from the matrix of the cytoplasm by membranous walls.

We shall begin our study of the organelles of cytoplasm by describing the membrane that segregates the matrix of the cytoplasm from tissue fluid.

The Cell Membrane (Also Called the Plasma Membrane or Plasmalemma)

Can the Cell Membrane Be Seen With the LM? In the usual diagram of a single cell it is customary to indicate the periphery of the cell with a dark line and this is sometimes labeled the "cell membrane." However, if the surface of a free cell is examined in a section there is no indication of a membrane at the free edge of the cell—all one sees is the edge of the cell. Next, in drawings of groups of cells the borders between adjacent ones are usually indicated by dark lines, as in Figure 2-3. Such illustrations, while useful in many respects, tend to give the impression of the existence of a cell membrane that can be seen readily with the LM is much more substantial than it really is. Actually, the cell membrane is only about 95 Å thick; hence, it is much too thin for a cross section of it to be resolved with the LM. Indeed, the borders between the cells of liver cords, as is shown in Figure 1-11 (see label: cell boundaries not apparent) are often not seen, as you will observe when H and E sections are studied in the laboratory. We are, therefore, led to ask what is responsible for the dark lines that are sometimes seen between adjacent cells.

Although it complicates the discussion somewhat, it should first be explained that the cell membranes of adjacent cells are not in *continuous* direct contact with one another. The space between them, which is somewhat wider than each of the membranes that border it, is generally filled with a carbohydrate-rich material, the nature of which will be described later, under "cell coat." This material constitutes the filling of a sandwich, with the slices of bread being represented by the cell membranes of adjacent cells. However, this sandwich made of cell membranes with its filling would still be too thin for a cross section of it to be resolved with the LM (Fig. 5-2, Invis.). Why is it then sometimes seen in a stained section? The reason is that it absorbs stain and, if the stained sandwich slants through the substance of the section, its slanting sides may provide large enough expanses of color to see (as is shown in Fig. 5-2, Vis.). It must be remembered that a paraffin section is roughly half as thick as the cells through which it is cut. There is then, speaking relatively, a considerable distance for a sandwich to pass as it extends from the top of a paraffin section to its bottom.

How Cell Membranes Appear in the EM. The EM easily allows a single cell membrane (which is around 95 Å in thickness) to be identified as a distinct entity when it is cut at an angle approaching a cross section. In the earlier days of electron microscopy, a cell membrane cut at right angles to the section, or even at an angle approaching a right angle, appeared in a micrograph as a single dark line. As methods of fixation were improved further and better electron microscopes were made, it became apparent that if a cell membrane passed from the top to the bottom of an

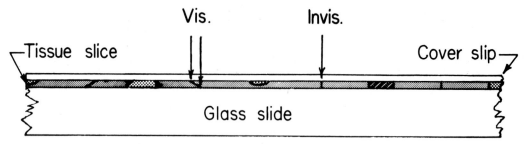

FIG. 5-2. Diagram to show that a stained cell membrane which is too thin for its cross section to be resolved (Invis.) can be seen in a section if it passes through the section at an angle other than a right angle, for then its stained side is seen over a large enough area for it to be visible (Vis.).

ultrathin section exactly at or approaching a right angle to the plane of section, it showed up in a micrograph as two dark lines with a light line between them as is shown in Figure 5-3. This appearance has been interpreted as indicating that the cell membrane has a trilamellar (*lamella,* a thin leaf or plate) structure with its outer and inner layers (lamellae) having a similar composition and its middle layer a different chemical composition.

Unit Membrane. The type of trilamellar membrane seen in the electron microscope became known as the *unit membrane.* The same trilamellar type of structure can be found in the membranes of all the membranous cytoplasmic organelles. The latter membranes, being about 70 Å thick, are somewhat thinner than the cell membrane, which is about 95 Å thick. They are also slightly different in their chemical composition and have different enzymes associated with them, depending on the organelle from which they come. Some of the enzymes that different organelle membranes contain are characteristic for the organelle and thus help-

ful in isolating, assaying and identifying various membranous organelles encountered after cell fractionation procedures.

The appearance of a unit membrane in an electron micrograph depends on the angle at which it passes from the top to the bottom of an ultrathin section. Depending on this angle, a membrane may be (1) almost invisible, or appear as (2) a fuzzy dark line, or (3) a fairly distinct dark line or (4) a trilamellar structure as in Figure 5-3.

In considering why this should be so it must be remembered that everything in a section examined in the EM is in focus at the same time, and that contrast is seen in the EM only because some things encountered in a section as the electron beam passes through it are more electron-dense and so scatter more electrons than other things that are beside them. With this in mind we shall now refer to the examples shown in Figure 5-4, in which it is assumed that an electron beam is directed from above and passes through a trilamellar membrane that is disposed at various angles to the

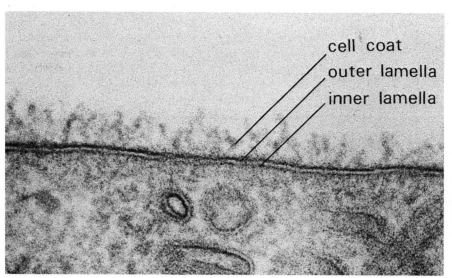

FIG. 5-3. High resolution electron micrograph of a cell membrane and cell coat. The trilaminar unit membrane structure consisting of a dense inner lamella, a dense outer lamella and a light staining lamella between the two is clearly visible. Cell coat covers the cell membrane on the outside. × 200,000. (From M. Weinstock, Dept. of Anatomy, McGill University)

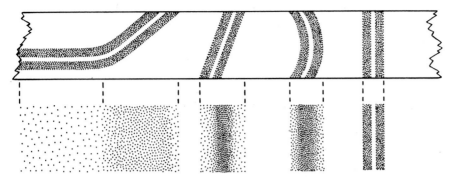

Fɪɢ. 5-4. Diagram illustrating why cell membranes seen in electron micrographs may not always show the trilaminar unit membrane structure. The upper part shows cell membranes passing through a section at various angles and the lower part shows the corresponding images seen in the electron microscope. Note that a typical unit membrane appearance is seen only when the membrane passes through the section at right angles to the plane of the section (far right). See text for more detailed explanation.

plane of the section. What is seen in a micrograph is shown immediately below each example.

First, at the left, the membrane is parallel with the section so that the electron beam would pass through just the thickness of the membrane. The membrane is so very thin that this would not scatter many electrons. The site of the membrane would, therefore, not appear greatly different from sites where a membrane was not present, as is shown beneath the section.

Next (moving to the right), the membrane is shown to slant through the section. Here electrons would have to pass through more membrane substance than where the membrane was flat. As is shown by moving still further to the right in Figure 5-4, more and more electrons are scattered as the angle of the membrane approaches 90°. A membrane that passes through the section at close to 90° could scatter enough electrons to appear as a single dark line. A membrane that passed from the top of the section to the bottom at approximately a right angle, but pursued a slightly curving course would also appear as a dark line but with fuzzy edges (Fig. 5-4). Finally only a straight membrane that passed through the section at a 90° angle to it would reveal its trilamellar structure, because in such a preparation the middle layer of the membrane would not scatter as many electrons as the more electron-dense layers on each of its sides (Fig. 5-4, *right*).

RELATION OF APPEARANCE OF MEMBRANES IN THE EM TO PRESENT-DAY CONCEPTS OF MEMBRANOUS STRUCTURES

Development of Knowledge. Early physiological experiments showed that cells in solutions of various osmotic pressures would swell or shrink in a fashion that indicated they must be surrounded by a membrane with special permeability properties. It was also noted that the cell membrane was in general permeable to materials that were soluble in lipid. Experimental data of many kinds, as well as theoretical considerations, led to the concept of the membrane for the most part being composed of an inner and an outer layer of protein separated by a middle layer of lipid, more specifically by two rows of phospholipid molecules arranged more or less perpendicular to the surface of the membrane so that their nonpolar or hydrophobic ends meet, and their polar ends are next to the protein layers.

The above described classic concept of the membrane was well established before cell membranes could be studied in the EM. When the EM became available cell membranes were seen as single black lines. Since osmium was used to blacken fats for LM studies, and since osmium tetroxide was the common fixative used for electron microscopy, it was assumed that the single black line seen with the EM was due to the middle lipid layer being rendered electron-dense by the osmium and that the protein layers on either side of it were probably not stained sufficiently by osmium to be made visible.

Consequently, as the EM and fixing and staining methods all improved, and the membrane was revealed as a trilamellar structure (Fig. 5-3), it was disturbing to find that even after osmium fixation it appeared to be the two outer protein layers that were electron-dense and not the middle layer, as had been assumed. The reasons for the electron density of the layers of the unit membrane after osmium fixation being more or less the opposite of what might be expected were not entirely clear. It seems perhaps that only the polar hydrophilic ends of the lipid molecules—that is, those in contact with the protein layers—combine with osmium. Or it may be that the osmium dissolves the lipid after it is stained and that it then is absorbed by the protein on either side of it, thus producing the two black lines.

Some Physical Attributes of the Cell Membrane. The cell membrane is not permeable to protein macromolecules; hence, the protein sols of the cell cannot escape into the tissue fluid. But the protein sols in the cell exert osmotic pressure, and this would continuously draw water into the cell if the tissue fluid did not contain other substances in solution to counterbalance the osmotic pressure generated by colloids within the cell. The counterbalancing factor is the osmotic pressure exerted by the greater concentration of inorganic ions outside the cell than inside it, and for this to be maintained requires that some mechanism must exist to maintain different concentrations of inorganic ions on the two sides of the membrane. The different concentration of inorganic ions on the two sides of the membrane brings up another factor—namely, that since ions bear electrical charges, there is a difference in electrical potential between the two sides of the membrane (in muscle cells this can be 85 millivolts), with the tissue fluid side being more positive than the cytoplasmic side. For a difference of electrical potential to exist, a cell membrane would have to possess dielectric properties. This property, as well as another property, namely that the membrane is relatively permeable to substances that dissolve in lipids, fitted with the concept of the membrane's having a substantial content of lipid, because lipid has good dielectric properties.

Whereas the amount of some dissolved substances present on either side of the membrane can be accounted for by the fact that the substances pass by virtue of diffusion from sites of high concentration to sites of low concentration, the passage of many dissolved substances and inorganic ions through the membrane cannot be explained in this way—as, for example, the higher concentration of Na ions on the outside of the membrane and the higher concentration of K ions on the inner side.

An important factor in accounting for the difference in the concentration of sodium and potassium ions inside and outside the cell is believed to be what is termed the *sodium pump.* In its operation, which requires energy supplied by the cell, it pumps sodium ions out through the cell membrane and hence keeps the concentration of sodium ions lower on the inner than on the outer side of the membrane. The sodium pump is believed to transport ions by means of carrier molecules located in the cell membrane. Carrier molecules likewise pick up K ions on the outside of the membrane and release these on the inner side of the membrane, but they may not carry as many K ions inward as they do Na ions outward.

It is also believed that glucose, amino acids and fatty acids also require special mechanisms to transport them from the tissue fluid into the cytoplasmic matrix, and that most of these mechanisms require the expenditure of energy. The mechanisms are believed to depend on carriers in the cell membrane. Such mechanisms are spoken of as *active transport mechanisms.*

If the middle layer of the membrane was a continuous layer of lipid it was, of course, difficult to understand how any substances not soluble in lipid could be transported through it. The existence of pores a few Å in diameter was proposed, and these were believed, for example, to permit the passage of water and small ions. But the regulated passage of substances not soluble in lipid through the cell membrane would be easily explained if there was continuity between two protein layers of the membrane so that substances would not necessarily have to pass through the lipid to gain entrance to the cell. In this connection modifica-

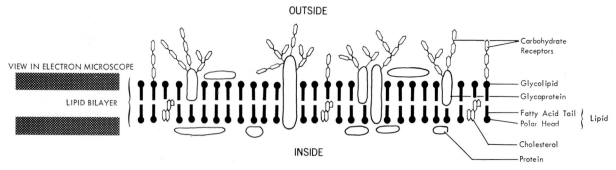

FIG. 5-5. Diagram of cell membrane. (Provided by V. Kalnins)

tions of the classic concept of the cell membrane have been proposed in which the position of some protein molecules is such that they run all the way from one side of the membrane right through to the other (Fig. 5-5). A number of findings that have been made recently indicate that protein molecules actually do extend through the membrane in this way. These findings were made by means of electron microscopy used in combination with the freeze-etch technic (see Footnote *) and by improvements in the technics of biochemical analysis of membrane structure. The former revealed small globular bodies embedded in the middle (lipid) layer of the membrane (Fig. 5-6) which are digested by trypsin (an enzyme that digests protein), and these little protein globular bodies could provide the protein continuity between the outer and inner protein layers of the membrane. Furthermore, recent biochemical studies have indicated that some of the same glycoproteins of the membrane become labeled when either the outer or the inner surface of the membrane is exposed to the label. This indicates that some of the glycoprotein molecules must pass right through the membrane and that parts of these molecules are exposed on either surface. Such molecules are illustrated in Figure 5-5. Some of these proteins could be the enzymes which participate in the active transport mechanisms that operate through the membrane.

Still another feature of the membrane has recently come to light—that is, there may be certain differences

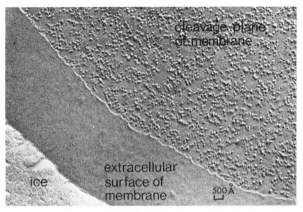

FIG. 5-6. An electron micrograph of a carbon-platinum replica of an erythrocyte membrane which had been frozen directly in liquid nitrogen, cleaved by a knife, and the ice allowed to sublime in a vacuum for a few seconds before the carbon-platinum replica was made. The residual extracellular water (now ice) is seen in the lower left; the smooth extracellular surface of the membrane is seen where the ice has sublimed away; the central plane of the membrane has been cleaved, exposing 90-Å-wide globules moving around in the plane of the membrane. These globules are protein, since they can be digested by proteinases; the smooth areas between the globules is mostly lipid arranged in a bilayer. (Preparation by P. Seeman)

* *The Freeze-Etch Technic.* It is possible to obtain a view of various cell surfaces by means of what is termed the freeze-etch or freeze-fracture-replica technic. Although the technic is elaborate, the essentials are that a small piece of tissue is frozen rapidly in liquid nitrogen and transferred to an apparatus in which a vacuum can be produced, and in which the piece of tissue can be fractured so that a tissue surface resulting from having a portion of frozen tissue split away from it is exposed. These fractures in the tissue usually occur along membranes in such a way that the membranes are split in half and the interior of membranes is exposed. The vacuum is then usually allowed to act on the surface of the still frozen fractured piece of tissue for a very brief period, during which it becomes etched because of the vacuum evaporating ice from it. This etching exposes the outside surface features of the membranes as well as the surfaces that were split in the fracturing step. All the surfaces thus exposed are then covered with a thin deposit obtained by evaporating a metal over them in the apparatus; this can be so done that the mist that evaporates from the metal is, as it were, sprayed from an angle onto the fractured and etched surface, and as a result more of the metallic mist is deposited on one side of any structure that projects from the surface than is deposited on the other side (the latter side is said to be in the shadow). After a shadowed replica of the fractured and etched surface is thus obtained, the tissue is then digested away and the metal replica, after washing and mounting on a grid, is examined in the EM. No fixation or sectioning is required with this method.

between the inner and the outer parts of the membrane. In other words, the cell membrane is not the symmetrical structure suggested by its appearance in electron micrographs as two stained dense lamellae with an unstained lamella between. For example, all of the carbohydrate portions of the glycoprotein and the glycolipid molecules are found on the outer surface of the membrane (Fig. 5-5) and form what is known as the cell coat, which will be described in greater detail later on. The outer surface of the membrane also contains various molecules or groups of molecules called receptors (Fig. 5-5) which interact with specific molecules in the environment of the cell so that the cell is triggered into action or shut down if it is already active. It has been found that besides proteins and lipids, most membranes contain a significant amount of cholesterol and most of this seems to be disposed in the inner half of the membrane (Fig. 5-5). More recent evidence indicates that the proteins of the outer and inner lamellae are different and hence that, in this respect as well, the two sides of the membrane are not identical (*see* Fox). Occasionally it can even be seen directly by electron microscopy that the membrane is asymmetrical. For example, the membrane of the cells that line the urinary bladder does not stain evenly, for the outer lamella of the membrane that abuts on the lumen of the bladder stains much more densely than the inner lamella that faces the cytoplasm of the lining cells.

With what has been said already about interpreting the appearances presented by membranes in ordinary electron micrographs, it will be appreciated that if a cell membrane was constructed according to the model described in Figure 5-5 and disposed in a section so that it passed through the section at right angles, an electron micrograph of the section would show a 3-layered structure as in Figure 5-3 because in this model most of the middle layer is lipid and the relatively small amount of protein in the middle layer would not constitute a sufficient amount of electron-dense material to scatter many electrons and so reveal its presence.

Phagocytosis. The term phagocytosis (*phagein,* to eat; *osis,* a process) refers to the process by which a cell takes a particle or macromolecular aggregate of some sort from its exterior into its substance. The way phagocytosis occurs is illustrated in Figure 5-7. Essentially what happens is that when the cell membrane comes into contact with a particle (Fig. 5-7, *left*), the particle becomes engulfed by it and thus becomes surrounded on all sides by membrane so that it is, in effect, contained within the cytoplasmic matrix in a little membranous bag that is called a *vesicle* (a little sac or bladder). The membranous vesicle with the particle it contains becomes detached from the cell membrane and sinks into the cytoplasmic matrix.

In Phagocytosis the Inner Lamella of the Cell Membrane Becomes the Outer Lamella of the

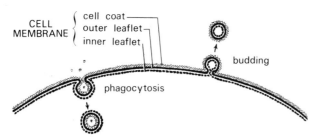

FIG. 5-7. Diagram illustrating the phagocytosis and budding. Pinocytosis, the uptake of fluid by the cell, occurs by a process similar to that of phagocytosis. Note that in phagocytosis or pinocytosis the outer lamella of the cell membrane becomes the inner lamella of the membrane of the vesicle that forms while the inner lamella of the cell membrane becomes the outer lamella of the membrane of the vesicle. But budding from the cell or any membranous structure within the cell does *not* result in a reversal of the lamellae of the membrane from which budding occurs.

Vesicular Membrane. The process of phagocytosis illustrates an important fact about the "sidedness" of any membranous structure that develops from the cell membrane as an invagination. This is illustrated in Figure 5-7 in which the outer lamella of the cell membrane is indicated by a solid line and the inner lamella of the cell membrane is indicated by a dotted line. It is readily apparent that it is the inner lamella of the cell membrane that becomes the outer lamella of the vesicular membrane. It should be noted that in the instance of both the cell membrane and the vesicular membrane the lamella of the membrane that faces the cytoplasm is the same lamella (the inner one of the cell membrane).

Pinocytosis. This term (*pinein,* to drink) refers to the phenomenon by which very tiny droplets of fluid are taken in through the cell membrane by a mechanism identical with that of phagocytosis (Fig. 5-7). The vesicles formed in this instance are termed *pinocytotic vesicles.* The importance of pinocytosis will be discussed in more detail when we later consider capillaries.

The Cell Coat

Development of Knowledge. Plant cells, it will be recalled, live in compartments. Carbohydrate is either an important component or the chief component of compartment walls. The cell membranes of bacteria are coated with a carbohydrate material which is of physiological importance; for example, if their cell coats are removed, the bacteria are affected by solutions of osmotic pressures that would not affect them if their coats were intact. In the 1930's Chambers demonstrated the existence of a coat of unknown nature on the cell membranes of egg cells and suggested that many body cells would be shown to possess similar coats. Ten years later he intimated that many of the physical properties hitherto believed to be attributes of the cell surface would be found to be due to extraneous coatings. Later, with the advent of the PA-Schiff technic and other methods for demonstrating glycoproteins, several observers found that many of the cells lining surfaces inside the body had on their free surface a thin layer of glycoprotein material. Such findings, however, did not necessarily prove the existence of a cell coat in these sites, for it is common for secreted mucus to adhere closely to epithelial cells. With the advent of the EM more convincing evidence appeared and many cell types were demonstrated to possess a cell coat (Fig. 5-3). The microvilli of the intestine (microvilli are tiny fingerlike processes covered with cell membrane, which project from the free surfaces of lining absorptive cells and thus increase the absorptive area of the free surface) are covered with a particularly thick and easily demonstrable cell coat which appears as a "fuzz" and is composed of a layer of material of low electron density containing numerous fine filaments (Fig. 5-8) which are very closely associated with the cell membrane.

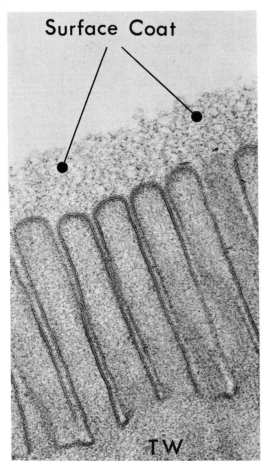

FIG. 5-8. Electron micrograph ($\times$ 75,000) of part of a section of an epithelial lining cell of cat small intestine. The unit membrane of the surface of the cell that abuts on the lumen of the intestine is thrown into fingerlike projections that are parallel and close to one another; these are microvilli. Between adjacent microvilli, and on the free surfaces of their tips, there is a coat of a fibrillar-appearing material that comprises the surface coat; this provides a covering for the unit membrane that in turn covers the microvilli. The three layers of the unit membrane may be seen in many sites. The cytoplasm of the cell at the bases of the microvilli is fibrillar and reveals no organelles; this part of the cytoplasm is termed the terminal web (TW). (Electron micrograph courtesy of Dr. Susumu Ito)

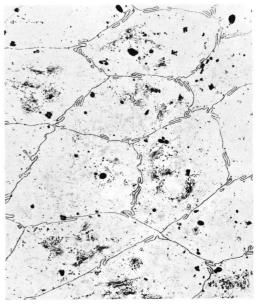

FIG. 5-9. Electron micrograph ($\times$ 2,600) of oblique section cut through epithelial cells of intestine and stained by the PA-silver methenamine technic for glycoproteins. The black lines between adjacent cells represent the staining of the material of the cell coats of the cells. Notice also how cells interdigitate with one another. The nuclei of cells are not visible in this type of preparation. (Preparation courtesy of C. P. Leblond and A. Rambourg)

It was one matter to accept the existence of a cell coat on free wet epithelial surfaces; it was another to accept the idea of a carbohydrate-containing cell coat being a heritage that all or almost all body cells demonstrate to some degree. Nevertheless, observations suggesting this began to accumulate and in 1967 Rambourg and Leblond undertook an extensive study inquiring into the possibilities of the universality of the coat in body cells. They examined over 50 different types of body cells in rats and found that all of the 50 types of cells examined had demonstrable cell coats which appeared as thin films along all their surfaces, whether these surfaces abutted on the surfaces of other cells (as is shown in Fig. 5-9) or basement membranes, or were free. One exception was found: the cell coat was not seen at sites between adjacent cells where they form special types of junctions (to be described in a later section). (It should be emphasized here that in most cases special technics are required to demonstrate the cell coat; hence, it is not seen in routine electron micrographs.)

Nature of the Cell Coat. The cell coat has been studied both by histochemical technics with both the

LM and the EM and by the biochemical analysis of material which can be obtained from cell surfaces after treatment of cells with various enzymes. The use of the PA-Schiff technic with the LM and the PA-silver technic with the EM indicates that the coat contains carbohydrate. Since it also stains with colloidal thorium, it is believed that the carbohydrate(s) it contains are rich in acidic groups. Chemical studies have led to the identification of sialic acid as one of the major components of the cell coat. The probable conclusion is that the cell coat is made up predominantly of sialic-acid-containing glycoproteins. Most of these glycoproteins are anchored in the cell membrane just below the cell coat as shown in Figure 5-5 so that their sialic-acid-rich carbohydrate chains and a part of the protein molecule to which they are anchored project out into the cell coat. The carbohydrate chains of glycolipids also seem to project into the cell coat area. Thus there appears to be a very intimate relationship between the cell coat and the cell membrane just below it.

Function of the Cell Coat. As will be described in more detail later, the cell coat probably acts as an adhesive, helping to hold cells together, often in very specific manner. It is interesting that most of the cell coat can be removed from the cells and they still remain viable and can regenerate it in a relatively short period of time. If, on the other hand, even small holes are made in the cell membrane, the cell dies. It probably plays an important role in the ability of cells to recognize cells of their own special kind and to form aggregates with them. As Moscona has shown, if cells of different kinds and from the same animal are dissociated and placed together in a culture medium, the cells of one special kind, such as cartilage cells, seek out each other and adhere to one another. Indeed, cells of the same specialized type but from different species recognize each other much better than the cells of the same species but of different specialized types, for cartilage cells from different species associate better together than they do with other kinds of specialized cells from the same animal.

Formation and Maintenance of the Cell Coat. This matter will be discussed in connection with the Golgi apparatus.

The Cell Surface: Definition and Properties. Before it was established that mammalian cells had cell coats, the term cell surface was used to refer to the outer surface of the outer lamella of the cell membrane. The fact that this surface is now known to be covered with a coat has led to the term now often being used to refer to a complex of what was formerly considered as the cell surface plus the cell coat. One

reason for this broad concept of a surface is that cells recognize one another and associate with one another as was described above because of their surface properties. It is also by their surfaces that foreign cells (for example, of transplants from other individuals) are recognized in the body so that immunological mechanisms are set into operation which can lead to their rejection. The surface by which a cell is recognized seems to depend on the molecules of the cell coat and those molecules of the cell membrane that are exposed at the surface. Both are responsible for the properties of the particular surfaces different cells present to other cells.

Surface Flow. It is possible experimentally to bring about fusions between two different kinds of cells and when this is done it has been found that certain characteristic molecules on the surface of one of the cells mix quickly with the molecules present on the surface of the other cell that fused with it (these can be identified by immunological means). Within an hour the molecules intermix to such an extent that it is impossible to tell which part of the cell surface had come from which cell. Experiments of this sort have been interpreted to indicate that the cell surface in at least a number of cells is normally not static but fluidlike in nature and that molecules can flow from one portion of it to another with ease.

The Order To Be Followed in Describing the Other Organelles. Many of the organelles function similarly to the different parts of a production line in that a basic product made at the beginning of the line is altered or modified in various ways as it is carried along the line and its branches—that is, to and through other organelles. Hence, so far as possible, we shall discuss the organelles in an order that will allow some of the products that are formed to be followed readily from their beginnings to their completion. We shall, however, begin with the one that provides the energy for the others to operate.

Mitochondria

Introduction. Near the beginning of this chapter it was noted that the energy required for the life and function of cells is almost entirely derived from the oxidation of nutrients—a process that takes place in cytoplasm; this therefore requires that nutrients and oxygen pass from the tissue fluid through the membranes of cells to enter the cytoplasm (Fig. 5-1). It should now be pointed out that the ability to oxidize nutrients is not an attribute of cytoplasm as a whole; instead it is a function that is delegated to the membranous organelles which were long ago termed *mito-*

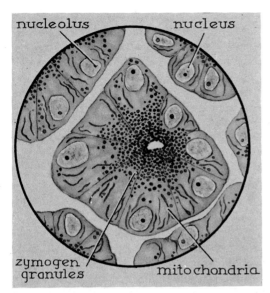

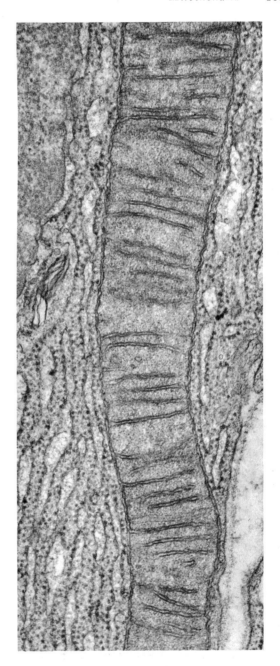

Fig. 5-10. (*Left*) A high-power drawing made with the LM of a pancreatic acinus stained with aniline acid fuchsin and methyl green. Long mitochondria are present toward the bases of the acinar cells. (Preparation courtesy of S. H. Bensley) (*Right*) An electron micrograph of a portion of an acinar cell near its base and beside the nucleus; this illustrates the fine structure of a part of one of the long mitochondria seen in this position. (Preparation courtesy of H. Warshawsky)

chondria because of their threadlike (*mitos,* thread) appearance in studies made with the LM (Fig. 5-10).

It is now known that mitochondria house the chains of enzymes responsible for what is termed *cell respiration*. These enzymes of mitochondria catalyze reactions that provide the cell as a whole with an energy-rich compound known as adenosine triphosphate (ATP). This compound accomplishes its energy-providing function in various parts of the cell by transplanting one of its energetic terminal phosphate groups to another molecule. The ATP is thereby changed to adenosine diphosphate (ADP). This reaction allows compounds to be synthesized which would not be made in the absence of an energy-providing reaction resulting from the breakdown of ATP. Within mitochondria ADP is, as it were, recharged by the addition of another phosphate group to become ATP again and so is able again to perform its energy-providing function.

Since mitochondria through their production of ATP are responsible for providing most (but not all, as will be explained presently) of the energy required for the cell, they are often referred to as the power-houses of the cell. Further details of their function in relation to their structure will be given later. Here, however, we must describe their structure, first as it was studied with the LM and later with the EM.

Early Studies With the LM. In the latter half of the last century a few microscopists sometimes noticed what seemed to be tiny bodies in cytoplasm, which varied from being round to rod-shaped. However, with the staining methods then available and even with most stains used today, including H and E, they were seldom demonstrable.

Near the end of the century Altmann managed to stain these little bodies regularly and selectively using acid fuchsin. A drawing (Fig. 5-10, *left*) of a portion of a section stained by a variation of this technic shows some rod-shaped mitochondria. Altmann was thus able to demonstrate the little bodies in a great variety of cells. He termed them bioblasts and suggested that they were of the nature of elementary forms of life that were present in all kinds of cells and that, like bacteria which they resemble, they were probably capable of independent existence. His contemporaries, however, were mostly antagonistic to his views and as a result he became so withdrawn that he avoided others to the point that he was referred to as "the ghost" in the laboratory. His career ended sadly. Curiously enough new evidence, soon to be described, and obtainable only with modern knowledge and methods, is providing support to some extent for his prophetic views.

Studies With Supravital Stains. In this century it was found that mitochondria could be demonstrated in fresh, unfixed tissue by what are known as supravital stains. For these to act, a cell must be alive, because the stain combines with a cell component selectively only because of a particular vital process occurring in the cell component with which it combines. The supravital stain most commonly used for mitochondria is a weak solution of Janus green and it imparts a transient blue-green color to the mitochondria which can be detected between the time the stain is applied and the time when the cell dies.

Studies With the Phase Microscope. By the time the phase contrast microscope became available, many laboratories had tissue culture facilities which provided single layers of flattened-out living cells which were very suitable for examination with this microscope. With this instrument, which enhances contrast between cell components that are roughly similar in optical densities, mitochondria can be seen readily and their behavior in a living cell investigated. Such studies showed that they constantly move and often change their shapes. This feature of the mitochondria is strikingly illustrated in the micrographs of living cells shown in Figure 5-11.

Separation From Cell Homogenates by Means of Differential Centrifugation. The revered cytologist R. R. Bensley, who had long ago been interested in mitochondria, with Hoerr in 1934, was able to separate mitochondria from homogenized cells by differential centrifugation. This technic has been greatly improved through the years and now almost all the cell organelles

seen inside cells by electron microscopy can be isolated in a relatively pure form by variations of this method. The basic method is illustrated in Figure 5-12 and summarized below (see Footnote *). The fact that this had become possible, plus the rapid development of knowledge in enzyme chemistry, enabled biochemists to study the enzymes of mitochondrial fractions and, as a result of studies made on separated mitochondria, it was established that they house the enzymes concerned in the oxidation of foodstuffs.

Studies With the EM. About the midpoint of this century both Palade and Sjostrand were able to prepare sections for the EM which showed mitochondria to be membranous structures. It was revealed that they were vesicles bounded by two membranes, and outer and an inner, separated by a space about 80 Å wide (Figs. 5-13 and 5-15 and in a diagrammatic form in Fig. 5-14). The membranes are of the unit type, about 70 Å thick and hence slightly thinner than the cell membrane (Fig. 5-13). The outer membrane is

* Cell fractionation illustrated in Figure 5-12 has become a potent technic for enabling biochemists to isolate the different cell organelles in a relatively pure form which allows them to determine their chemical composition and enzyme content and from these facts draw conclusions about their function in the cell. As a first step the cells are disrupted by homogenization in a suitable medium that preserves the organelles and prevents them from aggregating. Very often this is a sucrose solution. Although mitochondria and other cell organelles remain intact, interconnected networks of membranes as well as the cell membrane get broken into fragments which form rounded vesicles of variable size by this procedure. As a next step the cell homogenate is subjected to a series of centrifugations of increasing speed and duration, a process called differential centrifugation. Depending on their size, density and shape, different organelles sediment at the bottom of the centrifuge tube at different speeds. The structures that are large and dense, such as nuclei, sediment most rapidly, whereas smaller, less dense structures, such as vesicles of endoplasmic reticulum, require higher speeds and longer times to sediment. Therefore at the lower speeds nuclei will sediment while the other cell organelles remain in suspension. At higher speeds the mitochondria and lysosomes will be sedimented and at very high speeds and long periods of centrifugation even particles as small as ribosomes will form a pellet. The pellets thus obtained are then examined by electron microscopy to determine how pure the fractions are. All fractions are contaminated by other organelles to some extent. If sufficient purity has been achieved, the fractions can then be subjected to biochemical analysis to determine their chemical composition and enzymatic activities.

More recently a technic of cell fractionation called density gradient centrifugation has been introduced in which the centrifugation is done through layers of sucrose of increasing concentrations and therefore of increasing densities. During centrifugation the organelles of the homogenate position themselves at those levels in the centrifuge tubes where their density matches the density of the sucrose solution. This technic has enabled biochemists to separate organelles of similar size but of different densities.

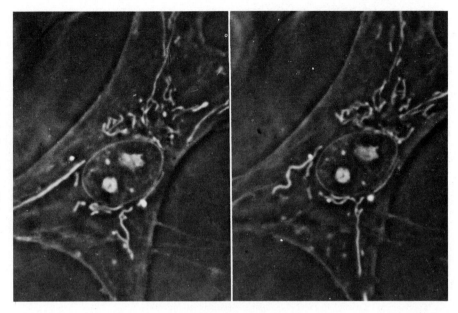

Fɪɢ. 5-11. Changes in the shape of mitochondria in living fibroblasts as seen by light microscopy using negative phase contrast. The two figures show the same cell photographed 4 minutes apart. The nucleus, easily recognizable, contains two nucleoli and is limited by the nuclear envelope. Note the remarkable changes in the shape of the mitochondria especially in the region below and to the left of the nucleus. × 2,440. (From M. Chèvremont, Cytologie et Histologie ed. 2. p. 142. Liège, Desoer, 1966)

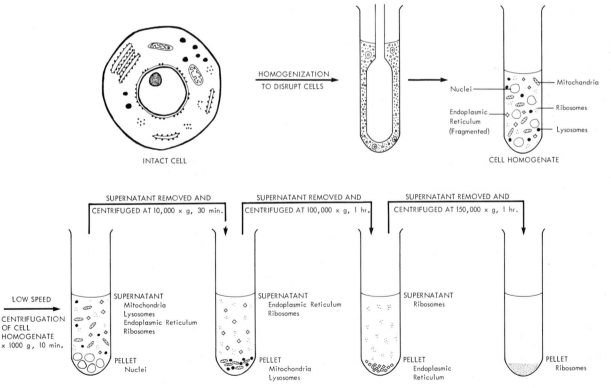

Fɪɢ. 5-12. Diagram illustrating steps in cell fractionation.

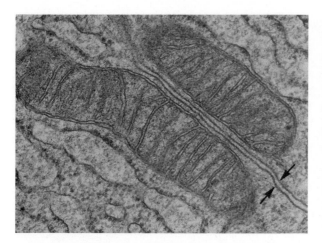

FIG. 5-13. Electron micrograph ($\times$ 86,000) of two mitochondria from the tracheal epithelium of the newborn rat, showing the cristae and matrix. The plasma membranes (arrows) of two adjacent cells are shown. There is a narrow intercellular space between them. Rough endoplasmic reticulum is seen at lower left. (Courtesy of M. Weinstock)

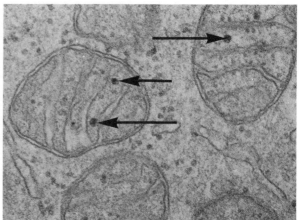

FIG. 5-15. Mitochondria in the epithelial cells of chick trachea, showing cristae and spherical dense granules (arrows) in the matrix between them. $\times$ 80,000 (From V. I. Kalnins)

thought to play a role in controlling the movement of substances in and out of the mitochondria, the uptake of substrates and the release of ATP.

The inner membrane is thrown into folds that project like shelves into the mitochondrion (Figs. 5-10 and 5-15); these projections, shown in a 3-dimensional diagram in Figure 5-14, are termed *cristae*. Obviously, in thin sections a mitochondrion will be cut only infrequently in longitudinal section throughout its whole length as is the one shown in Figure 5-10. Most will be cut in cross and oblique section (Figs. 5-13 and 5-15); hence, deciding on their size, shape and structure from thin sections would require mak-

ing reconstructions of them from serial sections or at least a thoughtful exercise in 3-dimensional visualization. Typical mitochondria usually vary in size considerably in any one cell type but most are from 0.4 to 1.0 μ (or μm) in diameter. In different cell types the size, shape and number of the cristae (internal shelves) vary considerably. In the liver cells, for example, the cristae are short and extend only about halfway across the mitochondria; in other cells, such as muscle cells, the cristae may extend completely across the mitochondria. Some cell types have mitochondria with very few cristae; other cell types have mitochondria with a large number of cristae. In the mitochondria of some kinds of cells the cristae are tubular in form instead of lying shelflike as is apparent when the cristae are cut in cross sections.

The interior of each mitochondrion is filled with a fluid which usually is slightly denser than the surrounding cytoplasm; this is sometimes termed the *mitochondrial matrix*. Occasional spherical or ovoid electron-dense granules are seen in it (Fig. 5-15). These granules are cations of metals such as calcium, and their presence testifies to the ability of mitochondria to concentrate cations to the point at which they precipitate in the form of solid granules. Some of these ions are required for the functioning of mitochondrial enzymes.

Numbers, Distribution and Renewal. Mitochondria are usually very numerous in cells. However, their numbers differ in relation to the energy requirements of different kinds of cells; thus some kinds of cells— for example, lymphocytes—have only a few, whereas

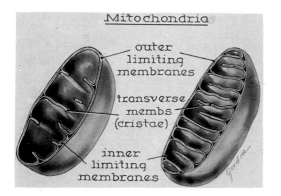

FIG. 5-14. Diagrammatic drawings to illustrate the structure of mitochondria in 3 dimensions.

a liver cell has around a thousand. The number of cristae in the mitochondria reflect the energy requirements of cells. Cells with mitochondria that have numerous cristae (such as those of muscle cells) have higher energy requirements than cells whose mitochondria have fewer cristae. Moreover, although mitochondria in general are suspended in the cytoplasmic matrix, in many kinds of cells they are aggregated particularly in those parts of the cell that have the highest energy requirements.

There is a continual renewal of mitochondria; in rat liver they turn over in about 10 days. All aspects of the formation of new mitochondria are not clear. However, it is believed that mitochondria may divide by fission, similar to that involved in the division of bacteria; that is, a partition develops across the middle of a mitochondrion and the two halves separate along this partition, as is suggested by Figure 5-16.

Relation of Structure to Enzymes Concerned in Cell Respiration

From early research it was believed that there were two pathways by which sugar could be metabolized to yield energy in mammalian cells: (1) an anaerobic (without air) pathway, now generally termed glycolysis, which enabled sugar to be metabolized in the absence of oxygen, and (2) an (aerobic) pathway in which oxygen was utilized, which yielded much more energy (ATP) than the anaerobic one. As more was learned it became established that although there were two pathways in the cell they were not side-by-side alternatives as was at first believed; instead, the two pathways are arranged in tandem, with the anaerobic pathway preceding the aerobic. It is now accepted that sugar absorbed by cells is, without the help of oxygen, degraded by a series of steps catalyzed by enzymes to a substance known as *pyruvic acid* or *pyruvate* and that the reactions involved occur in the cytoplasmic matrix and result in the formation of a small amount of ATP and a low energy yield as compared with that from the aerobic pathway which normally follows. It is the reactions of the second and aerobic pathway that accomplish what is known as *cell respiration,* and this takes place in mitochondria.

Detailed information on glycolysis and cell respiration is a matter dealt with in detail in biochemistry courses, and the brief and superficial comment on the subject that follows is given here only to relate certain of the processes involved to mitochondrial structure.

Sites of Enzymes. The end products of glycolysis (after being somewhat altered) are taken through the

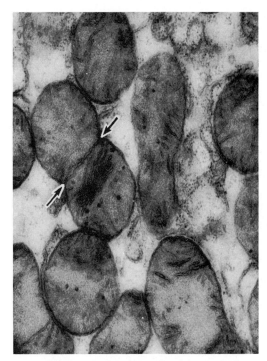

Fig. 5-16. Electron micrograph ($\times$ 30,000) of a section of a liver cell of a rat that was fed an azo dye that causes a great increase in the number of mitochondria in liver cells. The arrows indicate where a mitochondrion may be dividing. (Preparation by Dr. J.-G. Lafontaine)

mitochondrial membranes into the mitochondrial matrix where the enzymes of the Krebs cycle are located. These enzymes catalyze a host of different reactions concerned with the breakdown of the end products of glycolysis and of amino and fatty acid metabolism. Within mitochondria the end products of glycolysis are gradually broken down to CO_2 by the enzymes of the Krebs cycle. During this process there is a release of several hydrogen ions which are captured by the coenzyme nicotinamide adenine dinucleotide (NAD). The electrons of the hydrogen are then passed along a series of respiratory enzymes called flavoproteins and cytochromes and ultimately combine with protons and oxygen to form water. The energy obtained from this passage of electrons is utilized at several sites along the series to permit the phosphorylation that regenerates ATP from ADP and inorganic phosphate. For this reason the reactions involved in electron transport are closely coupled with those of phosphorylation and as a result ATP is produced in a very efficient manner. It is not surprising therefore to find that the enzymes concerned in electron transport and oxidative phos-

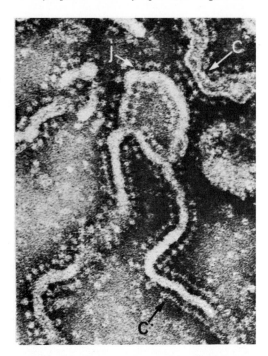

Fig. 5-17. Electron micrograph ($\times$ 192,000) of a negatively stained preparation, showing a number of mitochondrial white-appearing cristae which are covered on both surfaces by toadstool-like objects, whose heads are visible as small round white objects lined up at a specific distance from the cristae. The heads are attached to the membrane by thin stalks. (Parsons, D. F.: Science, *140*:985)

phorylation are arranged in extensive integrated complexes on the inner mitochondrial membrane and its cristae. This arrangement is believed to be one that would permit special step-by-step enzymatic processes to occur. The energy-rich ATP finally produced is made available to the cytoplasm outside the mitochondria.

Negative Staining of Mitochondria. In an attempt to obtain more precise information about the location of the various enzymes concerned in cell respiration, mitochondrial cristae have been examined in the EM by means of the negative staining technic—a technic which has also given much new information about the structure of various viruses. The negative staining procedure involves surrounding a particle with an electron-dense material. When a micrograph is prepared, the object itself is delineated by electron-dense material so that it appears light against a dark background. When the inner membranes of mitochondria

are studied in this way, they appear as shown in Figure 5-17. The surfaces on both sides of the cristae are seen to be covered with toadstool-like objects that have heads 90 Å in diameter and stems 35 Å wide. It is thought that these possess a special enzyme concerned in the reaction involving the phosphorylation of ADP to ATP.

Mitochondria As Symbionts—Nucleic Acid in Mitochondria. As already noted, Altmann in the last century was scorned for his beliefs about the nature of mitochondria. Recently Margulis described a similar fate for the concepts of an American physician, J. E. Wallin who, in the 1920's, conceived of mitochondria as being bacteria that had come to live as symbionts in animal cells. Unfortunately, he was unable to substantiate his concept with definitive proof and so his views were rejected. However, recent events have done much to vindicate both Altmann and Wallin, for mitochondria have now been shown to contain DNA, RNA and ribosomes which are slightly different from those found elsewhere in the cytoplasm and hence mitochondria possess the means for a considerable degree of independent existence. Their DNA, RNA and ribosomes are in forms similar to those found in bacteria. It is now accepted that mitochondrial DNA provides the information for the synthesis of many but not all of the proteins of a mitochondrion (the information for the rest being supplied by the nucleus); thus they are at least semi-autonomous. Hence the concept that long ago they originated from bacteria that invaded animal cells where they become symbionts and added much to the total metabolic capacity of the animal cell looks quite attractive at the present time.

Free Ribosomes

Although the synthesis of rRNA occurs in the nucleolus, ribosomes perform their chief function in the cytoplasm where they are considered as one type of cytoplasmic organelle and so must be dealt with from this aspect in this chapter.

Ribosomes are disposed in two general ways in the cytoplasm. First, they are scattered about diffusely in the somewhat viscous cytoplasmic matrix as free agents not attached to any membranous structures; these are the kind we shall discuss here. They are also found attached to the membranous walls of the organelle that we shall consider next, which is known as the rough-surfaced endoplasmic reticulum. This matter is mentioned here because it is important to realize that free ribosomes are organelles capable of functioning in their own right without being attached to a membrane. The structure of the ribosome was discussed in Chapter 4 and illustrated in Figure 4-5. It consists of two subunits, a large one and a small one. Both contain rRNA and protein. The units are difficult to see in ordinary electron micrographs of sectioned material and can be demonstrated clearly only if special technics such as negative staining are used.

THE RELATION OF FREE RIBOSOMES TO DIFFUSE CYTOPLASMIC BASOPHILIA

Although free ribosomes are present in every kind of living cell (except mature red blood cells) and although free ribosomes are basophilic because of their content of rRNA and although they are generally scattered about throughout the cytoplasmic matrix of cells, there are not enough of them in most kinds of cells for them to impart basophilia to the cytoplasm in H and E sections. There are, however, special situations (to be described shortly) in which there are enough free ribosomes in the cytoplasmic matrix to make the cytoplasm basophilic in H and E sections.

The Function of Free Ribosomes. The function of free ribosomes is to synthesize the protein of the cytoplasmic matrix. Since this is always being catabolized, it must be constantly renewed. In addition to its maintenance, the free ribosomes are essential for the extra amounts that are required when growth occurs. Free ribosomes are also responsible for the synthesis of many special cytoplasmic proteins found in various types of cells—for example, for the hemoglobin found in red blood cells.

Special Situations in Which There Are Enough Free Ribosomes in Cytoplasm To Make It Diffusely Basophilic

In Rapidly Growing Cells. It was observed long ago with the LM that the cytoplasm of rapidly growing cancer cells was often diffusely basophilic. In 1955 Howatson and the author made an early study with the EM of two types of rapidly growing cancer cells and showed (Fig. 5-18) that their cytoplasm revealed a much higher proportion of free ribosomes than could be seen in the types of cells from which these tumors

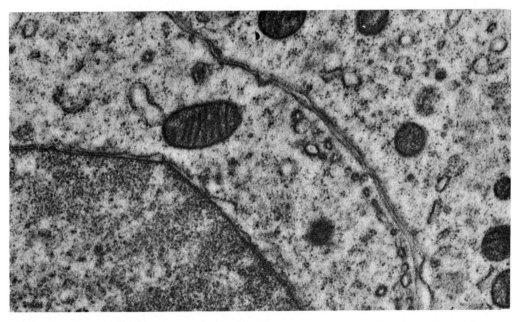

FIG. 5-18. This electron micrograph ($\times$ 30,000) shows parts of two cells of a malignant liver tumor of a rat. Part of a nucleus is seen at lower left. The membranes of the adjacent cells run from upper left to lower right. The cytoplasm of both cells shows a heavy content of fine dark particles which are ribosomes. This was one of the earlier electron micrographs published to show the nature of the cytoplasm of tumor cells, hence it was prepared before the present-day methods, which demarcate free ribosomes more clearly, were evolved. Nevertheless, it shows that the basophilia of rapidly growing tumor cells is to be explained by their content of free ribosomes. (Howatson, A. F., and Ham, A. W.: Cancer Res., *15*:62, 1955)

originated. (Figure 5-18 was one of the first micrographs that became available to illustrate this point. At that time modern fixation and staining methods for electron microscopy had not yet been developed and so in this micrograph the ribosomes are somewhat dustlike and not as individually prominent as they would be in modern micrographs.) As might be expected, diffuse basophilia of the cytoplasm is also seen in many types of rapidly growing normal cells of a developing embryo and, in postnatal life, in the cytoplasm of cells that are proliferating rapidly to bring about the repair of an injury.

In Connection With the Synthesis of Hemoglobin. Fully formed red blood cells have lost both their nuclei and almost all cytoplasmic components they had at an earlier stage of development. Indeed, mature red blood cells are not much more than little biconcave bags of cell membrane, filled with the protein hemoglobin (Fig. 11-1) which, as has already been mentioned, serves as an oxygen carrier. The cell that gives rise to a red blood cell is called an erythroblast (Fig. 5-19). At this stage of development the cell still possesses a nucleus, the DNA of which gives off information via mRNA to the cytoplasm which becomes diffusely basophilic as seen with the LM in stained sections or films because, as the EM shows, it comes to have a heavy content of free ribosomes (Fig. 5-19). Almost all the information given off by the DNA of the nucleus in an erythroblast is concerned with directing the synthesis of hemoglobin, which in due course will be the only major component left in the cytoplasm. So almost all of the free ribosomes that are both abundant and dispersed throughout the cytoplasm in erythroblasts represent sites of hemoglobin synthesis. This more or less special case shows that abundant and widely dispersed free ribosomes can be

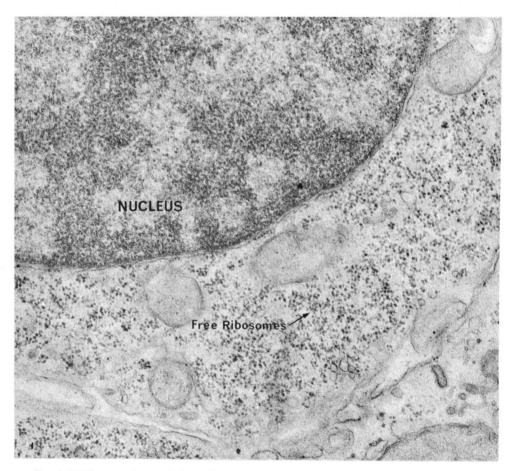

Fɪɢ. 5-19. Electron micrograph ($\times$ 40,000) showing part of an erythroblast of a rat. Notice that the cytoplasm has many free ribosomes that are arranged into groups forming polyribosomes for the synthesis of hemoglobin. (Preparation courtesy of A. M. Jézéquel)

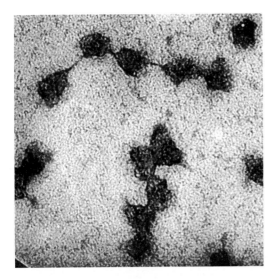

FIG. 5-20. Electron micrograph ($\times$ 400,000) of poly-ribosomes from red blood cell precursors, stained with uranylacetate. Note the thread of messenger RNA connecting the 5 ribosomes in the upper part of the picture. (Preparation by Henry S. Slater, supplied by Dr. Alexander Rich)

code that directs the particular amino acids that are to be joined together and determines the order in which they are to be joined, has to move along in relation to a ribosome so that the successive amino acids that are called for in its code can be joined to the end of the chain of amino acids that has already been assembled. If only a single ribosome were available for synthesis, a single long polypeptide molecule would have to be completed before another could be begun. However, if there were, say, five ribosomes located at different points along the same long mRNA molecule that moved along past them, five molecules of the long polypeptide could be in the process of assembly simultaneously and, as a result, five complete molecules could be finished in roughly the same time it would take to make one protein molecule if only one ribosome were available.

The ribosomes of polyribosomes may be arranged in whorls or spirals. Compared to other protein macro-

present in cells for synthesizing special proteins, i.e., proteins other than those required for normal cell maintenance or growth.

Free Polyribosomes. It was in connection with the synthesis of hemoglobin that the arrangement of ribosomes into functional units called polyribosomes or polysomes was first observed; this was done by Warner, Rich and Hall who devised special ways of extracting ribosomes from developing red blood cells. They found that the free ribosomes concerned in hemoglobin synthesis tended to be arranged in clusters, the average number of which (in the instance of hemoglobin synthesis) seemed to be five. Furthermore, as is shown in Figure 5-20, the free ribosomes in a polyribosome are connected by a fine thread which is the messenger RNA. Electron micrographs of sections of erythroblasts also show that the ribosomes are arranged in little groups or clusters, as is shown in Figure 5-19.

The advantage possessed by a group of ribosomes (a polyribosome) over a single ribosome in connection with the synthesis of hemoglobin (or any other protein) is to be explained as follows: in order for a particular polypeptide molecule to be synthesized, particular amino acids have to be linked together one at a time and in a certain order. One amino acid can be joined to another only at the site of a ribosome. Hence the long molecule of mRNA, which carries the

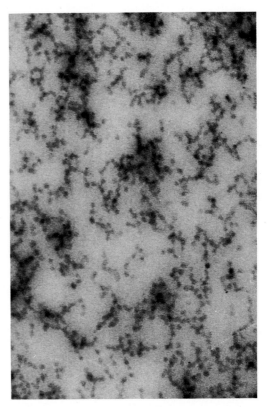

FIG. 5-21. Electron micrograph ($\times$ 80,000) of a section of a pellet of a fraction obtained by differential centrifugation from a homogenate of pancreas cells. The micrograph shows this fraction to be a very pure preparation of ribosomes. (Palade, G., and Siekevitz, P.: J. Biophys. Biochem. Cytol., *2*:671)

molecules, the hemoglobin molecule is relatively small. Therefore only a relatively small number of ribosomes form the polysomes along which it is synthesized. As might be expected, the polyribosomes that are concerned in the synthesis of the larger protein macromolecules have a larger number of ribosomes because their messenger RNA's are longer and there is room for more ribosomes. Indeed, the number of ribosomes seen in a polyribosome provides information about the size of the protein macromolecule with whose synthesis it is concerned. Ribosomes, polysomes of various sizes, and the large and small subunits of ribosomes can now be isolated in a relatively pure form by some of the cell fractionation procedures previously described in connection with Figure 5-12 and can be studied independently of other cell components. Ribosomes isolated in this way are shown in Figure 5-21.

The Rough-Surfaced Endoplasmic Reticulum

The term rough-surfaced endoplasmic reticulum was not coined until cytoplasm could be studied in sections with the EM. However, long before this happened something had been seen in cytoplasm with the LM, the precise nature of which was revealed only by the EM, and as a result when anyone now sees this particular something in the cytoplasm with his LM he is able to visualize the detailed picture that would be revealed if he were examining the same area with the EM. Since it is of the greatest importance for a microscopist to be able to translate mentally what is seen with the LM into what is seen with the EM, we shall first describe the development of knowledge about rough-surfaced endoplasmic reticulum that occurred before its name was coined and its intricate structure was elucidated with the EM.

Development of Knowledge With the LM. After the chromatin of the nucleus was seen in stained sections with the LM and given its name, microscopists noticed that the cytoplasm of many different kinds of cells often revealed localized deposits of a substance that had an affinity for basic stains similar to that of nuclear chromatin. Some called it *chromidial substance* while others named it *chromophil* substance to indicate its resemblance to chromatin. Still others preferred to refer to it as the *basophilic component of cytoplasm* so as to emphasize its different staining reaction from cytoplasm in general—which, of course, is acidophilic and hence pink to red. In 1900 Garnier made an extensive study of this same material and, because he was convinced that it must perform important work in the cell, he gave it still another name, *ergastoplasm* (*ergon,* work).

When the Feulgen reaction became available for specifically identifying DNA in cells, it was found that the basophilic material in cytoplasm was Feulgen-negative and hence not DNA. However, it was shown to absorb ultraviolet light of a band that indicated that it contained nucleic acid. When the enzymes DNA-ase and RNA-ase became available, it was shown to be digested by RNA-ase but not by DNA-ase and so it was given still another name, *cytoplasmic RNA.* The way it appears in a liver cell is shown in color at the upper left corner of Figure 1-14, where it is labeled by this last term, and the way it appears in black and white illustrations of liver cells is shown in Figure 5-22, *left,* where it is not labeled but is shown as irregular darkly staining areas in the cytoplasm which disappear after extraction with RNA-ase (Fig. 5-22, *right*).

Although this material with so many names can be seen in many kinds of cells, it is most commonly studied both with the LM and the EM in certain secretory cells of the pancreas and this is where we shall at this time describe its appearance in detail as seen with both the LM and the EM. However, until you have studied and become familiar with the structure of the pancreas as an organ, it may not be easy to locate the kinds of cells in this organ which reveal it so well, so we shall now describe enough about the microscopic structure of the pancreas to enable you to find the right kind of cells to study. For those who wish further information

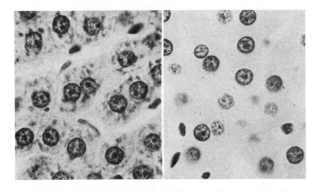

FIG. 5-22. Micrographs of liver cells stained with toluidine blue (*left*) before and (*right*) after extraction with RNAase. This enzyme which is specific for RNA has removed the irregular patches of basophilic material in the cytoplasm of liver cells (*left*), indicating that the basophilia in these regions is due to the presence of RNA. The staining of nuclei, on the other hand, is very little affected by this treatment, since most of their staining is due to DNA rather than to RNA. (From R. Daoust)

about the pancreas, it is described in detail as an organ later in this book.

Some Guidance for Finding the Cells in the Pancreas That Reveal Localized Basophilic Material. Most of the cells of the pancreas are of a type that produces a secretion of potent enzymatic protein. This secretion is delivered from secretory cells into a branch of a tube called the pancreatic duct which eventually empties into the intestine where the protein enzymes of the secretion act to digest certain foods. The cells of the pancreas that synthesize and secrete the enzymes of this secretion are arranged in little groups, and since each little group resembles a grape, it is called an *acinus (acinus,* grape). Each acinus has a minute central lumen that connects to a little duct which extends from it much as a stem extends from a grape and this duct carries the secretion away from the acinus to a branch of the pancreatic duct. The acini and their ducts are fitted into the pancreas in a random fashion so that a section that is cut through pancreatic tissue slices through acini and ducts at all sorts of angles. It generally takes a good deal of hunting with the low-power objective to find an acinus that is cut more or less in cross section like the one in the

rectangle in Figure 5-23, *left.* A high-power photomicrograph of a cross section of a similar acinus is shown in Figure 5-23, *right.* In the latter it will be seen that a cross section of an acinus resembles a pie that has been cut into pieces but not yet served. Each piece of pie represents a secretory cell. The secretion is made in several steps, soon to be described, and the final product passes through the tip of each cell into the central lumen of the acinus (arrow, Fig. 5-23, *right*) which connects with the duct that drains the secretion away. The nucleus of each secretory cell is located near the broad base of the cell and the basophilic component of the cytoplasm is disposed between the nucleus and the sides and base of each cell. In these sites it appears as blue-purple material in an H and E section (Fig. 5-23, *right,* lower arrow).

Development of Knowledge and Terminology From EM Studies. Before it was feasible to cut sections thin enough for the EM, Porter, Claude and Fullam grew cells in cultures in which their cytoplasm spread so very thin that they were able to examine it (after it was fixed) with the EM. In it they observed a lacelike network of what appeared to be strands and vesicles, which they named the *endoplasmic reticulum*

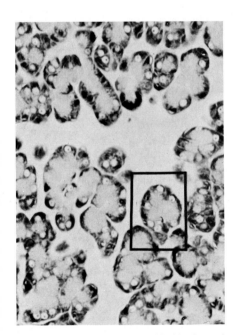 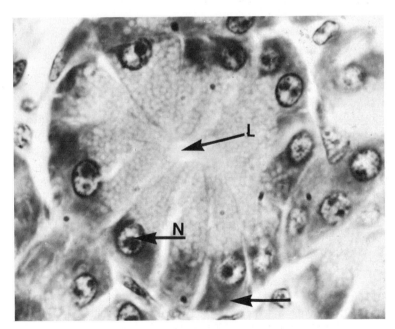

Fig. 5-23. (*Left*) A section of human pancreas stained with toluidine blue and seen under medium power. A cross section of a single acinus is seen in the rectangle. (*Right*) A high power photomicrograph of a single acinus. The central lumen of the acinus (L) and the unstained secretory granules which are going to be discharged into it fill those parts of the cells which are near the lumen. The nuclei of the cells (N) are located near the base of the cell, and the basophilic regions of the cell located between the nuclei and the bases and the sides of each cell are clearly visible (bottom arrow).

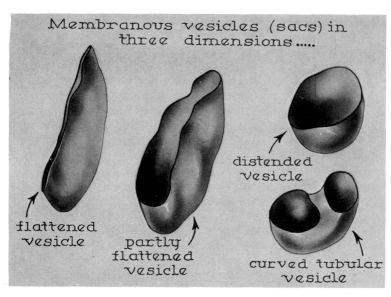

Membranous vesicles (sacs) in three dimensions.....

flattened vesicle

partly flattened vesicle

distended vesicle

curved tubular vesicle

Fig. 5-24. Diagrammatic drawings illustrating in 3 dimensions various forms assumed by cytoplasmic membranous vesicles. The cut surface of each vesicle shows how it would appear in a section. The large flattened vesicles (as at left) are termed cisternae.

(ER). The term *reticulum* indicated that the strands and vesicles were arranged in a network (*rete*, net). Since the student may be puzzled about it being called the "endoplasmic" reticulum, it should be explained that the adjective endoplasmic can be used with either of two meanings, to refer to the innermost cytoplasm of a cell (which is sometimes called the endoplasm) or to mean *within* the cytoplasm. When the reticulum was first seen it was thought that it was confined to the innermost cytoplasm, which probably accounted for the term endoplasmic being used; later, when it was found that the reticulum extended into the outermost cytoplasm, the term endoplasm was probably retained because of its second meaning.

When it became possible to study the ER in sections with the EM, the network was clearly shown to consist of hollow membranous structures—either *tubules*, or bladderlike structures termed *vesicles* (*vesicula*, a small bladder). Figure 5-24 illustrates some of the latter in 3 dimensions. Large flattened vesicles of the ER are commonly termed *cisternae*. Although there are different amounts of ER in different kinds of cells, all or nearly all kinds of cells contain at least a little of it. Furthermore, as it was studied in sections with the EM, it soon became apparent that there were two kinds of ER, the *rough* and the *smooth*. Here we shall deal only with the rough type (rER) because it possesses ribosomes which are responsible for the localized cytoplasmic basophilia seen with the LM which we have just described.

The discovery made with the EM of ER in cells did not immediately solve the problem of what was re-

sponsible for the basophilia seen in cytoplasm with the LM, because ribosomes had not yet been identified with the EM. At first it was thought that membranes in the cytoplasm must account for the basophilia. It was later established that the cytoplasmic basophilia seen in stained section with the LM was to be accounted for by the large numbers of ribosomes that are both attached to membranes and free in these areas. For a time what are now universally referred to as ribosomes were termed *Palade granules* in honor of Dr. George Palade, who contributed so much to establishing their existence and nature.

Appearance of Rough-Surfaced ER in Micrographs. As shown in Figures 5-25 (diagram) and 5-26 (electron micrograph), the rough-surfaced endoplasmic reticulum in pancreatic cells is seen with the EM to be in the form of membranous cisternae the outer walls of which are studded with ribosomes. These ribosome-studded cisternae are packed fairly close together and generally in parallel (Figs. 5-25 and 5-26). As shown in Figure 5-26, secretion can be seen in the lumens of the cisternae. It appears slightly more electron-dense than the cytoplasmic matrix between cisternae. Although most of the ribosomes in this area are attached to the outer surface of the flattened vesicles, there are also some free ribosomes between the adjacent flattened vesicles.

Function of the Rough-Surfaced Vesicles of the ER. The synthesis of protein occurs at the ribosomes which sit on the outer aspects of the membranous walls of cisternae. Here, amino acids, tRNA and mRNA are all available in the cytoplasm to participate with the ribosomes that adhere to the cisternae in the reactions by which amino acids are linked together according to the instructions coded in the mRNA that travels to this site, as illustrated in Figure 4-6. The reason for the close association of ribosomes and membranous vesicles or cisternae as occurs in the rough-surfaced ER is, of course, that proteins to be exported must, as they are synthesized, be segregated within membranous vesicles to prevent them from mixing with those which the cell has to retain. Moreover, some enzymes have to be kept segregated in membrane-bound vesicles because they could destroy the cytoplasm if they were released into the cytoplasmic matrix from the ribosomes instead of being released into the membrane-bound cisternae. This segregation is, of course, in contrast to proteins that are synthesized in association with free ribosomes. These proteins do not have to be segregated from the cytoplasmic matrix.

Polysomes of the Rough ER. The ribosomes of the rough ER, like most of the free ribosomes, are arranged

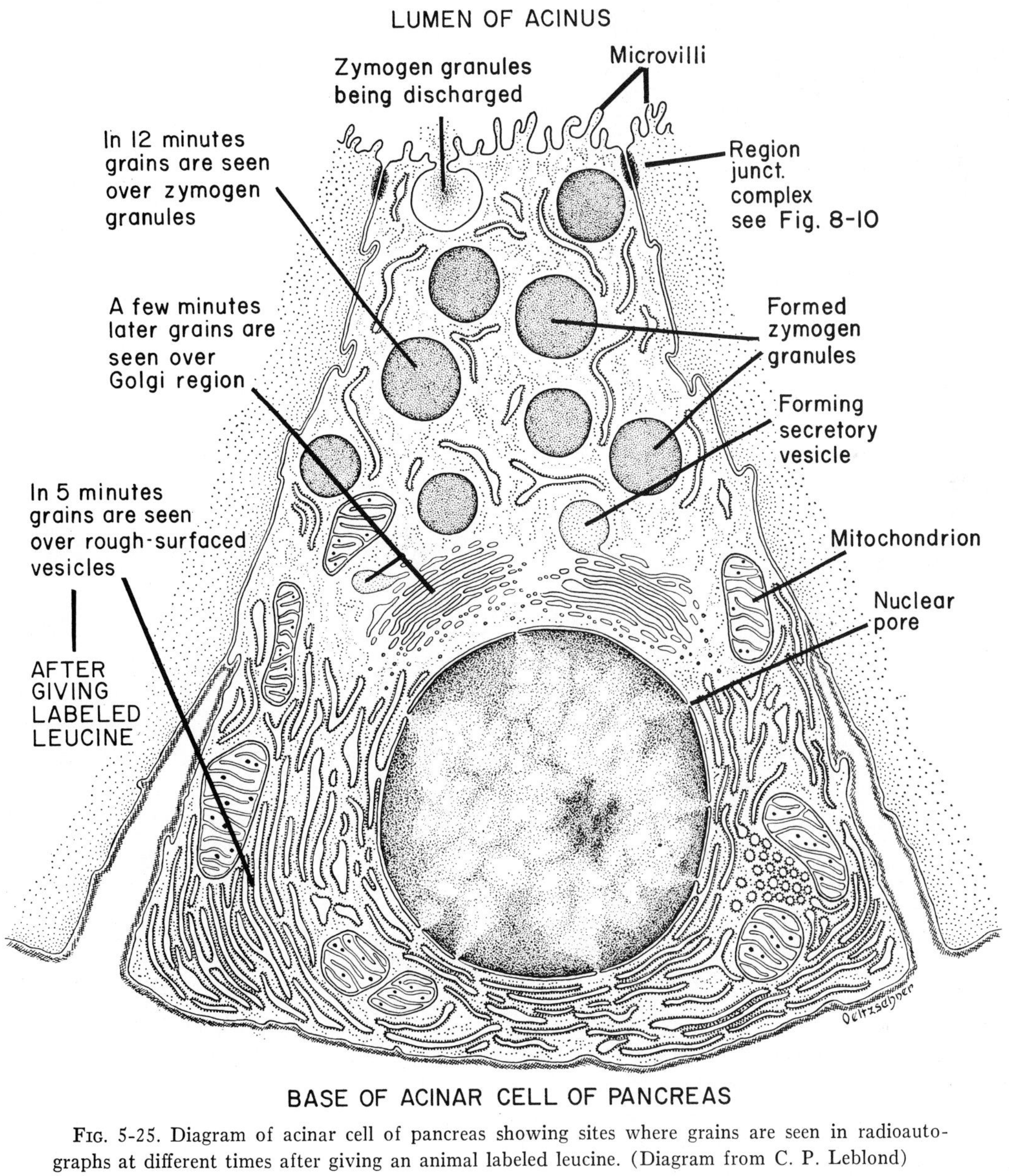

FIG. 5-25. Diagram of acinar cell of pancreas showing sites where grains are seen in radioautographs at different times after giving an animal labeled leucine. (Diagram from C. P. Leblond)

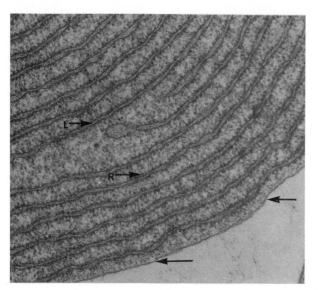

FIG. 5-26. Electron micrograph showing cisternae of rough endoplasmic reticulum in the basal part of an acinar cell of rat pancreas. The lumen of the cisternae (L) contains recently synthesized protein that will eventually be secreted. The outer surfaces of the cisternae are studded with ribosomes (R). The cell membrane runs along the bottom of the micrograph (arrows). × 65,000. (From V. I. Kalnins)

in clusters which often form whorls (Fig. 5-27) in association with mRNA molecules. The larger of the two subunits of a ribosome sits on the membrane itself; the smaller one projects out into the cytoplasmic matrix (Fig. 5-28). Since polysomes are on the outer surfaces of the cisternae, it seems reasonable to assume that as the amino acids are linked to form polypeptide chains the protein being synthesized is delivered through the membranous walls of the vesicles into the lumens of the vesicles (Fig. 5-28). Possibly there is something like a pore in the membrane through which the end of a newly forming macromolecule of protein could be pushed, as it were, as rapidly as it was being lengthened by the ribosomes on the exterior of the membrane. By cell fractionation (Fig. 5-12) rER can be isolated in a relatively pure form, although it does break up into little membrane-bound vesicles with ribosomes on the outside upon preparation of cell homogenates. Moreover, by using detergents it is now possible to remove the ribosomes from these vesicles. Thus the ribosomes of the rER, the membranes of the vesicles of rER and their contents can be separately analyzed by biochemical technics.

Distribution of Rough ER in Different Types of Cells. Some rough ER is necessarily present in every kind of nucleated cell because the outer membrane of

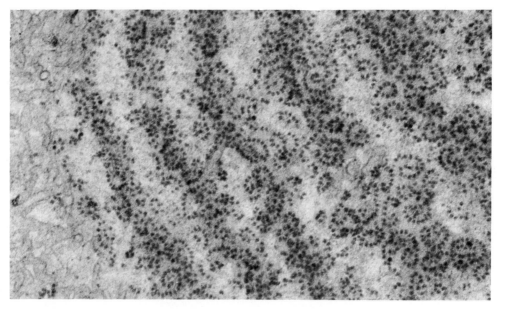

FIG. 5-27. Electron micrograph of section of cortex of adrenal gland of a human fetus. The right two thirds of the picture show polyribosomes that are attached to the outer surfaces of cisternae of endoplasmic reticulum. Notice how the individual ribosomes in a polyribosome are arranged to form spirals. At the left is some smooth-surfaced endoplasmic reticulum. (Preparation courtesy of E. Yamada)

the nuclear envelope is identical and often continuous with the membranes of the rough endoplasmic reticulum and has ribosomes attached to it, as is shown in Figure 2-7. The greatest amounts of rER are found in secretory cells such as the acinar cells of the pancreas (Figs. 5-25 and 5-26). However, many other kinds of cells that are not always thought of as secretory cells also release protein-containing substances through their membranes into their environment—for example, the cells termed the *fibroblasts* of connective tissues, which release proteins and other substances that form intercellular substances which occupy the spaces between the cells of connective tissue, or the *osteoblasts* of bone, which elaborate proteins that become part of the organic intercellular substance of bone, or the plasma cells that make and secrete a very important group of proteins that comprise the antibodies. Some of the hormones—i.e., those that are proteins—also are made by cells which have a well developed rough ER. And in all kinds of cells rough ER is required for the synthesis of the enzymes that come to be contained within the cell in little vesicles called *lysosomes* which we shall soon consider. Accordingly, although the rough ER is most highly developed in cells that are frankly secretory, it is a component of all nucleated cells; for it is required for synthesis and segregation of products required within the cell as well as for the production of products that will be secreted into the environment.

The Golgi Apparatus

Introduction. The elucidation of the structure and function of the Golgi apparatus only became possible with the development of the EM and the tracer technics of radioautography; hence, most of the definitive information about it is of relatively recent origin. It is now known that it is a very important membranous organelle and that it is different from and not part of the endoplasmic reticulum. It is present in all types of cells but its size varies greatly in different kinds of cells. To avoid repetition, we shall not describe further the many things that have been learned about it by modern methods until we have described what was learned about it with the LM.

Early Development of Knowledge With the LM. In 1898, Camillo Golgi, an Italian neurologist, working with a microscope and not much more equipment than might be found in a kitchen, made a discovery that started him on the path to sharing a Nobel prize many years later. When he examined with his microscope some sections of brain tissue that had been fixed in a bichromate solution and then impregnated with a silver salt, he noticed in the cytoplasm of the nerve cells

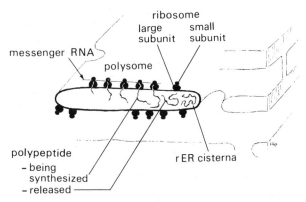

Fig. 5-28. Diagram illustrating the synthesis of protein by ribosomes on the surface of rough endoplasmic reticulum and the release of this protein into the cisterna. Note that it is the large subunit of the ribosome which is in contact with the membrane of the cisterna.

some dark material that seemed to be arranged in a network and so he named this the internal reticular apparatus of the cell. Subsequent studies on other kinds of cells confirmed its existence but did not confirm that it always seemed to form a network and so it became known as the *Golgi apparatus* or *Golgi complex*. In discussing it or writing about it many people refer to it simply as the *Golgi*.

During the many decades that preceded the EM and radioautography, the Golgi apparatus stimulated much study, speculation and controversy and was the subject of a relatively enormous number of scientific publications which yielded only a little definitive information about its nature. It was, for example, soon shown that it could be demonstrated in cells that have been immersed for several days in 2 percent osmium tetroxide. Many studies indicated that its position, and what seemed to be its form, were different in different kinds of specialized cells. In secretory cells, such as the acinar cells of the pancreas, the apparatus was shown to be located between the nucleus and the apex of the cell through which the secretion of the cell is delivered (Fig. 5-29). In other kinds of cells without such polarized secretory activities, parts of the apparatus were sometimes seen to be more or less distributed about in the cytoplasm, but generally fairly close to the nucleus. Finally, in light of what is now known, the prophetic views of both Bowen and Hirsch in the 20's and 30's respectively should be mentioned, for both concluded that the Golgi apparatus must function as site of aggregation and condensation for secretory products made elsewhere in the cell.

Negative Golgi Images. It is usual in laboratory work for the student to examine with the LM a section

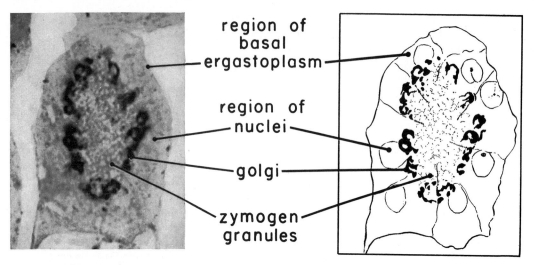

FIG. 5-29. (*Left*) A pancreatic acinus stained to demonstrate the Golgi apparatus in the acinar cells. (*Right*) A diagram for orientation. Note that the Golgi apparatus is between the nuclei and the aggregations of zymogen granules that are toward the apical parts of the cells. (Preparation by C. P. Leblond and H. Warshawsky)

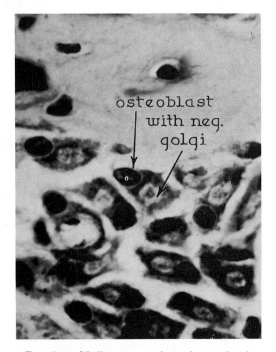

FIG. 5-30. Medium-power photomicrograph of a section of decalcified bone stained with azure-eosin-hematoxylin. It shows osteoblasts beginning to lay down bone near the site of a fracture. The osteoblasts show pale areas (negative Golgis) in their basophilic cytoplasm.

or two that have been prepared by one of the technics that demonstrate the Golgi apparatus in cells. Although routine methods such as H and E do not stain the apparatus itself, they do often reveal the existence of a little relatively clear area next to the nucleus which marks the site where it exists. These clear areas are termed *negative Golgi images,* and they are seen to best advantage in cells that are elaborating secretions (Fig. 5-30). The paleness results from the fact that the Golgi apparatus does not contain any ribosomes, since in secretory cells the cytoplasm adjacent to the apparatus generally has a heavy content of rough ER which makes it basophilic, the clear Golgi area appears in contrast to it.

THE FINE STRUCTURE OF THE GOLGI APPARATUS

General Features. The EM showed that the Golgi apparatus was a membranous structure. If the unit of structure of the rER is a flattened vesicle studded with ribosomes it could be said that the unit of structure of the Golgi apparatus is a flattened vesicle that is not studded with ribosomes. The flattened vesicles of the rER are termed cisternae but those of the Golgi apparatus are termed *saccules.* Golgi saccules are commonly arranged in stacks much in the same way as hotcakes, one above the other. But, unlike stacks of hotcakes, there is a little space between each rounded flattened saccule of a stack as is shown in Figure 5-31. Stacks commonly contain 3 to 8 saccules. A stack cut in sec-

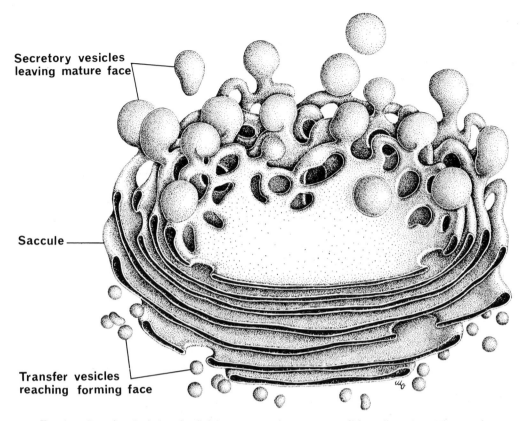

Secretory vesicles
leaving mature face

Saccule

Transfer vesicles
reaching forming face

FIG. 5-31. Drawing depicting the Golgi apparatus of a secretory cell in 3 dimensions. The transfer vesicles shown below are in this instance small enough to be termed microvesicles, but in some kinds of cells they are larger. The transfer vesicles bud off from rough-surfaced endoplasmic reticulum, which would be below. The secretory vesicles that bud off from saccules on the mature face become, in the instance of acinar cells, the so-called zymogen granules. (Drawn from a model by Joyce Kephart. Illustration courtesy of C. P. Leblond)

tion at right angles to its broad surface appears as is shown in Figure 5-25 where two are shown just above the nucleus, with one on each side. The way a stack appears in a micrograph is shown in Figure 5-32 where it can be seen that the contents of individual saccules may cause them to be swollen here and there.

General Function. In considering the rER we learned that it is concerned with the synthesis, primarily, of protein materials that are destined for export from the cell. The rER is, in a sense, the first step along the assembly line that results finally in secretions being elaborated by cells. The second step along the assembly line is the Golgi apparatus. But there are no direct connections between the cisternae of the rER and the saccules of a Golgi stack. The way that the products synthesized in the rER reach what is called the immature face of a stack of Golgi saccules is by means of what are termed transfer vesicles budding off from the cisternae of the rER as is shown in Figure

5-34. They lose their ribosomes as they leave the rER and move to the immature face of a Golgi stack (Fig. 5-31) where they fuse with a Golgi saccule and empty their contents into its lumen. As will be explained in detail shortly, at the same time vesicles are budding off from the mature face of the Golgi stack; these will become secretory granules or their counterparts. While it is in the Golgi stack the product formed originally in the rER is chemically modified, particularly with regard to its carbohydrate content, and the package that leaves the mature face of a Golgi stack as a secretory vesicle therefore contains a product somewhat different from that which was synthesized in the rER. The way that a product that reaches the immature face of a Golgi stack reaches the mature face will be described very shortly.

The general function of Golgi stacks as described above explains their position. In specialized secretory cells such as the acinar cells of the pancreas (Fig. 5-

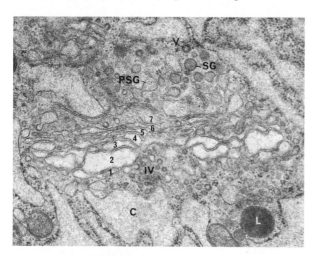

FIG. 5-32. Golgi apparatus of thyroid cell (× 40,000). The Golgi apparatus extends across the figure with the mature face above and the forming or immature face below. Immediately beneath the immature face, groups of intermediate vesicles (IV) may be seen, next to endoplasmic reticulum cisternae (C) which have only few ribosomes on the surface facing the Golgi apparatus. The first saccule on the immature face (labeled 1) is small and seems to arise from the fusion of intermediate vesicles. Successive saccules are numbered. The last one (labeled 7) is irregularly broken into presecretory granules which are scattered along the mature face (PSG). Next, several secretory granules may be seen (SG), as well as coated vesicles (V).

Outside the Golgi region, there are cisternae of rough endoplasmic reticulum, and a dense body presumed to be a lysosome (L). (Haddad, A., Smith, M. D., Herscovics, A., Nadler, N. J. and Leblond, C. P.: J. Cell Biol., *49*:856, 1971)

25) the Golgi apparatus is located between the rER and the apex of the cell through which the secretion of the cell is delivered. In cells in which secretory activity is not so definitely polarized, Golgi stacks do not have such a specific location, but, although they may be seen scattered about here and there in a few kinds of cells, in most types they are close to the centrioles. The number of stacks in a cell varies in relation to its type of function, frankly secretory cells having the most. But all kinds of cells have to have some representation of the Golgi apparatus because, as we shall soon see, it is essential for the maintenance of their cell membranes and cell coats. We shall now consider some of the features mentioned above in more detail.

The Two Faces of Stacks. A stack of saccules is said to have two faces, a *forming,* or *immature, face,* which is usually convex (but sometimes concave) and

a *mature face,* which is usually but not always concave. In Figure 5-31 the immature face seen at the base of the picture is associated with small rounded vesicles whereas the mature face at the top is associated with larger rounded vesicles. In Figure 5-25, the immature face is oriented toward the base of the cell (toward the nucleus) and is close to the rough-surfaced endoplasmic reticulum. The mature face, on the other hand, faces the apex of the cell, the direction in which secretion is delivered (Fig. 5-25).

The Loss of Saccules on the Mature Face by the Formation of Secretory Granules. Although the individual saccules of a stack are in general thin, the saccules close to the mature face, particularly around their periphery, demonstrate ovoid or rounded swellings caused by these portions of the saccules becoming distended from within by their contents (Figs. 5-25 and 5-31). The swollen portions of saccules bud off from the saccules and assume the form of membranous globules (Fig. 5-31). As soon as they become free they are called *secretory vesicles* (Fig. 5-31). They now go through some changes and as they do they are called by various names which need some explaining.

The secretory vesicles that bud off from Golgi saccules in actively secreting cells are filled with a protein-containing fluid. In the acinar cells of pancreas these vesicles soon become what are termed, from light microscopy, *zymogen* (*zymo,* ferment; *gennein,* to produce) *granules* (Fig. 5-25). The reason for the term zymogen being used was that it was shown that the granules, after being secreted and reaching the intestine, demonstrated potent enzymatic activity. The reason for the term granule was that the sections in which they were studied with the LM were fixed in solutions that coagulated the protein sols contained in the vesicles and hence with the LM they appeared as solid little bodies like granules.

However, a secretory vesicle is not termed a zymogen or a secretory granule immediately on its release from a saccule. It first goes through a stage in which its contents become increasingly condensed. To describe it at this stage some investigators refer to it as a *condensing vacuole* because its contents are being condensed. Since the term vacuole suggests a hole rather than a membranous structure, it seems better to denote it at this stage by another term that is often used, namely, a *presecretory granule;* then, after the concentration of its contents is complete it can be termed a *secretory granule* or, in the pancreas, a *zymogen granule* (but only with the realization that it is not really a granule in life, because its contents are fluid; it is only a granule when it has been fixed). Zymogen "granules" can be centrifuged from homogenates of unfixed fresh cells as shown in Figure 5-12 only under conditions that ensure that their membranous walls remain intact. Secretory granules are illustrated in the secretory cells of the thyroid gland (SG in Fig. 5-32) and in the acinar cells of the pancreas (Fig. 5-25).

Although the customary way for secretory vesicles to form is by their budding off from saccules as individual vesicles, it happens occasionally that a whole saccule on the mature face may break up into vesicles.

How the Saccules of a Stack Are Renewed. Since the process of secretion depends on secretory vesicles constantly budding off from saccules at the mature face of a stack, the membrane of the saccules of a stack would soon be used up and the stack would disappear if new saccules were not formed on the immature face at the same rate at which they are used up on the

mature face. To understand how stacks can remain a constant size it should first be realized that no new unit membrane is synthesized in the Golgi apparatus in a Golgi that remains the same size. Instead, new membrane is brought to it to form new saccules on its forming face at the same rate at which membrane is lost on the mature face. Differences between the two processes could account for a Golgi increasing or decreasing in size. The saccules on the forming face are being constantly supplied with new membrane which arrives there from the rough ER via what are termed intermediate or transfer vesicles, as will now be described.

Intermediate (Transfer) Vesicles. Intermediate vesicles bud off from the rough ER as fairly small ribosome-free vesicles (Fig. 5-33). They then move

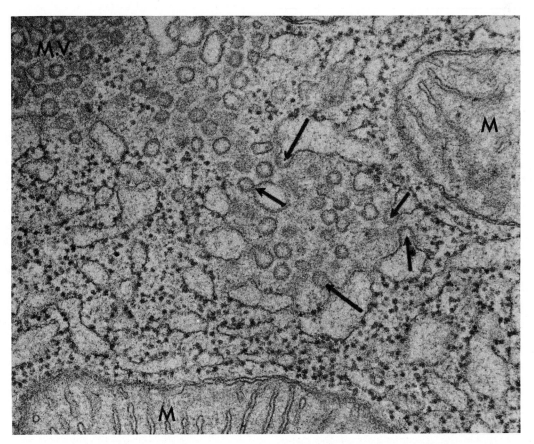

FIG. 5-33. Electron micrograph ($\times$ 70,000) showing the region in a secretory cell where rough-surfaced vesicles of endoplasmic reticulum abut on the periphery of the Golgi apparatus. Micro-vesicles of the Golgi apparatus are prominent in the center of the picture and also at the upper left corner where they are labeled M.V. In several sites, some of which are indicated by arrows, smooth-surfaced transfer or intermediate vesicles are probably budding off from rough-surfaced vesicles of endoplasmic reticulum. It is because of these vesicles becoming filled with secretion from rough-surfaced vesicles that protein secretion can be transported from rough-surfaced endoplasmic reticulum to the Golgi apparatus. (Palade, G. F.: Proc. Nat. Acad. Sci., *52*:613)

FIRST GOLGI SACCULE

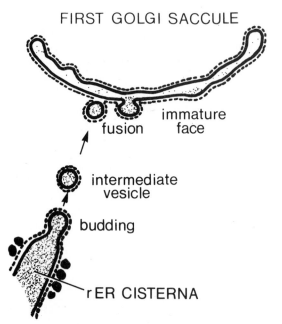

FIG. 5-34. Diagram illustrating the formation of transfer or intermediate vesicles from rER and their fusion later with the immature face of the Golgi apparatus, thus carrying the newly synthesized protein from the rER and releasing it into the first saccule of the Golgi.

toward the Golgi where they meet and fuse with a saccule on the forming face of a stack (Figs. 5-31, 5-32 and 5-33). Three steps seem to be involved in the fusion and emptying process; these are illustrated along the bottom of the Golgi saccule in Figure 5-34. First (at the left) the outer lamella of the unit membrane of the vesicle (dotted line) fuses with the outer lamella of the Golgi saccule, and at the point of fusion the fused lamella becomes discontinuous. Second, the inner lamella of the unit membrane fuses with the inner lamella of the unit membrane of the Golgi saccule and then it becomes discontinuous at this point; this permits the third step to occur, which is that the contents of the intermediate vesicle are emptied into the Golgi saccule. Note that the outer lamella of the intermediate vesicle becomes continuous with the outer lamella of the Golgi saccule. The inner lamellae of both also become continuous. The unit membrane of the intermediate vesicle thus becomes part of the membranous wall of the Golgi saccule and by this process it, of course, adds to the membrane of the saccule. This is how new membrane is supplied to the forming face at the same rate at which it is lost at the mature face.

In some cells intermediate vesicles may also be formed as a result of their budding off from the outer layer of the nuclear envelope which, as has already

been mentioned, is similar to the rough ER. Moreover, in some cells it is thought that intermediate vesicles may bypass the Golgi and fuse directly with secretory vesicles that have budded off from the Golgi.

Moreover, in some cells—for example, liver cells—there is also evidence of a close association of the smooth endoplasmic reticulum (to be described presently) and the Golgi apparatus, particularly with regard to the synthesis of lipoprotein particles whose lipid component seems to be added in passing through the smooth ER, as will be described shortly when the smooth ER is considered.

THE ROLE OF THE GOLGI APPARATUS IN ADDING A CARBOHYDRATE COMPONENT TO THE PROTEIN SECRETIONS BROUGHT TO IT BY INTERMEDIATE VESICLES

Goblet Cells. In order to discuss this matter, it is helpful to consider an interesting type of secretory cell that is highly specialized to elaborate a secretory product that is glycoprotein. All cells in the body manufacture glycoprotein to some extent but goblet cells are most highly developed in this respect. They abound in the lining of the small and large intestine and the larger tubes of the respiratory system. We shall now describe how their study by means of radioautography showed that most of the carbohydrate component of the glycoprotein that they produce and secrete is added in the Golgi apparatus.

The small intestine is lined by a single layer of cells that are taller than they are wide and are arranged side by side (Fig. 1-14, *center*). Some of these lining cells, called absorptive cells, are specialized to absorb the products of digestion while others (the goblet cells) are specialized to secrete mucus, which, as was explained in Chapter 1, is a thick slippery material made from glycoprotein and which stains magenta with the PA-Schiff technic as is shown in Figure 1-14, *center*. The mucus secreted by goblet cells flows over to cover and protect the naked free surfaces of the absorptive cells. The shape of a goblet cell is due to the basal part of the cell, which contains the nucleus, being narrow and, hence, appearing as the stem of a goblet while the part of the cell between the stem and the free surface (the bowl of the goblet) is so distended by bubblelike, membrane-enclosed globules of mucus that it bulges sideways, pressing into the sides of the absorptive cells beside it (Fig. 5-35).

The Role of the Golgi Apparatus in Adding Carbohydrate to Secretions. Clues indicating that the Golgi apparatus might have some function in this respect came from several sources. For example, the

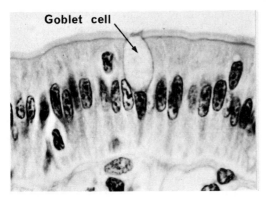

Fig. 5-35. Photomicrograph (× 800) of section of dog intestine, stained with H and E, and showing a goblet cell. Notice the nucleus of the goblet cell below the bowl part of the goblet.

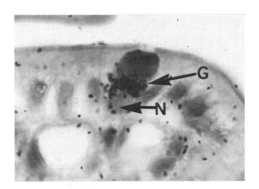

Fig. 5-36. Radioautograph of section of duodenal epithelium of rat 5 minutes after intravenous injection of ^{3}H glucose, showing grains over the Golgi region of the goblet cells. (Illustration courtesy G. C. Bennett)

PA-Schiff technic (which colors certain carbohydrates magenta) often revealed PA-Schiff positive material in the Golgi region of various types of cells. Badinez et al. showed that the Golgi region stains with the colloidal iron technic, a technic which detects the acidic groups of carbohydrates. Revel and Hay, using the EM, showed that the latter reaction occurred in the content of the distended portions of the flattened vesicles of the Golgi apparatus of cells that produce the intercellular substance of cartilage (which contains some carbohydrate). Peterson and Leblond then showed that when radioactive glucose was administered to animals, radioautographs of tissues containing goblet cells, prepared as previously explained in Chapter 3, revealed grains over the Golgi region of goblet cells and that this occurred in tissues fixed less than 5 minutes after the radioactive glucose was given (Fig. 5-36). These results indicated that the labeled glucose that is made available to goblet cells is almost immediately incorporated into carbohydrate macromolecules in the Golgi region which is located just above the nucleus. When the fate of this material was followed by radioautography, it was found that it subsequently enters the bowl portion of the goblet cell and later still is eliminated through the free surfaces of the cell in its mucous secretion.

The evidence available indicates that most of the carbohydrate component of the glycoprotein secretion is being continually added to the protein material in all Golgi saccules, the protein, of course, being derived from the rough ER. However, the addition of some of the sugar residues that make up the carbohydrate side-chains of glycoproteins already begins in the rough-surfaced endoplasmic reticulum, soon after the protein chains synthesized on ribosomes are released into the

cisternae. Usually, N-acetylglucosamine first and, later, mannose are added in the rER; then, later in the Golgi apparatus, galactose, fucose, sialic acid—and, in some cells, glucose—are added to complete the carbohydrate side-chains of the glycoproteins. This is done by certain enzymes called sugar transferases and, as expected, the Golgi is a rich source of these enzymes. It may be pointed out that, unlike the polypeptide chain of a protein that is synthesized by a single ribosome in one spot, the carbohydrate side-chains of glycoproteins are built up successively at different sites by various transferases adding sugars one at a time in a stepwise manner during the time it travels through the cisternae of the rough endoplasmic reticulum and from there through the Golgi apparatus.

Since much of the carbohydrate is added in Golgi saccules and since the saccules migrate from one face to the other at a steady rate, it is clear that the saccules nearer the mature face should contain more carbohydrate than the saccules near the forming face. Rambourg, Hernandez and Leblond showed that the contents of the first 2 or 3 saccules on the forming face of a stack give only a weak positive reaction for carbohydrate by the periodic acid-silver technic (this technic for electron microscopy corresponds to the PA-Schiff technic so commonly employed to demonstrate carbohydrate for light microscopy). These investigators also found that the reaction in the contents of saccules increased in intensity as the mature face was approached and that the most intense reaction was found in the last (the most mature) saccule of the stack. This saccule has been shown by Novikoff often to give also a positive reaction for acid phosphatase, an enzyme which is present in lysosomes—a point which will be of interest when we consider these organelles later on.

The Turnover of the Saccules of a Stack

From what has been said, it can now be appreciated that the stacks of saccules in the Golgi apparatus are not the static structures they were commonly visualized to be only a few years ago but, instead, are always undergoing changes in their structure and composition. A stack, however, exists in a steady state only because new saccules are added to its forming face as rapidly as they are lost on its maturing face to give rise to secretory vesicles and other membranous vesicles, including lysosomes. The rate at which the last saccule on the forming face becomes converted into secretory vesicles at the maturing face varies tremendously from one cell to another. An extremely rapid turnover of saccules is observed in the goblet cells of the colon, where Neutra and Leblond have shown that there is a complete turnover of the whole stack of saccules in less than 40 minutes.

The Role of the Golgi in the Maintenance of the Cell Membrane and the Cell Coat

How the Membrane of Zymogen Granules Could Add to the Cell Membrane. Before it was known that each zymogen granule is encased in a membrane it was thought that the discharge of zymogen granules through the apex of an acinar cell would be injurious to the cell membrane at the site through which they passed; indeed, many thought that the cytoplasm of the cell could probably not be effectively sealed off

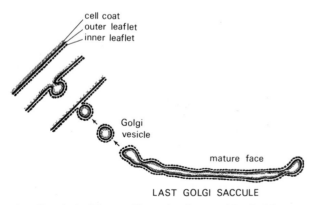

FIG. 5-37. Diagram illustrating how vesicles budding off from the Golgi saccules can contribute membrane and cell coat to the cell surface after fusing with it. Note that the outer lamella of the membrane of the vesicle becomes the inner lamella of the cell membrane.

from the lumen of the acinus at this site. However, when the EM became available, it was shown that each zymogen granule is encased in unit membrane, and in a relatively early study Palade showed that the membrane surrounding a granule remained intact until it reached and fused with the cell membrane that covered the apex of the cell (*see* Fig. 5-25). He then described how the granule breaks through the central part of the fused membranes in such a way that the membrane of the granule and the cell membrane remain fused all around the site at which the rupture occurs, so that the cytoplasm at all times is effectively sealed off from the lumen of the acinus—only the contents of the granules escape. The membrane which had surrounded the bulk of the granule would thus add additional membrane to the cell membrane (Fig. 5-25). Hence, the mechanism by which zymogen granules leave the apex of a cell does not cause a loss of cell membrane but instead provides a constant supply of new membrane.

How Special Secretory Vesicles Could Add Both Membrane and Cell Coat to the Cell Surface. Next, it is obvious that during the growth of any tissue by means of cell multiplication there is a need for the synthesis of new cell membrane because, following division, daughter cells quickly enlarge. There is also a need for more cell coat to cover the surfaces of the increased number of cells. How this is accomplished has been investigated by Bennett and Leblond by radioautography, using ^{3}H-fucose as a precursor to trace the formation of glycoprotein. They were working with the columnar (absorptive) cells lining the intestine, for these represent a type of cell that is enlarging rapidly after a recent division and, also, they have a prominent cell coat (Fig. 5-8). They showed that 2 minutes after ^{3}H-fucose injection, the radioactivity is in the Golgi apparatus where this sugar is taken up during glycoprotein synthesis. Presumably, fucose is the last sugar to be picked up by the glycoprotein molecules, since it is located at the end of the carbohydrate side chains. Within 20 minutes, most of this radioactivity had appeared on all the cell surfaces, thus indicating that the glycoprotein had migrated from the Golgi apparatus to the cell coat. The carrier involved seems to be a type of secretory vesicle whose membrane would provide additional cell membrane and whose glycoprotein content would provide additional cell coat as illustrated in Figure 5-37. Similar observations on nongrowing liver cells suggest that there may be a renewal of membrane and cell coat even in nongrowing cells by this same mechanism. It is interesting in this respect that the membranes of the saccules on the mature face of the Golgi, the face from which new membrane is added to the cell membrane, resemble the cell membrane in thickness whereas those of the saccules on the immature face are considerably thinner, i.e., more like those of the endoplasmic reticulum. This suggests that another function of the Golgi may be to modify the membranes assembled in the rER so that they become similar to and capable of fusion with the cell membrane. Phospholipids, sterols and proteins in the membrane of the Golgi are present in amounts intermediate to those of the ER and those of the cell membrane.

Possible mechanisms for getting rid of excess membrane will be considered after we deal with lysosomes.

The Mechanism by Which Unit Membranes Fuse and Its Implications. As is shown in Figure 5-34, *top*, when the unit membranes of two membranous structures touch each other and fuse, the outer lamellae of the unit membranes that touch are the first to fuse. After fusing so that the outer lamellae of the two unit membranes become continuous, they can open up sufficiently at the site of fusion for the inner lamellae of the two unit membranes to meet and fuse (Fig. 5-34, *top*). They too then open up at the site of fusion so that the contents of the two membranous structures can mix or be delivered from one to the other (Fig. 5-34, *top*). Since the outer lamellae of the unit membranes of structures that meet and fuse become continuous with one another, it might be thought that since, as is shown in Figure 5-37, the outer lamella of the unit membrane of a Golgi vesicle is the first to touch the inner lamella of the cell membrane, that the outer lamella of a unit membrane would have to fuse with the inner lamella of another. The fact is, however, that the outer lamella of an intracytoplasmic vesicle of any kind is the counterpart of the inner lamella of the cell membrane because it is the lamella that faces cytoplasm. As is shown in Figure 5-7, when intracytoplasmic vesicles arise from the cell membrane in phagocytosis or under any other circumstance, the inner lamella of the cell membrane becomes the outer lamella of the unit membrane of the vesicle. So, as is shown in Figure 5-37, when a Golgi vesicle meets and fuses with the cell membrane, the lamella of the cell membrane that faces cytoplasm and the lamella of the vesicular membrane that faces cytoplasm are the first to meet and fuse and, after the other lamellae have fused, the new membrane that is added to the cell membrane is "right side up."

The above is of significance with regard to the synthesis of the material of the cell coat, for it is formed partly in the rough ER and partly in the Golgi and is contained as it is formed within the cisternae or saccules of these representative structures. It is, therefore, gradually formed in association with the counterpart of the outer layer of the cell membrane (solid line in Figs. 5-34 and 5-37). It remains in association with the counterpart of the outer layer of the cell membrane in the vesicles that transport it to the cell membrane (Fig. 5-37), and as these vesicles fuse with the cell membrane and empty their contents onto it (Fig. 5-37) the layer of the membrane with which it has been in contact all this time becomes everted to become the outer layer of the cell membrane at this site (Fig. 5-37), where it is covered by the cell coat that it contained when it was a vesicle (Fig. 5-37).

Recent Evidence of Continuity Between Golgi Stacks. In Chapter 1 comment was made on the difficulties of determining three-dimensional structure of anything from the inspection of a single slice cut through it (Fig. 1-12). In studying the ultrathin sections required for electron microscopy a particular difficulty is presented as to whether or not there might be continuity between what appear in single sections to be individual patches of rER or individual stacks of Golgi saccules. Until now it has been generally assumed that Golgi stacks were isolated from one another. If it were possible to employ thicker sections, connections between what appear to be isolated structures in an ultrathin section might be seen to be connected at, for example, a level lower than the level at which an ultrathin section may have been cut. This has to some extent become possible with the development of the million volt electron microscope, because its great penetrating power permits much thicker sections to be studied than has been possible with instruments of the ordinary voltages used, as will now be described.

As already mentioned, osmium tetroxide will impregnate the Golgi apparatus of cells left standing in a solution of it. Friend showed that this stains only part of the apparatus, namely, the first saccule of the forming face. Rambourg and Clermont took advantage of this property to examine this saccule in 2-micron-thick sections in the million volt electron microscope. They found, in eight different cell types, that the first saccule was continuous from stack to stack and was in fact a ribbonlike structure arranged into an irregular network within the cell. Thus, in nerve cells, the picture they obtained was that of a reticulated internal apparatus very much like the one originally described by Golgi around the nucleus. In other cells, it was usually a single irregular network on one side of the nucleus.

At high magnifications, the first saccule appears fenestrated, as was already known, but the fenestrae are often so wide that Rambourg and Clermont describe it as being composed of a tubular network.

While the continuity of the first saccule throughout the cell has been demonstrated, the situation with regard to other saccules is not clear. It is probable, however, that those of each level are continuous. Hence, what has been described as a stack would only be what is seen in a slice cut through connected saccules.

With regard to function, it seems that what has been said of stacks should apply equally if saccules at each level are connected.

Lysosomes

Some General Features. Lysosomes are membranous organelles that are present in almost all kinds of body cells. Their numbers, however, vary greatly from one cell to another, depending on its type and function. They were given their name because they are little bodies (*soma,* body) (actually they are membranous vesicles) that contain various enzymes that are hydrolytic (*lysis,* dissolution) and are called hydrolases; these act to catalyze reactions in which H_2O is used to break down large molecules into smaller components—for example, peptides into amino acids.

Since the hydrolytic enzymes of lysosomes are capable of lysing the various components of the cytoplasmic matrix, it is fortunate that their content of enzymes is separated from the rest of the cytoplasm by their membranous walls.

In healthy cells lysosomes serve an important digestive function; they are concerned with digesting certain substances which may originate either from within or from without the cell. This function, as will be explained later, is the reason why they have a variety of appearances. Moreover, this work is accomplished without their enzymes escaping into the cytoplasmic matrix. But when a cell, because of oxygen lack or for some other reason, approaches death or dies, the lysosomes quickly liberate their enzymes into the surrounding cytoplasm and bring about the digestion of the cell and, thereafter, even some of the materials in the environment of the cell. Thus the enzymes of lysosomes are believed to be largely responsible for the profound changes that are initiated in cells and tissues after death and account for what is generally termed autolysis or *portmortem degeneration* of tissues.

As more is learned about lysosomes, it becomes increasingly evident that, as will be described later in this book, they not only carry out essential roles in regard to maintaining the health of normal cells; they are also of great importance in the defense of the body against certain bacterial invaders. Furthermore, they can also be the cause of certain *inflammatory lesions.*

Development of Knowledge About Lysosomes. In contrast to the organelles that we have already studied, the LM provided no direct evidence of the existence of lysosomes. That there were such organelles in cytoplasm was first postulated by Christian de Duve in 1955 from biochemical data. Shortly before this time, de Duve and his associates were examining by biochemical methods the enzyme content of various fractions that could be separated from homogenates of rat liver cells by the method of differential centrifugation discussed earlier in this chapter (Fig. 5-12). They were interested particularly in investigating the enzymes of the fractions that contained mitochondria. By refinements of the centrifugation procedures, they managed to obtain a fraction which, although similar to mitochondria in sedimentation characteristics, contained enzymes that were different from those of mitochondria. In this fraction they unexpectedly found a number of hydrolytic enzymes, including acid phosphatase. They then performed a number of biochemical experiments which led them to postulate that the hydrolytic enzymes in this fraction are contained in vesicles about 0.4 micron in diameter, and that each of these is surrounded by a membrane which kept the enzymes from reacting with substrates in the cytoplasm. Realizing that the little bodies in this fraction were not mitochondria but, instead, a new type of cytoplasmic organelle, they proposed the name *lysosomes* for these organelles.

Identification of Lysosomes With the EM. Subsequently, the fractions which contained the acid phosphatase were examined in the EM by Novikoff, Beaufay and de Duve. As was anticipated they proved to be membranous organelles about 0.5 μ in diameter. Since that time Novikoff and others have studied lysosomes in a great variety of cells, by combining the histochemical test for acid phosphatase with electron microscopy. Although lysosomes contain several other hydrolytic enzymes—namely proteases, nucleases, glycosidases, lipases, phospholipases, certain sulfatases and phosphatases—acid phosphatase is the most easily tested for by a histochemical technic (Fig. 5-38) and its demonstration in a membranous organelle is usually taken as proof that the organelle is a lysosome. The presence of a phosphatase can be determined by a procedure that indicates the location of the enzyme by the deposition of a black precipitate. The latter is electron dense and hence shows up as black material in an electron micrograph (Fig. 5-38).

Formation of Lysosomes. Lysosomes are similar to the so-called zymogen granules of the acinar cells of the pancreas, which we have just studied, in that they are membranous vesicles filled with digestive enzymes. It is therefore not surprising that they are formed in the same way. The enzymes of lysosomes, necessarily being protein, are synthesized in rough-

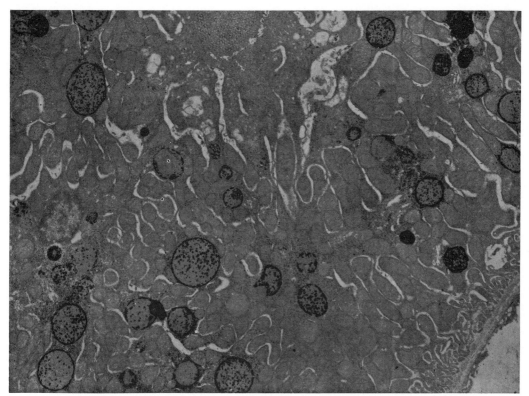

Fig. 5-38. Electron micrograph ($\times$ 7,600) of section of kidney of male rat. This section illustrates how lysosomes can be identified by and hence shown to contain acid phosphatase. The enzyme is demonstrated here by the Gomori technic. The end result of this histochemical procedure leads to the deposition of lead salts where acid phosphatase was present. Since lead salts are very electron-dense, the sites of their deposition are black in this illustration. (Novikoff, A. B.: Ciba Symposium on Lysosomes. p. 36. Boston, Little, Brown & Co., 1963)

surfaced vesicles of the endoplasmic reticulum and, from there, transferred via transfer vesicles to the saccules of the forming face of the Golgi apparatus, where the enzymes soon come to be contained in an expanded portion of the edge of a saccule on the mature face of the Golgi apparatus, which then bud off to constitute a membrane-surrounded vesicle filled with enzymes (Figs. 5-25 and 5-31). Lysosomes are rich in glycoprotein, and most of the carbohydrate component present in them is probably picked up during the passage of the protein through the Golgi apparatus.

TERMINOLOGY USED TO DESIGNATE THE DIFFERENT APPEARANCES OF LYSOSOMES IN VARIOUS STAGES OF FUNCTION

A lysosome that buds off from the maturing face of a stack of Golgi saccules is termed a primary lysosome (Figs. 5-39 and 5-40, *left*). A primary lysosome may interact with material that is brought into the cell from outside the cell, as will be described below, or it may interact with broken-down products which arise within the cell, as will also be described below. When the primary lysosome fuses with another vesicle containing material from either source, the resulting vesicle which contains both the material from another source and the enzymes of the lysosome is known as a secondary lysosome and also by other names.

There is some controversy about the morphologic features of primary lysosomes, since many morphologically different granules or vesicles have the enzymes characteristic of lysosomes (Fig. 5-39). They can be seen budding off from a Golgi saccule and then condensing in a way similar to that in which zymogen granules are formed. A primary lysosome is shown on the left side of Figure 5-40.

We shall now recall how particulate matter or non-particulate matter that is of macromolecular dimensions is brought into the cell from outside (phagocy-

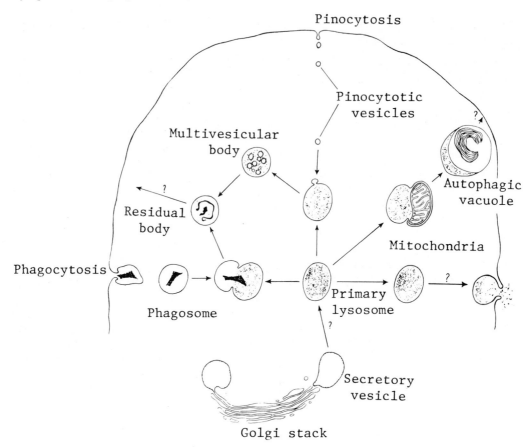

Fig. 5-39. Diagram showing phagocytosis at left and pinocytosis above and the formation of lysosomes from the Golgi apparatus. Various fates of ingested materials contained in vesicles that meet and fuse with lysosomes are depicted. Likewise, the various possible fates of lysosomes are depicted. Since much investigation is proceeding in this area, the terminology and concepts are subject to change.

tosis and pinocytosis); this was illustrated in Figure 5-7. As is shown on the left in Figure 5-39, the membranous vesicle containing the particle brought in from outside the cell is known as a *phagosome* because the process by which the little body is brought into the cell is, of course, phagocytosis. Cells very active in phagocytosis include macrophages and certain types of white blood cells. If the matter taken into the cell is a fluid that contains proteins or other substances in solution, the vesicles, which form at the surface in a similar way except that they are usually smaller, are called pinocytotic vesicles and the process is termed pinocytosis (Fig. 5-39, *top*). Pinocytotic vesicles thus differ from phagosomes in that they have no solid particles inside them. Such vesicles are particularly common in cells that line blood capillaries and in certain types of muscle cells. Both phagocytosis

and pinocytosis are processes that use up the cell membrane. When a phagosome containing, for example, a bacterium meets a lysosome, the surrounding membranes of the two vesicles fuse at their site of contact so that the lysosome discharges its contents into the phagosome. The membranous vesicle formed this way is termed a secondary lysosome. Additional primary lysosomes may meet with and fuse with this secondary lysosome, and several secondary lysosomes also may coalesce. The enzymes contributed by primary lysosomes act to digest the material that was carried into the cell by the phagosomes. Whatever is left over after digestion in the secondary lysosome becomes known as a residual body (Fig. 5-39). Residual bodies may finally be extruded from the cell (Fig. 5-39, *right*) by what is termed *exocytosis*.

If the foreign material that entered the cell is contained in pinocytotic vesicles, the course of events is not as clear. One hypothesis is that somehow the small pinocytotic vesicles get inside the lysosomes. These small, seemingly intact vesicles which appear within the lysosomes are surrounded by a solution containing the hydrolytic enzymes characteristic of lysosomes. This body thereupon becomes known as a multivesicular body (Figs. 5-39 and 5-40, *right*) and it, of course, is another type of secondary lysosome. Presumably, its contents are eventually digested.

Next, as a result of wear and tear, mitochondria and pieces of rough-surfaced endoplasmic reticulum and other cell organelles may become functionless and separated from the rest of the cytoplasm by a membrane. These organelle-containing membrane-bound bits of cytoplasm, like phagosomes, coalesce with lysosomes and undergo digestion (Fig. 5-39, *right*). The resulting structures may take on an endless variety of appearances because they can contain various kinds of cell organelles in different degrees of digestion (Fig. 5-41). Usually, parts of membranes can be recognized because they persist longer than the other components of the organelles (*see* Fig. 5-41). These bodies are referred to as autophagic vacuoles or cytolysosomes. Figure 5-41 shows one with a mitochondrion within it; Figure 5-42 shows one at a later stage, when only the relatively resistant whorls of lipid-containing membrane known as myelin figures can be demonstrated in it. Later the contents of these autophagic vacuoles

may be ejected from the cell. If they persist in the cells for long periods of time, they may accumulate in addition to lipid products a wear-and-tear pigment called *lipofuscin,* particularly in the cells of heart muscle, nervous tissue and liver. These granules will be described in more detail later on in this chapter. Lysosomes and their activities thus provide a type of demolition system that normally works in cells to do away with various cytoplasmic structures that wear out and begin to disintegrate. Normally, of course, the cytoplasmic structures thus disposed of have their places taken by new ones being formed at the same time.

Coated Vesicles

Discovery and Definition. As both the resolving power of the EM and methods for preparing sections for study with the instrument continued to improve, it became apparent that certain rounded free vesicles seen in cytoplasm each had what appeared to be a bristly or fuzzy coating applied to the outer or cytoplasmic matrix side of its membrane. Such vesicles thereupon came to be termed coated vesicles.

SITES OF FORMATION

Coated vesicles arise from several different membranous surfaces as follows:

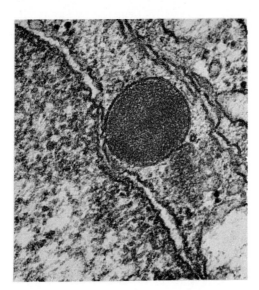 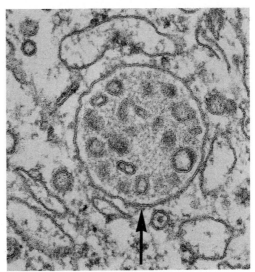

FIG. 5-40. (*Left*) Electron micrograph showing a primary lysosome in a thyroid cell. (Courtesy of C. P. Leblond) (*Right*) Electron micrograph ($\times$ 90,000) showing a multivesicular body. (Friend, D. S., and Farquhar, M. G.: J. Cell Biol., *35:*357, 1967)

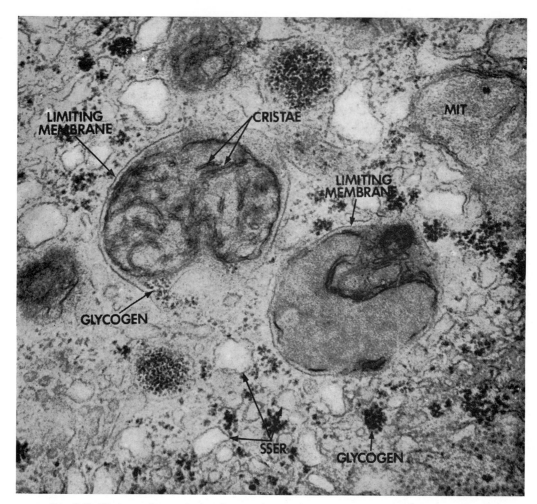

FIG. 5-41. Electron micrograph ($\times$ 57,000) of part of the cytoplasm of a hepatocyte of a rat 3 days after partial hepatectomy. In the center are 2 autophagic vacuoles. They are each surrounded by a membrane. The autophagic vacuole on the left contains a clearly recognizable, though markedly altered, mitochondrion, and some glycogen. The organelloid contents of the one on the right are no longer clearly recognizable. The autophagic vacuoles are thought to be specialized lysosomes in which obsolete cytoplasmic components are undergoing degradation. (Preparation by A. M. Jézéquel)

The Cell Membrane. An early study of coated vesicles that arise from this source was made by Friend and Farquhar in connection with the absorption of protein from the fluid in the lumen of the vas deferens of the male rat. The protein in the fluid of the lumen of the vas deferens (which is a tube) is not digested (as it would be in the intestine) but is taken up as such by the cells lining the tube as if it were a foreign body. The cell membrane that covers the free surfaces of the cells that line the vas deferens is thrown into many little folds and declivities, as is shown in Figure 5-43, *top*. Friend and Farquhar used a protein

that could be traced in electron micrographs and showed that the protein solution in the deepest parts of the folds became surrounded by membrane in a way similar to that in which bacteria became enclosed in a membrane during phagocytosis (Fig. 5-39). By this means a vesicle was formed that enclosed the protein. The vesicle then became detached from the cell membrane and made its way into the cytoplasmic matrix (Fig. 5-43). What is particularly interesting here, however, is that the inner (cytoplasmic) aspect of the cell membrane at these sites has a material which appears bristly in sections associated with it, with the

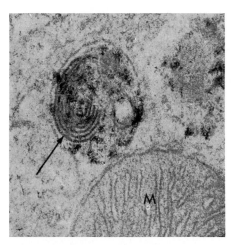

FIG. 5-42. Electron micrograph (× 41,000) showing myelin-like figure in lysosome that is identified by histochemical reaction. (Goldfischer, S., Essner, E., and Novikoff, A. B.: J. Histochem. Cytochem., *12:*72)

From the Rough-Surfaced Endoplasmic Reticulum. As already described, transfer or intermediate vesicles form from the ends of the cisternae of rough-surfaced endoplasmic reticulum that are close to the Golgi apparatus (Fig. 5-33). The outer surface of these little vesicles that bud off in this fashion are free of ribosomes. Some of them, however, develop a fuzzy coating.

Since fuzz-coated vesicles can arise from the Golgi apparatus and since some intermediate (transfer) vesicles that bud off from the rough ER are fuzz-coated and, like other transfer vesicles, fuse with one of the lower saccules of the Golgi apparatus, there may be some difficulty in deciding in some situations whether a coated vesicle is budding off from, or fusing with, a Golgi saccule. Whether vesicles are fusing

bristles projecting into the cytoplasmic matrix (Fig. 5-43). As these vesicles form at the cell membrane the bristly material that is on the inner cytoplasmic side of the cell membrane remains on the cytoplasmic matrix side of the resulting vesicle, with the bristles projecting outward from it into the cytoplasmic matrix (*see* Figure 5-43, arrow).

From the Golgi Apparatus. Small to moderate-sized coated vesicles are sometimes seen close to the edges or upper surface of the flattened saccules at the mature face of the Golgi apparatus. These seem to form in much the same manner as noncoated vesicles, by budding.

From Secretory Vesicles. As was described in connection with the Golgi apparatus, secretory vesicles bud off from the uppermost saccules on its mature face. On leaving the saccules, these secretory vesicles move into the cytoplasm, where they are termed *prosecretory granules* or *condensing vacuoles* as was described in connection with the Golgi. Weinstock and Leblond have found in a study of this phenomenon in ameloblasts that, as the secretory vesicles become smaller because of their contents becoming condensed, small portions of their membranous wall may develop a bristly appearance. They believe that these little bristly areas of membrane bud off as small coated vesicles from a secretory vesicle as it becomes smaller and, hence, requires less membrane to surround its contents than before because of its contents becoming condensed.

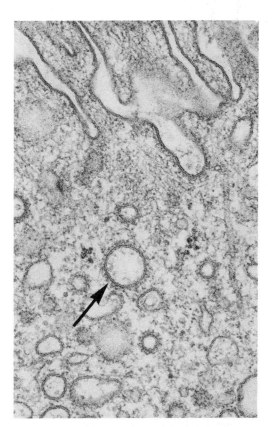

FIG. 5-43. Portion of an epithelial lining cell of the vas deferens close to its free surface. A large type of coated vesicle is seen close to the center of the illustration. Note its bristle coat, and also that the intermicrovillar pit closest to it and above it shows a similar bristle coat on the cytoplasmic side of the cell membrane. (Friend, D. S., and Farquhar, M. G.: J. Cell Biol., *35:*357, 1967)

with or forming from a saccule can often be determined by seeing if any of them are connected to the saccule by a stalk; if so, this is a site where vesicles are being formed. Moreover, vesicle formation occurs primarily from saccules at the mature face, fusion with saccules at the forming face of a stack of saccules.

To sum up, coated vesicles can arise from the cell membrane, the Golgi apparatus, and secretory vesicles (condensing vacuoles) that arise from the Golgi, and from the rough-surfaced endoplasmic reticulum.

The Nature of the Coat. In sections the coat may seem to be bristly on some vesicles and fuzzy on others. However, as the reader should now be well aware, the appearance of anything seen in a slice may be deceiving so far as its three-dimensional structure is concerned. Sections cut obliquely through the same object, or in a place close to and parallel with its surface, can help to determine three-dimensional structure, as can technics such as negative staining. From studies made by these methods it appears that the bristly outer surface of a coated vesicle is not due to actual bristles projecting from its outer surface (like the quills of an emotionally disturbed porcupine); instead, the appearance of a bristle in a slice has the same explanation as the bristle-like appearances that would be seen if a slice were cut longitudinally through the wax walls of the hexagons at the face of a honeycomb; for in such a section each wall would appear as a bristle.

The coat of a vesicle should not be confused with the cell coat. The cell coat is found on the outside of the cell membrane (Figs. 5-3 and 5-8), whereas the coat of a vesicle forms on the inner side, i.e., the cytoplasmic side of the cell membrane, and remains on the cytoplasmic side in the fully formed coated vesicle (Fig. 5-43). It is the content of a vesicle that adds to the cell coat as vesicles from the Golgi apparatus fuse with, and open their contents onto, the surface of a cell (Fig. 5-37). The coat of a coated vesicle, however, is not derived from the contents of a vesicle; it is derived from something that is in the cytoplasmic matrix, as is illustrated by the formation of coated vesicles from the cell membrane of the cells lining walls of the vas deferens (Fig. 5-43).

Function, Fate and Significance. In the instance of coated vesicles that form and are released from the secretory vesicles as their contents become increasingly condensed, the concept suggested by Weinstock and Leblond, namely that the formation and release of coated vesicles represent a means whereby excess membrane is disposed of, is attractive. In addition, as indicated before, there is a large amount of evidence

that those coated vesicles which form from the cell membrane (Fig. 5-43) allow many different types of cells to take up protein from their environment.

The Smooth-Surfaced Endoplasmic Reticulum (sER)

The amount of sER in cells varies in relation to their type and only in certain cell types is it prominent. It differs from the rER structurally in two ways: first, the outer surfaces of its membranes are not studded with ribosomes. Secondly, instead of consisting mostly of fairly large vesicles, flattened or otherwise, the sER consists almost entirely of tubules that are arranged in an anastomosing network and that individually pursue tortuous courses in the cytoplasm (Fig. 5-44). The tubules of the sER are often continuous with vesicles and cisternae of the rER. The kinds of cells in which the sER is prominent will be mentioned in the following.

FUNCTIONS

The sER carries out a wide variety of functions. Since it possesses no ribosomes, it is not concerned with the synthesis of protein; instead, it is concerned with the metabolism and/or segregation of other kinds of chemical entities as follows:

Lipids. The sER is concerned with the synthesis of lipids and compounds of the cholesterol family. Accordingly, sER is abundant in cells that synthesize and secrete lipids, lipoproteins and steroid hormones (Fig. 5-45). As will be described in the chapter dealing with endocrine glands, the steroid hormones are related chemically to cholesterol.

Liver cells probably produce most, if not all, of the lipoprotein that is found in blood. The protein component of this is synthesized in the rER of liver cells. From there, however, the protein passes to the sER, where lipid is added to it. The lipoprotein thus formed then passes through the Golgi, from which it is delivered to the cell surface in the usual manner and from which it is secreted into the bloodstream, as will be described when we consider the liver as an organ.

Another example of the sER having a function in relation to fat metabolism is provided by the cells that absorb fat from the intestine. As mentioned at the beginning of this chapter, fat is digested in the intestine, which results in its being broken down to simpler components which can be absorbed by the absorptive cells that line the small intestine. Within the cytoplasm of these cells, however, the simpler components are

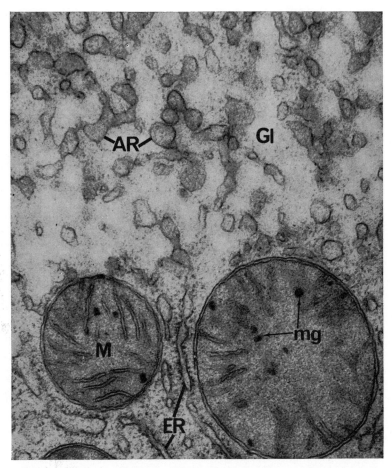

Fig. 5-44. Electron micrograph of liver cell of normal mouse, showing smooth-surfaced (agranular) endoplasmic reticulum (AR) and glycogen (Gl), which is unstained, disposed between the tubules and vesicles of the AR. Two mitochondria are present in the lower part of the illustration, one labeled M; in the other, mg indicates mitochondrial granules. A little rER is seen between them (labeled ER). (Trump, B. F.: Lab. Invest., *11*:986)

resynthesized into fat, and this occurs in the sER. The tiny droplets of fat thus formed are later secreted by the cells into the tissue fluid, where they are known as chylomicrons. From the tissue fluid they make their way into lymphatics and via this route eventually reach the bloodstream.

Relation to Drug Detoxification. That the liver can be concerned with the detoxification of certain drugs has been believed for a long time and studies with the EM indicate that the sER plays a significant role in the process involved. For example, there is a dye commonly known as "butter yellow" which, on being fed to experimental animals, has been shown to induce cancer of the liver. The EM shows that the

amount of sER becomes increased when this drug is fed and it is believed that this occurs because of the sER's becoming larger to function better in detoxifying this drug. It is believed that the sER functions in detoxifying many other drugs as well, including barbiturates.

Relation to Glycogen Formation. Glycogen, when present, lies as deposits in the cytoplasmic matrix; these are commonly found in close association with the sER (Fig. 5-44). Although the cytoplasm of liver cells contains patches of both rER and sER, glycogen is found in association only with the latter. As can be seen in Figure 5-44 where the glycogen is unstained and appears as a pale homogenous material, the tubules of the sER are scattered about in this pale material. The same kind of close association between the sER and glycogen can be seen in sections in which the glycogen has been stained (Fig. 5-46).

The close association of glycogen with the sER is also seen in striated muscle, in which tissue the sER is commonly referred to as the sarcoplasmic reticulum. The numerous tubules of this which permeate the muscle fiber to surround the contractile elements are, in turn, commonly surrounded by glycogen granules.

The premise that the sER is concerned with the synthesis of glycogen with which it is so closely associated receives support from the finding that sER that has been separated from cells by differential centrifugation contains several factors and enzymes that are concerned in the reactions by which glucose is converted to glycogen, and particularly glucose-6-phosphate which activates the enzyme glycogen synthetase.

Mineral Metabolism. In certain cells of the stomach which will be considered in detail later, the sER seems to be concerned in the mechanism by which chloride ions are concentrated in connection with the production of free hydrochloric acid.

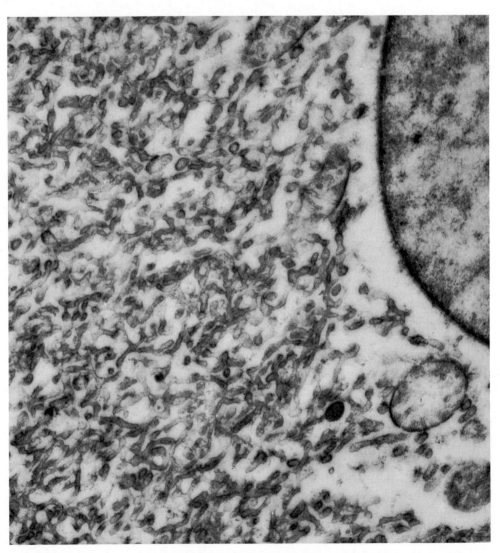

FIG. 5-45. This electron micrograph ($\times$ 33,000) is of a section of the testis of an opossum and shows part of an interstitial cell. Part of a nucleus is seen at top left, with 4 mitochondria adjacent to it. The remainder of the field is filled with a network of interconnected tubules of agranular endoplasmic reticulum. (From Drs. A. K. Christensen and D. W. Fawcett)

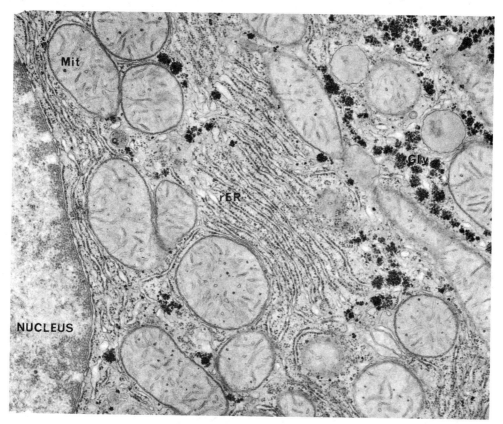

Fig. 5-46. A patch of granular endoplasmic reticulum (labeled rER) in the cytoplasm of a liver cell. Patches such as this in liver cells account for the spotty basophilia of cytoplasm seen with the LM. At the upper right some stained glycogen (Gly) associated with sER is present. Numerous mitochondria are scattered about in the cytoplasm. (Coimbra, A., and Leblond, C. P.: J. Cell Biol., *30:*151, 1966)

FORMATION

Since the sER is continuous with the rER in certain sites, and since there are no arrangements for protein synthesis along the smooth kind, it would seem reasonable to assume that the rough endoplasmic reticulum is formed first and then transforms, by losing its ribosomes, into endoplasmic reticulum of the smooth type. The fact that in many places the membranes of the sER remain continuous with those of the rER also supports this conclusion.

Microtubules, Cilia, Flagella and Centrioles

Development of Knowledge. Cilia, flagella and centrioles were all given their respective names when they were seen long ago with the LM. However, it was not until it became possible to study these structures with the EM that it was found that they were all composed basically of tiny tubules which were there-upon named *microtubules*. For a few years it was not known that microtubules could also exist as individual entities dispersed throughout the cytoplasm. The reason for microtubules being seen first in structures composed of them was that the methods used for fixing tissue for the EM at that time (osmium tetroxide) did not preserve microtubules unless a number of them were bunched together in structures. It was not until glutaraldehyde came to be used for fixation that it was found that single microtubules were dispersed throughout the cytoplasm. We shall comment on these first and then later consider the structures into which they may be organized.

DISPERSED MICROTUBULES

Morphology. Microtubules are present in all kinds of cells except those of bacteria and certain algae. They are slender filamentous structures about 250 Å in

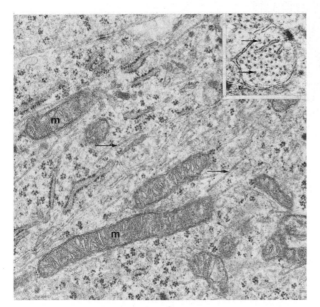

FIG. 5-47. Cytoplasm of rat ependymal cells showing numerous microtubules in longitudinal section (arrows). Mitochondria (M), short segments of rough endoplasmic reticulum and numerous polysomes are also present in the cytoplasm. (*Inset*) Nerve cell process showing numerous microtubules in cross section (arrows). × 40,000. (From V. I. Kalnins)

diameter and of variable length (Fig. 5-47). They can be very long and tend to be straight, which implies that they have a certain amount of rigidity, but they are sufficiently elastic to bend without breaking. When they are seen in cross section they appear as tiny circles because their walls are denser than their central parts (*see* inset, Fig. 5-47).

Functions. The free dispersed microtubules act to some extent as a skeleton for a cell. Cells are of many different shapes, some even being star-shaped, and the maintenance of these various shapes that characterize different kinds of cells is due substantially to the way microtubules are distributed within them. As an aid to their serving a skeletal function, most are anchored in a region near the centriole. Dispersed microtubules, however, are not the only organelle to serve a supportive role within the cell, for the cell web, to be described presently, also functions to some extent in this respect.

A second function of microtubules seems to be that of facilitating the transport of various particles and perhaps also large macromolecules throughout the cytoplasm. The paths along which they move seem to be related to the directions in which the microtubules are disposed. It is therefore thought that microtubules

exist in some sort of an arrangement whereby the movement of the particles is restricted to specific courses much as the movement of trains is restricted to tracks.

An interesting illustration of microtubules serving both of the above described functions has come from studies made by Tilney and Porter on the skin of fish which change their surface appearance quickly in order to blend in with their background. This helpful ability enables them to camouflage themselves from their enemies. This ability depends on their having in their skin certain cells called *melanocytes* (which we shall study in more detail when we describe skin). The melanocytes of these fish not only have the ability to produce melanin pigment (as our melanocytes have); they also, when stimulated by exposure to a light or dark background, can bring about rapid movements of the pigment-containing granules in their cytoplasm, as follows:

Melanocytes have a curious shape, roughly resembling octopuses because of their having long, wavy cytoplasmic processes that extend off from the region of their nuclei in many different directions, winding their way between other cells in the skin. When a fish swims from a light into a dark background, the melanin (which is in the form of granules) quickly migrates from the cytoplasm that is close to the nucleus into the processes and, since these lie between so many of the cells in the skin, the skin appears dark. When the fish enters an area where the background is light, the melanin granules quickly leave the processes to become grouped around the nucleus where they become concentrated and take up so little space that the skin appears light. Note that the mechanism depends, not on the withdrawal or extension of the cytoplasmic processes themselves but on the rapid movement of the pigment granules into and out of the processes. The EM has shown that microtubules extend off from the region around the centriole, which is close to the nucleus, into all of these processes, where they seem to serve two functions—that of providing internal support for the processes and also as a guidance system for the rapid movement of the melanin granules back and forth.

Another kind of cell which has cytoplasmic processes extending off from its main body of cytoplasm is the nerve cell; here a fine process (a nerve fiber) may be several feet in length. As shown in the inset of Figure 5-47, which is a cross section of a nerve fiber, these processes too have microtubules within them to provide support and here also they seem to give direction to the flow of material that is synthesized close to the nucleus and constantly moves toward the extremity of a long process as will be described in Chapter 17 under "Axon Flow."

A third function of microtubules is concerned with movements in which they are more directly involved. These movements, however, like those already described in connection with mitosis in Chapter 2, are not due to microtubules themselves being contractile. They can become longer, because of new microtubule subunits being added to their ends; thus they can spread two objects apart, as occurs when the continuous tubules grow in length and push the two pairs of centrioles apart to increase the length of the spindle in mitosis. In addition, they may be able to change their positions in relation to one another because of forces that act between them, as may occur in mitosis when the chromosomal microtubules (as some think) slide along the continuous tubules to move the chromatids from the equatorial plane toward the two poles of the dividing cell (*see* Chapter 2). Forces generated between adjacent microtubules can probably cause them to slide past each other as occurs when they bend in ciliary movement, as will be described shortly.

The Formation of Microtubules. As was described in connection with the formation of the spindle in mitosis, microtubules are assembled from a specific protein called tubulin that is present in cells. This protein has a molecular weight of around 55,000. In order for macromolecules of this protein (which are called monomers of tubulin and are about 40 Å in diameter) to form microtubules, the first step is for them to unite in pairs called *dimers;* these, in turn, become assembled into the walls of the microtubules. In cells tubulin is present in solution in considerable amounts and is in equilibrium with the microtubules as follows:

$$tubulin \rightleftharpoons microtubules$$

Microtubules, except those of cilia, centrioles and basal bodies (which are fairly stable), are always breaking down into tubulin and the latter is always being assembled into microtubules, which is of great interest in connection with the action of two drugs, *colchicine* and *vinblastine,* which affect the process of mitosis—indeed, the latter is used in the treatment of certain malignancies to arrest the division of tumor cells.

It has been found that one of these drugs, colchicine, acts by binding fairly specifically to the dimers of the tubulin that are in solution in a cell and, of course, form the pool of tubulin from which new microtubules would ordinarily be assembled. However, if this drug becomes bound to soluble tubulin, the latter can no longer aggregate into microtubules. Since microtubules are constantly breaking down into tubulin, and since, in the presence of this drug, tubulin becomes incapable of being aggregated into microtubules (which is why this drug interferes with mitosis and inhibits spindle formation), the action of the drug in interphase cells leads in due course to the disappearance of the free microtubules from the cytoplasm; only the microtubules that are organized into the more permanent structures such as centrioles and cilia persist. However, the process is reversible, for, if the drug is washed away from cells or metabolized, the assembling of new microtubules from the pool of soluble tubulin in the cell begins once more. Vinblastine, which acts in a slightly different manner on tubulin, also has the same effect, i.e., it prevents the microtubule subunits from polymerizing into microtubules.

It is thought that the assembly of microtubules is initiated at special sites distributed throughout the cytoplasm, called microtubule organizing centers (MTOC). These centers are particularly common near the centrioles and are also present at the ends of structures called basal feet which are attached to the basal bodies of cilia (Fig. 5-48) which are to be described later on. The kinetochore located on the chromosome (Figs. 2-19 and 2-20) is another structure that acts as a site for the assembly of microtubules or MTOC.

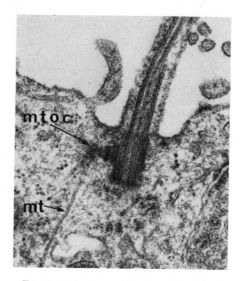

Fig. 5-48. A cilium of a rat ependymal cell. Attached to the left of the basal body of the cilium is a basal foot whose end serves as a microtubule organizing center (mtoc) to which the cytoplasmic microtubules (mt) are attached. × 40,000. (From V. I. Kalnins)

Cilia and Flagella

Cilia is plural of the Latin word for eyelid, which is *cilium*. Since eyelashes extend from the free border of the eyelid, it is not surprising that, when microscopes became available and it was noticed that certain unicellular organisms and cells in the body had hairlike processes extending from their free surfaces, the processes would be termed cilia.

General Distribution and Function of Ciliated Cells. Ciliated cells are found in certain parts of the respiratory system, in certain parts of the female reproductive tract and in one small part of the male reproductive tract, as follows:

The cells that line the cavities of the nose, the paranasal sinuses, nasopharynx, trachea, bronchi and bronchioles (all of which will be described when we study the respiratory system) are of two general types that are interspersed: (1) goblet cells that produce and secret mucus onto the free surface and (2) ciliated cells which have cilia on their free surfaces (Fig. 5-49).

This arrangement permits the free surface to be always covered with a film of mucus in which the cilia of the ciliated cells are immersed. The cilia beat in unison in such a way (as will be described shortly) as to move the film of mucus in one direction, with the result that particles inhaled in the air we breathe are caught in the mucus and moved along the tubes or cavities. Most of it is eventually swallowed (or "coughed up") although blowing one's nose does get rid of some of the mucus that might otherwise accumulate in the cavities of the nose. In other words, the upper respiratory tract offers an example of an air-conditioning mechanism for removing some of the contaminants from the air before they reach the more delicate respiratory portion of the lungs where gaseous interchange occurs between air and blood.

The other important site where there is a somewhat similar arrangement is in the lining cells of the oviducts. Here, although there are ciliated cells, they are interspersed with cells that secrete mucus but are not typical goblet cells. The mucus here is moved along

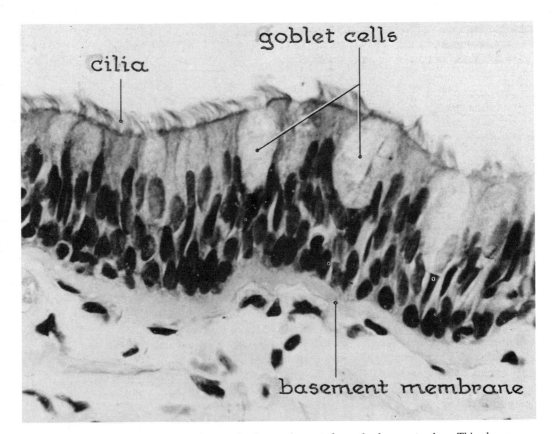

Fig. 5-49. High-power photomicrograph of a section cut from the human trachea. This shows pseudostratified ciliated columnar epithelium with goblet cells.

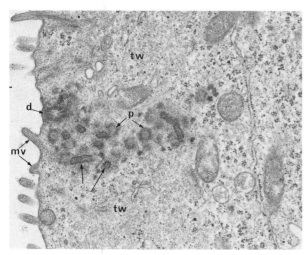

FIG. 5-50. A differentiating ciliated cell from the chick trachea, showing the assembly of centrioles. Clusters of immature centrioles (p) may be seen in a finely fibrous region in the apical portion of the cell known as the terminal web (tw). The procentrioles assemble around cylindrical structures known as "centriolar organizers" (arrows) near the diplosomal centrioles of the cell (d). Microtubules have not yet formed in these procentrioles. Microvilli (mv) project from the cell into the lumen of the trachea (L). Filaments similar to those of the terminal web may be seen inside the microvilli. × 40,000. (From J. D. Marshall and V. I. Kalnins)

the oviducts to the uterus as will be described in more detail in Chapter 26.

The small part of the male reproductive tract where cilia are present will be described in connection with the male reproductive system.

Structure of Ciliated Cells As Seen With the LM. Ciliated cells are commonly longer than they are wide (Fig. 5-49) and their sides are apposed to the sides of the cells that surround them. Cilia are found only on the free surface of each, the surface that abuts on a lumen or cavity (Fig. 5-49). There may be several hundred cilia on a single cell. Commonly cilia are from 5 to 15 μ long and around 0.2 μ in diameter. Accordingly, cilia can be discerned with the LM but their internal structure cannot be resolved with it (Fig. 5-49). However, the LM, used in conjunction with special staining, revealed that there was a little body in the cytoplasm beneath each cilium to which it appeared to be connected and this was called its *basal body*. It is these bodies arranged in a row which give the dense appearance to the cytoplasm just below the cell surface (Fig. 5-49).

The Development and Fine Structure of Cilia. The EM revealed that the cilia develop from centrioles

and indeed that the basal body of a cilium is a centriole.

It will be recalled that centrioles (described in Chapter 2 in connection with mitosis) are short cylindrical structures (Figs. 2-11, 2-12 and 2-18). The wall of each is composed of 9 longitudinally disposed parallel bundles of microtubules, each bundle containing 3 microtubules (Fig. 2-11). A bundle of 3 closely grouped microtubules is termed a *triplet*. The 9 triplets of a centriole are held in position by fibrillar material so that they form the wall of a cylinder. As noted previously, centrioles are commonly present in interphase cells in pairs which are located either close to the nucleus and near the Golgi apparatus or near the cell surface.

The Basal Body. To develop a ciliated surface, a cell must first assemble enough centrioles for there to be one for each of the several hundred cilia that will form. A cell in which such an assembly of centrioles is taking place is shown in Fig. 5-50. After the baby

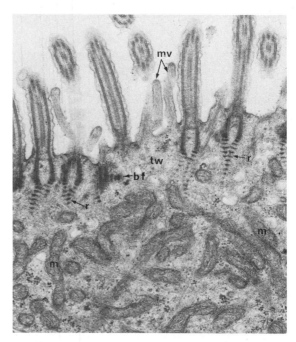

FIG. 5-51. Ciliated cell in the duck trachea, showing a number of cilia in longitudinal and oblique sections. The basal bodies of the cilia are embedded in the terminal web region of the cell (tw). Rootlets (r) are attached to their basal ends and a basal foot (bf) projects from their sides. Microtubules may be seen inside the ciliary shafts. Microvilli (mv) with cores composed of filaments are present between the cilia. Numerous mitochondria (m) are found in the region below the terminal web. (From J. D. Marshall and V. I. Kalnins)

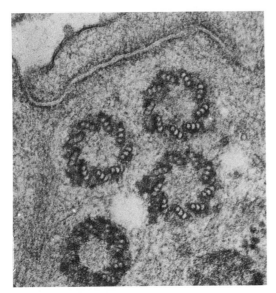

Fig. 5-52. Electron micrograph of a part of a ciliated cell from rat trachea, showing four basal bodies cut in cross section. The 9 triplets of microtubules in their walls are clearly visible. Note their resemblance to cross sections of centrioles (Fig. 2-11). × 74,000. (From V. I. Kalnins)

the order of waves of mucus that are propelled in one direction across a cell surface. Measurements made in the nose showed that a particle caught in the mucus is moved up to 6 mm or more per minute. A cilium, while fairly rigid, beats in one direction, then relaxes, and is pulled back to the starting position in the other direction to complete a cycle in about 1/25 of a second. It then beats forward again. The first is called the *effective stroke* (the stroke that propels the mucus) whereas the return stroke in the other direction is called the *recovery stroke*. The question arises, however, as to how this back and forth motion of cilia moves mucus in only one direction. This is due to the fact that on its effective stroke the cilium remains stiff and pushes mucus ahead of it. But on its return stroke it relaxes or bends and so it is, as it were, crouched down so that it eases back into position without disturbing the mucus to any great extent, whereupon it straightens and stiffens for its next forward stroke.

The mechanics of ciliary action are not clear. There are, however, a few features of, and findings about, cilia that deserve mention in this connection. First, the two singlets in the central core of a cilium are seen in cross section to be lined up perpendicularly to the direction of the beat. Next, there are short arms on the doublets (Fig. 5-53) and it has been found possible

centrioles develop to full size, they migrate toward the free surface of the cell and line up just below it. Next, microtubules of the ciliary shaft (called an axoneme) grow out from the distal end of each centriole (which now is called a basal body) and become the core of a cilium that will project, surrounded by a cell membrane, from the free surface of a ciliated cell (Fig. 5-51).

The Growth of the Shaft. An axoneme grows toward the surface as a result of the two innermost tubules of each triplet of the basal body increasing in length as new tubulin is added to their distal ends. A pair of microtubules such as this is called a *doublet*. Since the third microtubule of each triplet of the basal body does not increase in length, there is a difference in the cross section appearance of the basal body and the axoneme of the cilium, for a cross section of the former shows a ring of nine triplets (Fig. 5-52) whereas a cross section of the shaft reveals a ring of nine doublets (Fig. 5-53). There is another change also: two single microtubules develop in the central region of the shaft. These are termed *singlets* and they also grow toward the surface. They can be seen in a cross section of the shaft (Fig. 5-53) but not in a cross section of the basal body (Fig. 5-52).

The Movement of Cilia. Rows of cilia commonly beat in sequence so that they produce something of

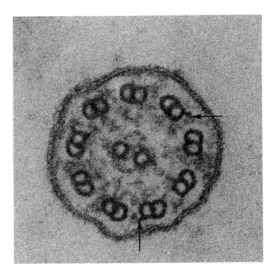

Fig. 5-53. A single cilium from a ciliated cell of rat trachea cut in cross section, showing the 9 peripheral doublets, and the 2 central singlet microtubules of the axoneme. On some of the doublets fine projections (arrows) which have ATPase activity may be observed. The unit membrane structure may be seen in the cell membrane which surrounds the cilium. × 220,000. (From V. I. Kalnins)

to remove these and study them by biochemical methods and this has revealed that they contain the enzyme ATPase. Presumably they are, therefore, involved in releasing energy from ATP so that work can be done in their immediate neighborhood. Since microtubules themselves are not contractile the work which results in ciliary movements would seem to involve the doublets of microtubules in the cilium (Fig. 5-53) somehow sliding in relation to one another. The arms containing the ATPase may provide the force for this sliding mechanism between adjacent doublets.

Cells That Develop a Single Cilium. In contrast to cells that develop hundreds of cilia there are many kinds in the body that develop only one and it is usually rudimentary or incomplete and probably nonmotile. For its formation the two centrioles of a cell migrate to the cell surface where only one of them gives rise to a ciliary shaft and hence becomes a basal body (Fig. 5-54). Single rudimentary cilia develop particularly in types of cells that have lost their ability to divide; their function is not clear at this time.

In certain other instances a single cilium may undergo extensive development (as occurs in the formation of certain of the organs of special sense) to become very important parts of the arrangement by which nervous impulses are initiated as a result of exposure to certain forms of energy. The rods and cones of the eye which are the light receptors provide examples of this, as will be described when these structures are dealt with later.

Flagella. Another example of a single cilium becoming highly developed is manifested in what are termed flagella. Like cilia, flagella are found on many kinds of unicellular organisms where they, like cilia, serve as means for propulsion for the organism. Cilia and flagella are much alike; they differ chiefly in that the flagella (*flagellum*, whip) are somewhat longer than cilia. Also, whereas a cell may have very large numbers of cilia, it usually has only one or two flagella. In mammals the only cells with flagella are the spermatozoa (the germ cells of the male), each of which has one. ·

Filaments

Definitions and General Features. The words fiber, fibril and filament from their derivation all mean an elongated threadlike structure. In practice these words are used in microscopy to refer, in the order given above, to threadlike structures of decreasing diameters. The words, however, do not have pre-

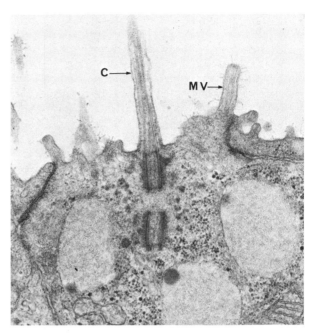

Fig. 5-54. Electron micrograph showing the apical part of a mucus secreting cell from the rat trachea with a single cilium (C), on one of the two diplosomal centrioles cut in longitudinal section. Microvilli (MV) project into the lumen of the trachea. The three pale staining areas in the cytoplasm are mucus granules. × 40,000. (From J. D. Marshall and V. I. Kalnins)

cise meanings with regard to size—for example, the fine wire readily seen with the naked eye in an electric light bulb is termed its filament. However, in histology a threadlike structure that can be seen with the naked eye or with the lower powers of the LM is generally termed a fiber. One that is resolved only by the higher power of the LM is in general termed a fibril while those that are resolved only with the EM are usually termed either fibrils or filaments. Filaments are generally in the range of from around 40 to 150 Å in diameter and of variable length. They are believed to be present, but not in equal numbers, in all kinds of body cells. In many kinds of cells they are arranged in networks or in bundles that are large enough to be seen with the higher powers of the LM in suitably stained preparations. The term fibril is used to denote a structure thicker than a filament in the EM.

To avoid possible confusion it should be emphasized that filaments constitute a category of threadlike structures completely different from microtubules. Though often associated, filaments and microtubules differ in their functions. An analogy is sometimes used to indicate their functional relationship, namely that microtubules form the "bones" of the cell whereas filaments are like the muscles of the body, since at least certain of the filaments provide for movement that occurs in the cell. The two, however, are not attached to each other.

DEVELOPMENT OF KNOWLEDGE

Tonofibrils. A couple of decades ago when most knowledge of microscopic structure was based on what could be resolved with the LM, it was usually thought that there were tiny fibrils within certain types of cells (particularly in the skin) which in contiguous cells passed from one cell to another at sites which were described as intercellular bridges (Fig. 5-55). They were termed *tonofibrils* (*tono,* related to tone or tension) and believed to play some sort of supportive role in the cytoplasm and also to be a factor in holding cells together. Then with the EM it was learned that (1) they were composed of filaments (now called tonofilaments) grouped together more or less side by side so that they formed bundles large enough to be seen with the LM and (2) they did not pass from one cell to the next, as they seem to do in Figure 5-55, but end inside cells at cell membranes in

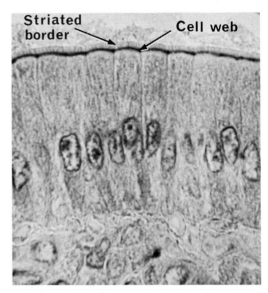

FIG. 5-56. Photomicrograph of absorptive cells of rat intestine stained (see text) to show the terminal webs of the cells. Note how the terminal web seems to dip down at sites where cells are contiguous. The striated border of the epithelial cells can be seen immediately above the terminal web.

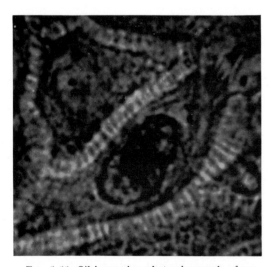

FIG. 5-55. Oil-immersion photomicrograph of section of thick human skin showing prickle cells. The fine lines that join adjacent cells, and which account for the prickly appearance of the cells, are tonofibrils. It was once believed that they passed from the cytoplasm of one cell into the cytoplasm of the next, and so anchored the cells together. It is now known that they do not pass between cells but are contained within their cytoplasm. They terminate at the cell membrane of the cell they are in at what are termed desmosomes (soon to be described; see Fig. 5-61).

structures called desmosomes, as will be described presently.

The Cell Web and the Terminal Web. Before these points about tonofibrils were clarified by EM studies, another finding was made from LM studies which was an important milestone along the development of knowledge about filaments. By developing a special staining method known as the tannic acid, phosphomolybdic acid and amido acid technic, Leblond, Puchtler and Clermont were able not only to stain tonofibrils to advantage but to show that there was a great deal more of the same sort of material distributed in various sites and in a less dense form in many different kinds of cells—enough, in fact, to indicate the existence of an internal supportive structure within cells. They termed this the *cell web.* Their method demonstrated very clearly that in particular there was a dense layer of this material immediately below the free surface of the absorptive cells of the small intestine (Fig. 5-56) (the cells that are intermingled with goblet cells in this part of the intestinal tract as has already been described). They termed this layer at the ends of the absorptive cells the *terminal web* (Fig. 5-56).

Striated Borders. Before describing the EM appearance of the terminal web, we should comment on another feature of the absorptive cells that was noted long ago, namely that the free surfaces of these cells did not appear to be smooth, even and sharply defined as do the free borders of cells in many other sites but instead they were covered with what seemed to be a layer of something that was striated, with the striations running at right angles to the free surfaces of these cells (Fig. 5-56). This was called a *striated border*. With the development of the EM the nature of the striated border and the cell web which lies immediately beneath it were both elucidated as follows.

Microvilli. The striated border seen with the LM proved to be the result of innumerable little fingerlike processes of cytoplasm, each covered with cell membrane, projecting from the cell surface into the lumen of the intestine (Fig. 5-8). These were termed *microvilli* (*villus*, a tuft of hair). (The reason for "micro" in this term is that there are much larger structures called villi that are easily visible with the LM in the lining of the small intestine, as will be described when this organ is considered later).

Microvilli enormously increase the surface through which absorption of nutrients can take place in the small intestine. Moreover, microvilli are found on almost all cells in the body (Figs. 5-50, MV, and 5-51, MV) although they rarely are found as large and as uniformly arranged as in the absorptive cells of small intestine as shown in Figure 5-8. Only when they are can a striated border be distinguished in the LM.

The Fine Structure of the Terminal Web. With the EM the terminal web (TW in Fig. 5-8) proved to be composed of a network of filaments (Fig. 5-50, TW) and in most instances to have a reduced amount of the other types of cytoplasmic organelles. Furthermore, it became evident that bundles of filaments extended from the terminal web up into the microvilli where they serve as cores for these structures (MV in Fig. 5-54). These cores extend down into the terminal web to provide anchorage for the microvilli.

THE RELATION OF FILAMENTS TO CONTRACTILITY

The next development of interest about microfilaments depended on evidence which began to accumulate to the effect that some of them at least were involved in contractile mechanisms. Before discussing this we should comment briefly on contractile mechanisms.

The Nature of Phenomena of Contraction in Striated Muscle. The contractile mechanism is most readily studied in striated muscle fibers which of course are specialized for this function and which will be dealt with in detail when we later consider muscle tissue. When the EM first became available it was found that the fibrils of muscle (which could be seen with the LM) were largely composed of filaments and for a time it was assumed that contraction depended on these shortening in length, which belief fitted in with the concept of the existence of threads consisting of proteins that were contractile. Chemical studies made on muscle indicated that the material involved was some sort of complex of two proteins, *actin* and *myosin*.

The Sliding Filament Hypothesis. The concept of individual protein threads shortening in length to account for muscular contraction was rudely shattered when the EM studies of Huxley and Hanson showed that this did not happen in striated muscle; instead the shortening occurred by filaments remaining the same length but sliding along one another, as will now be explained. Their beautiful studies showed that the contractile unit of a fibril of striated muscle (which is called a *sarcomere—sarcos*, flesh; *meros*, part) contained two kinds of filaments, thin ones made of actin and around 50 Å in diameter and thicker ones of myosin of about 100 Å in diameter and that these were arranged so that they interdigitated within the contractile unit in a complex way. Half of the actin filaments were found to be attached to one end of a contractile unit and the other half to the other end of the unit (Fig. 18-7). In a relaxed muscle, their free ends did not meet in the middle of the unit but were some distance apart. (Details are all given in Chapter 18 but reference to Figure 18-7 here will be helpful.) The thicker myosin filaments, in a relaxed unit, were found to lie in roughly the middle two thirds of the unit where they interdigitated with the free ends of the actin units attached to each end of the unit. Contraction of the unit was found to depend on forces that caused the actin filaments to slide past the myosin filaments until their ends reached the middle of the sarcomeres. Since the actin filaments were attached to the ends of the unit, the two ends of the unit were pulled closer together when they slid toward its middle.

Contractile Phenomena in Other Types of Cells. When it was shown that the contractile mechanism in muscle, where it is studied to best advantage, did not depend on filaments shortening, the question was raised as to whether contractile phenomena in other kinds of cells did not also depend on filaments sliding along one another instead of becoming thicker and shorter. In cells other than those that are highly specialized to contract, this constituted a problem that was much more difficult to study. Since it was obvious from studies on muscle that contraction somehow depended on actin having an attraction for myosin, it was of interest that it was found that there were filaments in many kinds of cells that will bind parts of myosin molecules if they are exposed to them and hence that actinlike filaments are present in many types of cell. Next, in describing the telophase of mitosis (Chapter 2) it was noted that the separation of the mother cell into two daughter cells depended on a contraction furrow developing in the midsection of the mother cell and deepening until the mother cell was pinched in two. It was pointed out also that at that time a bundle of filaments could be seen to encircle the cell like a ring at the bottom of the furrow just below the cell membrane (Fig. 2-22) and that the filaments of this ring were probably responsible for causing the furrow to deepen and eventually pinch the cell into two.

In 1969 Schroeder discovered that adding the drug cytochalasin (which is obtained from certain fungi) to dividing marine eggs in which a furrow was just developing would cause both the furrow and the ring of filaments just under the furrow to disappear. As a result two daughter cells did not develop; instead the mother cell ended up with two nuclei. Most likely cytochalasin indirectly caused a loss of filaments and thereby prevented the formation of the two daughter cells.

Contractile activities involving actinlike filaments are now thought to be responsible for many of the changes in shape and types of movement noted in many kinds of cells when living cells are directly observed in the body or in cell cultures. Another well known phenomenon, the retraction of a blood clot, which is an important factor in sealing off bleeding from various types of injuries, could be due to the actin filaments in little bodies termed platelets, as will be described later. Most of the filaments in the cell web as well as those forming the cores of microvilli have been found to be actinlike, in that they will bind parts of myosin molecules. Actinlike filaments have also been detected in cells capable of ameboid motion. Tonofilaments, however, are not actinlike.

A great amount of movement that occurs within cells could be explained readily if it were still believed that filaments of actinlike molecules are individually contractile. But the nature of the contractile process in muscle makes it seem more likely that movements in cells in general that are dependent on actin filaments must somehow involve their remaining the same length but moving in relation to something. In this connection it is of interest that it is only the actin filaments in the contractile unit of striated muscle (Fig. 18-7) that have to be anchored. The myosin in a contractile unit merely causes actin filaments to slide along it. The reason, of course, that the myosin fila-

ments are not shifted when the actin filaments pull is that the pull that is exerted on the myosin filaments is equalized; they are pulled as strongly toward one end of the unit as they are to the other and hence movement occurs only in the actin filaments. It is therefore conceivable that some less well organized arrangement exists in many kinds of cells wherein myosin molecules could cause adjacent actin filaments to slide along them in opposite directions and if the actin filaments had one of their ends anchored somewhere, movements within the cytoplasm could result. Whatever the contractile mechanism proves to be in cells other than muscle cells, there is evidence accumulating to the effect that, as in muscle cells, it is triggered by calcium ions and requires ATP.

It is of interest that the presence of myosin has now been detected in many cells other than muscle cells and where actinlike filaments are present.

Cell Junctions

INTRODUCTION

Cells are often fitted together side by side to form linings or coverings that are only one cell thick and in these only the sides of the cells are attached to one another (Fig. 5-1). In other sites cells may be aggregated to form thicker layers or structures and in these an individual cell is attached to other cells on all its surfaces.

Three features that would seem to be involved in holding cells together may be observed with the EM.

1. In some cellular arrangements the border between any two cells is often irregular because of the two contiguous cells possessing tongued and grooved surfaces, with the tongues from each cell extending into the grooves on the surface of its neighbor (Fig. 5-9). (Tongues and grooves have been used by carpenters for centuries to hold boards together.)

2. Where the membranes of adjacent cells abut on one another, with the exceptions to be described in the next paragraph, the membranes are separated from each other by what appears in ordinary electron micrographs to be an empty space around 200 to 250 Å wide (Fig. 5-13). However, if sections are stained by the P.A. silver methanamine technic, this space is blackened (Fig. 5-9), which indicates the presence of the glycoproteins of the cell coats of the contiguous cells. The apposition of the cell coats of contiguous cells could have an adhesive effect.

3. Here and there along the surfaces of cells there are specialized structural arrangements called *cell junctions* (*junction*, a place of joining or meeting). We shall now consider the various types.

There are three main types of junctions: (1) the occludens type, commonly called *tight junctions*, (2) the nexus or gap type, and (3) the adherens or desmosome type. These and their subtypes will be considered in this order.

Both occludens and adherens types are seen to advantage between the absorptive lining cells of the small intestine which have already been described (Fig. 5-56); we shall begin our description with those seen in this site.

JUNCTIONS OF THE OCCLUDENS TYPE (TIGHT JUNCTIONS)

There are three types:

A. **The Zonula Occludens.** The one-cell thick layer of cells that lines the intestine (Fig. 5-56) constitutes a barrier between the contents of the intestine and the internal environment of the body and it is of the greatest importance that only certain substances that are present in the lumen of the intestine be absorbed into any part of the living tissues of the body, and that other substances be prevented from gaining entrance to it. The ability to select what is to be absorbed is a property of the lining absorptive cells. It is, therefore, imperative that no separations should occur *between* the individual lining cells and, furthermore, that the *most perfect seal between the lining cells should be at their free margins,* which are in contact with the contents of the intestine. The nature of this seal was not ascertained until it was investigated with the EM. When this was done it was found that the membranes of the cells were actually fused at this site (Figs. 5-57, Z.O., and 5-58). This arrangement which holds cells together near their free mar-

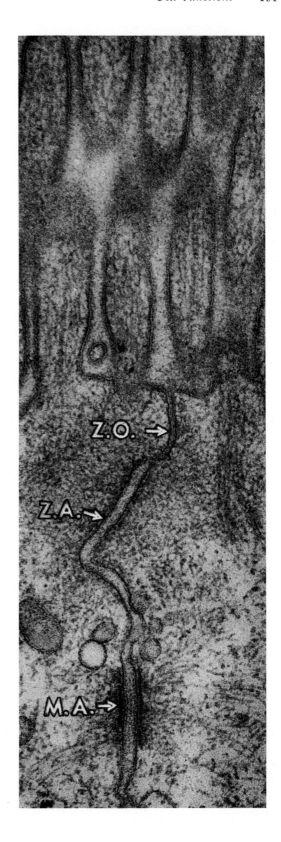

FIG. 5-57. If the reader is not clear as to the area encompassed by this electron micrograph of great magnification it may help to explain that the area involved is one about two or so millimeters in height and is located at the very point of the arrow in Figure 5-56 which points to "Cell web." The top half of the micrograph indicates the region of microvilli which project into the lumen of the intestine; these microvilli are mostly cut in oblique section. The arrow from Z.O. points to the site at which the cell membranes of the sides of two absorptive cells are in contact, and at this site the outer lamellae of their respective cell membranes are fused to form a zonula occludens. A little deeper down, but still within the region of the terminal web, the two membranes are joined by a zonula adherens (Z.A.), and, still farther down, be a macula adherens (a desmosome). (From Farquhar, M. G., and Palade, G. E.: J. Cell Biol., *17*:375)

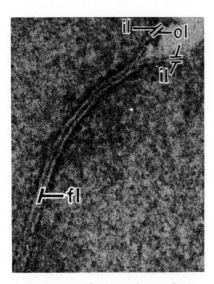

Fig. 5-58. Electron micrograph (×
230,000) of section passing through
zonula occludens of a junctional complex
between two cells of the gastric mucosa.
The line of fusion between the outer
layers of the cell membranes of the two
contiguous cells is marked fl; this appears as a dark line that is continuous
along this portion of the complex. Near
the top of the illustration the cell membranes of the two cells diverge. The
outer layer of the cell membrane of
each cell is here marked ol and the inner
layer, il. (Farquhar, M. G., and Palade,
G. E.: J. Cell Biol., *17*:375)

gins was first described clearly by Farquhar and
Palade and named by them the *zonula occludens.*

Since the term zone means a girdle and since a
girdle surrounds something, a zonula is a little girdle
that surrounds a cell. So a *zonula occludens* is a girdle
of fused membrane that surrounds each of the lining
cells of the intestine at their free margins (which are
just below the bases of the microvilli) and joins them
to surrounding contiguous cells.

The function of zonula occludens as a seal was confirmed experimentally when it was shown that these
junctions prevented dyes or marker molecules from
entering the lumen from the intercellular space or
from reaching the intercellular space from the lumen
of the intestine.

FINE STRUCTURE. In a zonula occludens (a tight
junction) it is the outer lamellae of the cell membranes of the contiguous cells that become fused; this
appears in a micrograph of great magnification as a
single faint dark line (Fig. 5-58). To each side of the

single dark line is a lighter line; these two lighter
lines represent the middle lamellae of the respective
cell membranes involved. The dark lines seen on the
cytoplasmic aspects of the lighter lines represent the
inner lamellae of the cell membranes of the two contiguous cells.

More recently it has been found using the freeze-
etching technic described in connection with Figure
5-6 that at tight junctions the outer lamellae of adjacent cell membranes, although very close together,
are not fused throughout the whole junction. Actual
fusion of the outer lamellae occurs only where match-
ing ridges that project from the adjacent cell surfaces
are present and meet in the middle, as illustrated in
the diagram (Fig. 5-59). There are enough of these,
however, to assure a perfect seal. It has been found
recently that the greater the number of such fused
ridges the better is the seal that such a junction makes.

B. The Fascia Occludens. From its origin, fascia
means band. The term fascia occludens is used to
denote patchy regions of such fusions of the outer
lamellae of the membranes of two adjacent cells.

As will be described later, blood vessels are lined
by a one-cell-thick pavement of what are termed the
endothelial cells; these are very thin. Furthermore,
the walls of capillaries consist of little more than this
single layer of these thin cells. Band-type occludens
junctions are found between the edges of adjacent
cells in this type of lining. Unlike the zonula type of
occludens junction, the band type does not produce a
perfect seal between contiguous cells because there
are gaps between sites at which the membranes of
adjacent cells are fused. As will be described in later
chapters, the gaps in this instance act more or less as
pores to permit fluid and sometimes even whole cells
to pass back and forth between the blood and tissue
fluid (to be explained in detail later).

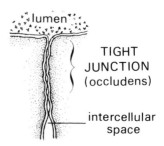

Fig. 5-59. Diagram of a tight junction
showing the ridges within the junction at
which the two unit membranes of adjacent
cells are fused.

C. **The Macula Occludens.** Macula means a spot; hence, a macula occludens junction is one in which the outer lamellae of the membranes of contiguous cells are fused in a small spotlike area. However, a spot of fusion seen in a section with the EM could be a cross section of a line of fusion that crossed the plane of the section; hence the existence of a true macula occludens type of cell junction would have to be established from three-dimensional data.

JUNCTIONS OF THE NEXUS TYPE—GAP JUNCTIONS

The word nexus means a bond. Since all types of junctions bond cells together it is not a very precise term. It is used for a type of junction that was believed a few years ago to be identical or almost identical to junctions of the occludens type. However, Revel and Karnovsky in 1967 showed that there was a 20-Å space or gap between the outer lamellae of the cell membranes that approached each other in this type of junction; this accounts for its also being called a *gap junction* and also for 7 lines being seen in one, 4 dark and 3 light, instead of the 5 seen in a tight junction (Fig. 5-60, *left*).

Fine Structure in Relation to Function. The 20-Å gap in the nexus is crossed by structures that are embedded, on both sides of the junction, into the membranes of the cells that abut on the gap. These structures became apparent when they were outlined as light regions against a black background; this was done by introducing lanthanum, an electron-dense material, through the extracellular space into the junctions (Fig. 5-60, *right*). Structures (Fig. 5-60, *right*) were also observed later inside the membranes at gap junctions in freeze-etched preparations (method described in connection with Fig. 5-5). The fracturing involved here splits the lipid bilayer of the cell membrane and exposes its internal structure. It is likely that these two technics show different portions of the same structure—the lanthanum the portion in the space between the cells and the freeze-etching technic the portions of the structures embedded in the cell membranes of adjacent cells. Furthermore it is believed that these structures (Fig. 5-60, *right*) have something of the nature of a central pore in them which allows ions and small molecules to pass from the cytoplasm of one cell into the cytoplasm of the adjacent cell. This enables a cell to communicate with its neighbors. Thus, for instance, the passage of nervous impulse from muscle cell to muscle cell in the heart requires a diffusion of ions from cell to cell; this takes place through the gap or nexus junctions connecting heart muscle cells, as will be described in Chapter 18. Likewise, for waves of contraction to sweep along the intestine, what are termed smooth muscle cells must contract successively in an orderly way and these too are connected together by nexus junctions. The precise function of these junctions in other types of cells is less clear at the present time.

JUNCTIONS OF THE ADHERENS TYPE

No direct contact occurs between the unit membranes of contiguous cells in junctions of the adherens type. However, they are called junctions because they are sites where the space between contiguous cell membranes is filled with a special type of cell coat material which joins the two cell membranes firmly together. Indeed, it has been shown that under conditions which tend to pull cells apart, it is this type

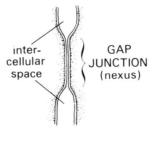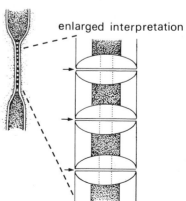

FIG. 5-60. Diagram illustrating the gap junction as it appears in sectional material (*left*) and after filling of intercellular spaces with lanthanum (*right*). At the left 7 lines can be identified because each of the two cell membranes has three lines, two dark and one light, and there is here a light line between the two cell membranes.

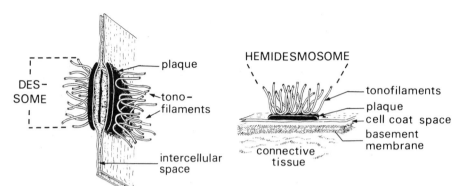

DESSOME

plaque

tono-filaments

intercellular space

HEMIDESMOSOME

tonofilaments
plaque
cell coat space
basement membrane

connective tissue

FIG. 5-61. Diagrams illustrating the structure of a desmosome (*left*) and of a hemidesmosome (*right*) and how tonofilaments are anchored in the electron dense plaques of these structures.

of junction which is the last to break. They also serve as sites where the tonofilaments of the cell web of a cell are anchored.

A. **The Zonula Adherens.** This type, like the zonula occludens, is disposed as a girdle around each cell that is joined. Zonulae adherentes are present just below the zonulae occludentes (Fig. 5-57) in the absorptive lining cells of the intestine. The two cell membranes participating in a zonula adherens are separated by a space of around 200 Å which is filled with a material that is not very electron dense. Electron-dense material, however, is found along the inner surfaces of those parts of the cell membranes that participate in forming this type of junction. In addition, the tonofilaments of the terminal web are anchored in the dense material at these junctions.

B. **The Macula Type of Adherens Junction (the Desmosome).** As already mentioned, it was once believed that tonofibrils, now known to be bundles of filaments, crossed from one cell to another to help hold them together. This view arose because observations with the LM indicated that in some body sites contiguous cells after fixation were clearly separated from one another except at the sites where tonofibrils were present (Fig. 5-55). The EM, however, showed that tonofilaments *did not cross;* instead, at these sites the tonofilaments in each cell entered the electron-dense material that was present on the cytoplasmic side of the cell membrane of each cell and then looped back out into the cytoplasm (Fig. 5-61). At these sites the cell membranes of the contiguous cells remained intact and adhered to one another instead of shrinking away from one another as occurred between sites of tonofilaments as in Figure 5-55. This type of cell junction was termed a macula type because examples of it appeared in sections as spots (*macula,* spot) along the cell membranes of contiguous cells. More commonly, however, these junctions came to be called *desmosomes* (*desmos,* bond or fastening). In the ab-

sorptive lining cells of the small intestine desmosomes (maculae adherentes) can be seen below the zonula adherens (Fig. 5-57, MA).

Desmosomes can be demonstrated in surface views of separated cells by the shadow-cast replica technic as follows.

Preparation and appearance of shadow-cast replicas showing desmosomes. The surface of a detached cell can be coated with a very thin layer of a tough material that follows all the contours of its surface. The cell is then digested away, leaving a thin covering of tough material which is a cast of the surface of the cell. A stream of molecules of high electron density is then shot at the surface of the cast from an oblique angle. Because this spraying is done from an angle, the regions in front of the high points get a thicker coating of the electron-dense molecules, and the areas behind these get a much thinner coating or none at all. The cast of the surface, thus treated, is now photographed in the electron microscope (Fig. 5-62).

Figure 5-62 shows that desmosomes on the cells of the deeper layers of epidermis appear in this kind of preparation as spotlike structures.

Even in ordinary ultrathin sections of tough cellular membranes a desmosome can often be seen with the EM to be larger than a small spot, as for example, the four that can be seen in Figure 5-63. If the attachment between cells is wide as well as long it is sometimes termed a fascia (*fascia,* band) type of adherens junction. In other words, the distinction between desmosomes and the fascia type of adherens junction is not sharp. A junction related to a desmosome known as an intercalated disc occurs in the cardiac muscle. We shall now describe the fine structure of a desmosome in the deeper layers of the epidermis (the outer layer of skin) in detail.

FINE STRUCTURE OF DESMOSOMES. In a section that cuts the adjacent cell membranes at right angles some dark parallel lines with lighter lines between them are seen as is shown in Figure 5-63 in the desmosomes labeled D. Farther out still, on each side there is a good deal of dark fibrillar material. What accounts for these various appearances will now be described.

The membranes of two contiguous cells do not come into direct contact at the site of a desmosome; at this site they are both separated and connected by a region composed of material of low electron density which is light in Figure 5-63, except for a dark line in its middle (Fig. 5-63, In). The dark line, which is really a thin layer, probably represents a condensation of the outer borders of the cell coats of the two cells that come into contact with each other in a desmosome. This dark line in the center of the extracellular space is more pronounced in desmosomes between cells in tough protective layers of cells as in the epidermis (Fig. 5-63) than in those between absorptive cells (MA in Fig. 5-57) where it is indistinct or absent. The origin and nature of the layer of low electron density that lies to either side of this dense line and constitutes the bulk of the extracellular space at the desmosome is not known but it is probably similar to cell coat. The next dark layer on each side is the outer lamella of the cell membrane of the cell that is on that side. Farther out on each side is a light layer, which is the middle layer of the cell membrane of the cell on that side and farther out still on either side is a thick dark layer. The latter in each case is due in part to the inner lamella of the cell membrane of the cell on that side and also in part to a condensation of electron-dense material on the cytoplasmic side of the cell membrane. This *thick* dark line is called a *plaque* (P in Fig. 5-63). The desmosome also includes bundles of tonofilaments which form part of the cell web. They may come from the cytoplasm toward the desmosome perpendicular to the cell membrane, enter the plaque and then loop outward again back into the cytoplasm (Fig. 5-61). In addition, bundles of tonfilaments running parallel to the cell membrane are often associated with the desmosomes on the cytoplasmic side of these plaques. Very often such bundles of tonofilaments join a long series of desmosomes which encircle the cell in a trainlike fashion. No tonofilament has yet been shown to terminate at a desmosome. Desmosomes are illustrated in the diagram on Figure 5-61 (*left*).

HEMIDESMOSOMES. Some areas of cell surface have the structures which have the appearance of half desmosomes (Fig. 5-61, *right*). They are appropriately called *hemidesmosomes* (*hemi,* half). They are found in sites where a cell, instead of being attached to a

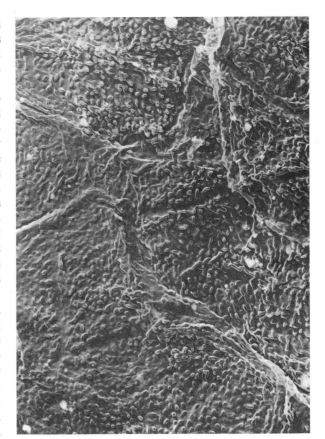

FIG. 5-62. Desmosomes on cells from the deeper layers of the epidermis demonstrated by the shadow cast replica technic. They appear as small projections on the cell surface. This technic indicates that there are about 160 desmosomes per 100 square microns of cell surface. (From R. C. Buck)

neighboring cell, is strongly attached to extracellular material such as a basement membrane, as will be described in a later chapter.

Cytoplasmic Inclusions

The term *inclusion* was coined to designate certain structures or materials, demonstrable in the cytoplasm with the LM, which were not considered to be part of the cytoplasm but of the order of inanimate materials or objects that had somehow become included in it.

So far as normal cells are concerned the term is used chiefly to denote such things as stored foods and certain pigments. Secretion granules were once placed in the category of inclusions because it was appre-

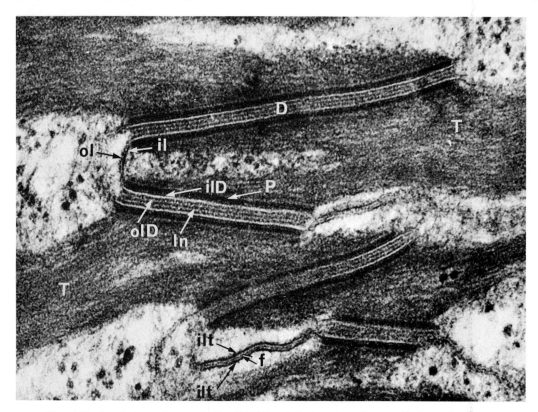

Fɪɢ. 5-63. An electron micrograph (× 114,000) of the junction of two cells from the stratum spinosum of epithelium from human palate showing desmosomes and tight junctions between the membrane of the cell at right and that of the cell at left, which come together along a zigzag line.

At the top a large desmosome (D) is seen. At its left end the two cell membranes which met in it diverge, and only the membrane of the cell on the right can be seen. Both the outer layer (ol) and the inner layer (il) of its cell membrane are apparent. After making a hairpin turn, the outer layer continues into one of the lines seen within the desmosome (olD). Similarly, the inner layer is continuous with another line (ilD), which is immediately adjacent to a thick band of cytoplasmic material, the attachment plaque (P). Bundles of tonofilaments forming tono-fibrils (T) seem to connect to the attachment plaque on either side of the desmosome. In the middle of the desmosome, a central line running parallel to the outer and inner layers of the cell membrane can be seen, the intermediate line (In). This line is situated in the middle of the intercellular space.

Continuing past the desmosome from left to right, the cell membranes fuse to form a tight junction which is not clearly visible due to the plane of section. Then the membranes turn down and back again toward the left and form a third desmosome. After another hairpin turn down and to the right, the membranes converge and fuse once more to form a second tight junction (*bottom, center*). The tight junction is characterized by two parallel thicker lines representing the inner layers (ilt), and a central, thinner fusion line (f), depicting the fused outer layers of adjacent cell membranes. Osmium fixation. (Wilgram, G. F., and Weinstock, A.: Arch. Derm., *94:*456, 1966)

ciated that they did not perform their function inside the cytoplasm but outside it. However, since we now know that secretion "granules" are membranous vesi-cles containing enzymes, they are now dealt with in connection with the organelles.

Stored Foods

Of the three basic foodstuffs—carbohydrate, protein and fat—only carbohydrate and fat are stored in cells as inclusions and these are stored only in certain cells.

Carbohydrate is stored chiefly in liver cells and to a lesser extent in muscle cells. In all instances it is stored in the form of glycogen that exists as deposits in the cytoplasmic matrix, as was described in connection with liver cells in Chapter 1 and illustrated in Figures 1-14 and 1-15. Although not a constant component of their cytoplasm, it is found in many other kinds of cells. The storage of glycogen in liver cells will be considered in more detail when we later describe the liver as an organ. When stained, glycogen appears in electron micrographs as in Figure 5-44.

Fat is stored as such in special cells known as adipose or fat cells. These are the basic cells of a special tissue known as fat or adipose tissue that will be considered in detail when we study the connective tissues. Fat sometimes accumulates in liver cells also, as was described in Chapter 1 and illustrated in Figures 1-14 and 1-16.

PIGMENTS

The value to the medical student of becoming interested in normal and abnormal color of various parts of the body, and the basis for the color, is very great. A most important factor and sometimes the chief one in the clinical diagnosis of some diseases is the changed color of some part of the body. Color is of even greater importance to the pathologist than to the clinician. A good part of the description of the gross appearance of diseased organs at operation or at autopsy relates to their changed color.

Color in any tissue is due chiefly to the kind and amount of pigment it contains. Pigments in cells have generally been classed as inclusions, but in the instance of some pigments this is debatable. In disease conditions certain pigments derived from cells may be found in extracellular spaces as well as in the cells in which they were formed.

It is important to realize what constitutes a pigment. There are many ingredients of cells that, while colorless in life, take on brilliant colors after they are treated with stains. These are not pigments. To qualify as a pigment a material must possess color in its natural state; hence, a pigment, to be seen, does not need to be treated with stains. However, pigments are sometimes colored further or differently by stains.

Fortunately, there are only a few broad groups of pigments with which the student should become familiar.

Classification. Pigments are usually classified into two groups, exogenous and endogenous. Exogenous (*ex,* out; *genein,* to produce) pigments are those that have been generated as such outside the body and

subsequently taken into it by one route or another. Endogenous (*endon,* within) pigments are generated inside the body from nonpigmented ingredients.

Exogenous Pigments

Lipochromes—Carotenoids. Carotene is a pigment formed in several kinds of vegetables. There are several types of carotene, and different vegetables form somewhat different kinds. Carotene is abundant in carrots, and the kind in carrots is predominantly yellow. In tomatoes the carotene is more of a red color. The carotenes are soluble in fat and so are taken up from the food eaten by animals to color certain body components that contain fat. For example, the coloring of egg yolks is caused by carotene absorbed by chickens from the vegetable food that they eat. Likewise the (natural) yellow color of butter is due to the carotene eaten by cows becoming dissolved into the fat of the cream they produce. The body fat of man often has a yellow tinge because of its content of carotene.

Since carotenes are soluble in fat, the carotenoid pigments are sometimes termed lipochrome pigments. However, the term *lipochrome* was in the past applied also to certain endogenous pigments which had some lipid in their ill-defined constitution, and so its use may cause some confusion. Carotenoids, however, are clearly lipochrome pigments because they are soluble in fat and can give color to fatty materials.

Several forms of carotene are provitamins and may be converted into vitamin A in the body, which is one reason for eating fresh vegetables or drinking vegetable juices. Occasionally individuals do not practice moderation in this respect. It is possible to eat so many carrots or tomatoes, or to drink so much vegetable juice, that the skin of the body takes on a yellow or even a reddish color due to its great content of carotene. The condition caused by excessive consumption of carotene is called carotenemia, and individuals with this clinical condition may at first glance be thought to have jaundice. It is, however, an unusual condition. Interested students will find "The Orange Man," an article which appeared in *The New Yorker* magazine (vol. 43, May 27, 1967), as intriguing as a good mystery story and very much more informative. Further comment would detract from the denouement.

Dusts. A second important group of exogenous pigments is provided by the various kinds of dusts that gain entrance to the respiratory system through inspired air. Pigmentation of parts of this system by this means is of course pathologic. We shall comment briefly on this matter later in the chapter on the Respiratory System.

Minerals. Certain minerals taken by mouth or absorbed through the surface of the body may lead to pigmentation. For example, too much silver applied to body surfaces in the treatment of certain diseases may lead to an accumulation of silver and hence a gray pigmentation of the body. Lead can be absorbed to give a blue line on the gums.

Tattoo Marks. These are due to pigments being driven deep into the skin by needles where they become fixed in position, as will be described when we consider skin.

Endogenous Pigments

The most important one is hemoglobin, the iron-containing coloring matter of red blood cells. This serves as the great oxygen carrier of the body. It will be discussed in detail in Chapter 11. Here it is enough to note that pink cheeks and red lips are due to this pigment which is in the red blood cells that are circulating in capillaries just below the surface of these parts of the body. Certain altered forms of hemoglobin of a different color from the normal will also be discussed in the same chapter.

Pigments From the Destruction of Hemoglobin. Under normal conditions, red blood cells do not survive for more than a few months in the circulatory system. As they wear out, they are phagocytosed by certain large cells in the spleen, the liver and the bone marrow. In the cytoplasm of these large cells, the iron-containing hemoglobin is broken down into an iron-containing pigment called hemosiderin and a noniron-containing one called hematoidin or bilirubin.

Hemosiderin. This is golden brown and is disposed in the cytoplasm of phagocytes in the form of granules or small irregular masses. By histochemical tests for iron, hemosiderin can be shown to contain this element; this permits it to be distinguished from the other golden and brown pigments of the body.

Whereas hemosiderin is normally present to some extent in the phagocytes of the spleen (where it will be described further), the liver and the bone marrow, it becomes greatly increased in these sites in diseases in which red blood corpuscles are broken down much more rapidly than usual. It may even appear in large quantities in certain other cells under certain pathologic conditions.

Hematoidin and Bilirubin. Bile is a yellow-to-brown fluid that is secreted by the liver, and stored and concentrated in a bag termed the gallbladder; eventually, it passes into the intestine, where it plays an important role in absorption and digestion. Its coloring matter is bilirubin, a yellow-to-brown pigment

which is easily oxidized to biliverdin, a green pigment. In some animals (birds), a considerable amount of biliverdin is present normally in their bile, enhancing the tendency of the bile to be green, but in man only a little biliverdin is normally present, so that human bile is yellow to brown.

For many years it was believed that bilirubin was manufactured by the liver cells that secrete it. With further studies it became apparent that bilirubin, like hemosiderin, is a breakdown product of hemoglobin and hence formed in the sites where old, worn-out red blood corpuscles are destroyed. Unlike hemosiderin, however, bilirubin contains no iron and is more soluble; hence it does not tend to remain in the cytoplasm of the phagocytes that destroy red blood cells but instead dissolves into the blood, from which it is continuously removed by the cells of the liver to be transferred into the bile.

The first tangible lead indicating that bilirubin was derived from hemoglobin was given by Virchow, the great pathologist, about 100 years ago. He observed that crystals of pigment tended to form in tissues of the body that were the sites of previous hemorrhages. He named the pigment that crystallized out among the old, breaking-down red blood corpuscles, hematoidin, and concluded that it was derived from hemoglobin. Not content with microscopic examinations alone, he subjected deposits of this pigment to chemical tests and made the remarkable discovery that hematoidin, so far as these tests would demonstrate, was the same thing as the pigment that colors bile (bilirubin). Yet for many years afterward, hemoglobin was not accepted as the origin of bile pigment, and many decades passed before his view gained general acceptance.

Melanin. This is usually a brown-to-black pigment found chiefly in the skin and its appendages and in the eye. In white races it appears in skin in appreciable amounts after exposure to sunlight (suntan). Melanin accounts for the dark color of the Negro; here, too, the degree of pigmentation is increased by sunlight. The color of brown eyes is due to melanin. Deep in the eye melanin is used as a light-proofing material much in the same way as photographers use black paper, black curtains and black paint.

Melanin is a nitrogenous substance that in pure form contains no sulfur or iron. The formation of melanin will be considered in detail and it will be illustrated in connection with skin in Chapter 20. Cells that make melanin are termed *melanocytes*. They contain an enzyme capable of acting on a colorless chromogen brought to the cell by blood and tissue fluid, converting it into melanin.

Lipofuscin. This is a pigment which contains some fatty material, permitting this pigment to be stained with certain fat stains. In its natural state it is of brownish color (*fuscus,* brown). Lipofuscin appears in the form of small clumps sometimes called granules (Fig. 5-64). It is more common in the muscle cells of the heart, nerve cells, and liver cells than in most other cell types. The amount of lipofuscin in these and other cell types increases with age. This latter fact has given rise to the concept that it is a pigment partaking of the nature of a "wear and tear" product which is not readily disposed of in the cytoplasm or excreted. The development of histochemical methods for the identification of certain of the enzymes of lysosomes has resulted in its having been shown that some hydrolase activity is commonly associated with deposits of lipofuscin, and that the pigment is contained in residual bodies.

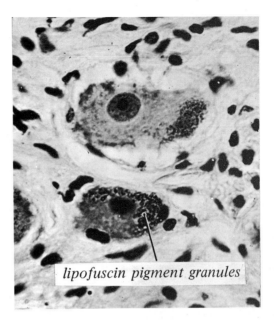

FIG. 5-64. High-power photomicrograph of a human nerve ganglion. Two ganglion cells may be seen in the picture; their cytoplasm contains numerous granules of lipofuscin pigment.

References

GENERAL REFERENCES INCLUDING ATLASES ON THE FINE STRUCTURE OF CELLS AND TISSUES

Fawcett, D. W.: The Cell: An Atlas of Fine Structure. Philadelphia, W. B. Saunders, 1966.

Fujita, T., Tokunaga, J., and Inoue, H.: Atlas of Scanning Electron Microscopy in Medicine. Amsterdam, Elsevier, 1971.

King, D. W. (ed.): Ultrastructural Aspects of Disease. New York, Harper & Row, 1966.

Lenz, T. L.: Cell Fine Structure. Philadelphia, W. B. Saunders, 1971.

Matthews, J., and Martin, J.: Atlas of Human Histology and Ultrastructure. Philadelphia, Lea & Febiger, 1971.

Porter, K. R., and Bonneville, M. A.: An Introduction to the Fine Structure of Cells and Tissues. ed. 4. Philadelphia, Lea & Febiger, 1973.

Rose, G. G.: Atlas of Vertebrate Cells in Tissue Culture. New York, Academic Press, 1970.

Sandborn, E. B.: Light and Electron Microscopy of Cells and Tissues. New York, Academic Press, 1972.

SPECIAL REFERENCES AND OTHER READING ON CYTOPLASM

Cell Membrane, Cell Surface and Cell Coats

Bangham, A. D.: Models of cell membranes. Hosp. Prac., March 1973.

Branton, D.: Membrane structure. Ann. Rev. Plant Physiol., 20:209, 1969.

Burger, M.: Surface properties of neoplastic cells. Hosp. Prac., July, 1973.

————: Surface changes in transformed cells detected by lectins. Fed. Proc., 32:91, 1973.

Chapman, D.: Lipid dynamics in cell membranes. Hosp. Prac., February, 1973.

————: The chemical and physical characteristics of biological membranes. Membranes and Ion Transport. vol. 1, p. 23. New York, Wiley-Interscience, 1970.

Curtis, A. S. G.: Cell contact and adhesion. Biol. Rev., 37:82, 1962.

Danielli, J. F.: The bilayer hypothesis of membrane structure. Hosp. Prac., January, 1973.

De Pierce, J. W., and Karnovsky, M. L.: Plasma membranes of mammalian cells. A review of methods for their characterization and isolation. J. Cell Biol., 56:275, 1973.

Fox, C. F.: The structure of cell membranes. Sci. Am., 226:30, 1972.

Fox, T. O., Sheppard, J. R., and Burger, M. M.: Cyclic membrane changes in animal cells: transformed cells permanently display a surface architecture detected in normal cells only during mitosis. Proc. Nat. Acad. Sci. (USA), 1968:244, 1971.

Frye, C. D., and Edidin, M.: The rapid intermixing of cell surface antigens after formation of mouse-human heterokaryons. J. Cell Sci., 7:319, 1970.

Guidotti, G.: Membrane proteins. Ann. Rev. Biochem., 41:731, 1972.

Haydon, D. A., and Hladky, S. B.: Ion transport across thin lipid membranes: a critical discussion of mechanisms in selected systems. Q. Rev. Biophys., 5:187, 1972.

Hendler, R. W.: Biological membrane ultrastructure. Physiol. Rev., 51:1, 66, 1971.

Hughes, R. C.: Glycoproteins as components of cellular membranes. Prog. Biophys. Molec. Biol., 26:189, 1973.

Lucy, J. A.: The fusion of cell membranes. Hosp. Prac., Sept., 1973.

Marchesi, V. T., Jackson, R. L., Segrest, J. P., and Kahane, I.: Molecular features of the major glycoprotein of the human erythrocyte membrane. Fed. Proc., 32:1833, 1973.

Martinez-Palomo, A.: The surface coats of animal cells. Int. Rev. Cytol., 29:29, 1970.

Moscona, A.: Analysis of cell recombinations in experimental synthesis of tissues in vitro. Symp. on Cell Differentiation and Interaction. p. 64. Philadelphia, Wistar Institute, 1962.

Pinto da Silva, P., and Branton, D.: Membrane splitting in freeze-etching. J. Cell Biol., *45:*598, 1970.

Porter, K. R., Prescott, D., and Frye, J.: Changes in surface morphology of Chinese hamster ovary cells during the cell cycle. J. Cell Biol., *57:*815, 1973.

Rambourg, A., and Leblond, C. P.: Electron microscope observations on the carbohydrate rich cell coat present at the surface of cells in the rat. J. Cell Biol., *32:*27, 1967.

Revel, J. P., and Ito, S.: The surface components of cells. *In* Davis, B. D., and Warren, L. (eds.): The Specificity of Cell Surfaces. Englewood Cliffs, N.J., Prentice-Hall, 1967.

Singer, S. J.: The molecular organization of biological membranes. *In* Rothfield, L. I. (ed.): Structure and Function of Biological Membranes. New York, Academic Press, 1971.

———: Proteins and membrane topography. Hosp. Prac., May, 1973.

Singer, S. J., and Nicolson, G. L.: The fluid mosaic model of the structure of cell membranes. Science, *175:*720, 1972.

Taylor, R. B., Duffus, P. H., Raff, M. C., and de Petris, S.: Redistribution and pinocytosis of lymphocyte surface immunoglobulin molecules induced by anti-immunoglobulin antibody. Nature (New Biol.), *233:*225, 1971.

Mitochondria

Baxter, R.: Origin and continuity of mitochondria. *In* Reinert, J., and Ursprung, H. (eds.): Origin and Continuity of Cell Organelles. p. 46. New York, Springer-Verlag, 1971.

Borst, P.: Mitochondrial DNA: structure, information content, replication and transcription. Symp. Soc. Exp. Biol., *24:*201, 1970.

Dawid, I. B.: The nature of mitochondrial RNA in oocytes of Xenopus and its relation to mitochondrial DNA. Symp. Soc. Exp. Biol., *24:*227, 1970.

Ernster, L., and Z. Drahota (eds.): Mitochondria, Structure and Function. New York, Academic Press, 1969.

Goodenough, U., and Levine, R.: The genetic activity of mitochondria and chloroplasts. Sci. Am. *223:*22, Nov., 1970.

Hackenbrock, C.: Ultrastructural bases for metabolically linked mechanical activity in mitochondria. J. Cell Biol., *37:*345, 1968.

Lehninger, A. L.: The Mitochondrion. 263 pp. New York, W. A. Benjamin, 1964.

Margulis, L.: Symbiosis and evolution. Sci. Am., *225:*48, August, 1971.

Nass, S.: Structural and functional similarities of bacteria and mitochondria. Internat. Rev. Cytol., *25:*55, 1969.

Parsons, D. F.: Recent advances correlating structure and function in mitochondria. Int. Rev. Exp. Path., *4:*1, 1965.

Peachey, L. D.: Electron microscope observations on the accumulation of divalent actions in intramitochondrial granules. J. Cell Biol., *20:*95, 1964.

Racker, E.: The membrane of the mitochondrion. Sci. Am., *218:*32, Feb. 1968.

Rouiller, C.: Physiological and morphological changes in mitochondrial morphology. Int. Rev. Cytol.: 9, 1960.

Van Dam, K., and Meyer, A.: Oxidation and energy conservation by mitochondria. Ann. Rev. Biochem., *40:*115, 1971.

Wainio, W.: The Mammalian Mitochondrial Respiratory Chain. New York, Academic Press, 1970.

Williams, C., and Vail, W.: Ultrastructural transitions in energized and de-energized mitochondria. Adv. Cell Molec. Biol., *2:*385, 1972.

Ribosomes, Rough Endoplasmic Reticulum, Protein Synthesis

Anderson-Cedergren, E., and Karlsson, V.: Polyribosomal organization in intact intrafusal muscle fibers. J. Ultrastruct. Res., *19:*409, 1967.

Andrews, T. M., and Tata, J. R.: Protein synthesis by membrane bound and free ribosomes of secretory and non-secretory tissues. Biochem. J., *121:*683, 1971.

Brenner, S.: RNA, ribosomes and protein synthesis. Cold Spring Harbor Symp. Quant. Biol., *26:*101, 1961.

Burka, E. R., and Bulova, S. I.: Heterogeneity of reticulocyte ribosomes. Biochem. Biophys. Res. Commun., *42:*801, 1971.

Clark, B. F. C., and Marcker, K. A.: How proteins start. Sci. Am., *218:*484, 1968.

Caro, L. G., and Palade, G. E.: Protein synthesis, storage and discharge in the pancreatic exocrine cell. An autoradiographic study. J. Cell Biol., *20:*473, 1964.

Campbell, P. N.: Functions of polyribosomes attached to membranes of animal cells. FEBS. Letters 7, 1, 1970.

Daliner, G., Siekevitz, P., and Palade, G. E.: Biogenesis of endoplasmic reticulum membrane. J. Cell Biol., *30:*73, 97, 1966.

Darnell, J. E.: Ribonucleic acids from animal cells. Bacteriol. Rev., *32:*262, 1968.

Haguenau, F.: The ergastoplasm. Its history, ultrastructure and biochemistry. Int. Rev. Cytol., *7:*425, 1958.

Holder, J. W., and Lingrel, J. B.: Localization of the hemoglobin mRNA on the 40S ribosomal subunit of rabbit reticulocyte ribosomes. Biochem. Biophys. Acta, *204:*210, 1970.

Jamieson, J. D., and Palade, G. E.: Intracellular transport of secretory proteins in the pancreatic exocrine cell. III. Dissociation of intracellular transport from protein synthesis. J. Cell Biol., *39:*580, 1968.

Labrie, F.: Isolation of an RNA with the properties of haemoglobin messenger. Nature, *221:*1217, 1969.

Leblond, C. P., and Warren, K. B.: The use of radioautography in investigation protein synthesis. New York, Academic Press, 1965.

Leduc, E. H., Avrameas, S., and Bouteille, M.: Ultrastructural localization of antibody in differentiating plasma cells. J. Exp. Med., *127:*109, 1968.

Lengyel, P., and Söll, D.: Mechanism of protein biosynthesis. Bact. Rev., *33:*264, 1969.

Lucas-Lenard, J., and Lipmann, E.: Protein biosynthesis. Ann. Rev. Biochem. *40:*409, 1971.

Maden, B. E. H.: The structure and formation of ribosomes in in animal cells. Progr. Biophys. Molec. Biol., *22:*127, 1971.

Meldolesi, J., Jamieson, J., and Palade, G. E.: Composition of cellular membranes in the pancreas of the guinea pig. J. Call Biol., *49:*109, 130, 150, 1971.

Ribosomes, Rough Endoplasmic Reticulum, Protein Synthesis

Nonomura, Y., Blobel, G., and Sabatini, D.: Structure of liver ribosomes studied by negative staining. J. Molec. Biol., *60:*303, 1971.

Nomura, M.: Ribosomes. Sci. Am., *221:*28, Oct. 1969.

Palade, G. E.: Structure and function at the cellular level. JAMA. *198*:815, 1966.

Perry, R. P.: On ribosome biogenesis. Monographs, U.S. Nat. Cancer Inst., *23*:527, 1966.

Porter, K. R.: Electron microscopy of basophilic components of cytoplasm. J. Histochem. Cytochem., *2*:346, 1954.

Rich, A.: Polyribosomes. Sci. Am., *209*:44, 1963.

Sabatini, D. D., Tashiro, Y., and Palade, G. E.: On the attachment of ribosomes to microsomal membrane. J. Molec. Biol., *19*:503, 1966.

Spirin, A. S.: Structure of the ribosome. Progr. Biophys. Molec. Biol., *19* (Part 1):133, 1969.

Stanners, C. P.: Polyribosomes of hamster cells; transit time measurements. Biophys. J., *8*:231, 1968.

Tata, J. R.: Ribosomal segregation as a possible function for the attachment of ribosomes to membranes. Sub. Cell Biochem., *1*:83, 1971.

Warner, J. R., Rich, A., and Hall, C. E.: Electron microscope studies of ribosomal clusters synthesizing hemoglobin. Science, *138*:1399, 1962.

Warner, J. R., Knoff, P., and Rich, A.: A multiple ribosomal structure in protein synthesis. Proc. Nat. Acad. Sci. (U.S.A.), *49*:122, 1963.

Warshawsky, H., Leblond, C. P., and Droz, B.: Synthesis and migration of proteins in the cells of exocrine pancreas as revealed by specific activity determination from radioautographs. J. Cell Biol., *16*:1, 1963.

The Golgi Apparatus

Beams, H. W., and Kessel, R. G.: The Golgi apparatus: structure and function. Int. Rev. Cytol., *23*:209, 1968.

Bennett, G., and Leblond, C. P.: Formation of cell coat materials for the whole surface of columnar cells in the rat small intestine as visualized by radioautography with L-fucose-³H. J. Cell Biol., *46*:409, 1970.

Carro, L. G., and Palade, G. E.: Protein synthesis, storage and discharge in the pancreatic exocrine cell. An autoradiographic study. J. Cell Biol., *20*:473, 1964.

Cheetham, R. D., Morre, D. J., and Yunghans, W. N.: Isolation of a Golgi apparatus–rich fraction from rat liver. J. Cell Biol., *44*:492, 1970.

Flickinger, C. I.: Fenestrated cisternae in the Golgi apparatus of the epididymis. Anat. Rec., *163*:39, 1969.

———: The pattern of growth of the Golgi complex during fetal and postnatal development of the rat epididymis. J. Ultrastr. Res., *27*:344, 1969.

Grove, S. N., Bracker, C. E., and Morre, D. J.: Cytomembrane differentiation in the endoplasmic reticulum–Golgi apparatus–vesicle complex. Science, *161*:171, 1968.

Jamieson, J. D., and Palade, G. E.: Intracellular transport of secretory proteins in the pancreatic exocrine cell. I. Role of the peripheral elements of Golgi complex. II. Transport to condensing vacuoles and zymogen granules. J. Cell Biol., *34*:577, 597, 1967.

Moe, H.: The goblet cells, Paneth cells and basal granular cells of the epithelium of the intestine. Int. Rev. Gen. Exp. Zool., *3*:241, 1968.

Morre, D. I., Merlin, L. L., and Keenan, T. W.: Localization of glycosyl transferase activities in a Golgi apparatus–rich fraction isolated from rat liver. Biochem. Biophys. Res. Commun., *37*:813, 1969.

Neutra, M., and Leblond, C. P.: Synthesis of the carbohydrate of mucus in the Golgi complex, as shown by electron microscope radioautography of goblet cells from rats injected with ³H-glucose. J. Cell Biol., *30*:119, 1966.

———: The Golgi apparatus. Sci. Am., *220*:100, February 1969. Northcote, D. H.: The Golgi apparatus. Endeavour, *30*:26, 1971.

———: The Golgi complex. *In* E. E. Bittar (ed.): Cell Biology in Medicine. New York, John Wiley & Sons, 1973.

Novikoff, P. M., Novikoff, A. B., Quintana, N., and Houw, I. I.: Golgi apparatus, GERL, and lysosomes of neurons in rat dorsal root ganglia studied by thick section and thin section cytochemistry. J. Cell Biol., *50*:859, 1971.

Rambourg, A., Clermont, Y., and Marraud, A.: Three-dimensional structure of the osmium-impregnated Golgi-apparatus as seen in the high voltage electron microscope. Am. J. Anat. 1973 (In press).

Rambourg, A., Hernandez, W., and Leblond, C. P.: Detection of periodic acid-reactive carbohydrate in Golgi saccules. J. Cell Biol., *40*:395, 1969.

Schenkein, I., and Uhr, J. W.: Immunoglobulin synthesis and secretion. I. Biosynthesis studies of the addition of the carbohydrate moieties. J. Cell Biol., *46*:42, 52, 1970.

Whaley, W. G., Dauwalder, M., and Kephart, J. E.: Golgi apparatus: influence on cell surfaces. Science, *175*:596, 1972.

Lysosomes

Allison, A.: Lysosomes and disease. Sci. Am., *217*:62, 1967.

Allison, A. C., and Paton, G. R.: Lysosomes, chromosomes and cancer. Biochem. J., *115*:31, 1969.

Arstila, A., Jauregui, H., Chang, J., and Trump, B.: Studies on cellular autophagocytosis. Lab. Invest., *27*:162, 1972.

Baggiolini, J., Hirsch, J. G., and De Duve, C.: Resolution of granules from rabbit heterophil leukocytes into distinct populations by zonal sedimentation. J. Cell Biol., *40*:529, 1969.

Bainton, D.: Sequential degranulation of the two types of polymorphonuclear granules during phagocytosis of microorganisms. J. Cell Biol., *58*:249, 1973.

Bainton, D., and Farquhar, M.: Origin of granules in polymorphonuclear leukocytes. J. Cell Biol., *28*:277, 1966.

Brady, R. O.: Hereditary fat metabolism diseases. Sci. Am., August 1973.

Brandes, D., and Bertini, F.: Role of Golgi apparatus in the formation of cytolysosomes. Exp. Cell Res., *35*:194, 1964.

Cohn, Z. A., and Benson, B.: The differentiation of mononuclear phagocytes. Morphology, cytochemistry and biochemistry. J. Exp. Med., *121*:153, 279, and 835, 1965.

———: The in vitro differentiation of mononuclear phagocytes. III. The reversibility of granule and hydrolytic enzyme formation and the turnover of granule constituents. J. Exp. Med., *122*:455, 1965.

Cohn, Z. A., and Hirsch, J. G.: Isolation and properties of specific cytoplasmic granules of rabbit polymorphonuclear leucocytes. J. Exp. Med., *112*:983, 1960.

Dauwalder, M., Whaley, W. G., and Kephard, J. E.: Phosphatases and differentiation in Golgi apparatus. J. Cell Sci., *4*:455, 1969.

De Duve, C.: The lysosome. Sci. Am., *208*(5):64, 1963.

———: Lysosomes and phagosomes. Protoplasma, *63*:95, 1967.

De Duve, C., and Wattiaux, R.: Function of lysosomes. Ann. Rev. Physiol., *28*:435, 1966.

De Reuck, A. V. S., and Cameron, M. P. (eds.): Lysosomes. Ciba Foundation Symposium. London, Churchill, 1963.

Dingle, J. T., and Fell, H. B. (eds.): Lysosomes in Biology and Pathology. Vols. 1, 2, and 3. Amsterdam, North Holland, 1969.

Gahan, P. B.: Histochemistry of lysosomes. Int. Rev. Cytol., *21:*1, 1967.

Graf, J., Kerjaschki, D., and Horandner, H.: Simultaneous demonstration of exogenous horse radish peroxidase and acid phosphatase activities in phagolysosomes. J. Histochem. Cytochem., *19:*569, 1971.

Hirsch, J. G.: Lysosomes and mental retardation. Quart. Rev. Biol., *47:*303, 1972.

Hirsch, J. G., and Cohn, Z. A.: Digestive and autolytic functions of lysosomes in phagocytic cells. Fed. Proc., *23:*1023, 1964.

Larsson, L., Maunsbach, A. B., Saxen, L., and Wartiovaara, J.: Lysosomes in developing kidney tubule cells in vitro. J. Ultrastruct. Res., *29:*570, 1969.

Novikoff, A. B., Esner, E., and Quintana, N.: Golgi apparatus and lysosomes. Fed. Proc., *23:*1010, 1964.

Rajan, K. T.: Lysosomes and gout. Nature, *210:*959, 1966.

Straus, W.: Occurrence of phagosomes and phagolysosomes in different segments of the nephron in relation to the reabsorption, transport, digestion, and extrusion of intravenously injected horse radish peroxidase. J. Cell Biol., *21:*295, 1964.

Weissmann, G.: Lysosomes. New Eng. J. Med., *273:*1084, 1143, 1965.

Zeja, H. I., and Spitznagel, J. K.: Isolation of polymorphonuclear leukocyte granules from rabbit bone marrow. Lab. Invest., *24:*237, 1971.

Zucker-Franklin, D., and Hirsch, J. G.: Electron microscope studies of the degranulation of rabbit peritoneal leukocytes during phagocytosis. J. Exp. Med., *120:*569, 1964.

Phagocytosis, Pinocytosis and Coated Vesicles

Bowers, B.: Coated vesicles in the pericardial cells of the aphid. Protoplasma, *59:*351, 1964.

Bowers, B., and Olszewski, T. E.: Pinocytosis in *Acanthamoeba castellanii*. Kinetics and morphology. J. Cell Biol., *53:*68, 1972.

Cohn, Z. A.: The fate of bacteria within phagocytic cells. J. Exp. Med., *117:*27, 1963.

Cornell, R., Walker, W. A., and Isselbacher, K. J.: Small intestine absorption of horse radish peroxidase. Lab. Invest., *25:*42, 1971.

Friend, D. S., and Farquhar, M. G.: Functions of coated vesicles during protein absorption in the rat vas deferens. J. Cell Biol., *35:*337, 1967.

Graham, R. C., and Karnovsky, M. J.: The early stages of absorption of injected horseradish peroxidase in the proximal tubules of mouse kidney: ultrastructural cytochemistry by a new technique. J. Histochem. Cytochem., *14:*291, 1966.

Gropp, A.: Phagocytosis and pinocytosis. *In* Rose, G. C. (ed.): Cinemicrography in Cell Biology. New York, Academic Press, 1963.

Hirsch, J. G., Fedorko, M. E., and Cohn, Z. A.: Vesicle fusion and formation at the surface of pinocytotic vacuoles in macrophages. J. Cell Biol., *38:*629, 1968.

Holter, H.: How things get into cells. Sci. Am., p. 167, September 1961.

Holtzman, E., and Peterson, E. R.: Protein uptake by mammalian neurons. J. Cell Biol., *40:*863, 1969.

Kanaseki, T., and Kadota, K.: The "vesicle in a basket." A morphological study of the coated vesicle isolated from the nerve endings of the guinea pig brain with special reference to the mechanism of membrane movements. J. Cell Biol., *42:*202, 1969.

Karnovsky, M. J.: The ultrastructural basis of capillary permeability studied with peroxidase as a tracer. J. Cell Biol., *35:*213, 1967.

Lagunoff, D.: Macrophage pinocytosis. The removal and resynthesis of a cell surface factor. Proc. Soc. Exp. Biol. Med., *138:*118, 1971.

Marshall, J. M., and Nachmias, V. T.: Cell surface and pinocytosis. J. Histochem. Cytochem., *13:*92, 1965.

North, R. J.: The uptake of particulate antigens. J. Reticuloendothel. Soc., *5:*203, 1968.

Rabinovitch, M.: The dissociation of the attachment and ingestion phases of phagocytosis by macrophages. Exp. Cell Res., *46:*19, 1967.

Rodewald, R.: Intestinal transport of antibodies in the newborn rat. J. Cell Biol., *58:*189, 1973.

Roth, T. F., and Porter, K. R.: Yolk protein uptake in the oocyte of the mosquito *Aedes aegypti* L. J. Cell Biol., *20:*313, 1964.

Rustad, R. C.: Pinocytosis. Sci. Am., p. 120, April 1961.

Simionescu, N., Simionescu, M., and Palade, G. E.: Permeability of muscle capillaries to exogenous myoglobin. *57:*424, 1973.

Werb, Z., and Cohn, Z. A.: Plasma membrane synthesis in the macrophage following phagocytosis of polystyrene latex particles. J. Biol. Chem., *247:*2439, 1972.

Williams, R. C., Jr., and Fudenberg, H. H. (eds.): Phagocytic Mechanisms in Health and Disease. New York, Intercontinental Medical Book, 1972.

Smooth Endoplasmic Reticulum

Black, W. H.: The development of smooth surfaced endoplasmic reticulum in adrenal cortical cells of fetal guinea pig. Am. J. Anat., *135:*381, 1972.

Black, W. H., and Christensen, A. K.: Differentiations of interstitial cells and Sertoli cells in fetal guinea pig testes. Am. J. Anat., *124:*211, 1969.

Cardell, R. R., Jr., Badenhausen, S., and Porter, K. R.: Intestinal triglyceride absorption in the rat. An electron microscopical study. J. Cell Biol., *34:*123, 1967.

Christensen, A. K.: Fine structure of testicular interstitial cells in humans. *In* Rosemberg E., and Paulsen, C. (eds.): The Human Testis. p. 75. New York, Plenum Press, 1970.

Emans, J. B., and Jones, A. L.: Hypertrophy of liver cell smooth surfaced reticulum following progesterone administration. J. Histochem. Cytochem., *16:*561, 1968.

Gillim, S. W., Christensen, A. K., and McLennan, M. E.: Fine structure of the human menstrual corpus luteum at its stage of maximum secretory activity. Am. J. Anat., *126:*409, 1969.

Higgins, J. A., and Barrnett, R. J.: Studies on the biogenesis of smooth endoplasmic reticulum membranes in livers of phenobarbital treated rats. J. Cell Biol., *55:*282, 1972.

Ito, S.: The endoplasmic reticulum of gastric parietal cells. J. Biophys. Biochem. Cytol., *11:*333, 1961.

Jones, A. L., and Fawcett, D. W.: Hypertrophy of the agranular reticulum in hamster liver induced by phenobarbital. J. Histochem. Cytochem., *24:*215, 1966.

Kelly, A. M.: Sarcoplasmic reticulum and T-tubules in differentiating rat skeletal muscle. J. Cell Biol., *49:*335, 1971.

McNutt, N. S., and Jones, A. L.: Observations on the ultra-structure of cytodifferentiation in the human fetal adrenal cortex. Lab. Invest., *22:*513, 1970.

Orrenius, S., and Ericsson, J. L. E.: Enzyme-membrane relationship in phenobarbital induction of synthesis of drug-metabolizing enzyme system and proliferation of endoplasmic membranes. J. Cell Biol., *28:*181, 1966.

Remmer, H., and Merker, J. J.: Effect of drugs on the formation of smooth endoplasmic reticulum and drug metabolizing enzymes. Ann. N.Y. Acad. Sci., *123:*79, 1965.

Microtubules

Adelman, M. R., Brisy, G. G., Shelanski, M. L., Weisenberg, R. C., and Taylor, E. W.: Cytoplasmic filaments and tubules. Fed. Proc., *27:*1186, 1968.

Behnke, O., and Forer, A.: Evidence for four classes of microtubules in individual cells. J. Cell Sci., *2:*169, 1967.

Bickle, D., Tilney, L. G., and Porter, K. R.: Microtubules and pigment migration in the melanophores of *Fundulus heteroclitus* L. Protoplasma, *61:*322, 1966.

Borisy, G. G., and Taylor, E. W.: The mechanism of action of colchicine. Binding of colchicine -H³ to cellular protein. J. Cell. Biol., *34:*525, 1967.

Brinkley, B. R., Stubblefield, E., and Hsu, T. C.: The effects of colcemid inhibition and reversal on the fine structure of the mitotic apparatus of Chinese hamster cells in vitro. J. Ultrastr. Res., *19:*1, 1967.

Olmsted, J. B., and Borisy, G. G.: Microtubules. Ann. Rev. Biochem, p. 507, 1973.

Olmsted, J. B., Witman, G., Carlson, K., and Rosinbaum, I.: Comparison of the microtubule proteins of neuroblastoma cells, brain, and chlamydomonas flagella. Proc. Nat. Acad. Sci. (U.S.A.), *68:*2273, 1971.

Porter, K. R.: Cytoplasmic microtubules and their functions. *In* Wolstenholme, G. E. W., and O'Connor, M. (eds.): Principles of Biomolecular Organization, Ciba Foundation Symposium. London, Churchill, 1966.

Tilney, L. G.: The assembly of microtubules. *In* Locke, M. (ed.): The Emergence of Order in Developing Systems, p. 63. New York, Academic Press, 1968.

———: Origin and continuity of microtubules. *In* Reinert, J., and Ursprung, H. (eds.): Origin and Continuity of Cell Organelles. New York, Springer-Verlag, *2:*222, 1971.

Tilney, L. G., Bryan, J., Busch, D. J., Fujiwara, K., Moosekar, M. S., Murphy, D. B., and Snyder, D. H.: Microtubules: evidence for 13 protofilaments. J. Cell Biol., *59:*267, 1973.

Yamada, K. M., Spooner, B. S., and Wessels, N. K.: Axon growth: roles of microfilaments and microtubules. Proc. Nat. Acad. Sci. (U.S.A.), *66:*1206, 1970.

Centrioles, Cilia and Flagella

Baba, S., and Hiramoto, Y.: A quantitative analysis of ciliary movement by high speed microcinematography. J. Exp. Biol., *52:*675, 1970.

Fawcett, D. W.: Cilia and flagella. *In* Brachet, J., and Mirsky, A. E. (eds.): The Cell. Vol. 2. New York, Academic Press, 1961.

Fulton, C.: Centrioles. *In* Reinert, J., and Ursprung, H. (eds.): Origin and Continuity of Cell Organelles. Vol. 2, p. 170. New York, Springer-Verlag, 1971.

Gibbons, I. R.: The relationship between the fine structure and direction of beat in gill cilia of a lamellibranch mollusc. J. Biophys. Biochem. Cytol., *11:*179, 1961.

———: Studies on the ATPase activity of 14 S and 30 S dynein from cilia of tetrahymena. J. Biol. Chem., *241:*5590, 1966.

———: The structure and composition of cilia. *In* Warren, K. B. (ed.): Formation and Fate of Cell Organelles. p. 99. New York, Academic Press, 1967.

Kalnins, V. I., and Porter, K. R.: Centriole replication during ciliogenesis in the chick tracheal epithelium. Z. Zellforsch., *100:*1, 1969.

Pederson, H.: Observations on the axial filament complex of the human spermatozoan. J. Ultrastr. Res., *33:*451, 1970.

Pickett-Heaps, J.: The autonomy of centriole: fact or fallacy. Cytobios, *3:*205, 1971.

Robbins, E., Jentzsch, G., and Micali, A.: The centriole cycle in synchronized HeLa cells. J. Cell Biol., *36:*329, 1968.

Satir, P.: Studies on cilia. II. Examination of the distal region of the ciliary shaft and the role of the filaments in motility. J. Cell Biol., *26:*805, 1965.

———: Studies on cilia. III. Further studies of the cilium tip and a sliding filament model of ciliary motility. J. Cell Biol., *39:*77, 1968.

Sleigh, M. A.: Patterns of ciliary beating. Symp. Soc. Exp. Biol., *22:*131, 1968.

———: Cilia. Endeavour, *30*(109):11, 1971.

Sorokin, S. P.: Reconstructions of centriole formation and ciliogenesis in mammalian lungs. J. Cell Sci., *3:*207, 1968.

Summers, K. E., and Gibbons, I. R.: Adenosine triphosphate-induced sliding of tubules in trypsin treated flagella of sea urchin sperm. Proc. Nat. Acad. Sci. (U.S.A.), *68:*3092, 1971.

Warner, F. D.: Macromolecular organization of eukaryotic cilia and flagella. Adv. Cell Molec. Biol, *2:*193, 1972.

Wolfe, J.: Basal body fine structure and chemistry. Adv. Cell Molec. Biol., *2:*151, 1972.

Cell Web—Filaments

Baker, P. F., and Schroeder, T. E.: Cytoplasmic filaments and morphogenetic movements in the amphibian neural tube. Develop. Biol., *15:*432, 1967.

Bhenke, O., Forer, A., and Emmerson, J.: Actin in sperm tails and meiotic spindle. Nature, *234:*408, 1971.

Bonneville, M. A., and Weinstock, M.: Brush border development in the intestinal absorptive cells of *Xenopus* during metamorphosis. J. Cell Biol., *44:*151, 1970.

Carter, S. B.: Effects of cytochalasins on mammalian cells. Nature, *213:*261, 1967.

Clermont, Y., and Pereira, G.: The cell web in epithelial cells of the rat kidney. Anat. Rec., *156:*215, 1966.

Crane, P. K.: Structure and functional organization of an epithelial cell brush border. *In* Warren, K. B. (ed.): Intracellular Transport. p. 71. New York, Academic Press, 1966.

Fine, R. E., and Bray, D.: Actin in growing nerve cells. Nature, New Biol., *234:*115, 1971.

Holtzer, H., and Sanger, I. W.: Cytochalasin B. Problems in interpreting its effect on cells. Develop. Biol., *27:*443, 1972.

Huxley, H. E.: The structural basis of muscular contraction. Proc. Roy. Soc. London [B]*178:*131, 1971.

———: Muscular contraction and cell motility. Nature, *243:*445, 1973.

Ishikawa, H., Bischoff, R., and Holtzer, H.: Formation of arrowhead complexes with heavy meromyosin in a variety of cell types. J. Cell Biol., *43:*312, 1969.

Leblond, C. P., and Clermont, Y.: The cell web, a fibrillar structure found in a variety of cells in animal tissues. Anat. Rec., *136:*230, 1960.

Lowey, J., and Small, J. V.: Organization of myosin and actin in vertebrate smooth muscle. Nature, *227:*46, 1970.

Perdue, J. F.: The distribution, ultrastructure and chemistry of microfilaments in cultured chick embryo fibroblasts. J. Cell Biol., *58:*265, 1973.

Rice, R., Moses, J., McManus, G., Brady, A., and Blasik, L.: The organization of contractile filaments in a mammalian smooth muscle J. Cell Biol., *47:*183, 1970.

Schroeder, T. E.: Cytokinesis: filaments in the cleavage furrow. Exp. Cell Res., *53:*272, 1968.

————: The contractile ring. I. Fine structure of dividing mamalian (Hela) cells and the effects of cytochalasin B. Z. Zellforsch., Mikroskop. Anat., *109:*431, 1970.

Spooner, B. S., Yamada, K. M., and Wessels, N. K.: Microfilaments and cell locomotion. J. Cell Biol., *49:*595, 1971.

Szollosi, D.: Cortical cytoplasmic filaments of cleaving eggs: a structural element corresponding to the contractile ring. J. Cell Biol., *44:*192, 1970.

Tilney, L. G., and Cardell, R. R., Jr.: Factors controlling the reassembly of the microvillous border of the small intestine of the salamander: J. Cell Biol., *97:*408, 1970.

Tilney, L. G., and Mooseker, M.: Actin in the brush border of epithelial cells of the chicken intestine. Proc. Nat. Acad. Sci. (U.S.A.), *68:*2611, 1971.

Tucker, J. B.: Microtubules and a contractile ring of microfilaments associated with a cleavage furrow. J. Cell Sci., *8:*557, 1971.

Wessels, N. K.: How living cells change their shape. Sci. Am., *225:*76, 1971.

Zucker, Franklin D., and Grusky, G. G.: The actin and myosin filaments of human and bovine blood platelets. J. Clin. Invest., *51:*419, 1972.

Cell Junctions

Claude, P., and Goodenough, D. A.: Fracture faces of zonulae occludentes from tight and leaky epithelia. J. Cell Biol., *58:*391, 1973.

Douglas, W. H. J., Ripley, R. C., and Ellis, R. A.: Enzymatic digestion of desmosomes and hemidesmosome plaques performed on ultrathin sections. J. Cell Biol., *44:*211, 1970.

Farquhar, M. G., and Palade, G. E.: Junctional complexes in various epithelia. J. Cell Biol., *17:*375, 1963.

Goodenough, D. A., and Revel, J. P.: A fine structural analysis of intercellular junctions in the mouse liver. J. Cell Biol., *45:*272, 1970.

Johnson, R. G., and Sheridan, J. D.: Junctions between cancer cells in culture—ultrastructure and permeability. Science, *174:*717, 1971.

Kanno, Y., and Lowenstein, W. R.: Cell-to-cell passage of large molecules. Nature (Lond.), *212:*629, 1967.

Keeter, J. S., and Pappas, G. D.: Gap junctions in embryonic skeletal muscle. Anat. Rec., *175(2):*355, 1973.

Kelly, D. Fine structure of desmosomes, hemidesmosomes and an adepidermal globular layer in developing newt epidermis. J. Cell Biol., *28:*51, 1966.

Lentz, T., and Trinkaus, J. P.: Differentiation of the junctional complex of surface cells. J. Cell Biol. *48:*455, 1971.

Loewenstein, W. R.: On the genesis of cellular communication. Dev. Biol., *15:*503, 1967.

————: Intercellular Communication. Sci. Am., *222:*79, May 1970.

McNutt, N. S., Hershberg, R. A., and Weinstein, R. S.: Further observations on the occurrence of nexuses in benign and malignant human cervical epithelium. J. Cell Biol., *51:*805, 1971.

————: Ultrastructure of intercellular junctions in adult and developing cardiac muscle. Am. J. Cardiol., *25:*169, 1970.

McNutt, N. S., and Weinstein, R. S.: The ultrastructure of the nexus. A correlated thin-section and freeze-cleave study. J. Cell Biol., *47:*666, 1970.

————: Membrane ultrastructure at mammalian intercellular junctions. Progr. Biophys. Molec. Biol., *26:*47, 1973.

Overton, J.: Experimental manipulation of desmosome formation. J. Cell Biol., *56:*636, 1973.

Pappas, G. D.: Junctions between cells. Hosp. Prac., August 1973.

Revel, J. P., and Karnovsky, M. J.: Hexagonal array of subunits in intercellular junctions of the mouse heart and liver. J. Cell Biol., *33(3):*C7, 1967.

Weinstein, R. S., McNutt, N. S., Nielsen, S. L., et al.: Intramembranous fibrils at tight junctions. Proc. Electron Micros. Soc. Am., *28:*108, 1970.

Weinstein, R. S., and McNutt, N. S.: Cell junctions. New Eng. J. Med., *286:*521, 1972.

Glycogen, Lipid, Pigment and Inclusions

Ashworth, C. T., Leonard, J. S., Eigenbrodt, E. H., and Wrightsman, F. J.: Hepatic intracellular osmiophilic droplets. Effect of lipid solvents during tissue preparation. J. Cell Biol., *31:*301, 1966.

Barnicot, N. A., and Birbeck, M. S. C.: The electron microscopy of human melanocytes and melanin granules. In Montagna, W., and Ellis, R. A. (eds.): The Biology of Hair Growth. p. 259. New York, Academic Press, 1958.

Biava, C.: Identification and structural forms of human particulate glycogen. Lab. Invest., *12:*1179, 1963.

Bissell, D. M., Hammaker, L., and Schmid, R.: Hemoglobin and erythrocyte catabolism in rat liver: the separate roles of parenchymal and sinusoidal cells. Blood J. Hematol., *40:*812, 1972.

————: Liver sinusoidal cells. Identification of a subpopulation for erythrocyte catabolism. J. Cell Biol., *54:*107, 1972.

Bjorkerud, S.: Isolation of lipofuscin granules from bovine cardiac muscle. J. Ultrastr. Res. (Suppl.), *5:*5, 1963.

Drochmans, P.: Morphologie du glycogène. J. Ultrastruct. Res., *6:*141, 1962.

Fitzpatrick, T. B., and Szabo, G.: The melanocyte: cytology and cytochemistry. J. Invest. Derm., *32:*197, 1959.

Frank, A. L., and Christensen, A. K.: Localization of acid phosphatase in lipofuchsin granules and possible autophagic vacuoles in interstitial cells of the guinea pig testis. J. Cell Biol., *36:*1, 1968.

Harrison, P.: Ferritin and haemosiderin. In Iron Metabolism. p. 148. Ciba International Symposium, Berlin, Springer-Verlag, 1964.

Karrer, H. E., and Cox, J.: Electron microscopic study of glycogen in chick embryo liver. J. Ultrastruct. Res., *4:*191, 1960.

Malkoff, D., and Strehler, B.: The ultrastructure of isolated and in situ human cardiac age pigment. J. Cell Biol., *16:*611, 1963.

Maul, G. G.: Golgi-melanosome relationships in human melanosomes *in vitro*. J. Ultrastr. Res., *26:*163, 1969.

Moyer, F. H.: Genetic effects on melanosome fine structure and ontogeny in normal and malignant cells. Ann. N.Y. Acad. Sci., *100:*584, 1963.

Napolitano, L.: The differentiation of white adipose cells. An electron microscope study. J. Cell Biol., *18:*663, 1963.

Napolitano, L., and Fawcett, D. W.: The fine structure of brown adipose tissue in newborn mice and rats. J. Biophys. Biochem. Cytol., *4:*685, 1958.

Novikoff, A. B., Albala, A., and Biempica, L.: Ultrastructural and cytochemical observations on B-16 and Harding-Passey mouse melanosomes. J. Histochem. Cytochem., *16:*299, 1968.

Palay, S. L., and Revel, J. P.: The morphology of fat absorption. *In* Meng, H. C. (ed.): Lipid Transport. pp. 33-43. Springfield, Illinois, Charles C Thomas, 1964.

Pictet, R., Orci, L., Forssmann, W. G., and Girardier, L.: An electron microscope study of the perfusion-fixed spleen. II. Nurse cells and erythrophagocytosis. Z. Zellforsch., *96:*400, 1969.

Revel, J. P.: Electron microscopy of glycogen. J. Histochem. Cytochem., *12:*104, 1964.

Richter, G. W.: A study of hemosiderosis with the aid of electron microscopy with observations on the relationship between hemosiderin and ferritin. J. Exp. Med., *106:*203, 1957.

Seiji, M., Birbeck, M. S. C., and Fitzpatrick, T. B.: Subcellular localization of melanin biosynthesis. Ann. N.Y. Acad. Sci., *100:*497, 1963.

Senior, J. R.: Intestinal absorption of fats. J. Lipid Res., *5:*495, 1964.

Silagi, S.: Control of pigment production in mouse melanoma cells *in vitro*. J. Cell Biol., *43:*263, 1969.

Wood, E. N.: An ordered complex of filaments surrounding the lipid droplets in developing adipose cells. Anat. Rec., *157:*437, 1967.

PART TWO

The Tissues

6 From Cells to Tissues

Cells, our topic until now, are the ultimate building blocks of the body just as atoms are the ultimate building blocks of all chemical compounds. However, in analyzing complex chemical compounds it often helps to deal with another order of larger building blocks, namely molecules. Similarly, in studying and describing the microscopic structure of various body parts it is a great help to deal with an order of building blocks that are larger than cells. These are called the *tissues* and from them all body parts are constructed. We shall now describe how the concept of tissues as building blocks developed and why it proved to be so helpful in understanding microscopic structure.

Development of Knowledge. The English word tissue was taken from the French *tissu* (weave or texture). Although long used with reference to cloth and fabric it was first employed as an anatomical term in the latter part of the 18th century by Bichat, a brilliant young French anatomist. As he dissected human bodies he became so conscious of the different textures of the various layers and structures he separated that he wrote a book describing what he termed the tissues of the body, classifying more than 20 varieties. He did not employ the microscope in making this classification because he thought it gave rise to misconceptions—and, indeed, at that time the instrument was far from perfect. But this soon changed, for during the 19th century improvements in the microscope and in methods for preparing materials for study with it led to its replacing the naked eye and the magnifying glass as the primary method for studying tissues. This engendered two developments:

First, 17 years after Bichat's death, the term *histology* (*histos,* web or tissue; *logos,* study of) was coined by a microscopist to designate the science of the tissues. Second, the microscope revealed in due course that there were not as many tissues as Bichat had thought and indeed it eventually became accepted that there were only four basic ones, with each of the four, however, having two or more subtypes. The important conclusion followed—that everything in the body is put together from four basic tissues and that

these building blocks can be distinguished from one another by their respective microscopic appearances and the particular roles they play. The names of the four basic tissues are:

1. Epithelial Tissue
2. Connective Tissue
3. Nervous Tissue
4. Muscle Tissue

The reasons for these names will be given in due course.

Why the Concept of Tissues Persisted Into the Era of Microscopy. The reader may be curious as to why it is necessary or helpful to learn about this second order of building blocks from which body parts are assembled. One very important reason is that cells are not the only components of the body, for one of the four basic tissues, *connective tissue,* consists not only of cells but also, and often to a far greater extent, of nonliving materials that are called *intercellular substances.* These are organic materials that are secreted by certain types of connective tissue cells so as to lie between these cells, where they thus have an intercellular (*inter,* between) position. Moreover in bone, which is one kind of connective tissue, the organic intercellular substance secreted by bone-forming cells normally absorbs calcium salts from the blood and tissue fluid to become calcified and stonelike. Even without becoming calcified much intercellular substance is strong and indeed it is only because of the intercellular substances of connective tissue that the human body has form and is able to stand erect. If it were composed solely of cells it would be as jellylike as they are. Accordingly, it is easy to understand why connective tissue must enter into the composition of innumerable body parts. However, the other tissues play equally important roles, so the point to be made here is that we shall find that all important organs and body parts are constructed from two, three or four of the basic tissues. Furthermore, the arrangements in which these exist in relation to one another are very similar in many body parts. *Hence, a knowledge of the four basic tissues and the ways in which they are so often arranged with one another enormously simpli-*

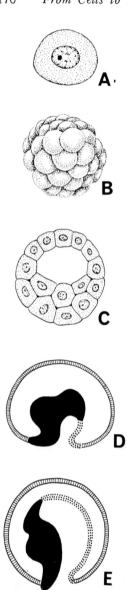

tology *and* microscopic anatomy; the book would deal first with *histology* as it was then defined—that is, with the study of tissues—and the second part of the book would deal with the *microscopic anatomy* of organs. The reason for this order was that learning about tissues first was recognized as an essential for learning about the microscopic structure of organs. This still holds true and explains why in this book we shall describe all the tissues before attacking the microscopic structure of the parts of the various organ systems. It should be noted that over the years the meaning of histology has become broadened to include the microscopic anatomy of the organ systems as well as the science of the tissues so there is no need to add microscopic anatomy to the title of this book.

Another reason for the tissue concept being retained was that it was of the greatest help in understanding how organs and various other body structures develop during embryonic life. As soon as microscopists had a knowledge of the four basic tissues they were able to study sections of successively older embryos and see where and how the four tissues developed and then how these tissues, retaining their respective identities, grew along with one another to form the various types of microscopic arrangements that are to be observed in the various organs of the postnatal body.

In order to understand the four tissues and how they become arranged with one another, it helps to have some knowledge of how they develop in the embryo. So, we shall next deal very briefly with this subject. (For detailed information on the development of the embryo, textbooks of embryology should be consulted.)

The Origin and Development of the Three Germ Layers of the Embryo— Predecessors of the Four Tissues

Since the human fertilized ovum not only forms an embryo but also certain membranes and a placenta (as will be described in Chapter 26), its early development is more difficult to describe at this time than is the development of the fertilized ovum of an amphibian. Furthermore, the amphibian embryo lends itself to experimental studies, the results of which are helpful to mention, and, since it illustrates the general principles involved in the development of the tissues, which is the topic with which we are concerned here, we shall describe briefly here the early development of the fertilized egg cell of the frog.

The fertilized egg cell of the frog (Fig. 6-1, A) undergoes a series of divisions called cleavages to develop into a morula (Fig. 6-1, B), so called because it resembles a mulberry (*morus,* mulberry). The cells of

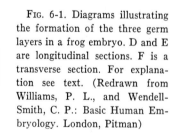

Fig. 6-1. Diagrams illustrating the formation of the three germ layers in a frog embryo. D and E are longitudinal sections. F is a transverse section. For explanation see text. (Redrawn from Williams, P. L., and Wendell-Smith, C. P.: Basic Human Embryology. London, Pitman)

fies the study of the microscopic anatomy of organs and other important body parts.

This became so obvious decades ago that textbooks such as this were sometimes termed textbooks of his-

the morula are not all of the same size because the large store of yolk in the cytoplasm of the fertilized ovum is divided up unequally as it divides to form the cells of the morula (Fig. 6-1, B). Those in its lower half obtain most of the yolk, which makes the cells there larger than those in the upper half. The morula at this time is described as having two poles, with the smaller cells surrounding the *animal pole* and the larger yolky cells aggregated toward the *vegetative pole.*

As a result of continuing mitosis, the morula enlarges, but, because no outside source of food is available, it can become larger only because a central cavity forms within it to make it into a hollow sphere (Fig. 6-1, C). It is now termed a *blastula* (*blastos*, germ) because it germinates an embryo, and so the cavity within it is termed a *blastocoele* (*coele*, cavity). At this time the cells of the wall nearer the animal pole become smaller and smaller because they continue to divide more rapidly than those nearer the vegetative pole. The wall of the blastula near its vegetative pole consists of several layers of yolk-containing cells. In due course the wall of the blastula at this site will become partly invaginated into the hollow sphere (black in Fig. 6-1, D). This process continues so that the invaginated portion of what was part of the wall of the blastula becomes an inner lining for the hollow sphere (Fig. 6-1, E). Since the invagination encroaches on the blastocoele, the latter becomes smaller and smaller, and in due course it becomes obliterated. The new cavity within the invagination (Fig. 6-1, E) is termed the *archenteron* (*arch,* first; *enteron*, intestine) and much of its wall of yolky cells will in due course give rise to the lining of the gut of the embryo.

The name given the stage of development when these changes occur is *gastrulation* (*gastro,* relating to the stomach or abdomen) which denotes that this is the stage at which the cells of the blastula begin to form the gut. However, there are other changes that occur at this stage.

The first indication that gastrulation is to begin is that a crack or groove appears on the surface of the blastula, close to its vegetative pole and, as already noted, most of the wall of the archenteron is derived from the yolk-laden cells that are near the vegetative pole and become invaginated at this site. However, while these cells are moving in to form most of the archenteron, smaller cells of the animal pole type move inward at the lip of the groove and proliferate to constitute, at first, a part of the wall of the archenteron. But some migrate and proliferate in such a way as to form a cellular filling (stippled in Fig. 6-1, F) that separates the cells of the outer wall of the blastula from the yolky cells that form the wall of the archenteron which presently becomes a tube (Fig. 6-1, F). Hence, the structure that at the blastula stage had only a single layer for its wall now has three layers in its wall, as shown in Figure 6-1, F. These are:

1. An outer layer (striped in Fig. 6-1, F) which is by now constituted almost entirely of cells of the animal pole type and is called *ectoderm* (*ektos*, outer; *derma*, skin).

2. The layer of cells that constitutes the wall of the archenteron and, in due course, forms a tube (black in Fig. 6-1, F). This layer of cells is termed the *entoderm* (*ento*, inner).

3. The cellular layer that lies between the ectoderm and the entoderm; this layer, stippled in Figure 6-1, F, is at first termed the *chorda-mesoderm* because its cells form (among other things) a long bar of cells disposed longitudinally in the developing embryo and called the *notochord*, around which the vertebrae subsequently form. The cells of this middle layer, which in due course is termed *mesoderm* (*mesos*, middle) are also responsible for forming most of the muscle of the embryo and also its skeleton and other connective tissue structures, as will be described presently.

Before long a stage is reached in which a cross section of the very young embryo appears more or less as an oval which is covered with a cellular layer of ectoderm (Fig. 6-1, F). Within the oval is the cross section of a tube and this is lined by the cellular layer that is the *entoderm*. Between the entoderm and the ectoderm there is a layer of cells which is more compact along the back of the developing embryo than it is closer to its ventral part and where the body cavity, the coelom, will form. All of this middle layer constitutes the *mesoderm*. At the upper part of the oval, which roughly represents the back of the embryo, the denser mesoderm around the notochord (not shown in Figure 6-1) forms the vertebrae and a little farther away the mesoderm will give rise to most of the muscles of the body. The remainder will give rise to various types of connective tissue components, as will soon be explained in more detail.

The Development of the Four Basic Tissues From the Three Germ Layers

EPITHELIAL TISSUE (EPITHELIUM)

Epithelium is a morphological (*morpho*, relating to form) term—that is, its definition is based on the form or particular construction of the tissue and *not on its origin from a particular germ layer.* Indeed the origin of epithelium in different sites in the body can be traced to ectoderm, entoderm and mesoderm. Most, however, comes from ectoderm and entoderm.

From its derivation the term epithelium (*epi*, upon; *thele*, nipple) refers to something that covers (is upon) nipples (the nipples referred to when the term was coined were the little capillary-containing connective tissue nipples in the lips). From this beginning the term epithelium came to be used for all covering and lining membranes in the body that are composed of cells. The epithelial part (which is the outer part) of the skin arises from ectoderm. That which lines the intestinal tract is derived from entoderm while that which lines the peritoneal (body) cavity is derived from mesoderm. However, while the latter is true epithelium because it is a cellular lining membrane, it is generally termed *mesothelium* because of its origin from mesoderm. Likewise, the epithelium that lines the blood vessels and the heart and is also derived from mesoderm is not generally called epithelium but *endothelium* to distinguish it from epithelium that arises from ectoderm and entoderm.

All covering and lining epithelial membranes are composed of cells joined together by cell junctions, the various types of which were described in the preceding chapter. Epithelial membranes are all supported by connective tissue, the capillaries of which are responsible for nourishing the epithelial cells of the membrane (Fig. 5-1). External epithelial membranes, however, except for those of the lips and a few other sites, are not translucent, so blood in capillaries cannot be seen through the epithelium of the skin except in special circumstances when the capillary bed of the underlying connective tissue becomes expanded—as, for example, in blushing or sunburn.

Glands. Some or all of the epithelial cells of some membranes elaborate a secretion onto the surface they cover. An example is the goblet cells (Fig. 7-5) of the epithelial membrane that lines the intestine. However, in many body sites the need for secretion is too great to be satisfied by the limited number of secretory cells that can be accommodated in a covering or lining membrane. To provide for extra secretion the cells of the epithelial membrane at these body sites, during the development of the embryo, grew into the underlying developing connective tissue as is illustrated in Figure 6-2 to form structures that were called *glands* (*glans*, acorn) because some of the first that were studied were shaped like acorns.

Exocrine and Endocrine Glands

The most common type of gland is the *exocrine* (*ex*, out or away from; *krinein*, to separate). As this name

suggests, an exocrine gland delivers its secretion onto the surface from which the gland originated and hence *outside* the substance of the body. To do this exocrine glands possess tubes called *ducts* that convey the secretion which is produced in the more deeply located secretory cells to the surface (Fig. 6-2, *lower left*).

The other type of gland is of the endocrine (*endo*, within; *krinein*, to separate) type. These develop in the same way as exocrine glands except that the cellular connection with the surface (which they at first have and which in an exocrine gland would become a duct) is lost; hence endocrine glands have no ducts (Fig. 6-2, *lower right*). Endocrine glands therefore are constituted of islands of epithelial secretory cells surrounded by connective tissue and hence have to deliver their secretions *into* the substance of the body. Most of their secretory cells have a close association with the blood capillaries of connective tissue (Fig. 6-2, *lower right*) into which their secretions gain entry and are thus carried all over the body. Most endocrine secretions are chemical substances called *hormones* (*hormaein*, to arouse to activity or spur on), which in very small amounts exert most important physiological effects in the various parts of the body to which they are carried by the blood, as will be described in a later chapter on the Endocrine System.

MESODERM AND CONNECTIVE TISSUE

Connective tissue develops from mesoderm. Thus connective tissue is in a good position to nourish and support epithelial membranes and glands that develop from ectoderm and entoderm. Blood cells, the heart and the blood vessels of various sizes through which blood is pumped all through the body, are all formed from cells that develop in the mesoderm and hence throughout life blood circulates in vessels that are confined to connective tissue. As might be expected in the development of any epithelial glandular structure, epithelial cells and mesodermal connective tissue develop in close association with one another (Fig. 6-2). Since the epithelial cells perform the special work of the gland and since the connective tissue supports and nourishes the epithelial part of the gland, the epithelial part of the composite structure is termed the *parenchyma* (which from its derivation means anything poured in beside) of the gland (or organ) while the connective tissue that supports and nourishes the parenchyma is termed the *stroma* (anything laid out for lying or sitting upon) of the gland (or organ).

As already mentioned, connective tissue is unique because many varieties of it consist chiefly of nonliving

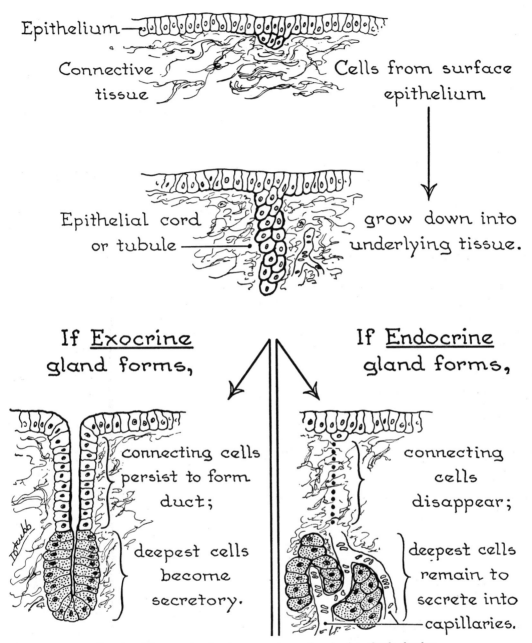

Fig. 6-2. Diagram showing how exocrine and endocrine glands develop.

material (called intercellular substances) produced by certain kinds of connective tissue cells. Details will be given in Chapters 8 and 9. The cartilage and bone of the skeleton as well as ligaments, fascia and tendons all develop from mesoderm and represent types of connective tissue that consist chiefly of intercellular substance. In these the chief role of connective tissue cells is to produce and maintain the intercellular substances. But there are other kinds of connective tissue which are essentially cellular and in these there are other kinds of connective tissue cells that are concerned, not with producing intercellular substances but with other functions—for example, defending the body against bacteria or other disease-producing organisms that gain entrance to it as will be described in subsequent chapters.

ECTODERM AND NERVOUS TISSUE

At a very early stage of development the ectoderm along the middle of the back of the embryo becomes depressed along its midline (Figs. 6-1, F and 6-3) to form the *neural plate*. This plate of ectodermal cells sinks more deeply into the back to form the *neural groove* (Fig. 6-3). The edges of the groove then come together and fuse so that the groove becomes a tube which lies just below the ectodermal surface (Fig. 6-3). This tube runs all the way from the head to the tail of the developing embryo. In the head region the walls of the tube thicken to develop into a brain (Fig. 6-3). Along the remainder of its course the wall of the tube thickens to become the spinal cord. As will be described in more detail in Chapter 17, the ectodermal cells of the walls of the tube give rise in both sites to nerve cells (called neurons) and cells which support them (called neuroglia [*glia*, glue] cells). As will be described in Chapter 17, little bits of nervous tissue

become detached along the tube where the edges of the groove become fused and these remain scattered along the tube on each side of its posterior aspect to become what are known as the cerebrospinal ganglia (*ganglion*, a knotlike mass). They are composed of nerve cells and supporting cells.

Cytoplasmic fibers grow out from the bodies of the nerve cells that develop in the ectodermal-derived tube of nervous tissue that becomes the brain and spinal cord, and other nerve fibers grow out from the bodies of the nerve cells of the ganglia. There is also some migration of nerve cells to certain body parts, as will be described later. The nerve fibers that grow from the tube and ganglia must, of course, enter the mesoderm that is becoming connective tissue. Here each of the nerve fibers with a special coating of their own becomes surrounded by a sheath of delicate connective tissue. Nerve fibers commonly become grouped together to become the nerves (Fig. 17-39) that are ensheathed with more connective tissue and are distributed to various parts of the body via connective tissue.

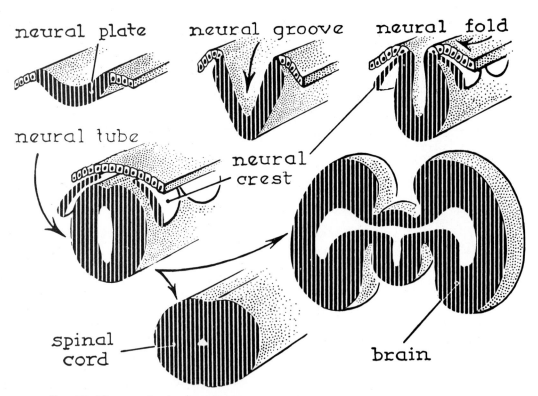

FIG. 6-3. Diagrams showing how the neural plate forms from ectoderm, and how it becomes the neural groove and then the neural tube. The diagrams also show that the neural tube, in different sites, turns into the spinal cord and the brain, respectively.

MESODERM AND MUSCLE TISSUE

Muscle cells, of which there are three types, which will be described in detail in Chapter 18, develop from the mesoderm. All types of muscle cells are elongated structures and for this reason they are called muscle *fibers*. When they contract they shorten in length, thus becoming somewhat thicker. Most muscle fibers are individually ensheathed in delicate connective tissue which contains capillaries; this arrangement is facilitated because both the fibers and the connective tissue components of muscle develop in the mesoderm. The connective tissue component of what are termed muscles in the dissecting room consists not only of the delicate capillary-containing sheathing between each fiber; in addition, there are connective tissue sheaths that contain more intercellular substance and surround bundles of fibers and even bundles of bundles. This stronger connective tissue becomes continuous with dense connective tissue structures such as tendons or aponeuroses which connect with the skeleton and through which muscles can move bones.

THE SIGNIFICANCE OF THE FOREGOING WITH REGARD TO THE STUDY OF SECTIONS FROM VARIOUS BODY PARTS

The fact that there are four basic tissues which play different roles in the formation of body parts and in the function of body parts means that, when a student examines a section from any part of the body, more than one basic tissue—and, often, representatives of all four—will be present. An important reason for there being more than one is that connective tissue has the exclusive function of carrying blood vessels to the vicinity of cells of the other tissues. It also has the exclusive function of carrying nerves to epithelial and muscle tissue. Furthermore, for all practical purposes connective tissue exclusively has the function of producing the intercellular substances of the body which provide support and strength for body structures. So, with the exception of the nervous tissue of the brain and spinal cord (which are special cases, as will be described later), a section taken from almost any part of the body will reveal (1) some connective tissue, consisting of (A) connective tissue cells and (B) intercellular substances which will contain (2) blood vessels and often (3) a few nerves. In addition, sections from many sites will also contain (4) epithelium or (5) muscle, or both.

Tissue Interactions During Development. The significance of there being four tissues and their developing in intimate association with each other during embryonic development is, however, not limited to enabling a student to interpret sections from various body parts more readily. Of great fundamental importance is the fact that during development they influence each other, in that one tissue seems to be responsible for organizing another, with which it is in contact, to become a special structure. Thus the development of many parts of the body is dependent to a great extent on interactions first between the cells of the three germ layers and later between the four tissues. We shall next discuss this fascinating topic.

Cell Differentiation—A Requisite for the Formation of the Different Tissues

By the time a human body has formed, the fertilized ovum has given rise to billions of cells and—what is much more interesting—the fertilized ovum has given rise to probably something over a hundred distinctly different kinds of cells that are variously allocated to the subdivisions of the four basic tissues. The formation of different kinds of cells and the disposition of different kinds to the different tissues is due to the occurrence of a process termed *cell differentiation*. This process operates during both embryonic development and postnatal life to cause cells to become different from the way they were before by acquiring new structural or functional characteristics. The change that a cell undergoes when it differentiates from one stage to another is associated with an increasing specialization and in mammalian cells this change in the nature of a normal diploid cell is generally regarded as being irreversible. In other words, in the process of normal differentiation, cells only go forward toward a state in which they are more specialized than they were before.

The Meaning of Potentiality. Any step in the differentiation of a cell is generally associated with a concomitant loss of some of the *potentiality* it previously possessed. This word is used in relation to cells with a special meaning. The potentiality of a cell is assessed by the number of various kinds of cells into which it can differentiate. Hence the fertilized ovum, because it can give rise to every kind of cell in the body, is said to possess great potentiality, indeed it is said to be a *totipotent* cell. However, as soon as cells derived from the ovum begin to differentiate, they lose some of the potentiality possessed by the ovum, and thereafter the number of different kinds of cells they can form becomes restricted. Any given cell that is becoming increasingly specialized becomes, with each further step in differentiation, less able to become specialized in other ways; hence, there is a general rule to the effect that there is a reciprocal relation in a cell between the extent to which it has differentiated and its potentiality.

Differentiation Involves Genes. We must next inquire into the basis for cells becoming different from one another and why this restricts their potentiality when they do. It was easier to theorize about this many decades ago when not so much was known about genes and how they acted and are duplicated in cell division. At that time it was easy to assume that the process of differentiation was associated with the genes of the fertilized ovum becoming more or less divided up among the cells that formed from it and hence that the special genes that, for example, were needed for nerve cells went to them and those for muscle cells to muscle cells and so on. This concept allowed the loss of potentiality observed in various types of specialized cells to be explained because of their having lost some of the genes they previously possessed. But when it was found that genes had their chemical basis in DNA and that the way DNA is duplicated leads always to daughter cells having exactly the same DNA and hence the same genes as a mother cell, it began to seem doubtful that differentiation, with a concomitant loss of potentiality of cell, could any longer be explained this way. Indeed it is now generally believed that every normal diploid body cell has the same complement of genes as every other body cell whether it is a nerve cell, a muscle cell, a secretory cell or any other kind of cell. It has been shown (*see* Gurndon) that when the nucleus of an epithelial lining cell of the intestine of a tadpole is transplanted to a frog's egg that has been enucleated, the nucleus from the epithelial lining cell of the tadpole can cause a complete embryo to develop from the egg. The nucleus of at least this type of differentiated cell is therefore totipotent but the differentiated cell in which it exists is not. How, therefore, is the differentiation of a cell with a concomitant loss of its potentiality to be explained?

Some Concepts. If the cells of a developing embryo all have the same genes in their nuclei, the only explanation for cells becoming different from one another must be that different sets of genes are turned on and off in different cells in the developing embryo. Next, since cells, when they become different from one another, not only remain different from one another but also reproduce their respective kinds, the same genes must be turned on (and off) in daughter cells as were turned on in the mother cells that divided. Furthermore, since cells differentiate along different lines in the body to become more and more specialized, further genes must be turned on as cells continue to differentiate along their respective lines to become more and more specialized and others must be successively

turned off to account for the cells' decreasing potentiality.

We shall first describe some morphological evidence indicating that different genes are indeed turned on in different kinds of cells and at different times in development.

Morphological Evidence for Genes Being Turned On in a Sequential Fashion. The fact that different genes are turned on and at different stages of development has been shown from studies on what are termed the giant chromosomes of certain insects. Giant chromosomes are formed because of the chromosomes continuing to duplicate in a cell without their halves separating so that after several duplications they become large and are thus profitably studied with the microscope. It has been found that what are called *puffs* appear at sites where genes become active. Puffs reflect sites where a chromatin thread (or threads) becomes uncondensed and sufficiently extended to give off information. The appearance of puffs at different sites (bands) along the chromosomes can be related to different events occurring in the tissues of the insect and the different events are of course believed to be due to the DNA of the chromosome at the site of a puff beginning to transcribe mRNA which directs the protein synthesis that causes the change observed in the tissue. What is of great interest also is the fact that the hormone *ecdysome,* which appears, relatively, in quantity in an insect when it undergoes a metamorphosis from a larva into a pupa and again when the pupa becomes an adult, has been shown to cause puffs to appear on certain chromosomes which presumably begin to transcribe on mRNA so that the proper proteins will be produced for its life in its new state.

The foregoing provides morphological evidence indicating that different genes are, in effect, turned on at different times in cells and that this is reflected in changes occurring in the tissue concerned. However, the turning on of specific genes in cells in one part of a body by a hormone requires the pre-existence of some sort of a circulatory system to carry the hormone from where it is produced to where it acts. Since there is no circulatory system, for example, at the gastrula stage of a frog embryo, there must be other mechanisms for turning on genes in the very early stages of the development of a mammal or an amphibian.

When, and Possible Ways, Genes Are Turned On in the Developing Embryo. Although all the cells of a morula have identical genes, there are differences in their cytoplasm. The cells at the vegetative pole are larger and contain much more stored food than those at the animal pole (Fig. 6-1, B). This could be a reason for metabolic differences existing in the cells of the two general areas of the morula. Next, the rate of cell division is not the same in all parts of the morula, for the cells closer to the animal pole have divided more often than those at the vegetative pole (Fig. 6-1, C); this also could cause metabolic differences between the cytoplasm of the two types of cells. However, *at this point metabolic differences in the cytoplasm would not have affected gene expression: there is much evidence indicating* that at and through the morula stage there is no transcription from the genes of the cell onto mRNA because all the mRNA in the cytoplasm at that time was left over from mRNA present in the egg cell that was fertilized and which, up to this point, has been directing such protein synthesis as has occurred in the cells of the morula.

Around the time of gastrulation, however, new mRNA begins to appear in the cytoplasm. Until this happens it could be assumed that all the genes of the cells of the morula have been turned off. But, as noted in the above paragraph, the metabolic reactions that were proceeding in the cytoplasm of the cells of, say, the animal pole type and the vegetative pole type could be different. As was described in Chapter 4, a substrate for an enzyme, or a similar substance, can act as an inducer which combines with the repressor of some particular operon so that the repressor no longer represses the operator gene of that operon and hence the operator turns on the structural gene or genes of that particular system so that it or they begin to transcribe mRNA which in turn directs the synthesis of the protein enzymes that metabolize the substrate that acted as the inducer. It was noted in Chapter 4 that in the instance of amino acid synthesis the abundance of the amino acid in the environment of the cell can cause the genes that control the synthesis of that particular amino acid to be turned off because an abundance of the end product can affect the repressor so that it combines with and inhibits the operator that controls the genes of the system concerned. Hence, differences in the metabolic patterns of the two general types of cells (animal and vegetative) could conceivably bring about the activation and maintain the repression of somewhat different genes in the two types of cells. Further, as cells of the animal pole type grow to form mesoderm between the cells that become ectoderm and those that become entoderm, the external environment of the cells thus sandwiched between the other two germ layers might be expected to play a part in causing still different chemical reactions to be set up which through negative feedback mechanisms could cause still different genes to become active. In other words, it is conceivable that phenomena similar to those

that have been shown to turn genes on or off in bacteria could cause different sets of genes to be turned on in the cells of the three germ layers of the early embryo.

Why Cells of a Particular Cell Lineage Remain of the Same Kind Through Divisions. In bacteria the genes that are turned on by, for example, lactose stay "turned on" only as long as lactose is available to them. In contrast, the genes that are turned on to account for the three different germ layers of the embryo seem—at least, for the most part—to stay turned on so as to modify thereafter the character of the cell lineages that are derived from them. In considering this matter it must be pointed out that bacteria are single cells, and the differentiation and specialization of cells that occur in the multicellular animal cannot as such be studied in them. It could of course be argued that differentiation has occurred in bacteria, because there are many different kinds of them that perpetuate their own kind. The explanation for these numerous varieties is that mutations occurred which explains their differences at the gene level. But if we assume that the genes of all the body cells of the multicellular animal are the same, we have to think of some way to explain why a mechanism that causes certain genes to be turned on temporarily in a bacterium stay turned on in the cells of a developing embryo and in their progeny, for the cells that develop from ectoderm, entoderm and mesoderm in general retain the characteristics of the germ layer from which they originated. Furthermore, as development proceeds, families or lines of different kinds of cells are established within which cells perpetuate their own special nature; in other words, the same genes that were turned on by some previous event are turned on again in daughter cells after every division while those that were not previously turned on but must act as templates for new DNA molecules in the S period (so in a sense they are turned on at this time) are immediately turned off and they stay turned off in daughter cells after cell division has been completed. A possible explanation for the inheritance of particular arrangements of gene expression from mother to daughter cells is that the internal environment of the cytoplasm remains the same long enough after DNA is duplicated for the same feedback mechanisms that caused certain genes to be activated with others remaining suppressed in the original differentiation process to be reinstated in the two daughter cells. There are probably two factors of importance in maintaining this internal environment in the cytoplasm: (1) the persistence for a time of the enzyme systems that were established in the mother cell and are divided up in the cytoplasm of the daughter cells and (2) persistence of the mRNA formed before DNA duplication begins which might function long enough to maintain these particular enzyme systems so that the feedback from the reactions they catalyze activates and suppresses the same genes in the daughter cells as were activated and suppressed in the mother cell. (Although much mRNA is relatively short-lived there are examples of it continuing to direct protein synthesis for some time even in cells that have lost their nuclei—for example, reticulocytes and the lens fibers of the eye.) In any event the hereditary nature of different cell lines is probably maintained through the S period (while DNA is duplicating) and mitosis (when all the chromatin of the chromosomes is condensed) by cytoplasmic factors. It would be difficult to understand how activated or suppressed genes could be duplicated as such.

The third problem we should discuss is that of different genes being turned on successively with others being seemingly permanently blocked as a cell differentiates through different stages to reach its final highly specialized state. In order to describe examples of this, we first have to comment on some terminology.

The Terms Determination and Commitment. The fact that cells do stay of the same family type even in a changed environment is easily demonstrated by transplanting them from one environment to another in an animal. If, for example, bone-forming cells are transplanted into a muscle, they do not begin to form muscle cells but instead retain their inherent nature and form bone. Hence the nature of cells of different family types that reproduce their own kind is said to be *determined*. Such cells are also referred to as being *committed*.

Competence. In contrast to cells that become determined (committed) so that they thereafter remain as members of a particular cell family type, the cells of an embryo before they become determined are described as being *competent,* which term means that their further development is not determined and hence they are susceptible to responding to an environmental stimulus of some sort by becoming different from what they were before. When they respond they of course become (at least to some extent) determined (committed).

Competence and determination, or commitment, are terms that are relative to the various stages of differentiation through which a cell may pass. At different stages of the development of the embryo its cells may successively become competent to respond to successively different environmental influences each of which causes it to become more specifically determined. The first environmental factor may determine

the nature of a cell within certain relatively broad limits so that it proceeds along a specific pathway of differentiation—as, for example, when a cell is influenced to become a mesodermal cell. But from there on it may become competent to respond to still different environmental factors which cause it to become the kind of connective tissue cell that can produce intercellular substance. This cell in turn is competent to respond to a factor that causes it to produce a specific type of intercellular substance, such as that of cartilage, or to a factor that causes it to form bone. Its nature is then fully determined.

Induction. This term denotes the process that takes place when some change is *caused* to occur, as for example, when some friend "induces" you to go to a movie instead of reading your textbook as you would otherwise have done. In the developing embryo, the term induction has a specific meaning denoting the effect of an environmental influence that results in competent cells undergoing some degree of differentiation whereby they attain at least some degree of determination. Induction plays an all-important role in the orderly development of an embryo and much of it depends on one developing tissue affecting an adjacent tissue. The phenomenon of induction is not limited to embryonic development; examples of it also occur in postnatal life. In all instances inductive phenomena can affect only competent cells; hence, since inductive phenomena occur in postnatal life, it follows that there are some kinds of cells in the postnatal body that are not fully determined and are still competent to respond to certain inductive influences.

All of the foregoing discussion will be placed in clearer perspective after we describe a few examples of induction that occur at different times and at different levels of differentiation.

Some Examples of Induction in Embryonic Development

Formation of the Neural Plate and Tube (Nervous Tissue). Many kinds of experiments have shown that it is contact with mesoderm that induces the formation of the neural plate (Fig. 6-3) and tube from the overlying ectoderm. For example, if an impervious membrane is placed between the ectoderm and the mesoderm, the neural tube does not form. However, if the membrane has pores of a certain size, the induction of a neural tube takes place. If the ectoderm that would form a neural tube is removed before the mesoderm comes into contact with it and is cultivated in a proper type of tissue culture, it does not show any indication of forming neural tissue. But if it is transplanted after mesoderm has come into contact with it, it differentiates into neural tissue. In other words, after its cells have been acted on by the inducer (mesoderm), their nature becomes determined; they will all form nerve cells and neuroglia cells.

The Formation of the Lens of the Eye. In this instance the inducer is developing neural tissue and the tissue that is competent to respond to the inductive influence exerted by this neural tissue is ectoderm. As the nervous system develops, the forebrain is a hollow structure (it is derived from the neural tube), and from its anterior wall two bulges called the optic vesicles will in due course develop into the retina (the light-sensitive portion of the eye), which requires that their anterior walls become invaginated as will be described in connection with the eye. The point to be made here, however, is that as the optic vesicles approach the overlying ectoderm, the latter tissue bulges inward to form a vesicle which in due course becomes closed over on its anterior aspect (to form the lens of the eye), with the cells of its posterior wall differentiating into cells termed lens fibers. The fact that the organization of the lens is dependent on the inducing influence of the optic vesicles is shown by the fact that optic vesicles of developing embryos can be removed and transplanted to other sites of the young embryos so as to underlie ectoderm and at these sites they induce ectodermal cells to differentiate into cells of the type that normally develop into lens fibers. Furthermore, if ectodermal epithelium from some other site on the body of the embryo is substituted for the ectodermal epithelium that normally covers the developing optic vesicles, the latter structures will induce a lens to form from the transplanted ectodermal epithelium.

Induction is not always a one-way street but instead tissue interactions may involve reciprocity between the two interacting tissues. This has been shown in experiments wherein ectoderm from an embryo of an animal which would have relatively small eyes is transplanted to an embryo of a related species that would normally have relatively large eyes; the formation of a lens is induced but the lens is larger than it would have been had it formed in its own species. What is of still greater interest is the fact that the eye that forms is smaller than it otherwise would have been and as a result the relative sizes of these two parts of the eye that develop are in proper proportion to one another (*see* Ebert Sussex).

Development of a Gland. An example of induction occurring at a later stage of prenatal development is provided by the development of the secretory cells of the pancreas; this has been intensively investigated by

Wessels and Rutter in the rat and the mouse. About halfway through prenatal life some lining cells of the developing intestine (which are epithelial in type and entoderm-derived) at the site where a pancreas will develop begin to bulge outward so as to constitute a small evagination. Close to the primitive intestine the evagination becomes narrowed, which is a preliminary to its becoming a tube that in due course will be the pancreatic duct. Farther out from the developing gut the cells of the evagination that are growing into the mesoderm-derived developing connective tissue begin to become arranged in the form of acini (which remain connected to the cells that will form the pancreatic duct). Some also differentiate into the cells of little islets that will later constitute the endocrine elements of the pancreas and produce hormones, one of them being insulin (the antidiabetic hormone, to be described in the chapter on the Endocrine System). Before long, zymogen granules begin to appear in the secretory cells of the acini, which indicates that the DNA of their nuclei is by then directing the synthesis of the special proteins that comprise the substance of zymogen granules. The appearance of these granules also indicates that they are being properly packaged in the Golgi apparatus, from which they become detached to enter the cytoplasm as prosecretory granules ready for later release from the cytoplasm into the duct system. In other words, the cells of the acini have by then differentiated into highly specialized types of secretory cells.

Wessels and Rutter found that there is a time in the development of the mouse embryo when the epithelial cells of the gut at the site where the pancreas would normally form become determined to form pancreas. Gut epithelium taken before this time and cultivated free from mesoderm does not form pancreatic tissue. However, gut epithelium taken a few days later forms pancreatic tissue under the same conditions (it is by then determined). In investigating what causes it to become determined they found that contact with mesoderm at the time in embryonic development when the gut epithelial cells had become competent to respond to an inductive stimulus was the factor and that, after contact had been sufficiently prolonged, the cells from the gut were then determined and would develop into pancreatic parenchyma independently. Curiously enough, the mesoderm that would cause this induction was found not to be limited to that which was normally at the site where the gut epithelium evaginated to form pancreatic parenchyma, for mesoderm from many different body sites had the same effect. Furthermore, mesoderm would exert this inductive effect on competent gut epithelium even if it was separated from the epithelium by a porous membrane if the pores were of a size that would permit fairly large molecules to pass through them. The precise chemical nature of the substance or substances that cause induction is, however, not yet established. Through the years both RNA and proteins have come under study.

Summary: Differentiation in the Early Embryo. The examples of induction in the early embryo described above, together with many others that could be cited, are in harmony with the concept that during the early stages of development different combinations of genes are turned on to account for the cells of the three germ layers becoming different from one another. It seems possible that different genes are turned on because the metabolic reactions in the cytoplasm of the cells that form the three layers are different. The cytoplasm of the egg is by no means homogeneous so that when it divides and continues to divide, different components in it, both organelles and stored food, are divided among the cells of the morula unequally. Furthermore, some of the cells of the morula have divided more often than others. Factors in the external environment could also perhaps play a part because of different cells of the morula not having equal access to oxygen. It is therefore conceivable that the metabolic differences in the cells of different areas of the morula could, by means of feedback mechanisms similar to those discussed in connection with the operon concept in Chapter 4 and briefly reviewed in this chapter, cause different genes to be turned on when transcription of mRNA begins in the gastrula stage.

The inductive phenomena that account for such things as the development of the nervous system, the lens of the eye, the formation of glands and still other events not mentioned in the above account are difficult to explain. A great deal of research has been directed at trying to ascertain the nature of the inducing agents that presumably diffuse (say) from mesoderm to ectoderm, to account, for example, for the induction of glands or other structures, but the results do not indicate the existence of various specific agents that would account for different examples of induction. Indeed, an inducing agent often seems to be relatively nonspecific and acts like a trigger that sets off a charge that was ready to be fired. Whereas it is commonly believed that one tissue would affect the differentiation of another by supplying it with some form of an inductive agent, the possibility should be kept in mind that one tissue may affect the differentiation of another by absorbing something from it. To help round out this discussion of a very complex problem we shall next consider some examples of how differentiation is affected in postnatal life.

Examples of Factors Affecting Differentiation in Later Prenatal and Postnatal Life

As an embryo continues to develop, more and more cells become specialized, and some of their various products are able to reach various parts of the body by way of the circulatory system which by this time has also developed. Hence, cells that are as yet relatively undifferentiated in various body parts are exposed to increased amounts of both oxygen and nutrients as well as to new substances that are of the general nature of chemical messengers, including hormones, which are synthesized by, and enter the bloodstream from, various types of specialized cells that develop in various body sites. We shall first comment on an example of how increased amounts of oxygen in the blood could affect cell differentiation.

Cartilage or Bone. Bones develop in the limb buds that grow out from an embryo. Here only mesoderm is involved. An early indication that a bone is to form in a limb bud is that the mesoderm-derived cells in the central part of the bud become packed together so as to form a structure that roughly denotes the form of the bone-to-be. The cells of this mass secrete enough intercellular substance to separate the cells from one another sufficiently for the shape and size of the bone-to-be to be more clearly outlined as a cartilaginous structure. However, at a certain time during development, the cells along the side of a cartilage model of a bone-to-be, which are of the same type that previously differentiated into cartilage cells, begin to form bone cells so that soon a shell of bone surrounds the cartilage model. (Eventually, as will be described in more detail later, most of the cartilage model degenerates and is replaced by bone.)

The point of interest to explore here is why the same kind of cells that at first form cartilage later in development begin to form bone. A clue in this connection came from the study of the repair of fractures, as follows: When a bone is broken in postnatal life, cells along the sides of the bone proliferate to form a mass called an external callus which bridges the broken ends together. In its formation embryonic history repeats itself, for some of the proliferating cells differentiate into cartilage cells while others become bone cells. The question arises as to why the same kind of cells should differentiate into cartilage in some sites and into bone in other sites. In this connection the author pointed out from his studies some decades ago that whether the proliferating cells differentiated into cartilage or into bone in the repair of fractures seemed to depend on how far they were from blood capillaries *as they differentiated*. When the proliferating cells were far away from capillaries, they differentiated into cartilage cells; if capillaries were close, they differentiated into bone cells. He pointed out also that when bone began to form along the sides of a cartilage model in an embryo, capillaries had appeared in the vicinity. The factor responsible for directing the differentiation of competent cells into either cartilage or bone both in the embryonic development of bones and in the repair of fractures seems most likely to be the concentration of oxygen in the tissue fluid in which the competent cells differentiate, and indeed in 1961 Bassett and Herrmann showed that a strain of cells with which they were working would, in cell cultures, form cartilage if the oxygen tension was low but would form bone if the oxygen tension in the culture was high.

Many Hormones Induce Cell Differentiation. To continue briefly with cell differentiation in bone, it should be mentioned here that the growth of any bone depends on cells called osteoblasts forming bone on an advancing front and cells called osteoclasts resorbing simultaneously pre-existing bone as the new bone is formed on the advancing front. It is a usual but not universal belief that both osteoblasts and osteoclasts arise from a common stem cell but what is well established is that under the influence of large amounts of the hormone of the parathyroid gland vast numbers of cells in growing bones differentiate into osteoclasts so that bone resorption far exceeds bone formation. This matter will receive detailed comment in Chapter 15.

An example of an insect hormone affecting cell differentiation has already been mentioned. An interesting example of a hormone affecting cell differentiation in the human embryo is provided by male sex hormone being produced in male embryos. The human embryo at any early stage develops the forerunners of what could become either male or female reproductive organs. Which set develops depends on whether or not a normal embryo possesses a Y chromosome. If it does, two male sex glands (testes) develop in it instead of two female sex glands (ovaries). In fetal life the male sex glands secrete male sex hormone and this causes the forerunners of the reproductive system to develop into male reproductive organs. In the absence of male hormone reproductive organs of the female type develop (oviducts, uterus and vagina, etc.).

Hormones and Genes. One question that arises is how different hormones can cause different genes to be turned on and off in competent cells. One possible way different genes could be turned on by different environments was described in Chapter 4 in connection with the operon concept. Since it is now well known that many different hormones can profoundly stimulate the function and growth of the particular kind of

specialized cells that are their special targets, it is obvious that they must at least indirectly affect certain genes in their target cells if the target cell increases its secretory function and grows. Information on this matter could be of interest with regard to how hormones might affect the process of differentiation in competent cells.

Cyclic AMP. The first hormone that was successfully extracted from an endocrine gland and shown to exert its effects when it was injected into animals was adrenaline (epinephrine); this was accomplished in 1894. In 1901 a pure crystalline preparation of the hormone was obtained. Epinephrine is produced as will be described in Chapter 25 by the inner parts of the adrenal glands. Curiously enough, it was found that this hormone was not secreted into the bloodstream in sufficient quantities under restful conditions to exert much effect. However, increased and effective amounts of it were found to be secreted into the blood under conditions which profoundly arouse emotions such as fear or rage. The general idea gained ground that this mechanism had survival value, because it helped animals including *Homo sapiens* to either run away faster or fight harder when these emotions were aroused; for epinephrine, under these conditions, exerted numerous physiological effects that would aid an individual to run faster or fight harder. For example, it causes the heart to beat faster and harder, the blood pressure to be increased, more blood to be diverted to muscles and less to the intestines and so on. Among other effects it was also found that it caused glycogen in liver cells to be broken down to glucose which entered the bloodstream; this of course led to muscles having more fuel for either flight or fight. For many decades how it caused glycogen to be quickly broken down to glucose which then entered the blood was not understood. The final solving of this mystery was of such great importance that it led to Sutherland's receiving the Nobel prize for Physiology and Medicine in 1971, for it led to the discovery of what is now known as cyclic AMP, a substance now known to be involved in the effects produced by many hormones on their target cells.

Cyclic AMP is the short term for cyclic 3′5′-adenosine monophosphate. It is a small molecule and is formed from ATP (which was described in connection with mitochondria in Chapter 5) in small quantities by a special enzyme, adenylate cyclase, which is located in the cell membrane. It is now believed that the hormones in general are able to affect the special cells that they stimulate (their target cells) because the latter have special receptors on their cell membranes to which the specific hormone that affects that particular kind of cell becomes attached. When a hormone from the bloodstream finds and becomes attached to its special receptors on a cell membrane, it causes the enzyme adenylate cyclase that is in the cell membrane to be activated which causes increased amounts of cyclic AMP to be formed from ATP. The cyclic AMP diffuses throughout the cell. In the instance of liver cells affected by epinephrine, the increased content of cyclic AMP activates an enzyme which triggers further reactions that result in glycogen being converted to glucose. This is how epinephrine causes more glucose to be released into the blood when an individual experiences a profound emotional reaction such as fear or rage.

There is another interesting assortment of hormones which are secreted by the cells of the anterior pituitary gland (as will be described in detail in Chapter 25) and are called trophic (*trophikos,* nourishing) hormones because they stimulate the growth and function of the cells of various other endocrine glands. For example, the anterior pituitary gland secretes the hormone *thyrotrophin,* and target cells of this hormone are the cells of the thyroid gland, whose number, size and function it controls. To produce this effect thyrotrophin must somehow exert some influence in regulating the activity of the genes of the cells of the thyroid that control the synthesis of the protein of its hormone and the growth of its cells. Thyrotrophin has been shown to bring about an increase in the level of cyclic AMP in thyroid cells, and the question arises as to whether this could bring about the gene activation required.

Cyclic AMP and Gene Regulation. Here again studies in *E. coli* have indicated a way by which genes are affected by cytoplasmic factors in the working cell. It has been shown by most ingenious experiments that cyclic AMP in *E. coli* combines with a particular protein called AMP receptor protein and that the complex so formed becomes bound to DNA at a site that is close to the operator gene and called the promotor, the activation of which is essential if transcription of mRNA is to occur. Transcription, however, does not occur if the operator gene is repressed by repressor protein. Moreover, even if an inducer has combined with the repressor so that it does not block the activity of the operator gene, transcription does not occur in the absence of the complex of cyclic AMP and AMP receptor protein. Accordingly, cyclic AMP is a factor in regulating gene function. The presence or absence of cyclic AMP in the cells that develop in and from the fertilized ovum is therefore another factor that has

to be considered in connection with differentiation (*see* Pastan).

The Control of Cell Multiplication and Its Relation to Differentiation

Different species of mammals grow to different sizes. The particular size range attained by members of different species must of course be determined by the genes in their cells. But the problem we are concerned with here is another that hinges on the regulation of gene activity: it relates to how cell division is regulated in the various tissues and organs of any given mammal so that the cellular content of the various tissues and organs of the adult remain fairly constant in health. A second and related problem is why the partial removal or loss of any tissue or organ, in which cell division can occur, is followed by an increased rate of cell division in that tissue or organ which continues until the size or function of the part is restored. Still another and very important problem is presented by cancer (briefly described in Chapter 2), in which some genetic change seems to take place in a cell or cells so that it or they continue to multiply under circumstances in which the multiplication of normal cells of the same type is controlled. It should be emphasized that the problem in cancer is not a breakdown of an external control mechanism but an alteration of some sort in a cell or cells so that they are no longer normally responsive to the factors that ordinarily control cell populations.

In order to consider the control of cell populations it is important to recall (from Chapter 2) that, so far as their reproductive capacities are concerned, there are three categories of cells in the human body. Those of Category 1 are unable after the first year or so of life to undergo mitosis. Nerve cells are the important representatives of this type. In the second category there are various families of cells, with the members of each ranging from highly specialized functioning cells (which are unable to divide) to relatively undifferentiated but determined cells that are able to divide and, when it is required, differentiate into the highly specialized cells to take the place of those that wear out or are lost from a surface. The blood cell family provides good examples of arrangements of this type. Finally, cells of Category 3 are represented mostly by parenchyma cells of organs, where they exist generally as fully differentiated specialized cells which normally seldom divide but which under certain conditions are able to divide to restore that particular organ to its normal functioning size. The cells of the thyroid gland and the liver are in this category.

CHALONES

To begin discussing the problem of the control of cell multiplication we shall first consider cells of the Category 3 variety and in particular the cells of the liver. If a large portion of the liver of an animal is surgically removed, its contents of epithelial parenchymal cells is restored close to normal in less than a week. Sections of the liver taken 36 hours after the operation will reveal many liver cells in mitosis (Fig. 2-8 was prepared from such a section). Why liver cells should almost immediately begin to divide after a part of the liver is removed has long been an intriguing mystery. It seemed reasonable to assume that some substance must be liberated from the injured organ to stimulate mitosis in the part that remained, and many attempts were made to find such a substance. However, as matters turned out, the situation may be more or less the reverse of what had been previously assumed, for it was discovered that liver cells normally elaborate small quantities of a substance called a *chalone* (which is derived from a Greek word that refers to something that restrains or slows some action). Since they do this continuously, it has been suggested that a certain concentration of liver chalone is maintained in the blood, enough to constantly restrain the cells of the liver from undergoing division. If, however, a large portion of a liver is removed there are not enough liver cells to maintain a normal concentration of liver chalone in the blood and the level of it falls until there is not enough of it to keep the liver cells that remain from dividing. Hence liver cells under these conditions would, according to this concept, divide not because they are particularly stimulated to do so but because they are no longer restrained from dividing (to divide seems to be their natural inclination). According to the chalone concept, when an adequate number of cells have accumulated in the liver because of the active division of liver cells to produce enough liver chalone for it to reach its normal concentration in the blood, further cell division is restrained; so when the liver reaches its normal size again, cell multiplication in it ceases.

Various studies on the control of the cell population of other body parts suggest the possibility of there being a separate chalone that controls cell population in many of them. However, the development of knowledge about chalones is at a stage at which most of the work done to indicate their existence and function has

been done with extracts prepared from body parts supposed to produce them. Since pure preparations of chalones have not been available, the results obtained from using tissue extracts cannot of course be attributed to chalones alone because of other components being present in the extracts. So until it becomes possible to prepare chalones in pure form and test them with a knowledge of their precise chemical nature, some caution must be used in interpreting some of the results obtained. Probably the greatest progress toward obtaining a pure chalone and in assaying its activity has been made (at the time of writing) in connection with the liver chalone by Verly et al.

Such experimental evidence as exists, however, suggests that chalones are tissue or organ specific but are not species specific, which means that they can be prepared from various species and used in others. They do not seem to be long lasting in their effects and hence new chalone must be more or less constantly produced if it is to exert its proper control of specific cell populations. They are effective in restraining cell division in cell cultures and also in tissue slices that are maintained under proper conditions. In connection with the latter, Verly et al. use liver slices for their assay of their material.

The Control of Cell Populations of the Category 2 Type by Chalones. The way the cell population is controlled by chalones in cell families of the Category 2 type, the members of which range from relatively undifferentiated cells (that can divide) to mature differentiated cells (that cannot divide) appears to be different from that observed in cells of the Category 3 type. In cell families of Category 2, chalone seems to be made by the fully differentiated cells of a given family and this inhibits cell division in the less differentiated cells of the same family type that ordinarily divide to maintain the line with some differentiating to take the place of such fully differentiated cells as are worn out or die. For example, experiments indicate that certain white cells of the blood (granular leukocytes, to be described in Chapter 10) produce a chalone that suppresses division in the younger, less differentiated cells that multiply to provide cells to differentiate into mature granular leukocytes. Thus in the cell lines of Category 2, cell populations seem to be controlled by the older members of the cell family who themselves are unable to reproduce.

The Epidermal Chalone. This is the one that was first discovered and which has been studied the most. The epidermis, as will be described in the next chapter, is the epithelial portion of the skin and always at least a few layers of cells in thickness. The cells of the deepest layer (or layers, if it is thick) more or less constantly divide to supply cells that, as they are pushed toward the surface, lose their ability to divide and are finally lost from the surface. Evidence for an epidermal chalone was obtained by Bullough and Lawrence in 1960. Since then many experiments seem to have confirmed their observations; a unique one showed that if the epidermis is removed from one side of the wing of an African fruit bat, the rate of cell division is greatly increased in the epidermis on the other side of the wing. The action of the epidermal chalone, however, is somewhat more complicated than that of others, for it seems to require the help of a hormone (which is probably epinephrine) to form a complex stable enough to inhibit cell division. This may explain why it is difficult to obtain a section of epidermis that demonstrates mitotic figures if the tissue is taken during the day (cell division in the epidermis generally occurs at night—a phenomenon termed diurnal mitotic rhythm). The suggested reason for it is that daytime is associated with activity and stress, which accounts for more epinephrine being secreted than is secreted during the night when sleep is the rule. Hence, during the day there is enough epinephrine in the blood to form a complex with epidermal chalone stable enough to block cell division in the epidermis. Another possibility is that there is a chalone-neutralizing factor which epinephrine blocks during the day so that it is only during the day that chalone can effectively block cell division.

Possible Role in Repair. Why there should be a local proliferation of cells around the site of a wound or injury which in due course restores the continuity of the tissue involved has puzzled investigators for decades. Most investigations have been based on the concept that some substances must be liberated locally from the injured tissue which affect nearby cells so as to stimulate their growth. In view of the effects of chalones demonstrated, for example, in connection with the regeneration of the liver, some attention must now be paid to the possibility that another factor in repair could be that the cells at and near the site of a wound bring about its repair because of their being released from the effect of their specific chalone. It has been shown that sprinkling epidermal chalone on an epidermal injury slows its repair. Cells that are close enough to suffer the direct effects of an injury are believed to lose their chalone. However, since cells far enough away from the site of a wound to not have been physically injured commonly participate in the repair process, it seems possible that they too could find themselves in a relatively chalone-free environment. Two possibilities come to mind. Injured breaking-down

tissue might inhibit or inactivate chalone locally. Secondly, wounds sever smaller blood vessels which then become sealed off, so that for a time there is stagnation of the circulation in and about a wound and less bloodborne chalone could reach the cells that usually does.

The Stage in the Cell Cycle at Which Chalones Would Act. Some confusion has been caused by references which have been made to chalones being mitotic inhibitors. Actually they have no direct effect on the mitotic process. As has been pointed out in Chapter 2, cell division is a longer process than mitosis, for the process of cell division begins with the S phase of the cell cycle. Once DNA duplication is triggered in a cell, the cell (with certain exceptions) seems to be inexorably committed to proceed through the S and G_2 phases of the cell cycle and on through mitosis. What chalones seem to do is to act on cells when they have entered the G_1 stage of the cell cycle so that their stay in this stage of the cycle is perpetuated as long as sufficient chalone is available. It seems therefore that chalones must be essential if the relatively undifferentiated cells of a given cell family are to be enabled to differentiate into mature specialized cells that perform their specific function. It could be argued that if no chalone was present undifferentiated cells would merely continue in cycle just as certain cell types can do in certain types of cell cultures. It seems that the natural tendency of cells is to multiply; hence, for them to differentiate requires that they be prevented from multiplying and for this reason chalones may be involved in the differentiation process.

Verly et al. have suggested a most interesting explanation of how a chalone could prevent a cell from entering the S phase. There is evidence to indicate that a cell enters the S phase because of the action of an initiation protein or initiation proteins triggering DNA duplication in the chromosomes. DNA duplication seems to begin, in bacteria, where a chromosome touches the cell membrane and, in mammalian cells, where chromosomes touch the nuclear envelope. In mammalian cells the initiation proteins seem to act at the nuclear envelope, but it may be that they are formed at the cell membrane, and if chalone is present at the cell membrane in sufficient concentration, it might possibly combine with the initiation protein and thus keep it from being able to initiate DNA replication at the nuclear envelope. In the absence of sufficient chalone the initiation protein would trigger DNA duplication.

Comparison With Hormones. From what is known it is conceivable but not yet proven that most types of specialized cells in the body liberate into the blood-stream a specific chalone that retards the beginning of cell division in the cells of that particular family that can divide. In the instance of cells of the Category 3 type, the chalone liberated by specialized cells into the bloodstream seem to return to the same kind of cells that liberated it, to retard their division. In the instance of cells of the Category 2 type, the chalone liberated by the mature specialized cells of a given cell lineage into the bloodstream would have to act on the less differentiated cells of that family type. That cells of different types should liberate a specific chemical messenger into the bloodstream that controls the rate at which new cells of the same type are formed has led to the suggestion that each cell line makes its own hormone to control its population. However, the word hormone from its derivation (*hormaein,* to set in motion or spur on) refers to a chemical messenger that arouses certain body cells to activity whereas chalones (if they exist and act as indicated) do the opposite. Hence to refer to chalones as hormones can only cause confusion.

References and Other Reading

GENERAL

Ebert, J. D. and Sussex, I. M.: Interacting Systems in Development, ed. 2. New York, Holt, Rinehart and Winston, 1970.

SPECIAL

For references about influences on cell differentiation in Bone and Cartilage see Chapter 15.

Gurndon, J. B.: Transplanted nuclei and cell differentiation. Sci. Am., *219:*24, 1968.

Pastan, I.: Cyclic AMP. Sci. Am., *227:*97, 1972.

Wessells, N. K., and Rutter, W. J.: Phases in cell differentiation. Sci. Am., *220:*36, 1969.

CHALONES

Bullough, W. S., and Rytomaa, T.: Mitotic homeostasis. Nature, *205:*573, 1965.

Maugh, T. H., II: Chalones: Chemical regulation of cell division. Science, *176:*1407, 1972.

Verly, W. G., Deschamps, Y., Pushpathadam, J., and Desrosiers.: The hepatic chalone. I. Assay method for the hormone and purification of the rabbit liver chalone. Canad. J. Biochem., *49:*1376, 1971.

7 *Epithelial Tissue (Epithelium)*

The origin and general nature of epithelial tissue were described in the previous chapter. As was noted, it is helpful to classify epithelium into two divisions, as follows:

Epithelial Tissue $\begin{cases} 1. \text{ Covering and Lining Membranes} \\ 2. \text{ Glands} \end{cases}$

Some Features of Covering and Lining Epithelial Membranes

The Terms Covering and Lining. Great care should be taken in using the terms covering and lining, for, used more or less indiscriminately, they cause a lot of confusion. In general the outer surface of a given structure is said to be covered while the interior surface of a given structure is said to be lined. The skin is covered with epithelium; the great body cavities are lined with mesothelium. However, a piece of intestine is covered (not lined) with mesothelium and lined with epithelium. A tennis ball provides a good example of a given structure used for reference; it is covered with fuzzy felt (so that spin will affect its flight) but it is lined with rubber (so that it will retain air under pressure).

Epithelial Membranes Are Composed of Cells. With a few exceptions such as the surfaces that are exposed within freely moveable joints, all body surfaces, whether they are external or internal, are covered or lined with some type of epithelial membrane. As is shown in a, b and c of Figure 7-1, epithelial membranes consist entirely of cells. The cells are fitted together closely and joined firmly together by one or more of the types of cell junctions described in Chapter 5. The kinds found in different epithelial membranes will be described as they are individually considered. Cell junctions of the desmosome type hold epithelial cells of the skin so tightly together that an epithelial membrane that is detached from the underlying connective tissue—as can happen in a small blister—remains unbroken (unless someone meddles with it).

The Terms Simple, Stratified and Pseudostratified Epithelium. If an epithelial membrane consists of only a single layer of cells it is said to be a *simple epithelium* (Fig. 7-1, a, b and c). If, however, it is two or more layers of cells in thickness, as is shown in e and f of Figure 7-1, it is said to be *stratified epithelium*. If some of the cells of a membrane reach from its bottom to its surface and others extend from the bottom of the membrane only partway to its outer surface, it is said to be *pseudostratified*, an example of which is shown in d, Figure 7-1. The reason for this name is that in a section an observer can see two rows of nuclei, due to the nuclei of the shorter cells forming a row closer to the bottom of the membrane than the row of nuclei that are in the longer cells; this gives the false impression of there being two rows of cells.

Epithelial Membranes Are Avascular. Epithelial membranes contain no capillaries. They receive oxygen and nourishment from capillaries that are close to them in the connective tissue on which the epithelial membrane rests, as illustrated in Figure 5-1 in which arrows indicate the passage of oxygen and nutrients from the capillary, through the intercellular substance of the connective tissue, to the cells of the epithelial membrane. Other arrows indicate the route taken by waste products from the epithelium back to the capillary.

Basement Membranes Between Epithelial Membranes and Connective Tissue. Commonly there is a layer of special nonliving material between an epithelial membrane and the connective tissue on which it lies. This is called a *basement membrane*. The components of a basement membrane are colored by the P.A.-Schiff technic as shown in Figure 7-2. The origin and components of basement membranes will be described in the next chapter, which deals with connective tissue.

Epithelium on Wet and Dry Surfaces. The outer surface of every epithelial membrane within the body must be kept wet if the cells of the membrane are to remain alive. For example, the outer surface of the epithelium in Figure 7-5 is wet with a layer of mucus which is P.A.-Schiff-positive and hence dark in this illustration. The various ways epithelial surfaces are kept wet in various parts of the body will be explained as these different parts are described later. The epithelium of the skin, however, has to exist in a dry world and this requires that the epithelium that covers the

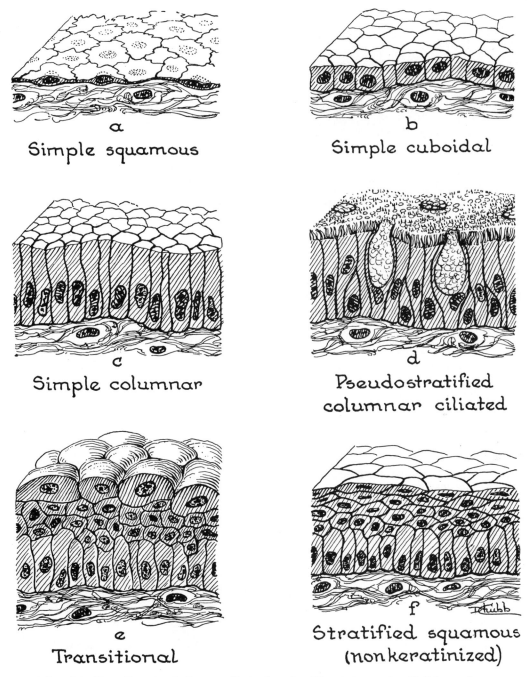

FIG. 7-1. Three-dimensional diagrams illustrating the different types of epithelial membranes found on wet surfaces.

body must possess some special feature which allows its deeper cells to remain healthy even though the outer surface of the membrane is exposed to dry air. This is accomplished as follows: First, all the membranes present on dry surfaces are stratified. Next, as is shown in Figure 7-9, their outermost cells become converted to a nonliving tough waterproof protein material called *keratin* which prevents evaporation from the deeper living cells of the epithelial membrane. If it were not for keratin, the deeper cells of the

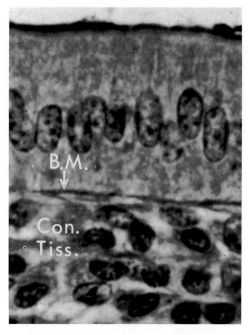

FIG. 7-2. Photomicrograph of section of mouse intestinal epithelium stained by the PA-Schiff method. Mucus on the free surfaces of the cells is stained by this method, as is the basement membrane (B.M.) that is seen between the bases of the epithelial cells and the connective tissue (Con. Tiss.) on which the epithelial membrane rests.

epithelial part of the skin could not be maintained in a fluid environment. The formation of keratin will be described later in this chapter.

CLASSIFICATION OF EPITHELIAL MEMBRANES

Epithelial membranes are classified not only as to whether they are simple, stratified or pseudostratified but also according to the kinds of cells they contain. We shall first describe the classes of epithelium found on wet surfaces.

Simple Squamous Epithelium

An epithelial membrane that is composed of a single layer of very thin cells as is illustrated in three dimensions in Figure 7-1, a, is termed a *simple squamous epithelium* (squamous means scalelike). Simple squamous epithelium generally does not appear to advantage in sections that cut through it at right angles (Fig. 7-3). As can be seen at the top of this figure, the nuclei of the individual cells can be seen, but since the nuclei are thicker than the cytoplasm of the

squamous cells they create bulges along the membrane. In this kind of a preparation (a section of fixed tissue cut at right angles to the membrane) the cytoplasm of simple squamous cells is so thin that in some sections it cannot be seen at all with the LM. Only the somewhat flattened nuclei distributed at fairly regular intervals along the surface may be visible.

Because simple squamous epithelium is so difficult to study in sections, the endothelium that lines blood vessels and the mesothelium that lines the great body cavities (pleural, pericardial and peritoneal) are often studied in mounts that allow the flat surface of the membrane to be examined directly. In this type of preparation it appears like the flat surface seen in Figure 7-1, a, after a suitable stain is applied to it (for example, silver nitrate darkens the borders between adjacent cells). There are more refined methods for making mounts of pieces of blood vessels in order to investigate early changes in arterial disease which sometimes begins at the endothelial lining surface of the vessel.

The medulla of the kidney is a good site for studying simple squamous epithelium in sections but it may be difficult for the inexperienced to find good examples of it (like the one in Figure 7-3) until the kidney is studied as an organ.

Simple Cuboidal Epithelium

The cells of simple cuboidal epithelium are not actually cubes. Like so many other things in the body cuboidal epithelium was given its name because of the way it appeared in a section cut through it at right

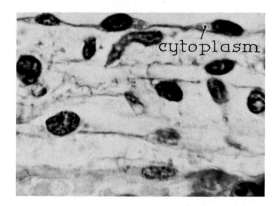

FIG. 7-3. Simple squamous epithelium runs across the top from one side to the other. This is how it appears in sections cut at right angles to its flat surface. Note how the nuclei bulge to form small bumps on its free surface, and that the cytoplasm is very thin.

angles. As is shown in Figure 7-1, b, the cut surfaces of the cells in such a section are indeed roughly squares. But in the surface view provided by Figure 7-1, b, the cells have an irregular hexagonal appearance so they are not true cubes.

Simple cuboidal epithelium is not found in very many sites in the body. The student can probably find an example of it most easily in a section of the ovary of a young adult animal where it forms a covering for that organ.

Simple Columnar Epithelium and the Various Ways Its Structure Is Modified for Special Functions

There are several sub-types of simple columnar epithelium. In all the basic structure is similar in that the cells are taller than they are wide and are joined together side by side by means of cell junctions of the occludens and adherens types as illustrated in Figure 5-57 and described in the accompanying text. As is shown in Figure 7-1, c, the cells of simple columnar epithelium tend to be hexagonal, which permits them to be fitted closely together on all their sides.

Unmodified Simple Columnar Epithelium. Examples of this are not very numerous, being found only in sites where the chief function of the epithelium is to provide protection along some wet surface and not to engage to any great extent in secretory or absorptive activities. In such epithelium the cells all resemble one another, and their cytoplasm is of an even texture and stains somewhat lightly in H and E sections. One place to find epithelium of this type is in some of the ducts of glands (Fig. 7-17, *left*). Here, however, the simple columnar cells may be secretory to some extent, elaborating watery secretions.

Most simple columnar epithelium, however, is modified to perform, in addition to a protective function, either specialized secretory or absorptive functions. We shall now consider some examples.

Secretory Simple Columnar Epithelium. In this type of simple columnar epithelium all the cells are specialized to secrete mucus. Since they cannot individually bulge they all appear alike with an ordinary columnar form. Two sites where this type of epithelium can be found are (1) the surface lining of the stomach and (2) the lining of the cervical canal (Fig. 7-4). Both will be described again when the organs concerned are studied later. In H and E sections the cytoplasm of all the cells in an epithelial membrane of this type have much the same light and somewhat frothy appearance which is caused by the cytoplasm being packed with membrane-surrounded globules of

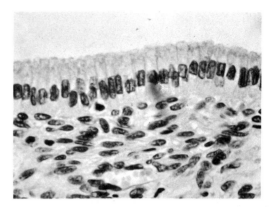

Fig. 7-4. Photomicrograph of columnar secretory epithelium in which cells are all alike. Cervical canal.

mucus destined for secretion from the free end of the cell; since globules of mucus do not stain well with H and E, the cytoplasm superficial to the nucleus in cells of simple columnar epithelium of this type appears pale and vacuolated (Fig. 7-4). With the PA-Schiff technic the cytoplasm stains similarly to that of goblet cells.

Simple Columnar Epithelium That Is Composed of Both Secretory and Absorptive Cells. Epithelium of this type is ideal for a lining for the small intestine, because, if effective absorption is to occur, the membrane can be only one cell thick and, since this membrane is subjected to a good deal of wear and tear, it helps to have its surface coated with mucus, which is a protective slippery fluid. Since absorptive cells (cells specialized for absorption) are interspersed with mucus-secreting goblet cells, there are enough goblet cells to provide a protective coating of mucus over the whole inner surface of the membrane as is shown in the PA-Schiff preparation in Figure 7-5.

Goblet Cells. Goblet cells, with their mucus content stained by the PA-Schiff technic, are shown in Figure 7-5. As already described in Chapter 5 and illustrated in Figures 5-35 and 5-36, where mucus-secreting cells are interspersed with some other kind of cell—in this instance, absorptive cells—a mucus-secreting cell can assume the form of a goblet because the portion of the cell which is packed with membranous vesicles filled with mucus can expand to assume a bowl-like shape by indenting the cytoplasm of the absorptive cells beside it.

The nuclei of goblet cells, as is shown in Figure 7-5, are in the narrow stemlike portions of the cells, close to their bases.

Absorptive Cells, Striated Borders and Microvilli. The absorptive cells between the goblet cells of in-

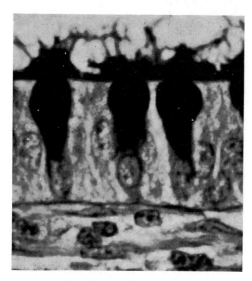

FIG. 7-5. Intestinal epithelium of mouse stained by the PAS technic. Three goblet cells are evident, with their secretion flowing over the free surfaces of adjacent cells. The basement membrane also can be seen.

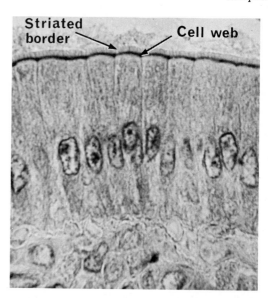

FIG. 7-6. Photomicrograph of absorptive cells of rat intestine stained (see text) to show the terminal webs of the cells. Note how the terminal web seems to dip down at sites where cells are contiguous. The striated border of the epithelial cells can be seen immediately above the terminal web.

testinal epithelium may be seen with the LM to be covered with a thin layer of some material with a refractive index different from that of the underlying cytoplasm (Fig. 7-6). This thin layer was at first believed to be of the nature of a protective cuticle. In good preparations it was possible with the LM to demonstrate fine striations in this layer; these roughly paralleled the long axes of the underlying cells. So this thin layer was termed a *striated border*. When thin sectioning methods improved to the point at which this border could be studied with the EM, it was shown that the appearance of striations was due to the cytoplasm, at the free surface of the cells, being arranged in multitudinous adjacent and very minute fingerlike projections termed microvilli (Figs. 5-8), which were described in Chapter 5 in the section on Filaments in association with Figure 5-56.

Cell Junctions Between the Cells of Epithelial Membranes That Are Both Absorptive and Secretory. These are of four main types—zonulae occludentes, zonulae adherentes, desmosomes and some patches of the gap type, all of which are described in Chapter 5 and illustrated in Figures 5-57, 5-58, 5-59, 5-60 and 5-61. The bases of the cells are attached to the basement membrane by hemidesmosomes (Fig. 5-61, *right*).

Simple Columnar Ciliated Epithelium. Another combination of cells found in a simple columnar epithelial membrane is that of goblet cells intermixed with ciliated cells. The fine structure of the latter was

described in Chapter 5 and illustrated in Figures 5-48 to 5-54 inclusive. The cilia beat in such a way as to move mucus along the membrane as was described in Chapter 5. This type of epithelium is found in some parts of the upper respiratory tract, but it is not as common here as another type which is called pseudostratified columnar ciliated epithelium which will now be described.

Pseudostratified Columnar Ciliated Epithelium With Goblet Cells

As already described, some of the cells in contact with the basement membrane do not reach the surface in pseudostratified epithelium (Fig. 7-1, d), but many do. It gives the appearance of being stratified because sections cut at right angles to its surface show nuclei at two levels. Pseudostratified columnar epithelium with goblet cells forms the lining for most of the upper respiratory tract and it is to be seen to advantage in a section cut from the trachea (Fig. 7-7). As can be seen in this illustration, the cells that reach the surface are either ciliated or goblet cells. The mucus secreted by the latter forms a film on the inner surface of the respiratory passages and this serves as a dust-catcher to prevent dusts being inhaled into the lungs; it also moistens the dry air that is inspired. The cilia

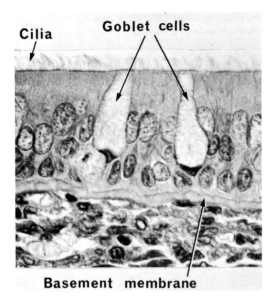

Cilia   **Goblet cells**

Basement membrane

FIG. 7-7. Photomicrograph of H and E section of pseudostratified columnar ciliated epithelium (dog trachea).

serve a very useful function by moving the mucus that contains the dust particles upward to a point at which it can be swallowed or otherwise eliminated from the body. The function of the cells that do not reach the surface is probably that of serving as a type of progenitor cell to produce new cells of the long type that are lost from the membrane.

Stratified Epithelial Membranes

Stratified epithelial membranes—membranes of two or more cells in thickness—can withstand more wear and tear than membranes of the simple type. But because they are stratified, they cannot serve efficiently as absorptive membranes; furthermore, their stratified structure makes them ill adapted to the performance of secretory functions. Hence such secretion as is found on stratified membranes is provided by glands that are situated below the epithelial membrane and open through the membrane by way of ducts. Therefore, stratified membranes serve chiefly to protect, and they differ from one another because they provide different kinds and degrees of protection in different places.

Stratified Squamous Nonkeratinizing Epithelium. This type of membrane (f, in Fig. 7-1) is found on wet surfaces that are subjected to considerable wear and tear, surfaces where absorptive function is not needed. The fluid required to keep such a surface wet is provided not by cells of the membrane but by glands. The inside of the mouth and the esophagus (Fig. 21-22) are both lined with this type of epithe-

lium as are the crypts of the palatine tonsil (Fig. 21-19) where the epithelium is kept wet by saliva and provides protection from coarse foods. Part of the epiglottis is covered with it, and the vagina is also lined with it (Fig. 26-31).

Stratified squamous nonkeratinizing epithelium is not, as its name implies, composed of successive layers of squamous cells. As is shown in Figure 7-1, f, the deepest cells in such a membrane (the basal layer that abuts on the basement membrane) are columnar. Just above this layer the cells are *polyhedral* (many sided), and it is only toward the surface that the cells assume a squamous shape; so only the more superficial cells in stratified squamous nonkeratinizing epithelium are actually squamous.

Stratified Columnar Epithelium. This type of epithelium is found on only a very few wet surfaces in the body where presumably more protection is required than would be afforded by simple columnar epithelium and where some slight absorption of fluid from the surface is required so that stratified squamous nonkeratinizing epithelium could not be used. For example, whereas ducts of moderate size are usually lined with simple columnar epithelium, the larger ducts of glands are commonly lined by stratified columnar epithelium. In a few sites stratified columnar epithelium is ciliated.

Transitional Epithelium. This is somewhat similar to stratified squamous nonkeratinizing epithelium when it is stretched but when it is not stretched the more superficial cells of transitional epithelium become rounded instead of squamous in shape (Fig. 7-1, e).

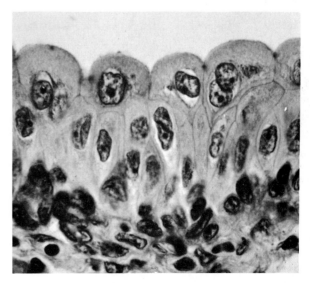

FIG. 7-8. Photomicrograph of H and E section of transitional epithelium from bladder of dog.

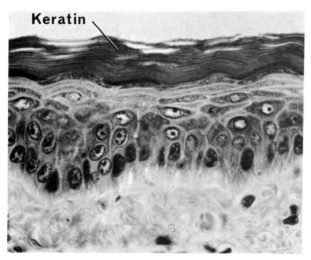

Keratin

FIG. 7-9. Photomicrograph of H and E section of skin of ear of monkey showing stratified squamous keratinizing epithelium.

Such a membrane can be stretched without the superficial cells breaking apart from one another; they merely become drawn out into broader, thinner cells. Hence transitional epithelium is well adapted to lining tubes and hollow structures that are subjected to being expanded from within—such as the urinary bladder, in which it is best studied (Fig. 7-8). What happens at the level of fine structure when these cells are stretched is explained in connection with Figure 24-22.

It was observed some years ago that such mitotic figures as were seen in the surface cells in the transitional epithelium of rodents were very large. Subsequently, Leuchtenberger, Leuchtenberger and Davis found that the nuclei of the surface cells of the transitional epithelium in the urinary bladder of man contained multiple amounts of DNA; in other words, these cells demonstrated polyploidy. Walker has studied the development of this condition in the mouse and has found that about the 16th to the 17th day of embryonic life both binucleate cells and polyploid nuclei become evident in the superficial layers of the epithelium lining of the urinary bladder. Walker suggests that the chromosomes of binucleated cells entering division become grouped together, and consequently each of the two daughter cells that results has double the previous number of chromosomes.

Stratified Squamous Keratinizing Epithelium (*The Usual Covering of Dry Surfaces*)

Stratified squamous keratinizing epithelium resembles stratified squamous nonkeratinizing epithelium except that the more superficial cells of the membrane undergo a metamorphosis into a tough nonliving layer of *keratin* which is tightly attached to the underlying living cells of the epithelial membrane. The epithelial part of the skin (the epidermis) provides a good example of stratified squamous keratinizing epithelium (Fig. 7-9). In skin, keratin serves several purposes. It is relatively waterproof; hence it prevents fluid from evaporating from the living cells that lie beneath it; likewise it keeps the body from imbibing water when one has a bath. Since it is tough and resilient, it protects the underlying living epithelial cells from being injured by the ordinary wear and tear to which skin is exposed. It is relatively impervious to bacteria and hence is a first line of defense against infection. Over the soles of the feet and the palms of the hands the stratified squamous epithelium of the skin becomes thicker, and, in particular, the keratin becomes very thick; this enables it to withstand the great wear to which these particular surfaces are exposed.

The Formation of Keratin in Stratified Squamous Epithelium. Keratin is a tough fibrous protein, highly resistant to chemical change. From what has been said in previous chapters about the syntheses of proteins that are to remain within a cell or are to be exported from it, it might be thought that keratin would be synthesized in cells as keratin either in association with free polyribosomes or even perhaps in association with rough-surfaced endoplasmic reticulum. However, the production of keratin seems to be more complex, for part of it at least does not seem to be synthesized as keratin but to result from the transformation of other cell constituents into keratin, as will now be described briefly. More will be said about the formation of keratin in Chapter 20, which deals with skin, hair and nails.

The deepest cells of a stratified squamous epithelial membrane are generally more or less columnar in shape, and they constitute the *stratum basale* which is often called the germinal layer of the membrane (Figs. 7-9 and 7-10), because mitosis occurs frequently in this layer. The latter phenomenon accounts for cells being pushed from this layer into the next one above.

The cells in the germinal layer (Fig. 7-10) have a good content of free polyribosomes which are probably concerned in the synthesis of the considerable content of fibrillar material (tonofilaments) that forms the cell webs in the cells of this layer and eventually becomes part of the keratin. As the cells pass into the next layer above, the fibrillar material of the cell web shows many condensations, which results in bundles of fibrils becoming large enough to be seen with the LM. These bundles are called tonofibrils. Tonofibrils in this layer

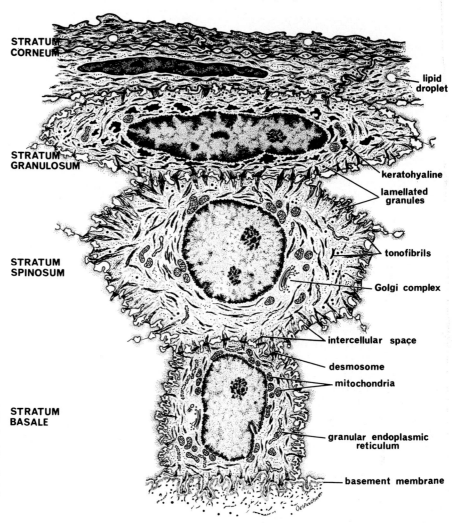

STRATUM
CORNEUM

lipid
droplet

STRATUM
GRANULOSUM

keratohyaline

lamellated
granules

tonofibrils

STRATUM
SPINOSUM

Golgi complex

intercellular space

desmosome

mitochondria

STRATUM
BASALE

granular endoplasmic
reticulum

basement membrane

FIG. 7-10. Drawing based on electron micrographs of stratified squamous keratinizing epithelium. Shown are a representative cell of each layer and the keratin of the stratum corneum. Note in particular desmosomes and tonofibrils. (Preparation courtesy of A. Weinstock)

are commonly attached to desmosomes (Figs. 5-61 and 7-10), and at these sites there tend to be little spikelike projections of the cytoplasm that extend between adjacent cells and can be seen with the LM (Fig. 5-55). This appearance is probably due in part to the fact that the cytoplasm of contiguous cells at these sites cannot shrink away during fixation from the site where it is attached to the next cell by means of a desmosome. These little projections account for the cells of this layer having a prickly appearance, and this layer is called the prickle-cell layer, or stratum spinosum (Fig. 7-10).

As cells from the stratum spinosum are pushed farther toward the surface, they become somewhat flattened so that they are more or less diamond-shaped. They accumulate in their cytoplasm granules of a material that stains blue with hematoxylin. This material

is called keratohyalin (Fig. 7-11). With the EM the granules of keratohyalin, which are about a few microns in diameter, are seen to be mixed intimately with cell fibrillar material (Fig. 7-10). Because of the granules this layer of more or less diamond-shaped cells is called the granular layer of the membrane, or *stratum granulosum* (Fig. 7-11).

As cells are pushed more superficially into the *stratum corneum* (which is the name for the layer of keratin), their nuclei and all cytoplasmic organelles seemingly disappear. Even their keratohyalin granules seemingly disappear. Nevertheless, desmosomes connecting the drawn-out squames which were formerly living cells can still be distinguished in the EM. There are different points of view as to what happens. One view is that the keratohyalin granules turn into a homogeneous matrix in which all the previously formed

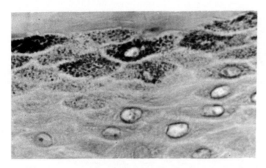

Fig. 7-11. Photomicrograph of H and E section of thick skin of man showing the stratum granulosum at higher magnification so that keratohyalin granules may be discerned.

fibrillar material of the cell web is embedded and which also infiltrates nuclei and other organelles. In this manner, each cell is transformed into one of the squames of keratin that constitute the keratin layer (stratum corneum). Not everything in the cells become keratin, because there is still some other protein and a few other materials that can be recovered from the keratinized layer of the epithelium.

It should perhaps be noted that keratohyalin granules are not essential for keratinization. Some species have keratinized skin in which keratohyalin granules are not visible.

In Chapter 20 two kinds of keratin will be described.

The Maintenance of Cell Populations in Epithelial Membranes

The site of the formation of new cells required for the maintenance or repair of an epithelial membrane varies in different types of membranes as will now be described.

Simple Squamous, Cuboidal and Columnar Epithelia. The degree of specialization attained by cells of these membranes is not very great and does not seem to result in any diminution of their capacity to divide. The cells of membranes of these types are representative of our Category 3 type of cell. Perhaps the best example of cell growth in a simple epithelial membrane is manifested when there is an injury to tissue containing capillaries, because in these instances new tubes of endothelium grow out from pre-existing endothelium to form new capillaries, a phenomenon that can be observed with the LM in living preparations.

Simple Columnar Epithelia Composed of Only Secretory Cells As in the Surface Lining of the Stomach, or of a Combination of Secretory Cells and Absorptive Cells, As in the Small Intestine. In these instances the cells of the membrane have all undergone a degree of specialization which seems to be sufficient to have caused them to have lost their ability to divide; hence, their replacement in maintenance and repair is due to stem cells differentiating to take the place of those specialized cells that die or are lost from the surface. Thus the membranes of these types provide examples of our Category 2 type of cells.

In these membranes the stem cells are all located in some sort of a gland that projects from the membrane into the connective tissue on which the membrane rests. In the instance of the intestine the glands are short little structures called crypts of Lieberkuhn. In other sites the glands are longer structures and the stem cells that account for the replacement cells originate from the ducts (or the counterparts of ducts) of glands whose lumens empty onto the membrane surface. In these various locations the stem cells multiply, and as new surface cells are required some of the stem cells migrate toward the surface and differentiate to take the place of the cells that are lost. Thus the membrane is kept intact. Details will be given in Chapter 21.

Pseudostratified Epithelia. It is believed that the stem cells responsible for dividing and able to differentiate into either goblet or ciliated cells to take the place of those that wear out are the short cells that lie between the bases of the goblet or other taller cells such as ciliated cells. In this instance the stem cell lies at the base of the membrane between the kinds of cells that it replaces.

Stratified Epithelia. In this cells are continuously lost from the free surface of the membrane. In thick stratified membranes the cells of the deepest layers of the membrane are sufficiently unspecialized to be able to divide, which they do and thus they serve as stem cells. The proliferation of these cells in the deepest layers pushes cells toward the free surface of the membrane; as they move toward the surface they become more specialized to provide protection and lose their ability to divide. A most interesting study by Marques-Pereira and Leblond revealed that in the rat esophagus (which is lined by stratified squamous epithelium) the only cells of the membrane that divided were those of the basal layer. They showed, moreover, that when a cell of the basal layer divided there was no set rule as to what happened to the two daughter cells. Both could move toward the surface and differentiate into cells of the outer layers. Or both could remain in the basal layer to provide for more stem cells. Or one could move up and differentiate and leave the other to serve as a stem cell. Their results indicated that it is a matter of chance as to whether a daughter cell of a stem cell differentiates or remains as a stem cell; they all have the capacity to do either.

Migration of Cells of Epithelial Membranes. Although the cells of epithelial membranes are firmly attached to the surfaces they cover, they manifest a surprising degree of plasticity and behave as if they had a mission to immediately cover any site that is normally covered with epithelium should it become uncovered for some reason. Although ultimately the proper covering of any bare spot depends on mitosis occurring in epithelial cells to provide new ones to take the place of those that were lost, the epithelial cells adjacent to a site where membrane has been lost do not wait for mitosis to occur but almost immediately begin to migrate toward and over the bare area. They remain attached to each other but become thinner so that in the form of a wedge they can project over as much of the bare area as possible. This is the first step in epithelial migration; the second is that mitosis occurs behind the advancing edge of the migrating epithelium to provide more cells which push the advancing edge along to help cover the entire surface where membrane is required. Details and illustrations will be available later, when we study the repair of skin wounds and burns.

A Second Source of Stem Cells for Stratified Epithelial Membranes. It might be thought that, if a scrape or a burn removed or destroyed a large patch of epithelium from the skin, for it to be re-covered with epithelium the basal cells of the surrounding epithelium would have to proliferate to supply new cells that would continue to proliferate so as to spread over the denuded area and cover it again with epithelium. If the area to be re-covered is very small, this method of repair suffices. But if this were the only method for repair, it would take a very long time for a sizeable scrape or a burn to be re-covered, and while this was taking place the uncovered connective tissue of the part would form a nasty scar.

Fortunately, there is a second source of stem cells for providing new epithelium for sizeable areas that are denuded. The cells of the numerous hair follicles and sweat glands (both of which structures extend deep into the connective tissue below the epidermis; hence, their deeper parts commonly escape injury) undergo division, and cells from this source multiply and migrate onto the surface and serve as stem cells to form a new stratified epithelium. As a result a localized scrape or burn that destroys the surface epithelium over a given area heals from myriad foci and infinitely

more quickly than it would if epithelium had to grow from the edges of the injury in order for the denuded area to be re-covered (and with the formation of far less scar). Details are given in Chapter 20.

Glands

As already described, there are two main divisions of epithelial tissue:

1. Covering and Lining Membranes, which were discussed in the preceding sections, and
2. Glands.

The way in which glands develop from epithelial membranes was described and illustrated (Fig. 6-2) in the previous chapter.

Classification of Glands. Glands are classified on several different bases. First they are divided into two broad groups, depending on whether they are (1) *exocrine* glands, which type are provided with ducts that convey their secretions to the epithelial surface from which they originated and hence *out of* the substance of the body or (2) *endocrine* glands, which have no ducts and so have to secrete *into* body substance (generally capillaries) and are therefore called ductless glands. Exocrine glands are classified further as follows.

Exocrine Glands

Simple and Compound Glands. Any exocrine gland with an unbranched duct is said to be a *simple gland* (Fig. 7-12, *bottom, left*). The sweat glands of the skin are simple glands (Figs. 20-3 and 20-5). If the duct branches so as to form a duct system, the gland is known as a *compound gland* (Fig. 7-12, *bottom, right*).

As the trunk of a tree branches first into a few fairly large branches and then into smaller and smaller and increasingly numerous ones, eventually to supply twigs for the leaves, so the main duct branches into smaller and smaller and more numerous branches to supply all of the almost innumerable secretory units of large compound glands. Large glands such as the pancreas, parotid and other important compound glands have extensive branching duct systems.

Tubular, Acinous and Alveolar Glands. This classification is chiefly of academic interest. If the clusters of cells that constitute the secretory unit or units of a gland are tubular in shape (Fig. 7-12), the gland is said to be a tubular gland. But if the secretory units are more rounded in shape, the gland is said to be an *acinous* (*acinus*, grape, berry) or an *alveolar* (*alveolus*, a little hollow or a little hollow vessel)

If secretory portion is :

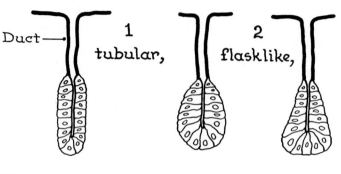

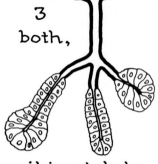

Duct —

1 tubular,

2 flasklike,

3 both,

it is a tubular exocrine gland.

it is an alveolar or acinous gland.

it is a tubulo-alveolar gland.

If duct doesn't branch :

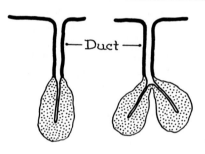

—Duct—

it is a simple gland.

If duct branches :

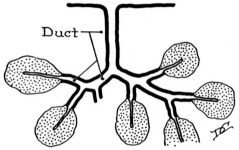

Duct—

it is a compound gland.

Fig. 7-12. Diagram showing the different kinds of secretory units of exocrine glands and the difference between simple and compound glands.

gland. Although in the past some distinction was made between acini and alveoli, it is now usual to call them all alveoli except those in the pancreas which are still, because of custom, termed acini. If glands contain both tubular and alveolar secretory units, or units that have some characteristics of each, they are called tubulo-alveolar glands (Fig. 7-12).

Serous, Mucous or Mixed Glands. It is important to learn how to recognize these different types in sections of them examined with the LM.

This classification is based on the character of the secretion made by the gland. The word serous means *wheylike;* whey is a clear, watery fluid, and glands whose secretion is of this nature (and contains enzyme) are termed *serous glands.* Mucus is a slightly more viscid fluid. The glands that secrete the glycoprotein called mucus are termed *mucous glands.* Any

gland that produces a mixture of serous and mucous fluids is called a *mixed gland.*

These types of glands can be distinguished from each other by examining sections cut from them, because the cells of the secretory units that produce serous (enzyme-containing) secretion have a different appearance from those that make mucous secretions, as follows:

Serous Secretory Units. How to locate a secretory unit with the LM in a section of the pancreas, a gland in which the secretory units are all of the serous type, was described in connection with Figure 5-23.

An H and E section of a serous secretory unit that is cut in cross section and seen with the oil-immersion objective, as already noted in Chapter 5, resembles a pie that has been cut into pieces and not yet served (Figs. 5-10 and 5-23). Each piece of pie corresponds to a single secretory cell; the secretory cells thus have, roughly, a triangular appearance. A lumen is present in the center of an acinus where the apices of the secretory cells meet. However, in fixed tissue preparation this is so small it is difficult to see with the LM; indeed, it is often impossible to see a lumen of a serous acinus with the LM.

The cytoplasm at the base of each cell is basophilic because of its content of free ribosomes and cisternae of rough-surface endoplasmic reticulum. The nucleus of a secretory cell is rounded and close to the base of the cell but not directly against it. In properly fixed preparations the cytoplasm toward the apex of each cell can be seen with the LM to contain eosinophilic granules which are called zymogen granules (Fig. 5-25). As described in Chapter 5, these are membrane-surrounded vesicles which in life contain a semifluid material. On fixation this is coagulated. The fine structure and the mechanism of secretion in these cells are described in detail in Chapter 5.

Mucous Secretory Units. The appearance of a cross section of a mucous secretory unit differs from that of a serous secretory unit. Whereas the nuclei of serous cells are rounded, the nuclei of the cells of mucous secretory units are flattened, almost to the point of appearing disklike; furthermore, they are crowded against the bases of the cells that contain them (Fig. 7-13). The cytoplasm of mucous cells is also different from that of serous cells. There is less basophilia at the bases of the cells than there is in serous cells. That portion of the cytoplasm situated between the nucleus and the apex of a mucous cell, like that of a goblet cell, contains membrane-surrounded droplets of mucus.

The glycoprotein in the membrane-surrounded droplets in the cytoplasm of mucous cells does not stain well with H and E; hence in H and E sections the cytoplasm of mucous cells appears pale and vacuolated. The contents of the droplets, however, stain brilliantly with the PA-Schiff technic, which is so useful for demonstrating glycoproteins.

Radioautographic Studies. Belanger has shown that in suitable preparations radioactive sulfur given by injection into animals enters and can be demonstrated by radioautographs in many tissues. Of interest to us here is that the secretory cells of some mucous glands take up the labeled sulfur in considerable amounts; indeed, in low-power radioautographs, some mucous glands stand out as a sprinkling of black ink drops on a white page. This uptake of radioactive

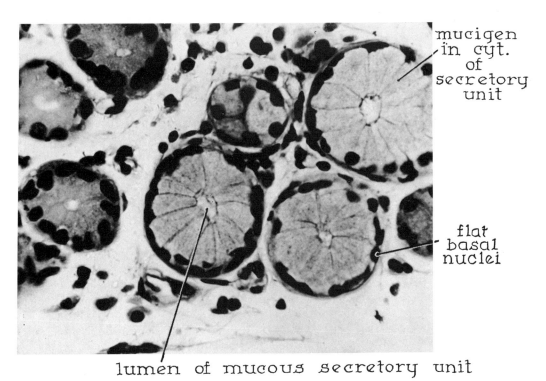

mucigen in cyt. of secretory unit

flat basal nuclei

lumen of mucous secretory unit

Fig. 7-13. High-power photomicrograph of a section of trachea, showing mucous secretory units cut in cross section.

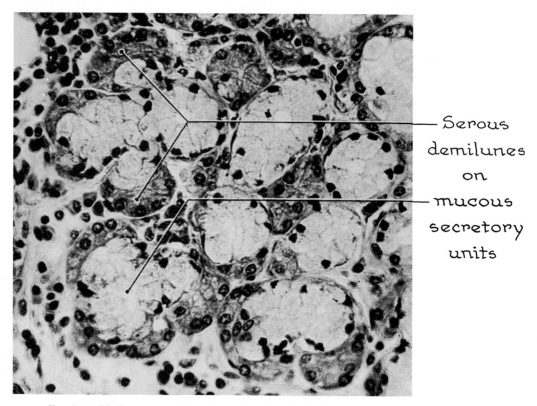

Serous
demilunes
on
mucous
secretory
units

Fɪɢ. 7-14. Medium-power photomicrograph of a mixed gland, showing mucous secretory units with serous demilunes.

sulfur is to be explained by the fact that some glyco-proteins synthesized by mucous cells contain sulfur. Radioautographic studies on the formation of the glycoprotein secretion of goblet cells by the use of glucose labeled with tritium are described in Chapter 5.

Mixed Glands. Some exocrine glands deliver both serous and mucous secretions through their ducts. This is due to these glands possessing both serous and mucous secretory units and/or secretory units that are assembled from both mucous and serous secreting cells (Fig. 7-14). The latter type of secretory unit usually consists of mucous units capped by crescent-shaped aggregations of serous cells called *serous demilunes* (half moons) (Fig. 7-14). Obviously there must be passageways for the secretion of these serous cells to gain entrance between the mucous cells which separate them from the lumen of the mucous unit. These passageways are probably in the nature of tiny intercellular canals situated between adjacent cells of the mucous secretory unit and between the walls of the serous and mucous cells. They are not usually seen in the ordinary preparation.

Myoepithelial Basket Cells. Secretory units of either the mucous or the serous type can be shown by special technics to be cradled in a loose basket made of the cytoplasmic processes of special cells that lie between the bases of the secretory cells and the basement membrane. These cells have a central body and many long cytoplasmic processes that encircle and so grasp the secretory unit (Fig. 7-15). Although these cells are of epithelial origin, it seems very probable that their cytoplasm is contractile, not only because of their shape and position, but also because myofibrils have been seen in them with the EM. Therefore it is assumed that these cells function in some way to encourage the expression of secretion from secretory units into ducts. These cells can be demonstrated to advantage by the histochemical method employed for the demonstration of alkaline phosphatase (Fig. 7-15).

Capsule, Septa, Lobes and Lobules of Glands. The secretory units and the ducts of glands are epithelial in nature and constitute the parenchyma of the gland. The parenchyma, being soft, must be supported by a connective tissue stroma, which is also required to bring capillaries into close contact with the secretory units and ducts to provide their cells with oxygen and nutrients.

Support for a gland is provided by (1) a capsule of connective tissue which surrounds the gland as a whole, and (2) partitions of connective tissue that extend into the gland from the capsule and divide the substances of the gland into areas that are thus "fenced off" in 3 dimensions by connective tissue. The capsule and the partitions both contain enough intercellular substance to make them strong. In some glands large areas so fenced off, particularly if cleavage has occurred in the partition so that the fenced-off areas are somewhat separated from one another, are termed *lobes;* if the fenced-off areas are not very large and are close to one another, they are called *lobules* (little lobes).

A connective tissue partition of the sort described above is termed a *septum*. Hence connective tissue partitions between lobes are termed *interlobar septa,* and those between lobules, *interlobular septa* (Fig. 7-16).

Interlobular and Intralobular Ducts. The septa in some glands converge toward the point at which the main duct leaves the gland. Hence, septa provide an excellent means whereby the main branches of the duct may be conveyed and supported as they pass from the gland's interior to its exterior. The larger branches of the duct system conveyed in interlobular septa are termed *interlobular ducts;* they are easily recognized because they are large, have a thick epithelial lining and a large lumen and are surrounded by the connective tissue of the partition that conveys them (Fig. 7-16). Branches of the duct system that are smaller and lie *within* lobules are termed intralobular ducts; they drain into the interlobular ducts of the septa. Intralobular ducts (Fig. 7-17) are smaller than interlobular ducts (Fig. 7-16). Furthermore, they are not surrounded by as much connective tissue as are the interlobular ducts because they do not run in partitions (Fig. 7-17). However, they may be surrounded by a certain amount of connective tissue which connects with that of the partition that the intralobular duct enters; this provides some support for ducts within the substance of lobules.

Blood Vessels in the Stroma. The larger blood vessels that supply a gland usually enter and leave it by way of the connective tissue septa where they can easily be distinguished from ducts because they are lined by squamous cells whereas the ducts are lined by columnar epithelial cells. The blood vessels within lobules give rise to capillary networks which lie in the delicate connective tissue in which the epithelial secretory units are embedded. These capillary nets provide

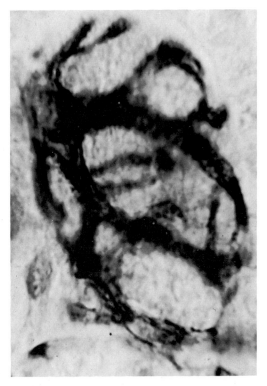

FIG. 7-15. Photomicrograph (× 2,250) of myo-epithelial (basket) cell in submaxillary gland of rat. The material was fixed in acetone and stained by the Gomori method for alkaline phosphatase. The cytoplasmic arms of the cell appear black in the illustration. (Leeson, C. R.: Nature, *178:*858)

the secretory cells with oxygen and nutrients. In fixed tissue they are often collapsed and so difficult to see.

MEROCRINE, APOCRINE AND HOLOCRINE GLANDS

This is a classification based on the manner by which glands produce their secretion.

Merocrine Glands. These have secretory cells of the type the fine structure of which we have already discussed in Chapter 5—for example, the acinar cells of the pancreas, and goblet cells. In secretory cells of this type the secretion is a product of the cell and is delivered through the cell membrane in membranous vesicles in such a way as to keep the cell membrane intact (Fig. 5-25), so that there is no loss of cytoplasm in the secretory process.

Apocrine Glands. When only the LM was available it was thought that whereas the main part of the secretion of the cells of some glands was a cell product, its delivery into the lumen of a secretory unit required

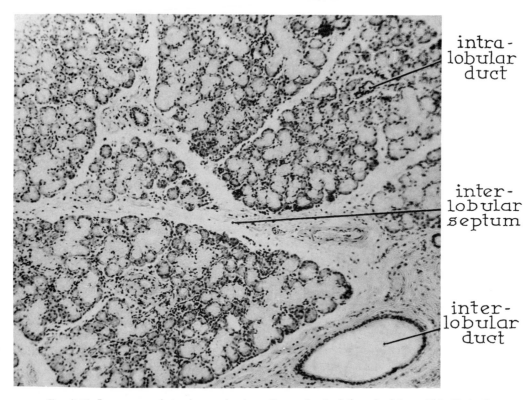

FIG. 7-16. Low-power photomicrograph of a salivary gland of the mixed type. This illustration shows interlobular septa, interlobular and intralobular ducts and secretory units.

intra-
lobular
duct

inter-
lobular
septum

inter-
lobular
duct

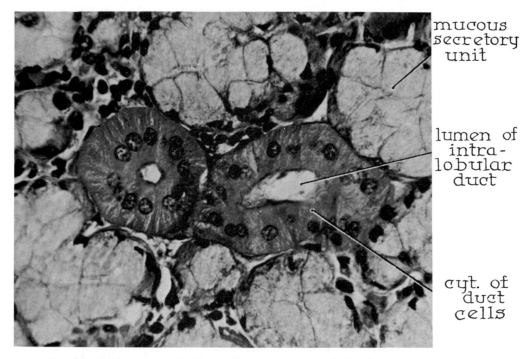

FIG. 7-17. High-power photomicrograph of a mucous gland, showing two ducts cut more or less in cross section.

mucous
secretory
unit

lumen of
intra-
lobular
duct

cyt. of
duct
cells

that some of the superficial cytoplasm of the secretory cell be lost in the process so that it became part of the secretion. However, the EM has shown that the concept of cells losing some of their cytoplasm in the secretory process is not nearly as likely as was believed from LM studies and indeed it is probable that most glands that have in the past been termed apocrine are really merocrine glands.

Holocrine Glands. Holocrine (*holos,* all) is fortunately a very specific term. It means that in order for a holocrine gland to secrete, whole cells must become detached and die and become the secretion of the gland. This of course is a very drastic process and holocrine glands are far from common. The sebaceous glands of the skin are the only ones we shall mention. A sebaceous gland is a little sac (Fig. 7-18) with a lining of epithelial cells that multiply; by this process more and more cells are forced into the interior of the sac while at the same time their cytoplasm becomes filled with a pale fatty material (Fig. 7-18) termed *sebum* which the cells manufacture as they move from the wall toward the interior of the saclike gland. Here they die and break down (Fig. 7-18) to constitute the secretion of the gland which is squeezed out of the body via hair follicles (Fig. 20-15) to lubricate the skin. Details are given in Chapter 20.

THE CONTROL OF THE SECRETORY ACTIVITY OF EXOCRINE GLANDS

There are two kinds of control mechanisms; one is mediated by the nervous system and the other by hormones. Some exocrine glands are under the control primarily of the first and the others of the second.

The secretory activity of glands, unlike the activity of one's muscles, is not under voluntary nervous control. People by taking thought can neither prevent themselves from sweating nor prevent their mouths from becoming dry if they become nervous while making a speech. The nervous control of the secretory activity of exocrine glands is mediated by what is termed the involuntary division of the nervous system, which normally runs automatically, except that its functioning is affected by emotional states—which explains why the functioning of certain glands can be affected enough by frustrations to cause symptoms. To avoid further repetition, discussion of the nervous control of the secretory activity of exocrine glands will be post-

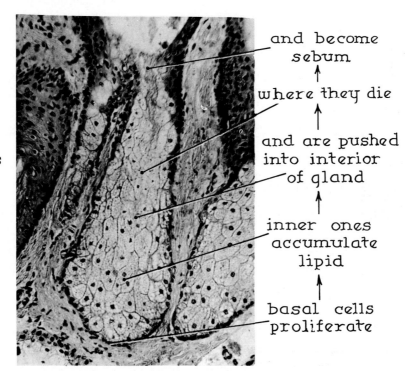

sebaceous gland (holocrine type)

and become sebum
↑
where they die
↑
and are pushed into interior of gland
↑
inner ones accumulate lipid
↑
basal cells proliferate

FIG. 7-18. A medium-power photomicrograph of a sebaceous gland of the skin. These glands generally open into hair follicles, and they make the fatty secretion, sebum. For details of structure see Chapter 20.

poned until we can consider the Nervous System in sufficient detail in Chapter 17.

The hormone control of the secretory activity of exocrine glands is best observed in connection with the gastrointestinal tract where the presence of certain foods in the stomach cause a hormone to be secreted into the bloodstream which causes certain glands that make digestive juices farther down the tract to secrete so that when the contents of the intestinal tract arrive at this point in the tract they will be further digested. Further comment on this matter will be given when we deal with the Digestive System in Chapter 21.

Endocrine Glands

The development of endocrine glands was described in the previous chapter and illustrated in Figure 6-2. Their structure is considerably simpler than that of exocrine glands because they possess no ducts. Since their secretory cells discharge their secretions into capillaries, the secretory cells must be arranged in such a fashion that all abut on capillaries. This is accomplished by the secretory cells being disposed in either straight or irregular cords separated from one another by capillaries, or in little clumps surrounded by capillaries (Fig. 6-2, *bottom right*).

Intracellular Storage. All endocrine glands store their secretion to some extent. This is accomplished in most of them by intracellular storage. In the cells of many of the endocrine glands it is possible to demonstrate secretion granules in specially stained sections examined with the LM. The secretion granules are stored in the cytoplasm temporarily before they are secreted. For example, the beta cells of the islets of Langerhans of the pancreas—the cells that produce the hormone insulin, which regulates the level of the sugar in the blood—store enough of their secretion in their cytoplasm to kill a person if it were all released into the blood at a given time; it would have this effect because it would cause the level of sugar in the blood to fall to a level incompatible with life.

Extracellular Storage. Another way secretion or its precursor can be stored is provided by the thyroid gland. In it the cells of what would otherwise be a clump, secrete inwardly to form a pool of secretion or its precursor in the central part of the clump, where the secretion or its precursor is stored extracellularly in what is termed a *follicle* (a small bag), as is shown in Figure 7-19, *right*.

Capsules, Trabeculae and Blood Supply. Endocrine glands are enclosed by capsules of connective tissue, and usually some projections from these extend into the substance of the gland as trabeculae (little beams) to provide it with internal support and to carry blood vessels into it. The trabeculae account for the

ENDOCRINE GLANDS

How a clump of cells can become a follicle

Capillaries

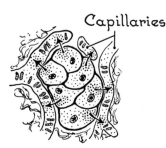
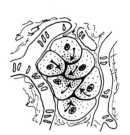
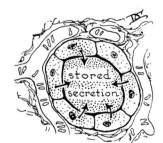

Endocrine cells commonly secrete into capillaries,

but, to store secretion, cells may secrete in opposite direction.

Then they expand the clump into a follicle.

FIG. 7-19. Diagram showing how different types of endocrine glands store secretion and how a clump of cells can become a follicle.

lobulated appearance that sections of some endocrine glands present under the microscope. Capillaries are abundant in the delicate connective tissue that lies between cords or clumps of secretory cells (Fig. 7-19).

Functions of Endocrine Glands. Although most endocrine glands make hormones, a gland can properly be termed endocrine even if it does not make a hormone provided that it secretes a useful product into the substance of the body. The liver, for example, secretes sugar into the bloodstream and for this reason it can be included in a list of endocrine glands.

Glands That Are Both Exocrine and Endocrine

The liver, as just mentioned, secretes a useful substance into the bloodstream; in addition it possesses a duct system into which its cells secrete bile. So it is both an endocrine and an exocrine gland. The pancreas provides even a better example. It arises from an epithelial ingrowth that comes from the epithelial lining of the intestine. This epithelial ingrowth branches and branches to become a duct system, but it also gives rise to two kinds of secretory units: serous ones, in which the lumina of the secretory portions remain connected with the end branches of the duct system, and little groups of cells, called islets of Langerhans, that do not develop a lumen but become arranged into irregular cords and clumps richly provided with capillaries. These islands of cells, which arise from the same source as the developing duct system, secrete their hormones directly into the many capillaries with which they are provided. They thus constitute the endocrine element of the pancreas.

The Control of the Secretory Activity of Endocrine Glands

When we study the endocrine system in detail in Chapter 25 and discuss each gland and the hormone or hormones it makes in some detail, it will be possible to discuss how the secretion of hormones is normally controlled within narrow limits. For those who are curious about this matter at this time, however, we can say that one very important factor in regulating the secretion of most hormones is termed *feedback inhibition;* this will now be described briefly.

Feedback Inhibition. The term *feedback* originated to designate an arrangement whereby some of the output of a circuit—for example, in a radio receiver—is fed back into the input of the circuit. When the term *inhibition* was combined with *feedback,* a term was evolved that seemed useful to describe many of the regulatory mechanisms operating in the body, in which

the final product of some reaction is fed back, not into the input but, instead, to depress the output of the reaction. (This kind of reaction has already been mentioned in connection with the turning off of genes, in Chapter 4.) In other words, feedback inhibition mechanisms can operate so that when the product from some reaction begins to increase over normal levels, the increased product automatically inhibits the reaction that produces the product. Then, as the product continues to be utilized, the amount of it will begin to fall below normal levels, at which point there is no longer enough product to inhibit the reaction, which then automatically increases the production of the product. Such mechanisms can be very sensitive and regulate within narrow limits the concentration in the bloodstream of various products, including hormones and the products whose levels hormones control. The concept of feedback inhibition helps a good deal in understanding the control of the secretion of most endocrine glands (and a lot of other regulatory mechanisms in the body). But the matter is complicated with regard to endocrine glands, because in some instances, as will be described in Chapter 25, two or more endocrine glands and their hormones are sometimes involved in a chainlike way in the feedback mechanism that controls the secretion of some one hormone. We shall here describe a relatively simple example of a control mechanism involving negative feedback.

A very direct type operates in connection with the parathyroid gland, the secretion of whose hormone controls the level of calcium in the bloodstream. If the concentration of calcium in blood falls below a certain level, the cells of the parathyroid gland are released from inhibition control and begin to secrete hormone more rapidly; this hormone, probably by acting on cells associated with bone so as to make them release some calcium from bone into the blood, causes the blood calcium level to increase. When the amount of calcium in the blood reaches a normal level, it inhibits the secretion of extra hormone by the gland. In other words, a product of the effect of the hormone (increased calcium in the blood) feeds back, as it were, to inhibit the production of undue amounts of a hormone which, if secreted, would increase the level of the blood calcium to levels not compatible with health.

A discussion of the more complicated negative feedback control mechanisms in relation to hormones is given in Chapter 25.

References and Other Reading for Chapter 7

Since the general purpose of this chapter was to enumerate and describe the various arrangements in which epithelial cells are disposed in various types of covering or lining membranes and in various types and parts of glands, the information presented has been of such a general nature that it scarcely justifies listing references and other reading. Furthermore, to do so would entail needless repetition, because as we study the various systems of the body we shall encounter all of these types of epithelial arrangements in their relation to their functions in different systems. For example, pseudostratified columnar ciliated epithelium will be dealt with again in connection with the respiratory system, simple columnar cells of the absorptive type and goblet cells will be dealt with in connection with the small intestine, transitional epithelium in connection with the urinary system and stratified squamous keratinizing epithelium in connection with skin (Integumentary System). References and Other Reading will be given at the ends of these various chapters.

It should be pointed out, moreover, that the fine structure of various types of epithelial cells has already been described in connection with cytoplasmic organelles in Chapter 5. For example, striated borders and cilia are both described in this chapter and the account of cell junctions between contiguous cells given in Chapter 5 applies to epithelial cells. The secretory process in the cells of exocrine glands is also described. References and Other Reading on all of these and other features of epithelial cells will be found at the end of Chapter 5.

References regarding the maintenance of epithelial cell populations were given at the end of Chapter 2. References on the repair of epithelial membranes will be given at the end of the chapter on the Integumentary System.

8   Connective Tissue

As was described in Chapter 6, connective tissue was given its name because it connects, and thus holds, the other tissues together. The other tissues are composed almost entirely of cells which, of course, are soft; connective tissue is necessary to hold these tissues in place and give the body form, which it can do because it consists not only of cells but also of nonliving intercellular substances some of which are very strong. The intercellular substances are made by certain of the cells of connective tissue.

Although it is customary to speak of connective tissue as being one of the four basic tissues it should be said immediately that it contains many subtypes that differ from each other in one way or another and it could be argued that they should not all be classed under the one heading of connective tissue. Certainly some of them are not very strong, because they contain very little intercellular substance and consist almost entirely of cells that are not even attached to one another. Nevertheless, the subtypes of connective tissue, even though they may seem to differ, are all related as will become apparent as we discuss them in turn.

Since the subtypes of connective tissue represent a somewhat heterogenous collection of tissues, but with a common thread running through them, it is difficult to determine the best order to describe them. There are advantages and disadvantages associated with almost any order in which they are considered. However, since connective tissue is unique among the four tissues because it consists of intercellular substances as well as cells, we should begin with some kind of connective tissue that will allow us to introduce the study of intercellular substances and to show in particular that in addition to providing strength intercellular substances serve another extremely important function in the body: they provide the means whereby nutrients are transported from the capillaries that lie in intercellular substances to the cells of other tissues that are connected to the capillaries by the intercellular substances of connective tissue. Probably the most representative subtype of connective tissue, so far as illustrating the various kinds and functions of intercellular substances

and the various kinds of cells that exist in connective tissue is concerned, is the subtype called *loose connective tissue*. So we shall begin with it and then take up the others in the following order:

Loose Connective Tissue
- Its Intercellular Substances (This Chapter)
- Its Cells (Chapter 9)

The Hemopoietic Types of Connective Tissue
- Blood Cells (Leukocytes, Chapter 10)
- Blood Cells (Erythrocytes, Chapter 11)
- Myeloid Tissue (Chapter 12)
- Lymphatic Tissue—Thymus, Lymph Nodules and Nodes and Spleen (Chapter 13)

The Strong Supporting Types of Connective Tissue
- Dense Regularly and Irregularly Arranged Connective Tissue and Cartilage (Chapter 14)
- Bone (Chapter 15)
- Joints (Chapter 16)

Loose Connective Tissue

Distribution. Loose connective tissue is called loose because it is soft, pliable and somewhat elastic; these are qualities imparted to it by its intercellular substances. Loose connective tissue with its capillaries is distributed widely throughout the body, mostly in layers to provide the bedding on which the cells of epithelial membranes rest (as, for example, in Figure 8-2) and in which glands lie. It also provides intimate support and nutrients for the cells of much muscle tissue. It is also found in and around peripheral nerves. Loose connective tissue is not strong enough to withstand much strain and so it is often supported by, and continuous with, denser kinds of connective tissue with which it merges. One kind of its cells can synthesize and store fat (as will be described in the next chapter) and in sites where loose connective tissue penetrates into crevices or fills up spaces between other structures, part of its bulk may be due to the presence of globules of fat contained in these cells. In most sites, however, it is disposed as a thin film between other structures. It is loose connective tissue that is so often torn apart as layers and structures are separated from one another in the dissecting room. It is not easy to study in *sections* because it is so commonly disposed in the form of thin films which, in sections, appear as relatively thin lines. So if there is enough time in a laboratory course, a better perspective of this tissue can be obtained by studying it in little pieces of fresh tissue that are spread and mounted in saline as will be described shortly.

Development. Loose connective tissue originates from a primitive kind of connective tissue that develops in the embryo and was named *mesenchyme* (*mesos,* middle, *enchyma,* infusion) because it was believed that it all developed from the mesoderm. Most of it does but some, particularly in the head region, develops from ectoderm. Mesenchyme (Fig. 8-1) consists chiefly of a jellylike amorphous type of intercellular substance which is made by the mesenchymal cells that are distributed throughout it (Fig. 8-1). However, as the embryo continues to develop, the mesenchymal cells in sites where loose connective tissue will appear differentiate into different cell types,

forming most of the kinds illustrated in Figure 9-1. Certain of these cells, called fibroblasts, produce the intercellular substances that are indicated in this diagram (Fig. 9-1), namely collagenic fibers and elastic fibers, as well as amorphous intercellular substance, the site of which is labeled in this figure, although it is not seen in ordinary sections (its existence is demonstrated in other ways).

The Two Main Components of Intercellular Substance. There are two main components of the intercellular substances of connective tissue and both are represented in the loose variety. They are (1) fibers and (2) an amorphous material. The fibers are of three types: (1) collagenic, which are composed of the protein collagen and are strong; (2) elastic, which are physically elastic and made of the tough protein elastin, and (3) reticular, which are very fine fibers which contain a form of collagen and also some carbohydrate-containing material, and are called reticular fibers because they are generally arranged in networks (*rete,* a net).

The second main type of intercellular substance does not present any particular structural form as seen with the LM so it was termed amorphous (without form). This component, like many colloids, exists either as a gel or as a sol, both of which were described

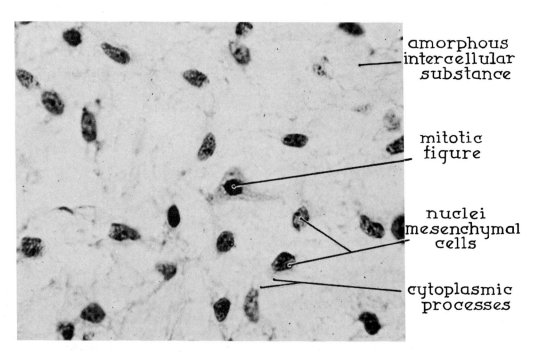

amorphous
intercellular
substance

mitotic
figure

nuclei
mesenchymal
cells

cytoplasmic
processes

Fig. 8-1. High-power photomicrograph of a section cut through developing connective tissue (mesenchyme) of an embryo. This tissue is characteristically soft because the cells are separated by a jellylike, amorphous type of intercellular substance.

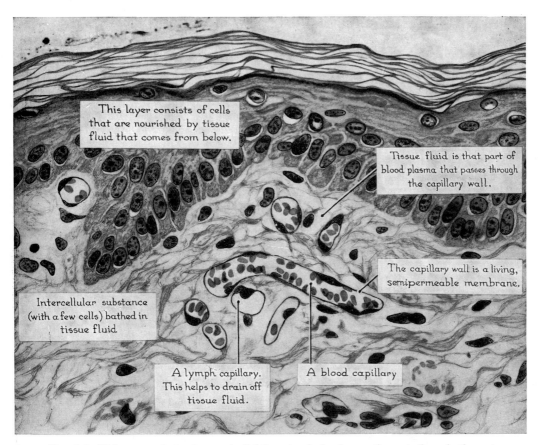

This layer consists of cells that are nourished by tissue fluid that comes from below.

Tissue fluid is that part of blood plasma that passes through the capillary wall.

Intercellular substance (with a few cells) bathed in tissue fluid

The capillary wall is a living, semipermeable membrane.

A lymph capillary. This helps to drain off tissue fluid.

A blood capillary

Fɪɢ. 8-2. High-power photomicrograph, lightly retouched, of a section cut through the outer part of the skin of a pig. This illustration shows the cellular epidermis above and capillaries surrounded by intercellular substance below. It shows how tissue fluid must migrate from capillaries to nourish adjacent cells. Wavy collagenic fibers of various diameters, but generally slightly narrower or wider than the red blood cells in the capillaries, pass in various directions through the intercellular substance. The relatively clear areas between collagenic fibers represent sites occupied by amorphous ground substance which is mostly hyaluronic acid.

in Chapter 1. In other words, amorphous intercellular substances vary from being very firm jellies to fluids of varying viscosity. In some types of connective tissue, for example in cartilage, the amorphous intercellular substance is a firm gel. In loose connective tissue the amorphous component of intercellular substance is a semifluid jellylike material as will be described in more detail presently.

The Functions of the Two Main Types of Intercellular Substance. The collagenic fibers provide strength and elastic fibers, elasticity, as well as strength. Reticular fibers often form lattice-like networks which provide attachments for cells much in the same way that lattice fences in gardens provide attachments for plants such as climbing roses. The amorphous intercellular substance of loose connective tissue

does not provide any strength to the tissue but it does provide substance because it permeates between all the cells and fibers that are in the tissue. The amorphous component, however, serves another very important function which is described in the following section.

The Role of Amorphous Intercellular Substance in the Transport of Nutrients. The blood capillaries that bring oxygen and nutrients to the cells of all parts of the body are confined to loose connective tissue as was shown in Figure 5-1. They are shown also in Figure 8-2 where the epithelium of the skin (which is above) is seen to be some little distance away from the capillaries that underlie it in the loose connective tissue. Accordingly nutrients and oxygen, to supply the epithelial cells of the skin, would have to diffuse from the capillary through the intercellular substance of loose connective tissue to reach the epithelial cells. The substance through which they diffuse is chiefly the amorphous component of the intercellular substance of loose connective tissue, and the ability of the amorphous material to serve as an excellent medium for diffusion is due to its very considerable content of water (which is termed tissue fluid) which is held in position by its macromolecules. When we later study cartilage we shall see that, although its amorphous intercellular substance is a firm gel, the bound water of its gelled amorphous component permits such efficient diffusion of nutrients through it that cartilage cells buried in this intercellular substance are kept alive over long distances. We shall give details later but the point to be made here is that the water-containing amorphous intercellular substances serve the very important role of permitting diffusion mechanisms to act between capillaries and cells that are some distance off from capillaries.

The Study of Loose Connective Tissue in Spreads

As already mentioned, loose connective tissue is commonly disposed in relatively thin layers, and it is difficult to study its cells and intercellular substances in sections because the thin layers in which it exists are so often cut in cross or oblique section that there is little expanse of it to study. If there is time in a histology course it is therefore usual to obtain some fresh loose connective tissue from a freshly killed labo-

ratory animal and make some spreads from it. Tissue for making spreads is easily obtained by reflecting the skin and the subcutaneous tissue from the muscles of the thigh of the animal and then cutting tiny pieces of the loose connective tissue that is torn apart along the plane of cleavage. These are mounted on a slide in a little saline and covered with a coverslip.

Unstained spreads reveal both *collagenic* and *elastic* fibers. The amorphous type of intercellular substance is not visible in a fresh unstained preparation. To see the fibers it helps to cut down the diaphragm of a condenser. Any clear spherical bodies seen are either fat cells or air bubbles; the latter can be avoided by making the preparation with care.

Collagenic Fibers. Collagenic fibers appear as wavy structures that weave their way about in the preparation as is shown in Figure 8-3. The refractive index of these fibers is so similar to that of the fluid in which they are immersed that they do not, with the ordinary LM, stand out in very great contrast to their environment. They consist of the fibrous protein, collagen. Collagen (*kolla*, glue) was given its name because it is used to produce glue. It is also used to make gelatin.

Elastic Fibers. Thinner darker fibers that are of a more constant diameter than collagenic fibers, and sometimes branch, can be seen much less frequently than collagenic fibers in a preparation of this type; these are elastic fibers (Fig. 8-3). They consist of the protein elastin which is not only an elastic material but extraordinarily tough and long-lasting.

Some Features of Fibers

The Difference Between Fibers and Fibrils. If a fresh preparation of collagenic fibers is suitably treated and examined preferably with a phase microscope, the individual fibrils that run parallel to make collagenic fibers come apart sufficiently to be seen under high power (Fig. 8-4). The fibrils are about 0.3 to 0.5 micron in diameter. Collagenic *fibers* vary in diameter, since their diameter depends on the number of fibrils within the fiber. In different connective tissues, fibers range from being only a few fibrils thick to a dozen or more microns in diameter. Elastic fibers do not break up into fibrils.

Flexibility of Loose Connective Tissue. Since collagenic fibers have great tensile strength, it might be thought that loose connective tissue would not be as flexible as it is. The reason for its flexibility is that such collagenic fibers as it contains are generally disposed in various directions in a loose irregular weave; hence loose connective tissue can be stretched slightly without having to stretch individual fibers longitudi-

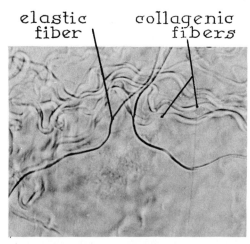

FIG. 8-3. Collagenic and elastic fibers as seen in a fresh, unstained, teased preparation of loose connective tissue with the light cut down. The elastic fibers are more refractile than the collagenic.

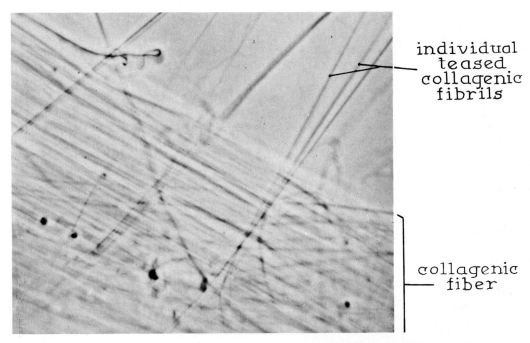

individual
teased
collagenic
fibrils

collagenic
fiber

FIG. 8-4. Oil-immersion photomicrograph, taken with the phase microscope, of collagenic fibers which had been treated with a mild alkali and then teased apart. Individual collagenic fibrils may be seen (*upper right*), and in the lower part of the photograph a collagenic fiber, having a longitudinally striated appearance due to its fibrils, is present.

nally. The elastic fibers in loose connective tissue help to restore it to its usual state when a stretching force is removed from the tissue, for unlike collagenic fibers, straight elastic fibers can be stretched longitudinally, after which they will snap back like rubber bands to their original lengths.

Color of Fresh Fibers. Fresh collagenic fibers are white and so are termed *white fibers*. Fresh elastic fibers are slightly yellow and hence are termed *yellow fibers*. Since collagen is such a tough protein, a considerable content of it in meat makes meat tough. If collagen is boiled in water, it becomes hydrated and this makes it into gelatin, which is soft; this is the reason why tough (collagen-rich) meats are cooked in a stew for a long time. Collagen can be made into leather; this is done by digesting off the epithelium from the hides of animals and then treating the dense connective tissue of the hide (the part remaining) with tanning agents which make the collagen even more resistant to chemical change than before. Before World War Two, burns were often treated by painting them with tannic acid which acted to more or less tan the collagen of the affected skin and this made a sort of impervious dressing. However, this treatment was abandoned when it became apparent that patients

treated this way sometimes absorbed enough tannic acid from the painted area to seriously damage their livers. Histological studies also showed that the tannic acid penetrated the collagen of the skin so deeply that it added to the damage of the skin that was caused by the burn.

Fine Structure. The synthesis of collagen and the fine structure of collagenic fibers are described in detail in the next chapter in connection with the fine structure of fibroblasts. The synthesis and fine structure of elastin are described in Chapter 19 in connection with arteries.

THE AMORPHOUS COMPONENT OF THE
INTERCELLUAR SUBSTANCE OF LOOSE
CONNECTIVE TISSUE

Development of Knowledge. An appreciation of the existence of the amorphous component (also called ground substance) in which the fibers and cells of loose connective tissue are embedded was relatively late in developing, probably because this component is not demonstrable in ordinary sections. Important support for its existence was provided by Sylvia Bensley in 1934 who showed by ingenious experiments performed on living tissue that there was indeed some-

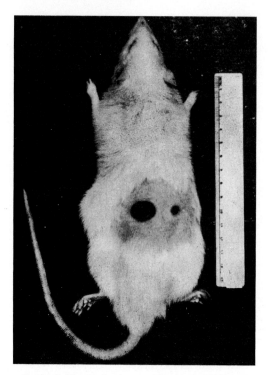

FIG. 8-5. The back of a rat, showing the spreading phenomenon. Two dark spots may be seen. The one at the right is the result of the injection of 0.1 ml of saline and India ink into the site; the spot at the left is due to the injection of 0.1 of ml of India ink and an aqueous extract of rat testicle. The extract of testicle contains a spreading factor which permits the India ink to spread much more widely and much more quickly in the tissues than occurs when India ink is injected by itself. (W. R. Harris)

investigating the chemistry of the intercellular substances, including the amorphous "ground substance" of loose connective tissue. His researches led to identification of the chief component of the amorphous intercellular substance as a type of carbohydrate that he called *acid mucopolysaccharides* (*muco,* because ground substance seemed to be somewhat similar to mucus). (A later term for them which is more accurate is glycosaminoglycans.) Two kinds of acid mucopolysaccharides, (1) a nonsulfated type called *hyaluronic acid* and (2) a sulfated type termed *chondroitin sulfuric acid,* constitute the amorphous intercellular substance of most loose connective tissue, but hyaluronic acid is predominant.

Hyaluronidase. As research on the mucopolysaccharides continued the mystery of the spreading factor was solved. Meyer found that certain kinds of bacteria produced an enzyme that could cause the depolymerization of hyaluronic acid. He named this enzyme *hyaluronidase.* Subsequently, Chain and Duthie showed that this enzyme was responsible for the spreading effect of testicular extracts. By depolymerizing hyaluronic acid it removes the chief obstacle to the spread of particulate or dissolved matter widely through the intercellular substances of loose connective tissue.

Mucopolysaccharides and Their Staining. Some Differences Between Them and Glycoproteins. The acidic side chains of tissue polysaccharides may be either simple organic groups (as in hyaluronic acid) or sulfuric acid groups (as in sulfated types).

Hyaluronic acid varies from being a slightly viscid fluid as it is in the cavities of synovial joints (e.g., the knee joint) where it serves as a lubricant, to a soft jellylike material that fills up the interstices between the collagenic and elastic fibers of the intercellular substances of loose connective tissue. It has a profound ability to hold water (tissue fluid), probably because of its carbohydrate molecules being long and feathery and having a vast surface area within their meshes which can hold, within certain limits, varying amounts of water without the physical properties of the material being greatly altered.

There are several types of sulfated mucopolysaccharides which differ from one another in minor ways. At least three of them are termed chondroitin sulfuric acid. They are abundant in the intercellular substance of cartilage and are present in smaller amounts in certain other connective tissues. The chondroitin sulfates impart cohesiveness to tissues; when abundant, they constitute a solid mass as in cartilage, as will be described later. When hyaluronic acid predominates as in the skin, the tissue remains soft and pliable.

thing between the fibers and cells of loose connective tissue that restricted the free movement of particles as would occur in free fluid. About this time another discovery was made which proved to have an important bearing on this matter. In 1928 Duran-Reynals had noted that when he injected rabbits' skins with an extract that had been made from a testis infected with a certain disease, the disease *spread* very rapidly in the connective tissue of the infected skin. Later studies showed that the rapid spread was not due to the disease agent; for it was found that an extract of normal testis tissue would cause dye that was injected with it into the connective tissue of the skin to spread rapidly (Fig. 8-5). From these experiments Duran-Reynals postulated the existence of a *spreading factor* that could be extracted from the testicular tissue. For many years the nature of the spreading factor remained a mystery. In the meantime, Karl Meyer was

Since both glycoproteins and mucopolysaccharides can exist as soft, water-containing jellies in the body and since both contain protein and carbohydrate, there can be some confusion involved in distinguishing one from the other. Mucopolysaccharides are distinguished from glycoproteins mainly by chemical methods. The former usually contain more carbohydrate and the latter more protein, but this is not a universal rule. In both the carbohydrates are arranged as side chains along a polypeptide main chain. The side chains are short in glycoproteins and composed of several hexoses and hexosamines ending with fucose or sialic acid, whereas they are long in mucopolysaccharides and composed of numerous repeating pairs of a uronic acid and a hexosamine. Histochemically, as was described in Chapter 1, the glycoproteins of mucus are colored magenta by the P.A.-Schiff reaction (Fig. 1-14) as is glycogen. The mucopolysaccharides, however, usually give no P.A.-Schiff reaction. Sites containing hyaluronic acid are not stained in an H and E section. Body depots of hyaluronic acid are difficult to stain in any event, for the very important reason that hyaluronic acid holds so much water that there is very little substance (aside from water) in the sites where it is present. While hyaluronic acid does not stain with either H or E, the sulfated mucopolysaccharides are somewhat denser and their presence may be indicated (particularly in cartilage) in H and E sections because of their combining with hematoxylin sufficiently to give a blue color to the intercellular substance.

Hyaluronic acid, and sulfated mucopolysaccharides as well, can be stained by (1) metachromatic methods, (2) alcian blue, and (3) Hale's colloidal iron method. Metachromatic (*meta*, beyond; *chroma*, a color) methods involve using certain dyes that color a tissue differently from the color of the dye itself. Toluidine blue is a common dye of this sort. It is blue but it colors mucopolysaccharides red, pink or purple. Another method for staining mucopolysaccharides is to use alcian blue; this is a copper phthalocyanin dye. It becomes linked to acidic groups of mucopolysaccharides and thus colors the mucopolysaccharides blue. Hale's colloidal iron technic takes advantage of the fact that, at a pH of 2.5, the acidic groups of the mucopolysaccharides bind colloidal iron which can then be stained with a specific method for iron.

Other Components of Ground Substance. Although the ground substance of loose connective tissue consists chiefly of hyaluronic acid plus some sulfated mucopolysaccharides, it contains also in a few body sites a glycoprotein that is P.A.-Schiff positive and fairly uniformly distributed. Furthermore, apart from the protein that is in the form of fibers in loose con-

nective tissue, there is also present in ground substance some protein that is in the form of a sol; this is sometimes referred to as the soluble protein of loose connective tissue. Some of this may be molecules of the precursor of collagen which have not yet been polymerized into fibrils. Another portion of it is derived from the blood (the extravascular pool of blood proteins is considerable; see the review by Mancini). As will be described in the next section, blood plasma contains macromolecules of protein, and some of these normally leak through the walls of blood capillaries to enter the ground substance of loose connective tissue, although in health their concentration in the intercellular substance is kept at a low level compared with their concentration in blood.

It is of interest that the amount of amorphous intercellular substance relative to fibrous types of intercellular substance diminishes with age, which at least partly explains why the skin tends to become wrinkled and seems to be thinner as a person ages.

THE FLUID COMPONENT OF THE INTERCELLULAR SUBSTANCE OF LOOSE CONNECTIVE TISSUE

The study of histology is not limited to the materials that can be fixed, stained and seen in sections suitable for the LM or the EM; it is also concerned with components of tissue that are not seen with the microscope but are present in tissue. The most notable of these is water. This component of intercellular material is represented in sections of loose connective tissue (as in Fig. 8-2) by empty spaces, for this water is all removed in preparing paraffin sections. Actually, although the fluid component of intercellular substance is water, it contains some soluble materials that are all in the process of diffusing back and forth between capillaries and cells, and so it is termed *tissue* or *extracellular fluid*. We prefer the term tissue fluid and we shall now describe this very important watery fluid in some detail. In our discussion of it we shall deal briefly with its origin, its circulation and some common basic causes of edema—the clinical condition characterized by the amount of tissue fluid becoming increased over normal.

The Formation and Absorption of Fluid

Tissue Fluid Is Derived From Blood. Arteries have relatively thick and strong walls because they carry blood away from the heart under considerable pressure. Arteries branch and rebranch and finally empty their blood through arterioles (which act as pressure-reduction valves) into capillary beds under relatively low pressure. Capillaries are narrow tubes

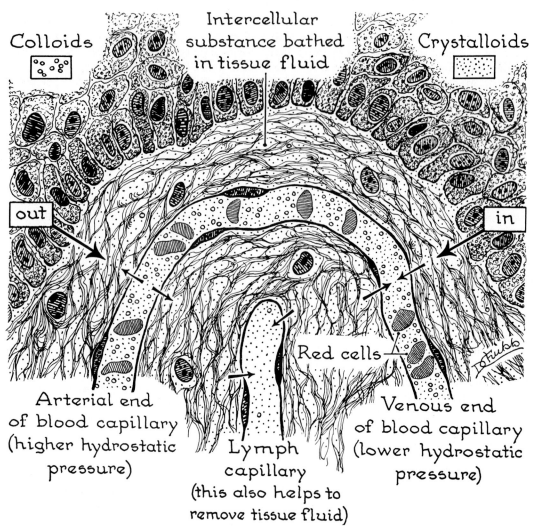

Colloids

Intercellular substance bathed in tissue fluid

Crystalloids

out

in

Red cells

Arterial end of blood capillary (higher hydrostatic pressure)

Lymph capillary (this also helps to remove tissue fluid)

Venous end of blood capillary (lower hydrostatic pressure)

Fig. 8-6. A diagram to show how tissue fluid is formed by capillaries and absorbed by capillaries and lymphatics. The proteins of the blood are represented as small circles and the crystalloids of blood and tissue fluid as dots. Under normal conditions only a very little colloid escapes from most capillaries, and such colloid as escapes is returned to the circulation by way of the lymphatics.

with thin delicate walls (Figs. 8-2, 8-6 and 8-7); their structure will be described in detail presently. Capillaries generally pursue a curving course through the intercellular substance (hence the term capillary loops) and then drain into veins (Fig. 8-6) which carry the blood back to the heart. Blood in the veins is not under much pressure.

Tissue fluid is basically a watery simple solution of nutrients and gases. It is derived from the fluid portion of blood which is called *blood plasma* and in which the cells of the blood are suspended. Plasma contains both substances that dissolve in simple solu-

tion and colloidal particles (macromolecules of protein). Both the substances in simple solution (such as salts and glucose) and the colloids (protein macromolecules) of blood exert osmotic pressure, so if blood plasma is separated from pure water by a membrane that does not allow the passage of either crystalloids or colloids, blood plasma would attract water through the membrane because of the osmotic pressure exerted by its crystalloids and colloids. The membrane that separates blood plasma from tissue fluid is the endothelium that constitutes the thin walls of the blood capillaries. This membrane, however, is permeable to crystalloids as well as to water; hence there are crystalloids on both sides of the membrane to exert osmotic pressure. But the colloids of blood cannot pass (except in very minute quantities) through the endothelial membrane. Hence the colloids of the blood plasma account for a marginal difference existing between the osmotic pressure exerted by blood within the capillaries and that exerted by the tissue fluid outside the capillaries. The result is that blood, by means of its greater osmotic pressure, is always trying, as it were, to draw the tissue fluid back into the capillaries. However, it is only able to do this at the venous ends of capillaries. At the arterial ends of capillaries the hydrostatic pressure within the capillary, which is caused by the pumping action of the heart, exceeds the difference between the osmotic pressure of blood and that of tissue fluid by a sufficient margin to force water in which gases and crystalloids are dissolved to pass through the capillary wall into the adjacent intercellular substance as tissue fluid (Fig. 8-6). However, because blood is viscous and a capillary is so narrow, the hydrostatic pressure gradually falls as blood passes along a capillary loop, so by the time blood reaches the venous end of a capillary the hydrostatic pressure within the capillary can no longer overcome the attraction that blood has for tissue fluid because of the osmotic attraction of its colloids (protein). Hence the protein macromolecules of the blood plasma are responsible for drawing tissue fluid back through the endothelial wall of the venous end of a capillary into the blood, as is shown in Figure 8-6. Thus there is to some degree a circulation of tissue fluid, with formation of tissue fluid occurring at the arterial ends of capillaries and absorption at the venous ends of capillaries.

The Origin of Lymph—Lymphatic Capillaries. More tissue fluid is usually produced at the arterial ends of capillaries than is absorbed at their venous ends. However, loose connective tissue does not normally become swollen with tissue fluid because the extra amount that is produced over that which is absorbed is drained away from the tissue by a second set of capillaries which are called lymphatic capillaries (*see* Fig. 8-6) because the tissue fluid that seeps into them is called lymph (*lympha,* water).

Lymphatic capillaries originate in tissue, frequently from blind ends (Fig. 8-6) and, because they branch freely, they commonly form networks of great complexity. Lymphatic capillaries drain into larger lymph vessels, to be described later, and these, connecting with still other lymph vessels, eventually form two chief lymphatic trunks that return the lymph collected from the whole body into large veins near the heart.

Hence that part of the tissue fluid absorbed by lymphatic capillaries eventually reaches the confines of the blood circulatory system again, but by a somewhat circuitous route.

Lymphatic capillaries are useful in regulating the quality of the tissue fluid as well as its quantity. At present it is generally agreed that the endothelium of blood capillaries normally allows a little blood protein to escape into intercellular substances. It is also generally agreed that the escaped protein macromolecules cannot pass back into blood capillaries. However, it seems that macromolecules of protein can pass from intercellular substances back through the endothelial walls of lymphatics. The studies of Drinker and his associates have shown that if it were not for the lymphatic drainage of tissue fluid, blood protein would accumulate in tissue fluid and by virtue of its osmotic pressure would tend to hold increasing amounts of water in the tissue. By more or less continually draining away protein from tissue fluid, lymphatic capillaries keep tissue fluid from accumulating protein from the blood.

How Fluid Passes In and Out Through Capillary Walls

The Fine Structure of Blood Capillaries. This topic will be considered in detail in Chapter 19 (Circulatory System); however, a few points about capillaries must be made here. There are two kinds: In one kind, called *continuous* capillaries (Fig. 8-7, *left*), it is believed that tissue fluid (but not protein macromolecules) leaves and enters the capillary between the borders of contiguous endothelial cells in the wall of the capillary. The junctional complexes that connect the edges of the contiguous endothelial cells of most capillaries are of the fascia type of occludens junction; hence, there are spaces between the sites where the outer laminae of the cell membranes of contiguous endothelial cells are fused. These intercellular spaces are believed to be small enough to hold back protein macromolecules but large enough to permit water and substances in simple solution to pass. In the second type of capillary, called *fenestrated* (Fig. 8-7, *right*), there is a second way for tissue fluid to enter and leave because in these capillaries the cytoplasm of the endothelial cells at certain sites becomes so greatly thinned that there are tiny holes (fenestrae) which are somewhat less than 1,000 Å (100 nm) in diameter. These tiny holes seem for the most part to each be closed over by a diaphragm which is thinner than a cell membrane and hence is presumably sufficiently porous for water and dissolved substances to pass through it.

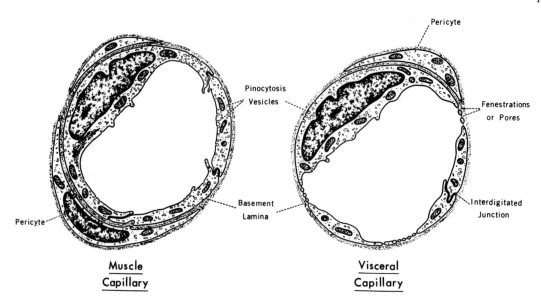

FIG. 8-7. The muscle capillary is of the continuous type whereas the visceral capillary shown is of the fenestrated type. (Fawcett, D. W.: *In* Orbison, J. L., and Smith, D. (eds.): Peripheral Blood Vessels. Baltimore, Williams & Wilkins, 1963)

Fenestrated capillaries are the type usually found where the production and absorption of tissue fluid is most rapid.

The circulation of tissue fluid is one thing; diffusion through it is another.

Diffusion. So far as diffusion mechanisms are concerned, the continuity of fluid between the tissue fluid and the blood via the spaces between the cell membranes of contiguous endothelial cells and via the fenestrae of fenestrated capillaries would allow for diffusion mechanisms to operate between tissue fluid and blood so that various dissolved substances could pass in both directions between blood and tissue fluid from sites of high to sites of low concentration. Thus tissue fluid is of vast importance because it is the medium through which cells are fed and oxygenated.

Pinocytosis. The EM shows that the endothelial cytoplasm, except where it is very thin in fenestrated capillaries, commonly reveals abundant pinocytotic vesicles within its substance (Fig. 8-7). Vesicles, for example, could fill with plasma and then bud off from the inner membrane of an endothelial cell, traverse the endothelium, and deliver their contents through the outer membrane of the endothelial cell into the region occupied by tissue fluid. It does not seem probable that pinocytosis is important in the formation of tissue fluid; physiological data indicate that its formation and absorption can be so rapid that it is difficult to conceive of pinocytosis accounting for more than a

fraction of the tissue fluid that can be produced by the previously described mechanism. Pinocytosis, however, could account for macromolecules—for example, of protein—being transported through the endothelial wall from blood to tissue fluid, or vice versa.

The endothelial wall of a capillary is surrounded by a thin basement membrane; the latter structure will be described presently.

Edema (*oedema,* a swelling) is a condition that is much encountered clinically. It is due to there being an excess over normal of tissue fluid in regions normally occupied by intercellular substance. It can be local or more or less general.

The amount of tissue fluid that can accumulate in tissue varies in relation to the type of tissue. Some tissues—for example, loose connective or adipose tissue—offer little resistance to being spread apart from within; others, such as dense connective tissue, as in a tendon, resist expansion. In most sites edema tends to be self-limiting because the more a tissue becomes swollen, the more resistance it offers to becoming stretched further. When a certain point is reached, the hydrostatic pressure of the fluid in the stretched tissue is almost as great as that within the capillaries and, as a result, the production of tissue fluid in the part almost ceases.

It might be thought that the increased hydrostatic pressure of the tissue fluid in swollen tissue would cause the collapse of its lymphatic vessels and so interfere with lymph drainage. However, the studies of Pullinger and Florey indicate the opposite. The walls of lymphatic vessels are attached to fibers of intercellular substance that extend through the tissue. As tissues become spread apart by fluid, these fibers are put on the stretch, with the result that they pull on the walls of lymphatic vessels in various directions and so hold them open.

For the medical or paramedically oriented student, four basic causes of edema are described briefly below and all are illustrated in Figure 8-8.

Some Basic Causes of Edema

1. **Obstruction to the Return of Blood Via Veins.** As is shown in Figure 8-8, *top left,* if venous drainage from capillaries is obstructed, the hydrostatic pressure rises all along the length of the capillaries involved so that more tissue fluid is produced and at the same time less or none is absorbed at their venous ends because the greater osmotic pressure within the capillary at its venous end is no longer sufficient to overcome the increased hydrostatic pressure present within the capillary (Fig. 8-8, *upper left*). This condition can arise in a more or less localized area because of the veins draining that part of the body becoming obstructed, or it can be generalized when a diseased heart becomes unable to pump blood into the arterial system as rapidly as it is being returned to the heart via the veins.

2. **Lymphatic Obstruction.** As is shown in Figure 8-8, *top right,* obstructed lymphatics can cause edema for two reasons: First, they do not return their usual quota of tissue fluid to the venous system; secondly, obstructed lymphatics cannot drain away such blood protein as normally escapes from blood capillaries; hence the tissue fluid comes to contain more and more protein, which raises its osmotic pressure so that the differential between the osmotic pressure in the tissue fluid and the venous ends of capillaries become less and less, which results in less and less tissue fluid being returned to the blood at the venous ends of capillaries. This type of edema is most dramatically illustrated in a tropical disease called elephantiasis, in which parasites may invade and obstruct the lymphatics of parts of the body which thereupon become enormously swollen.

3. **Insufficient Protein in the Blood Plasma.** As is illustrated in Figure 8-8, *bottom left,* if there is too little protein in the blood plasma, its osmotic pressure in the venous ends of capillaries is too little to draw tissue fluid produced at their arterial ends back into them. This condition can arise from plasma protein being lost from the body more rapidly than it is formed

because of some disease condition—for example, a large weeping wound, or kidney disease, which permits protein to leak into urine or as a result of insufficient production of blood protein as occurs in starvation or in malnutrition caused by a lack of protein in the diet.

4. **Increased Permeability of Capillaries.** This can occur at or close to sites where a part of the body suffers an extensive burn or is crushed in an accident. In and around injured sites the injured capillaries tend to leak plasma, and this can be extensive enough to result in the amount of fluid in the circulatory system being reduced to such an extent that the amount of fluid being returned to the heart is too little for it to act as an efficient pump. This in turn leads to further complications, as the student will find when the problem of shock is described in later courses. One feature of plasma loss is shown in Figure 8-8, *lower right.* Because the red cells of the blood are not lost along with the plasma, they become relatively concentrated in such plasma as is left. This is called *hemoconcentration* and it is treated—or, better still, prevented—by the intravenous administration of blood plasma.

Basement Membranes

The structures called basement membranes were given their name because they were seen at the bases of the cells of epithelial membranes or glands, between the epithelium and the loose connective tissue on which the bases of the epithelial cells would otherwise have been in direct contact. With the light microscope a basement membrane appeared as a layer of what appeared to be a seemingly structureless kind of intercellular substance that stained poorly with ordinary methods (labeled in Fig. 7-7).

It was at first assumed that, since basement membranes were composed of some type of intercellular substance, they were produced by the cells of connective tissue that produced the other kinds of intercellular substance and, hence, were connective tissue structures. This view was supported by the observations that were made after silver impregnation technics became available; for the use of these showed that what appeared to be networks of delicate fibers, called reticular or argyrophilic fibers, were present in close association with the deeper aspect of many basement membranes—and, indeed, at that time it was generally considered that they were part of the membrane. They differed from ordinary collagenic fibers because they were finer and, unlike collagenic fibers, they could be stained by the silver technics. When the PA-Schiff method became available it was found that basement membranes reacted positively to

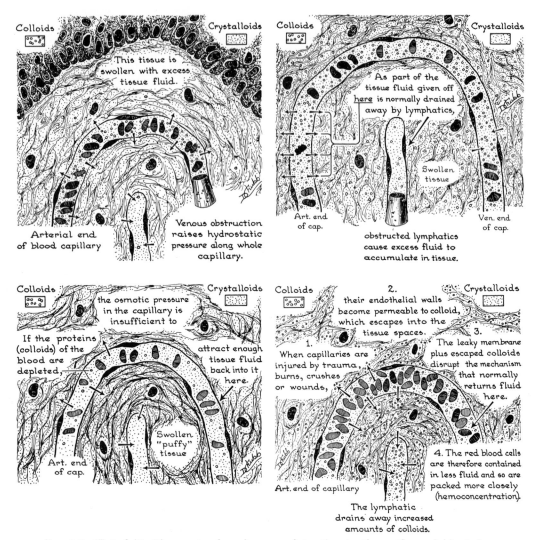

Fig. 8-8. (*Top, left*) Diagram to show how an obstruction to the outflow of blood from capillaries (back pressure on veins) can cause an increased amount of tissue fluid to form from the capillaries and also interfere with its absorption.

(*Top, right*) Diagram to show how the obstruction of lymphatics may cause an increased amount of tissue fluid to be present in the tissues they normally drain. It should be observed also that the amount of colloid in the tissue fluid becomes increased when lymphatics are obstructed because such colloid as normally escapes from capillaries is normally drained away by the lymphatics.

(*Bottom, left*) Diagram shows how a lack of colloid in the blood increases the amount of tissue fluid.

(*Bottom, right*) Diagram shows how plasma escapes when the endothelial walls of capillaries are injured by burns, crushes, nearby wounds or other means. Notice that as plasma leaks away from the capillary, the number of red blood cells in relation to plasma in it becomes increased. This is called hemoconcentration. Observe also how, under conditions of this sort, increased amounts of colloid are drained away by the lymphatic capillaries.

it (Fig. 7-2, B.M.), which of course suggested that basement membranes contained glycoprotein. However, since reticular fibers are PA-Schiff positive it was somewhat confusing as to whether the PA-Schiff staining was due to the reticular fibers being present in the basement membrane or whether the amorphous material of the membrane was also PA-Schiff positive. In other words, the PA-Schiff technic did not indicate whether or not reticular fibers were part of the basement membrane or, if they were not part of it, present immediately beneath it.

When basement membranes were investigated by increasingly modern methods, new information became available. For example, ingenious immunological experiments showed that the antigens (a term that will become familiar when the next chapter is read) of basement membrane material were related to those of the epithelial cells, and this of course raised the possibility of the epithelial cells producing the seemingly structureless intercellular substance that made up the membrane. Firm evidence proving that membrane was indeed an epithelial product and not of connective tissue origin later became available (Hay and Revel).

With the new evidence it became customary to regard the reticular fibers, which previously had been believed by some to be part of the membrane, as not actually belonging to what was then commonly defined as the *basement membrane* or *basal lamina*. The reticular fibers are now regarded as a specialized part of the connective tissue present directly beneath the true basement membrane, as is shown in Figure 8-9.

Fine Structure. With the advent of the EM, basement membranes were found to also exist between the endothelial walls of capillaries and the intercellular substance that contains the capillaries (labeled basement lamina in Fig. 8-7). These will be discussed in Chapter 20. However, the study of the basement membranes of ordinary epithelial origin with the EM has not revealed much detail. They seem to consist of a fine feltwork of fibers 30 to 40 Å (3 to 4 nm) which are not orientated in any particular way and which lie in some amorphous type of matrix. In some special basement membranes the fibrils have been shown to be orientated and to demonstrate what is termed banding (banding will be described in the next chapter in connection with collagenic fibers). However, any banding seen in normal basement membranes is not that which characterizes the collagen of connective tissue. It can, however, be shown chemically that there is a form of collagen in basement membranes, as will next be described.

Chemically, basement membranes are composed of three types of substance. One of these, as mentioned above, is a form of collagen. The other two are glycoproteins, one of high and one of low molecular weight. This is of interest because basement membranes can be demonstrated by the PA-Schiff technic (Fig. 7-2, B.M.), and this would seem to be due not only to the glycoprotein of the membrane but also to the fact that the form of collagen present within basement membranes contains a great deal more sugar in certain of its side chains than is present in ordinary collagen. As will be described in the next chapter, the banding of ordinary collagen is due to molecules of tropocollagen becoming arranged in a staggered fashion in the collagenic fibrils that form. This step does not seem to occur in basement membrane collagen.

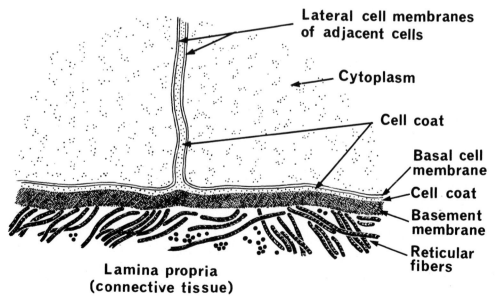

FIG. 8-9. Diagram of a basement membrane and associated structures at a magnification at which the various structures shown could only be seen as such with the EM and suitable technics.

Summary of Structure. As is shown in Figure 8-9, there are three layers of material between the cell membranes of epithelial cells and the loose connective tissue that is deep to them. Only one of these is now considered to be the basement membrane or, as it is sometimes termed, the basal lamina.

The first layer is the cell coat of the epithelial cells, labeled Cell Coat in Figure 8-9. With routine staining technics this appears in the EM as a light space separating the base of the cell from the basement membrane proper. By staining with PA-silver, this space was shown to contain the cell coat of the epithelial cells (Fig. 8-9). The second layer is the basement membrane proper (basal lamina) (Fig. 8-9). Below this is a third layer of more or less specialized connective tissue rich in reticular fibers (Fig. 8-9). This is not now regarded as part of the basement membrane proper, and it is of connective tissue origin. This layer of reticular fibers is lacking under some basement membranes. In some locations, e.g., the gingiva, there are instead discrete groups of fibers, known as anchoring fibers, which pierce the basement membrane and insert on the basal cell membrane.

Functions. Kefalides indicates that basement membranes may function in two ways: (a) to provide elastic support, and (b) to act as filtration or diffusion barriers. The first property is best exemplified by the capsule that surrounds the lens of the eye and which is of the order of a basement membrane. The lens capsule must not only support the lens; it must also possess elasticity because it must expand when the lens accommodates for distant vision and then returns to its original shape when this process has terminated. Other examples of basement membrane material providing an elastic type of support will be encountered as we study different body parts; this role of basement membrane material has only become adequately appreciated in recent years.

Basement membranes must permit both the passage of fluid and the diffusion of ions. They can, however, probably act as a barrier to macromolecules but their role as barriers is a complex matter under investigation.

For **References and Other Reading** see lists at end of Chapter 9.

9 The Cells of Loose Connective Tissue and Their Functions

As was described in Chapter 6, cells that are morphologically similar but possess great potentiality can be induced by different cellular environments to differentiate along different pathways to become cells that have very different appearances and perform very different specialized functions. This happens in connection with the mesenchymal cells that in prenatal life occupy the sites where the loose connective tissue of the body develops, for in these various sites mesenchymal cells such as those shown in Figure 8-1 variously differentiate into all of the cells shown in Figure 9-1 (except for the plasma cell). The student, however, should not expect to see all these cells in any particular loose connective tissue he examines. But if enough loose connective tissue from a sufficient number of different parts of the body is studied, some examples of each kind will of course be encountered.

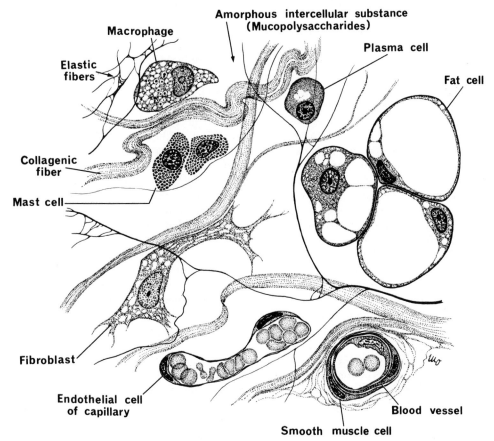

FIG. 9-1. Diagrammatic representation of the cells that may be seen in loose connective tissue. The cells lie in intercellular substance which is bathed in tissue fluid that originates from capillaries.

CAPILLARY DEVELOPING IN MESENCHYME

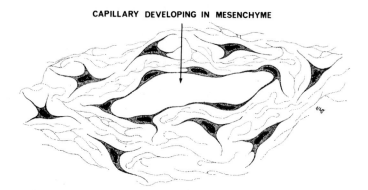

Fɪɢ. 9-2. Diagrammatic drawing to illustrate how mesenchymal cells can form the lining for a space which can become a capillary, and how the mesenchymal cells that line the space can become more flattened to become endothelial cells.

A Preview of the Cells of Loose Connective Tissue

In various sites where loose connective tissue develops in the embryo some mesenchymal cells become *fibroblasts* (Fig. 9-1), the cells that synthesize and otherwise account for the intercellular substances of loose connective tissue. Some become *fat* cells and store fat (Fig. 9-1). Some become the *endothelial lining cells* of the blood vessels that form in mesenchyme (Fig. 9-2) and later exist in loose connective tissue (Fig. 9-1). Some become *smooth muscle cells* to become parts of the walls of larger blood vessels (Fig. 9-1). Others become *mast* cells, the cells that produce heparin and histamine (Fig. 9-1). Still others develop into cells that have phagocytic properties but have been given various names—for example, histiocytes and clasmatocytes—because they seem to have had somewhat different appearances or occupied somewhat different positions. However, in the presence of suitable foreign material these cells not only exhibit phagocytic properties but come to have a similar appearance, and it is now customary to term them all macrophages (Fig. 9-1). Although some of the macrophages of loose connective tissue may develop in prenatal life from the original mesenchymal cells of the part they later inhabit, most of those seen in postnatal life develop from blood cells termed monocytes which arrive in the part via the bloodstream.

It is usual for cells termed plasma cells (Fig. 9-1) to be seen in loose connective tissue in many parts of the body. Plasma cells are not seen until after birth and they develop from cells that enter loose connective tissue from the blood. However, they are common enough in loose connective tissue (but only in restricted parts of the body—for example, in the loose connective tissue that is immediately beneath the epithelial lining of the intestine) to be considered as one of the cells of loose connective tissue.

Finally, there is some opinion to the effect that certain mesenchymal cells (not illustrated in Fig. 9-1)

may persist in loose connective tissue without differentiating sufficiently to lose very much of their original potentiality; these are termed undifferentiated mesenchymal cells. In this connection it should be mentioned that there are cells associated with small blood vessels called *perivascular cells* which seem to retain a good deal of potentiality, so this is where the least differentiated mesenchymal cells probably persist.

Fibroblasts and the Synthesis of Intercellular Substances

Terminology. The term fibroblast, which means fiber-forming (*blastos,* a sprout) cell, was coined before it was known that these cells, as well as giving rise to fibers, secrete a ground substance. It is possible that there may be some specialization among fibroblasts, for it has been reported that some strains of fibroblasts on being grown in tissue cultures make only amorphous intercellular substances; but it is generally believed that under in-vivo conditions any fibroblast can produce both kinds of intercellular substance. As described in the second paragraph below, old fibroblasts are often termed fibrocytes. It is now known moreover that fibroblasts are not the only kind of cell that can make fibrous types of intercellular substances; for example, it has been shown that both collagen and elastin can be produced by smooth muscle cells in at least certain parts of the body.

Appearance in Stained Spreads. If teased spreads of freshly obtained loose connective tissue prepared similarly to those used to study fibers (Fig. 8-3) are stained lightly with a basic dye such as methylene blue, cells similar to the one illustrated in Figure 9-3 are readily seen, because the fibroblast is probably the most numerous cell in most of the loose connective tissue of the body. The pale cytoplasm of these cells is probably drawn out into processes by the teasing procedure so that the processes of the cells are more prominent than they would be in life. Some fibroblasts are fusiform. The nuclei of the fibroblasts in this type

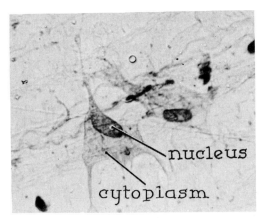

FIG. 9-3. A teased preparation of areolar tissue stained lightly with methylene blue, and showing two fibroblasts.

of preparation are generally ovoid and pale. Their chromatin is finely granular and nucleoli can generally be seen in them.

Fibroblasts As Seen in H and E Sections. Tissues in different states of activity or development reveal fibroblasts of somewhat different appearances. Although both young cells and old cells of this type are commonly referred to by the same term, i.e., *fibro-*

blast, many authors termed the older ones *fibrocytes.*

Fibrocytes (old fibroblasts) are seen in stained sections to be surrounded by intercellular substances most of which was made some time previously (Fig. 9-4, *right*). Little or no cytoplasm can be seen in these old cells whose presence is revealed only by their pale nuclei (Fig. 9-4, *right*). Their nuclei are more or less flattened ovoids; so, if cut in some planes, they appear much thinner than they do in others, and if they are cut in cross section, they appear smaller than if they are cut in longitudinal section.

In an H and E section a young fibroblast differs from a fibrocyte in that it has an abundant amount of basophilic cytoplasm surrounding its nucleus as is shown in Figure 9-4, *left*. From the main cell body, processes that are not so basophilic as the cytoplasm closer to the nucleus, extend for considerable distances (Fig. 9-4, *left*). Furthermore, the nucleus of a young active fibroblast can generally be seen to have a prominent nucleolus (Fig. 9-4, *left*). Thus the appearance (abundant basophilic cytoplasm and a large nucleolus) of a young fibroblast as seen under the LM is that of a cell that is *actively synthesizing protein*. The protein synthesized by active fibroblasts could be either protein for growth (for the formation of more fibroblasts, because fibroblasts can divide)

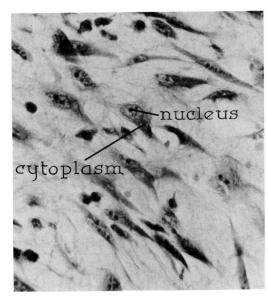
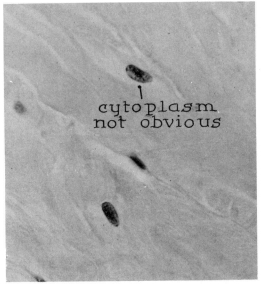

FIG. 9-4. (*Left*) A medium-power photomicrograph of a section cut through a healing wound, where young fibroblasts are growing rapidly. Observe that the cytoplasm of young, actively growing fibroblasts is apparent in H and E sections. (*Right*) Picture taken from a section of mature connective tissue in the deeper part of the skin. Most of the tissue in this illustration consists of collagenic fibers. Only the nuclei of the old fibroblasts present in such tissue can be seen to advantage.

or protein destined for secretion (the production of intercellular substances), or both. In this connection it seems probable that after a fibroblast has made its quota of intercellular substances, its cytoplasm becomes pale and scanty so that only its nucleus is apparent in H and E sections (Fig. 9-4, *right*); it has then become a relatively non-active fibrocyte. Fibrocytes have been shown to take up labeled proline, an amino acid required for the synthesis of collagen, which would indicate that they could still secrete some intercellular substance; however, it seems improbable that a fibrocyte could dedifferentiate into a young fibroblast that can, for example, undergo mitosis, as will become apparent in the next section.

The Origin of Fibroblasts. In embryonic development fibroblasts are believed to develop from the mesenchymal cells of the area. Experiments on the repair of connective tissue wounds in postnatal life indicate the mitoses that result in the formation of new fibroblasts to repair the tissue occur not in the old fibrocytes but in less differentiated cells that are closely associated with small blood vessels and are in general termed perivascular cells. Over the years there has been controversy as to whether certain cells (monocytes) present in the bloodstream enter areas where connective tissue has been injured and there differentiate into fibroblasts to assist in the repair process. Ross et al., using parabiotic rats (rats joined together so that they share a common bloodstream), have shown in a most ingenious experiment that monocytes or any other blood cells that become labeled with thymidine do not become fibroblasts in the repair of a wound. They believe that the fibroblasts that repair a wound are of local origin, arising mostly from perivascular cells, which cells are somewhat less differentiated than fibroblasts and can serve as their precursors.

The Fine Structure of Fibroblasts. From having read the chapters on cytoplasm, in which the mechanism of secretion was described, and about epithelium, in which many examples of epithelial secretory cells were given, the student may assume that secretion is a property possessed only by epithelial cells. In the present chapter we shall find that several kinds of connective tissue cells are also secretory, and later we shall find that certain kinds of muscle cells and nerve cells also perform secretory functions. So in beginning our study of the fine structure of the fibroblast it is most important to realize that it is a secretory cell and that what has been said previously about secretion in Chapters 5 and 7 is relevant. The only difference between a fibroblast and an epithelial secretory cell is that the fibroblast does not secrete its

product onto a free surface through a particular segment of its cell surface. It secretes its products into the substance of the body and probably through different sites around its surface. Fibroblasts secrete two main products, procollagen and mucopolysaccharides; some also produce and secrete elastin.

As might be expected in a secretory cell, a secreting fibroblast contains abundant rough-surfaced vesicles of endoplasmic reticulum and several well developed Golgi stacks in its cytoplasm, and transfer vesicles are present between the rER and Golgi stacks and secretory vesicles between Golgi stacks and the cell surface (Fig. 9-5).

Steps in the Formation of Collagen. In Chapter 3 the way the amino acids are strung together to form the long polypeptide chains of a protein was outlined, and the process was illustrated in Figure 4-6. Collagen molecules are very long (about 2,800 Å) and about 15 Å thick. Each consists of three polypeptide chains that are wound together in the form of a triple helix. The chains are termed alpha chains and each consists of sequences of 3 amino acids which are repeated along its course. The first amino acid of a sequence of three may be any of a variety of amino acids other than the next two to be mentioned. The second amino acid of a sequence is either proline or lysine and the last one is always glycine.

Collagen is unusual because it contains a high percentage of proline and glycine and it is unique because a considerable amount of the proline and the lysine it contains is hydroxylated. The particular function of the hydroxyproline in collagen is not known but advantage can be taken of the fact that it is present (to any great extent) only in collagen. First, whether or not cells are capable of producing collagen can be determined by showing whether or not they contain the enzymes required for hydroxylating proline. Second, and of clinical significance, is the fact that whether collagen is being broken down in the body at an excessive rate can be determined, for hydroxyproline then appears in quantity in the urine. Since bone contains a good deal of collagen, conditions in which excessive amounts of bone are being resorbed can be detected by this means.

The function of the hydroxylysine is better known. Its first function is that the hydroxylysine of one collagen molecule can attach to the hydroxylysine of other collagen molecules and thus account for the strong cross linking of collagen molecules that gives collagenic fibers their strength. The second function is that the hydroxylysine molecules provide for the attachment of the short carbohydrate chains of col-

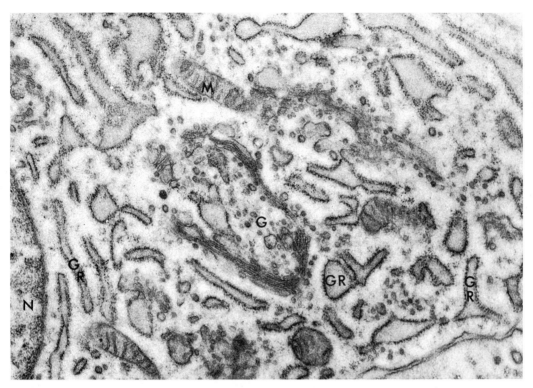

FIG. 9-5. Electron micrograph showing portion of an active fibroblast. A small portion of the nucleus is evident (*lower left*, N). The cytoplasm constitutes the remainder of the illustration and contains very numerous rough-surfaced vesicles of endoplasmic reticulum (labeled GR for granular reticulum); the presence of so many indicate the synthesis of much protein destined for secretion. A well-developed Golgi (G) is seen in the central region; here a group of flattened smooth-surfaced vesicles are arranged in the shape of a horseshoe. Mitochondria are present; one is labeled M. (Movat, H. Z., and Fernando, N. V. P.: Exp. Mol. Path., *1*:509)

lagen (which are usually composed of galactose and glucose).

Collagen is synthesized in the form of a precursor known as procollagen. The synthesis of the alpha chains of procollagen occurs in association with the polyribosomes of the rough endoplasmic reticulum. When first synthesized these are longer than they are later because a tail piece of about 130 Å is added to each as it is produced. A number of the proline and lysine residues present in the chains become hydroxylated within 3 minutes after they are incorporated into an alpha chain that is being synthesized. It takes around 5 to 6 minutes for a complete chain to be synthesized. These facts have been established by biochemical investigations. Further information was derived from radioautographic studies using ^{3}H-proline as a marker in both fibroblasts and odontoblasts. There are certain advantages for studying the synthesis of collagen in the latter type of cell because it is polarized as will now be described.

Dentin is the kind of intercellular substance that constitutes most of the hard substance of the tooth. The cells that produce it are called odontoblasts, and they, like fibroblasts, produce collagen. (In dentin calcium is subsequently deposited to make dentin hard.) Odontoblasts are more or less columnar in form and are lined up beside each other around the inner surface of the shell of the tooth (Fig. 21-8). The latter becomes steadily thicker because collagen and other intercellular substances are laid down at the ends of the odontoblasts that abut on the inner surface of the shell. Since collagen appears at only one end of each odontoblast (the end that abuts on the shell of dentin), its formation is relatively easy to follow. In studying collagen formation at this site, Weinstock and Leblond found labeled proline in the rough-surfaced endoplasmic reticulum in 2 to 5 minutes after its injection, which time would be in accord with the concept of the alpha chains being synthesized at this site (Fig. 9-6, *left* and *bottom*). After 10 minutes they found

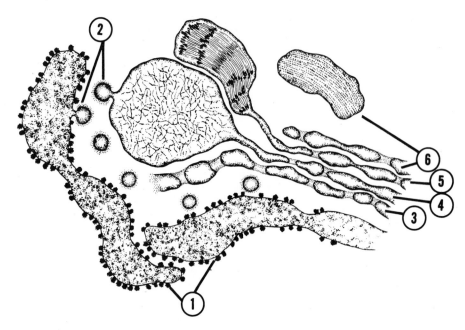

FIG. 9-6. Part of Golgi region of collagen-secreting cell. From base to top, it is possible to see: (1) the cisternae of rough ER with their coating of ribosomes; (2) a few intermediate or transfer vesicles, one of which, at left, is being released from a cisterna, while another is connected to the distended portion of a Golgi saccule; (3) part of a stack of Golgi saccules at right, the first saccule of which shows the pattern characteristic of fenestrations; (4) the second saccule ending in a distended portion filled with entangled threads; (5) the third saccule ending in a distended portion filled with parallel threads; (6) the fourth saccule showing no connection in the figure; but, above it, a solid structure with discrete striation, which is believed to come from a distended portion which has been separated from it; the parallel threads have aggregated. This is a secretory vesicle (also called secretory granule) which carried its content for release at the cell surface. (Illustration courtesy of M. Weinstock and C. P. Leblond)

label in spherical portions located at the periphery of the Golgi saccules (Fig. 9-6). Here the saccules contained thin entangled threads (Fig. 9-6) in no organized arrangements. Somewhat later the threads became arranged so that they were parallel and, after 20 minutes had elapsed, label was found over saccules that contained rigid parallel threads (Fig. 9-6). Physical chemical work revealed that alpha chains have a variable shape, whereas the triple helix is a rigid structure. Their interpretation is that alpha chains have a variable shape when they enter saccules at the forming face of the stack so they appear as entangled threads (Fig. 9-6, large dilation of part of saccule in approximately the center of the illustration), but within the Golgi saccules they become combined into the triple helices of procollagen and, when this has occurred, they appear as rigid parallel threads (Fig. 9-6, upper right). These threads aggregate into one to three thick rods. By 35 minutes the rods are within free vesicles presumably derived from Golgi saccules and in which the label is located (Fig. 9-6, farthest upper right).

These are secretory vesicles which contain aggregates of procollagen and in due course deliver this material onto the cell surface. It is suggested that at the cell surface the tail piece formerly attached to each alpha chain is split off by enzymatic action (a peptidase) and thus the procollagen molecules are converted to what is generally termed tropocollagen molecules which become arranged into what are termed collagenic fibrils.

THE STRUCTURE OF COLLAGENIC FIBRILS

The Fine Structure of Collagen. The EM showed that the fibrils seen under high magnification with the LM (Fig. 8-4) are not the finest fibrils present in collagen. The EM disclosed smaller ones that vary in size from some at the limit of visibility with the LM, that is, 2,000 Å, to some visible only in the EM (depending on the different body sources from which the collagen was obtained).

The fibrils seen with the EM exhibit *axial periodic-*

ity, which means that along their lengths they exhibit units of structure that repeat themselves every 640 Å (Fig. 9-7). This feature of collagen was first seen with the EM, not in sections, but in shadow cast mounts of collagen that was treated to break it up into its fibrils. When the periodicity of collagenic fibrils was discovered a search was almost immediately begun to find an explanation for it. First, it was found that collagen could be dissociated into the molecules of which fibrils and fibers are composed, and next, that the basic molecules of collagen could then be reassembled by biochemical procedures into fibrils that showed the same axial periodicity as natural collagen. The basic molecules into which collagen could be dissociated were termed *tropocollagen molecules;* these are what appear just outside of fibroblasts. An interesting question then arose; namely, how mole-cules of tropocollagen 2,800 Å long were assembled so as to account for the 640-Å periodicity of collagenic fibrils.

The attainment of a 640-Å periodicity in fibrils constituted of molecules 2,800 Å in length could be explained if the 2,800-Å molecules in a fibril were arranged in a parallel but staggered fashion, with each molecule overlapping the one *beside* it by one quarter of its length but not meeting the end of the molecules ahead or behind it end to end (Fig. 9-8). This hypothesis was proposed by Hodge and Petruska and it explains how molecules 2,800 Å in length could be fitted together side by side in a staggered fashion in a fibril so as to cause a fibril to have less dense and more dense crossbands that alternate along the length of the fibril. To be more specific: along the length of a negatively stained fibril (Fig. 9-8) there are light

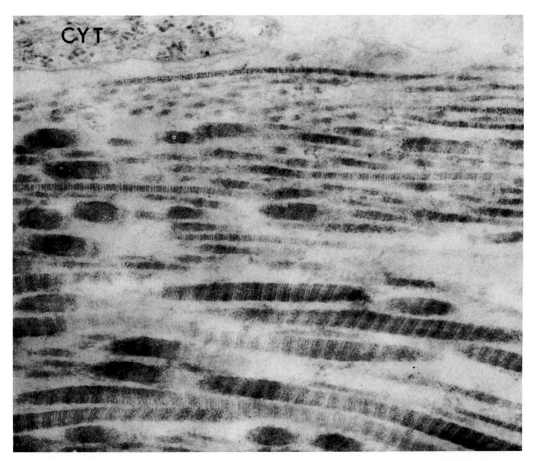

Fig. 9-7. Electron micrograph (× 76,000) of newly polymerized microfibrils of collagen beside a fibroblast, the edge of whose cytoplasm is seen at the top (CYT). Note that the microfibrils closest to the cytoplasm are finer than those that are farther away, showing how microfibrils can increase in diameter after they are first polymerized outside of fibroblasts. (Fernando, N. V. P., and Movat, H. Z.: Lab. Invest., *12:*214)

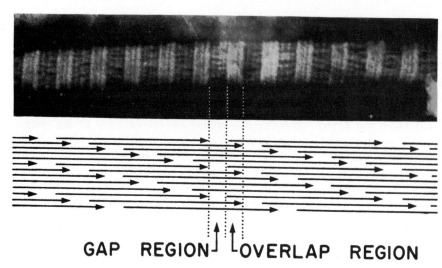

GAP REGION⏌ ⎿OVERLAP REGION

FIG. 9-8. Electron micrograph (× 175,000) of an isolated negatively stained collagenic microfibril showing alternating light and dark regions. One dark and one light segment represents one 640 Å period. The diagram below is based on the arrangement of tropocollagen molecules suggested by Hodge and Petruska to account for the 640 Å periodicity (see explanation in text). (Electron micrograph by A. F. Howatson and J. D. Almeida)

and dark segments which repeat themselves. One dark plus one light segment accounts for one period. Each light segment accounts for slightly less than half a period. Next, the tropocollagen molecules are assembled side by side and in a staggered arrangement, but they are staggered so that the gaps between the ends of tropocollagen molecules always fall in a dark segment (see diagram at bottom of Fig. 9-8). Hence the dark segments are not as dense as the light segments, for each light segment has 5 macromolecules passing through it to every 4 that pass through a dark segment. By this arrangement each 2,800-Å tropocollagen macromolecule extends over approximately 4½ periods, always over 5 light segments and over only 4 dark segments (Fig. 9-8, *bottom*). The existence of alternating light and dark segments accounts for the periodicity.

The longitudinal striations that can be seen in the negatively stained microfibril illustrated in Figure 9-8 probably represent small (and perhaps unit) bundles of staggered tropocollagen molecules.

Still finer crossbanding can be seen in the 640-Å units (Fig. 9-9). It is known that some sequences along the tropocollagen molecules repeat themselves several times. When these sequences are in register, they may cause the fine banding seen within the main bands.

The Synthesis and Secretion of Mucopolysaccharides. The rough endoplasmic reticulum is responsible for synthesizing the protein components of the mucopolysaccharides of ground substance, and the carbohydrate components are probably attached to this protein to some extent in the rough-surfaced endoplasmic reticulum and to a greater extent in the Golgi apparatus, from where the mucopolysaccharides are also delivered to the cell surface by secretory vesicles.

Whether or not there is any chemical association between the two types of intercellular substance before they are delivered to the cell surface is not known. Furthermore whether or not there is some chemical interaction between the tropocollagen and mucopolysaccharides as collagenic fibrils are assembled or, later, as fibrils are bundled into the types of fibrils and fibers that can be seen with the LM is not known, but such interaction seems improbable.

Formation of Elastic Fibers. The formation of most of the elastin in the body occurs in connection with the formation of blood vessels, particularly the larger arteries, and here it is formed primarily by smooth muscle cells. A discussion of the formation and chemistry of elastin will be given in connection with arteries in Chapter 19. Here it is enough to say that fibroblasts probably synthesize elastin in much the same way as collagen but it is secreted as an amorphous and not a fibrillar material. In connection with its formation, fibroblasts secrete some microfibrils that are not elastin but function to mold the shape of the amorphous material into fibers.

Reticular Fibers. These were discussed briefly in the previous chapter in connection with basement membranes. They will be discussed in more detail in connection with the hemopoietic tissues, where they are relatively prominent.

Fat Cells and Adipose Tissue

Fat cells are also known as *adipocytes*. Although single or small groups of fat cells are normal constituents of loose connective tissue, when a tissue consists almost entirely of fat cells that are organized into lobules, the tissue is termed *adipose tissue*.

Fat Cells As Representatives of a Special Cell

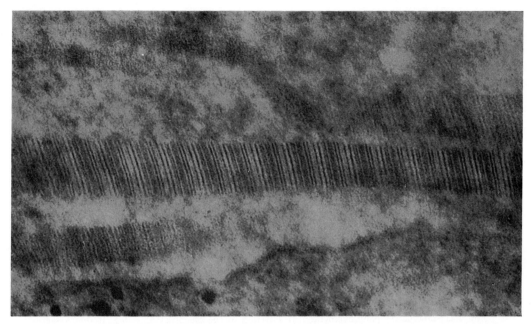

Fɪɢ. 9-9. Electron micrograph, approximately of the same magnification as Figure 9-8, showing the appearance presented by a fibril of collagen in a thin section. Although traversed by finer cross banding, the gap and overlap regions illustrated in Figure 9-8 can be identified. For an explanation of the finer cross banding, the article by Hodge and Petruska should be consulted. (Preparation by H. Warshawsky)

Lineage. Since fat cells seem to appear more or less haphazardly in loose connective tissue, it was often assumed that they could develop from fibroblasts. However, there is evidence indicating that they represent a special line of connective tissue cells. If fat is transplanted from one part of a body where fat normally accumulates to a site where fat does not ordinarily accumulate, the transplanted cells do not revert to fibroblasts in their new location but instead continue to function as fat cells. Accordingly, it seems reasonable to conclude that the reason for fat accumulating in certain sites—e.g., over the belly or buttocks—is that, instead of developing into fibroblasts, the mesenchymal cells in the developing con-

nective tissue of these parts of the body differentiate along a different line and that fat cells represent a special type of cell.

Morphology of Fat Cells As Seen With the LM. The first indication of a mesenchymal-derived cell taking on the function of a fat cell that can be seen with the LM is the appearance of droplets of fat in its cytoplasm. In H and E sections these are seen as little holes. But in frozen sections the fat is retained and can be stained as was described in Chapter 1 and illustrated in Figure 1-14, *bottom.* In Figure 9-10, the droplets are indicated in black. As this illustration shows, going from left to right, the droplets as they increase in number fuse with one another and, even-

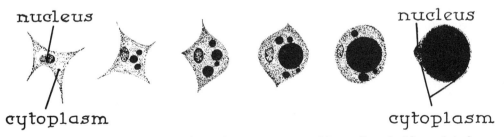

Fɪɢ. 9-10. Diagrams showing the changes in appearance caused by a cell synthesizing and storing fat. It finally becomes a typical fat cell with a "signet-ring" appearance.

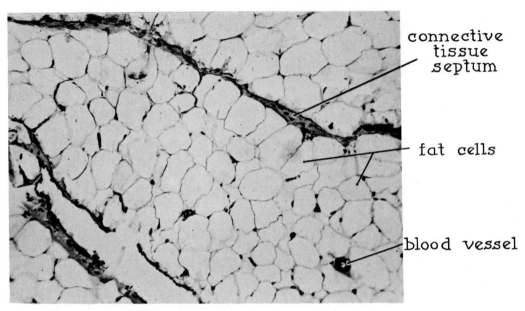

Fig. 9-11. Low-power photomicrograph of a section of the omentum of a dog. It shows aggregations of fat cells (small lobules) separated from one another by partitions of connective tissue which carry blood vessels throughout the tissue.

tually, one relatively huge droplet of fat so expands the cell from within that the cytoplasm is reduced over most of it to a thin film, and even the nucleus becomes somewhat stretched. The appearance of such a cell in cross section (if the section passes through the region of the nucleus) is of a signet ring worn on a finger of fat; the nucleus accounts for the signet and the ring is composed of the greatly thinned cytoplasm that surrounds the fat (Fig. 9-10, *right*). Even though the cytoplasm is thinned its total amount is believed not to be reduced.

Morphology of Adipose Tissue. This variety of connective tissue consists of fat cells that are organized into groups called lobules. The lobules of fat cells are separated from each other and supported by partitions of loose connective tissue called septa which extend between them and support them (Fig. 9-11). This connective tissue stroma also conducts blood vessels and nerves into the adipose tissue. Within a lobule the individual fat cells are supported by a stroma that consists of nets of delicate reticular and collagenic fibers which contain abundant capillaries in their meshes, and by this means capillaries are brought into intimate contact with fat cells. Mast cells are also present in the connective tissue stroma. About 50 percent of the cells of adipose tissue are not fat cells but cells of the stroma. In H and E sections the fat cells are of course empty of fat and the capil-

laries between them have had their content of blood mostly squeezed out because of the procedures involved in preparing the section.

The way that fat cells are packed together in lobules can be illustrated in a striking manner by means of scanning electron microscopy. By this technic a 3-dimensional surface view of a structure can be obtained (see Footnote * for method). A micrograph of this type (Fig. 9-12) shows that the rounded individual fat

* SCANNING ELECTRON MICROSCOPY. This technic is a relatively recent development. It does not depend on electrons passing through the object that is being examined; hence, it differs fundamentally from transmission electron microscopy (the kind described in Chapter 2). What it reveals is a 3-dimensional picture of the surface of the object that is examined. For example, Figure 9-12 is a scanning electron micrograph which shows a 3-dimensional surface view of part of a lobule of fat tissue, with individual fat cells, which are rounded globular bodies, bulging from the surface, like the outer grapes of a bunch.

In order to prepare a micrograph of the surface of an object by the scanning electron microscope the specimen does not, of course, have to be cut into sections. Instead, the specimen is prepared so that its surface can be scanned. This entails fixing the specimen and then dehydrating it by special procedures. It is then mounted in a specimen holder and its surface is coated with a very thin layer of a metal—for example, gold. In the microscope it is then scanned, back and forth, by a focused thin pencil-like electron beam about 100 Å in diameter. As the beam passes over the specimen it sets electrons on the surface of the specimen in motion. These electrons that are generated

cells, each containing a fat droplet, are packed together in a lobule much as grapes are packed together in bunches for shipment.

Types of Fat and General Functions. There are two main types of adipose tissue—white, and brown. White adipose tissue is the common type in mammals and comprises almost all of the adipose tissue of man. Its color may sometimes be an off-white because of its containing carotene. Brown adipose tissue is very scanty in man but is relatively abundant in some mammalian species. It appears brown in life because it has a very rich capillary blood supply and, also, because its cells contain many mitochondria and are therefore rich in cytochromes (mitochondrial enzymes that, like hemoglobin, contain a colored component). Brown adipose tissue serves a special purpose, being mainly concerned with regulating body temperature in newborn animals and serving as a source of heat production in members of certain species during arousal from hibernation.

White adipose tissue comprises 15 to 20 percent of the body weight of adult males and 20 to 25 percent of that of females. In a sense it can be spoken of as a large organ which is metabolically active, being primarily engaged in the uptake, synthesis, storage and mobilization (mobilization means to make mobile so its calories can be used for fuel in other parts of the body) of neutral lipid (fat). In fat cells at body temperature, fat is in the form of oil. It consists of triglycerides, which consist of three molecules of fatty acid esterified to glycerol. Triglycerides have the highest calorie content of all food, hence the fat in fat cells constitutes a store of high calorie fuel that is relatively light in weight. Moreover, fat is an excellent insulating material, and in those who live in cold countries fat helps insulate those parts of the body that lie beneath it. In addition, fat serves as an excellent filler of various crevices in the body and provides cushions on which various parts of the body can rest comfortably.

The Fine Structure of Fat Cells. As is shown in the insert in the upper right corner of Figure 9-13, the cytoplasm of a fat cell that has stored its complement of fat is so thin that the organelles it contains

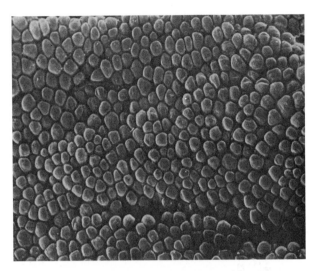

Fɪɢ. 9-12. The surface of part of a lobule of adipose tissue as shown by the scanning electron microscope. Fat cells are very large, fairly uniform in shape, and globular in conformation. Ninety-five percent of their mass is stored lipid. (From A. Angel, R. H. Mills and M. J. Hollenburg)

are to some extent displaced to the region closer to the nucleus, where there is more cytoplasm. As can be seen in the main illustration in Figure 9-13, which is a micrograph of a fat cell that as yet has stored only a small amount of fat, some organelles can be seen, particularly in the cytoplasm adjacent to the nucleus. Free ribosomes, both kinds of endoplasmic reticulum, a Golgi apparatus and mitochondria can all be found in fat cells. Mitochondria are the most prominent organelles; in Figure 9-3 they appear as rods because of the low magnification. They serve an important function in fat cells, as will soon be described.

The Ingredients From Which Fat Cells Synthesize Fat. The fat in a fat cell has been synthesized within the cell in which it appears. The fat in a person's diet, as well as carbohydrate and even protein, can provide the building blocks from which fat is synthesized in fat cells, as will now be described.

Fate of Fat in the Diet. Triglycerides (neutral fat) consumed in the diet are digested chiefly by an

at the point where the fine electron beam strikes the surface are picked up by a detector and the resulting electrical signals are displayed on a T.V. cathode ray tube. A scanning electron micrograph is a photograph of the image thus produced on the face of the television tube.

In a general way it might be said that scanning electron micrographs are easier to interpret than those made by transmission microscopy because we are accustomed to seeing irregular surfaces in three dimensions with the naked eye. The scanning electron microscope achieves the same kind of result, but in infinitely greater detail, that can be obtained by examining, say, the surface of the skin with a good magnifying glass. Interpreting transmission type electron micrographs is more difficult for several reasons, an important one being that we are not accustomed to visualizing the 3-dimensional structure of objects from 2-dimensional slices that are cut through them.

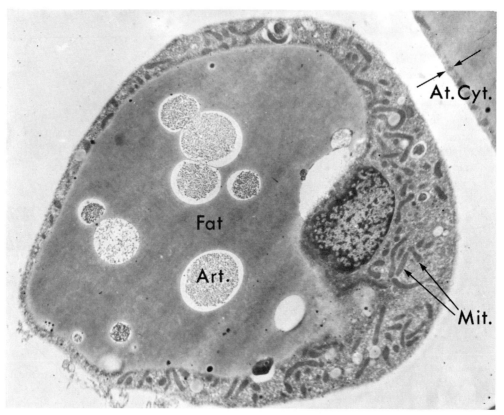

FIG. 9-13. Electron micrograph (× 3,000) of a fat cell in a preparation of free adipose cells, fixed in glutaraldehyde and postfixed in osmium tetroxide for 2 hours. The cell shown contains less lipid than most cells; otherwise the cytoplasm would be so attenuated it would be difficult to see organelles in it, as is evident at the upper right, where part of the cytoplasm of another cell which has a larger lipid content is shown, and in which the cytoplasm is very attenuated (At. Cyt.). The clear granular areas in the lipid are due to artifact (Art.). Mitochondria (Mit.) are numerous. (Angel, A., and Sheldon, H.: Ann. N.Y. Acad. Sci., *131:*157, 1965)

enzyme termed lipase which is secreted by the pancreas into the duodenum. Its action is facilitated by the presence of bile which is secreted by the liver into the same site. Bile helps to emulsify the fat so that the action of the lipase is more effective. As a result, most of the fat in the intestine is broken down to fatty acids and glycerol while up to about 30 percent may be broken down only to monoglycerides. The fatty acids are absorbed through the membranes of the epithelial cells lining the small intestine. Within the cytoplasm of these cells glycerol-phosphate is synthesized and combined with the fatty acids so that new triglycerides are formed. The monoglycerides are readily absorbed into the lining cells and there they are recombined with fatty acids to form triglycerides (this is termed the monoglyceride pathway). The newly formed fat appears as submicroscopic droplets of fat

called chylomicrons which are coated with protein. These make their way out of the epithelial cells to gain entrance to the tissue fluid at the bases of the epithelial cells, and from there into the lymphatic capillaries. After a fatty meal the chylomicrons in the lymphatics may be numerous enough to make the lymph milky; indeed, if there is a heavy enough content of chylomicrons in lymph it can make the plasma of the blood milky when the lymph reaches the bloodstream. As the blood containing chylomicrons circulates it passes through capillaries in several tissues and organs where the chylomicrons close to the endothelium of the capillaries are exposed to an enzyme called *lipoprotein lipase* which is secreted by cells along the sides of the capillaries. This enzyme breaks down the triglycerides of the chylomicrons to fatty acids and glycerol again. If this happens in a capillary in fat tissue, the fatty acid may be immediately absorbed by a fat cell where it will be combined with glycerol-phosphate synthesized by the fat cell, as will be described presently.

After the chylomicrons have been cleared from the blood there is still lipid in the blood in the form of what are called *lipoproteins*. These are complex particles believed to be produced in the liver, in part from lipid obtained from chylomicrons absorbed by that organ. The lipoproteins serve as a source of fatty acids for cells; these are obtained locally by cells because of the local action of lipoprotein lipase on the lipoproteins that are brought to cells via the capillaries.

The Synthesis of Triglycerides in Fat Cells From the Fatty Acids of the Chylomicrons and Lipoproteins of the Blood. Most of the lipid in fat cells is derived from this source, as follows: Under the action of lipoprotein lipase, free fatty acids are released from the chylomicrons or lipoproteins of blood and pass into the cells of adipose tissue. Within the fat cells the fatty acids are rapidly reconverted into triglycerides by means of a coupling reaction involving glycerol-phosphate and this substance is available only from the metabolism of glucose that is occurring in the fat cell. The glycerol released from the breakdown of the triglycerides that come to the cell cannot be recombined with the fatty acids because adipose tissue lacks the enzyme (glycerol kinase) that would be essential for this to happen; hence, the glycerol-phosphate required for producing triglycerides within fat cells is dependent on carbohydrate being metabolized in the same cell. The new fat commonly appears in the form of very tiny droplets that resemble chylomicrons but are not ensheathed with a protein coat, but instead with an electron-dense single-layer limiting membrane. They are called liposomes (Fig. 9-14). The liposomes fuse with one another to form a single droplet. Sometimes the newly formed fat is synthesized so close to the main droplet of fat that it does not have to move to it in the form of liposomes.

Fates of Carbohydrate and Protein in the Diet. In the intestine carbohydrates are broken down by enzymes to monosaccharides and proteins are broken down to amino acids. These products are absorbed through the epithelial cells of the intestine and reach the blood circulation and they too (particularly glucose) can serve as building blocks for fat. Both glucose and amino acids pass through the cell membranes of fat cells by means of specific transport mechanisms.

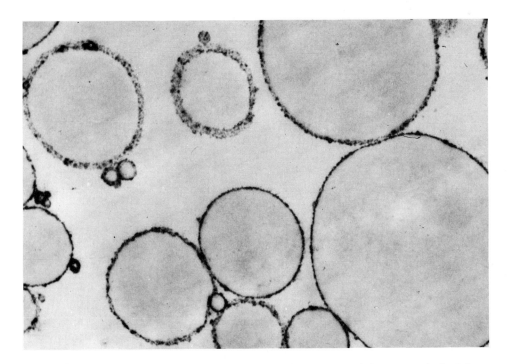

Fig. 9-14. Electron micrograph ($\times$ 22,000) of a preparation of a homogenate obtained from free adipose cells, fixed in osmium tetroxide for 2 hours. The droplets vary in size from about 0.5 μ to 2.5 μ and are termed liposomes. They resemble chylomicrons. Their role is discussed in the text. (Angel, A., and Sheldon, H.: Ann. N.Y. Acad. Sci., *131*:157, 1965)

The Formation of Fat From Glucose or Amino Acids. As was mentioned in Chapter 5 in connection with mitochondria, glucose is broken down in the cytoplasmic matrix by a series of reactions termed glycolysis and the products of this are oxidized by enzymes within the mitochondria to provide most of the energy required by the cell. However, certain of the products of the breakdown of both glucose and amino acids that occur in the cytoplasmic matrix can be converted to long chain fatty acids which, as has already been explained, are combined with newly synthesized glycerol-phosphate to become triglycerides.

How Fat Is Broken Down in Fat Cells, With the Release of Fatty Acids Into the Bloodstream So That Other Body Cells Can Use Them for Fuel. When a person's calorie intake is restricted for any reason the energy requirements of the cells of the body are met by drawing on the food reserve that is stored in fat cells. Furthermore, under the influence of a lack or an excess of certain hormones (to be described shortly) fatty acids are released from fat cells and used for fuel. The mechanism by which fat is broken down is dependent on the action of an enzyme called *tissue lipase,* which is distinct from the lipoprotein lipase system. The tissue lipase system consists of a hormone-sensitive triglyceride lipase and a monoglyceride lipase.

Under ordinary conditions the triglyceride lipase remains dormant and must be activated before it is able to break down triglyceride molecules. This activation occurs following the interaction of a lipolytic hormone—e.g., epinephrine or norepinephrine—with its specific receptor on the cell surface. As a result of this interaction, the levels of intracellular cyclic AMP (described in Chapter 6) rise and this rise is thought to be responsible for the ultimate activation of tissue lipase. The functioning of this system breaks down the triglyceride stored in the fat globule at its surface and the fatty acids thus released either are metabolized or pass through the membrane of the fat cell to enter the circulation where they bind to albumin which acts as a carrier and they are thus transported to other cells to supply them with fuel.

EFFECTS OF CERTAIN HORMONES AND OF
NERVE STIMULATION ON ADIPOSE TISSUE

Several hormones have effects on adipose tissue. For example, the different distribution of fat in males and females suggests that sex hormones affect the site at which fat cells will develop. It is also known that hormones from the adrenal cortex can affect fat distribution. In fact many hormones either indirectly or, perhaps, directly affect adipose tissue one way or another. The two most important are *insulin* and the hormone from the adrenal medulla called *epinephrine.* The effect of the latter is mimicked by stimulation of the sympathetic fibers of the autonomic nervous system which terminate around fat cells and release the substance norepinephrine locally, as will be described later. But first we shall consider the effects of insulin.

Effects of Insulin. As will be described in detail later, the hormone insulin is produced by cells in the islets of Langerhans of the pancreas and the amount that is secreted is regulated by the amount of glucose that is present in blood. Hence, when a person eats a lot of carbohydrate it leads to more insulin being secreted into the bloodstream, whereas under conditions of fasting or a reducing diet, insulin secretion by the pancreas is greatly reduced. Insulin, in addition to other effects, greatly influences fat cells. The latter have what are termed insulin receptors on their surface membranes and when the amount of insulin in blood becomes sufficiently abundant, insulin can combine with enough of these receptors on fat cells to cause several different reactions to be triggered in fat cells which makes them synthesize and store fat. The reactions that are triggered include an increase in the uptake of glucose and the synthesis of fat from it and an increased activity of the enzyme lipoprotein lipase and hence an increased delivery into the fat cells of fatty acid from chylomicrons and lipoprotein lipid. At the same time insulin slows the mobilization of fat from fat cells by depressing the action of the enzymes concerned in breaking down the fat stored in the cell.

It is of interest that the capacity of the cells that produce insulin to respond to the increased amounts of glucose in the blood varies in people and, if these cells are overstrained by the demands for increased function, which can occur in people who have limited capacities in this regard, the cells that produce insulin may undergo degeneration. Thus people with limited capacities to produce insulin are prone to develop diabetes and should live on regulated diets if they are to avoid diminishing their limited capacity to produce insulin. It is easily understood why people with diabetes become thin, because insulin is so important in facilitating both the synthesis and storage of fat in fat cells as well as blocking its breakdown. Under conditions of a limited carbohydrate intake less insulin is produced in the body and so it is easy to understand why limiting their carbohydrate intake keeps normal people from becoming fat and why those who have cells that are competent to produce lots of insulin and who cannot resist sweets and starches become fat.

Effects of Epinephrine and Nerve Stimulation

Information about the effects of epinephrine and of stimulation of the nerves of the sympathetic division of the autonomic nervous system (to be described in Chapter 17) on adipose tissue was facilitated by the study of brown fat which was formerly termed hibernating gland because of its superficial resemblance to glandular tissue.

Brown Fat. This type of fat is characterized histologically by the fact that the fat exists as multiple droplets in the cytoplasm of its cells. Since they do not coalesce into one large droplet, this arrangement of lipid is termed "multilocular" (Fig. 9-15), in contrast to that of white fat cells, in which, since they contain a single droplet, the arrangement is unilocular. Brown adipose cells are about one tenth the size of white fat cells and differ also by having more and larger mitochondria. The larger content of mitochondria in brown fat is important in its role as a heat-producing tissue. Brown adipose tissue is commonly found in the mediastinum, along the aorta and under the skin between the scapulae. The cells in brown fat have an excellent supply of nerve fibers from the sympathetic division of the autonomic nervous system, a system which will be described in Chapter 17.

The hormone epinephrine (produced by the medulla of the adrenal gland in amounts that differ in relation to different conditions—as, for example, in emotional states), and a similar substance termed norepinephrine, which is liberated at the periphery of fat cells by the endings of those fibers of the sympathetic division of the autonomic nervous system that innervate fat tissue when these fibers are stimulated, both cause the formation of more cyclic AMP which augments the activity of tissue lipase. In connection with the arousal of hibernating animals (in which state their metabolism has been very sluggish), epinephrine and norepinephrine appear to be involved. They activate tissue lipase which causes the release of fatty acids from the stored triglycerides. Some of the fatty acids which accumulate in the fat cell affect the mitochondria in such a way as to uncouple the oxidation process from the production of ATP so that a large proportion of the energy generated appears as heat. This controlled inefficiency is a very important part of the mechanism of heat production and is a property unique to brown adipose tissue and is vital in survival of the newborn human infant and in the warming-up process of hibernating animals.

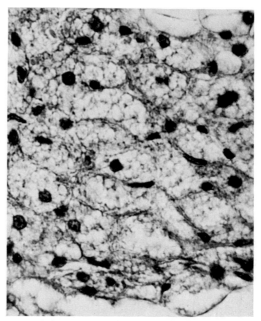

Fig. 9-15. Medium-power photomicrograph of a section cut from the brown fat of a rat. In this type of fat the nuclei of the fat cells tend to be located more centrally, and the globules of fat do not all fuse together. Therefore such cytoplasm as is present has a vacuolated appearance.

Plasma Cells and the Formation of Antibodies

Cellular Aspects of Immunology. Immunology is an exceedingly important branch of medical science. Like so many other subjects related to medicine various aspects of it extend into many other disciplines. Since this book deals with cells, tissues and organs and since immunological phenomena have their bases in cellular activities, it is within our scope to describe and discuss in some detail the cells of the body that are concerned with immunological phenomena. To avoid having information on this matter scattered, we shall try to more or less localize it by beginning here and interspersing the remainder of the material dealing with the cellular aspects of immunology in the rest of this chapter and in the chapters immediately following, which deal with blood cells and the hemopoietic tissues.

It is impossible to present meaningful information about the cells that are concerned in immunological reactions unless it is accompanied by some information about immunology in general. This will be done at more or less of an elementary level because this material is dealt with in other courses and books.

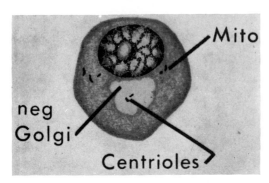

FIG. 9-16. A mature plasma cell as it appears in a stained section under oil immersion. Note the large negative Golgi; this area is sometimes crescentic. Compare Figure 9-18. (Preparation from C. P. Leblond)

The Term Immunology. The word immunity from its origin means *safe*. The study of immunity began long ago when it was observed that individuals who had recovered from an attack of any of a variety of communicable diseases were in most instances safe from ever suffering another attack of the same disease even though they were exposed to conditions similar to those in which they developed their original attack. The question arose, "Why did one attack make them safe from having a second attack?"

In due course it was established that the reason for a person developing immunity to a disease from having had an attack of it was that his blood thereafter contained antibodies which reacted specifically with the kind of disease organism that was responsible for that disease and in such a way as to render these organisms innocuous should they again enter his body.

A great deal was learned about antibodies before their cellular origin was determined. For example, it was first learned that they were of the nature of globulins, a particular type of protein found in the blood. Antibodies are now generally referred to as immunoglobulins. It was learned that they were specific for the kind of disease organism that incited their formation, and tests were devised by which the presence of different ones in blood plasma could be established. It was learned that their formation could be induced in some instances by injecting killed disease organisms, or organisms treated some other way which prevented them from propagating, into the body of an individual as *vaccines* and hence that it was possible to artificially immunize individuals against certain communicable diseases. However, all this time the cellular source of antibodies was unknown, which may seem surprising because all this time pathologists and his-

tologists were very familiar with the morphology of cells known as plasma cells and also with the fact that these cells were seen in sites which might be expected to be sites of reaction to infection, notably in the loose connective tissue that is disposed immediately beneath the wet epithelial membranes that line the intestine, and in the respiratory tract including the tonsils as well as in lymph nodes and the spleen (as will be described in following chapters). However, in 1948, Fagraeus assembled and published indirect but very convincing evidence to the effect that plasma cells were responsible for the production of antibodies. That plasma cells did indeed produce antibodies was subsequently proved by direct means in 1955 when Coons and his associates achieved this aim by means of the immunofluorescence technic, which will be described presently.

Morphology of Plasma Cells in H and E Sections. Plasma cells are easily distinguished with the LM in sections stained by ordinary methods. If they are lying free in tissue they are generally rounded (Fig. 9-16), but if they are pressed upon by other cells, their outlines may be angular (Fig. 9-17). A plasma cell has

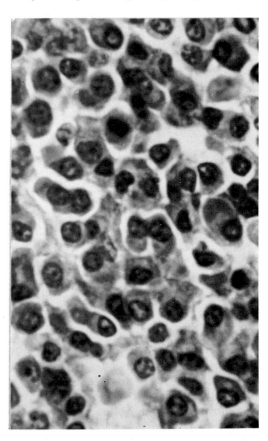

FIG. 9-17. Many plasma cells in the loose connective tissue immediately below the epithelium of a tonsil.

much cytoplasm in relation to the size of its nucleus which is commonly round and placed eccentrically (Fig. 9-16). The nuclei of some plasma cells may seem to be roughly in their centers but it must be appreciated that this appearance would be seen if a plasma cell with an eccentric nucleus was present in a section with its eccentric nucleus at its upper part. The chromatin of the nucleus is mostly condensed. Sometimes it is arranged in dense-staining flakes distributed as are the spokes of a wheel to give the nucleus a "clock-face" appearance (Fig. 9-16). The cytoplasm is generally strongly basophilic but often reveals a pale area (a negative Golgi) in the region where the centrioles and the Golgi apparatus are located (Figs. 9-16 and 9-17).

MATURE PLASMOCYTE

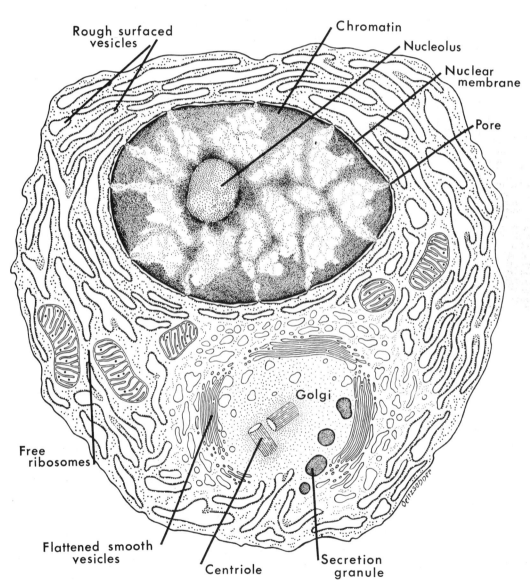

FIG. 9-18. Semidiagrammatic drawing to illustrate the fine structure of a plasma cell. The abundance of rough-surfaced vesicles of endoplasmic reticulum is characteristic and indicates the synthesis of protein destined for secretion. The extremely well developed Golgi region suggest that the secretion is delivered via this organelle. (Drawing supplied by C. P. Leblond)

The pale area sometimes is rounded with ill defined edges, but it may be crescentic, following the curved border of the nucleus but removed from it by a very short distance. A heavy content of plasma cells in loose connective tissue beneath with epithelium in a tonsil is shown in Figure 9-17. The pronounced basophilia of the cytoplasm of plasma cells is due to its great abundance of RNA.

Rounded bodies or droplets of acidophilic material are sometimes seen in mature plasma cells with the LM. These are termed Russell bodies.

The Fine Structure of Mature Plasma Cells. The plasma proteins referred to as the immunoglobulins are synthesized in and secreted by plasma cells. Hence, as might be expected, the cytoplasm of plasma cells shows a great specialization for the synthesis of a protein secretion, being replete with rough-surfaced cisternae of endoplasmic reticulum (Fig. 9-18) which may be flattened or somewhat dilated. In sections cut at appropriate angles the ribosomes on the endoplasmic reticulum can be seen to be arranged in the form of spirals; these are polyribosomal units.

The Golgi region of plasma cells is customarily large (Fig. 9-18). Centrioles are seen in this region, close to the nucleus (Fig. 9-18). The apparatus itself consists of the usual three components, flattened smooth-surfaced saccules and transfer and secretory vesicles. Immunoglobulins contain some carbohydrate; some of this is probably added to protein in the rER and the remainder is added in the Golgi. The secretory vesicles would seem to originate in the same manner as they do in the acinar cells of the pancreas; namely, secretion first accumulates at the edge of a flattened saccule so that at this site a localized expanded vesicular structure is formed which then buds off from the edge of the flattened vesicle to become a free secretory vesicle. Secretory vesicles reach and deliver their contents through the cell surface as occurs in connection with the secretion of zymogen granules (Fig. 9-18). The rounded dark bodies shown in Figure 9-18 are suggestive of secretory vesicles. These bodies are smaller than the Russell bodies which are sometimes seen in rough-surfaced vesicles of the endoplasmic reticulum. Accordingly, Russell bodies seen with the LM seem to represent abnormally large accumulations of secretion in rough-surfaced cisternae. One opinion about them is that they signify the beginning of degeneration of the plasma cell.

The other features of plasma cells, as seen with the EM, are not unusual except that the cell membrane of plasma cells often extends from the cell in fingerlike processes. The fine structure of plasma cells will be further illustrated in Chapter 13.

The immunoglobulins secreted by the plasma cells of loose connective tissue and those secreted by the plasma cells of lymphatic tissue would have to reach the bloodstream by way of lymph. Plasma cells in the spleen, as we shall learn in Chapter 13, have a more direct access to blood.

WHY PLASMA CELLS DEVELOP IN THE BODY TO SECRETE SPECIFIC ANTIBODIES IN RESPONSE TO DISEASE ORGANISMS AND OTHER FOREIGN MACROMOLECULES

What Is an Antigen? Plasma cells develop in the body in response to the entry into the body of what are termed *antigens*. There are two aspects to be considered in explaining what constitutes an antigen. First, an antigen is a protein or carbohydrate macromolecule or a small molecule known as a hapten attached to a macromolecule with a molecular weight of at least several thousand. Second, for large macromolecules to act as antigens in *any given body*, they must be different from any of the macromolecules that developed normally in that particular body and were exposed to the body fluids during embryonic and fetal life. It must be understood that as a body develops, countless different macromolecules are synthesized in it. These do not act as antigens in that body. When the work of producing a body (and all the great variety of macromolecules that are in it) is finished—and this is generally close to the time of birth—the body develops the ability to recognize further (different) macromolecules that get into it and to react to them by developing plasma cells. These foreign macromolecules are antigens and the plasma cells that develop in response to the presence of each new kind produce specific antibody that combines specifically with them. With very few exceptions, disease organisms do not gain entrance to a body until after birth, and since their macromolecules are different from those with which the body is familiar, disease organisms are regarded as antigens by the body. In addition to the antigens of viruses, bacteria, protozoa and other types of disease organisms, foreign macromolecules of certain inert materials that may gain entrance to the body—for example, dusts and pollens that somehow get through epithelial covering and lining membranes to enter the connective tissues—may also act as antigens. Furthermore, certain chemical substances—for example, certain drugs—that are absorbed in a normal way by the body may as haptens become combined with body proteins to constitute macromolecules having configurations different from those normally present in the body and so these too become antigens and incite the formation of antibodies.

Plasma cells are responsible for producing antibodies that circulate in the blood; these antibodies are termed *humoral* antibodies (*humoral* means liquid). There is, however, another kind of cellular mechanism concerned in immunity that does not depend primarily on humoral antibodies. This other kind (to be described in the next chapter) is seen, for example, in connection with the rejection of transplants of tissue from one person to another and is mediated not by plasma cells but by cells of another type that go directly to transplants of foreign tissue (which are antigenic), where they react with the foreign antigens of the transplant in such a way as to destroy its cells (described in the next chapter).

Natural and Acquired Immunological Tolerance. The fact that a body does not react to its own macromolecules is expressed by saying that the body has a *natural immunological tolerance* to its own macromolecules. It is obvious that the time at which macromolecules appear in the developing body is an important factor in whether or not the body will regard any given kind of macromolecules as antigenic or not. If enough *foreign* macromolecules are suitably injected into a body before birth, or in many instances immediately after birth, the body, having not yet learned to distinguish foreign macromolecules from its own macromolecules, will accept these foreign macromolecules as part of its own constitution, and as long as some of these foreign macromolecules remain in the body it does not react to them by producing plasma cells to make antibodies that would combine with them. In such an instance a body is said to have *acquired immunological tolerance* to these particular foreign macromolecules. If, however, the foreign macromolecules do not persist, the body will regain its ability to react immunologically to them on another encounter with them.

One of the reasons for it being possible to induce tolerance to an antigen so readily just before or after birth has become apparent from attempts to produce tolerance to antigens in later postnatal life. Here it was found that the amount of antigen in relation to the number of body cells that could react to the antigen being tested was important. If the amount of antigen was very great in relation to the number of cells that could react, the result tended to be tolerance; if the amount of antigen was small in relation to the number of reactive cells, an immunological response occurred. Hence one of the reasons for it being possible to induce tolerance so readily just before or after birth is that the number of cells in the body at that time that can

react to a specific antigen is very small for reasons that will be explained when we consider the thymus gland in a subsequent chapter.

So there are three aspects to be considered with regard to a particular body regarding anything as an antigen and reacting to it. First, it must be in the form of a macromolecule of a certain size. Second, it must be of a different chemical structure from all other macromolecules that are present in a body up to the time of birth, or very shortly after the time of birth. Third, its concentration must not be too high relative to the number of host cells capable of reacting with it.

At this point the interested student might wonder what would happen if some disease organism that was not very virulent managed to gain entrance to an embryo or fetus so that the offspring when born was tolerant to the antigens of this organism. There are some examples of this happening, for there are a few examples of animals being born with disease organisms with which they had become infected in prenatal life, and to which they remained immunologically tolerant. An interesting one is lymphocytic choriomeningitis in mice. Mice born with the virus responsible for this condition do not react to the virus later in life; and since the virus is not very virulent, the mice ordinarily lead lives in a seemingly good state of health. But if mice that were free of this virus in prenatal life and are, therefore, not tolerant to it, are injected with it (in the brain) when they are adults, they have a profound reaction to the virus and die, presumably as a result of the body's recognizing the virus as a disease agent and reacting against it. It would seem that in this instance (which is a great exception) the operation of the defense mechanisms of the body against infection do much more damage than the disease agent would have caused had it not been recognized as being antigenic.

HOW IT WAS ESTABLISHED THAT PLASMA CELLS PRODUCE ANTIBODIES

The technic by which this was done is termed the immunofluorescence technic and it has subsequently been used for so many purposes it requires description.

Fluorescence Microscopy

The wavelength of ultraviolet light or of x-rays is too short to register on the eye as light. However, certain unique substances are fluorescent in that they have the property of giving off visible light (light of a longer wavelength) when they are exposed to ultraviolet light or even to x-rays. This is taken advantage of in the technic known as fluorescence microscopy. Its use for studying plasma cells and antibodies hinges on certain fluorescent dyes being used to combine selectively with certain specific body components so that these can be identified in sections exposed to ultraviolet light because they fluoresce.

The Immunofluorescent Sandwich Technic. If a particular antigen is injected into an animal every few days over a certain period of time, the animal produces increasing amounts of a specific antibody to the injected antigen, and blood collected at a suitable time after the injections have ceased will contain a high titer of antibody to this antigen. Antibody can be separated from the rest of the blood in a reasonably concentrated state. It can then be conjugated with a fluorescent dye.

Next, to locate the particular cells that produced the antibody, the animal is killed and sections are prepared from pieces of tissue taken from its various parts and fixed in a special manner. Frozen or paraffin sections can be used (*see* Sainte-Marie). Sections containing the antibody-forming cells (Fig. 9-19, *top*) are flooded with the antigen used to induce the formation of antibody (Fig. 9-19, *center*). Since antibody is still in the cells that were producing it and since it has an affinity for the specific antigen with which the sections are flooded, the antigen adheres to those cells that were making the specific antibody (Fig. 9-19, *center*). The sections are then washed to remove antigen that has *not* combined with antibody. The sections are then flooded with some of the antibody that was conjugated with a fluorescent dye and this fluorescent antibody in

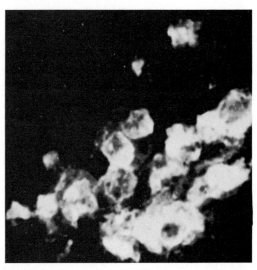

FIG. 9-19A. High-power photomicrograph (taken with a dark-field condenser) of a section of a kidney of a hamster that was infected at birth with polyoma virus. The section was treated with antibody that was prepared by injecting polyoma virus into a rabbit. The antibody to polyoma virus was then conjugated with a fluorescent dye. Since the fluorescent antibody combines specifically with polyoma virus, the cells that contain virus fluoresce under ultraviolet light and appear white against a dark background of cells that do not contain virus and hence do not attach fluorescent dye.

turn sticks to the antigen that has adhered to the cells that were producing the antibody to this antigen (see bottom illustration, Fig. 9-19). In the fluorescence microscope the cells that have fluorescent antibody attached to them (these are the cells that originally made the antibody) can be identified (Fig. 13-15, *left, right*). This is referred to as the sandwich technic because it necessitates making a sandwich with a layer of antigen between two layers of antibody. By using it, Coons and his associates showed in 1955 that antibody produced in response to a specific antigen appeared in the cytoplasm of plasma cells.

Equipment Required for Fluorescence Microscopy. The wavelengths in the ultraviolet spectrum that are used for illumination in fluorescence microscopy are generally long enough to pass through the glass lenses of an ordinary condenser in appreciable amounts; hence a condenser of the ordinary dark-field type generally is employed which allows fluorescent sites to be seen easily against a dark background (Fig. 9-19A). Since light of relatively long wavelengths in the ultraviolet spectrum is employed, some of it, after passing through the nonfluorescing parts of the sec-

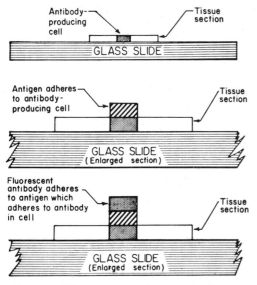

FIG. 9-19. Diagram representing steps in the sandwich technic. Sizes of objects illustrated are of course greatly out of proportion.

tion, may continue on through the glass lenses of the objectives and eyepieces. Accordingly, *to prevent injury to the eyes from this invisible light,* filters that exclude ultraviolet rays but permit the passage of light in the visible spectrum must be inserted in the eyepiece for inspecting sections. Moreover, a filter that excludes ultraviolet light but permits the passage of visible light must also be used in the eyepiece for photographing sites of fluorescence in sections; otherwise, enough ultraviolet light may pass through the nonfluorescing parts of the section to fog the photographic film.

THE ORIGIN OF PLASMA CELLS

As previously noted, the plasma cells of loose connective tissue do not develop from the original mesenchyme of the part of the body in which they subsequently appear. They arise from a type of blood cell termed B lymphocytes that enter that part of the body where they form (which is mostly in lymph nodes and spleen) from the bloodstream. The factors and processes involved will be described in succeeding chapters.

Mast Cells: Their Relation to Heparin, Histamine, Anaphylaxis and Allergies

The word *mast* from its derivation relates to feeding and was applied by Ehrlich in 1879 to certain cells that he thought were overnourished kinds of connective tissue cells because they were large and stuffed with granules (Fig. 9-20). The granules, however, do not show up well in H and E sections, so the numbers of mast cells, as seen in routine sections of connective tissue, may be underestimated. The easiest way to see mast cells in abundance is to inject some methylene blue into the loose connective tissue or adipose tissue of a rodent and then make a whole mount of some of the teased injected tissue. In this, many large mast cells will be seen lying along blood vessels and in other sites, as is shown in Figure 9-20, *left*. Under higher power the mast cells are seen to be blue because they

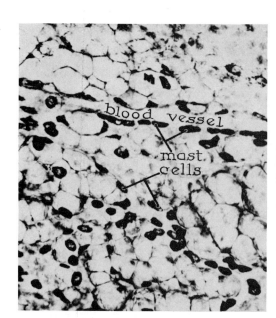 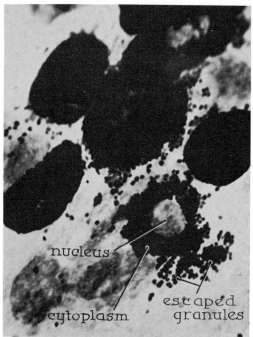

FIG. 9-20. (*Left*) Low-power photomicrograph of a spread of fat tissue (from a rat) containing a blood vessel. It was stained lightly with methylene blue. At this magnification the mast cells show as dark-blue blotches. It is to be observed that many of them are distributed along the blood vessel, which courses across the tissue. (*Right*) Oil-immersion photomicrograph of a spread of areolar tissue (from a rat) stained with methylene blue. Several dark-stained mast cells may be seen. Granules are so densely packed in most that no details can be seen. However, the lowermost one is broken up, and some of its granules can be seen to have escaped into the adjacent area. Its nucleus is also apparent.

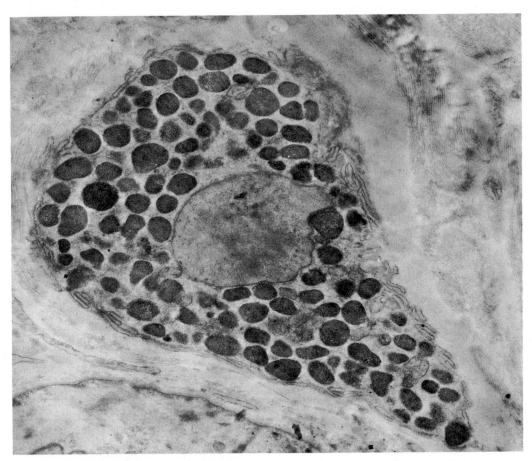

Fig. 9-21. Electron micrograph ($\times$ 12,000) of a mast cell in a section of a rat's tongue. The cytoplasm is well filled with specific granules. (Fernando, N. V. P., and Movat, H. Z.: Exp. Mol. Path., *2*:450)

are stuffed with blue-staining granules. In such a preparation, the cells are often ruptured, and so granules are strewn about (Fig. 9-20, *right*).

In whole mounts the nuclei of the cells may be difficult to see because whole cells are present and the nuclei are, of course, covered with the cytoplasmic granules. However, nuclei can be seen in sections (Fig. 9-21).

Since mast cells are so common and so large and so easily demonstrated in the rat, there is danger of thinking that the mast cells of other species are as large, of the same shape and as numerous. The shape of mast cells varies with different species, and it may even vary within the same species. In the skin of man, mast cells may be rounded or spindle shaped, and their granules are relatively small.

The granules of mast cells are known to contain two substances of physiological and pharmacological interest: (1) heparin and (2) histamine. In some spe-

cies (rat and mouse) they contain a third substance, serotonin. Before discussing the fine structure of mast cells we shall comment on heparin.

Heparin. About 50 years ago it was discovered that extracts of liver would keep blood from clotting. The active principle in such extracts was called *heparin* (*hepar*, liver). Subsequently it was found that heparin can be extracted from many different organs and tissues and that the relative amount in different organs and tissues varies considerably with regard to species.

Since many deaths are caused by thrombosis (thrombosis is caused by platelets aggregating and blood clotting so that they block the lumen of a blood vessel, as will be described in the following chapter), the discovery of heparin aroused hopes that it might find a role in preventing thrombosis—and, indeed, this hope was realized; for it was shown that, in addition to preventing clotting, it also helps to keep platelets from agglutinating.

The administration of heparin to individuals threatened with fatal thrombosis has saved many lives. It also introduced the era of blood-vessel surgery, for operations on blood vessels involve a great risk of thrombi forming. Other anticoagulants also are now available.

Heparin Found To Be a Sulfated Mucopolysaccharide. As already mentioned, mucopolysaccharides stain metachromatically. In the late 30's Jorpes found that heparin was metachromatic and it became known that heparin is a *sulfated mucopolysaccharide*. Since the cytoplasmic granules of mast cells were by this time also known to be metachromatic, they soon were suspected of being the source of the heparin that could be extracted from tissues. It was soon shown that the amount of heparin that could be extracted from an organ or tissue was related to the number of mast cells it contained and so, as matters turned out, heparin extracted from liver was found to be not a product of liver cells themselves but of the mast cells that lie in the connective tissue component of the liver.

Next, there was much suspicion to the effect that mast cells did not synthesize sulfated mucopolysaccharide but phagocytosed it from the intercellular substance of loose connective tissue in which they resided. However, two solid pieces of evidence soon indicated that mast cells actually produce the heparin they contain. The first came from the study of mast cell tumors, which are not uncommon in dogs. Bits of mast cell tumors have been grown in tissue cultures and transferred from one culture to another many times, and all the while the cells of the tumors continued to produce heparin. The second type of evidence has come from radioautographic studies in which radioactive sulfur given to animals was shown to be taken up very quickly by mast cells, an indication that the mast cell itself is the site where the precursor sulfur becomes integrated into macromolecules of sulfated mucopolysaccharide.

Possible Normal Functions of the Heparin in the Granules of Mast Cells. It is somewhat surprising that, from the evidence that is available, there is no indication that heparin normally plays a role in keeping blood from clotting in the vascular system. It has not been possible to demonstrate enough heparin in the blood of normal people to suggest that it serves any normal function in this respect. It therefore becomes a problem to know what purpose mast cells serve in producing heparin. Two possibilities may be considered.

First, it might be thought that mast cells secrete the sulfated mucopolysaccharide that is a normal component of ground substance. But this differs chemically from heparin, so the evidence does not suggest that mast cells have anything to do with the formation of intercellular substance.

Second, it has been shown that injecting heparin into the bloodstream causes the fat that is in the form of chylomicrons (which, when numerous enough, can make plasma milky) to be quickly dissipated so that the plasma becomes clear. Hence, heparin is said to have a *clearing action* on blood plasma. Subsequent work has shown that an enzyme is responsible for breaking down chylomicrons in plasma; this has been called *lipoprotein lipase,* an enzyme described under adipose tissue. Heparin is closely related to this enzyme in some manner not yet thoroughly understood. It may activate lipoprotein lipase, stimulate its production, or act as a cofactor with it, and it is not improbable that at least some of the components of heparin enter into the formation of the enzyme. Since the operation of this enzyme along capillaries, particularly in some parts of the body, is a normal function, and since heparin seems to be required for the production or function of this enzyme, perhaps a normal function for the heparin secreted by mast cells may be to participate in the production or functioning of lipoprotein lipase.

Fine Structure of Mast Cells. The nuclei of mast cells are generally centrally disposed and are not unusual in any respect (Fig. 9-21). The main feature of the cytoplasm is its great content of large granules, around 0.5 μ in diameter, each of which is enclosed by a membrane. The granules vary from being solid and dense to being less electron dense and having a finely granular texture (Fig. 9-22). The endoplasmic reticulum is not very prominent in mast cells but the Golgi is well developed (Fig. 9-22, *left*). Secretory vesicles containing electron-dense material can be seen budding off from Golgi saccules so that it would seem that the Golgi plays the chief role in the synthesis of the sulfated mucopolysaccharide. The mitochondria of mast cells are relatively inconspicuous (Fig. 9-22).

The Relation of Mast Cells to Histamine, Anaphylaxis and Allergy

Immunology was born, as already noted, when it was observed that those who recovered from certain infectious diseases were immune from further attacks of the same disease. In due course vaccines were made from the causative organisms, modified in some way (but not enough to prevent the vaccine from being antigenic) and given to people *before* they were exposed to the disease in order to immunize them so that they would not develop the disease when they

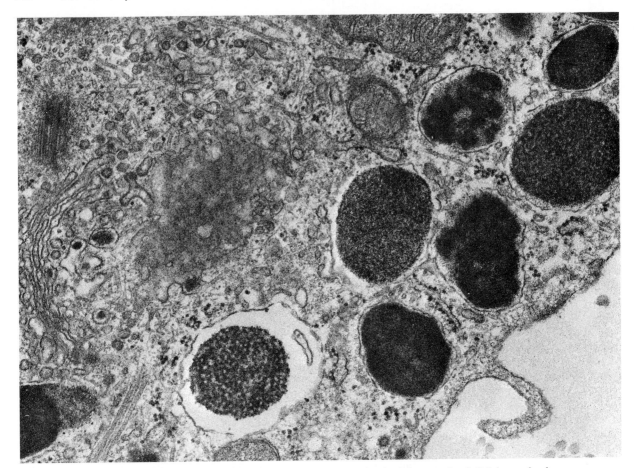

Fig. 9-22. Electron micrograph of part of a mast cell. At the left a stack of Golgi saccules is present and above it a centriole can be seen. At the right of the Golgi stack some small granules enclosed by membranes can be seen. Farther right and below there are typical large mast cell granules each enclosed by a membrane from which the granule in most instances seems to have shrunken away so as to leave a space between it and its surrounding membrane. One mitochondrion and parts of two others can be seen; these are lighter than the granules and show cristae. A little rER and some free ribosomes are scattered about. Note a microvillus. (Micrograph courtesy of C. P. Leblond)

were exposed to it. As we all know, this approach has been successful in many instances. Procedures such as this that are designed to *prevent disease* are said to be *prophylactic* (the word from its origin means "to be on guard").

Late in the last century, however, it was found that the second injection of an antigen given to an animal sometimes had a deleterious effect, and indeed it could be fatal. Richet in 1893 gave a name to the phenomenon that was observed; he termed it *anaphylaxis* because he thought it was the opposite of prophylaxis. Actually it turned out that the individual is put very much "on guard" by the first injection.

Anaphylaxis is easily demonstrated in guinea pigs. If a guinea pig is injected with a suitable antigen and then after 10 to 14 days is injected with a second dose of the same antigen, the guinea pig goes into anaphylactic shock. It manifests difficulty in breathing and a rapid pulse rate and it may die from an inability to breathe. The reason for its respiratory failure is that the smooth muscle cells that encircle the tubes through which it draws air into the lungs become contracted to such an extent that the lumens of these tubes become too narrow to permit air to enter and, in particular, to leave the lungs.

Another effect observed in anaphylactic phenomena

is that blood capillaries become dilated, congested and leaky, so that plasma escapes from them. This can give rise (in man) to blebs of plasma forming from the capillaries of the loose connective tissue directly under the epithelium of the skin.

Attempts to determine why smooth muscle cells in the bronchioles of the lung should contract and why capillaries should leak after a second injection of an antigen were greatly facilitated by the discovery, around 1914, that most of the events noticed in anaphylaxis could be duplicated in guinea pigs by giving them a substance that had just been discovered, called *histamine*. Histamine, a base derived from the amino acid histidine, exerts a profound effect on most smooth muscle, causing it to contract; in most species it also causes blood capillaries to dilate and leak plasma. It has other deleterious effects.

Relation of Histamine to Mast Cells. In 1955, West and Riley introduced the concept of mast cells containing histamine as well as heparin. Many of the same kinds of experiments were done with histamine as had been done with heparin, to show that mast cells are the chief repositories of histamine in tissue. For example, Riley and West found that there was a correlation between the histamine content and the mast cell content of various tissues in various animals. By means of certain procedures it became possible to separate fractions from mast cells that contained the granules, and these were shown to contain histamine. Certain chemicals which can be injected into animals to cause the liberation of histamine became available, and it was found that giving these caused mast cells to more or less disintegrate and liberate their granules into the tissues. As proof that the histamine in them was not absorbed, it was shown that mast cells have enzymes that would be involved in producing histamine from its precursor, and that the content of histamine in the cells of mast cell tumors that were transferred many times became increased, instead of becoming decreased, as it would if mast cells did not synthesize the histamine that they contain.

Relation of Histamine Release to Antigens and Antibodies. From the knowledge available it therefore seemed most probable that giving a guinea pig a properly timed second dose of the same antigen somehow caused its mast cells to release histamine which in turn caused the symptoms and signs of anaphylaxis (Fig. 9-23). This came to be explained as follows: the first dose of antigen given the animal incited the formation of specific antibodies to that antigen. Next, some of the antibodies thus formed became attached to cells and, in particular, to the mast cells of the animal. Then, when the second dose of antigen was given

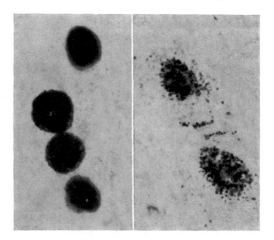

FIG. 9-23. Mast cells from a rat (*left*) before and (*right*) after an antigen-antibody reaction. Toluidine blue stain. Note that the mast cells on the right are disrupted and their granules scattered. The process is accompanied by the release of histamine. (Humphrey, J. H., and White, R. G.: Immunology for Medical Students. Oxford, England, Blackwell, 1963)

and circulated in the blood, it quickly contacted the specific antibody on the mast cells and there formed an antigen-antibody complex. Antigen-antibody complexes seem to have some curious effects in the body; in any event, those that form on mast cells cause the cells to release their granules (Fig. 9-23), and, since these contain histamine, the signs of anaphylaxis are produced. (It should be noted here that species differ and that other substances in addition to histamine are probably also released in many and from platelets as well as from mast cells.)

True anaphylaxis sometimes occurs in man and it has accounted for a fair number of deaths. It has occurred chiefly in persons who were sensitized by an earlier dose being given a second injection of some substance, two successive doses of which would not disturb most people. Sometimes people do not know or remember that they have had an injection of this substance or other effective contact with it before; hence, the physician carefully watches individuals who, for example, are given injections of penicillin or tetanus antitoxin, for if they begin to develop anaphylactic shock *very* prompt treatment is essential.

Allergy. All of us absorb some macromolecules that could serve as antigens through little breaks in the epithelium of our respiratory tracts or intestines. Pollens, dusts and so on, absorbed this way, can act as antigens and incite the formation of specific antibodies, with the result that subsequent absorption of these antigens may set off antigen-antibody reactions.

Those people who react to antigens absorbed into the body in normal life by manifesting reactions to them are said to be *sensitive* to these antigens, or *allergic* to them, and in general such people are said to be *hypersensitive*. Hay fever is a common manifestation of an allergy; people who suffer from hay fever are commonly sensitive to the pollen from ragweed, which is prevalent in the air at the time of year when hay is cut. There are literally hundreds of possible allergy-causing antigens to which people may be exposed in everyday life.

Allergic disease, which affects one of every five persons, is now known to be mediated by one class of antibody, the immunoglobulin IgE (there are other classes, as will be described in Chapter 13). IgE is produced in response to certain antigens that enter the body and are called allergens. Plasma cells which produce IgE specifically are found mainly beneath the wet epithelial linings of the respiratory and gastrointestinal tracts through whose linings the antigens gain entrance to the underlying loose connective tissue.

While much remains to be learned about the mechanism of allergic disease, it is known that mast cells (and the basophils of blood, which will be described later) have a high affinity for IgE antibodies. This type of antibody becomes attached to the surface of mast cells in such a way as to leave the antigen combining sites of the antibody exposed, so that if the proper antigen in due course enters the body, it can readily react with these sites. The combination between the antigen and IgE antibody that is bound to the cells triggers the release of histamine and other chemical mediators of the allergic response, producing the familiar symptoms of allergic disease. The symptoms depend upon the part of the body involved.

In general *antihistamines* do not act by preventing histamine from being liberated from mast cells but instead they seem to act by occupying the receptor sites for histamine on cells that would ordinarily respond to it, so that histamine that is liberated from mast or other cells is prevented from having as great an effect on cells that would ordinarily respond to it as it would if the antihistamine were not there.

The treatment of allergies by lengthy desensitization procedures is based at least partly on the concept that if very minute and then gradually increasing doses of the antigens to which they are allergic are very cautiously injected into patients, they will eventually produce an increasingly higher percentage of another class of antibody (IgG—to be described in Chapter 13) in relation to IgE antibody. The IgG class of antibody is the type most commonly produced during any sustained immunization procedure and it

does not stick to the surface of mast cells or basophils. Therefore, it cannot cause the release of histamine. However, it can compete with IgE antibody for antigens and thus block the reaction of IgE antibody with the allergen. When the hypersensitive individuals are producing enough blocking antibody, it combines with the minute quantities of antigen they absorb from the outside world so that these never reach and react with the IgE antibody that is present on their mast cells and basophils. The release of histamine and the consequent allergic symptoms may in this way be prevented.

The question arises as to why some people are hypersensitive to antigens which do not cause difficulty in other people. There is probably a genetic basis for this state of affairs but its mechanism is still not clear. It may be that certain individuals inherit the tendency to make more IgE antibody than others (and indeed the level of circulating IgE antibody is higher in hypersensitive than in normal individuals), or these people inherit the tendency to respond to certain antigens that happen to be allergenic. Perhaps both occur. Certain other cells beside mast cells may contain some histamine; in particular, the blood platelets of some species contain appreciable amounts of it. At least in some species mast cells may contain other substances which on being released act something like histamine. One of these is serotonin; this acts like histamine in many respects but differently in others. It is found in the mast cells of some species (not in man) but is more usually a constituent of blood platelets. Its release from platelets can be triggered by antigen reacting with antibody on the platelets.

ORIGIN AND MAINTENANCE OF THE MAST CELL POPULATION

Mitotic figures are not commonly seen in mast cells; however, Walker has shown that DNA duplication occurs in their nuclei, and so perhaps mitosis, when it occurs, is obscured by their granules. There is normally a very slow turnover of the mast cell population. Whether any stem cell assists in maintaining their population is not known.

Macrophages

The concept of phagocytosis (Fig. 5-7) was first elaborated by Metchnikoff, a Russian zoologist and anatomist. In 1882 he pushed some rose thorns through the skin of some transplant starfish larvae and followed the course of events with his microscope, and microscopes at that time were far from perfect. He found that on the second day certain mobile cells had gathered around the foreign material. Subsequently it was shown that comparable cells in vertebrates could phagocytose and digest foreign material. It was found that a special kind of cell that lived in loose connective tissue could perform this particular kind of phagocytic function. Different names were given to it—clasmatocyte, histiocyte and macrophage. The latter term, which means "big eater," is the most widely used. Macrophages are not the only kind of phagocytes; in the next chapter we shall describe the "little eaters" (microphage was the early name given to the blood cell now known as a polymorph).

Morphology. Macrophages that are relatively free and active tend to assume an oval shape, like those illustrated in Figure 9-24. The shape of older ones will be described under Fine Structure. When they are compressed by other tissue elements and resting, they may be elongated and have angular contours, which is probably the reason for macrophages having been given different names. In oval macrophages the nucleus is commonly disposed toward one end. The nucleus itself is generally in the form of an indented oval with its convex aspect directed toward the end of the cell closest to it. The chromatin of the nucleus is more condensed than that of the nucleus of a fibroblast and less condensed than that of a plasma cell. The nucleus as a whole is smaller than that of a fibroblast but somewhat larger than that of a plasma cell.

The Vital Staining of Macrophages. The identification of macrophages under experimental conditions was greatly facilitated by the development of vital staining. As the name implies, this term refers to a method whereby cells are stained during life because of their possessing some particular vital activity which causes them and not other cells to selectively take up a stain and not be destroyed in the process.

That it was possible to identify certain types of phagocytic cells by this method was shown shortly after the turn of this century and in the next few decades the method became highly developed, in particular by Aschoff, a famous German pathologist. The dye that was first found to be phagocytosed when it was injected into the body was lithium carmine. However, several other dyes were found to act in a similar way and produce better results than the one first used. Trypan blue is perhaps the most used and, as is shown in Figure 9-24, it is phagocytosed by macrophages and thereafter appears in their cytoplasm as a blue material. The dyes that act as vital stains are colloidal and it is because of their macromolecules that they are phagocytosed. Colloidal particles in suspension

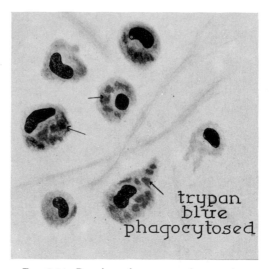

Fig. 9-24. Drawing of a group of macrophages (under oil immersion) which have phagocytosed trypan blue in an area of loose connective tissue into which trypan blue and some bacteria were injected. Observe that the nuclei of macrophages tend to be indented, smaller and more deeply stained than those of fibroblasts.

are also used as vital stains; for example, colloidal silver is phagocytosed by macrophages, as are the particles of india ink which is also much used for vital staining.

The Reticuloendothelial or Macrophage System. When vital stains are injected locally into loose connective tissue they are taken up mostly by local macrophages; this was what was done to provide Figure 9-24. However, if given intravenously (or into the peritoneal cavity), the vital dye is carried by the blood all over the body. When this is done, as Aschoff showed some decades ago, cells with a function similar to that of the macrophages of loose connective tissue were found in great numbers, particularly in the spleen, liver, bone marrow and lymph nodes. Accordingly, Aschoff conceived of a system of cells in the body that have the same particular type of phagocytic function. He called it the reticuloendothelial system. The reason for the "endothelial" part of the name seems to have been that in the liver, spleen and bone marrow the counterparts of the blood capillaries present in most tissues are wider channels called sinusoids, and observations with the LM seemed to show that the cells that lined sinusoids were not the same as the endothelial cells that line ordinary blood capillaries because they seemed to be much more phagocytic with regard to vital dyes than ordinary endothelium. However, on being studied with the EM, the sinusoids of the bone marrow and spleen have been shown to be lined by cells that are probably no more phagocytic than ordinary endothelium, but they are associated so closely with macrophages that are just outside their walls and often project between them into the sinusoids that it is easy to see how the impression that the lining cells themselves were phagocytic arose when only the LM was available. Even so, the phagocytic cells of the spleen, liver and bone marrow manage to rid the blood of a great deal of debris that would otherwise accumulate in the vascular system; this debris is derived mostly from the cells of the blood which, having only a limited life span, begin to disintegrate, and this is when they are normally phagocytosed.

The reason for the "reticulo" part of the name for the system was that in all these organs Aschoff found the phagocytic cells to be intimately associated with reticular fibers. It is generally believed that these are produced by cells that are commonly associated with the phagocytic cells and have cytoplasm that is often spread out over the reticular fibers they are believed to produce. Cells of the latter type are commonly termed reticular cells. Whether or not these are of the same cell lineage as macrophages will be discussed later. However, it is usual to include reticular cells along with macrophages as part of the reticuloendothelial system.

Another Function in Addition to Phagocytosis. Over the last decade it has become increasingly apparent that cells of the reticuloendothelial system may serve a role in the complicated process whereby an antigen that gains entrance to the body induces a particular lymphocyte to become a plasma cell and produce specific antibody against that antigen. This matter will be considered in Chapter 13.

Foreign Body Giant Cells. Any particles or masses of foreign material in loose connective tissue that are too large to be phagocytosed by individual macrophages may incite the formation of foreign body giant cells. These are very large and contain from two to a great many nuclei (Fig. 9-25). They originate from the fusion of monocytes or macrophages; this has been observed in tissue cultures. Their purpose seems to be that of providing a cell large enough to enclose or wall off masses of debris that cannot be incorporated into a single phagocyte.

Giant cells of this type are common in the lesions of tuberculosis (Fig. 9-25, *left*), where they are probably incited to form because of the tubercle bacilli's causing a curious type of tissue death called *caseous necrosis*. It is very easy to produce foreign body giant

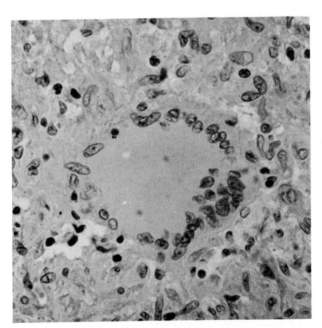 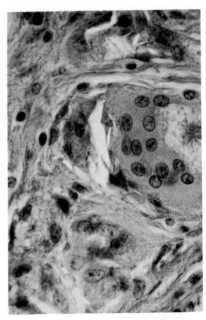

Fig. 9-25. Photomicrographs of two giant cells. The one on the left is typical of the kind that forms in sites infected with the tubercle bacillus. The one on the right, of which only a portion is shown, was present in what is termed a nonspecific granuloma. (Preparation courtesy of Dr. T. Brown)

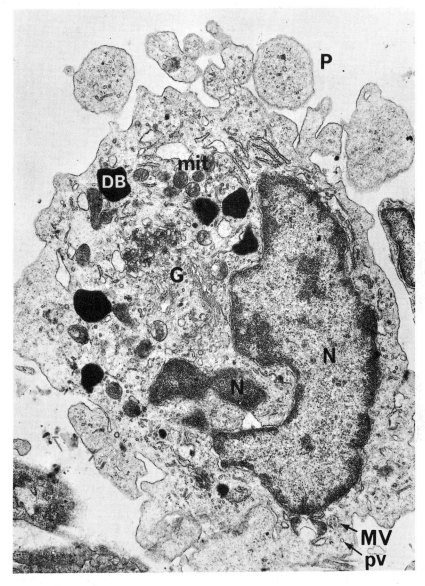

FIG. 9-26. Electron micrograph ($\times$ 8,000) of a macrophage found in connective tissue. The following structures are labeled: N, nucleus: because of irregularity of nuclear surface, the nucleus is cut in several places; P, pseudopods; Mit, mitochondria; the light space over the letter *m* may be a cross section of the groove between pseudopods; G, Golgi apparatus; DB, dense body, of which there are several; MV, multivesicular body; pv, probably a pinocytotic vesicle; many other small vesicles are seen in the cytoplasm. (Illustration courtesy of C. P. Leblond)

cells experimentally by injecting foreign material, such as agar, into the loose connective tissue; they soon form around the margins of the larger masses of injected foreign material and completely surround the smaller masses. If this procedure is performed in animals that are given vital stains such as trypan blue before the foreign material is introduced into them, the vital stain can be found later in some of the foreign body giant cells. Sometimes this leads to the assumption that foreign body giant cells themselves are phagocytic. However, if vital stains have been given, the cells that fused to form the giant cells could have accumulated vital stain in their cytoplasm before they fused. In our experience foreign body giant cells,

once they have formed, do not seem to be very active so far as further phagocytosis of vital stain is concerned. They could, of course, perform functions dependent on the action of the hydrolytic enzymes of their lysosomes.

Fine Structure. The boundaries of a free macrophage of loose connective tissue are seen with the EM to be very irregular because of numerous pseudopodia projecting from them in various directions (Fig. 9-26). Furthermore, there are invaginations of the surface membrane that may extend deeply into the cytoplasm and which, if cut in oblique or cross section, may appear as vacuoles in a thin section; there is one, for example, just above **mit** in Figure 9-26. It has

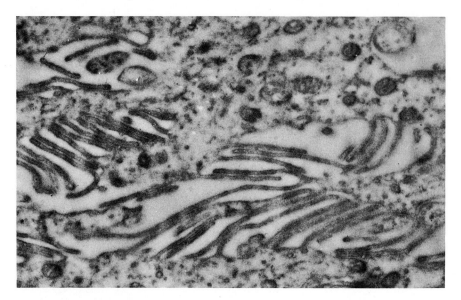

FIG. 9-27. Electron micrograph (× 24,000) of a section cut from tissue adjacent to where agar-agar had been injected into the subcutaneous tissue of a rabbit. This picture shows the cell borders of macrophages that in all probability are fusing to form a giant cell. Note the thin plate-like processes that extend from the surfaces of the macrophages, and how they interdigitate with one another. (Preparation by A. F. Howatson)

been shown that most, but not all, of these invaginations retain their connection with the cell surface. Those that do not may assume the form of closed tubules within the cytoplasm. The fact that what might appear to be a vacuole or a tubule in a section is an invagination of the cell membrane is indicated by the fact both are lined by a cell coat.

The rER is not very well developed in macrophages but the Golgi stacks are at least of moderate size (G in Fig. 9-26). Some macrophages have numerous free ribosomes, others have only a few. All contain a relative abundance of lysosomes of the types described in connection with lysosomes in Chapter 5; for example, there are dense bodies (DB) in Figure 9-26. Various types of phagosomes are often seen.

Fine Structure of Developing Foreign Body Giant Cells. From some thin sections that we have studied with the EM, there is evidence to suggest that, as a prelude to fusion, the cytoplasmic processes of adjacent macrophages may become sheetlike and interdigitate in a very extensive manner (Fig. 9-27).

Origin of Macrophages. It has generally been assumed that a normal complement of macrophages of loose connective tissue develop from the original mesenchyme in prenatal life. However, it seems improbable that these could divide to maintain the macrophage population of loose connective tissue in postnatal life. There is now evidence showing that in postnatal life the population of macrophages in loose connective tissue is maintained and, in times of need, augmented by monocytes (which are blood cells to be described in the next chapter) entering loose connective tissue and there differentiating into macrophages.

Potentialities of Macrophages. It was commonly believed in the past that macrophages (or monocytes) could develop into fibroblasts. In connection with fibroblasts evidence was cited early in this chapter that indicated this belief is no longer tenable. It therefore might be concluded that fully developed macrophages are highly specialized end-of-line cells.

Do Mesenchymal Cells of Great Potentiality Persist in the Loose Connective Tissue Throughout Postnatal Life?

Occasionally some curious things happen in loose or even in dense connective tissue which are difficult to explain. For example after an abdominal operation a piece of bone may develop in the connective tissue scar that repairs the incision. When the cell type and the nature of any tissue becomes different from that which normally exists in that part of the body, the phenomenon is called *metaplasia* (*meta* is a prefix which means, among other things, a change, and *plasia* means to form). So, for example, when bone is found in an operation scar it is said to be a result of metaplasia having occurred. Why and how does this occur? Long ago it was often assumed that one kind of tissue could actually change into another kind. But as Adami, a distinguished pathologist of many decades ago pointed out so clearly, one adult tissue never changes directly into another kind. For metaplasia to occur a new tissue must develop within the kind that previously existed in the area. This means, of course, that for metaplasia to occur, some new type of cell must have migrated into the area to form the new kind of tissue or that the local environment becomes changed in some way so that some of the pre-existing cells of the part are induced to differentiate along another pathway from that along which they differentiated before.

Several decades ago Huggins performed a most interesting experiment that showed that environmental factors could induce bone to form in ordinary connective tissue: he found that, if he transplanted some of the lining of the urinary bladder of an animal into its abdominal wall, bone would develop in the connective tissue beside it. This seems to indicate that a new environmental influence had been brought to bear on certain cells of the area which caused them to form bone instead of ordinary connective tissue of the abdominal wall. But what kind of cell of loose connective tissue could respond?

Since fibroblasts produce intercellular substance which is only somewhat different from that of bone, one view that arose, and with which we do not agree, was that a special environmental influence could induce fibroblasts to become bone-forming cells (which are called osteoblasts). However, others believed that fibroblasts are committed cells that do not possess the potentiality to become osteoblasts, and so, to explain the phenomenon, they made the very logical assumption that in any ordinary connective tissue there must be some cells that have not become committed but persist as relatively uncommitted undifferentiated mesenchymal cells possessing enough potentiality to respond under the proper circumstances to a new environmental influence by differentiating into a type of cell not normally found in that site. Huggins leans to this view to explain his results and, indeed, the concept of the persistence into postnatal life of some undifferentiated mesenchymal cells in the ordinary connective tissue, supported decades ago by Maximow, seems to be a most logical one.

As was suggested in connection with the repair of ordinary connective tissue, the cells that have the greatest potentiality for division and give rise to most of the fibroblasts that appear in a repair process seem to be cells that are closely associated with the smaller blood vessels. These are called perivascular cells. These have the capacity to form fibroblasts and it seems probable that some have the potentiality to form other types of cells that develop in mesenchyme —for example, smooth muscle cells and, under exceptional environmental changes, even osteoblasts.

There is, therefore, evidence indicating that normal loose connective tissue, in association with its smaller blood vessels, contains in postnatal life, some relatively uncommitted mesenchymal cells which, under

normal circumstances, can give rise to the normal cell types found in loose connective tissue but under unusual environmental influences can give rise to other types of cells that form in mesenchyme in other body sites. However, it should be noted that there is some evidence to the effect that certain undifferentiated free cells that circulate in blood (to be discussed in Chapter 12) may account for some of the metaplastic phenomena that occur in connective tissue; this possibility will be discussed in Chapter 15.

Immigrant Cells in Loose Connective Tissue

In the next chapter we shall deal with the white cells of the blood (leukocytes). As will be described, certain of these emigrate from blood into loose connective tissue under different conditions to serve various purposes.

References and Other Reading for Chapters 8 and 9

Fibroblasts and Collagenic, Elastic and Reticular Fibers

Asboe-Hansen, G. (ed.): Connective Tissue in Health and Disease. Copenhagen, Munksgaard, 1954.
———: Hormonal effects on connective tissue. Physiol. Rev., *38*:446, 1958.
Carneiro, J., and Leblond, C. P.: Role of osteoblasts and odontoblasts in secreting the collagen of bone and dentine as shown by radioautography in mice given tritium-labelled glycin. Exp. Cell Res., *18*:291, 1959.
Fernando, N. V. P., and Movat, H. Z.: Fibrillogenesis in regenerating tendon. Lab. Invest., *12*:214, 1963.
Fullmer, H. M.: The histochemistry of the connective tissues. Internat. Rev. Connective Tissue Res., *3*:1, 1965.
Gillman, T.: The Dermis. *In* Champion, R. H., Gillman, T., Rook, A. J., and Sims, R. T. (eds.): An Introduction to the Biology of the Skin. Oxford, Blackwell Scientific Publications, 1970.
Hodge, A. J., and Petruska, J. A.: Recent studies with the electron microscope on ordered aggregates of the tropocollagen macromolecules. *In* Aspects of Protein Structure. p. 289. New York, Academic Press, 1964.
Hodge, A. J., and Schmitt, F. O.: The tropocollagen macromolecule and its properties of ordered interaction. *In* Edds, M. V., Jr. (ed.): Macromolecular Complexes. pp. 19-51. New York, Ronald Press, 1961.
Jackson, S. F.: Connective tissue cells. *In* Brachet, J., and Mirsky, A. E. (eds.): The Cell. vol. 6, p. 387. New York, Academic Press, 1964.
Lewis, M. R.: Development of connective tissue fibers in tissue culture of chick embryos. Contrib. Embryol., *6*:45, 1917.
Maximow, A.: The development of argyrophile and collagenous fibers in tissue cultures. Proc. Soc. Exp. Biol. Med. *25*:439, 1928.

Movat, H. Z., and Fernando, N. V. P.: The fine structure of connective tissue. I. The fibroblast. Exp. Molec. Path., *1*:509, 1962.

Peacock, E. E., Jr., and Van Winkle, W., Jr.: Surgery and Biology of Wound Repair. Philadelphia, W. B. Saunders, 1970.

Porter, K. R., and Pappas, G. D.: Collagen formation of fibroblasts of the chick embryo dermis. J. Biophys. Biochem. Cytol., *5*:153, 1959.

Revel, J. P., and Hay, E. D.: An autoradiographic and electron microscopic study of collagen synthesis in differentiating cartilage. Z. Zellforsch., *61*:110, 1963.

Ross, R.: Collagen formation in healing wounds. *In* Montagna, W., and Billingham, R. E. (eds.): Advances in Biology of Skin: Wound Healing. p. 144. London, Pergamon Press, 1964.

Ross, R., Everett, N. B., and Tyler, R.: Wound healing and collagen formation. V. The origin of the wound fibroblast studied in parabiosis. J. Cell Biol., *44*:645, 1970.

Stearns, M. L.: Studies on the development of connective tissue in transparent chambers in the rabbit's ear. Am. J. Anat., *66*:133, 1939; *67*:55, 1940.

Weinstock, M., and Leblond, C. P.: Synthesis, migration and release of precursor collagen by odontoblasts as visualized by radioautography after ^{3}H-proline administration. J. Cell Biol., *60*:92, 1974.

Wolfe, J. M., Burack, E., Lansing, W., and Wright, A. W.: The effect of advancing age on the connective tissue of the uterus, cervix, and vagina of the rat. Am. J. Anat., *70*:135, 1942.

ELASTIC FIBERS

(*See also* references on Elastin in Chapter 19)

Fahrenbach, W. H., Sandberg, L. B., and Eleary, E. G.: Ultrastructural studies on early elastogenesis. Anat. Rec., *155*:563, 1966.

Greenlee, T. K., Ross, R., and Hartman, J. L.: The fine structure of elastic fibers. J. Cell Biol., *30*:59, 1966.

Hashimoto, K., and DiBella, R. J.: Electron microscopic studies of normal and abnormal elastic fibers of the skin. J. Invest. Derm., *48*:405, 1967.

Kirkaldy-Willis, W. H., Murakami, H., Emery, M. A., Mungai, J., and Shnitka, T. K.: Elastogenesis in the cranial patagium of the wing of the chick. Canad. J. Surg., *10*:348, 1967.

Low, F. W.: Microfibrils, fine filamentous components of the tissue space. Anat. Rec., *142*:131, 1962.

Ross, R., and Bernstein, P.: Elastic fibers in the body. Sci. Am., *224*:44, 1971.

Taylor, J. J., and Yeager, V. L.: The fine structure of elastin fibers in the fibrous periosteum of the rat femur. Anat. Rec., *156*:129, 1966.

GROUND SUBSTANCE AND THE AMORPHOUS INTERCELLULAR SUBSTANCES—METACHROMASIA

Bensley, S. H.: On the presence, properties and distribution of the intercellular ground substance of loose connective tissue. Anat. Rec., *60*:93, 1934.

Bergeron, J. A., and Singer, M.: Metachromasy: an experimental and theoretical re-evaluation. J. Biophys. Biochem. Cytol., *4*:433, 1958.

Chain, E., and Duthie, E. S.: Identity of hyaluronidase and the spreading factor. Brit. J. Exp. Path., *21*:324, 1940.

Curran, R. C.: The histochemistry of mucopolysaccharides. Int. Rev. Cytol., *17*:149, 1964.

Davies, D. V.: Specificity of staining methods for mucopolysaccharides of the hyaluronic acid type. Stain Techn., *27*:65, 1952.

Dempsey, E. W., Bunting, H., Singer, M., and Wislocki, G. B.: The dye-binding capacity and other chemohistological properties of mammalian mucopolysaccharides. Anat. Rec., *98*:417, 1947.

Duran-Reynals, F.: Some remarks on the spreading reaction. *In* Asboe-Hansen, G. (ed.): Connective Tissue in Health and Disease. p. 103, Copenhagen, Munksgaard, 1954.

Edds, M. V., Jr.: Origin and structure of intercellular matrix. *In* McElroy, W. D., and Glass, B. (eds.): The Chemical Basis of Development. p. 157, Baltimore, Johns Hopkins Press, 1958.

Glegg, R. E., Clermont, Y., and Leblond, C. P.: The use of lead tetraacetate, benzidine, o-dianisidine and a "film test" to investigate the significance of the "periodic acid sulfurous acid" technique in carbohydrate histochemistry. Stain Tech., *27*:277, 1952.

Glegg, R. E., Eidinger, D., and Leblond, C. P.: Some carbohydrate components of reticular fibers. Science, *118*:614, 1953.

————: Presence of carbohydrates distinct from acid mucopolysaccharides in connective tissue. Science, *120*:839, 1954.

Hale, C. W.: Histochemical demonstration of acid polysaccharides in animal tissue. Nature, *157*:802, 1946.

Hoffman, D. C., and Duran-Reynals, F.: Influence of testicle extract on intradermal spread of injected fluids and particles. J. Exp. Med., *53*:387, 1931.

Lillie, R. D.: Connective tissue staining. *In* Connective Tissues. p. 11, New York, Macy Foundation, 1952.

————: Further exploration of the H10$_4$ Schiff reaction with remarks on its significance. Anat. Rec., *108*:239, 1950.

————: Histochemistry of connective tissues. Lab. Invest., *1*:30, 1952.

McManus, J. F. A.: Histochemistry of connective tissue. *In* Asboe-Hansen, G. (ed.): Connective Tissue in Health and Disease. p. 31. Copenhagen, Munksgaard, 1954.

Mancini, R. E.: Connective tissue and serum proteins. Int. Rev. Cytol., *14*:193, 1963.

Meyer, K.: The biological significance of hyaluronic acid and hyaluronidase. Physiol. Rev., *27*:335, 1947.

————: The chemistry of the ground substances of connective tissue. *In* Asboe-Hansen, G. (ed.): Connective Tissue in Health and Disease. p. 54, Copenhagen, Munksgaard, 1954.

————: Mucoids and glycoproteins. Advances Protein Chem., *2*, 1945.

————: The chemistry of the mesodermal ground substance. Harvey Lect., Ser. 51, p. 88, 1955.

Revel, J. P.: Role of the Golgi apparatus of cartilage cells in the elaboration of matrix glycosaminoglycans. *In* Balasz, E. A. (ed.): Chemistry and Molecular Biology of the Intercellular Matrix. p. 1485, New York, Academic Press, 1970.

Sobel, H.: Ageing of the ground substance in connective tissue. Advances Geront. Res., *2*:205, 1967.

Strauss, J., and Necheles, H.: Variations in dermal absorption with age. J. Lab. Clin. Med., *33*:612, 1948.

BASEMENT MEMBRANES

Kefalides, N. A.: Chemical properties of basement membranes. Intern. Rev. Exp. Path., *10*:1, 1971.

Rambourg, A., and Leblond, C. P.: Staining of basement membranes and associated structures by the periodic acid-Schiff and periodic acid-silver methenamine techniques. J. Ultrastruct. Res., *20*:306, 1967.

Tissue Fluid, Lymph and Lymphatic Capillaries

(*See also* References for Chapters 14 and 19)

Drinker, C. K., and Field, M. E.: Lymphatics, Lymph and Tissue Fluid. Baltimore, Williams & Wilkins, 1933.

Leak, L. V.: Electron microscopic observations on lymphatic capillaries and the structural components of the connective tissue-lymph interface. Microvascular Res., *2*:391, 1970.

Pullinger, B. D., and Florey, H. W.: Some observations on the structure and function of lymphatics. Brit. J. Exp. Path., *16*:49, 1935.

————: Proliferation of lymphatics in inflammation. J. Path. Bact., *45*:157, 1937.

Rouviere, H.: Anatomy of the Human Lymphatic System. Translated by M. J. Tobias. Ann Arbor, Edwards Bros., 1938.

(*See also* textbooks of physiology and pathology.)

Blood Capillaries

References for their connections and fine structure are given in Chapter 19.

Edema

For references see textbooks of physiology, pathology and medicine.

Adipose Tissue

Angel, A., and Sheldon, H.: Adipose tissue organelles: isolation, morphology and possible relation to intracellular lipid transport. Ann. N.Y. Acad, Sci., *131*:157, 1965.

Angel, A., Desai, K., and Halperin, M. L.: Free fatty acids and ATP levels in adipocytes during lipolysis. Metabolism, *20*:87, 1971.

Clark E. R., and Clark, E. L.: Microscopic studies of the new formation of fat in living adult rabbits. Am. J. Anat., *67*:255, 1940.

Fawcett, D. W.: A comparison of the histological organization and histochemical reactions of brown fat and ordinary adipose tissue. J. Morph., *90*:363, 1952.

Hausberger, F. X.: Quantitative studies on the development of autotransplants of immature adipose tissue of fats. Anat. Rec., *122*:507, 1955.

Hayward, J. S., Lyman, C. P., and Taylor, C. R.: The possible role of brown fat as a source of heat during arousal from hibernation. Ann. N.Y. Acad. Sci., *131*:441, 1965.

Menschik, Z.: Histochemical comparison of brown and white adipose tissue in guinea pigs. Anat. Rec., *116*:439, 1953.

Napolitano, L., and Fawcett, D.: The fine structure of brown adipose tissue in the newborn mouse and rat. J. Biophys. Biochem. Cytol., *4*:685, 1958.

Napolitano, L.: The differentiation of white adipose cells. J. Cell Biol., *18*:663, 1963.

Sheldon, H.: The fine structure of adipose tissue. *In* Rodahl, K., and Issekutz, B. (eds.): Fat as a Tissue. p. 41, New York, McGraw-Hill, 1964.

Sheldon, H., and Angel, A.: Some considerations on the morphology of adipose tissue. *In* Meng, H. C. (ed.): Proc. Internat. Symp. on Lipid Transport. p. 155, Springfield, Ill., Charles C Thomas, 1964.

Sheldon, H., Hollenberg, C. H., and Winegrad, A. I.: Observations on the morphology of adipose tissue. Diabetes, *11*:378, 1962.

Sidman, R. L., and Fawcett, D. W.: The effect of peripheral nerve section on some metabolic responses of brown adipose tissue in mice. Anat. Rec., *118*:487, 1964.

Sidman, R. L., Perkins, M., and Weiner, N.: Noradrenaline and adrenaline content of adipose tissue. Nature, *193*:36, 1962.

Smith, R. E., and Hock, R. J.: Brown fat: thermogenic effector of arousal in hibernation. Science, *140*:199, 1963.

Thompson, J. F., Habeck, D. A., Nance, S. L., and Beetham, K. L.: Ultrastructural and biochemical changes in brown fat in cold exposed rats. J. Cell Biol., *41*:312, 1969.

See also References and Other Reading at the end of Chapter 5 under "Glycogen, Lipid, Pigment and Inclusions."

Plasma Cells and Immunofluorescence Technics

(*See also* References and Other Reading for Chapters 10 and 13)

Coons, A. H.: Histochemistry with labeled antibody. Int. Rev. Cytol., *5*:1, 1956.

————: Fluorescent antibody methods. *In* Danielli, J. F. (ed.): General Cytochemical Methods. pp. 399-422. New York, Academic Press, 1958.

Coons, A. H., Leduc, E. H., and Connolly, J. M.: Studies on antibody production: I. A. method for the histochemical demonstration of specific antibody and its application to a study of the hyperimmune rabbit. J. Exp. Med., *102*:49, 1955.

dePetris, S., Karlsbad, G., and Pernis, B.: Localization of antibodies in plasma cells by electron microscopy. J. Exp. Med., *117*:849, 1963.

Fagraeus, A.: Antibody production in relation to development of plasma cells; in vivo and in vitro experiments. Acta Med. Scand., *130*:3, 1948.

Humphrey, J. H., and White, R. G.: Immunology for Students of Medicine. ed. 2. Oxford, Blackwell, 1964.

Leduc, E. H., Coons, A. H., and Connolly, J. M.: Studies on antibody production: II. The primary and secondary responses in the popliteal lymph node of the rabbit. J. Exp. Med., *102*:61, 1955.

Movat, H. Z., and Fernando, N. V. P.: The fine structure of connective tissue. II. The plasma cells. Exp. Molec. Path., *1*:535, 1962.

Rifkind, R. A., Osserman, E. F., Hsu, K. C., and Morgan, C.: The intracellular distribution of gamma globulin in a mouse plasma cell tumor as revealed by fluorescence and electron microscopy. J. Exp. Med., *116*:423, 1962.

Sainte-Marie, G.: A paraffin embedding technic for studies employing immunofluorescence. J. Histochem. Cytochem., *10*:250, 1962.

————: Study on plasmocytopoiesis. I. Description of plasmocytes and of their mitoses in the mediastinal lymph nodes of ten-week-old rats. Am. J. Anat., *114*:207, 1964.

Some References on Induced Immunologic Tolerance

(*See also* references for Thymus in Chapter 13)

Billingham, R. E.: Actively acquired tolerance and its role in development. *In* McElroy, W. D., and Glass, B. (eds.): The

Chemical Basis of Development. p. 575. Baltimore, Johns Hopkins Press, 1958.

Billingham, R. E., and Brent, L.: A simple method for inducing tolerance of skin homografts in mice. Transplan. Bull., 4:67, 1957.

Billingham, R. E., Brent, L., and Medawar, P. B.: Quantitative studies on tissue transplantation immunity. III. Actively acquired tolerance. Phil. Tr. Roy. Soc. London, Ser. B., 15:357, 1956.

Billingham, R. E., Lampkin, G. H., Medawar, P. B., and Williams, H. L.: Tolerance to homografts, twin diagnosis, and the freemartin condition in cattle. Heredity, 6:201, 1952.

Burnet, Sir MacFarlane: The Clonal Selection Theory of Acquired Immunity. Nashville, Tenn., Vanderbilt University Press, and Cambridge, England, University Press, 1959.

Humphrey, J. H., and White, R. G.: Immunology for Students of Medicine. ed. 2. Oxford, Blackwell, 1964.

Medawar, P. B.: A discussion of immunological tolerance—introductory remarks. Proc. Roy. Soc., Series B, November 1956.

Owen, R. D.: Immunogenetic consequences of vascular anastomoses between bovine twins. Science, 102:400, 1945; Fed. Proc., 16:581, 1957.

Macrophages and Foreign Body Giant Cells

Clark, E. R., and Clark, E. L.: Relations on monocytes of the blood to tissue macrophages. Am. J. Anat., 46:149, 1930.

Evans, H. M.: The macrophages of mammals. Am. J. Physiol., 37:243, 1915.

Evans, H. M., and Scott, K.: On the differential reactions to vital dyes exhibited by the two great groups of connective tissue cells. Contrib. Embryol., 10:1, 1921.

Felix, M. D., and Dalton, A. J.: A comparison of mesothelial cells and macrophages in mice after the intraperitoneal inoculation of melanin granules. J. Biophys. Biochem. Cytol. (Suppl.), 2:109, 1956.

Haythorn, S. R.: Multinucleated giant cells with particular reference to the foreign body giant cell. Arch. Path. Lab. Med., 7:651, 1929.

Maximow, A.: Relation of blood cells to connective tissue and endothelium. Physiol. Rev., 4:533, 1924.

Osmond, D. G.: The origin of peritoneal macrophages from the bone marrow. Anat. Rec., 154:397, 1966.

Palade, G. E.: Relations between the endoplasmic reticulum and the plasma membrane in macrophages. Anat. Rec., 121:445, 1955.

Pearsall, N. N., and Weiser, R. S.: The Macrophage. Philadelphia, Lea and Febiger, 1970.

Sampaio, M. M.: The use of Thorotrast for the electron microscopic study of phagocytosis. Anat. Rec., 124:501, 1956.

Volkman, A., and Gowans, J. H.: The origin of macrophages from bone marrow in the rat. Brit. J. Exp. Path., 46:62, 1965.

See also References and Other Reading for Chapter 5 under "Phagocytosis, Pinocytosis and Coated Vesicles" and under "Lysosomes."

Mast Cells

(For references on heparin see textbooks of physiology)

Asboe-Hansen, G.: The mast cell. Int. Rev. Cytol., 3:399, 1954.

Bloom, F.: Spontaneous solitary and multiple mast cell tumors (mastocytomata). Arch. Path., 33:661, 1942.

Combs, J. W.: Maturation of rat mast cells. An electron microscope study. J. Cell Biol., 31:563, 1966.

Fawcett, D. W.: An experimental study of mast cell degranulation and regeneration. Anat. Rec., 121:29, 1955.

Fernando, N. V. P., and Movat, H. Z.: The fine structure of connective tissue. III. The mast cell. Exp. Molec. Path., 2:450, 1963.

Humphrey, J. H., and White, R. G.: Immunology for Students of Medicine. ed. 2. Oxford, Blackwell, 1964.

Mota, Ivan: The behaviour of mast cells in anaphylaxis. Int. Rev. Cytol., 15:363, 1963.

Padawer, J.: Studies on mammalian mast cells. Trans. N.Y. Acad. Sci., Ser. II, 19:690, 1957.

Paff, G. H., and Bloom, F.: Vacuolation and the release of heparin in mast cells cultivated in vitro. Anat. Rec., 104:45, 1949.

Paff, G. H., and Mergenthaler, D. D.: Vacuolation in normal mast cells and in mast cells treated with protamine sulfate. Anat. Rec., 121:579, 1955.

Riley, J. F.: The Mast Cells. Edinburgh, Livingstone, 1959.

Selye, H.: The Mast Cells. Washington, Butterworth, 1965.

Smith, D. E.: The tissue mast cell. Int. Rev. Cytol., 14:327, 1963.

Weinstock, A., and Albright, J. T.: The fine structure of mast cells in normal human gingiva. J. Ultrastruct. Res., 17:245, 1967.

10 *Blood Cells: Leukocytes*

Introduction. Blood cells represent a category of *free* connective tissue cells; they are free in the sense that they are not normally attached to each other or any other kinds of cells and they are not held more or less in position by intercellular substance, as are most kinds of connective tissue cells. They are formed in the hemopoietic tissues as will be described in following chapters. When they enter the bloodstream they are suspended by, and carried along in, blood plasma which is the fluid portion of blood. They are of two types—red, and white. Although fresh isolated red cells seen under the microscope are straw colored, the large numbers present in blood make it red. They are commonly called erythrocytes (*erythros,* red). White cells are called leukocytes (*leukos,* white) even though fresh ones are colorless; when they are packed together they appear white.

Erythrocytes perform their function in the blood whereas most leukocytes perform theirs only when they leave blood to enter the loose connective tissue or other tissues of the body. Thus leukocytes are blood cells chiefly in the sense that they use the blood as a means of transport, from the time they enter the bloodstream until they leave it to perform their work. We shall, therefore, consider leukocytes more or less as a continuation of the study of cells of loose connective tissue. Also, because they are involved in immunological reactions, this permits us to continue with this topic as well.

Leukocytes

Their Study in Blood Films. Blood cells are commonly studied in "blood films," also called "blood smears." They must be prepared on very clean slides.

To obtain blood for making a blood film the cleaned earlobe or finger is punctured lightly, and the first drop or two that well up are wiped away with sterile gauze. Then, a tiny drop (the first drops are too large) wells up from the puncture. Blood films (smears) are made differently in different laboratories. One way is to touch the tiny drop with one surface of a very

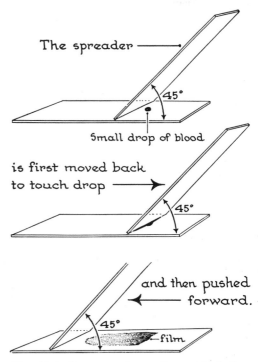

Fig. 10-1. One way of spreading a blood film.

clean slide (held by its edges and avoiding contact of the slide with the skin) so that most of the drop adheres to the slide midway between its sides and a short distance from one end (Fig. 10-1, *top*). A second very clean slide, hereafter called the spreader, is now put in the position indicated in Figure 10-1 (many consider that a spreader should be at an angle of 30° to the slide). The edge of the spreader should be pressed against the other slide, not firmly, but rather lightly. The spreader is now drawn back until the edge that is in contact with the first slide touches the drop of blood, which thereupon spreads quickly along the line of contact between the slides. The spreader is then pushed steadily forward, still without putting more than light pressure on it, and by this means the drop of blood is spread out into a thin film.

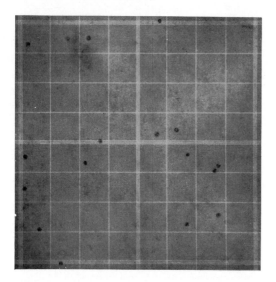

FIG. 10-2. The appearance presented by leukocytes in a counting chamber. Leukocytes are counted in representative squares enclosed by triple lines. When erythrocytes (not seen here) are counted, they are counted over the smaller squares at higher magnification. (Photomicrograph from R. Hasselback)

The angle at which the spreader is held in relation to the first slide determines to some extent the thickness of the film. The greater the angle, the thicker the film. Furthermore, a film is thicker if the spreading is done rapidly. A film is usually thicker toward the end of the slide from which the film is spread.

After a film has dried in air, it is generally stained with what is often called a "blood stain." (Glance at Fig. 10-4 to see the result.) Although there are different varieties of blood stains, each commonly exists as a single solution. Enough blood stain is added to a slide to cover the film, and then after a very short time twice as much distilled water, adjusted to a pH 6.4 to 6.6 with a phosphate buffer, is added to dilute the stain. After the diluted solution has been allowed to act for a few minutes, the slide is rinsed in tap water and dried in air. Then it can be studied with the oil-immersion objective, through oil, either with or without a coverslip.

Development of Blood Stains. In 1891 Romanovsky tried the effect of mixing an acid stain (eosin) with a basic stain (methylene blue). Curiously enough, the mixture acted as a better stain for blood than if the ingredients were applied separately. With it he was able to stain malarial parasites inside red blood cells (a great help in diagnosing malaria); indeed, one part of the parasite was colored a violet shade, which could

not be attributed directly to eosin or methylene blue. Another dye seemed to have been produced. Then Unna found if he treated methylene blue with alkali and heat, it would impart a violet color to tissues. Methylene blue treated to produce this new dye (or dyes) was said to be polychromed. Next, polychromed methylene blue was mixed with eosin and this was better still. But such mixtures soon precipitate. So, for convenience, they are allowed to do so, and the precipitate is then dissolved in methyl alcohol; this is roughly what is in the bottle of blood stain kept in the laboratory. However, in alcoholic solution, it is not an effective stain. But when water is added to it on the slide, the compound previously in solution in methyl alcohol partly passes into aqueous solution, and some dissociation occurs into anions and cations, and both carry color. So for a brief period the stain acts as if the ingredients had just been freshly mixed. Later on, of course, it tends to form a precipitate again, but by this time staining has been completed, and the slide has been washed.

Leukocytes are studied in films with the LM for two main purposes: First, the presence of abnormal leukocytes is associated with various disease states. Second, the relative percentages of the different kinds of normal leukocytes that are present in an individual's blood (this is called making a differential count) is important, because certain shifts in the percentages of the different kinds are of diagnostic significance.

Leukocyte Counts. It is also very important to know whether or not the total number of leukocytes in a patient's blood is increased or decreased; this is determined by making a leukocyte count. For this a known small amount of blood is mixed in a special pipette with a known large amount of counting fluid, which acts to destroy red cells and stain the nuclei of leukocytes. A little of the mixture is then floated over ruled squares on a special glass slide called a hemocytometer and a special type of coverslip is placed on it so that there is a known depth of fluid over the squares. The number of leukocytes seen over a given number of squares (Fig. 10-2) is counted and then, by knowing the dilution of the blood in counting fluid and the depth of the fluid over the squares, a calculation can be made of how many leukocytes are present in a cubic millimeter of blood. In normal adults counts vary from about 5,000 to 9,000. There are variations within this range that are dependent on time of day and other factors. Leukocyte counts must be interpreted in relation to what is found in the differential count.

Figure 10-3
and
Figure 10-4

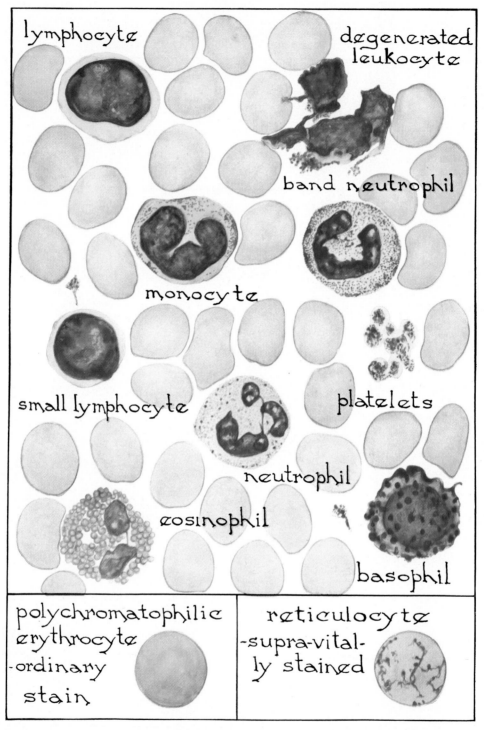

FIG. 10-3. The erythrocytes and the leukocytes of normal blood as they appear in a film stained with Hastings' stain.

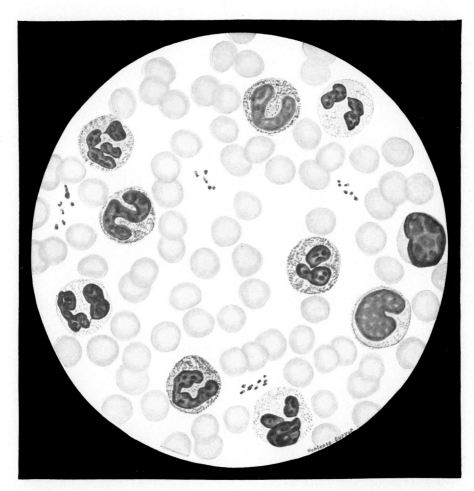

FIG. 10-4. Segmented band and juvenile neutrophils as they appear in a neutrophilic leukocytosis. A juvenile neutrophil may be seen at about 4 o'clock. Band neutrophils may be seen at 6:30, 9:30 and 12:30, respectively. With the exception of a lymphocyte present at 3 o'clock, the remaining leukocytes are segmented neutrophils. Several of the neutrophils in this illustration show toxic granulation. (Kracke, R. R.: Diseases of the Blood, ed. 2. Philadelphia, Lippincott)

The Basis for Classifying Leukocytes

There are five kinds of leukocytes. These in the past were believed to represent only two morphological types. Those of one were said to have granular cytoplasm; those of the other, nongranular cytoplasm. Hence leukocytes were classed as either *granular* or *nongranular*. Because of custom we shall adhere to this terminology but, as we shall see, nongranular leukocytes can have granules.

There are three kinds of granular leukocytes, so named because they differ from each other by the size and, in particular, the staining reaction of their cytoplasmic granules. Those with granules that stain avidly with acid dyes are called acidophilic granular leukocytes, or, since eosin is the dye generally used to color them, eosinophilic granular leukocytes. The short name most commonly used for a cell of this type is eosinophil (Fig. 10-3, *lower left*).

Those with granules that stain avidly with basophilic dyes are termed basophilic granular leukocytes or *basophils* (Fig. 10-3, *lower right*).

Those with granules that are neither markedly acidophilic nor basophilic in solutions of a normal pH are termed neutrophilic granular leukocytes (Fig. 10-3, just above and between the eosinophil and the basophil). The term neutrophil was probably based on the old and incorrect idea that when an acid dye was mixed with a basic dye, a neutral dye was formed and that this stained the granules of neutrophils. The short term for a cell of this type is, most commonly, *polymorph,* or even PMN; this term has no reference to their granules but to their nuclei which have many different forms (anywhere from 1 to 5 lobes). The cell labeled neurophil in Figure 10-3 has three lobes.

There are two kinds of nongranular leukocytes. The more numerous and usually smaller ones are called lymphocytes (Fig. 10-3, *middle and upper left*) because they are found in lymph as well as in blood. The larger and less numerous ones are called monocytes (Fig. 10-3, *left, above center*) for some unknown reason.

To summarize:

Leukocytes
- Granular leukocytes
  - Neutrophils (Polymorphs)
  - Eosinophils
  - Basophils
- Nongranular leukocytes
  - Lymphocytes
  - Monocytes

How To Find and Study Leukocytes in a Stained Blood Film

As preparation for studying a blood film with the LM it should be realized that there are about 1,000 red cells to every leukocyte in normal blood and, since both kinds of blood cells are spread over the slide, it may take some hunting around among red cells to find a leukocyte. However, it is easy to find one with the low-power objective because leukocytes, in contrast to red cells, have nuclei and these at this magnification appear as blue dots scattered around in a background of red cells.

Blood films are sometimes provided with a coverslip and sometimes not. A film with no coverslip can be seen fairly clearly with the low-power objective but not with the high-power (dry) objective. They can, however, be studied with the oil immersion objective by putting a drop of oil directly on the film. A common procedure is to spot the nucleus of a leukocyte in a film with the low-power objective, then center it and switch to oil immersion.

A film usually is thicker at the end from which it is spread. Leukocytes are more numerous and easier to find in the thicker part. But wherever the film is thick (and this is indicated by red cells being superimposed on one another to a great degree) the leukocytes do not stain sharply and hence are difficult to study. They appear to much better advantage in the thinner part of the film, but here they are not as numerous as might be anticipated, because, being somewhat larger than erythrocytes, they tend to be drawn to the edges of the film as well as toward the very end of it. In either of these positions (the edge or the end), they may become distorted and their cytoplasm may be broken and scattered about them. Therefore it is best to learn the appearance of normal leukocytes from the regions where they are most difficult to find, and in order to find here good examples of each kind the student may have to study not only one film but several.

The Differential Count. Since leukocytes are larger than red cells, and are of different sizes, they are distributed unevenly in a film. This creates a problem in attempting to ascertain the relative percentages of the different leukocytes present in a film. A proper sampling cannot be obtained from examining the leukocytes in only one small part of the film. A significant sample requires including in one's count the leukocytes from some of the poorer parts of the film as well as cells from the good parts.

In learning to distinguish the five different kinds of

leukocytes in films much time can be saved if the following traps are avoided:

(1) *Examining a Degenerating Leukocyte.* In every blood film there are many examples of partly broken-down leukocytes (Fig. 10-3, *top, right*), and it is a waste of time to try to identify their nature. So examine only well-formed and well-stained examples.

(2) *Confusing Clumps of Platelets With Leukocytes.* In every film there are many little bodies, called platelets, that commonly clump together (Fig. 10-3, *center, right*). Most of each platelet is pale blue, but its central part may contain a dark-staining granule or granules. Platelets will be considered in detail later.

(3) *Examining Cells That Are Difficult To Classify.* At first the student should examine only leukocytes that are easily recognized and should disregard those that seem difficult to classify until he has more experience.

In the following description of the five kinds of leukocytes, the student will learn that both the nuclei and the cytoplasm give important information that is useful in identifying them.

Granular Leukocytes: Neutrophils (Polymorphs)

Since the terms *neutrophil* and *polymorph* are both commonly used for the same cell, we shall use them indiscriminately to encourage familiarity with both.

Numbers. In normal blood, from 60 to 70 percent of the leukocytes are polymorphs. In absolute numbers, 3,000 to 6,000 per cubic millimeter of blood is considered a normal range. The reader can readily calculate that an individual with 5 liters of blood has 15 to 30 billion polymorphs in his circulation. Polymorphs are the first kind of leukocyte generally seen in a normal film.

Appearance. Polymorphs develop in myeloid tissue (the bone marrow), where they go through many developmental changes before they finally assume their mature form, and then they are liberated into the bloodstream. In health only an occasional polymorph is released into the bloodstream before it is mature. Under conditions of disease, however, some immature ones may be released and so are seen in films made from the peripheral blood. It is, therefore, necessary for the student to learn the appearance of both mature and immature polymorphs.

Motility. Polymorphs have great ameboid activity, as will be described presently.

Mature Polymorphs. These are from 10 to 12 μ in diameter; this is slightly less than half as wide again as the erythrocytes in a film.

The nucleus is in the form of lobes that appear in a film to be either completely separated from one another or connected to others by no more than very delicate strands. The nucleus of a mature polymorph has from 2 to 5, or even more, lobes (Figs. 10-3 and 10-4). The substance of the lobes is made up of coarse chromatin that is rather densely packed (Figs. 10-3 and 10-4). As a consequence, the nuclear material stains fairly deeply with basic dyes, being colored a blue or blue-purple in the usual preparation. The nucleoli cannot be distinguished.

Barr Bodies in Polymorphs. A few years after Barr and Bertram showed there was a sex difference in the chromatin of cells, Davidson and Smith demonstrated that it was possible to identify the chromosomal sex of an individual by the examination of blood films. The Barr body in a mature polymorph of a female is generally contained in one of the lobes of the nucleus, where it is very difficult, if not impossible, to identify because the chromatin is so packed; however, a Barr body sometimes appears as a separate tiny lobe which has the form of a drumstick (Fig. 10-5). According to Davidson and Smith, this happens in about 1 out of every 38 neutrophils of females. Somewhat similar little bodies very occasionally are seen in the neutrophils of males. Furthermore, as many as 6 never are seen in a series of 500 neutrophils from males and at least 6 always can be seen in 500 neutrophils obtained from females.

Cytoplasm of Mature Polymorphs. This occupies more space than the nucleus and reveals little structural detail except that it is fairly heavily sprinkled with granules (Fig. 10-4). There are two kinds often seen. The true neutrophilic granules in many preparations are so fine that they are difficult to resolve with the LM; hence all that may be seen is that the cytoplasm has a granular appearance. Commonly, these granules either have or impart to the cytoplasm a lavender (lilac) color. Granules that are larger than the specific neutrophilic granules are also seen; these are reddish-purple in color (Fig. 10-3, neutrophil). Since this color is imparted to them by the methylene azure, which is one of the basic dyes in a blood stain, they are called *azurophilic granules.* As we shall see when we study the formation of granular leukocytes, the first granules that appear in cells of this lineage are of the azurophilic type; only later do true neutrophilic granules appear and, when they do appear, they are first seen in the Golgi region of the developing cells.

Immature Polymorphs. In the development of polymorphs, the nuclei at first have the form of indented ovoids (Fig. 10-4, *4 o'clock*). At this stage of development the cell is called a neutrophilic metamyelocyte (or a juvenile neutrophil). As this cell develops further, its nucleus becomes increasingly indented until it becomes frankly horseshoe shaped, and at this stage of development it is termed a band or a stab neutrophil (Fig. 10-3, *band neutrophil* and Fig. 10-4, *7 o'clock*). Under normal conditions the horseshoe-shaped nucleus of the band form becomes segmented to divide the nucleus into 2 or more lobes before the cell is released into the bloodstream from bone marrow where it is formed, for under normal conditions not more than 1 or 2 percent of band forms are seen in films. But if there is a great need for neutrophils in the blood (as will be explained under The Functions of Neutrophils), some band and even some juvenile forms are released into the bloodstream, and so these are seen in blood films.

The nuclei of juvenile neutrophils do not stain as deeply as those of band forms (Fig. 10-4), and those of band forms do not stain as deeply as those of mature forms. Both juvenile and band neutrophils have cytoplasmic granules similar to those of mature neutrophils (Fig. 10-4), and both may contain some azurophilic granules in addition to their specific neutrophilic granules.

From the above it is evident that the maturity of a neutrophil is revealed chiefly by the shape of its nucleus and to a lesser extent by how heavily the nucleus stains.

Fine Structure. This must be studied by looking at very thin slices cut through neutrophils and not at whole cells as is done when examining a blood film with the LM.

Leukocytes may be obtained for sectioning by obtaining tiny pieces of bone marrow from a sternal puncture; these are fixed and sectioned. In these sections there are, of course, many immature cells of various kinds, but there are also many mature polymorphs. If whole blood is allowed to settle or if it is centrifuged in a tube, the erythrocytes are packed into a reddish layer in the bottom half of the tube, and the leukocytes form a whitish layer (called the buffy coat) just above them. Bits of this can be fixed and sectioned for electron microscopy. Still another way to see neutrophils in sections is to cut sections of the tissues of an animal where there has been the kind of injury that makes neutrophils migrate through the walls of postcapillary venules into the tissues; this is the way in which Figure 10-8 was obtained.

A thin section cut through a mature neutrophil passes through only some of the lobes of the nucleus. Hence, in electron micrographs, neutrophils do not reveal as many lobes as they do in blood films in which the whole cell is spread out for view. In sections viewed

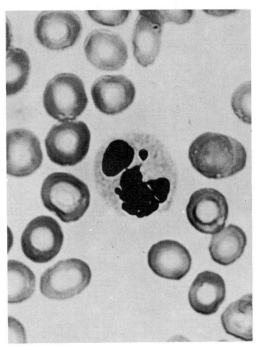

FIG. 10-5. Photomicrograph ($\times$ 1,750) of a stained film of the blood of a human female. The neutrophil in the center illustrates a characteristic "drumstick." (Davidson, W. M., and Smith, D. R.: Brit. Med. J., 2:6, 1954)

with the EM the lobes of a nucleus are seen to have condensed chromatin distributed along the inner surface of the nuclear envelope (Fig. 10-6). In the more central part of a lobe the chromatin is very extended, so the central parts of the lobes are pale (Fig. 10-6).

The cytoplasm of a mature polymorph does not contain a very good representation of the usual organelles. A few mitochondria and a small Golgi apparatus can often be seen. Granules of glycogen are often scattered about in it. However, the salient feature of the cytoplasm is its great content of granules; it has been estimated that there may be from 50 to 200 in each cell. The granules are of two types, *azurophilic* and *specific*. The azurophilic granules are the larger (around 700 nm in diameter) and less numerous, amounting to around a third of the total. They are round or oval in shape and denser in the EM than the specific granules. As is shown in Figures 10-6 and 12-9, they are most easily identified by the peroxidases which are enzymes that catalyze the transfer of oxygen from hydrogen peroxide to acceptors and thus they facilitate more rapid oxidation than would occur without them. As will be described in Chapter 12, they are formed at an earlier stage of development than the

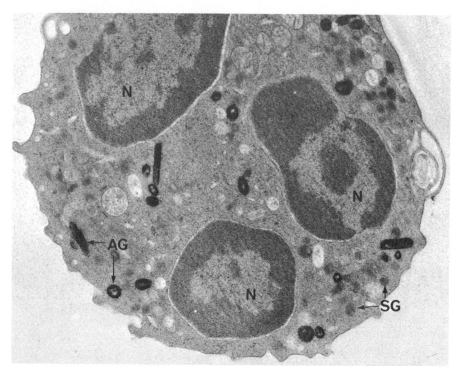

FIG. 10-6. Electron micrograph of a mature neutrophil from mouse bone marrow reacted for the enzyme peroxidase. The peroxidase-positive electron-dense azurophilic granules (AG) related to lysosomes and the peroxidase-negative and therefore lighter staining specific granules (SG) can be seen in the cytoplasm. Several lobes of the nucleus (N) with condensed chromatin along the nuclear envelope are also shown in the micrograph. (From V. I. Kalnins)

specific granules. The smaller specific granules (Fig. 10-6) are around 400 nm in diameter and are found later as the cell develops.

It has long been known that polymorphs contain enzymes that are concerned in the destruction of bacteria they phagocytose. With the development of knowledge about lysosomes, discussed in Chapter 5, it soon became apparent that polymorphs were rich in them. Bainton and Farquhar have shown that the azurophilic granules are the lysosomes of polymorphs, and Farquhar and Bainton have shown that they contain at least 6 hydrolytic enzymes as well as peroxidase. In contrast the more numerous specific granules were found to contain no lysosomal enzymes but instead a bactericidal substance and also the enzyme alkaline phosphatase. It has been shown that, after a polymorph has phagocytosed certain bacteria (*E. coli*), a specific granule quickly fuses with the membranous sac containing the phagocytosed bacterium and empties its alkaline phosphatase into the sac. About 3 minutes later, azurophilic granules fuse with the sac and release their content of hydrolytic enzymes and peroxidase into it and this soon destroys the bacterium.

INFLAMMATION AND THE FUNCTIONS OF POLYMORPHS

The process that is set in motion when living tissue is affected by an injurious agent is termed inflamma-

tion. The process operates to eliminate or neutralize the injurious agent and its effects and to repair the damaged tissue. It is sometimes described as having three phases—injury, reaction, and repair.

Polymorphs are of great importance in acute inflammation.

Although any of the body tissues can be injured by various means, the reaction to injury that tends to limit its spread and to overcome it, involves both the leukocytes and plasma of blood, the cells and intercellular substances of connective tissue and in particular, what is called the *terminal vascular bed* which includes the arterioles that supply the capillary bed and the venules that drain it as will be described in more detail presently.

The kinds of injurious agents that can induce inflammation in a part of the body are many and varied. Much is caused because body tissue is invaded by bacteria, viruses, protozoa or other kinds of pathogenic organisms. Inflammation can also occur when body tissue is injured by heat, radiation, cold or chemicals. Furthermore, certain substances formed within the body can cause inflammation or participate in causing inflammation, sometimes in a complex way as will be learned in pathology courses.

The classic signs and symptoms of inflammation in some part of the body, which are still often recited by students, were listed by A.D. 200 as redness, heat, swelling, pain and loss or impairment of function. We shall presently describe the microscopic changes in tissue that cause these signs and symptoms.

The presence of inflammation in any body part is denoted in medical language by adding the word termination "itis" to the body part in which inflammation is diagnosed as being present. Since almost any part of the body can be the seat of inflammation, a patient may be said to be suffering from (for example):

nasopharyngitis—inflammation of the lining of the nose and throat

sinusitis—inflammation of the lining of the nasal sinuses

tonsillitis—inflammation of the tonsils

laryngitis—inflammation of the larynx

arthritis—inflammation of joints

appendicitis—inflammation of the wall of the appendix

colitis—inflammation of the lining of the colon

cystitis—inflammation of the urinary bladder

cholecystitis—inflammation of the gallbladder

glomerulonephritis—inflammation of the glomeruli of the kidneys.

The above examples illustrate that much illness in man involves inflammation in some parts of his body and hence an understanding of inflammation is of prime importance for the medical or paramedical student. The details of the process constitute a large part of a course of instruction in pathology. We shall here give only an elementary account of it. However, before doing this it should be mentioned that inflammation can be described as being acute, subacute or chronic. The classic symptoms and signs of inflammation refer to the acute variety. Chronic inflammation occurs when the battle between the inducer and the defenses of the body is not quickly and decisively settled and as a result a subdued contest between injury and reaction continues for a long period. Subacute inflammation is not a very clear-cut type; it illustrates some of the features of both the acute and the chronic kinds.

SOME HISTOLOGICAL FEATURES OF THE INFLAMMATORY PROCESS

Almost everyone has run a dirty splinter through the protective epithelium of the skin into the connective tissue of a finger and found that unless it was properly treated the tissue around the sides of the sliver became inflamed. The presence of the inflammation is indicated by the area becoming red and swollen and by its feeling warm and painful, and, as a result,

one would be disinclined to use the finger for playing the piano or typing a letter (impairment of function). The microscopic bases for these changes will now be described.

An ordinary sliver either carries pathogenic bacteria or pushes them from the surface of the skin into the connective tissue that lies beneath the epithelium (Fig. 10-7). In the nutritive wet intercellular substance the bacteria can at first multiply. They and any noxious substances they produce, together with the physical presence of a foreign object (the sliver) soon bring about changes in the vascular bed of the part. The mechanisms involved will be discussed presently.

Changes in Flow in the Vascular Bed. In previous discussions we have described capillary loops and mentioned that they are supplied by arterioles and drained by venules. Actually a vascular bed is somewhat more complicated; for, as is shown in Figure 19-10, arterioles and venules are connected primarily by what are termed preferred channels or A-V bridges which have enough smooth muscle cells along their walls to permit the regulation of their diameters and hence the flow of blood through them. It is primarily from these preferred channels that capillary loops and networks arise. Capillaries themselves do not possess surrounding cells that control flow through them. Hence the amount of blood that passes through a terminal capillary bed is regulated primarily by the muscle cells that surround arterioles and portions of the preferred channels. (Details will be given in Chapter 19.) Circulation through the terminal vascular bed normally fluctuates; this phenomenon is termed *vasomotion*.

Following an injury there is at first an opening up of, and increased flow through, the vascular bed and this in turn is followed by a slowing of the flow. When the latter phase of the reaction is reached another phenomenon makes its appearance—the endothelium that lines the venules becomes leaky and allows increased amounts of plasma to escape into the adjacent intercellular substance. The leakage occurs between the cell membranes of contiguous endothelial cells. Leakage may also occur through the cytoplasm of the endothelial cells if the capillary walls have been directly injured by the agent that induced the inflammation as, for example, might occur in thermal burns. The leakage that occurs through the walls of the venules, and is not due to direct injury to them, is to be explained, to some extent at least, by the fact that the injury or its immediate sequelae have led to histamine being liberated from mast cells or other sources. The liberation, from other sources, of substances called in general *vasoactive amines* (histamine is one of them) that have the same type of effect may also be involved. The

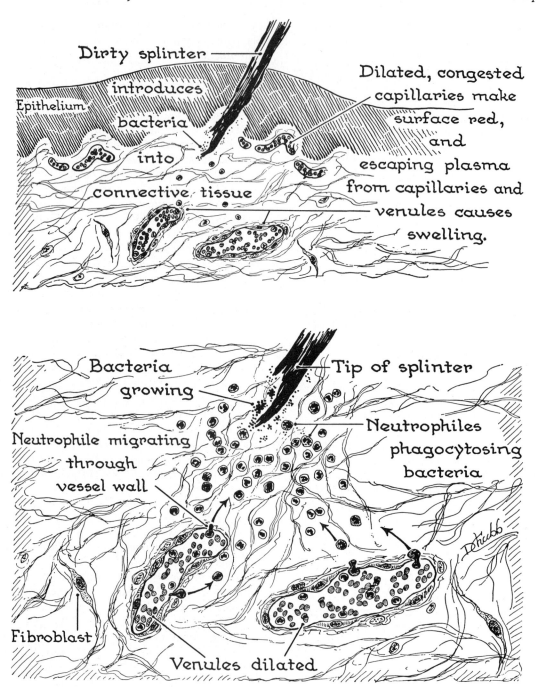

FIG. 10-7. Diagrams to show how neutrophils migrate from congested, dilated small blood vessels to combat bacteria introduced into the tissues by means of an injury.

leakage of plasma from venules into the intercellular substance is called *exudation*.

Almost as soon as the blood flow becomes slowed, and exudation has occurred, polymorphs can be seen sticking to the lining endothelium of the venules through which they were passing and, soon after, some examples of their cytoplasm extending in the form of pseudopodia between the cell membranes of contiguous endothelial cells can be found as is shown in Figure 10-8. Having found an opening with a pseudopodium,

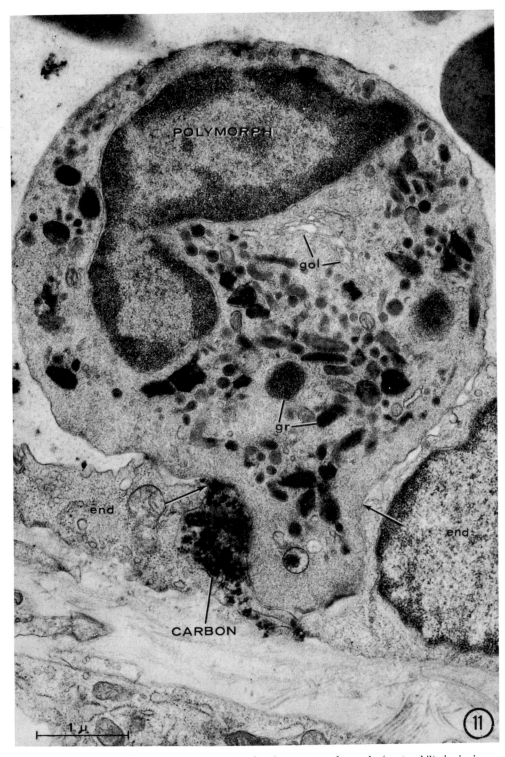

FIG. 10-8. Electron micrograph ($\times$ 23,500) showing a rat polymorph (neutrophil) beginning to migrate between two endothelial cells (*end*) in early inflammation. The nucleus is labeled *polymorph*, the Golgi apparatus *gol*, and the specific granules of the polymorph *gr*. Inflammation was produced before giving carbon particles intravenously; a clump of these can be seen to the left of the pseudopodium of the neutrophil that is projecting downward through the site of attachment between two endothelial cells in the lining of this small blood vessel. Notice the variation in size of the granules of the neutrophil. (Movat, H. Z., and Fernando, N. V. P., Lab. Invest., *12:*895)

the rest of the polymorph then squeezes through it to enter the intercellular substance outside the venule, and from there the polymorphs, which of course are motile, migrate to the site of the injurious agent which, in this instance, would be the site where bacteria were multiplying (Fig. 10-7). The question then arises as to what attracts polymorphs to leave the blood, migrate through a venule and move toward the noxious agents they are to phagocytose. The attraction bacteria have for polymorphs has been described for years as an example of *chemotaxis* which infers there is some sort of a chemical concentration gradient which attracts the polymorph to the bacteria. Bacteria probably elaborate some substances which have this effect. But there is now much evidence indicating that polymorphs are attracted by sites where antibodies have become fixed to antigens of the infective agent and have formed antigen-antibody complexes. But antigen-antibody complexes only attract polymorphs because they fix what is called *complement* which will now be described briefly.

The term complement refers to a group of proteins that are present in normal blood serum and become activated when an antibody reacts to an antigen. The various components of complement then combine with the antigen-antibody complex in an ordered sequence and, as they do, various biological effects are produced.

A given body identifies only certain sites on foreign cells as antigenic, and these (termed antigenic sites) are the sites with which antibody combines. If these sites on a foreign cell are not too far apart, as would be the case with bacteria and cells from other individuals such as erythrocytes, the combining of antibody with these antigenic sites initiates the binding of complement to them. First one component of complement becomes attached to the site; then other components of complement become activated and combine with the first in a cascadelike manner until finally an active lipase is produced which acts on the cell membrane of the foreign cells so that their contents are no longer retained by their membranes and they die by what is called *lysis*. During the process of complement activation several biologically active substances are released from the different components of the complement. Some of these are responsible for chemotaxis and others for other effects. For example, for a long time it has been known that there was something in blood that became attached to bacteria and made them easier for polymorphs to phagocytose and destroy; these were termed *opsonins*. It was, of course, known that antibody became attached to bacteria and for a time it was thought that the antibody itself was responsible for the opsonin effect. But it is now conceded that the

opsonin effect is to be explained by split products released from complement that becomes attached to the antigen antibody site. Complement is, therefore, of great importance in the inflammatory reaction and in facilitating the phagocytosis and killing of bacteria. It should, perhaps, also be noted that viruses are inactivated by antibody alone, without complement having to be involved in the reaction.

If the injurious agent is a form of pathogenic bacteria that attracts polymorphs, the bacteria are engulfed by the cell membrane of the polymorph and so come to lie in a membranous sac within the cytoplasm. This kind of membranous sac is called a phagosome. As was described a few pages back, the specific neutrophilic granules of the polymorph fuse with the sac containing the injurious agent and this is followed by the azurophilic granules fusing with it, and by this means the agent is destroyed by the lysosomes of the azurophilic granules.

It is of interest that the role of the lysosomes of polymorphs is not always limited to the destruction of phagocytosed bacteria. Under certain conditions they may be released from polymorphs and either assist in causing, or by themselves cause, an inflammatory reaction. An example of the latter is encountered in an acute attack of gout. This disease is basically due to a defect in the metabolism of nucleic acids in the body so that an end product, uric acid, tends to increase in the blood and to precipitate as a urate in joint tissues. Urates themselves are probably not very irritating but it seems that, in the tissue around a joint, polymorphs may somehow become involved in attempting to phagocytose certain crystals of urate, with the result that their lysosomes are liberated and these then cause an intense acute inflammation. Commonly this happens in association with the metatarso-phalangeal joint of the big toe and when it does the swelling around this joint becomes extensive, the skin becomes a dusky red and the pain can be so excruciating and the part so sensitive to touch that it is said that a sufferer from an acute attack of gout watches apprehensively lest a fly hovering over his uncovered toe should light on it. The curious thing about this inflammation is that after an acute attack has subsided it leaves little or no trace of damage and indeed it has been reported that one year a race was won at the Olympic Games by an individual between two acute attacks of gout. Nowadays acute attacks can be prevented by proper medication or, if they are not, they can be effectively ameliorated.

Gout thus provides an example of something that is formed within the body initiating an acute inflammation. Another example is provided by certain complexes that form between antigens and antibodies. These may circulate and become fixed in some site where, if they attract complement, they will attract polymorphs which break down and release their lysosomes which injure tissue and incite an acute inflammatory response.

The Cause of the Classic Signs and Symptoms of Acute Inflammation

The redness and increased local temperature noted at the site of an acute inflammation is to be explained by an increased amount of blood flowing through the terminal vascular bed. This in turn is due to the dilation of the arterioles and venules that normally control the circulation through the bed. The swelling at the site of an acute inflammation (unless it is severe enough to have caused local hemorrhage) is due to the exudation of plasma that takes place between the endothelial cells that line the dilated venules. The question arises as to how these changes occur in these vessels which are not actually being affected directly by (say) bacteria which may be some microscopic distance away from them.

Experiments have shown that if an animal is depleted of its leukocytes and infected at some site with bacteria, inflammation does not occur at the site where the bacteria were injected. (Under these conditions, however, the bacteria grow and spread all through the body.) Hence it is obvious that the heat, redness and swelling observed in a local inflammatory response is due to something produced by the body and not by the bacteria. The substances that are produced or elaborated and that act at, for example, a site in infection, to produce the changes that account for heat, redness and swelling are called the *chemical mediators of the acute inflammatory response*. There are different kinds of these. One kind is referred to as the vasoactive amines; histamine is one of these and this is released by mast cells in the vicinity. Another is serotonin; this is released from platelets but its role in man is uncertain. It is assumed that bacteria can produce enough toxin to cause enough histamine release to initiate enough exudation and emigration of polymorphs to launch the acute inflammatory process which, for reasons already described, would then be self-sustaining until the infection is overcome. There are other chemical mediators also involved; their formation involves interactions between plasma peptides and proteins that would be far beyond the scope of this book to describe. An important one is termed the kinin system. Complement is also involved. For a full

and recent discussion of inflammation and chemical mediators see Movat.

The pain involved in acute inflammation is probably due to the stretching of nerve endings by the swelling and also to the irritation of nerve endings by products of the inflammatory process. In particular, lysosomes released from polymorphs could act this way.

The Role of Monocytes and Macrophages. The migration of polymorphs through the walls of venules either is accompanied by the migration of monocytes, or is quickly followed by such a migration, from the blood into the tissues by the same means as that employed by the polymorphs. Monocytes, on entering the tissues, become macrophages. At first they participate with the polymorphs in phagocytic activities but soon they dominate the picture because the polymorphs have a very short life span and when their work is over they cease to enter the area. The macrophages remain longer. Polymorphs and macrophages seem to be attracted by different types of antigens; there are some forms of bacteria that do not attract polymorphs but do attract macrophages. Macrophages, moreover, are adapted to phagocytosing such debris as is left in an area when the inflammation subsides.

The phase of repair requires the formation of fibroblasts which in most areas are probably derived from the relatively undifferentiated cells that are scattered along the smaller blood vessels. As was described in the previous chapter, they synthesize and elaborate collagen to restore so far as possible the intercellular substances of the part. New capillaries bud off from pre-existing vessels to provide such blood supply as is needed. Epithelial membranes regenerate as was described in Chapter 7.

Pus and Pyrogens. Accumulations of dead polymorphs together with some breakdown products of infected tissue can account for the formation of a creamy-yellow semifluid material in infected wounds called *pus*. In infected wounds that are open to the surface pus can drain away or be absorbed into dressings. If, however, an accumulation forms in an area below, and not open to, the surface, it is called an abscess and surgical means may be adopted to drain it.

Certain products formed from the breakdown of polymorphs and also from bacterial toxins and breakdown protein products are termed *pyrogens,* because if they are absorbed into the body and carried to the thermostatlike temperature control center in the brain, they affect it so that the body temperature is raised. The same or similar substances can also have an effect on the bone marrow, as will next be described.

Leukocytosis. The effect of substances that are probably similar to those that induce fever somehow stimulates the release of mature polymorphs from the bone marrow, so that severe infections of many types are associated with a *leukocytosis*. Although there is a large pool of mature polymorphs in the bone marrow, the bone marrow stimulation also results in increased numbers of immature polymorphs being released into the circulation. Accordingly, in patients suffering from many types of acute infections, the leukocyte count rises, and a differential count made on a blood film reveals increased percentages of band and juvenile polymorphs. In tabulating the types of polymorphs seen in a film it is customary to enter the band and juvenile kinds on the left-hand side of the sheet of paper, and those that are more mature (those that have two to five lobes) on the right-hand side of the paper. Accordingly, if in any patient the examination of regularly obtained blood films show that the percentage of immature cells is increasing, it is said that a shift to the left is occurring. If, however, it is found in regularly obtained films that the percentage of immature forms is decreasing, it is said that there is a shift to the right. So, in a very general way, a shift to the left indicates that an infection is progressing, and a shift to the right indicates that it is subsiding.

Eosinophils

Numbers. Eosinophils constitute from 1 to 4 percent of the leukocytes seen in a film of normal blood. In absolute figures, 150 to 450 per cu mm of blood is considered normal.

Morphology. Eosinophils are from 10 to 15 microns in diameter; they tend to be slightly larger than neutrophils. Their nuclei are commonly composed of only 2 lobes (Fig. 10-3) which may or may not be connected with a strand of nuclear material. The coarse clumps of chromatin are not so densely packed in the nuclei of eosinophils as they are in neutrophils; hence eosinophil nuclei do not stain as deeply (Fig. 10-3).

The cytoplasm of eosinophils has a somewhat irregular outline because of occasional pseudopodia and characteristically is packed with large refractile granules that in well-stained blood films are colored red or orange (Fig. 10-3). In poorly stained films their color may veer toward pink or a muddy blue. Even in poorly stained preparations they can be distinguished from the granules of neutrophils because they are more numerous—the cell seems to be packed with them—and be-

cause they are distinctly larger and more refractile (Fig. 10-3).

Fine Structure. The EM reveals no special features in the nuclei except that, as in neutrophils, condensed chromatin is distributed on the inner surface of the nuclear envelope (Fig. 10-9). The chief feature of the cytoplasm is its content of specific membrane-surrounded granules.

These have a striking appearance, being dense and from 0.5 to 1 μ in diameter (Fig. 10-9). In immature eosinophils they are composed of a homogeneous material of considerable density. In mature eosinophils some of the granules are seen to contain still denser bodies in their more central parts (Fig. 10-9) which are crystalline in structure and may have the form of rough squares or rectangles. The shape of these bodies differs in different species. They sometimes occupy more and sometimes less than half of a granule.

The granules contain large amounts of a stable peroxidase and most, but not all, of the enzymes that are found in the granules of polymorphs; hence, the granules are regarded as lysosomes.

The Golgi is the only organelle that is at all prominent in eosinophils; the others have minimal representation.

Functions of Eosinophils. Like polymorphs, eosinophils perform their function when they leave the bloodstream and enter the tissues. They are normally found in the lining of the intestine, in the lungs, in the dermis of the skin and in the tissue of the external genitalia. However, unlike polymorphs, they are not very phagocytic so far as bacteria are concerned, nor are they as motile. However, it has been recognized for a long time that eosinophils are somehow concerned in anaphylactic phenomena, because they are more numerous both in the tissues that are the sites of allergic reactions and in the blood of people who suffer from allergies. The hormone hydrocortisone, which depresses allergic reactions, causes eosinophils to disappear from the blood. Indeed, the number of eosinophils in blood varies over each 24-hour period, probably because the secretion of hydrocortisone by the adrenal gland varies over the same period. In some species eosinophils have been shown to contain histamine, and so it has been thought that they might either liberate histamine or perhaps absorb histamine and neutralize it, or release antihistaminelike substances from their cytoplasmic granules. Eosinophils are found in nasal secretions of allergic individuals during seasonal hay fever and in the sputum of most patients with asthma. It is of interest that haptens (which are small molecules capable of

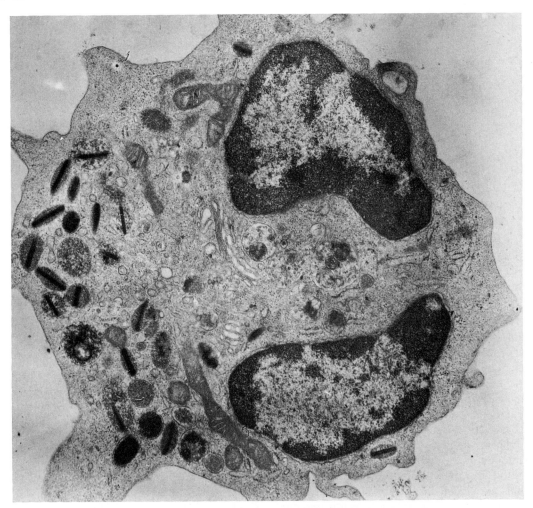

FIG. 10-9. Electron micrograph ($\times$ 18,500) of eosinophil of mouse. Note the bilobed nucleus. Golgi saccules can be seen slightly left of the center as well as some free rounded vesicles filled with pale secretory material. The specific granules in the cytoplasm vary in size; many show the dark disks that characterize the specific granules of eosinophils. Only a few mitochondria are visible. (Preparation from A. F. Howatson)

conferring antigenic activity on otherwise nonantigenic proteins with which they combine), if injected into the lungs of experimental animals, can nonspecifically induce the accumulation of eosinophils locally. Moreover, it has been shown experimentally that eosinophils are attracted to free antigen-antibody complexes and can phagocytose them. However, although it is clear that they are involved in immunological responses, their precise role is not yet entirely clear. Perhaps they serve to diminish the deleterious effects of allergic reactions.

A fact that can be of some diagnostic importance is that the number of eosinophils becomes increased in the blood of people who have become infected with certain types of parasites.

Basophils

Basophils comprise only about 0.5 percent of the blood leukocytes; hence, to find a good example of one, it may be necessary to examine several hundred leukocytes and perhaps several different blood films. However, even if they constitute only one half of one percent of the leukocytes in the blood, this still allows for there being enormous numbers of them in the body so their possible role and importance deserve attention.

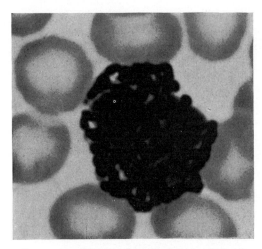

FIG. 10-10. Oil-immersion photomicrograph of a basophil from human blood. Prominent granules are darker than the nucleus and tend to obscure it. (Preparation from C. P. Leblond and Y. Clermont)

Basophils are usually from 10 to 12 μ in diameter; they are of about the same size as neutrophils (Fig. 10-3). About half of the cell consists of nucleus, which may be segmented and, in any event, often presents a very irregular shape. It is colored much less intensely than the nucleus of the neutrophil or the eosinophil and, in blood films stained with blood stains, the nucleus is overshadowed by the large, dark, blue-stained granules of the cytoplasm, which may be seen lying over the paler nucleus (Fig. 10-10). The granules of basophils are similar in many respects to those of mast cells and, like them, are metachromatic and contain heparin. The EM has shown that the granules are enclosed by membrane. The function of basophils has not been clearly established. Basophils are phagocytic and are reported to contain about half of the histamine that is present in blood. Furthermore, basophils, like eosinophils, tend to leave the bloodstream under the influence of certain hormones of the adrenal gland. In many respects they seem to be involved in allergic and inflammatory phenomena in much the same way as eosinophils.

Circulating immunoglobulin IgE (described in connection with allergy) readily becomes attached to the surface of basophils. Thus an encounter between basophils in this condition and the allergen that called forth the production of the IgE antibody by plasma cells can result in discharge of the granules from the basophils, with release of substances that affect blood vessels in a manner similar to that of substances liberated by mast cells. If the reaction is of great magnitude and systemic, it can result in vascular collapse and death.

Lymphocytes

Although the general function of polymorphs has been known since the time of Metchnikoff, almost nothing was known about the function of lymphocytes until recently. However, over the last decade and a half, lymphocytes have become the focus of a vast amount of research that has been facilitated by modern methods and it has become apparent that they are the cells that endow the body with its immunological defenses. If these cells that were named lymphocytes long ago, because they were found in lymph as well as in blood, were given a name today they would probably be called preimmunocytes or some such name to indicate what is now known to be their roles, which will soon be described in detail.

Numbers. Next to neutrophils, lymphocytes are the commonest leukocytes seen in a normal blood film. In absolute numbers, there are 2,000, plus or minus 1,000, per cu mm of blood. From about 20 to 30 percent of the leukocytes seen in a normal blood film are lymphocytes. The percentage of lymphocytes in the blood of many experimental animals differs considerably from that in man; those beginning experimental work can obtain precise information about the normal range of leukocytes in different species from Albritton's *Standard Values in Blood.*

Appearance in Blood Films and H and E Sections. The common lymphocyte is termed a small lymphocyte and it is the smallest of all the 5 kinds of leukocytes (Fig. 10-3, *small lymphocyte*). The chromatin of their nuclei is almost all condensed so their nuclei are very small and they have very little cytoplasm. Even in films where their cytoplasm is spread out, it is no more than a narrow rim of material that exhibits varying degrees of basophilia with blood stains (Fig. 10-3, *small lymphocyte*). In sections, the normal globular shape of the lymphocyte is preserved and the rim of unspread cytoplasm is so thin and stains so poorly with H and E that it can be seen only with difficulty. The rounded or ovoid nucleus generally exhibits a little indentation of one of its sides.

Nucleoli are not seen in lymphocyte nuclei in films because they are obscured by the condensed chromatin. Even in the usual section they are not seen, for the same reason. Nucleoli can be seen if *very thin* sections are cut from lymphocytes, because individual slices that cut through nucleoli have no chromatin above or below them to obscure them.

The cytoplasm of about 10 percent of lymphocytes

seen in stained films contains reddish-purple azuro-philic granules which are probably lysosomes.

Living Lymphocytes. Living lymphocytes studied with the phase microscope (Fig. 10-11) are seen to be very active, moving about at what seems to be a great rate (it must be remembered that their speed is magnified as much as their size). They can insinuate themselves between other cells and thus pass through endothelial membranes. A moving lymphocyte has a head end and a tail end; the head end consists of its nucleus, covered with a little cytoplasm, and its tail, of drawn-out cytoplasm. In life a lymphocyte that is on the move thus has a shape like a tennis racquet.

Fine Structure. Their cytoplasm has only a few mitochondria (Fig. 10-12)—perhaps not more than 25, which suggests that their metabolic rate is low. In suitable sections a pair of centrioles can be seen close to the indentation in the nucleus (Fig. 10-12). A Golgi exists to the outer side of the centriole. Endoplasmic reticulum of either type is very scarce but free ribosomes are present in sufficient numbers to account for the basophilia of the cytoplasm observed in blood films (Fig. 10-3).

Lymphocytes of Two Sizes. Although most are small, some have both larger nuclei and more cytoplasm than the smaller kind (Fig. 10-3, *upper left*). In deciding whether some lymphocytes are larger than others one must take into account the fact that the size of cells seen in films depends to a considerable extent on how thin the cells are spread and this differs in different parts of a film. If two lymphocytes are found close together and one is obviously larger than the other, it can be assumed that they have been

spread to the same extent. However, the safest way to draw conclusions about lymphocytes being of different sizes is to study them in sections and measure their nuclei. This will show that the nuclei of most lymphocytes are about 5 microns in diameter whereas 8 percent have nuclei that are about 7 microns in diameter. If examples of these two types of cells were seen side by side in a blood film, the smaller would have an over-all diameter of from 7 to 8 microns and the larger a diameter of about 12 microns. The volume of the larger lymphocytes is about 3 times that of the smaller. The smaller kind are termed small lymphocytes and the larger, large lymphocytes.

(Some confusion is caused by still larger cells which are seen in lymphatic tissue, but do not enter the blood under normal conditions, also being termed large lymphocytes by some authors; these, however, are not circulating blood cells, and there are other names for them.)

WHY LYMPHOCYTES ARE FOUND IN LYMPH

As described in Chapter 8, some of the tissue fluid formed from capillaries is returned to the blood circulatory system via lymphatic capillaries (Fig. 8-6). *As soon as tissue fluid penetrates into lymphatic capillaries, it is called lymph.* Lymph, as it is formed, is almost cell free (if there are many lymphocytes in the loose connective tissue in which it forms, some may get into the lymphatic capillaries).

As lymphatic capillaries pass inward, they join together to form larger vessels called *lymphatics,* which are very similar to small veins except that they contain

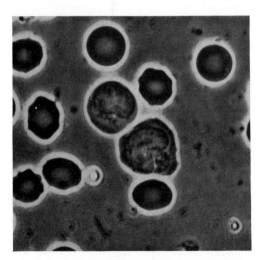
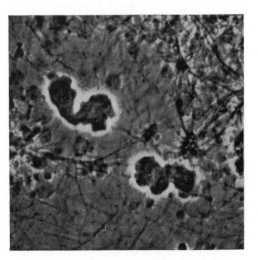

FIG. 10-11. Oil-immersion phase photomicrographs of living lymphocytes in cell cultures. The two at the left are resting, and the two on the right are moving. (Preparation from D. M. Whitelaw)

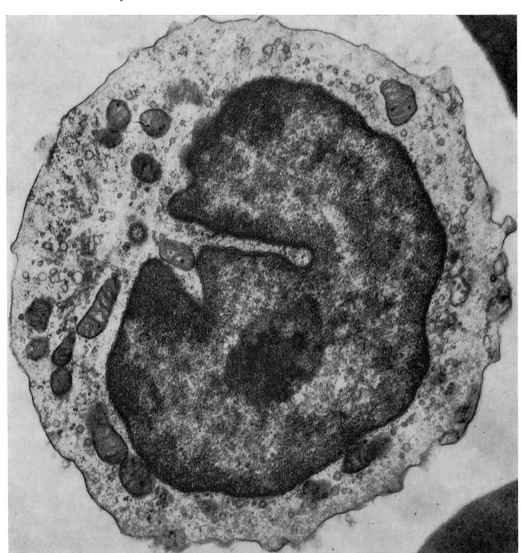

Fig. 10-12. Electron micrograph (approximately × 30,000) of section of small lymphocyte from thoracic duct lymph. Note the deep indentation of the nucleus, below which can be seen the nucleolus. Close to the open end of the indentation is a centriole cut in cross section; to its left, components of the Golgi apparatus are visible. About a dozen mitochondria can be seen. Note that free ribosomes are only sparsely distributed in the cytoplasm. (Preparation by Dorothea Zucker-Franklin)

lymph instead of blood. Sooner or later along their course the lymphatics reach little organs called *lymph nodes*. As can be seen in Figure 13-8, which should be referred to briefly here, lymphatics enter the convex surface of the bean-shaped lymph nodes as *afferent* lymphatics. Lymph nodes contain many lymphocytes (their origins will be described later); so, as lymph percolates through a node it picks up many lymphocytes. Hence the lymph that leaves a node by way of *efferent* lymphatics, which drain away from the concave hilus of the node (Fig. 13-8), contains *many* lymphocytes in suspension. Efferent lymphatics from one node commonly join with lymphatics from other nodes, and eventually lymph from the lower part of the body, including the intestine, empties into a main lymphatic duct called the *thoracic duct*. The thoracic duct and another large lymph duct which drains lymph from the rest of the body (mainly the upper right part of the body) both empty into large veins near the heart, and so by means of these two large lymph ducts all the lymph formed in the body, with the lymphocytes it has picked up by passing through lymph nodes, is emptied back into the blood circulatory system. *Thus the lymph that is returned* to the bloodstream differs from the lymph that forms in association with capillaries because it contains abundant lymphocytes.

The thoracic duct in an experimental animal is large enough to permit a cannula to be inserted into it, and by this means the lymph that flows along it may be collected. By this means it is possible to obtain fairly large numbers of lymphocytes for study. We can now describe some of the experiments that have been performed in connection with thoracic duct lymph and the cells it contains.

The Development of Knowledge About The Relation of Lymphocytes to Immunological Reactions

Establishing the Life Span of Lymphocytes. This began with the pioneer work of Yoffey and his associates, who counted the number of lymphocytes that were carried by the thoracic duct back to the blood circulatory system over given periods of time in experimental animals. They found that enormous numbers of lymphocytes were added to the bloodstream every day by the thoracic duct, so many that it would be impossible for them to remain in the bloodstream for more than part of a day without their numbers mounting rapidly instead of their numbers remaining relatively constant as they do. The question arose as to what happened to them.

Since it had been shown that lymphocytes are motile, and since many studies with the LM had shown lymphocytes in the act of migrating from small blood vessels into tissues in many body sites and even migrating through the epithelium of the intestine to enter its lumen, it was more or less assumed that lymphocytes had a very short life-span and after they left the blood to enter the tissues they mostly died or passed into the intestine.

However, in 1959, Gowans showed that if lymph (with its contents of lymphocytes) was continuously drained away from the thoracic duct, the number of lymphocytes present in the lymph that was draining away became fewer and fewer. Hitherto it had been assumed that the lymphocytes in the thoracic duct had all been newly formed in the lymph nodes through which the lymph had drained. Gowans' experiments showed that this could not be true and that some lymphocytes must recirculate from blood back to

lymph again. He proved this conclusively by showing that if he injected the lymphocytes collected from the thoracic duct back into the bloodstream the numbers in the thoracic duct lymph returned to normal. Hence it was established that some lymphocytes recirculate from blood back to lymph. Precisely where this happens will be described later, in connection with lymph nodes.

Previous to this work, it had been assumed that lymphocytes must have a very short life span. Gowans' findings of course led to this assumption being tested. Soon after radioactive tracers became available the life span of lymphocytes was investigated by this method. First, it was found by Hamilton that when lymphocytes that had been formed in people suffering from chronic lymphatic leukemia had been labeled with radioactive adenine over a short period, labeled cells could be found in the circulation as long as 300 days afterward. This seemed to show that at least some lymphocytes live as long as 300 days. However, these experiments did not prove that the labeled cells seen at 300 days were necessarily the cells that were labeled at the time when the labeled adenine was administered, for it was possible that cells labeled at that time might have died, with the result that their radioactive label was taken up by new cells that were forming. To rule out this possibility, Little, Brecher, Bradley and Rose continuously infused animals with labeled thymidine for 90 days, so that all the lymphocytes that formed during the 90 days would be labeled. They found that at the end of 90 days there were still some circulating lymphocytes that were not labeled and concluded that these must have formed before the experiment was begun, more than 90 days before. As a result of all these experiments, it was obvious that at least some lymphocytes have a long life-span (and the length of this long life-span varies), circulating back and forth between the lymph stream and the bloodstream.

Two Kinds of Small Lymphocytes. Another development was the establishing that there are two kinds of small lymphocytes, only one of which has a long life-span; this span, in rats, is probably months, but in man it is probably years or, in some instances, might even be a lifetime. The other kind are short-lived. Next, the long-lived small lymphocytes were found to be derived from the thymus gland (to be described in a following chapter), and for this reason they are termed T lymphocytes. They account for most of the recirculating lymphocytes. It was also shown from studying birds that the short-lived lymphocytes are formed in a structure called the bursa of Fabricius (a bursa is a saclike structure; Fabricius

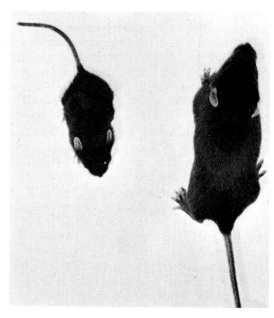

FIG. 10-13. Photograph of two 13-day-old mice from the same litter that resulted from mating a male of one inbred strain with a female of another inbred strain. The mouse on the left (the runt) received an intraperitoneal injection within the first 24 hours of life of 10^7 spleen cells from an adult of one of the parental strains. (From experiments by R. Escoffery and the author)

was the Italian anatomist who was first to show that veins have valves). This bursa develops from the epithelium of the hind gut and it is seeded by hemopoietic cells that come to it by the bloodstream and these form lymphocytes in this environment. The short-lived lymphocytes were therefore called B lymphocytes. The origin of all B lymphocytes in man is not established with certainty. There have been some thoughts to the effect that certain gut-associated lymphocyte depots may act like the bursa of Fabricius and form some B lymphocytes but it seems more probable that the B lymphocytes in mammals are derived from the bone marrow.

As will be described shortly, the T and B lymphocytes differ from each other in their immunological functions. But first we shall describe how it was found that lymphocytes have immunological functions.

How It Was Established That Lymphocytes Are Immunologically Competent Cells

That lymphocytes were immunologically competent cells was established before it was known that there were the T and B kinds. In order to explain how this

was done and how many other facts were elicited about lymphocytes, we must first describe the development and use of inbred strains of laboratory animals.

Inbred Strains. It is possible to inbreed mice, rats and animals with short lives by brother-to-sister matings through so many generations that for all practical purposes the members of the inbred strains all come to have exactly the same genes. In this way they resemble identical twins. Having the same genes, the proteins formed in their bodies are all alike. Hence when tissue—for example, skin—is transplanted from one animal to another within any inbred strain, the transplanted skin has no antigens that are foreign to those of the animal onto which the skin is transplanted, and so the skin graft "takes" readily and becomes part of the host.

Crossing Inbred Strains. If a male from one inbred strain is mated with a female of the same species but of a different inbred strain, their offspring, called F_1 hybrids, will have derived half of their genes from their mothers and half from their fathers. But since all their body cells will contain one *full set of chromosomes* from their mothers and one full set from their fathers, the body cells of the F_1 hybrids will have *all* the genes that directed the formation of proteins in both their mothers and their fathers. Hence, tissue from either their mother or their father will not contain any proteins to which the F_1 hybrids are not immunologically tolerant. (The above statement holds true only for inbred animals and not for randomly bred individuals such as man.)

Production of the Runting Syndrome and Wasting Disease. Whereas an F_1 hybrid from two inbred strains recognizes no antigens in a transplant from either its father or its mother as being foreign, any lymphocytes in the transplant will find foreign antigens in the F_1 hybrid into which they have been transferred. The reason is that the host (the F_1 hybrid), having genes from *both* its father and mother, possesses those proteins whose synthesis was directed by the genes of both its mother and father. So, if the transplant is from the father, any lymphocytes that are in it will find some of the proteins, whose formation was directed by the genes derived from the mother, foreign to them. This is strikingly illustrated if lymphatic tissue from either the mother or the father is injected into an F_1 hybrid when it is still very young. The F_1 hybrid does not react against the injected cells but the injected lymphocytes react immunologically against some of the proteins of their new host, with the result that the injected hybrid does not grow properly and is termed a *runt* (Fig. 10-13), and it soon dies. If the same experiment is done with older

F_1 hybrids in rats, the reaction produced by the transplant causes what is termed "wasting disease," which is often fatal. The phenomenon is called the *graft-versus-host reaction.*

In order to find out if lymphocytes were the cells that caused the graft-versus-host reaction, Gowans, in the early 60's, collected lymphocytes from the thoracic duct of fathers or mothers of hybrid rats and injected these into the hybrids and found that wasting disease occurred. Thus it was established that lymphocytes can recognize foreign antigens and react to living foreign cells sufficiently to cause wasting disease.

Lymphocytes Shown To Develop Into Larger Cells Which Divide and Form Clones. Another finding of Gowans, and Gowans and McGregor, was that small lymphocytes, under circumstances such as those described above, developed into larger cells which contain large numbers of free ribosomes in their cytoplasm (Fig. 10-14). This type of cell is often termed a *pyroninophilic cell* because the abundant RNA of its cytoplasm stains well and fairly distinctly with pyronin, which allows it to be distinguished with the LM. These cells have been shown to be able to divide

and hence are a type of blast cell because they "germinate" other cells. It was also shown, first by Nowell, that the addition of a substance known as phytohemagglutinin (PHA) to cultures of blood leukocytes stimulated small lymphocytes to turn into larger cells which divided. The kind of cell into which small lymphocytes develop in vitro under these conditions is similar to the large pyroninophilic cell described previously and illustrated in Figure 10-14.

It was next discovered that, if leukocytes from two different individuals were mixed in a cell culture, many lymphocytes would enlarge and divide without any phytohemagglutinin being added. It was also noticed that, if leukocytes from identical twins were mixed, no mitosis occurred without phytohemagglutinin being added. Accordingly, it became established that the lymphocytes in cell cultures could be stimulated at least sometimes to increase in size and to divide if they were exposed to antigens.

It thus became apparent that lymphocytes were not end-of-line cells, as had been so commonly believed in the past; rather, when suitably exposed to the right antigen, they became blast cells that produced progeny.

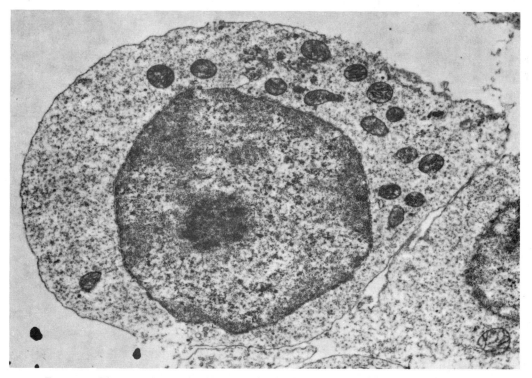

Fig. 10-14. Electron micrograph of an example of a large pyroninophilic cell that formed in the spleen of a mouse that had received lethal x-irradiation and had then been injected with small lymphocytes obtained from a rat. Note the abundance of free ribosomes in the abundant cytoplasm and the absence of endoplasmic reticulum. (Illustration courtesy of Prof. J. L. Gowans)

Where T and B Lymphocytes Become Blast Cells. As will be described in following chapters, T and B lymphocytes are from the thymus and bone marrow respectively and are fed chiefly into lymph nodes and the spleen. Some also are fed into lymphatic nodules present in loose connective tissue. It is in these sites that the T or B lymphocytes become activated and turn into blast cells and give rise to progeny. The latter transformations occur in different areas in the structures just mentioned, as will be described in Chapter 13. The progeny of activated B lymphocytes differentiate into cells of the plasma cell series (Fig. 13-17), and when they do this they can be recognized most easily by their great abundance of rER and a prominent Golgi (Fig. 13-16, *right*), for they become fairly typical secretory cells. Activated T lymphocytes become blast cells that are probably similar in appearance to those that first form from B lymphocytes, but they do not differentiate into plasma cells. Instead as such they can serve as killer cells in graft rejection phenomena, as will soon be described. They can also give rise to progeny with the appearance of small lymphocytes which are programmed to react to the antigen that caused their mother cell to become a blast cell. These are sometimes termed memory cells. Some of them remain in lymphatic tissue, particularly in lymph nodes, while others enter the circulation where they recirculate for a relatively long time.

Are Lymphocytes Programmed When They Are Formed? After it was shown that lymphocytes could react to antigens, an intriguing question received much consideration. In discussing this we shall first consider B lymphocytes. The question was whether or not a virgin B lymphocyte (that is, a B lymphocyte born of a precursor cell that had had no contact with an antigen) had the potentiality to react to the first antigen it met by forming plasma cells that would produce the specific antibody required to react with the particular antigen the B lymphocyte had encountered. In other words, can any antigen induce any virgin B lymphocyte to form plasma cells that will produce the specific antibody that reacts with that antigen? This view would more or less assume that virgin B lymphocytes are uncommitted competent cells of such great potentiality that they can be induced to develop along a specialized differentiation pathway by the first antigen they encounter. An alternative concept, which is now generally accepted, is that virgin B lymphocytes are not born alike but instead are each programmed for a particular antigen when they are formed. Thus the virgin B lymphocytes of the body represent a vast assembly of B lymphocytes already programmed to re-act with different particular antigens so that there will be at least a few in the population that are programmed to react specifically with any particular antigen that may enter the body.

How Lymphocytes Become Programmed

To understand how B lymphocytes become programmed, each with a particular specificity, something must be said first about the structure of antibody and how its specificity is determined. An antibody molecule is composed of 4 polypeptide chains; two are identical heavy chains and two are identical light chains. Each chain is made up of amino acids, the heavier having many more amino acids than the light chains. The molecule is symmetrical and Y-shaped. The stem of the Y consists only of parts of the 2 heavy chains. The arms each consist of the remainder of one heavy chain with each having a light chain lying alongside and associated with it.

There are 2 identical sites that can combine with antigen in each antibody molecule. These are at the free ends of the 2 arms of the Y. Thus each antigen combining site is constructed of the end of a heavy chain and the end of a light chain. The specificity of the antibody for a particular antigen resides in these combining sites and is determined by the particular amino acid sequences at the ends of the light and the heavy chains. Variations in amino acid sequence among different antibody molecules are confined to the regions of the chains that include these ends. The remainder of the light and the heavy chains have constant amino acid sequences.

For antibody molecules, as well as for other proteins, the amino acid sequences are determined by structural genes. The constant region of the antibody molecules are coded for by genes that are transmitted in stable fashion from one generation to the next in the usual way. But the variable regions, which determine the enormous diversity of antibodies, potentially capable of reacting with practically any antigen in the universe, must also be coded for by genes. How is this diversity accomplished?

Two views might be considered. First, in the formation of B lymphocytes, which in mammals probably occurs in the bone marrow, many mitoses are involved and it can be argued that enough gene mutations could occur during these mitoses to account for the variation that occurs in the genes that control the synthesis of antibody molecules.

A second view is that there are, in each progenitor cell that will differentiate into a B lymphocyte, a very large assortment of different genes that could code for the variable part of the immunoglobulin molecule. Which of these are turned on to participate with the gene or genes that direct the synthesis of the constant part of immunoglobulin molecules in developing B lymphocytes is a matter of chance. This haphazard arrangement results in the amino acid sequences present at the combining sites of the immunoglobulin molecules produced by different B lymphocytes being so different from one another that among the B lymphocyte population there would be at least a few that would produce immunoglobulin molecules with combining sites that would fit those of any antigen that gained entrance to the body.

After the choice of genes is made, even though it is made by chance, the lymphocyte thereafter remains stable so that the cell is committed to producing immunoglobulin molecules of only one specificity. The cell is now a programmed B lymphocyte. Encounter with an antigen of that specificity, and that specificity only, will activate the lymphocyte to become a blast cell and proliferate. All the cells of the clone that formed from it would be identically programmed to produce antibody molecules of the same single specificity. The subject of immunoglobulins and their production by plasma cells in lymph nodes and spleen will be considered further in Chapter 13.

Recognition Sites. The next point to make is that each B lymphocyte, after it becomes programmed, but before it or its progeny ever develop into full-fledged antibody-producing plasma cells, makes just enough of the specific immunoglobulin that it is programmed to make for this specific immunoglobulin to be present in small patches on the surface of the cell. These tiny surface patches are called recognition sites, surface receptors or epitopes (*epi*, upon; *topos*, place). It is by means of these that a B lymphocyte recognizes the particular antigen to which it is programmed to react. We might next ask what happens if such a meeting occurs and this brings up some more or less related problems.

T Lymphocytes As Helper Cells. First, although there are certain kinds of antigens which, on combining with a recognition site on a B lymphocyte directly, are able to activate the B lymphocyte so that it becomes a blast cell and forms a clone of cells which differentiate into plasma cells and produce specific antibody directed against that particular antigen, this is not the rule. In general, for a B lymphocyte to be activated by an antigen that antigen must have first been picked up by a recognition site (surface receptor) on a T lymphocyte that was programmed to react with it and subsequently delivered to a properly programmed

B lymphocyte. This can be done either directly or indirectly as is shown in Figure 13-14 which should be consulted at this point as well as later in connection with the text in Chapter 13. The role of T lymphocytes in bringing specific antigens to specifically programmed B lymphocytes, either directly or indirectly via the surface of reticular cells (Fig. 13-14) is spoken of as their role as helper cells. Thus, T lymphocytes are concerned in the immunological reactions that involve the production of antibodies as well as with cell-mediated immunological reactions which will be described next. But before commenting on the cell-mediated type of immunological reaction we must discuss another point.

Theories as to Why Antibodies Are Not Formed To React With Self. If B lymphocytes become programmed by mechanisms that depend on chance so that a vast variety of specifically programmed B lymphoctyes are produced in the body, it might be asked why some of these B lymphocytes are not programmed to react against the macromolecules of the body in which they develop. Or, if they are formed, we might ask why they do not become activated and develop into clones of plasma cells that produce antibodies that react with, and bring about the destruction of, the cells of the body of which they form a part. Answers to these questions are not as yet as satisfactory as might be wished. However, as will be explained when we discuss the thymus in Chapter 13, there is evidence to suggest that the premature contact of an antigen with a lymphocyte that is just developing its specificity probably leads to the lymphocyte being destroyed instead of activated. It might be thought that a B lymphocyte that develops in the bone marrow would prematurely meet so many body antigens that those that were becoming programmed to react to body antigens would be eliminated. Another point might also be mentioned. There is some reason to believe, as will be described in Chapter 13, that any T lymphocytes that are programmed to react against body macromolecules are weeded out before they are liberated from the thymus into the blood. Accordingly, since B lymphocytes generally do not become activated unless they receive antigen by way of helper T lymphocytes, and since T lymphocytes programmed to pick up body antigens are probably not present normally in the circulation, B lymphocytes programmed to react against body proteins would not become activated by T lymphocytes acting in a helper role.

The whole problem involving inquiry into why the immune system does not destroy the cells of the body in which it exists, and why there is sometimes the development of autoimmune disease in which the immune system does attack some body part, will be discussed further in connection with the thymus in Chapter 13 and in connection with the thyroid gland in Chapter 25. We shall here continue with our discussion of T lymphocytes and their role in what are termed cell-mediated immunological reactions.

T Lymphocytes and Cell-Mediated Immunological Reactions

The formation of T lymphocytes in, and their delivery from, the thymus will be described in detail in Chapter 13. T lymphocytes are the long-living kind that keep circulating back and forth between blood and lymph and so they are widely exposed to any antigens that might be present in any part of the body. Like B lymphocytes each T lymphocyte is programmed to react with a specific antigen. Furthermore, like B lymphocytes, T lymphocytes have surface receptors by which they recognize the antigen with which they are programmed to react. On meeting a foreign antigen, a T lymphocyte may act as a helper cell as was just described. Or on becoming activated it can give rise to a clone of cells, often called killer cells, that will react specifically with foreign cells that have gained entrance to the body and possess the proper antigen.

However, the only way these activated T lymphocytes can do anything about destroying a cell that bears the antigen it recognizes, is by discharging a chemical substance into it. This can be done only if the killer cells actually contact the foreign cells bearing the antigen they recognize. Contact with the antigen on the foreign cells triggers the release from them of a cytotoxic substance that destroys the cells they contact. The cytotoxic substance itself is nonspecific (but the recognition is specific). This type of immunological reaction which involves direct contact between foreign cells and killer cells is described as a cell-mediated type of reaction.

The above explains why T lymphocytes are the chief cause for the rejection of transplants of tissue or organs from one person to another, as will be described shortly under a separate heading. Moreover, it is now believed that T lymphocytes serve a very important function by exercising constant surveillance in the body for the appearance of cancer cells and destroying them almost as soon as they appear. This concept is based on two kinds of evidence. First, experiments made on cancer induced in animals either by chemical carcinogens or by viruses have revealed that the cancer cells, which of course develop from the animal's own

body cells, possess some antigens that are different from those of the body cells from which they developed. This was to be expected, in the light of the general belief to the effect that for a body cell to become a cancer cell a gene mutation or its equivalent must occur in it. However, it required elaborate modern methods to prove that experimentally induced cancers actually possessed some different antigens from normal body cells. The second kind of evidence appeared when people who were given organ transplants were extensively treated with agents designed to reduce the numbers or effectiveness of the T lymphocytes; this measure was of course designed to prevent the T lymphocytes from rejecting the transplant. It was found, however, that the incidence of cancer increased in people so treated. However, more remains to be learned before too definite conclusions about the cause of this can be drawn.

THE ROLE OF LYMPHOCYTES IN REJECTING TRANSPLANTS OF FOREIGN TISSUES OR ORGANS

The Homograft Reaction. Tissue or organ transplants are commonly called grafts. Tissue transplantation (grafting) has been much studied in experimental animals. A graft that is made from one part of an animal to another is called an *autograft* (*auto*, self). A graft made from one member of an inbred strain to another of the same strain is termed an *isograft* (*isos*, equal). A graft attempted from one member of a species to another of the same species (but not between two members of the same inbred strain) is called a *homograft* (*homos*, same) because of its being made between two members of the *same* species, or an *allograft* (*allos*, another) because it is made to *another* member of the species. A graft attempted between members of different species is called a *heterograft*.

What Is Meant by a Graft "Taking." Much confusion has existed for decades because there has been no clear definition of what is meant by a graft taking. Most of this confusion has been caused by a lack of appreciation of the fact that many tissues that are grafted consist chiefly of intercellular substances which of course are nonliving and, moreover, are not very antigenic. Hence grafts of fascia or bone made from one person to another (homografts) have often been described as "taking." Indeed, there is no question that they have often served useful purposes—for example, Macewen, a Scottish surgeon, in 1880 restored the use of an arm in a child by a large homograft of bone. The fact is, however, that the cells in these grafts, which are, of course, foreign to their hosts, die, but the nonliving intercellular substances survive and provide a scaffolding on and into which cells of the host can proliferate and form new living tissue as will be described when we consider bone. Such grafts are often described as "taking," but it would be better if this term was used for grafts in which the cells of the graft are compatible with the host so that they continue to live and function, as for example, is essential if kidney transplants are to be successful.

In experimental studies the kind of tissue commonly used for studying whether grafts "take" or are rejected is skin, probably because skin is easily transplanted and the surgical operation does not require, as transplanting organs does, that the blood vessels of the graft be surgically connected to those of the host. Skin is thin enough for its cells to be nourished by tissue fluid seeping from its bed into its substance, and, if the transplanted skin is compatible with that of its host, blood vessels of the host will by themselves become connected with those of the graft to provide it with a more permanent type of nourishment.

Skin autografts made from one part of an animal (or person) to another part take readily. In animals of pure strains skin grafts made from one animal to another (isografts) also take. However, if skin is transplanted from one animal to another of the same species but not a member of the same pure strain, a homograft reaction soon appears in the host along its site of contact with the graft. This can be seen to advantage if the graft is a very thin shaving cut from the surface of the skin so that it consists almost entirely of the epidermis (the epithelium) which, of course, is cellular. The connective tissue bed on which an epidermal graft is placed soon becomes infiltrated with what are generally termed *graft rejection cells* (Fig. 10-15); these are T lymphocytes that have become activated to become killer cells as will next be described. These make direct contact with the epidermal cells and elaborate a cytotoxic substance which destroys both the epidermal cell and usually also themselves.

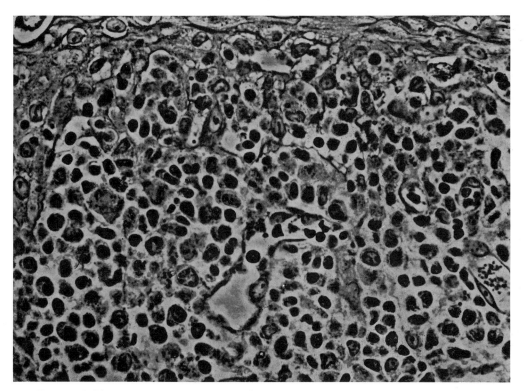

Fig. 10-15. Phase contrast photomicrograph of section of site of implantation of homograft of epidermis in a rabbit. The transplanted epidermis can be seen extending across the top of the picture. The bed of the transplant which is host tissue is heavily infiltrated with mononuclear cells, many of which have pyroninophilic cytoplasm and are graft rejection cells. Some of the latter have infiltrated into the epidermal transplant. This picture illustrates what is known as a homograft reaction. (Weiner, Joseph, Spiro, David, and Russel, P. S.: Am. J. Path., *44:*319)

The Source and Nature of Graft Rejection Cells

The operative procedure involved even in transplanting skin incites some degree of an inflammatory response in the graft bed and so there is some dilation of small blood vessels in the bed and some exudation and increased lymphatic drainage from it. In autografts and isografts the inflammation subsides in a few days. In homografts, however, the inflammatory reaction persists because a new factor enters the picture to maintain the inflammatory process.

Because there is an early inflammation it would be quite possible for T lymphocytes to leave small blood vessels of the graft bed and enter the tissues at the site of a homograft and meet an antigen with which they were programmed to react. These lymphocytes could then enter a lymphatic and then pass to the closest lymph node where they could settle out and develop into blast cells and produce progeny. Another possibility is that antigens from the graft might seep into the tissue of the bed and from there into lymphatic capillaries and thus reach the nearest lymph node where they would encounter properly programmed T lymphocytes which they would activate, causing them to become blast cells. As already described these are larger and have more basophilic cytoplasm (due to RNA) than ordinary lymphocytes. From a lymph node these would reach the graft bed by entering efferent lymphatics and from lymph they enter the bloodstream and, being motile, they leave it to attack the cells of the homograft. It requires energy for them to form and elaborate cytotoxic substance that kills the cells of the homograft.

T Lymphocytes as Memory Cells. As well as becoming killer cells activated T lymphocytes can take another pathway. They can stay within a lymph node and proliferate, with their progeny having the morphological appearance of small lymphocytes. Since these small lymphocytes are programmed to respond to only one particular antigen and since their numbers have been increased because of the mitoses of their progenitor blast cell, there are now a lot more of them than there were before their progenitor was first exposed to the particular antigen with which it was programmed to react. These lymphocytes are termed *memory cells* and many of them recirculate. Their persistence after a first homograft explains why a second homograft from the same donor is rejected much more quickly and more energetically than the first graft.

When a first homograft is made there may be only a rare T lymphocyte or only a few T lymphocytes in the regional lymph node that are programmed to react with the antigen it bears. So to mount a proper offensive against it, the few T lymphocytes that are activated have to undergo numerous mitoses as blast cells to produce enough killer cells to reject the graft, and all this takes time. However, on a second homograft there would be numerous memory cells ready to become activated by the antigen of the homograft to become blast cells, so, instead of beginning from a few cells, the second response could begin from many cells; hence the rate of production of killer cells would be much greater and the rejection of the graft much quicker.

Relation of Blood Supply to the Take or Rejection of Grafts. An interesting feature of the take of skin autografts of pigs which we once studied and whose skin and blood supply is similar to that of man is that the blood vessels of the graft become reconnected via capillaries to the blood vessels of the graft bed as soon as the fifth day after the autograft has been in place, so that by five days blood has begun to circulate again through the pre-existing vessels of the graft. But in homografts made every few days in a pig we found that the blood vessels of the homograft and those of the host did *not* become connected. Since the series of homografts were all made on the same pig, it would have begun to have a second set response by the end of the experiment when the grafts were removed for examination. These findings suggested that the homograft reaction is in part directed against the endothelial cells of the vessels of the homograft. Nevertheless, because its cells are nourished for a time by tissue fluid, many cells in the substance of a homograft survive for a few days, for mitotic figures can be found in them. (For illustrations of blood supply of skin grafts *see* reference to Ham, 1952 in Chap. 15.)

Why Humoral Antibodies Are Not the Cause of Graft Rejection. The antigens of homografts also incite the formation of some plasma cells in their hosts from B lymphocytes. These produce antibodies that react specifically with these antigens. But this does not necessarily affect transplanted tissue cells deleteriously. Antibody combining with antigen on body cells does damage to them only if the combining of the antibody with antigen on the cells fixes complement. Only some kinds of body cells—that is, those cells on whom antigenic sites are close together—fix complement under these conditions, and this exists chiefly on erythrocytes and leukocytes.

The antigens on the surface of most body cells, however, are not close enough together for complement to be fixed if humoral antibody combines with their surface antigens; this is the reason why humoral antibody, even if it is formed in response to a foreign transplant, may not have any deleterious effect on the cells of the transplant. Indeed humoral antibody combining with the antigens on the cells of a foreign transplant may have an opposite effect; it may hide these antigens, and so keep them from disclosing their presence to the activated T lymphocytes that would be concerned with their destruction. Another possibility is that the antigen-antibody complex may have the effect of inhibiting the immunological activity of the graft rejection cells (this effect of humoral antibody is termed the "enhancement" effect because antibodies may actually enhance the survival of a foreign transplant).

Rationale of Measures Taken in Attempts To Prevent the Homograft Reaction. The homograft reaction is the chief obstacle to overcome in making it possible to successfully transplant tissues and organs from one person to another. One basic measure that can be taken toward preventing the reaction has to do with the selection of donors. People who are not identical twins may have many genes and antigens in common but they also have some different genes and so their tissues contain different antigens; this is the inevitable result in species of animals (including man) that practice random breeding. So, aside from taking into account the fact that the children within a family may generally have fewer discordant genes among them so far as transplantation is concerned than would those of a similar but random group, the selection of a suitable donor for a transplant hinges on employing tests that depend essentially on showing the extent to which the lymphocytes of the host are going to react with the antigens of the donor, and laboratory methods are available for making such tests. Next, when a donor is selected and a transplantation effected, efforts may be directed at suppressing the homograft reaction in two ways. One method involves the use of immunosuppressive measures including radiation and certain drugs, both of which inhibit the formation of new lymphocytes. However, attempting to suppress the graft rejection response by radiation or drugs is not without consequences, for the measures taken may suppress also the capability of the host to combat antigens of all kinds, and so the host becomes less able to cope with infections. Another approach to the problem is directed toward injecting lymphocytes from the host into animals and then preparing a serum (antilymphocyte serum) from the animals. The serum is purified so that it contains only antibodies that combine with the host's lymphocytes. The serum is injected into the host. This procedure destroys host lymphocytes to some extent and in addition it may also adhere to host lymphocytes in such a way as to make them less able to attach themselves specifically to graft cells and destroy them.

Role of T Lymphocytes in Delayed Hypersensitivity Reactions. So far we have discussed two roles for T lymphocytes: (1) to act as helper cells in connection with activating B lymphocytes so that they develop into plasma cells and make specific antibodies, and (2) to develop into killer cells that destroy foreign cells by direct contact in cell-mediated reactions. A third effect they have in the body is in connection with a phenomenon described as delayed hypersensitivity reactions. Their role in this is described briefly at the end of the section on lymph nodes in Chapter 13.

Morphological Differences Between T and B Lymphocytes. It has recently been shown that with the scanning EM, they can be distinguished from one another morphologically. See Figure 10-15 A in which their appearances with this instrument are shown. Details are given in its caption.

Monocytes

Numbers. Monocytes comprise from 3 to 8 percent of the leukocytes of normal blood; hence, a great many leukocytes may have to be examined before a good example of a monocyte is found. A typical monocyte can be distinguished without undue difficulty. However, there are some difficulties associated with deciding whether some cells are monocytes or large lymphocytes, and whether others are monocytes or juvenile neutrophils.

Appearance. The largest leukocytes seen in blood films are generally monocytes (Fig. 10-3). They are from 12 to 15 microns in diameter when suspended in fluid (Fig. 10-16) where they assume a more or less spherical shape. When flattened in dried films, they measure up to 20 microns in diameter.

Nuclei. Some are ovoid, some indented ovals, and some have an indentation that is great enough for the shape of the nucleus to be that of a thick horseshoe (Fig. 10-3). Sometimes nuclei of the latter type appear as if they had been twisted or folded in preparing the film. The chromatin of the nucleus is in the form of granules and flakes; hence the chromatin is less condensed than in lymphocyte nuclei. It is colored a blue-violet shade in the usual preparation, and, since it is finer and more spread out than that of lymphocytes, it does not stain as intensely as that of lymphocytes. Nucleoli are not visible in the usual stained

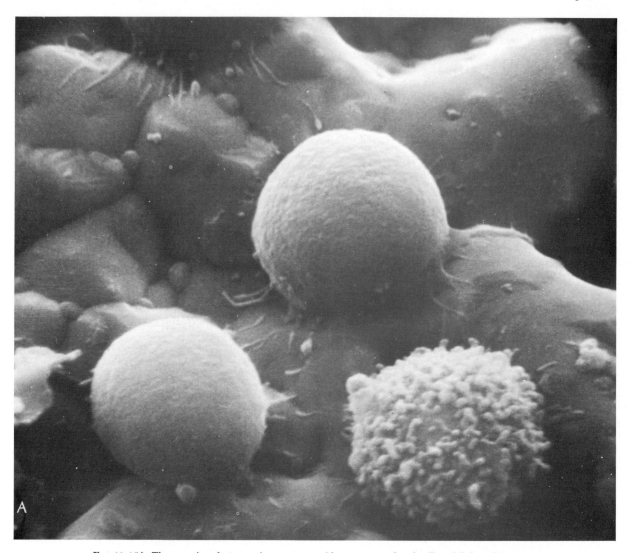

FIG. 10-15A. The scanning electron microscope provides a means whereby T and B lymphocytes can be distinguished from one another morphologically. This micrograph is of leukocytes from human blood, fixed in glutaraldehyde and osmium tetroxide, and dried by the critical point method. Three lymphocytes are shown. Two (above and at left) have a smooth surface which is characteristic of T lymphocytes. One has a surface studded with little villuslike projections which is characteristic of B lymphocytes. In human peripheral blood about 75 percent are of the T variety and about 25 percent are of the B type. $\times$ 14,000 approx. (From Drs. A. Polliack and E. de Harven, Sloan-Kettering Institute for Cancer Research. For further information *see* J. Exp. Med., *138:*607, 1973).

film but can be seen in monocytes examined with the phase microscope. There are often two in each nucleus.

Cytoplasm. This comprises the larger part of the cell. In stained blood films it is a pale blue-gray in color (Fig. 10-3). Fine azurophilic granules can often be seen in it (Fig. 10-3). With the EM these appear as lysosomes (Fig. 10-17). They have been shown to contain acid phosphatase and other enzymes; in man and the guinea pig the granules are peroxidase positive.

Mobility. They can extend and withdraw pseudopodia. Monocytes can readily migrate through capillaries or small venules to enter loose connective tissue and move within it.

Function. The monocyte reaches its full development and attains its full capacity for function when it leaves the bloodstream and enters the tissues. In the tissues monocytes cope with certain bacteria in a way similar to polymorphs and they also develop into ma-

FIG. 10-15B. Scanning electron micrograph of a normal human lymphocyte after separation of mononuclear cells by Ficoll-Hypaque gradient. This lymphocyte shows an intermediate type of surface morphology and would be difficult to classify exclusively on the basis of scanning electron microscopy. Cells fixed in glutaraldehyde and osmium tetroxide and dried by the critical point method. Magnification: approximately 31,500 ×. (Courtesy of Drs. A. Polliack and E. de Harven, Sloan-Kettering Institute for Cancer Research. For further information *see* J. Exp. Med., *138*:607, 1973.)

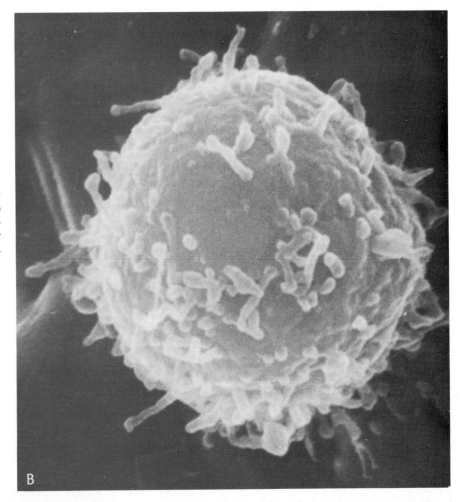

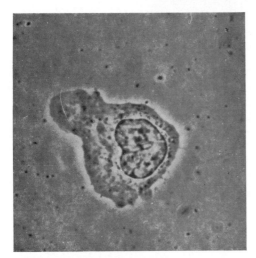

FIG. 10-16. Oil-immersion (phase) photomicrograph of a monocyte in a cell culture. (Preparation by D. A. Whitelaw)

crophages. The monocytes of the blood provide a force of cells that can be marshalled from the bloodstream into any tissue where more macrophages are needed. It seems improbable that monocytes can also serve as a source of fibroblasts as is sometimes suspected; evidence indicating they cannot was given in connection with the origin of fibroblasts earlier in this chapter.

Fine Structure. Their fine structure is illustrated in Figure 10-17. The peripheral chromatin of the nucleus is condensed. Golgi stacks are present toward the concavity of the nucleus and many dense granules which are primary lysosomes appear from this region (black in Fig. 10-17). Mitochondria are scattered about. Rough endoplasmic reticulum is not very prominent. Monocytes have ragged borders.

Origin. Over the years there have been several different theories about this matter. It has been postulated that they developed from lymphocytes, from reticuloendothelial cells or from special precursor cells

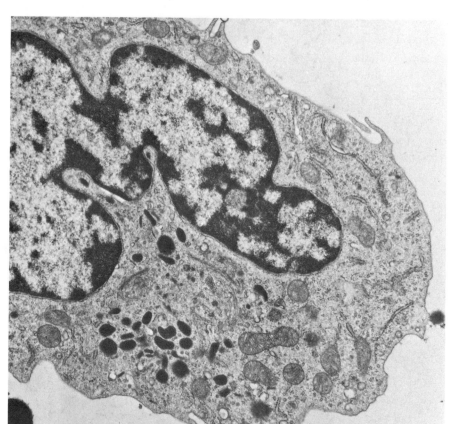

FIG. 10-17. Electron micrograph of mature rabbit monocyte from bone marrow. (From Nichols, B. A., Bainton, D. F., and Farquhar, M. G.: J. Cell Biol., *50:*498, 1971)

termed monoblasts that were present in bone marrow. A few years ago Osmond devised a method that labels, over a brief period, only cells that are undergoing DNA duplication in bone marrow (the method will be described in detail in Chapter 12). When the circulation is restored through the bone marrow (where label was available for a short period), labeled monocytes begin to appear in the blood, from 12 hours on. Furthermore, if measures are taken to institute an inflammation of the peritoneal cavity, labeled macrophages are seen in the exudate from 17 to 72 hours after the cells in the bone marrow have been labeled. Osmond's studies therefore prove that monocytes are formed in the bone marrow, and when we discuss bone marrow later their origin will be described more precisely.

Length of Life of Monocytes in the Circulation. This matter has been investigated by Whitelaw, who has shown by labeling experiments that monocytes leave the bloodstream in a random fashion under normal conditions, and that the average life of a monocyte in the bloodstream is about 3 days.

References and Other Reading

GENERAL

Good, R. A., and Fisher, D. W. (eds.): Immunobiology. Stamford, Connecticut. Sinaver Associates, 1971.

Jerne, N. K.: The Immune System. Sci. Am., *229:*52, 1973.

Low, F. N., and Freeman, J. A.: Electron Microscopic Atlas of Normal and Leukemic Human Blood. New York, Blakiston, 1958.

Metcalf, D., and Moore, M. A. S.: Haemopoietic Cells. Amsterdam, North-Holland Publishing Co., 1971.

Movat, H. Z. (ed.): Inflammation, Immunity and Hypersensitivity, ed. 2. New York, Harper and Row, In press, 1974.

Nossal, G. J. V.: Antibodies and Immunity. New York, Basic Books, 1969.

Nossal, G. J. V., and Ada, G. L.: Antigen, Lymphoid Cells and the Immune Response. New York and London, Academic Press, 1971.

Schwartz, M. R. (ed.): Proceedings of the Sixth Leucocyte Conference. New York and London, Academic Press, 1972.

Weiss, L.: The Cells and Tissues of the Immune System. Englewood Cliffs, New Jersey, Prentice-Hall, 1972.

(*See also* References and Other Reading for Chapters 12 and 13.)

INFLAMMATION

Movat, H. Z.: The acute inflammatory reaction. In Movat, H. Z., ed. 2 (listed under general references).

GRANULAR LEUKOCYTES

Ackerman, G. A.: Cytochemical properties of the blood basophilic granulocyte. Ann. N.Y. Acad. Sci., 103:376, 1963.

Anderson, D. R.: Ultrastructure of normal leukemic leukocytes in human peripheral blood. J. Ultrastruct. Res., Suppl. 9, 1966.

Bainton, D. F., and Farquhar, M. C.: Origin of granules in polymorphonuclear leucocytes: two types derived from opposite faces of the Golgi apparatus in developing leucocytes. J. Cell Biol., 28:277, 1966.

————: Differences in enzyme content of azurophil and specific granules of polymorphonuclear leucocytes: cytochemistry and electron microscopy of bone marrow cells. J. Cell Biol., 39:299, 1968.

————: Segregation and packaging of granules in eosinophilic leucocytes. J. Cell Biol., 45:54, 1970.

Bainton, D. F., Ullyot, J. L., and Farquhar, M. C.: The development of neutrophilic polymorphonuclear leucocytes in human bone marrow: origin and content of azurophil and specific granules. J. Exp. Med., 134:907, 1971.

Davidson, W. M., and Smith, D. R.: A morphological sex difference in the polymorphonuclear neutrophil leucocytes. Brit. Med. J., 2:6, 1954.

De Castro, N. M.: Frequency variations of "drumsticks" of peripheral blood neutrophils in the rabbit in different alimentary conditions. Acta anat., 52:341, 1963.

Farquhar, M. C., and Bainton, D. F.: Cytochemical Studies on Leucocyte Granules. Proc. 4th Internat. Congr. Histochemistry and Cytochemistry, Kyoto, Japan. p. 25-26. Published by the Soc. Histochemistry and Cytochemistry, 1972.

Garrey, W. S., and Bryan, W. R.: Variations in white blood cell counts. Physiol. Rev., 15:597, 1935.

Lillie, R. D.: Factors influencing the Romanovsky staining of blood films and the role of methylene violet. J. Lab. Clin. Med., 29:1181, 1944.

Litt, M.: Eosinophils and antigen-antibody reaction. Ann. N.Y. Acad. Sci., 116:964, 1964.

Sieracki, J. C.: The neutrophilic leukocyte. Ann. N.Y. Acad. Sci., 59:690, 1955.

Spiers, R. S.: Physiological approaches to an understanding of the function of eosinophils and basophils. Ann N.Y. Acad. Sci., 59:706, 1955.

Visscher, M. B., and Halberg, F.: Daily rhythms in numbers of circulating eosinophils and some related phenomena. Ann. N.Y. Acad. Sci., 59:834, 1955.

LYMPHOCYTES

(*See also* Special References on B and T Lymphocytes which follow this section.)

Dougherty, T. F.: Adrenal cortical control of lymphatic tissue mass. In Stohlman, F., Jr. (ed.): The Kinetic of Cellular Proliferation. p. 264. New York, Grune & Stratton, 1959.

Everett, N. B., Caffrey, R. W., and Rieke, W. O.: The small lymphocyte of the rat: rate of formation, extent of recirculation and circulating life span. In Proc. IX Congr. International Soc. Hematology, Mexico City. vol. 3, p. 345, 1962.

Everett, N. B., and Caffrey, R. W.: Radioautographic studies of bone marrow small lymphocytes. In Yoffey, J. M. (ed.): The Lymphocyte in Immunology and Haemopoiesis. p. 109.

Gesner, B. M., and Gowans, J. L.: The fate of lethally irradiated mice given isologous and heterologous thoracic duct lymphocytes. Brit. J. Exp. Path., 43:431, 1962.

Gowans, J. L.: The recirculation of lymphocytes from blood to lymph in the rat. J. Physiol., 146:54, 1959.

————: The life history of the lymphocytes. Brit. Med. Bull., 15:50, 1959.

————: The fate of parental strain small lymphocytes in F1 hybrid rats. Ann. N.Y. Acad. Sci., 99:432, 1962.

————: Life span, recirculation and transformation of lymphocytes. Int. Rev. Exp. Path., 5, 1967.

Gowans, J. L., and McGregor, D. D.: The origin of antibody forming cells. In Graber, P., and Miescher, P. A. (eds.): Immunopathology, IIIrd International Symposium. p. 89. Basel, Schwabe, 1963.

————: The immunological activities of lymphocytes. Progr. Allergy, 9:1, 1965.

Gowans, J. L., McGregor, D. D., and Cowen, D. M.: Initiation of immune response by small lymphocytes. Nature, 196:651, 1962.

————: The role of small lymphocytes in the rejection of homografts of skin. In Wolstenholme, G. E., and Knight, Julie (eds.): The Immunologically Competent Cell, Ciba Foundation Study Group No. 16. p. 20. London, Churchill, 1963.

Little, J. R., Brecher, G., Bradley, T. R., and Rose, S.: Determination of lymphocyte turnover by continuous infusion of triated thymidine. Blood, 19:236, 1962.

Marshall, W. H., and Roberts, K. B.: The growth and mitosis of human small lymphocytes after incubation with a phytohemagglutinin. Quart. J. Exp. Physiol., 48:146, 1963.

Martin, W. J., and Miller, J. F. A. P.: Site of action of antilymphocyte globulin. Lancet, p. 1285, December 16, 1967.

Medawar, P. B.: Zoologic laws of transplantation. In Peer, L. A. (ed.): Transplantation of Tissues. vol. 2, p. 41, Baltimore, Williams & Wilkins, 1959.

Merrill, J. P.: Transplantation of normal tissues. Physiol. Rev., 39:860, 1959.

Najarian, J. S., and Feldman, J. D.: Passive transfer of tuberculin sensitivity by tritiated thymidine-labeled lymphoid cells. J. Exp. Med., 114:779, 1961.

Nowell, P. C., Phytohemagglutinin: an initiator of mitosis in cultures of normal human leukocytes. Cancer Res., 20:462, 1960.

Osmond, D. G., and Everett, N. B.: Radioautographic studies of bone marrow lymphocytes in vivo and in diffusion chamber cultures. Blood, 23:1, 1964.

Peer, L. A.: Transplantation of Tissue. vols. 1 and 2. Baltimore, Williams & Wilkins, 1955, 1959.

Porter, K. A. (ed.): Tissue and Organ Transplantation: Immunological Society Symposium Organized by the College of Pathologists. London, British Medical Association House, 1967.

Rosenau, W., and Moon, H.: Lysis of homologous cells by sensitized lymphocytes in tissue culture. J. Nat. Cancer Inst., 27:471, 1961.

Trowell, O. A.: The sensitivity of lymphocytes to ionizing radiation. J. Path. Bact., 64:687, 1952.

Wiener, J., Spiro, D., and Russel, P. S.: An electron microscopy study of the homograft reaction. Am. J. Path., 44:319, 1964.

Yoffey, J. M. (ed.): The Lymphocyte in Immunology and Haemopoiesis. London, Edward Arnold, 1966. (This volume contains 43 reports by various investigators.)

SPECIAL REFERENCES
ON T AND B LYMPHOCYTES

Gutman, G. A., and Weissman, I. L.: Lymphoid tissue architecture: Experimental analysis of the origin and distribution of T-cells and B-cells. Immunology, *23:*465, 1972.
Möller, G. (ed.): Lymphocyte immunoglobulin: synthesis and surface representation. Transplantation Rev. *14,* 1973.
Polliack, A., Lampen, N., Clarkson, B. D., de Harven, E., Bentwich, Z., Siegal, F. P., and Kunkel, H. G.: Identification of human B and T lymphocytes by scanning electron microscopy. J. Exp. Med., *138:*607, 1973.

T and B Lymphocyte Interactions

Claman, H. N., and Chaperon, E. A.: Immunologic complementation between thymus and marrow cells—a model for the two cell theory of immunocompetence. Transplantation Rev., *1:*92, 1969.
Claman, H. N., and Mosier, D. E.: Cell-cell interactions in antibody production. Prog. Allergy, *16:*40, 1972.
Feldmann, M., and Nossal, G. V. V.: Cellular basis of antibody production. Quart. Rev. Biol., *47:*269, 1972.
Miller, J. F. A. P.: Lymphocyte interactions in antibody responses. Internat. Rev. Cytol., *33:*77, 1972.
Mitchison, N. A.: Cell cooperation in the immune response: the hypothesis of an antigen preservation mechanism. Immunopathology, *6:*52, 1971.

Raff, M. C.: T and B lymphocytes and immune responses. Nature, *242:*19, 1973.

Killer Cells

Able, M. D., Lee, J. C., and Rosenau, W.: Lymphocyte-target cell interaction in vitro. Ultrastructural and cinematographic studies. Am. J. Path., *60:*421, 1970.
Bloom, B. R.: In vitro approaches to the mechanism of cell-mediated immune reactions. Advances Immunol. *13:*101, 1971.

SOME REFERENCES ON MONOCYTES

Brahim, F., and Osmond, D. G.: Radioautographic studies on the production and fate of bone marrow lymphocytes and monocytes. Proc. Canad. Fed. Biol. Soc., *136,* 1967.
Clark, E. R., and Clark, E. L.: Relation of monocytes of the blood to tissue macrophages. Am. J. Anat., *46:*149, 1930.
van Furth, R. (ed.): Mononuclear Phagocytes. Philadelphia, F. A. Davis, 1970.
Nichols, B. A., Bainton, D. F., and Farquhar, M. G.: Differentiation of monocytes. Origin, nature and fate of their azurophil granules. J. Cell Biol., *50:*498, 1971.
Tompkins, E. H.: The monocyte. Ann. N.Y. Acad. Sci., *59:*732, 1955.
Volkman, A., and Gowans, J. H.: The origin of macrophages from bone marrow in the rat. Brit. J. Exp. Patho., *46:*62, 1965.
Whitelaw, D. M.: The intravascular lifespan of monocytes. Blood, *28:*455, 1966.

11 Erythrocytes and Platelets

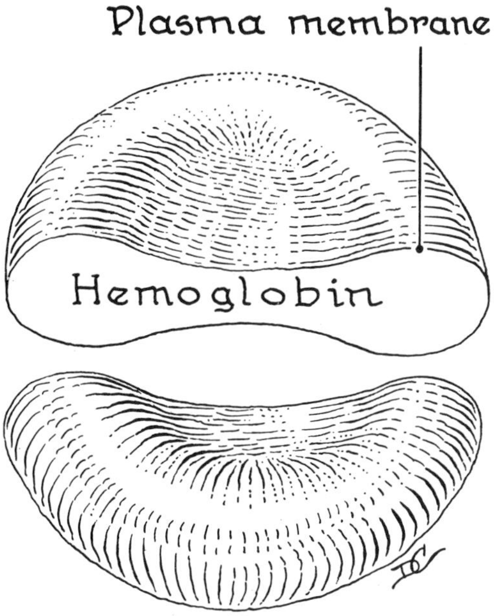

Plasma membrane

Hemoglobin

Fig. 11-1. Diagram of a red blood corpuscle that has been cut in half.

In order to complete our account of blood cells we must here consider red blood cells and platelets. Our secondary theme (the cellular basis for immunological reactions) will be resumed in the following chapters on hemopoietic tissues.

Erythrocytes

Erythrocytes (red blood cells) are from 500 to 1,000 times more numerous in blood than leukocytes. Their number in blood averages around 5 million per cubic millimeter.

Shape. The human erythrocyte is a *biconcave* disk (Fig. 11-1). The animal kingdom presents examples of other shapes. In certain diseases human erythrocytes of altered shape make their appearance in the circulation (Fig. 11-2, *right*); hence the determination of the shape of erythrocytes in any given sample of blood can be of diagnostic importance.

Size. Their diameter is usually determined from a blood film (Fig. 10-1) by measuring the dried cells under high magnification by means of a micrometer eyepiece. Since erythrocytes are biconcave disks, they lie flat on a slide, and drying does not affect their diameters greatly. If blood is normal, the erythrocytes in a film are of an almost uniform diameter, not differing from one another by more than 1 μ (Fig. 11-3). If the size of each is ticked off on a properly prepared piece of graph paper, it will be found that the greatest number are 7.2 μ wide, and that almost all are within half a micron of this either way. If the sizes seen in a large sample are all indicated on graph paper, a curve can be drawn which shows at a glance whether the size range is normal, or whether the size of the cells as a whole is greater or less than normal, or whether the size range within the sample is greater than it should be. Such a curve is called a Price-Jones curve. An abnormal curve can be of diagnostic significance.

Cells smaller than 6 μ are termed *microcytes* (*mikros,* small) (Fig. 11-2, *right*). Cells moderately larger than the normal, from 9 to 12 μ are termed *macrocytes* (*makros,* large) (Fig. 11-4, *right*). The shift in size that occurs in certain blood diseases is usually either to the smaller or the larger side; when the average is smaller, the condition is termed *microcytic* (Fig. 11-4, *left*), and when larger, *macrocytic* (Fig. 11-4, *right*). In some conditions both microcytes and macrocytes may be present (Fig. 11-2, *right*).

Structure and Composition. Although it has been shown with the EM that there are some microtubules in the peripheral part of the erythrocytes of some species, it seems that the chief supporting factor in the erythrocyte, so far as determining its shape is concerned, is the particular molecular constitution of the homogeneous colloidal complex with which it is filled. This results in the cell being soft and elastic.

More than half of the erythrocyte consists of water (60%), the rest of solids. About 33 percent of the erythrocyte is the conjugated protein hemoglobin. This is said to be a conjugated protein because it consists of the protein *globin* joined to the pigment *heme.* Al-

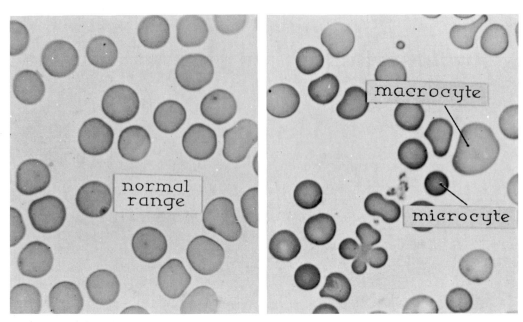

Fig. 11-2. Oil-immersion photomicrographs of stained films of rabbit's blood. (*Left*) Normal blood with the cells varying in size only slightly and, except where they have been pressed upon by other cells in the film, having a normal shape. (*Right*) Blood that was obtained from an animal with TNT poisoning. It shows a great range in the size of the red blood cells, with both microcytes and macrocytes present. It also shows red blood cells of different shapes.

though only 4 percent of hemoglobin actually consists of pigment (heme), its combination with globin results in the combined entity (hemoglobin) being colored; hence hemoglobin is spoken of as a pigment. A little other protein and some lipid also exist in the cell along with hemoglobin.

It may seem curious that erythrocytes containing only a soft jelly would maintain their biconcave shape, and that the molecular constitution of the jelly could be such as to be an important factor in making the cell assume this shape. However, the fact is that a change in the chemical constitution of hemoglobin can be responsible for the cells taking on a different shape. For example, there is a curious disease in which the erythrocytes may assume the form of sickles. In this form they are destroyed easily, and so individuals with this disease do not have enough erythrocytes. In 1949 Pauling and his colleagues discovered that hemoglobin in sickle cells was of a slightly different composition from the normal, but the difference was sufficient to make the cells assume a shape different from that of biconcave disks. Hereditary factors are responsible for the condition; hence this disease provides an example of how an altered sequence in a DNA molecule which results in one amino acid being substituted

for the usual one in the hemoglobin molecule can cause a disease.

Each erythrocyte is surrounded by a *cell (plasma) membrane*. As explained in Chapter 5, a cell membrane acts to prevent the escape of the colloidal protein material of the cell into the plasma. It also exhibits great selectivity with regard to the passage of ions. Features of the cell membrane are illustrated in Figures 5-5 and 5-6.

Rouleaux Formation. If fresh blood is placed on a slide and covered with a coverslip, the broad surfaces of erythrocytes often adhere to one another, with the result that numbers of erythrocytes may become arranged together like coins in a pile. These arrangements of adherent erythrocytes are termed *rouleaux formations* and they are probably manifestations of surface tension forces. If circulating blood is examined under the microscope, rouleaux formations are sometimes seen in areas where the circulation is not rapid. Rouleaux formations are not permanent, and the erythrocytes in them can become separated from one another again, with presumably no harm having been done to them.

Behavior in Solutions of Different Osmotic Pressure. The osmotic pressure of plasma equals that of erythrocytes, and so plasma is said to be *isotonic* (*iso,* equal; *tonos,* tension) with regard to them. In plasma, then, there is no tendency for the erythrocytes to absorb water from the plasma or vice versa. It is possible to prepare salt solutions that are *isotonic* with erythrocytes. If a salt concentration of a solution is below that of erythrocytes, it is said to be *hypotonic* (*hypo,* under), if above it, *hypertonic* (*hyper,* above, over), in relation to them.

Hemolysis. Erythrocytes are fairly resistant to slight changes in osmotic pressure, but in a solution that is sufficiently hypotonic, they swell and assume a spherical shape. Another phenomenon then occurs: their membranes become incapable of retaining hemoglobin, and this escapes into the surrounding fluid, coloring it. This is known as *hemolysis* (*lysis,* solution). Not all the substance of the erythrocyte escapes

when hemolysis occurs; enough remains to leave a "shadow" or "ghost" of the cell.

Hemolysis can be induced by means other than hypotonic solutions. Certain chemicals, particularly lipoid solvents, exert a hemolytic effect. Snake venom is a hemolytic agent. The plasma of some species hemolyzes the erythrocytes of others. Antibodies made by injecting the erythrocytes of one animal into a dissimilar one will hemolyze the erythrocytes of the first; this phenomenon involves the fixing of complement as described in the previous chapter.

Fragility. The erythrocytes in any given sample of blood are not equally susceptible to hemolysis. For instance, a solution of saline may be prepared in a concentration that will hemolyze only some cells; for all to be hemolyzed, the strength of the solution must be reduced further. Hence erythrocytes are said to vary

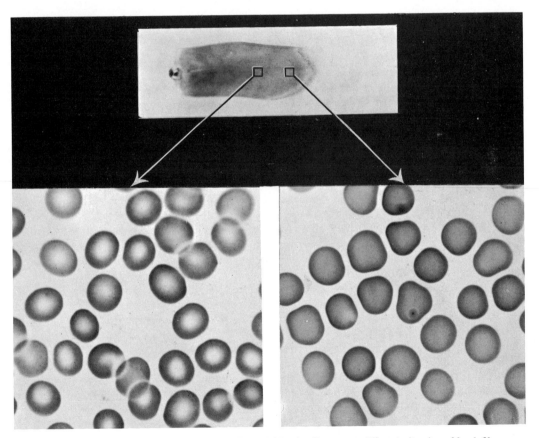

Fig. 11-3. Oil-immersion appearance of the red blood cells at two different sites in a blood film. (*Lower left*) These cells show the pale areas characteristic of normal cells. These pale areas show up only when the film is thick enough for occasional red cells to be superimposed on one another. (*Lower right*) Appearance of red cells at a place in the film where they are spread very thin. Notice that no cells here are superimposed and that in areas like this the central pale areas, characteristic of the normal red cell, cannot be seen.

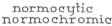

microcytic
hypochromic

normocytic
normochromic

macrocytic
hyperchromic

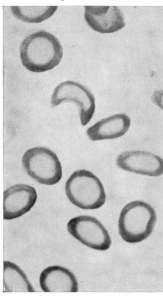
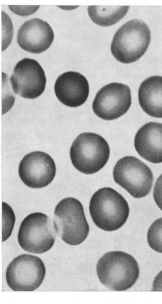
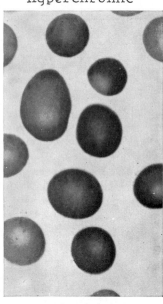

Fig. 11-4. Oil-immersion photomicrographs taken at the same magnification of 3 different films of human blood. (*Left*) This blood was obtained from a patient who had a microcytic hypochromic anemia due to iron deficiency, and the cells are seen to be small and their central pale areas greatly enlarged. (*Center*) Normal blood. (*Right*) Blood obtained from a person with pernicious anemia. In this condition the red blood cells, though fewer than normal, tend to be larger than usual and so they *appear* to be overfilled with hemoglobin.

in their *fragility* (their susceptibility to hemolysis). The fragility of erythrocytes becomes altered in certain diseases; hence fragility tests are of use in diagnosis.

Crenation. If erythrocytes are immersed in a hypertonic solution, water is drawn from them into the solution. This results in the shrinkage of the erythrocytes, and because they shrink irregularly, so that their outlines contain notches and indentations, they are said to be *crenated* (*crena*, a notch).

Function. Oxygen (at atmospheric pressure) does not dissolve to any great extent in water, or even in plasma. Hence, if the circulatory system contained nothing more than plasma, only a small fraction of the amount of oxygen needed by the cells of the body would dissolve into it as it was pumped through the capillaries of the lungs which are exposed to freshly inspired air. Blood is enabled to pick up large amounts of oxygen in the lungs because of the hemoglobin contained in erythrocytes. Hemoglobin is able to combine rapidly with oxygen to form the compound *oxyhemoglobin*. So because of the hemoglobin in erythrocytes blood can absorb enough oxygen as it passes through the lungs to constantly supply oxygen to all the cells of the body.

Hemoglobin, fortunately, does not bind oxygen firmly. So when oxyhemoglobin reaches the various tissues of the body, where the cells are constantly using oxygen, the hemoglobin releases a good part of its oxygen. When oxygen is thus divorced from oxyhemoglobin, the hemoglobin that remains is usually called the *reduced hemoglobin;* this, on reaching the lungs, as it continues on its route through the circulatory system, is again in contact with a high concentration of oxygen, and is prepared to unite with it and become oxyhemoglobin again.

Why Hemoglobin Must Be Confined in Cells. Hemoglobin macromolecules are relatively small and, if they were free in plasma, they would leak through the endothelial membranes of the blood vascular system. Hence, if hemoglobin becomes free in plasma, it escapes into the tissues and into the urine. This gave the name "red-water fever" to a disease of cattle in which a minute parasite invades the erythrocytes and so injures them that their hemoglobin escapes first into the plasma and then into the urine, which becomes colored. In certain human diseases—for example, in "black-water fever," which is a virulent type of malaria—enough erythrocytes may be injured to produce a like condition. There are other advantages in having hemoglobin enclosed by the cell membranes of erythrocytes. For example, erythrocytes are involved in the carriage of carbon dioxide from the tissues to the lungs where it escapes into the air. Their use in this respect is dependent on their containing an enzyme, carbonic anhydrase, which, like hemoglobin, is confined within the erythrocyte.

How the Structure of Erythrocytes Is Adapted to Their Function. Erythrocytes must absorb and release oxygen and carbon dioxide very quickly. The absorption and the release of gases between the cell and plasma occur at the surface of the cell membrane. Therefore it is desirable that the interface between each erythrocyte and plasma should be as extensive as possible per unit of hemoglobin, and this desirable end is obtained by the biconcave form of the erythrocyte, which gives a surface area from 20 to 30 percent greater than that of a sphere containing the same amount of hemoglobin. Furthermore, if erythrocytes were spheres, the average distance over which a gas would have to diffuse to reach the surface from the interior of the cell would be greatly increased. Hence the biconcave shape is an ideal one for providing a large interface at which gases can be absorbed and released quickly.

The non-nucleated state of the erythrocyte is also advantageous in that it allows the whole cell to contain hemoglobin and so be more efficient per unit volume.

The rounded edges of the erythrocyte protect it from injury, and its resilient elastic structure allows it to bend rather than break as it strikes bifurcations in capillaries. This phenomenon may be watched under the microscope in the web of a living frog's foot, suitably mounted.

Pink Cheeks and Red Lips. It is the oxyhemoglobin in the erythrocytes in capillaries below the surface that imparts pinkness to cheeks and varying degrees of redness to lips and mucous membranes. The degree of color so imparted depends on many factors: the number of capillaries in operation, their closeness to the surface, the transparency of the overlying tissue and finally, the percentage of oxyhemoglobin in the blood.

Blue Lips. Reduced hemoglobin is blue rather than red. Normally, as blood passes through capillaries, not enough reduced hemoglobin is formed for the blue color to show. However, in a normal person exposed to severe cold, the local circulation in the lips may be closed down sufficiently for the amount of reduced hemoglobin to be increased in the superficial capillaries so the blue shows. In certain diseases the oxygenation of blood in the lungs is seriously impaired so that blood containing a considerable amount of reduced hemoglobin is delivered to capillaries all over the body. A sufficient amount of reduced hemoglobin (absolute amount —not percentage) may under certain disease conditions be present to impart a blue color to all surfaces of the body that are ordinarily pink or red. This is termed *cyanosis* (*kyanos,* blue).

Carbon Monoxide Poisoning. Hemoglobin has a great affinity for certain other gases besides oxygen, most notably carbon monoxide. This gas forms a firm union with hemoglobin and so oxygen is not released to the tissues. Hence a person breathing air containing even a low percentage of carbon monoxide gradually comes to have more and more of his hemoglobin bound to it and therefore valueless for the transport of oxygen. (This happens all too often on cold nights in parked cars in which the motor is kept running to keep the heater on.) Carbon monoxide hemoglobin is a bright red color, and the cherry-red lips of the carbon monoxide victim, whose tissues are in reality starved for oxygen, provide a sad paradox.

How the Oxygen-Carrying Capacity of the Blood of a Person Is Determined

In the practice of medicine it is frequently necessary to determine whether or not a patient is suffering from the inability of his or her blood to properly transport oxygen. Aside from the relatively rare instances in which hemoglobin is chemically altered, it is obvious that the oxygen-carrying capacity of the blood could be diminished, by there not being (1) a proper number of erythrocytes in the blood, or (2) not enough hemoglobin in the red cells, or (3) both. The usual routine tests that are made are (1) counting the number of erythrocytes present per cubic millimeter of blood and (2) estimating the amount of hemoglobin in a given quantity of blood by a colorimetric method.

Erythrocyte Counts. These can be made by the same general method used for making leukocyte counts. Blood is diluted and mixed in a pipette with erythrocyte counting fluid and then some is used to flood a special type of glass slide on which there are ruled squares. The thickness of the fluid over the ruled squares is controlled by a special coverslip which is separated for a known distance from the ruled squares and the space between it and the ruled squares is taken up by the fluid. By counting the number of cells seen over several ruled squares a calculation can be made as to the number of erythrocytes per cubic millimeter of blood. Normal women have between 4,500,000 and 5,000,000 erythrocytes per cubic millimeter of blood while men have from 5,000,000 to 5,500,000.

Hemoglobin Estimations. Several methods allow the amounts of hemoglobin per cubic millimeter of blood to be determined from one drop. The amount used to be expressed in percentages of what was considered to be normal; for example, a person was said to have a hemoglobin of 100 (normal) or say 80 or some other percentage of the normal. However, it is best to express hemoglobin content in gm per 100 ml The normal is around 15 gm.

ANEMIA

If the amount of hemoglobin in circulating blood is significantly reduced, the condition is said to constitute anemia (without blood). A lack of hemoglobin can be due primarily either to a lack of erythrocytes or a lack of hemoglobin itself.

In order to consider the problem further, certain facts must be taken into consideration.

Life Span of Erythrocytes. Erythrocytes normally have a limited life span; in man this probably ranges from 100 to 120 days. After having lived their lives in the circulatory system, they must be removed from it to prevent their disintegrating bodies from cluttering up the circulatory system. Worn-out erythrocytes are removed from the bloodstream by cells of the macrophage type in the spleen, bone marow and liver. Details will be given in later chapters.

Since erythrocytes are constantly removed from the circulation as they wear out, their numbers in the blood would steadily fall if new ones were not delivered into the blood at a corresponding rate. Hence anemia could occur primarily as a result of an uncompensated increase in the rate of removal of erythrocytes from blood or a decrease in the rate at which they are formed and liberated into blood. In other words, some anemias are due primarily to an increased rate of erythrocyte destruction or loss from the body that is not compensated for by just as great an increase in the rate of their production, while other anemias could be due primarily to a deficient rate of production.

In order to ascertain whether the rate of erythrocyte production or the rate of erythrocyte destruction is at fault much useful information can be obtained by making what is termed a reticulocyte count.

The Reticulocyte Count. In a normal blood film, stained with an ordinary blood stain, and examined with the oil-immersion objective, almost all the erythrocytes are of a clear pink color. But occasionally an erythrocyte—anywhere from 1 in 100 to 1 in 1,000—will be slightly different, in that, while fundamentally pink, it demonstrates a blue tinge. Such an erythrocyte is said to demonstrate basophilia and to be a *polychro-*

matophilic erythrocyte (a red cell that loves many colors) (Fig. 10-3). The reason for a blue tinge is as follows:

The nucleated precursor cells that give rise to erythrocytes are larger cells called erythroblasts, and they synthesize the hemoglobin that is later found in their offspring the erythrocytes. In order to synthesize the protein hemoglobin they have a heavy content of free ribosomes (Fig. 5-19), which of course makes their cytoplasm basophilic in films or sections seen with the LM. In forming erythrocytes they divide several times and, generally, by the time they have formed smaller cells which have lost their nuclei to become non-nucleated erythrocytes the previously abundant polyribosomes have either faded away or become so divided up that they no longer impart any cytoplasmic basophilia to the cytoplasm of erythrocytes. Under normal conditions relatively few erythrocytes which are young enough to retain enough ribosomes to make their cytoplasm polychromatophilic, are released as such into the circulation.

Polychromatophilic erythrocytes can be extremely difficult to identify in blood films stained with ordinary neutral blood stains. A better way to detect rRNA in erythrocytes in a film is by utilizing a supravital staining method. The dye used is brilliant cresyl blue. This may be mixed with erythrocytes from a freshly obtained drop of blood by various methods (see books on technic) and a blood film prepared, which may be subsequently stained with an ordinary blood stain.

Brilliant cresyl blue reacts with such rRNA that still persists in erythrocytes in a curious manner so that it comes to appear as a threadlike blue structure, which, if abundant, may assume the form of a wreath (Fig. 11-5) or, if scanty, may be no more than a few scattered blue dots (Fig. 11-5). It was at first thought that the network appearance was due to the staining of a previously existing reticular network inside the cell and so the cells exhibiting it were termed *reticulocytes*. It is now agreed that the network is an artifact due to the staining procedure. The reticulocyte is, of course, the same cell that would be termed a polychromatophilic erythrocyte if it were stained with an ordinary blood stain (Fig. 10-3). Using a labeled amino acid and radioautography, reticulocytes have been shown to synthesize protein, so they must contain also some mRNA and tRNA.

The rRNA in those few erythrocytes that are liberated with enough in them to stain as reticulocytes soon fades away. Exactly how long it lasts in circulating reticulocytes has been estimated by different procedures with different results; but it is probably only for one, two or three days, depending on how much rRNA they contain.

The precise percentage of reticulocytes released from the bone marrow into the circulation under normal conditions is difficult to ascertain. However, when erythrocyte production is increased, the storage space in marrow is not increased proportionally, and so more erythrocytes are liberated into the blood, with the result that many of these have not had enough time to mature properly before they enter the blood. Probably both the fact that more erythrocytes are being made and the fact that more of these are released as reticulocytes contribute to the increased percentage of reticulocytes seen when erythrocyte production is increased. Hence reticulocyte counts provide information about the rate of erythrocyte production.

Under otherwise normal circumstances, any condition that causes an increased rate of erythrocyte destruction (or loss by hemorrhage) is compensated for, at least to some extent, by an increase in the rate of erythrocyte production. So if, for example, the reticulocyte count remains high day after day with no increase in the total number of erythrocytes in blood, it can be safely assumed that the rate of destruction of erythrocytes is increased, or that erythrocytes are being lost from the circulation in some other fashion. In other words, the reticulocyte count can often be used not only to provide information about the rate of erythrocyte production but also, in conjunction with daily erythrocyte counts, to give information indirectly about the rate of erythrocyte destruction or loss. For example, some explosives are toxic to erythrocytes. In experimental studies on TNT absorption in rabbits, we found that reticulocyte counts became greatly increased. Hence reticulocyte counts can be sometimes used to indirectly detect whether products toxic to erythrocytes are being absorbed by those who handle them.

How Anemias Are Classified. Sooner or later, the student must learn to examine a blood film and say whether it indicates a *hypochromic microcytic anemia* or a *macrocytic anemia* or some other kind designated by this type of terminology. What do these terms mean?

Macrocytes and microcytes have already been defined. If in any anemia the erythrocytes tend to be substantially larger than normal, the anemia is said to be macrocytic; if they tend to be smaller than normal, microcytic; and if of normal size, normocytic. The terms *hyperchromic, normochromic* and *hypochromatic* refer to the amount of hemoglobin in the red cells, which of course is what accounts for their depth of color in films. We shall elaborate.

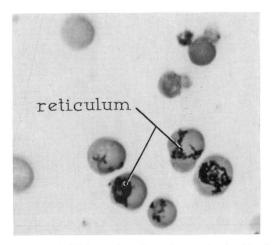

Fig. 11-5. Oil-immersion photomicrograph of a blood film stained with brilliant cresyl blue to show the so-called reticulum of the reticulocytes. The blood used was obtained from an animal which was regenerating large numbers of new erythrocytes.

Since the erythrocyte is a biconcave disk, it is thinner in its central portion than at its periphery. When stained and viewed from above, as is done when a dried film is examined, the thinness of its central portion is manifested by lighter staining than that which characterizes the peripheral zone of the cell (Fig. 11-3, *left*). Indeed, if the *proper part of a properly made film* is examined, the normal erythrocyte is seen to contain a central clear area that merges insensibly into the deeper-staining peripheral zone of the cell. In our experience, however, this clear portion is not to be seen in areas on a film where the erythrocytes are spread too thin (Fig. 11-3, *right*). It is best seen in areas where they are spread fairly thin but not so thin that no cells are superimposed on others (Fig. 11-3, *left*).

If the central pale area is not wider than a third, or slightly more, of the diameter of the erythrocyte, and if the peripheral zone of the cell stains reasonably well, the erythrocytes are said to be *normochromatic* (normal color) (Fig. 11-4, *center*). Some anemias are characterized by a reduction in the number of erythrocytes, but such cells as are present are normochromatic; hence they are said to be *normochromic anemias*. However, in a much more common type of anemia, the erythrocytes exhibit enlarged central pale areas and poorly stained peripheral zones (Fig. 11-4, *left*). The cells so altered are said to be *hypochromic* (undercolored); hence the anemias with which they are associated are called *hypochromic anemias*. In still other anemias there are fewer cells than normal but

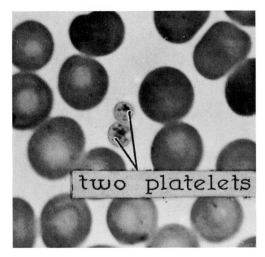

Fɪɢ. 11-6. Oil-immersion photomicrograph of a stained film of human blood. Two platelets may be seen adherent to one another in the center of the picture.

those are well filled with hemoglobin. It is doubtful if red cells can be overfilled, and so the reason these anemias have sometimes been called *hyperchromic* is that the cells are generally larger and, since they are well filled, they take on a deeper color (Fig. 11-4, *right*).

Films of normal blood usually exhibit an occasional erythrocyte of abnormal shape. The general term for such a cell is *poikilocyte* (*poikilis*, manifold). In the anemias, poikilocytes are common; hence, anemic blood is often said to exhibit poikilocytosis (Fig. 11-2, *right*). In some anemias the cells of abnormal shape are named more specifically—for example, the type in which erythrocytes tend to be shaped like sickles, which has already been mentioned.

The Different Effects of a Deficiency of Iron and of Vitamin B-12. In any given anemia, knowing whether the hemoglobin content is reduced more or less than the erythrocyte count is helpful in indicating the possible cause of the anemia. For example, iron is an essential ingredient of hemoglobin, and so when iron is deficient, the production of hemoglobin is reduced. However, iron is not as necessary for the production of erythrocytes as it is for hemoglobin, so in iron-deficiency anemias the hemoglobin content of blood is reduced more than the number of erythrocytes; hence the cells are poorly filled with hemoglobin, and the anemia is said to be of the hypochromic type (Fig. 11-4, *left*). On the other hand, certain chemicals (vitamin B-12 and folic acid) seem to be more necessary to the production of erythrocytes than

the production of hemoglobin, so that, when either one of these substances is lacking, there is more difficulty in producing cells than in producing hemoglobin; hence those cells that are produced under these conditions are filled to capacity with hemoglobin, and the anemia is of the *hyperchromic macrocytic* type (Fig. 11-4, *right*). The most important kind of this type is called *pernicious anemia,* and it is caused by an inability to absorb vitamin B-12 from the stomach and the intestine. If the vitamin is injected into persons with pernicious anemia, they recover, and the condition recurs only if injections are discontinued. There is no point in feeding the vitamin by mouth because those afflicted cannot absorb it. (Vitamin B-12 is present in liver extracts, and for those who might be interested it is a substance that, in the past, was called the extrinsic factor of Castle.)

Control of Erythrocyte Production by Erythropoietin. A substance produced in the body and known as erythropoietin affects the production of cells of the erythrocyte series. It will be discussed in the next chapter.

Platelets

Pʟᴀᴛᴇʟᴇᴛs, Fɪʙʀɪɴ ᴀɴᴅ ᴛʜᴇ Hᴇᴍᴏsᴛᴀᴛɪᴄ Mᴇᴄʜᴀɴɪsᴍ

Some Introductory Considerations. Platelets are not cells. They are little ovoid fragments of cytoplasm, 2 to 5 μ in diameter (Fig. 11-6) that, as will be described in the next chapter, become detached from the cytoplasm of very large cells (called megakaryocytes) in the bone marrow in such a way that each platelet is completely covered with cell membrane. *They have no nuclear components.* In this respect the blood of mammals differs from that of birds, for in the latter there are very small nucleated cells, called thrombocytes, that serve the same type of function as the platelets of man. Platelets are present in circulating blood in numbers that have been estimated at 250,000 to 350,000 per cubic millimeter.

The Basic Role of Platelets. When a person cuts himself, blood will flow from blood vessels that are severed at the site of the injury. But unless the vessels are relatively large the flow of blood from them soon ceases. Although other factors operate to achieve this end—for example, the circular muscle of the vessel walls become constricted so as to narrow the lumens of the bleeding vessels—the primary reason for the cessation of bleeding is that as blood flows out through the cut end of a vessel, platelets in the flowing blood continuously settle out to adhere to the inner surface of the vessel at, and close to, the site of the cut. This, of course, narrows the opening through which blood can escape, and as blood continues to flow through the narrowed opening more and more platelets adhere to those that have become attached to the lining of the vessel so that the lumen of the cut vessel soon becomes completely occluded by what is termed a *platelet plug*. The clumping of platelets that occurs when platelets pile up on, and adhere to, one another is termed *agglutination* and it is almost invariably associated with the formation of threads of fibrin that are derived from blood by a mechanism termed *coagulation* which will be described shortly.

A blood vessel does not have to be severed in order for platelets to adhere to its lining. The arteries of many people, as they become older, undergo degenerative changes (the condition is referred to as arteriosclerosis) which often affect the lining of the arteries in such a way that it no longer presents a smooth normal surface to the blood that flows along the lumen of the vessel and, as a consequence, platelets may begin to adhere to the lining of the vessel at affected sites. If platelets continue to accumulate from the blood that passes by such a site, they, together with fibrin that forms in association with them, may eventually occlude the lumen of the vessel. If the vessel in which this occurs is a coronary artery of the heart, part of the heart muscle would be deprived of a supply of oxygen and the person involved would experience what is commonly termed an acute coronary attack. If the same phenomenon occurs in an artery supplying the brain, a person is commonly said to have suffered a stroke.

Coagulation. In contrast to agglutination, which is a phenomenon that occurs in flowing blood, coagulation is a phenomenon more commonly associated with stagnant blood. Coagulation is responsible for the clots that form when blood is drawn from a living body and placed in a test tube. Coagulation also occurs in blood that escapes from vessels and becomes pooled in a tissue space in the body. For example, when a bone is broken, blood vessels are torn, and some blood leaks into the tissue in and around the fracture. In this blood which has escaped from the vascular system, just as in blood that is put in a test tube, an extensive mesh of fine fibers composed of a material termed *fibrin* (Fig. 11-7) materializes. The erythrocytes present in this blood become trapped in a network of fibrin fibers and can be seen there for a short time (Fig. 11-7), after which they disintegrate. Blood in which fibrin forms as above is said to have *clotted*.

Why blood should stay fluid when it is in the blood vessels of the body but clot when it is removed has always been a fascinating problem and it is now known that there are a host of factors involved, a thorough discussion of which is more the subject matter of physiology, clinical hematology and biochemistry than histology. However, in order to discuss platelets in any detail, we must give at least a very abbreviated account of the process of coagulation, because platelets are involved in it.

The Clotting Mechanism. One of the proteins of blood is fibrinogen. Under normal conditions fibrinogen, being a hydrophilic colloid, exists in solution. Also, there is in blood a substance called *prothrombin,* which under ordinary conditions is inactive. However, at sites of injury a substance commonly called tissue *thromboplastin* is liberated, and (although many factors are involved) the net result is that the release of tissue thromboplastin triggers the conversion of prothrombin to thrombin, which acts to cause soluble fibrinogen to become polymerized into insoluble threads of fibrin. These threads, seen with the EM, show axial periodicity (Fig. 11-8). The repeating periods, however, are shorter than those seen in collagen, being about 250 Å. Since the substance that triggers the coagulation that occurs in blood that— for example—escapes into the tissues at the site of a fracture comes from the tissue that was injured, it (tissue thromboplastin) is said to be an *extrinsic* factor; that is, it is a factor not originating in blood.

The coagulation mechanism, however, can be triggered by an *intrinsic* factor, a substance that originates in blood. Platelets can play a part in leading to the formation of this substance. It is an intrinsic factor that triggers coagulation when blood comes into contact with a foreign substance, as it does if it is put in a test tube with no precautions.

It should now be clear that, as a platelet plug begins to form on the inner surface of a diseased artery or at the edge of a cut vessel, both extrinsic and intrinsic factors could operate to trigger the coagulation phenomenon so that the formation of fibrin (coagulation) commonly occurs at sites of platelet agglutination.

Thrombosis—White and Red Thrombi. An agglutinated mass of platelets adhering to the inner surface of a blood vessel is known as a white thrombus (*thrombus,* a clot) because masses of platelets, in their fresh state, are white in color. A white thrombus can form only in flowing blood; it grows by abstracting fresh supplies of platelets from the blood that passes over it. Furthermore, it is very different in nature from the red clot that forms when still blood coagulates. Agglutination, then, tends to form a white clot, which con-

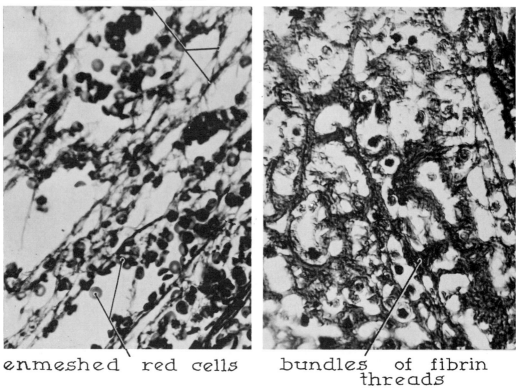

FIG. 11-7. High-power photomicrographs of sections cut through an area into which bleeding has occurred. (*Left*) Fine threads of fibrin which are forming a mesh entangling many cells. (*Right*) Fibrin threads arranged into coarser bundles.

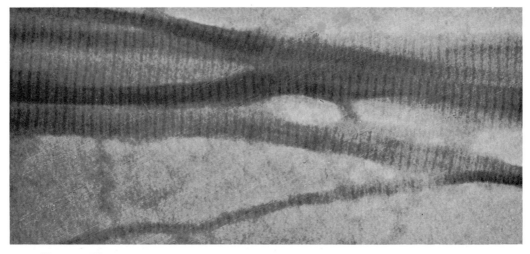

FIG. 11-8. Electron micrograph ($\times$ 115,000) of bovine fibrin, clotted in vitro by the addition of thrombin to fibrinogen solution, stained with phosphotungstic acid. (Preparation by C. E. Hall)

sists primarily of fused platelets; coagulation, a red clot that consists primarily of strands of fibrin that enmesh innumerable erythrocytes. Since platelets, when they agglutinate, liberate a substance which triggers the formation of thromboplastin, it is easy to see why red thrombi are often associated with white thrombi.

THE STUDY OF PLATELETS IN THE LABORATORY WITH THE LM

In living preparations of capillaries in which blood is circulating, platelets appear as oval biconvex disks. In ordinary blood films, platelets tend to clump together and so are usually seen in clumps (Fig. 10-3). However, sufficient searching will usually reveal occasional single platelets, and with the oil-immersion objective these generally have a flat rounded appearance (because platelets tend to spread out on surfaces, Fig. 11-6) and reveal two components. First, most of a platelet consists of a fairly clear ground substance which is colored only a pale blue with a blood stain and is called its *hyalomere* (*hyalos*, glass; *meros*, part) (Fig. 11-6). The second part of a platelet is generally disposed toward its central part and stains prominently (blue, purple to red) (Fig. 10-3); this component is termed its granulomere because the colored material is often in the form of granules (Fig. 11-6). Sometimes the granulomere appears as a solid clump of material which, in normal blood, may be due to a change having occurred before the platelet was fixed and stained. Sometimes platelets have spike-like pseudopodia extending from the periphery of the hyalomere. If blood is normal, this appearance also may be due to changes that occurred after the blood was drawn but before the platelet was fixed. Nevertheless, in abnormal conditions platelets may present different appearances. It has been suggested that younger platelets differ somewhat in appearance from older platelets. However, the amount of platelet morphology that can be learned with the LM is not very great compared to what can be learned with the EM, as will become apparent shortly.

How Platelets Are Counted

This is done with the LM. To keep them apart so that they may be counted as individual entities, it is necessary to mix blood taken from the body with an antiagglutinant immediately. The platelets in blood that contains antiagglutinant can be counted by either the indirect or the direct method. In the former, a drop of sterile antiagglutinating solution is placed on clean skin and a puncture is made through the drop so that the blood wells up into the antiagglutinant. A film of the mixture is then made on a slide and stained as is a blood film. The number of platelets in relation to the number of erythrocytes is then determined in several areas of the film. For example, if representative areas show there is an average of 6 platelets to every 100 erythrocytes and a proper erythrocyte count is then made from a fresh drop of blood, the number of platelets per cubic millimeter of blood can then be estimated; for example, if the erythrocyte count was 4,000,000 per cubic millimeter, the platelet count would be $\frac{6}{100}$ of 4,000,000, which is 240,000 per cubic millimeter.

With the direct method no agglutinating fluid is placed over the puncture site. Instead, a measured amount of blood is drawn up into a pipette containing a measured amount of antiagglutinant, and they are thoroughly mixed. A little dye is added to the antiagglutinant to stain the platelets so that they may be seen and distinguished from the erythrocytes when a portion of the mixture is examined in a counting chamber where both an erythrocyte and a platelet count may be made from the same preparation with the LM.

The phase microscope is very useful for counting platelets, and probably the best method now available is a direct count made with this instrument. Automatic (electronic) cell counters are also employed.

THE FINE STRUCTURE OF PLATELETS

Sections of platelets are commonly prepared from material fixed in glutaraldehyde followed by osmium tetroxide. Other special methods can be used to show certain inclusions more clearly but only at the cost of obscuring certain other components.

Seen with the EM, platelets are somewhat irregular in shape and vary from ovoid to round (Fig. 11-9); the difference probably depends on the plane in which an ovoid platelet is sectioned. Each platelet is enclosed by a membrane of the same kind that covers cells (unit membrane) and the membrane in turn is covered with a thin film of carbohydrate-containing cell coat amorphous material of low electron density (Fig. 11-9).

The Hyalomere, Microtubules and Filaments. The hyalomere appears as a homogeneous and generally fine granular material (Fig. 11-9) but contains, close to its periphery, both microtubules and filaments (Fig. 11-10). The former, seen in cross section, appears as compact bundles at opposite ends of the platelet. When sectioned longitudinally, they may be seen arching parallel to the plasma membrane, just beneath it. They probably function as a skeleton to maintain

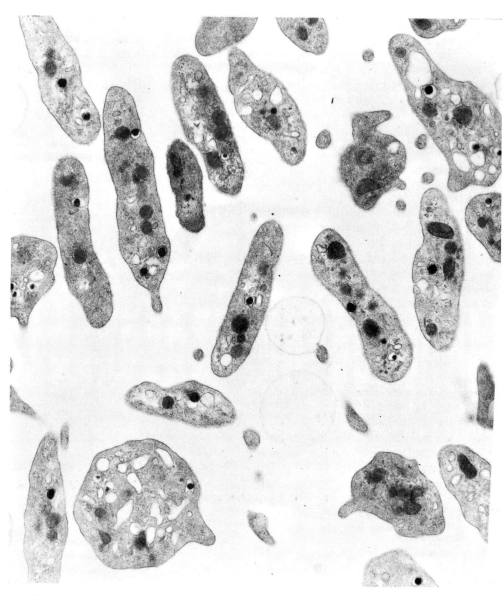

FIG. 11-9. Electron micrograph ($\times$ 15,500) of section of group of platelets prepared from platelet-rich rabbit plasma. The material was fixed in glutaraldehyde and postfixed in osmium tetroxide. Sections were stained with uranyl acetate and then with lead citrate. (Illustration courtesy of Dr. H. A. Gardner)

the platelet's ovoid shape. Filaments are thought to be associated with microtubules, either lying just superficial to them or being actually dispersed among them. Filaments are believed to account for platelets having contractile properties and thus being able to change their shapes.

Somewhat deeper in the platelet various components of the granulomere of light microscopy are encountered; these will now be described.

THE FINE STRUCTURE OF THE COMPONENTS OF THE GRANULOMERE

1. **Alpha Granules.** These account for most of what appear as colored granules with the LM. Seen with the EM, alpha granules are round to oval and measure 0.2 to 0.3 μ in diameter (Fig. 11-10). Their content of fine particulate matter is more or less aggregated in the more central part of the granule so that

there is a less electron dense zone between the main mass of the substance of the granule and its surrounding membrane. Alpha granules contain many substances that are concerned in platelet function. These granules are inherited from the cytoplasm of the megakaryocytes from which platelets become detached. Since they are covered with membrane, and since they contain enzymes, they are of the nature of intracytoplasmic secretory vesicles or lysosomes.

2. **Mitochondria.** These are sometimes referred to in platelets as beta granules, a terminology the use of which should be discouraged. Only 1 or 2 mitochondria are seen in a thin section of a platelet; these are small and generally have only 2 or 3 cristae (Fig. 11-10).

3. **Sydersomes.** These are rounded vesicles with clear contents except that the inner surface of the surrounding membrane of each is lined with small dense granules 55 Å in diameter. Since this is the size of ferritin particles, the vesicles containing these granules were termed sydersomes, but there is no indication that they contain iron. Sydersomes are also called delta granules.

4. **Very Dense Granules.** In rabbit platelets, Silver and Gardner have recently demonstrated a granule that is denser than any of the other granules so far seen in platelets, and so they have termed it the VDG (very dense granule). Frequently, the contents of this membrane-bound granule have a more or less eccentric position, leaving a wide, seemingly empty space between the granule and the unit membrane that contains it (Figs. 11-9 and 11-10). The number of these granules seen in platelets obtained from different species varies, in general, in proportion to the serotonin content of platelets. (Serotonin is a substance that can cause the muscle of arterioles and arteries to contract, or in some instances to relax.) Histochemical tests employable with the EM support the view that serotonin is located in the very dense granules. Human platelets do not contain very much serotonin, and as a consequence these granules are not as numerous as in rabbit platelets, which contain a great deal of serotonin.

5. **Glycogen Granules.** These are very small granules distributed in platelets in small groups or sometimes in aggregates of some hundreds (Fig. 11-10).

6. **Ribosomes.** These are not common in platelets but when present are thought to indicate that the platelet was recently enough formed to have carried away some ribosomes of the megakaryocyte cytoplasm.

7. **A System of Tubules and Vesicles.** This system is commonly described as also containing vacuoles; but as vacuoles are essentially holes, and since those described in platelets have membranous walls, they are therefore structures.

The system of tubules and vesicles is believed to

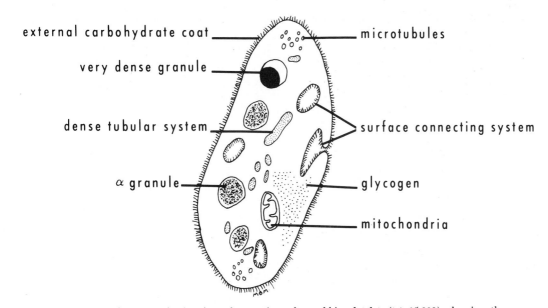

FIG. 11-10. Diagrammatic drawing of a section of a rabbit platelet (× 35,000) showing the various components that can be seen in rabbit platelets that are fixed in glutaraldehyde and postfixed in osmium tetroxide. (Modified slightly from an illustration in the master's thesis of Dr. H. A. Gardner, Department of Pathology, University of Toronto, 1968)

have two main divisions. The first part is described as a *surface-connecting system,* which means the tubules and vesicles that belong to it communicate with the surface (Fig. 11-10). Furthermore, the inner surface of the membranes of the vesicles of this system reveal the presence of the same kind of carbohydrate-containing coat as that seen on the membrane surrounding the platelets (Figs. 11-10). Since platelets have been shown to be phagocytic, it seems logical to think that the surface-connecting system represents invaginations of the covering membrane of the platelet and is concerned with taking substances into the interior of a platelet.

The second part of the system is termed the *dense tubular system* because the membranous tubules of this system contain a material that is moderately electron-dense (Fig. 11-10). It seems probable that the components of this system came from the Golgi apparatus of the megakaryocytes. It would be interesting to know the function of the components of this system.

EM STUDIES OF PLATELET PLUG FORMATION

Studies with the EM have shown that platelets pass through two stages in the formation of a plug. First, in agglutination they come together and adhere to each other. Their organelles become grouped toward their centers and pseudopodia form at their surfaces. Second, in the next stage, called thrombocytolysis (also called viscous metamorphosis), their various granules disintegrate, as do their surrounding plasma membranes. Eventually platelets as individual structures disappear, and they melt into a cohesive mass (Figs. 11-11 and 11-12).

Factors Involved in Platelet Plug Formation. Investigations have revealed 2 substances of importance in platelet plug formation, viz., ADP (adenosine diphosphate) and collagen. The former substance is formed from the breakdown of ATP, which is present in all cells. The enzyme responsible for this breakdown is present in the plasma. Therefore, one sequence of events in platelet plug formation may be that injury

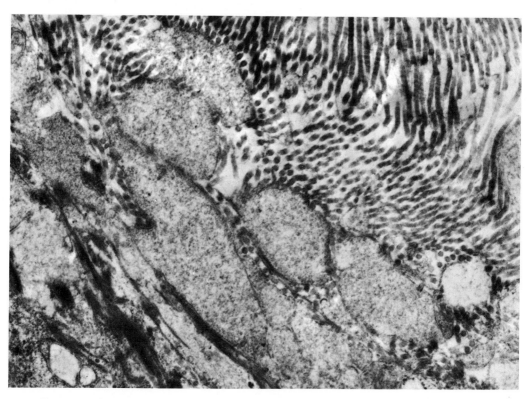

FIG. 11-11. Electron micrograph (approx. $\times$ 25,000) of platelets that have aggregated beside some exposed collagen in an injured vessel. It is to be noted that the normal constituents of the platelets that have aggregated in this forming plug or thrombus can no longer be discerned, and that the platelets are beginning to melt into an amorphous mass. See also Figure 11-12. (Illustration courtesy of J. F. Mustard)

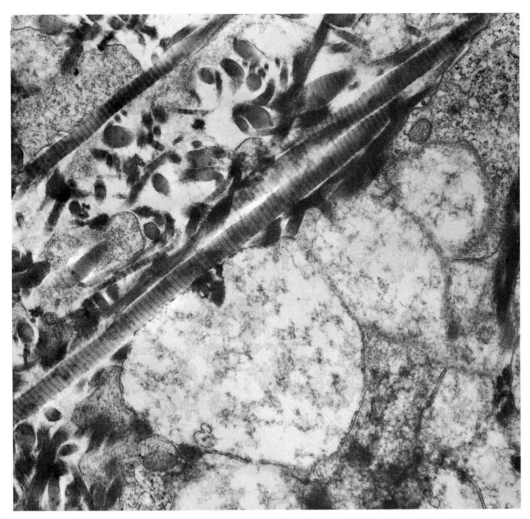

F ɪɢ. 11-12. Electron micrograph (approx. $\times$ 30,000) of platelets that have adhered to collagen that was inserted into a flow chamber. Note the intimate association between the large platelet (just below center) and the collagenic microfibril, which shows typical banding, just above it. Here again the constituents of the platelets have disappeared, and they are melting into an amorphous mass. (Illustration courtesy of J. F. Mustard)

to a blood vessel, with damage to its cells, releases ATP, which is broken down to ADP. The latter substance stimulates the aggregation of platelets. It is interesting that in-vitro experiments with platelet-rich plasma and ADP indicate that only the stage of agglutination occurs. Plasma denatures ADP, and, when none is left, the platelets separate and, for all intents and purposes, resume their natural state. The action of collagen, the second important aggregating substance, probably complements that of ADP. However, collagen induces thrombocytolysis following the stage of agglutination (Figs. 11-11 and 11-12). In other words, in contrast to the action of ADP, that of col-

lagen is irreversible. Under normal conditions platelets in circulating blood do not come into contact with collagen. Although there is collagen in the walls of the blood vessels, the platelets of blood are separated from it by the continuous endothelium that lines blood vessels. Although elastin is much more prevalent in artery walls than collagen (see Chapter 19), platelets could come into direct contact with collagen if an artery wall is severed. Moreover, in degenerative disease of arteries there is often an attempt at a repair process in which collagen may be formed. It is easily conceivable that endothelium would be deficient on occasion in such sites and that platelets could come into contact with collagen so that a white thrombus would form.

During the stage of thrombocytolysis (viscous metamorphosis), the platelets continue to take an active part in the thrombotic process. A phospholipid associated with platelets known as platelet factor 3 is released when platelets disintegrate. This reacts with other substances in plasma to form thromboplastin, which in turn stimulates the change of prothrombin to thrombin. Thrombin causes fibrinogen to become fibrin so that this is deposited in association with the platelets. In addition to the latter effect thrombin acts directly on platelets similarly to collagen, viz., it induces more aggregation and thrombocytolysis.

PLATELETS AND CLOT RETRACTION

A phenomenon somewhat loosely termed clot retraction occurs in connection with a platelet plug that forms in a cut vessel, a thrombus that forms in an artery or vein or in the clot that forms when blood is put into a test tube. One result of it is to make the total mass of the plug, thrombus or clot, smaller and more dense. It is dependent on there being both platelets and fibrin in the contracting material. It is believed that there is a contractile protein in platelets called thrombosthenin which has its physical basis in platelets in the form of the filaments which have already been mentioned. It has been suggested that, when thrombolysis occurs, this protein is released, and that ATP from damaged tissue and from platelets is essential for the contraction to occur because the process requires energy. It is known that platelets must be present in sufficient numbers if clot retraction is to occur, because it does not take place under conditions of platelet deficiency. However, a detailed understanding of what might be termed the mechanics of clot retraction is not yet available.

Also released when platelets disintegrate are serotonin (stored in the very dense granule), epinephrine, norepinephrine, and in some species, histamine. It is doubtful, however, if the small concentrations in human platelets play a major role in blood coagulation.

CONTROL OF PLATELET PRODUCTION— THROMBOPOIETIN

Experiments have shown that the blood serum of animals that have suffered a severe blood loss will, if it is injected into normal animals, cause an increase in the platelet count. It is therefore visualized that, when animals experience a severe hemorrhage, a substance must be produced in them that enters the bloodstream and stimulates the formation of platelets. Sufficient

work on this substance has been done to merit its being given the name thrombopoietin, and to indicate that it is probably a glycoprotein and is closely related to erythropoietin. Its source has not been established. Its action is not thoroughly understood; it probably results in increased numbers of megakaryocytes and a speed-up in the maturation of platelets from megakaryocytes. It takes a few days for thrombopoietin to manifest its full effects.

ABNORMALITIES OF THE CLOTTING MECHANISM

Platelets have a life span of around 5 to 9 days, after which they are probably phagocytosed by cells of the reticuloendothelial (macrophage) system. It follows that if there is a decreased rate of production of platelets, their numbers in blood would gradually fall. Such a state of affairs occurs, for example, when the normal, functioning cells of bone marrow are crowded out of the bone marrow by an invasion of, and/or a proliferation within, the bone marrow of tumor cells; for, under these conditions, there are not enough megakaryocytes to maintain the normal production of platelets. There are other conditions in which the production of platelets is normal but platelets are removed too quickly from the circulation. To relieve this condition, the spleen, which is the most important site for the phagocytosis of platelets, is removed surgically so that the platelets can have a longer lifespan. A platelet deficiency is associated with hemorrhages occurring for no apparent reason; these may appear in the skin, a mucous membrane or other sites. As will be explained in more advanced courses, there are, in addition to the hemorrhagic diseases due to platelet deficiencies, a host of hemorrhagic diseases that result from an inability to form fibrin from fibrinogen. Since the formation of fibrin depends on a large number of factors, and since any of this large number may be implicated in a deficiency, there are several different bleeding diseases caused by an inability to form fibrin normally. Many have a genetic basis. Hemophilia is probably the best known example of a disease of this type.

References and Other Reading

RED BLOOD CELLS

Berlin, N. I., Waldmann, T. A., and Weissman, S. M.: Life span of the red blood cell. Physiol. Rev., *39:*577, 1959.

Bishop, C. W., and Surgenor, D. M. (eds.): The Red Blood Cell; a Comprehensive Treatise. New York, Academic Press, 1964.

Haden, R. L.: Factors affecting the size and shape of the red blood cell. *In* Moulton, F. R. (ed.): Blood, Heart and Circulation, A.A.A.S. Publication No. 13. Lancaster, Pa., Science Press, 1940.

Harris, J. W.: The Red Cell, Production, Metabolism, Destruction: Normal and Abnormal. Cambridge, Mass., Harvard University Press, 1963.

Ingram, V.: The Hemoglobins in Genetics and Evolution. New York, Columbia University Press, 1963.

Isaacs, R.: The erythrocytes. *In* Downey's Handbook of Hematology. vol. 1, p. 1. New York, Hoeber, 1938.

Jones, O. P.: The influence of disturbed metabolism on the morphology of blood cells. *In* Macfarlane, R. G., and Robb-Smith, A. H. T. (eds.): Functions of the Blood. New York, Academic Press, 1961.

Jordan, H. E.: Comparative hematology. *In* Downey's Handbook of Hematology. vol. 2, p. 699. New York, Hoeber, 1938.

Lowenstein, L. M.: The mammalian erythrocyte. Internat. Rev. Cytol., *8,* 1959.

PLATELETS

A General Reference

Mustard, J. F., and Packham, M. A.: The reaction of the blood to injury. *In* Movat, H. Z. (ed.): Inflammation, Immunity and Hypersensitivity. ed. 2. New York, Harper and Row, In Press, 1974.

Special References

Aschoff, L.: Lectures on Pathology, XI. Thrombosis. New York, Hoeber, 1924.

Bak, I. J., Hassler, R., May, B., and Westerman, E.: Morphological and biochemical studies on the storage of serotonin and histamine in blood platelets of the rabbit. Life Sciences, *6:*1133, 1967.

Behnke, O.: Electron microscopic observations on the membrane systems of the rat blood platelet. Anat. Rec., *158:*121, 1967.

————: An electron microscope study of the megacaryocyte of the rat bone marrow. J. Ultrastruct. Res., *24:*412, 1968.

Behnke, O., and Zelander, T.: Filamentous substructure of microtubules of the marginal bundle of mammalian blood platelets. J. Ultrastruct. Res., *19:*147, 1967.

David-Ferreira, J. F.: The blood platelet: electron microscope studies. Int. Rev. Cytol., *14,* 1964.

French, J. E.: Blood platelets: morphological studies on their properties and life cycle. Brit. J. Haemat., *13:*595, 1967.

Gardner, H. A.: Studies on platelet fine structure. Thesis for M.Sc., Dept. of Pathology, University of Toronto, Toronto, Canada, 1967.

Hovig, T., Jørgensen, L., Packham, M. A., and Mustard, J. F.: Platelet adherence to fibrin and collagen. J. Lab. Clin. Med., *71:*29, 1968.

Hovig, T., Rowsell, H. C., Dodds, W. J., Jørgensen, L., and Mustard, J. F.: Experimental hemostasis in normal dogs and dogs with congenital disorders of blood coagulation. Blood, *30:*636, 1967.

Jørgensen, L., Rowsell, H. C., Hovig, T., and Mustard, J. F.: Resolution and organization of platelet-rich mural thrombi in carotid arteries of swine. Am. J. Path., *51:*681, 1967.

Jørgensen, L., Rowsell, H. C., Hovig, T., Glynn, M. F., and Mustard, J. F.: Adenosine diphosphate-induced platelet aggregation and myocardial infarcts in swine. Lab. Invest., *17:*616, 1967.

Miescher, P. A., and Jaffé, E. R. (eds.): Hemostasis and Thrombosis, Seminars in Hematology V. Nashville, Tenn., Henry M. Stratton, 1968.

Mustard, J. F., Glynn, M. F., Nishizawa, E. E., and Packham, M. A.: Platelet-surface interactions: relationship to thrombosis and hemostasis. Fed. Proc., *26:*106, 1967.

Nathaniel, E. J. H., and Chandler, A. B.: Electron microscopic study of adenosine diphosphate-induced platelet thrombi in the rat. J. Ultrastruct. Res., *22:*348, 1968.

Osler, W.: The third corpuscle of the blood. Medical News, *43:*701, 1883.

Sandborn, E. B., LeBuis, J., and Bois, P.: Cytoplasmic microtubules in blood platelets. Blood, *27:*247, 1966.

Silberberg, M.: The causes and mechanism of thrombosis. Physiol. Rev., *18:*197, 1938.

Silver, M. D.: Cytoplasmic microtubules in rabbit platelets. Z. Zellforsch., *68:*474, 1965.

Silver, M. D., and McKinstry, J. E.: Morphology of microtubules in rabbit platelets. Z. Zellforsch., *81:*12, 1967.

Stehbens, W. E., and Biscoe, T. J.: The ultrastructure of early platelet aggregation in vivo. Am. J. Path., *50:*219, 1967.

Tocantins, L. M.: The mammalian blood platelet in health and disease. Medicine, *17:*155, 1938.

Wright, J. H.: The histogenesis of the blood platelets. J. Morph., *21:*263, 1910.

Zucker-Franklin, D., Nachman, R. L., and Marcus, A. J.: Ultrastructure of thrombosthenin, the contractile protein of human blood platelets. Science, *157:*945, 1967.

12 The Hemopoietic Tissues: (1) Myeloid Tissue

What are termed the hemocytopoietic (*hemo,* blood; *cyto,* cell; *poiesis,* a forming) tissues of the postnatal body, or, for short, the hemopoietic tissues, were given their name because they were the tissues in which the various cells of the blood are formed in postnatal life. In man the hemopoietic tissues are divided into two main types:

| | 1. Myeloid Tissue (Bone Marrow) |
| Hemopoietic Tissue | 2. Lymphatic Tissue; in man |

this includes (1) nonencapsulated lymph nodules disposed generally in single or confluent masses beneath wet epithelial lining membranes, (2) lymph nodes, encapsulated lymphatic tissue scattered along lymphatics, and through which lymph drains, (3) the spleen, an organ in the upper left part of the abdomen, through which blood circulates and is filtered, and (4) the thymus, a paired organ that in most mammals lies in the chest below the sternum close to the neck.

The Division of Labor in Hemopoietic Tissues in Postnatal Life. Microscopic studies of myeloid tissue with the LM established clearly that its substance contained large numbers of erythrocytes and granular leukocytes in various stages of formation and maturation. It also was shown that in man it was the sole repository of megakaryocytes. Hence in man myeloid tissue came to be regarded as being specialized to produce the erythrocytes, granular leukocytes and platelets of the body. It is now known, moreover, that the myeloid tissue produces other kinds of blood cells, as will be described presently. Lymphatic nodules in loose connective tissue, lymph nodes, spleen and thymus were all shown to contain an abundance of lymphocytes; moreover, it was noted that mitotic figures were common in these tissues, which suggested that lymphocytes were produced in them. However, as was noted in the previous section on lymphocytes, it is now believed that they are also produced in myeloid tissue.

As will be described later, the lymphatic tissues are deeply involved in defense reactions.

In this chapter we shall deal with Myeloid Tissue.

Myeloid Tissue

Kinds and Distribution. Myeloid tissue in postnatal life is confined to the cavities of bones; this is the reason that it is called myeloid tissue (*myelos,* marrow). In the normal, the terms *myeloid tissue* and *bone marrow* are used more or less synonymously. Under certain pathological conditions, myeloid tissue may develop elsewhere and produce the kinds of blood cells that are produced in bone marrow; if this happens the phenomenon is termed *extramedullary myelopoiesis.*

Red and Yellow Bone Marrow. In the adult there are two kinds of bone marrow—red, and yellow. Red marrow derives its color from the vast number of red blood cells it is producing. Yellow marrow derives its color from the large quantity of fat it contains. Although yellow marrow has the potentiality to manufacture red blood cells, the fact that it is not red indicates that it is not very actively engaged in doing so, and the fact that it is yellow indicates that it has taken on the more leisurely work of storing fat.

In the fetus the marrow of most bones is red. But during the growing period in postnatal life the marrow of most bones becomes yellow so that in adult man red marrow is found only in the diploe of the bones of the vault of the skull, in the ribs and the sternum, in the bodies of the vertebrae and in the cancellous bone of some of the short bones, and at the ends of long bones. The marrow in all other sites is yellow. Under conditions in which there is an urgent and prolonged need for increased red blood cell production, a portion of the yellow marrow can become reconverted to red marrow.

TWO BASIC COMPONENTS OF MYELOID TISSUE

Myeloid tissue consists of two main components: (1) a connective tissue *stroma* which, though delicate, provides a three-dimensional bed, in which a great abundance of (2) free (unattached) cells which are blood cells in various stages of formation and maturation can lie. *It is now believed that the stroma cells and the free cells of myeloid tissue are derived from different sources, as will soon be described.*

The Development and Structure of the Stroma. The development of the stroma of bone marrow cannot be treated as a separate subject because its development is part of the story of the development of the bone in whose marrow cavity it forms. The development of bone will be dealt with in detail in Chapter 15 but we must describe it here briefly if we are to explain the nature of many of the cells of marrow stroma.

Most of the bones develop as a result of a two-step process. For example, leg or arm bones develop in what are termed limb buds that extend from the body of the embryo in the sites where arms and legs will later exist. The buds are composed of mesenchyme. In the more central part of a limb bud the mesenchymal cells begin to differentiate into cartilage cells which form intercellular substance around them, and soon a cartilage model having the outline of the bone-to-be in this location becomes evident (glance at Fig. 15-21). Most of the cartilage model of the bone-to-be has only a temporary existence because, beginning in its middle, its intercellular substance becomes calcified and its cells die for reasons to be explained in Chapters 14 and 15. Irregular cavities then begin to form in it (Fig. 15-23).

In the meantime, the mesenchymal cells that immediately surround the cartilaginous model of the bone-to-be have become arranged into a cellular membrane that is called the perichondrium (*peri,* around; *chondrium,* cartilage). However, about the same time that cavities begin to appear in the cartilage model the deepest cells of the perichondrium turn into bone-forming cells and lay down a shell of bone around the cartilage. Since the membrane now surrounds a shell of bone, the name of the membrane is changed from perichondrium to periosteum (around bone). The deepest cells of this membrane are called osteogenic cells and, as we shall see, they are competent to differentiate into either cartilage or bone-forming cells, depending on whether their environment is avascular or vascular. The shell of subperiosteal bone that is now present supports the cartilage model while its more central part is becoming riddled with irregular holes. However, at one or a few points, depending on the particular bone involved, a bud of osteogenic cells from the periosteum together with some capillaries (the combination is called a periosteal bud) grow through a hole in the layer of subperiosteal bone to enter the substance of the cartilage model which, by this time, as mentioned, is becoming riddled with holes.

As a result of the foregoing events two kinds of cells have gained access to the developing marrow cavity in the cartilage model of the bone-to-be; these are osteogenic cells, and the endothelial cells of capillaries. However, it is usual for perivascular cells to be associated with capillaries and at this stage of development it could be expected that the perivascular cells that grow into the future marrow cavity along with the capillaries of the periosteal bud would be relatively undifferentiated and so be able to differentiate into fat cells, reticular cells, fibroblasts and also the smooth muscle cells of the larger blood vessels which develop in the marrow cavity from the cells of the periosteal bud.

So there are three kinds of cells that enter what will be the marrow cavity that develops in the cartilaginous model of the bone-to-be to give rise to the stroma of the myeloid tissue that forms. These are (1) osteogenic cells, (2) endothelial cells (of capillaries) and (3) perivascular cells of considerable potentiality. These form the stroma of marrow, as follows:

A backbone for the otherwise delicate bone marrow stroma is provided by its blood vessels. The development and arrangement of the larger ones which develop from the periosteal bud are described in connection with the blood supply of bone in Chapter 15 because these vessels provide most of the blood supply of the surrounding bone as well as that of the marrow. Some perivascular cells become fibroblasts and form collagen around the larger blood vessels. Thus supported, the blood vessels provide the main skeleton for the bone marrow.

Next, connecting the arterial and venous sides of the circulation in marrow there are almost innumerable wide tubular channels lined by endothelial cells, called sinusoids. Their relatively great diameter allows for a slow circulation of the blood along them. They are difficult to see in ordinary H and E sections of red bone marrow, as is shown in Figure 12-1, because the stroma between them is packed with developing erythrocytes and leukocytes which press on their sides to such an extent that their borders of endothelial walls are difficult to discern. They are easier to see in the red bone marrow of an animal given total body radiation because this stops cell division in the developing red and white cells; as a consequence there are fewer of them in a few days and under these conditions the endothelial cells of the walls of the sinusoids are more readily seen (Fig. 12-2).

The Fine Structure of Sinusoids. The LM study of bone marrow in vitally stained animals gave rise to the concept that the sinusoids of bone marrow were lined by reticuloendothelial cells. These were regarded as being thicker and much more phagocytic than ordinary endothelial cells. They were also thought to

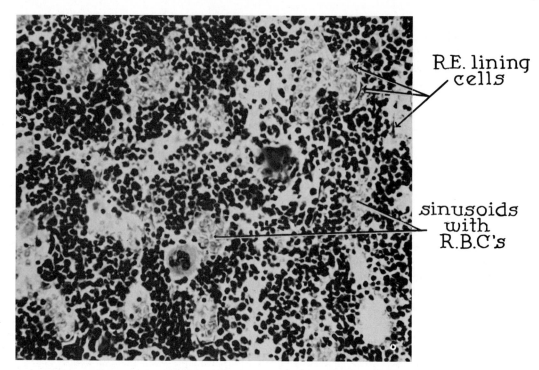

R.E. lining cells

sinusoids with R.B.C's

Fig. 12-1. Low-power photomicrograph of a section of red bone marrow. This section shows numerous sinusoids, most of which contain red blood cells. These are the lighter areas in the photograph. Between them are innumerable cells of the red blood cell and granular leukocyte series. One megakaryocyte is present in the lower middle part of the picture. In a few sites the thin, flattened endothelial lining cells of the sinusoids may be seen.

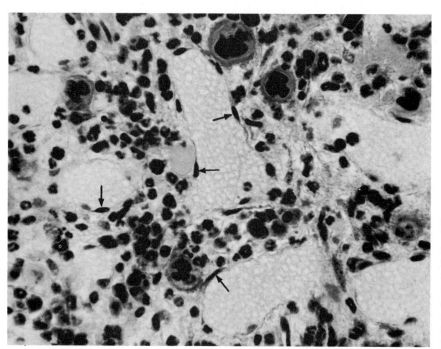

Fig. 12-2. High-power photomicrograph of an H and E section of the bone marrow of a mouse 24 hours after the mouse was given a dose of radiation sufficient to kill most of the mice so treated. Notice that the various cells between sinusoids are undergoing pyknotic changes, and that the sinusoids are congested. The arrows point to the nuclei of endothelial cells that are lining sinusoids.

Fig. 12-3. Electron micrograph (× 1,700) of bone marrow of rat 10 minutes after intravenous injection of colloidal carbon. One of the marrow macrophages (M) sends a large pseudopod (large arrow) into the sinus (S) through a large gap in its wall. Islands of erythroid cells (E) are present. One normoblast (asterisk) is undergoing mitosis. Another (⇑) is in the process of extruding its nucleus. One extruded nucleus (⇑⇑) is phagocytosed by a macrophage. Cells of the granulocytic series (my), megakaryocytes (meg), and fat cell (F) are all present. (Illustration courtesy of S. C. Luk and G. T. Simon)

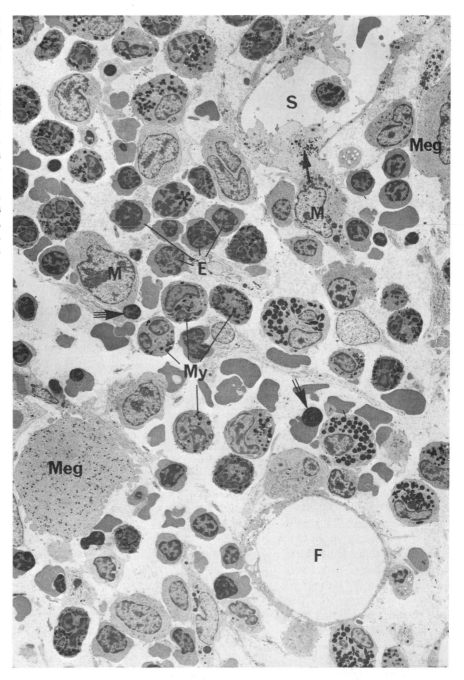

be fitted very loosely together so that fully developed free cells could pass between them from the stroma into the lumen of a sinusoid with ease. However, the greater resolving power of the EM used with thinner sections has disclosed that the sinusoids of marrow are lined by endothelium which differs little from that which lines the rest of the vascular system. The impression gained from LM studies in vitally stained animals to the effect that the lining cells were markedly phagocytic was probably due to the fact that macrophages are common on the outer aspect of the sinusoidal endothelium and, furthermore, they often extend pseudopodia between the endothelial lining cells of the sinusoids into the lumen where they phagocytose particulate matter from the bloodstream, as is shown in Figure 12-3 where at the upper right a macrophage

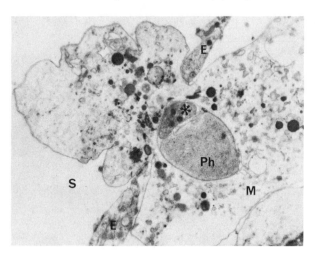

Fɪɢ. 12-4. Electron micrograph (× 13,500) of a macrophage (M) that has sent a pseudopod into a marrow sinus (S) through a gap in its wall. Numerous cytoplasmic inclusions are present in the macrophage. One large phagosome (ph) contains platelets (asterisk). Endothelial cells (E). (Illustration courtesy of S. C. Luk and G. T. Simon)

(labeled M) illustrates this phenomenon. It is easy to understand that with the LM and much thicker sections it might be concluded from appearances such as this that the lining cells of the sinusoids were thicker than ordinary endothelium and markedly phagocytic.

In a micrograph of greater magnification (Fig. 12-4) a large pseudopodium can be seen projecting between the endothelial cells (labeled E) which are of the usual thickness of endothelium in general.

As well as being much wider, sinusoids differ from ordinary capillaries in not possessing a relatively well developed continuous basement membrane. Such basement membrane as seen on the outer aspects of their endothelial cells is thin and discontinuous.

How the Marrow in a Bone Is Supported. From the foregoing description the stroma of bone marrow can be visualized as having a backbone of arteries with branches passing out sideways to the bone. The arteries are supported by a little connective tissue. Blood from the arterial vessels is delivered into sinusoids along which it flows to reach a vein. However, the support provided by these various blood vessel components, while helpful, is greatly augmented by bone marrow's being encased by bone. Furthermore, some of the stroma cells of marrow are continuous with the cells that line the bone that surrounds the marrow cavity and with the cells that cover any trabeculae (little beams) of bone that are present

within the marrow. This arrangement provides peripheral anchorage for the delicate marrow.

Some Implications That Result From Marrow Being Encased by Bone. Since both the cells and the blood of marrow are incompressible, the fact that marrow is contained in bony chambers with solid walls has some interesting implications. For example, the only way there can be room in the marrow for any kind of blood cells being made at a more rapid rate than normal is for older cells to leave the marrow at the same rate or, failing that, for less blood to be contained in the blood vessels of marrow. It therefore seems that the wide sinusoids filled with blood could serve to some extent as cushions that could expand or contract to allow for fewer or more cells to be present in marrow at different times. The formation of more fat or the mobilization of fat from marrow could also serve as a slower acting cushion to permit reduction or expansion of blood cell formation of longer duration. Finally, under conditions under which the cell bulk of marrow remains constant, more, or less, blood cannot enter or leave marrow than is leaving or entering it at that time. It seems, moreover, that edema, as we visualize it in soft tissues, could not occur in marrow because it cannot expand.

Tʜᴇ Tʏᴘᴇs ᴏꜰ Cᴇʟʟs Tʜᴀᴛ Aʀᴇ Cᴏɴsᴛɪᴛᴜᴇɴᴛs ᴏꜰ Sᴛʀᴏᴍᴀ

1. **Osteogenic Cells.** There is a great deal of evidence that osteogenic cells, similar in potentiality to those that invade the cartilage model of the bone-to-be, remain scattered about in the stroma of the marrow as well as lining the surface of the bony wall of the marrow cavity. For example, if adult bone marrow is transplanted to any of various body sites, it will form islands of bone. Furthermore, if a bone is broken, new bone materializes *in the marrow* close to the site of the fracture. It has also been shown that autologous transplants of cancellous bone (which are much used in orthopedic procedures to set up islands of new bone formation in sites where new bone is needed) give rise to more bone if the red marrow with which the cancellous fragments of bone are associated is left on them. These facts indicate that the stroma of normal red bone marrow contains many cells of the type we describe in more detail as osteogenic cells in Chapter 15.

2. **Fibroblasts and Fat Cells.** The perivascular (mesenchymal) cells that are associated with the capillaries of the periosteal bud seem to be relatively uncommitted and in different sites give rise to different cell types. Some, it is assumed, give rise to the

fibroblasts that are associated with the larger blood vessels, and others to the fat cells.

3. **Reticular Cells.** Still other perivascular cells are believed to form reticular cells which produce the delicate reticular fibers which have been described in marrow. Reticular cells have large pale nuclei but their cytoplasm is indistinct in H and E sections. Moreover, their cytoplasm seems to extend off from the region around the nucleus in irregular prolongations some of which are associated with reticular fibers. Such a cell is very difficult to outline in three dimensions and in general the information about what is termed the reticular cell of hemopoietic tissue is much less precise than that which exists about other cell types. It is believed that in addition to forming some reticular fibers the reticular cell is also mildly phagocytic and when we study the lymphatic type of hemopoietic tissue we shall see that there is evidence that reticular cells provide surfaces on which antigen-antibody complexes from T lymphocytes become attached and thus available for B lymphocytes to encounter. In the past it was believed that the reticular cell gave rise to the free cells of marrow but, as will be described shortly, this view has now been generally abandoned.

Relation of Reticular Cells to Macrophages. It was believed in the past that the macrophages of marrow (which will be described later as one of the types of free cells of marrow) differentiated from the reticular cells, during which differentiation they became increasingly phagocytic and lost their ability to produce reticular fibers. It is now believed that macrophages in postnatal life are formed from monocytes. Since monocytes are free cells produced in marrow, it now seems probable that they, and not reticular cells, are the source of marrow macrophages and hence that macrophages are free cells instead of being one of the components of the marrow stroma that develop from the periosteal bud. However, distinctions between reticular cells and macrophages are not always as clear as might be desired; for example, what might be termed a dendritic macrophage by one author might be termed a reticular cell by another.

To sum up: Three types of cells grow into the cavity of a bone-to-be via the periosteal bud to form the stroma of marrow; these are (1) osteogenic cells, (2) endothelial cells, and (3) perivascular (relatively uncommitted mesenchymal) cells. The last named give rise to fibroblasts, fat cells, reticular cells and the smooth muscle cells of the blood vessels. All these cell types are regarded as constituent cells of the stroma. The chief support for the delicate stroma is its backbone of blood vessels and its attachment to the lining of the marrow cavity.

The Formation of Blood Cells in the Stroma of Myeloid Tissue

The stroma of red marrow is packed with free cells that represent blood cells of various kinds in various stages of development (Fig. 12-3). Over many decades these were studied in sections stained with various stains and in imprints or films stained with blood stains. In the last two decades they have been studied with the EM in thin sections. Over the years certain assumptions were made and became so ingrained in the literature and so familiar to everyone who learned about the formation of blood cells only a few years ago that before we explain how new experimental methods have changed much of what seemed to have been established in the past, it may be helpful to inquire into why some of the previous assumptions that were made, and are now regarded as incorrect, were so generally accepted.

The Difficulties of Establishing Cell Lineages From Morphological Studies. Trying to establish by morphological methods which kind of cell gives rise to which depends primarily on finding that cells in approximately the same grouping or location are very similar in many respects but nevertheless slightly different from one another. It is then assumed that one of any such two is either the immediate precursor or descendant of the other and hence less or more mature than the other. This method of establishing cell lineages and cell maturation is generally reliable when the *cytoplasm* of the cells that are studied shows clear-cut evidence of increasing specialization along some particular line of differentiation and maturation. By studying the various cells seen in bone marrow with this kind of thinking it became possible to arrange certain cells that were encountered in marrow (as, for example, in Figure 12-3) into the lines of differentiation and maturation shown in Figure 12-5 which illustrates the successive changes that occur in cells as they become the erythrocytes and the three kinds of granular leukocytes of the blood.

The fact that the cells of the erythrocyte and granular leukocyte series of cells could be arranged so convincingly in a developmental sequence probably led most of us in past years into the trap of assuming that it was possible to trace these two cell lineages to a common ancestor by morphological means. The common ancestor chosen by morphological studies was a cell similar in appearance to the proerythroblast in Figure 12-5, but larger and having more extensive pale blue cytoplasm. It was termed by some a hemocytoblast and by others a myeloblast. The appearance attributed to it in the past is not illustrated in Figure

12-5 because it is now known that this appearance was incorrect. It has been established by new experimental methods that the common ancestor of cells of the erythrocyte and granular leukocyte series is a much smaller cell than was generally believed. This was not determined from morphological studies and even yet ascertaining the morphology of this cell presents certain problems. How the recent information on the common ancestor of erythrocytes was established will be described shortly. But first it is of interest to comment on how morphological studies probably went astray in attempting to identify the stem cell of blood cells.

Limitations of Morphology for Identifying Stem Cells. The basis for establishing cell lineages by cell morphology disappears when there are no specific cytoplasmic features in a cell to indicate that it has become committed to proceeding along some particular line of differentiation. Accordingly, morphology provided no certainty with regard to identifying, for example, the stem cell from which both the cells of the erythrocyte series and the granular leukocyte cell lineage series shown in Figure 12-5 are derived, because indications of specialization for production of hemoglobin or of granules would not as yet have manifested themselves in the cytoplasm of the stem cell. Although a *lack* of development of any cytoplasmic specialization in a free cell of marrow might suggest the possibility of its being a stem cell, a lack of cytoplasmic criteria provides no clue in regard to the direction in which the potentiality of the cell will be expressed. How, then, was it more or less agreed in the past that a cell with a certain morphology was the free stem cell of marrow?

An important reason would seem to be that morphologists turned from the cytoplasm to the nucleus for guidance. As is shown in Figure 12-5, the nuclei of cells along the lines that lead to the formation of erythrocytes and polymorphs become smaller and darker as the cells become increasingly specialized while at the heads of these lines the proerythroblast and the promyelocyte both have large pale nuclei. This seems to have led to the concept that, in connection with the formation of blood cells, a cell's potentiality was indicated by how large and pale its nucleus was and that its degree of differentiation and lack of potentiality could be judged by how small and dark its nucleus was. This same reasoning gave support to the widely held incorrect belief to the effect that lymphocytes were end-of-line cells (because of their small dark nuclei) as well as to the idea that the stem cell of marrow must have a large pale nucleus. Since cells in bone marrow were found which had large pale

nuclei and nondescript blue cytoplasm, they were termed myeloblasts or hemocytoblasts and considered to be the free stem cells of marrow. Moreover, the assumptions that cell lineages could be traced by nuclei and that large pale nuclei indicated potentiality seem to have led to a further incorrect conclusion—that is, that a free stem cell must in turn be derived from some fixed cell of marrow stroma that had a large pale nucleus, and so it was generally accepted that the free stem cells of marrow were derived from the reticular cells of marrow stroma which have large pale nuclei.

Actually, there is no basis for the generalization that the potentiality of a cell can be determined by the size of its nucleus and the extent to which its chromatin is extended. For example, nerve cells, which are as highly specialized as any body cells, have extremely large nuclei in which the chromatin is almost all extended (Fig. 4-1), yet they have no potentiality to form other cells and they are even unable to divide. At the other end of the scale, the nucleus of a male germ cell is the smallest nucleus in a body, with its chromatin extremely condensed and yet it has total potentiality. Furthermore, it is of course now known that lymphocytes are not end-of-line cells; for, under conditions of proper stimulation, they can develop into larger cells which divide and give rise to cells that, for example, are highly specialized to produce and secrete antibodies.

With the paucity of either cytoplasmic or nuclear criteria to enable the existence of free stem cells to be determined by morphological means, the situation became somewhat similar to what occurred in connection with the development of knowledge about viruses. Even though viruses were too small to be seen with the LM and hence characterized by their morphology, their existence was proven by what they could do. Only later, when the EM was developed, could they be seen. Somewhat similarly, the existence of the stem cell of blood cells was established not by determining its morphology but by showing by the means next to be described that a cell (whose numbers could be assayed) existed that could give rise to all the blood cells that can be recognized by morphological means.

THE DEVELOPMENT OF THE SPLEEN COLONY TECHNIC FOR ESTABLISHING THE EXISTENCE OF FREE STEM CELLS IN MARROW AND ASSAYING THEIR NUMBERS

This technic was an outcome of studies that Till and McCulloch were making on the regeneration of blood cells in animals given total body x-irradiation

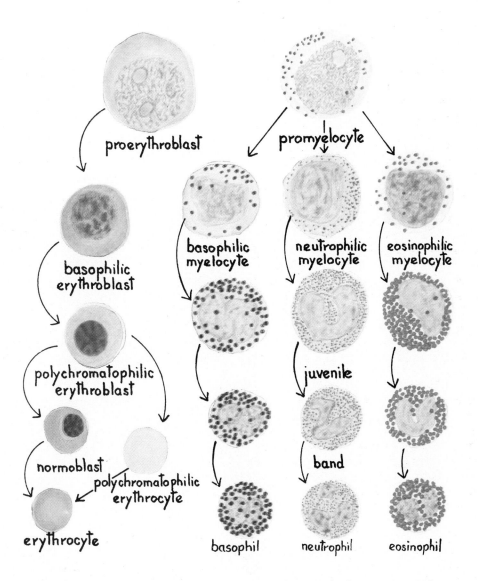

F<small>IG</small>. 12-5. Cells of the erythrocytic and granular leukocyte series from marrow as they appear in films stained with a Romanovsky-type stain (Hastings).

in the lethal range; the effects of the latter will first be described.

Effects of Total-Body Radiation in the Lethal Range. Following the advent of atomic energy and in particular the atom bomb, a great deal of research was devoted to the way in which exposure to sufficient amounts of radiation causes illness or death. Depending on the dose received, effects may be manifested quickly or over the long term. The short term effects can easily be investigated in small animals such as mice by exposing them to whole body x-irradiation in the lethal range. As was described in Chapter 2, the most important effect of radiation on cells is exerted on their chromosomes, and the damage done in this way may not become apparent until a cell attempts to undergo mitosis in which process the damage done is manifested by the mitosis being abnormal and generally unsuccessful. As a result, the parts of the body that are most severely affected by total body radiation, such as might occur from severe atomic fallout, are those parts in which there is a rapid rate of cell turnover. Since granular leukocytes have a lifespan of only a few days, they must be produced in the bone marrow as rapidly as they are lost from the bloodstream if the number of them in the blood is not to fall quickly. The same thing is true of platelets. Since erythrocytes live for a few months, interference with their production after total body radiation does not become apparent immediately. Accordingly, after total body radiation in the lethal range, the polymorphs and platelets mostly disappear from the blood in a few days. Likewise the proliferation and development *both* of T and B lymphocytes is halted and hence the formation of new killer cells or plasma cells in response to antigens is quickly diminished. Primarily because of the failure of the production of new polymorphs and new antibody-forming cells, the body becomes relatively unable to resist infection (and also, because of its inability to form new killer cells in response to new antigens, it becomes receptive to transplanted cells that it would ordinarily reject). Finally, since the lining cells of the intestine are normally lost at a rapid rate and must be replaced at the same rapid rate, another serious effect of total body radiation is that intestinal lining cells are not replaced as they are lost, so that patches of the intestine become denuded even though cells that persist stretch out and become relatively flat in an attempt to cover such areas. Denuded areas are soon invaded by bacteria and, since the body has lost its chief means for resisting infection and also its capacity to make platelets for preventing hemorrhages from the

infected denuded sites along the intestine, death soon occurs.

Effects of Transfusions of Bone Marrow Cells. If, however, an irradiated mouse after receiving a lethal dose of whole body radiation is given an intravenous transfusion of marrow cells from another— preferably identical—animal, it will recover. The reason for this is that certain cells in the transfused marrow settle out in the hemopoietic tissues of the host and repopulate them with new cells, which, of course, are of the donor animal type. The grafted cells soon produce enough granular leukocytes and platelets to prevent the infection and hemorrhages that would ordinarily kill the animal. Furthermore, the ability of the animal to produce new antibody-forming cells is restored. It is assumed that enough lining cells of the intestine survive and are able to multiply and so provide a complete lining for the intestine again if the *immunological* defenses of the body are restored and if the remaining lining cells have enough time to do it.

The Spleen Colony Technic. An unexpected dividend of such proportions that it transformed future research on the stem cells of bone marrow emerged from the series of studies made by Till and McCulloch and McCulloch and Till on the biological effects of radiation. Mice that had received total-body radiation in the lethal range were transfused with marrow cells from normal mice of the same pure strain. In the course of these experiments these investigators performed autopsies on animals in different stages of recovery and observed that the spleens of recovering animals developed little nodules that projected from the spleen surface (Fig. 12-6). Their histological studies of these nodules indicated that they were colonies of new cells of the erythrocyte and granulocyte series, sometimes with megakaryocytes. The relative percentages of cells of these 3 series were found to differ in relation to the time when the nodules were allowed to develop and also to other factors that need not be described here. They termed the nodules colonies and immediately questioned whether or not each colony was a clone, that is, whether it arose from a single cell that had the potentiality to give rise to the cells of the erythrocyte, granulocyte and megakaryocyte lines of differentiation. To determine this it was decided to employ marrow cells with radiation-induced chromosomal markers: this technic will next be described.

Chromosomal Markers. If cells with proliferative capacity are lightly irradiated, some of the cells may suffer an injury to some chromosomes which may involve their DNA but not DNA that is employed in that particular kind of cell for transcribing information

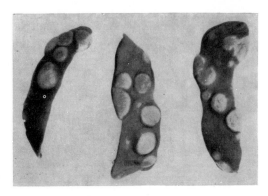

FIG. 12-6. Photograph of 3 mouse spleens with clones of cells derived from mouse marrow. The mice from which these spleens were taken had received 950 rads of x-ray followed by the injection of small numbers of nucleated bone marrow cells. After 10 days the spleens were removed and fixed in Bouin's solution. Each of the nodules visible in the spleens is a colony of proliferating and differentiating cells, each derived from a single hemopoietic stem cell. (Preparation by E. A. McCulloch)

that is necessary for survival of the cell. Nevertheless the structure, and hence the appearance, of some chromosome may be sufficiently altered for it to be identified as being abnormal in a karyotype. If a cell with a chromosome of this kind is allowed to multiply in vitro or in vivo, karyotypes of all its progeny will reveal the chromosomal defect that was created in the cell that gives rise to the clone.

Spleen Colonies Shown To Be Clones. Becker, McCulloch and Till then prepared marrow suspensions that were irradiated enough to produce some chromosomal markers in the marrow cells of the suspension and used these to transfuse irradiated hosts. The dividing cells in each spleen colony that developed nearly all showed the same marker. So it was concluded that each colony originated from a single cell and hence it represented a clone. This work, therefore, provided not conjecture but proof to the effect that there is a cell in bone marrow which can give rise to cells of the erythrocyte series, cells of the granular leukocyte series, and megakaryocytes. They decided to term this pluripotential stem cell a colony-forming unit (CFU), a term that has now become well established.

Effects of the Discovery of the CFU on Concepts of Maintenance of Blood Cell Populations—Necessity for Stem Cells. Before the existence of the CFU was established it was of course known that erythrocytes and granular leukocytes lack the capacity for cell division and that their numbers had to be maintained

by cell division occurring in less differentiated cells of the cell lineage to which they belonged, which cells in turn would differentiate into more specialized cells. But it was not appreciated that the erythrocyte line of differentiation could not be maintained by cell division occurring at the erythroblast or proerythroblast level or that the granulocyte lines of differentiation could not be maintained by cell division occurring at the level of, say, myelocytes. Accordingly, showing that the way that these cell lines are re-established in an irradiated animal by transfused marrow cells was by proliferation of a stem cell whose progeny could differentiate along either the erythrocyte or the granulocyte or the megakaryocyte line strongly suggested that the beginning of differentiation along any of these specialized lines was associated with some loss of proliferative capacity and hence that none of the cells forming along any of these three lines of differentiation could all through life maintain the population of that line of cells. As was pointed out in Chapter 2, there are many examples in the body of populations of highly specialized cells, which have lost their ability to divide, being maintained by the proliferation of relatively undifferentiated cells of the same family type—that is, by cells that are committed to forming only the cells of a certain cell family but have not begun to differentiate into specialized functioning cells of that family type. As soon as they do begin to differentiate along the line that will lead them to becoming functioning specialized cells they lose some degree of proliferative capacity. The cell that is committed to forming cells of a certain family, such as blood cells, but has not as yet begun to differentiate into any particular type of blood cell, retains close to unlimited proliferative capacity and is thus able to maintain a pool of cells that can differentiate under the right circumstances to form the members of some line of blood cells. Such cells are commonly termed *stem cells,* for it is from them that the more differentiated cells of a family all stem. Thus stem cells are cells that, although they are committed (restricted) to differentiating into a particular family of cells (which may have several branches), manifest no indication of having begun to differentiate into any of the cells they have the potentiality to form, and while they remain in this state they possess, for all practical purposes, unlimited proliferative capacity. It follows that for a stem cell to differentiate along a particular pathway requires that it be induced to do so by an environmental factor, and once influenced it ceases to be a stem cell. So we conclude that the CFU is a stem cell responsible for maintaining a pool of cells that are committed to forming blood cells (but not any particular kind) and, under the right circumstances, can differentiate into cells of the erythrocyte, the granular leukocyte or the megakaryocyte series and, as will be described shortly, the monocyte line as well. That it possesses the potentiality to form cells of the lymphocyte series as well will be discussed in due course.

The Use of the Spleen Colony Method for Demonstrating the Circulation of Stem Cells. Until the spleen colony technic was evolved to demonstrate the presence, and assay the numbers, of stem cells in various hemopoietic tissues and in blood, there was little thought given to the possibility that, under normal conditions, stem cells might circulate so that, having originated in one site, they could pass by the bloodstream to another site and seed it with stem cells. However, by means of the spleen colony technic it was possible to show that CFU's could be recovered from circulating blood, although in relatively small numbers, and that, although they were present in greater concentration in bone marrow, they were also present, in adult mice, in certain other hemopoietic organs. Thus the spleen colony technic (by determining the number of colonies formed by the number of cells injected) provided a means for assaying the relative numbers of stem cells in any given cell preparation despite the fact that the morphology of the CFU was not known.

The development of a technic whereby the presence and numbers of the free stem cells that give rise to the erythrocytes, the granular leukocytes and the megakaryocytes of marrow could be determined—in other words, an assay technic for stem cells—was bound to facilitate research on trying to find out where and how these stem cells are formed in the body. As mentioned, until this time it was a common assumption that the free stem cells of marrow arose from the reticular cells of marrow stroma. That this was highly improbable was shown by a series of extremely ingenious and informative experiments performed by Moore, Metcalf and their associates, in which the spleen colony technic played a very important role. These investigators traced the origin of the free stem cells of hemopoietic tissues to free stem cells that develop in the yolk sac of the embryo. They postulated that the formation of blood cells in other sites in embryonic, fetal and postnatal life is due to the stroma of these other hemopoietic tissues being seeded from free stem cells that originate in the yolk sac of the embryo. To explain this concept in more detail we first have to discuss the formation of blood cells in the embryo.

Blood Cell Formation in the Embryo. In Chapter 9 we described how mesenchymal cells become somewhat more flattened and connected with one another to surround a lumen and so become a primitive capil-

lary as shown in Figure 9-2. The cells constituting the walls of such vessels become endothelial cells and they proliferate so as to send out hollow buds which join up with other primitive vessels that form in mesenchyme to form the circulatory system.

In the mesenchyme of the yolk sacs of most mammalian embryos certain mesenchymal cells persist in what might otherwise become the empty lumen of a primitive capillary. The mesenchymal cells that persist in the lumen become free cells, and so a section cut across a developing blood vessel of this type will reveal a group of free cells lying in its lumen. This appearance gave rise to the name *blood island*. It was originally believed that the endothelium of the developing capillary gave rise to the blood cells that were in its lumen but it is now believed that the primitive blood cells within the island and the endothelium that surrounds the blood cells are independently derived.

Hemopoiesis in Other Organs Traced to Yolk Sacs. The great many experiments involved in providing proof for the hypothesis that the stem cells and blood cells are derived from the yolk sac are brought together and described in the most informative book *Hemopoietic Cells* by Metcalf and Moore (see "References and Other Reading"). Only a few will be mentioned here; these indicate that this hypothesis was proven by new methods and could not have been proven by purely morphological studies.

The hypothesis, in short, is that the stem cell for blood cells develops from mesenchymal cells in the blood islands of the yolk sac of the embryo, and that for a time the proliferation of the stem cell of blood cells occurs in the yolk sac. In the yolk sac there is, moreover, some differentiation that leads in particular to the formation of cells that synthesize hemoglobin (of the fetal type). Moore and Metcalf showed by means of the spleen colony technic that, almost as soon as these cells appeared in the blood islands, CFU's were present among them. They also showed that cells from the yolk sac could repopulate the hemopoietic tissues of a mouse given radiation in the lethal range. Moreover, it was shown by parabiotic experiments with chick embryos, in which the circulation of males and females was crossed, that the hemopoietic organs of the chicks in due course revealed the karyotypes of both male and female cells; this of course showed that there was circulation of stem cells. Experiments in which embryos were cultured for brief periods showed that, if the yolk sac was removed, the organs that otherwise would have become hemopoietic did not do so. It was also shown that hemopoiesis in the yolk sac was soon superseded by hemopoiesis that occurred in the liver because of that organ having been seeded by stem cells from the yolk sac, and that subsequently the spleen and bone marrow of the embryo were seeded with stem cells from the liver. After birth the bone marrow and spleen have become the chief sites where the population of stem cells is maintained. In mice, both erythrocytes and granulocytes are produced in the spleen after birth; this does not normally occur in man, and hence it might be expected that the relative percentages of stem cells in the bone marrow and spleen in man would differ from those of the mouse.

How the Newer Findings Affect the Traditional Concepts About Hemopoiesis

There have been two schools of thought about whether or not free stem cells of more than one type existed in postnatal life to account for the various lines of differentiation that lead to the several types of blood cells. One, termed the monophyletic (single tribe) school, maintained that all types of blood cells were derived ultimately from a single type of cell which they termed *hemocytoblasts,* and to these cells they ascribed a particular morphology. The other school maintained that there was more than one type stem cell and so was termed the polyphyletic school. Proponents of the polyphyletic school variously maintained that there were two or even more stem cells involved in maintaining the blood cell lineages in postnatal life, but most believe only two types of stem cells were required. Stem cells of one kind were believed to reside in myeloid tissue, where they were responsible for the erythrocyte and granulocyte lines of differentiation and the production of megakaryocytes; these stem cells were termed *myeloblasts* because they were thought to germinate (*blastos,* germ) all the cells of marrow. Cells of the other kind were believed to reside in the lymphatic types of hemopoietic tissue and to give rise to lymphocytes, so these were termed *lymphoblasts.* Although this was not always spelled out by them, the members of the monophyletic school would have to reason that the cellular environment would be the deciding factor as to whether or not a hemocytoblast would give rise to the lymphocyte series of cells or the series seen in marrow. The members of the polyphyletic school, on the other hand, would have to subscribe to the hypothesis that lymphoblasts were committed to form cells of the lymphatic series and myeloblasts, cells of the erythrocyte and granulocyte series and megakaryocytes, no matter where they were located. Many arguments arose as to whether or not the cells given these various names could be distinguished from one another on morphological grounds but none was convincing enough to settle the matter. Both types of cells

were described as having relatively large, pale nuclei and a good deal of basophilic cytoplasm. But there was another type of evidence suggesting that there might be two types of stem cells and this probably had greater influence than any suggested morphological descriptions: There seemed to be at least two main types of leukemia (lymphatic and myeloid), with cells of the lymphocyte series being mainly involved in the lymphatic type and cells of the granulocyte series in the myeloid type. Leukemia is a disease characterized by a more or less unrestrained production of some type of leukocyte and caused by a malignant transformation occurring in some cell concerned in the production of leukocytes. The existence of at least two types was thought to give some support to the concept of there being at least two different stem cells, with one stem cell being involved in one variety of the disease and the other in the other. It is of interest in this connection that in the early 1960's it was discovered that in most instances of the chronic form of the myelogenous (myeloid) type of leukemia, the chromosome abnormality termed the Philadelphia chromosome (described in Chapter 2) was found to be present in the leukemic cells as well as in the precursors of the erythrocytes and also in the megakaryocytes. This finding therefore tended to give support to the concept that there was a stem cell that gave rise to these three lines of cells (megakaryocytes, granulocytes and erythrocytes) and another stem cell for lymphocytes, because the latter cells did not reveal the Philadelphia chromosome. However, the problem presently became more complicated when it was established that lymphocytes, as well as the series of cells already mentioned, could be produced in myeloid tissue, and this gave rise to the question of the progenitor of the lymphocytes, particularly as to whether or not it was the same cell that gave rise to erythrocytes and granulocytes. The formation of lymphocytes in myeloid tissue will therefore be discussed to see what bearing this has on the problem of whether there is a cell that is the ultimate source of all blood cells.

The Source of Lymphocytes in Myeloid Tissue

Since it was for so long commonly accepted in man that lymphocytes were produced in the lymphatic division of hemopoietic tissue and erythrocytes, granular leukocytes and platelets in the myeloid division, little attention seems to have been paid to the presence of lymphocytes in myeloid tissue. It was not until Yoffey, who contributed so much to the study of lymph and lymphocytes, called attention to the fact that in normal laboratory animals there were large numbers of lymphocytes present in bone marrow that interest was taken in this matter. With the rigid view held in the past, the presence of lymphocytes in marrow was at first explained as being due to large numbers of lymphocytes, formed in lymphatic tissue, being strained from circulating blood as it passed through the marrow. And, indeed, there is evidence that some lymphocytes may be strained from the blood as it passes through marrow. However, as modern methods became available it was shown by ingenious labeling experiments that lymphocytes were indeed produced in the marrow of experimental animals in considerable numbers, as will now be described.

Osmond and Everett investigated the problem of preparing radioautographs of marrow obtained at different times after giving guinea pigs a dose of tritiated thymidine intravenously. They found that in the first 4 hours only about 0.4 percent of the lymphocytes of marrow had become labeled but that after 3 days about 40 percent of marrow lymphocytes were labeled, which of course suggested that some precursor cell of lymphocytes was dividing and taking up the label that was found later in the lymphocytes. To rule out the possibility that labeled lymphocytes found in the marrow might have been lymphocytes that were labeled elsewhere and then strained out by the marrow instead of having been formed in the marrow, Osmond and Everett, before administering a single dose of thymidine, put a tourniquet around one hind limb of each guinea pig to shut off temporarily the circulation in it. The tourniquet was released 20 minutes after the thymidine was given, at which time the labeled thymidine would have almost entirely disappeared from the circulation. If the labeled lymphocytes seen in marrow represented lymphocytes that had been labeled elsewhere and then filtered out by the marrow, just as many would subsequently accumulate in the marrow of the leg in which the circulation was shut off while the thymidine was available as in the marrow of the other leg because lymphocytes labeled, say, in the thymus or lymph nodes would be strained out in that leg as well as in the other. However, they found that relatively few labeled lymphocytes accumulated in the marrow of the leg in which the circulation had been cut off while the tritiated thymidine was available in the remainder of the animal.

Estimating the Rate of Production of Lymphocytes in Marrow. Subsequently Everett and Chaffrey, as well as Osmond independently, performed similar experiments on rats, with much the same results. However, they used a further technic, placing a tourniquet around one leg and, while the tourniquet was in place,

injecting labeled thymidine directly into the marrow of the tibia of that leg. In such an experiment the remainder of the body can be flooded with unlabeled thymidine, which makes so much unlabeled thymidine available in the rest of the body that any labeled thymidine that might escape from the tibia into the general circulation after the tourniquet is removed cannot compete with the much larger quantity of unlabeled thymidine in being taken up by cells undergoing DNA duplication. Hence the finding of labeled cells in the blood or in any other part of the body after the tourniquet is removed would indicate that those cells obtained their label while they were in marrow.

It is, of course, difficult to label very many marrow lymphocytes by giving a single injection of tritiated thymidine into the bone marrow through a small hole in the cortex of the bone, because the thymidine would tend to remain fairly localized. However, one way in which lymphocyte production in the marrow can be determined by labeling cells in such a very small part of the marrow is to take advantage of the fact that granulocytes produced in the same region will also be labeled. Since the rate of entry of granular leukocytes into the bloodstream is known, the number of labeled lymphocytes entering the blood in an experiment of this kind can be compared with the number of labeled granular leukocytes that appear in the blood over the same time period. Subsequently Osmond, in an experiment of this kind, found that the number of labeled lymphocytes appearing in the blood was at least 25 percent the number of labeled granular leukocytes appearing over the same period. In the usual experimental animal the rate of production and entry of lymphocytes into the blood is therefore very substantial.

When it was established that lymphocytes were actually produced in myeloid tissue the problem arose as to the type of stem cell from which they arose and what bearing a decision on this matter would have on the monophyletic/polyphyletic school controversy. Of still greater interest in this area, however, was the problem of whether or not the lymphocytes originated from the CFU, which, if proven, would indicate it to be the ultimate source of all types of blood cells.

THE CFU AS A POSSIBLE SOURCE OF LYMPHOCYTES

It will be recalled that marrow cells injected into irradiated recipients bring about the repopulation of all the hemopoietic tissues of their host, both myeloid and lymphatic and that they also cause spleen colonies to form in their hosts. Cytological studies of the colonies allow the cells of the erythrocyte and granulocyte cell lineages to be distinguished, as well as megakaryocytes. By using chromosomal markers it was shown that colonies are clones; thus all the cells mentioned above arise from a single stem cell. It has also been shown that yolk sac cells will bring about the repopulation of *all* the hemopoietic tissues of an irradiated mouse and that they too will bring about the formation of spleen colonies in their hosts. The question that immediately arises is whether the CFU is responsible for bringing about the repopulation of the lymphatic tissues of the irradiated host; for, if so, the formation of marrow lymphocytes could be attributed to it.

Very substantial evidence to the effect that the cells of the lymphocyte series arise from the CFU's that give rise to spleen colonies has been obtained. In 1962 Trentin and Fahlberg, by means of repeated transfers through irradiated animals, showed that cells obtained from an original single spleen colony could completely repopulate all the hemopoietic tissues of an irradiated mouse, which suggests that the CFU from which the original spleen colony developed had the potentiality to form cells of the lymphocyte series. Furthermore, Wu et al. showed that radiation-induced markers produced in CFU's could be traced into cells of the lymphatic division of the hemopoietic system. In order to show this, large numbers of CFU's with markers had to be obtained. This was done in a most ingenious manner in a three-step experiment that for the second step utilized a special strain of mice that have an inherited defect that prevents their own CFU's from forming colonies but allows the proliferation of CFU's from a related normal strain in which markers have been produced by proper doses of radiation. This thus permits large numbers of CFU's with markers to multiply in their marrow, and the marrow cells thus obtained after some months contain many CFU's with markers which can then be injected into irradiated normal mice. In due course the markers are found in the cells of the lymphatic tissues as well as in the myeloid tissue. The evidence from these experiments again strongly suggests that the CFU gives rise to cells of the lymphocyte series as well as the myeloid and hence that the lymphocytes of marrow could be formed from CFU's.

If the CFU has the potentiality to form lymphocytes, it might be asked, why could not this be established readily by examining spleen colonies and determining whether or not lymphocytes are present in them as well as cells of the erythrocyte and granulocyte series? This method presents several problems. With the LM it would be very difficult in ordinary sections to distinguish lymphocytes from certain of the cells of the erythrocyte series that develop in a colony. Secondly, since colonies develop in the spleen and since, by the time they have formed, there are lots of lymphocytes in the spleen stroma, the observer could not be certain that the presence of any lymphocyte identified in a colony was not due to the developing colony having enveloped it. Finally, chromosomal markers would be of no help in identifying a lymphocyte and proving it developed in a colony, because chromosomal markers are detectable only at mitosis, and small lymphocytes as such do not undergo mitosis. To see chromosomal markers in cells of the lymphocyte series small lymphocytes have to be stimulated, whereupon they become a type of blast cell that divides to form more lymphocytes. It is not improbable that lymphocytes are indeed produced in spleen colonies, but it is difficult to prove this by morphological criteria.

There is, however, another way of determining whether or not lymphocytes appear in spleen colonies, namely by testing colony cells to see if any cells present possess any immunological properties. This is also difficult because, as was explained in connection with lymphocytes, both T and B lymphocytes usually must collaborate to produce immunologically active cells. Furthermore, the lymphocytes that function as T lymphocytes can do so only after they have been processed in the thymus. Nevertheless, ingenious experiments have shown that cells obtained from spleen colonies, under the right circumstances, can be shown to possess immunological properties.

Conclusions. From all the above described experiments and others it would seem to be established that all types of blood cells are derived from a common ancestor which is a free cell and that this cell is the CFU. It is of interest that although modern methods thus support the concept of the monophyletic school— that there is, in fact, a cell with the potentiality they ascribed to the hemocytoblast—the above described studies provide no support for the concept that the CFU exhibits the morphology commonly ascribed to the hemocytoblast in the past with regard to its being a large cell.

How It Was Shown That the CFU Is a Smaller Cell than the Free Cells of Marrow Commonly Designated in the Past As Hemocytoblasts or Myeloblasts and Believed To Be Stem Cells. Although the morphology of the CFU was not established, its size could be determined indirectly by unit gravity sedimentation measurements; this method will now be described.

Unit Gravity Sedimentation is a method by which it is possible to distinguish between cells even if they are not distinguishable by morphological means, on the basis of differences in their size. The relative sizes of cells are obtained by this method from their relative rates of fall through a stationary liquid, since the rate of fall of a spherical body that is denser than its surrounding medium is known to be proportional to the square of its diameter. The principle on which this method is based is illustrated whenever one watches bubbles that form on the bottom of a glass of a carbonated beverage rise to the surface, for the bubbles of larger diameter get to the surface before the bubbles of smaller diameter. Bubbles rise because their density is lower than that of their surrounding medium but their rates of rise are determined mainly by their diameters. The same, only upside down, happens with cells; their density being greater than that of the surrounding medium makes them fall rather than rise. Here again, though, their rates of fall are determined mainly by their diameters. To carry out a determination, samples are taken at various depths throughout the length of the column of medium through which the cells have fallen in a fixed time, and these samples can be assayed by the spleen colony technic. By this method the size of cells that gave rise to colonies was found to be clearly too small for them to be identified with the cells described from their morphology as myeloblasts (or hemocytoblasts). Moreover, the frequency of the CFU in marrow, as determined by quantitative assay, was also found too low for it to be equated with the cells that were described as myeloblasts and are seen in bone marrow preparations. The latter have an average frequency of around 2 percent; the CFU, from spleen colony assays, constitutes only around 1 per 1,000 nucleated bone marrow cells.

STUDIES DIRECTED TOWARD DETERMINING THE MORPHOLOGY OF THE CFU

It is to be appreciated that all that has been described about the CFU up to this point was determined without any knowledge of its morphology except that, since it is a body cell, it must have a nucleus and some cytoplasm. Its morphology has been difficult to establish, because there is only about 1 CFU to every 1,000 nucleated cells in marrow and, second, as was previously explained, it should theoretically not possess any special positive cytoplasmic features by which it could be easily distinguished. However, the problem is not insurmountable and much progress has been made, as will now be described.

A logical first step in attempting to learn the appearance of CFU's would be to concentrate them in marrow preparations so that they might constitute a more substantial class of cells that differed in morphology from the other cells present. Van Bekkum et al. were able to concentrate CFU's in a cell preparation by two successive steps. First, they administered two different drugs to the mice from which they planned to obtain marrow cells. The drugs were of a type that are sometimes used in the treatment of cancer or leukemia and act on cells as they attempt to enter or pass through mitosis; thus in a sufficient dosage they kill cells that are regularly passing through cell cycles when they are administered. One interesting feature of stem cells is that they generally have relatively long resting periods between divisions; hence they are relatively unaffected by the temporary use of the kinds of drugs mentioned above. But the destruction of other cells in their vicinity somehow triggers them into proliferating. Hence, after this drug treatment the relative percentage of stem cells in marrow is greatly increased and so it is possible to get cell preparations that are relatively rich in stem cells.

Next, by means of density gradient centrifugation it is possible to separate from cell preparations different fractions in which the cells are of much the same specific density. By using this procedure it is possible to test the different fractions obtained from cell preparations of marrow by the spleen colony method and find out which fraction contains most of the CFU's. By using this procedure after the one described above, van Bekkum et al. obtained from cell suspensions of bone marrow a fraction containing, they believed, around 20 percent of stem cells. They then studied cells from this fraction in stained films with the LM and in sections with the EM. They found that around 20 percent of the cells seen were of a morphological type that differed from that of the other cells present and fitted the concept of the kind of morphology a stem cell should possess, which will next be described.

As has already been mentioned, both in earlier chapters and in this section on the hemopoietic tissues, cells of different types can be identified with assurance if they possess cytoplasmic criteria that indicate that they are specialized or are becoming specialized to perform some particular function. But a stem cell in any given cell preparation could be expected to reveal no indications of the development of any cytoplasmic organelles except mitochondria and free ribosomes, which organelles are essential for respiration and synthesizing protein for growth (multiplication), and only a very little rER and a small Golgi for producing and maintaining the cell membrane and cell coat. One further criterion that could be looked for in the stem cell of blood cells would be its size because this, as

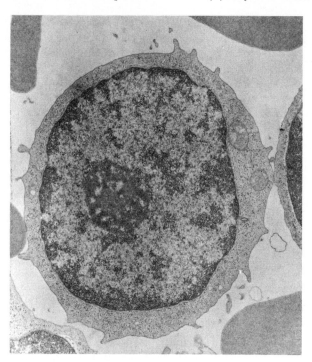

Fig. 12-7. Electron micrograph of a section of a cell obtained from guinea pig marrow which is of a type observed in the marrow of several species by Dr. Bainton in numbers commensurate with what is known of the incidence of the stem cell in marrow. The morphology of the cell is in harmony with that which could be expected on theoretical and other grounds for the stem cell, as is explained in the text. (Illustration courtesy of Dr. Dorothy Bainton)

size, and their nuclei, though roughly round, were more irregular in shape than those of lymphocytes and had less deep indentations. The chromatin of their nuclei was more finely dispersed than that of the lymphocytes; much of the chromatin in the latter was densely clumped. However, in our opinion, what is more important than nuclear differences is that although they could demonstrate a Golgi apparatus, some endoplasmic reticulum and lysosomes in lymphocytes, they did not observe any of these organelles in the prospective stem cell, which would indicate minimal development of them. The mitochondria, though few in both types of cells, were more numerous but smaller in the prospective stem cell than in lymphocytes. Finally, free ribosomes though present in lymphocytes were *abundant* in prospective stem cells while clustered ribosomes present in lymphocytes were few or absent in the prospective stem cell. An electron micrograph kindly provided by Dr. Dorothy Bainton, of a type of cell she has observed in the marrow of several species roughly in percentages that might be expected for the stem cell and possessing the fine structure that might be expected both on theoretical grounds and from the description of van Bekkum et al. is shown in Figure 12-7.

Our next problem is to attempt to visualize the cells that intervene between the CFU and other members of the various lines and types of cells that develop in marrow and for which morphological criteria are well established. To bridge the gap between the stem cell and these requires that we introduce some findings that have been made utilizing cell cultures.

Cell Cultures. Technics and media have been devised in which certain cells from bone marrow multiply in vitro (*vitrum,* glass) and give rise to colonies. The common type of colony that forms has been traced to a type of cell which is termed a CFU-C, the C in this instance implying that the cell from which this type of colony develops is one that multiplies and differentiates *in a culture.* Since both the CFU and the CFU-C give rise to colonies, it is necessary in instances where confusion might arise to designate the CFU as a CFU-S, with the S referring to spleen colonies and indicating that the colonies that develop from it do so in the spleens of *living animals.* The more differentiated cells that develop in a colony that develops from a CFU-C are of the granulocyte series and hence it is believed that the CFU-C represents a type of cell that is of the nature of a progenitor cell that is committed to forming this series of cells. It has been found furthermore that for colonies of this type to grow well in vitro the medium in which the cells are nourished must be "con-

already noted, has shown that the CFU is a relatively small free cell.

Van Bekkum et al. found in their concentrated preparations a class of cells that constituted about 20 percent of the total; these were from 7 to 10 microns in diameter and their cytoplasm demonstrated no organelles to speak of except free ribosomes and a few mitochondria. These cells did not give a peroxidase reaction as did the cells of the granulocyte and monocyte series present in the same preparations. A more important distinction, however, had to be made because the prospective stem cells bore a superficial resemblance to lymphocytes. Small lymphocytes are in the same size range, being about 8 microns in diameter. Furthermore, their cytoplasm, like that of the prospective stem cell, exists as little more than a rim around their nucleus. However, van Bekkum et al. listed several differences between their prospective stem cells and lymphocytes. The former varied a little more in

ditioned" by a particular factor which gives every evidence of being a special substance which specifically stimulates the growth and maturation of cells of the granulocyte series.

By using hemopoietic cells obtained from livers of 13-day mouse embryos, Stephenson, Axelrad, McLeod and Shreeve were able to grow colonies of a different type in cultures. To do this they added erythropoietin to the cultures. The discovery of erythropoietin was due to its being noticed that the blood of people who lived in high altitudes (where there is less oxygen) had greater amounts of hemoglobin and more erythrocytes in their blood than is normal. This state of affairs was shown to be due to a substance which was given the name *erythropoietin,* being produced in their bodies (the precursor molecule is made in the kidney) in response to a relative lack of oxygen in the blood passing through this organ. It was at first believed that erythropoietin exerted its effect by inducing more stem cells to differentiate into the progenitor cells of the erythrocyte series. But further studies showed that the content or proliferation of CFU's was not altered by erythropoietin and so it is now believed that it acts on a cell that is derived from the CFU which has proliferative capacity and is committed to forming cells of the erythrocyte series. Its action on this cell is probably that of stimulating hemoglobin synthesis and increased cell formation simultaneously. Since Stephenson et al. have shown that this cell produces colonies of cells of the erythrocyte line in cultures, they suggested that the name given the CFU-C, which hitherto was the only marrow cell that produced colonies in cultures, be changed to CFU-G (G for granulocyte series) and that the erythropoietin-sensitive cell from which erythrocytic colonies develop be termed the CFU-E (E for erythrocyte series). Hence when a preparation rich in hemopoietic cells is cultured, two different descendants of the CFU can be shown to proliferate and differentiate to form colonies under in vitro conditions. The fact that these two types of colonies will develop in vitro provides assay methods for erythropoietin, and what is probably granulopoietin, respectively. Moreover, colonies from CFU-G's can be grown from bone marrow cells of man, which fact can be put to use in studying the effects of certain drugs used in the treatment of leukemia.

The use of cell cultures has therefore shown that two types of committed cells arise from the CFU's, one the CFU-C (CFU-G) which can both proliferate and differentiate into the cells of the granulocyte series (and as will be described later, into monocytes as well) and the CFU-E which can proliferate and differentiate into cells of the erythrocyte series. The next question that arises is whether or not the CFU-C is the cell that is morphologically recognized in bone marrow films as the promyelocyte (Fig. 12-5) and if the CFU-E is the cell morphologically recognized as the proerythroblast (Fig. 12-5). The evidence indicates otherwise. It seems there are probably ten times as many promyelocytes in marrow as there are CFU-C's; furthermore, the CFU-C gives evidence of being a somewhat smaller cell than the promyelocyte. With regard to the CFU-E it appears that it is only about one tenth as common in marrow as proerythroblasts. So it appears that culture methods have disclosed the existence of two cell types which are more committed than the CFU-S and are the progenitor cells of the two series of morphologically identifiable cells commonly included in the erythrocyte and granulocyte leukocyte lines of differentiation. A tentative chart of the respective positions of the cell just discussed would therefore appear as below.

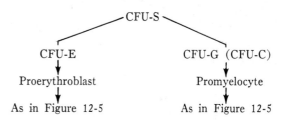

THE MORPHOLOGY OF THE CELLS OF THE LINEAGE LEADING TO THE FORMATION OF ERYTHROCYTES

The progenitor cell for this cell lineage seems to be the erythropoietin-sensitive cell—the CFU-E already described. We shall, in the following, deal only with the cells whose morphology has been established over the years, beginning with the proerythroblast.

The proerythroblast is described as being from 12 to 15 μ in diameter. In stained films the chromatin of the nucleus is finely granular and the nucleus commonly contains two nucleoli. The cytoplasm is mildly basophilic (Fig. 12-5).

With the EM one important feature discerned in this cell and those that evolve from it is the relative lack of development of endoplasmic reticulum and the Golgi. Another is that as the proerythroblast differentiates more and more free ribosomes and polyribosomes appear; these are diffusely distributed throughout the cytoplasm. In the cytoplasm, moreover, there are some bundles of microtubules which are peripherally arranged more or less parallel with the cell surface.

The proerythroblast can proliferate, and on differentiation its progeny become what are termed *basophilic erythroblasts*. In stained films these are somewhat smaller than proerythroblasts. Their nuclei are smaller and their chromatin is more condensed (Fig. 12-5). Their cytoplasm is more basophilic because of an increased amount of rRNA.

With the EM the salient feature of the cytoplasm is that it now has a great content of polyribosomes (Figs. 5-19 and 12-8). The development of the other organelles ordinarily seen in the cytoplasm of cells is minimal.

The next step in differentiation along this line leads to the basophilic erythroblasts becoming *polychromatophilic erythroblasts* (Fig. 12-5). The polychromatophilia observed in films stained with blood stains is due to the polyribosomes (which are basophilic) combining with the basic stains in the blood stain while the hemoglobin which is now being synthesized along polyribosomes (Fig. 5-20) is acidophilic and combines with the eosin of the blood stain. The net result is that the cytoplasm takes on a muddy-gray or green-violet color. The nucleus of the polychromatophilic erythroblast is somewhat smaller than that of the basophilic variety, and its chromatin is in the form of coarse granules which commonly are clumped so that the nucleus as a whole is very basophilic. No nucleoli can be seen in it. Polychromatophilic erythroblasts experience one of two different fates. Occasionally, under ordinary circumstances (probably less than one in 100 times), and more often when erythroid activity is increased because of a need for more red cells, the nucleus of the polychromatophilic erythroblast becomes pyknotic and is extruded while the cytoplasm is still polychromatophilic. This results in the formation of a polychromatophilic erythrocyte, as is shown in Figure 10-3. As has been described already, the polychromatophilic erythrocyte is called a reticulocyte (Fig. 10-3) when it is stained by supravital technics because polyribosomes still present in its cytoplasm show up under these conditions as if they were in the form of a reticulum.

The other and common fate of polychromatophilic erythroblasts is for them, as they continue to divide, to lose their cytoplasmic basophilia. When this has happened, the cell is termed a *normoblast* (also called orthochromatic erythroblast) because it is going to give rise to a normocytic erythrocyte. By this time a normoblast has a small spherical dark-staining pyknotic nucleus (Fig. 12-5). Normally, this is lost by extrusion (Fig. 12-3). The many extruded nuclei of normoblasts are mostly phagocytosed by the macrophages of the stroma (Fig. 12-3). Occasionally, small particles of the nucleus are left behind in erythrocytes; these are called Howell-Jolly bodies.

The Fine Structure of Erythroblasts. Several erythroblasts are seen in Figure 12-8. Their most interesting feature is their great content of ribosomes and polyribosomes. Since basophilic erythroblasts multiply to some extent, their free ribosomes are essential for synthesizing more cell substance. However, their numbers decrease as the cells mature, as fewer are then required for cell multiplication. The polyribosomes are required because hemoglobin molecules are synthesized along them in the cytoplasm (Fig. 5-20).

The increasing electron density of the cytoplasm of maturing erythroblasts is to be explained by the hemoglobin that is accumulating in their cytoplasm. Hemoglobin of course contains iron, and for other reasons as well it is very electron-dense, and this accounts for the fact that the electron density of the next stage along the red blood cell route—the reticulocyte—is electron-dense (Fig. 12-8) as are erythrocytes themselves (Fig. 12-8). Under normal conditions, the body is very economical of iron and uses that obtained from old, wornout red cells that are phagocytosed by macrophages of spleen and bone marrow for the synthesis of hemoglobin in new ones. But, under certain conditions, the body may suffer from a deficiency of iron, and as a result, an iron-deficiency anemia can occur. This is commonly of the hypochromic type (Fig. 11-4, *left*).

Regulation of Normal Erythrocyte Production. A lack of a proper supply of oxygen to the tissues stimulates the production of erythrocytes in the marrow and this effect is mediated by erythropoietin which exerts its effect at the level of the CFU-E. Erythrocyte production becomes greatly depressed if animals are transfused so as to raise the erythrocyte count far above normal.

Pathway By Which Erythrocytes Enter the Bloodstream. Different views have been held on this matter. The lack of a basement membrane along the endothelial cells of sinusoids makes it relatively easy for erythrocytes to enter through the endothelial cells themselves which are often attenuated. Tavassoli and Crosby from a recent study suggest that erythrocytes pass through the cytoplasm of the endothelial cells of sinusoids by way of pores, which are of a size that allows only erythrocytes to pass through them and

Fig. 12-8. Electron micrograph (× 6,000) of extramedullary hematopoiesis in the liver of a 5-day-old mouse. Three stages in the maturation of red blood cells can be seen. Erythroblasts (labeled as such) are lying in close apposition to liver cells. Their nuclear chromatin is clumped, and their cytoplasm contains large numbers of randomly dispersed free ribosomes. Adjacent to the erythroblasts is a reticulocyte. The nucleus has been extruded from this cell, but at least 1 small mitochondrion can still be seen in the cytoplasm. Ribosomes are present in the cytoplasm, but the greater density of the cytoplasm is due to its content of hemoglobin. Adjacent to the reticulocyte is a mature erythrocyte. Its cytoplasm is extremely electron-dense owing to the high content of hemoglobin. Neither ribosomes nor any other organelles can be recognized in the cytoplasm of the mature erythrocyte. (Preparation from K. Arakawa)

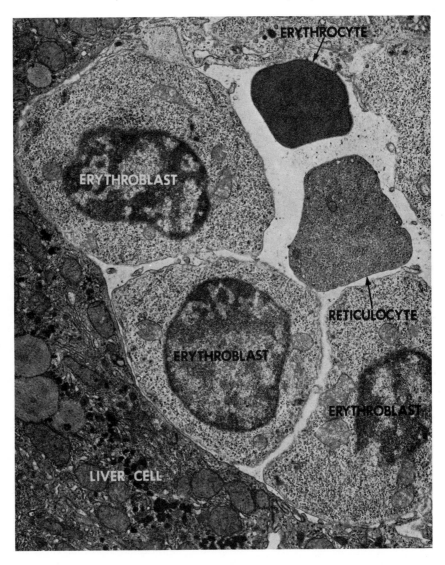

even then only because erythrocytes are elastic. They suggest that when nucleated erythrocytes attempt a passage through a pore the cytoplasm is elastic enough for it to squeeze through but the nucleus is left behind, so that the erythrocyte that enters the circulation is enucleated. The naked nucleus is ingested by a macrophage.

THE FORMATION OF GRANULAR LEUKOCYTES (GRANULOPOIESIS)

The three kinds of granular leukocytes that develop in the stroma of red marrow are all descendants of a common progenitor cell, the CFU-C (CFU-G) which is probably the immediate precursor of the promyelo-

cyte of the traditional terminology (Fig. 12-5). Since the granules that are first formed in cells of the granulocyte series are not of different specific types, it is impractical to attempt to distinguish 3 types of promyelocytes.

The second step in differentiation along this cell lineage (Fig. 12-5) is represented by the formation of myelocytes from promyelocytes. This step involves changes in both the nuclei and the cytoplasm of the cells and a reduction in the size of the cells concerned (Fig. 12-5). Whereas the nucleus of the promyelocyte is only slightly indented, the nucleus of the myelocyte begins to appear as an indented oval (Fig. 12-5). Generally, a cell is not called a myelocyte unless it

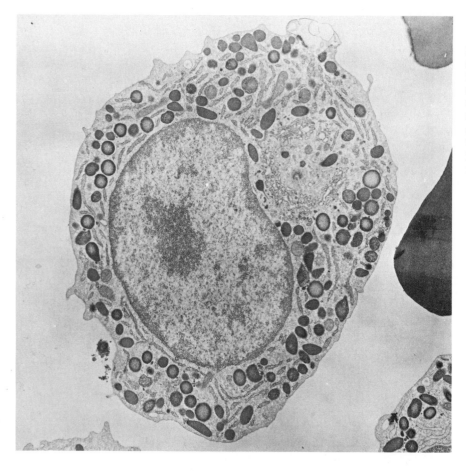

Fig. 12-9. Electron micrograph (× 15,000) of a promyelocyte, peroxidase reaction. The only granules formed at this time are peroxidase positive; these are the azurophilic granules seen with the LM. Note the well developed Golgi at the indentation of the nucleus. (From Bainton, D. F., Ullyot, J. L., and Farquhar, M. G.: J. Exp. Med., *134:*907, 1971)

has at least a dozen granules in its cytoplasm. However, myelocytes may be loaded with granules. The granules that appear in the cell at this time may permit different kinds of myelocytes to be distinguished. The 3 kinds of myelocytes mature to form the 3 kinds of granular leukocytes (Fig. 12-5) and in the maturation process they pass through a metamyelocyte stage.

EM Studies of the Development of Polymorphs

The fine structure of the cells leading to the formation of neutrophils has been investigated in detail by Bainton, Ullgot and Farquhar (see "References and Other Reading").

At the promyelocyte stage the granules that have developed are of the azurophilic type (Figs. 12-9 and 12-10): these are either spherical or ovoid in shape and are peroxidase positive. Rough ER can be seen scattered about in the cytoplasm and the Golgi is very prominent just to the right of the hilus of the nucleus

in Figure 12-9. Bainton, Ullgot and Farquhar have shown that these azurophilic granules bud off from the Golgi saccules that are on the concave side of a stack. The production of these granules soon ends. The large number of them found at the promyelocyte stage decreases in the course of the cellular evolution to the mature granulocyte. From the myelocyte stage onward granules of a new type begin to form; these arise from the *convex* surface of the Golgi (Farquhar and Bainton). These granules are smaller and less dense than those produced earlier. They are the specific neutrophilic granules (circles in Fig. 12-10). The specific granules of developing neutrophils vary somewhat in size but are smaller and rounder than the azurophilic granules (Fig. 10-6). They are not peroxidase positive as are the azurophilic granules. The nature and contents of the two types of granules in polymorphs was described in the chapter on leukocytes.

The development and maturation of a polymorph in relation to time is shown in Figure 12-10. It develops from a progenitor cell (labeled myeloblast in Fig. 12-10), but in view of the cell culture studies which indicate the CFU-G as the immediate precursor of promyelocytes it might be referred to by this term. At the promyelocyte stage the cell develops the azurophilic granules as already described (black in Fig. 12-10). At the myelocyte stage it develops specific neutrophilic granules (circles in Fig. 12-10) and the azurophilic granules become diminished in number. The cell then loses its ability to proliferate. Its subsequent maturation involves some reduction in size and the nucleus changing from the indented oval to the band (horseshoe) type and finally to the lobed type. It then enters the bloodstream from which it enters tissue where required. The times taken for the various stages are given in Figure 12-10.

Development of Eosinophils. In forming an eosinophilic leukocyte the slightly indented nucleus of the eosinophilic myelocyte generally develops a deep constriction at the metamyelocyte stage of development (Fig. 12-5). This deepens to divide the nucleus of the eosinophil into two lobes that usually remain joined together only by a strand of nucleoplasm (Fig. 10-3). As the constriction develops, the chromatin of the nucleus becomes somewhat condensed, and as a result the chromatin takes up a little more stain than the nucleus of a myelocyte. But the condensation of

chromatin that occurs is not so great as that which occurs in the neutrophil; hence the nuclei of eosinophils are paler than those of neutrophils (Fig. 10-3).

The fine structure of the granules is shown in Figure 10-9. Bainton and Farquhar have studied the formation of the granules and have shown that they are lysosomal in nature and develop similarly to lysosomes in other kinds of cells.

Formation of Basophils. In forming a basophilic leukocyte the nucleus of a basophilic myelocyte undergoes less change than occurs in the formation of either a neutrophil or an eosinophil. Irregular constrictions may appear in it to give it an irregular outline. But, in general, it does not become broken up into lobes to the same extent as neutrophils or eosinophils. Since its chromatin does not become condensed, it stains only very lightly. In contrast, its granules stain deeply, and as a result, those that lie in the cytoplasm that is spread over the nucleus tend to obscure it (Fig. 12-4). The granules of the basophil, unlike those of the eosinophils and the azurophilic granules of neutrophils, are not lysosomal in nature. Since they contain heparin it could be assumed that they develop similarly to the secretory granules of other kinds of cells that secrete mucopolysaccharides.

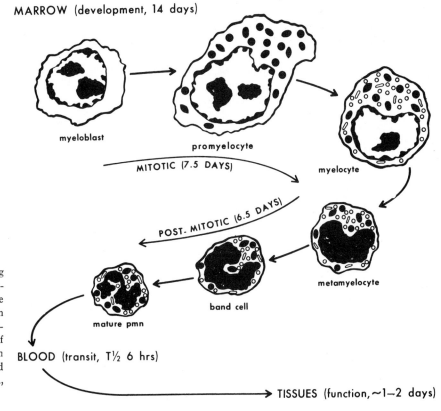

MARROW (development, 14 days)

myeloblast

promyelocyte

MITOTIC (7.5 DAYS)

myelocyte

POST-MITOTIC (6.5 DAYS)

metamyelocyte

band cell

mature pmn

BLOOD (transit, T½ 6 hrs)

TISSUES (function, ~1–2 days)

Fig. 12-10. Diagram illustrating the development of a polymorphonuclear neutrophilic myelocyte. In the text it is suggested that the term CFU-C could be used as an alternative for myeloblast. Description of stages is given in the text. (From Bainton, D. F., Ullyot, J. L., and Farquhar, M. G.: J. Exp. Med., *134:*907, 1971)

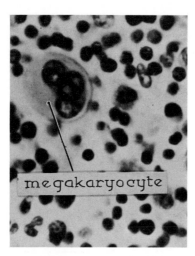

FIG. 12-11. High-power photomicrograph of a section of red bone marrow obtained from an infant. The cells in this specimen are less tightly packed than is usual. Note the great size of the megakaryocyte as compared with other free cells of marrow.

MEGAKARYOCYTES AND THE FORMATION OF PLATELETS (SUBLINE 8)

Megakaryocytes (*mega*, big; *karyon*, nucleus; *cyte*, cell) are so called because they are cells with huge nuclei (Figs. 12-11 and 12-12). The latter are the result of polyploidy described in connection with Figure 2-26. As well as having a huge nucleus, a megakaryocyte has also a great deal of cytoplasm (Figs. 12-11 and 12-12). The function of the cell is to produce the platelets of the blood which it does by liberating fragments of cytoplasm which enter the circulation as platelets. In H and E sections of red marrow, megakaryocytes are much larger than any other marrow cells (Figs. 12-1 and 12-11). The nucleus is colored a deep blue with hematoxylin. It may be ovoid in shape or lobulated. A megakaryocyte with a lobulated nucleus may, at the focus at which it is first examined, seem to be a multinucleated cell. But careful focusing of the microscope will show that what at first appear to be separate nuclei are in reality connected to one another. The only cell with which a megakaryocyte can be confused is an osteoclast which is an equally large cell often seen on bone surfaces (Fig. 15-10). However, by focusing up and down, osteoclasts can be seen to be multinucleated cells. So while osteoclasts and megakaryocytes can usually be distinguished by the fact that osteoclasts are seen on the surface of bone that surrounds marrow, focusing on nuclei permits osteoclasts, which for one reason or another, seem

to be in marrow, to be distinguished from megakaryocytes.

In 1906 Wright discovered the origin of platelets. He devised a special stain (a variation of the polychrome methylene blue and eosin mixture) and stained thin sections of red marrow, particularly that of kittens and puppies, with it. Figure 12-13 is a black and white picture of his original colored drawing. He observed that megakaryocytes often extended cytoplasmic pseudopodia into the sinusoids of the marrow and, further, that the cytoplasmic pseudopodia stained identically with platelets in that the red granules with which the pseudopodia were stippled resembled the granulomeres of platelets and the remaining substance of the pseudopodia stained similarly to the hyalomer of a platelet (Fig. 12-13). Moreover, as a clincher he pointed out that only those animals that possess megakaryocytes have platelets. The stippling of the cytoplasm of megakaryocyte cytoplasm can be seen in the low power micrograph, Figure 12-3, where the cell is labeled Meg.

Verification that platelets are detached portions of megakaryocyte cytoplasm came from EM studies of

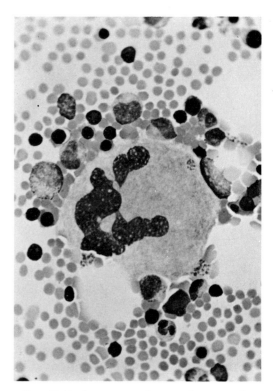

FIG. 12-12. Appearance of a megakaryocyte in a stained smear of bone marrow.

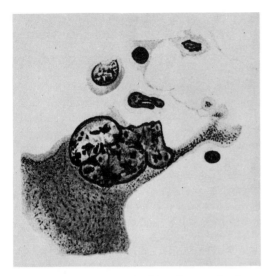

FIG. 12-13. A black-and-white photograph of one of Wright's colored illustrations of the appearance of megakaryocytes forming platelets in a section of the bone marrow of a kitten, stained with Wright's special stain. The picture shows a pseudopodium extending through a thin-walled blood vessel and liberating 2 platelets. (Wright, J. H.: J. Morphol., 21:263)

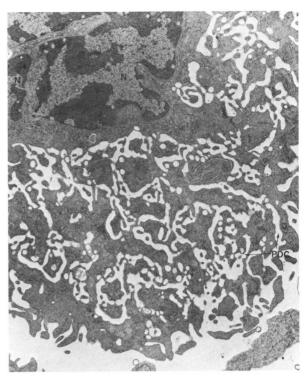

FIG. 12-15. Electron micrograph of a part of a megakaryocyte from mouse bone marrow showing the subdivision of its cytoplasm around the periphery of the cell into smaller regions by a complex network of channels. These platelet demarcation channels (PDC) originate by elongation and coalescence of smaller vesicles and become continuous with the cell surface. Platelets form when these fragments of cytoplasm become detached from the cell and are released into the circulation. Part of the multilobed nucleus (N) is also shown. (From V. I. Kalnins)

great magnification. The EM revealed that each platelet is surrounded by a membrane of the unit type. Studies of megakaryocyte cytoplasm have shown how each fragment of cytoplasm becomes completely surrounded with unit membrane while the cytoplasm from

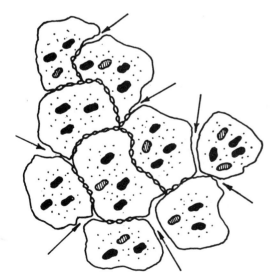

FIG. 12-14. Rows of membranous vesicles are sometimes seen in electron micrographs along the lines where the cytoplasm of megakaryocytes will separate into platelets.

which the fragments become detached remains covered with unit membrane, as will now be explained.

Yamada in 1955 described how the cytoplasm of megakaryocytes becomes divided up into small compartments by an extensive development within the cytoplasm of smooth-surfaced membranous vesicles (see Diagram, Fig. 12-14). Micrographs show that usually the peripheral cytoplasm of megakaryocytes is divided up by strings or sheets of these vesicles. The areas so divided are about the same size as platelets (Figs. 12-14 and 12-15). The vesicles fuse with one another and with invaginations of the cell membrane. Thus each future platelet becomes surrounded with unit membrane (Fig. 12-14); this accounts for cell coat material on the surfaces of platelets. By the mechanism illustrated in Figure 12-14 platelets can be separated from the main body of the cytoplasm of a megakaryocyte and yet be completely covered with unit membrane and cell coat, and the cytoplasm from which the platelet separated is left with an intact covering membrane and coat.

Formation and Maturation of Megakaryocytes. Since megakaryocytes are characterized by mitotic divisions occurring without the two sets of daughter chromosomes that arise becoming separated from one another into two daughter nuclei, mitosis in megakaryocytes results, not in the formation of more megakaryocytes but in polyploidy. Megakaryocytes, therefore, would seem to be end products. Hence for their numbers to be maintained new cells must appear on the scene to differentiate into the type in which future mitoses will result not in more cells but only in polyploidy. Some precursor cell—a promegakaryocyte—must therefore be able to divide normally to form more megakaryocytes. Since megakaryocytes in chronic myelogenous leukemia have been shown to carry the Philadelphia chromosome which serves as a marker to characterize also the erythrocyte and granulocyte cell lineages in this type of leukemia, it would seem that the promegakaryocyte would have to arise from the same precursor cell as those that give rise to the erythrocyte and granulocyte lines of differentiation. Such a cell would be the immediate progenitor of the CFU-E and the CFU-G. It seems probable that this cell is not the CFU-S, because there are other cell types derived from the CFU-S (lymphocytes) which do not reveal the Philadelphia chromosome as they would if it was present in the CFU-S. The cell at the level at which the Philadelphia chromosome is thought to arise is sometimes termed the myeloblast but this term should perhaps be avoided because it has so long been associated with a special morphology which the cell we have been discussing would probably not possess.

It has been shown that the maturation of megakaryocytes which leads to the cytoplasmic development that permits platelets to be produced is not dependent on increasing ploidy occurring in the cells but is a later development; in other words, the development of the huge nucleus can be a prelude to the maturation in the cytoplasm which permits the cell to perform its particular function.

As was described in connection with platelets in Chapter 11, there is evidence indicating that a humoral factor, thrombopoietin, exists which controls the processes involved in increasing the production of platelets by megakaryocytes, probably by stimulating their maturation.

THE CELL LINEAGE INVOLVED IN THE FORMATION OF MONOCYTES

As noted previously, one method used in the past in trying to determine the positions of different cells along a particular blood cell lineage was to assume that one of any two cells seen with the LM in stained films or sections that resemble each other closely was either the immediate precursor or the immediate descendant of the other. Perhaps nowhere did this method lead to so much confusion as in trying to work out the cell lineage involved in the formation of monocytes. Any student who examined enough blood films would sooner or later find what seem to be examples representing enough intermediate appearances between lymphocytes and monocytes to suggest that the former can transform into the latter. Second, if he examined enough films of both blood and marrow cells he could easily find examples of developing granulocytes that had appearances similar enough to monocytes to suggest they had a common progenitor, particularly because monocytes, like neutrophils, contain azurophilic granules. Still other views were held.

The evidence from in-vitro studies indicates that monocytes as such do not incorporate tritiated thymidine. However, in-vivo experiments have shown that, after animals are given tritiated thymidine, labeled monocytes appear in the body in considerable numbers, which strongly suggests that the label is taken up by a precursor cell that multiplies rapidly and gives rise to labeled progeny which immediately differentiate into monocytes. This finding in itself suggests the existence of a committed precursor cell with considerable proliferative capacity.

Metcalf and Moore have reviewed the extensive literature dealing with the many kinds of newer evidence that has accumulated over the more recent years which might suggest that lymphocytes, at least under some conditions, could give rise to cells which might be termed monocytes. However, they present very convincing evidence to the effect that monocytes arise along a cell lineage that begins from the CFU-C (CFU-G), for they have observed colonies of cells that arise from this cell which contain both granulocytes and monocytes. Furthermore, they cite examples of a type of leukemia which they have studied that occurs in certain mice and involves an overproduction of both monocytes and granulocytes, which again suggests that both types of cell evolve from a common progenitor cell which seems to be the CFU-C. This, however, would not necessarily mean that monocytes are just another type of granular leukocyte. It seems to be more probable that just as the CFU-C gives rise to promyelocytes it also gives rise to a cell which has the ability to proliferate and from its commitment could be termed a monoblast and that its progeny differentiate into monocytes.

STEPS IN THE FORMATION OF LYMPHOCYTES IN MYELOID TISSUE

The members of the cell lineage that arises from the CFU to give rise to small lymphocytes in myeloid tissue of the mouse have not been as clearly established as those of cell lineages that give rise to erythrocytes and granular leukocytes. The problem of attempting to work out this lineage by morphology is complicated by the fact that small lymphocytes and CFU's are probably in the same size range and it would be impossible to distinguish them from one another with the LM in stained films with accuracy. Of interest, however, is the finding by Osmond and Everett, who prepared radioautographs of bone marrow at intervals after giving guinea pigs an intravenous injection of tritiated thymidine. They found that in the first 4 hours only about 0.4 percent of the small lymphocytes of the marrow had become labeled. They found however that after 3 days around 40 percent of the marrow lymphocytes were labeled. Since small lymphocytes as such do not take up labeled thymidine because, as such, small lymphocytes do not undergo division, the fact that they become labeled in due course suggests there must be a type of blast cell in marrow which undergoes mitosis and hence takes up label that is inherited by its progeny which are small lymphocytes. Such a cell has been described on morphological grounds as existing in marrow where it has been termed a transitional cell. This cell is somewhat larger than a small lymphocyte and so could be thought of as being more or less of the order of a blast cell and it would seem logical to conceive of it as being derived from the CFU. It therefore seems probable that the cell lineage involved in the formation of lymphocytes in mouse marrow is as follows: a blast type of cell develops from the CFU and proliferates, with its progeny differentiating into small lymphocytes which soon leave the marrow to be replaced by new ones that are constantly being formed.

The small lymphocytes formed in the marrow of mammals are B lymphocytes which enter the blood and are filtered out mostly in the spleen but also in all the various types of lymphatic tissue except the thymus. In these tissues they are available for becoming blast cells of a type that divide and differentiate into plasma cells. As was noted in the section on lymphocytes in Chapter 10, these B lymphocytes are preprogrammed to react to different antigens. A possible way by which lymphocytes become differently preprogrammed was described in Chapter 10. Because of the substantial production of B lymphocytes constantly taking place, B lymphocytes variously preprogrammed to react with a vast variety of different antigens are provided to take up their residence in the various lymphatic tissues (except the thymus, as explained in next chapter). As was described in connection with lymphocytes in Chapter 10, a B lymphocyte generally produces only a trace of the specific antibody that it is programmed to make but, after contact with an antigen under appropriate conditions, they become blast cells and give rise to clones of plasma cells. For most antigens the appropriate conditions are simultaneous contact with a T lymphocyte or another type of cell studded with a product of the T lymphocyte, either one bearing the antigen in a special configuration (see Fig. 13-14).

References and Other Reading

THE STROMA AND BLOOD SUPPLY OF MYELOID TISSUE

Weiss, L.: The structure of bone marrow. Functional interrelationships of vascular hematopoietic compartments in experimental hemolytic anemia: an electron microscope study. J. Morphol., *117*:467, 1965.
———: Histophysiology of bone marrow. Clin. Orthop., *52:* 13, 1967.
Yoffey, J. M.: A note on the thick-walled and thin-walled arteries of bone marrow. J. Anat., *96*:425, 1962.
Zamboni, L., and Pease, D.: The vascular bed of the red bone marrow. J. Ultrastruct. Res., *5*:65, 1961.

For references and data on the osteogenic capacities of bone marrow *see* Ham, A. W., and Harris, W. R.: The repair and transplantation of bone. *In* Bourne, G. H. (ed.): The Biochemistry and Physiology of Bone. vol. 3, ed. 2. New York, Academic Press, 1971.

THE FORMATION OF BLOOD CELLS IN MYELOID TISSUE

General—Older Concepts

A good source book for the older literature is *Downey's Handbook of Hematology,* edited by H. Downey and containing numerous chapters by different authors. It was published in 1938 by Paul B. Hoeber, New York.

General—The Newer Concepts

A most informative and comprehensive book on the modern concepts by authors who were responsible for much of the new knowledge is that by Metcalf, D., and Moore, M. A. S. It is entitled *Haemopoietic Cells* and was published in 1971 by North-Holland Publishing Co., Amsterdam.

References and Other Reading Related Particularly to Stem Cells

General

Haemopoietic Stem Cells. Ciba Foundation Symposium, 13, New Series. London, Elsevier, 1973.

Special

Barnes, D. W. H., Ford, C. E., Gray, S. M., and Loutit, J. F.: Spontaneous and induced cell populations in heavily irradiated mice. *In* Burgher, J. G., Coursaget, J., and Loutit, J. F. (eds.): Progress in Nuclear Energy. Series VI, vol. 2, p. 1. London, Pergamon Press, 1959.

Becker, A. J., McCullough, E. A., and Till, J. E.: Cytological demonstration of the clonal nature of spleen colonies derived from transplanted mouse marrow cells. Nature, *197:*452, 1963.

van Bekkum, D. W., van Noord, M. J., Maat, B., and Dicke, K. A.: Attempts at identification of hemopoietic stem cell in mouse. J. Hematol., *38:*547, 1971.

Ford, C. E., Hamerton, J. L., Barnes, D. W. H., and Loutit, J. F.: Cytological identification of radiation-chimeras. Nature, *177:*452, 1965.

Ford, C. E., Micklem, H. S., Evans, E. P., Gray, J. C., and Ogden, D. A.: The inflow of bone marow cells to the thymus: Studies with part-body irradiated mice injected with chromosome-marked bone marrow and subjected to antigenic stimulation. Proc. 7th Internat. Transplantation Conf. Ann. N.Y. Acad. Sci., *129:*283, 1966.

Fowler, J. H., Wu, A. M., Till, J. E., McCulloch, E. A., and Siminovitch, L.: The cellular composition of hemopoietic spleen colonies. J. Cell Physiol., *69:*65, 1967.

Loutit, J. F.: Transplantation of haemopoietic tissues. Brit. Med. Bull., *21:*118, 1965.

————: Grafts of haemopoietic tissue: the nature of haemopoietic stem cells. Symp. Tissue and Organ Transplantation (Suppl.) J. Clin. Path., *20:*535, 1967.

McCulloch, E. A.: Differentiation of hemopoietic stem cells. *In* Plenary Session Papers, XII Congress of International Society of Hematology. p. 260. New York, International Society of Hematology, 1968.

McCulloch, E. A., and Till, J. E.: The sensitivity of cells from normal mouse bone marrow to gamma radiation in vitro and in vivo. Radiat. Res., *16:*822, 1962.

Micklem, H. S., Ford, C. E., Evans, E. P., and Gray, J.: Interrelationships of myeloid and lymphoid cells: studies with chromosome-marked cells transfused into lethally irradiated mice. Proc. Roy. Soc. (Biol.), *165:*78, 1966.

Moore, M. A. S., and Metcalf, D.: Ontogeny of the haemopoietic system: yolk sac origin of in vivo and in vitro colony-forming cells in the developing mouse embryo. Brit. J. Haematol., *18:*279, 1970.

Siminovitch, L., Till, J. E., and McCulloch, E. A.: Decline in colony-forming ability of marrow cells subjected to serial transplantation into irradiated mice. J. Cell Comp. Physiol., *64:*23, 1964.

Till, J. E., and McCulloch, E. A.: Initial stages of cellular differentiation in the blood forming system of the mouse. *In* Cameron, I. L., Padilla, G. M., and Zimmerman, A. M. (eds.): Developmental Aspects of the Cell Cycle. p. 297. New York, Academic Press, 1971.

Till, J. E., and McCulloch, E. A.: A direct measurement of the radiation sensitivity of normal mouse bone marow cells. Radiat. Res., *14:*213, 1961.

Wu, A. M., Till, J. E., Siminovitch, L., and McCulloch, E. A.: A cytological study of the capacity for differentiation of normal hemopoietic colony-forming cells. J. Cell. Physiol., *69:*177, 1967.

Hemopoiesis in Vitro

van Bekkum, D. W., and Dicke, K. A. (eds.): In Vitro Culture of Hemopoietic Cells. Rijswijk, The Radiobiological Institute TNO, 1972.

Robinson, W. A. (ed.): Proceedings of the Second International Workshop on Hemopoiesis in Culture. New York, Grune and Stratton, 1974.

Stephenson, J. R., Axelrad, A. A., McLeod, D. L., and Shreeve, M. M.: Induction of colonies of hemoglobin-synthesizing cells by erythropoietin in vitro. Proc. Nat. Acad. Sci. USA, *68:*1542, 1971.

The Formation of Erythrocytes

Grasso, J. A.: Cytoplasmic microtubules in mammalian erythropoietic cells. Anat. Rec., *156:*397, 1966.

Krantz, S. B., and Jacobson, L. O. (eds.): Erythropoietin and the Regulation of Erythropoiesis. Chicago, University of Chicago Press, 1970.

See also General Reference, Metcalf and Moore.

The Formation of Granular Leucocytes

See "References and Other Reading" on Granular Leucocytes at the end of Chapter 10.

The Formation of Monocytes

Brahim, F., and Osmond, D. G.: Radioautographic studies of the production and fate of bone marrow lymphocytes and monocytes. Proc. Canad. Fed. Biol. Soc., pp. 136-137, 1967.

Osmond, D. G.: The origin of peritoneal macrophages from the bone marrow. Anat. Rec., *154:*397, 1966.

Nichols, B. A., Bainton, D. F., and Farquhar, M. G.: Differentiation of monocytes. Origin, nature and fate of their azurophilic granules. J. Cell Biol., *50:*498, 1971.

See also General Reference, Metcalf and Moore.

The Formation of Lymphocytes in Myeloid Tissue

Hudson, G., Osmond, D. G., and Roylance, P. J.: Cell-populations in the bone marrow of the normal guinea pig. Acta Anat., *52:*234, 1963.

Osmond, D. G.: Lymphocyte production in the bone marrow: radioautographic studies in polycythaemic guinea pigs. *In* Yoffey, J. M. (ed.): The Lymphocyte in Immunology and Haemopoiesis. pp. 120-130. London, Edward Arnold, 1967.

Osmond, D. G., and Everett, N. B.: Radioautographic studies of bone marrow lymphocytes in vivo and in diffusion chamber cultures. Blood, *23:*1, 1964.

Osmond, D. G., Miller, S. C., and Yoshida, Y.: Kinetic and hemopoietic properties of lymphoid cells in the bone marrow. *In* Haemopoietic Stem Cells. Ciba Foundation Symposium 13 (new series). Amsterdam, ASP (Elsevier. Excerpta Medica. North-Holland), 1973.

Yoffey, J. M., Hudson, G., and Osmond, D. G.: The lymphocyte in guinea pig bone marow. J. Anat., *99*:841, 1965.

Yoshida, Y., and Osmond, D. G.: Identity and proliferation of small lymphocyte precursors in cultures of lymphocyte-rich fractions of guinea pig bone marow. Blood, *37*:73, 1971.

See also References for Chapter 10.

Megakaryocytes and the Formation of Platelets

Behnke, O.: An electron microscope study of the megakaryocyte of the rat bone marrow. 1. The development of the demarcation membrane system and the platelet surface coat. J. Ultrastruct. Res., *24*:412, 1968. 2. Some aspects of platelet release and microtubules. J. Ultrastruct. Res., *26*:111, 1969.

Garcia, A. M.: Feulgen-DNA values in megakaryocytes. J. Cell Biol., *20*:342, 1964.

Wright, J. H.: The histogenesis of the blood platelets. J. Morph., *21*:263, 1910.

Yamada, E.: The fine structure of the megakaryocyte in the mouse spleen. Acta Anat., *29*:267, 1957.

See also General Reference, Metcalf and Moore.

13 Lymphatic Tissue

As already mentioned, there are two main divisions of the hemopoietic tissues, myeloid and lymphatic. In this chapter we shall deal with the lymphatic division. It consists of four main parts: (1) the thymus, (2) the nonencapsulated lymphatic nodules of loose connective tissue, (3) lymph nodes, and (4) the spleen.

Lymphatic tissue is fundamental for the immunological defenses of the body. Its four main parts perform different functions but also work together in certain respects, as will be described as we discuss them in turn. We shall begin with the thymus.

The Thymus

The thymus is a lymphatic organ most of which lies in the thorax immediately beneath the upper part of

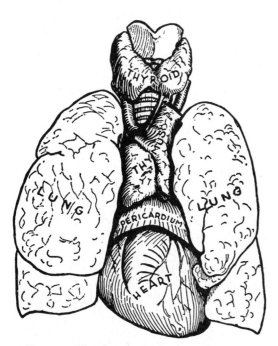

Fig. 13-1. The thymus gland of a child. (Grant, J. C. B., and Basmajian, J. V.: Grant's Method of Anatomy. ed. 7. Baltimore, Williams & Wilkins)

the sternum (Fig. 13-1). It is a flattened pinkish-gray mass that is roughly triangular. Its base lies below and is not as wide as its sides are long. Its apex extends into the neck and points toward the head. Its shape probably reminded some early anatomist of a thyme leaf, hence its name. In most species it probably consists of two parts, one on each side, that are not actually fused. In man it is generally considered to be a bilobed single structure because its two lobes which lie to either side are in apposition along the midline. Later we shall give some further details about its size and its weight at different ages.

General Functions and Importance. Until the beginning of the last decade almost nothing was known about the function of the thymus except that it produced lymphocytes (often called *thymocytes*) but these were not thought to have any special function. It was generally assumed that the thymus was not essential to life, for removing the organ from mature animals did not seem to have any untoward effect on them. However, early in the last decade it was shown that if the thymus was removed in a newborn animal it subsequently did not develop immunological competence and soon died. In particular it was unable to reject transplants of foreign tissue, but its capacity to make antibodies was also diminished. Experimental evidence was soon obtained which suggested that the thymus normally made an internal secretion that was essential if the other lymphatic organs were to function normally. However, it was subsequently shown that the effects of its removal at birth were due, perhaps mostly, to the fact that it normally makes a special kind of lymphocyte which it feeds to the body and which are vital for immunological reactions (T lymphocytes). Hence it is now accepted as an organ that is one of the keystones of the defense mechanisms of the body. All this development of knowledge has come about in a relatively short space of time and much of it is due to modern methodology, as will soon be described. However, there are very important problems yet to be solved about the thymus, as will also become obvious.

Size in Relation to Age. The size of the thymus varies greatly in relation to age. It is largest—in relation to the remainder of the body—during fetal life and in the first 2 years of postnatal life. From the 2nd year onward and until the time of puberty it continues to increase in size but not so rapidly as the remainder of the body. After puberty it begins to involute (*involvere*, to roll up), and as a consequence, it slowly becomes smaller as an individual ages.

For many years the size and weight of a normal thymus gland particularly in childhood was underestimated because, as it was found later, serious diseases in childhood tend to bring about its premature involution. Since so many children and adults from whom surveys were made in the relatively distant past had suffered serious attacks of the communicable diseases of childhood (which are now largely preventable) the average figure compiled from them was then not representative of what was really normal. According to modern views, the thymus gland weighs about 10 to 15 gm at the time of birth, and at the time of puberty, 30 to 40 gm. From then onward its weight slowly declines, but it still retains a reasonably substantial identity in old individuals. However, its size in normal middleaged

and older people has probably been underestimated because data are largely from autopsies made on people who died in hospitals after long illnesses. It has been noticed in autopsies of middleaged and older people who are killed in motor accidents that the thymuses are larger than those from patients of a comparable age that died from disease.

Development. The thymus gland develops as a result of tubes of epithelial cells growing out into mesenchyme from the third pharyngeal pouches, of which there are 2, one on each side of the body. These epithelial tubes soon become solid cords, which in due course are pulled down into the thorax and lose their connections with their points of origin. At this stage of development the thymus resembles an endocrine gland, because it is composed of cords of epithelial cells. These proliferate and send out side branches which are the forerunners of the cores (medullas) of lobules. The arrangement of the epithelial cells then begins to change! Here and there little groups of epithelial cells become arranged around a central point, much as football players pile up around and over a loose ball. These

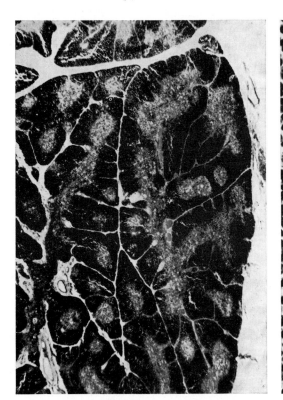 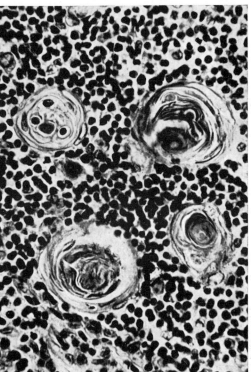

Fᴵɢ. 13-2. (*Left*) Very low-power photomicrograph of a section of the thymus gland of a child. The septa appear as clear lines. The cortex of the lobules is dark; the medulla is light. Observe that the medulla of one lobule is continuous with that of another. (*Right*) High-power photomicrograph of an area of medulla. Four Hassall's corpuscles are shown.

little groups of cells are known as Hassall's corpuscles (Fig. 13-2, *right*). The other cells of the epithelial cords become less densely arranged, tending to spread apart but remaining connected with one another because the processes of one adhere to the processes of other epithelial cells. This makes a 3-dimensional solid but spongelike structure. This unusual shape and arrangement of the epithelial cells gave rise to the term "epithelial reticular" cells (*rete,* a net).

The Development of the Lymphatic Component of the Thymus. The epithelium is enveloped by mesenchyme. The epithelium, in blunt thumblike protrusions, grows into a mass of doughlike mesenchyme which later forms a thin capsule around the organ. In the regions between the epithelial protrusions, the mesenchyme remains and forms thin partitions or septa which do not extend all the way to the center of the thymus but remain incomplete. The central epithelial part of the organ is thus continuous but it extends outward in all directions and peripherally it appears as the medulla of what appear as lobules (Fig. 13-2, *left*). Cells of the lymphocyte series fill the interstices between the epithelial cells and soon become the most prominent cells in the thymus (dark in Fig. 13-2) as it continues to develop; there have been several theories about where they come from. One theory was that they were derived from the epithelial cells. Another was that they were formed from the local mesenchyme. Still another was that they were derived from lymphocytes that came to the thymus by way of the bloodstream. One argument used against the last-mentioned concept was that they seemed to appear in the thymus before the mesenchyme of the part contained capillaries. Relatively recently, however, it seems to have become clearly established that the thymus is seeded with hemopoietic stem cells of the type described in the previous chapter which originate in the yolk sac and later seed the liver and spleen and finally the bone marrow. In the thymus they develop into larger cells of the lymphoblast type in the peripheral part of the cortex where they both proliferate and differentiate to produce small lymphocytes continuously, as will be described presently.

It should be mentioned that there is a very rapid turnover of the lymphocyte population of the thymus. If animals are given enough total body radiation, the lymphocyte content of the thymus, as might be expected, mostly disappears, as do the leukocytes being produced in the bone marrow. However, an animal treated this way can generally be saved if it is immediately injected intravenously with a suspension of bone marrow cells obtained from a nonirradiated ani-

mal of the same strain. Certain of the injected bone marrow cells bring about the repopulation of the bone marrow of the host and also of the thymus. Moreover, by using chromosome markers it has been shown that the lymphocytes in the repopulated thymus of the irradiated animal are derived from the donor marrow cells and not from the host. Other evidence makes it clear that in postnatal life in normal unirradiated animals as well, there are cells from bone marrow that circulate and take up residence in the thymus gland and there serve as progenitor cells for lymphocytes. So the origin of the lymphocytes of the thymus seems settled.

It seems more probable that CFU's are the cells from bone marrow that migrate to the thymus and serve as stem cells for the progenitor cells of the lymphatic series in postnatal life than it is that blast cells of the lymphatic type and formed from CFU's in the marrow migrate to the thymus to serve this purpose.

Microscopic Structure. Each of the two lobes of the thymus is surrounded by a capsule of connective tissue derived from mesenchyme. This extends into the substance of each lobe to form septa and to divide the two lobes into incomplete lobules which are usually from 1 to 2 mm in width (Fig. 13-2, *left*). The septa, although they penetrate deeply into the organ, do not partition the thymic tissue completely into lobules because in the central part of each lobe the thymic tissue of a given lobule is continuous with that of other lobules (Fig. 13-2, *left*). If, however, a lobule is sectioned parallel to and near the surface, it may appear as if it were completely surrounded by septa. As the thymus involutes, fat cells accumulate in the septa.

Cortex and Medulla. Cells of the lymphatic series are not spread evenly throughout the substance of each lobule; instead, they tend to be concentrated toward those borders of each lobule that abut on the capsule or on interlobular septa. The peripheral part of each lobule, heavily infiltrated with lymphocytes, is termed its *cortex* (Fig. 13-2, *left*) while the more central and much paler part of the lobule that does not contain so many lymphocytes is called its *medulla* (Fig. 13-2, *left*).

THE MICROSCOPIC STRUCTURE OF THE CORTEX
AND THE FORMATION AND MIGRATION
THROUGH IT OF T LYMPHOCYTES

The cortex is covered by a connective tissue capsule; this is thin in the rat and mouse (Fig. 13-3, Cs). The capsule may contain some small blood vessels but although they may supply the cortex in some animals, they do not do so in the mouse, as will be described later. An important point about the capsule is that, unlike lymph nodes, no lymphatics enter it. *No lymph drains into the thymus.*

The epithelial cells are arranged in a network that has spaces between the processes of the cells which are linked by desmosomes. An epithelial reticular cell is indicated by an arrow in Figure 13-3. The interstices between the epithelial cells is, for the most part, packed with cells of the lymphocyte series; these are of three orders of size (Fig. 13-3). In addition there is a capillary blood supply, which will be described presently.

As can be seen in Figure 13-3, the nuclei of the cells of the lymphocyte series in the part indicated as O. CORTEX (outer cortex) are large. These could be called lymphoblasts. Deeper in the cortex (I COR-TEX) the nuclei of the cells of the lymphocyte series are somewhat smaller, and more centrally they are mostly the size of ordinary small lymphocytes.

Some years ago Sainte-Marie and Leblond, from studies with the LM, classified the cells of lymphocyte series in the cortex of rats into 3 groups, depending on the diameters of their nuclei as measured in sections. From counting mitotic figures they estimated that each of the largest probably gives rise to 128 small lymphocytes. A mitotic figure is indicated by an asterisk in Figure 13-3. Mitosis occurs in the largest and the medium-sized cells. As the cells multiply and differentiate to form small lymphocytes, the latter move through the interstices of the epithelial network toward and into the medulla. Since the progenitor cells that give rise to the lymphocytes of the thymus must ordinarily enter the thymus in small numbers, they cannot be recognized.

The microscopic structure of the cortex described above applies to what is seen after lymphoblasts have already been produced in large numbers. Morphological details of the earlier events which involve the entry of CFU's (which are smaller than lymphoblasts) into the thymus and the production of lymphoblasts from these cells are unknown.

THE BLOOD SUPPLY OF THE CORTEX AND THE QUESTION OF A CORTICAL BARRIER TO ANTIGENS

The role of T lymphocytes was explained in part in Chapter 10. As will be described later in connection with lymph nodes and spleen, the T lymphocytes circulate via the bloodstream and from the thymus to take up positions in certain areas of lymph nodes and spleen; there, for reasons to be explained later, they are in a position to come into contact with antigens

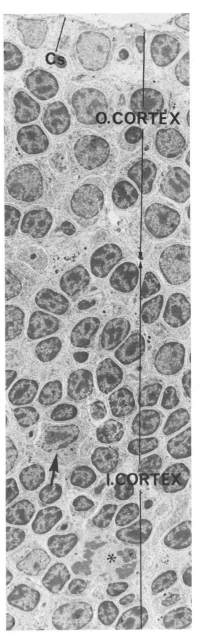

FIG. 13-3. Electron micrograph ($\times$ 2,000) of the thymic cortex. The outer part is indicated by O. Cortex and the inner by I. Cortex. The lymphocytes in the outer cortex are large. In the outer part of the inner cortex they are of a smaller size but not as small as in the deepest part of the inner cortex. The capsule can be seen at the surface (Cs). An arrow points to an epithelial cell and an asterisk indicates a lymphocyte in mitosis. (From W. S. Hwang and G. T. Simon)

which individual T lymphocytes will variously recognize because, when they leave the thymus, they are each programmed to react with a particular antigen. There can be a vast number of possible antigens, and there have to be as many differently programmed lymphocytes as there are possible antigens. Since T lymphocytes are formed in the cortex of the thymus, the problem arises as to how they become variously programmed. It seems that this must somehow occur in the cortex, with the result that the small lymphocytes that enter the medulla are different from one another with regard to their specificities for reacting to antigens.

As a background for attempting to visualize how T lymphocytes of an enormous number of different specificities for particular antigens could be produced in the thymus, it may help to realize that the thymus is the seat of enormous and continuous production of lymphocytes—a situation that would lend itself to the occurrence of genetic variations. Next, a T lymphocyte that is formed in the thymus and takes up its residence somewhere else in the body, where it meets an antigen with which it is specifically programmed to react, becomes a blast cell and gives rise to a clone of cells all programmed the same way it was; this indicates that basis for its specificity must be at the level of its genes. Although T lymphocytes do not become antibody-forming cells in the sense that B lymphocytes do, they each make a little antibody which is revealed on their surface as recognition sites. Hence the way they develop specificity for particular antigens is probably similar to that of B lymphocytes. In discussing the latter in Chapter 10 it was noted that the specificity of an immunoglobulin molecule is due to only one part of it being different from this part of other immunoglobulin molecules; the part that is different is called the variable part. In this there are sites where the amino acid sequences are different in different molecules and this accounts for the great variation of specificity that occurs. The reasons for the amino acids not being the same in certain parts of the variable part of all immunoglobulin molecules is of course that the presence of the particular amino acids in the variable part of any molecule was dictated by the genes of the cell in which it was produced, so what is dictated in different T lymphocytes in this respect must be different. This could suggest a high mutation rate, or perhaps some kind of a random turning on, of the genes that control amino acid selection in certain parts of the variable portion of the immunoglobulin molecules formed in T lymphocytes so as to provide them with different specificities with regard to antigens as was described in Chapter 10.

There are, however, complications that must be thought of in connection with this concept. First, if lymphocytes are variously programmed in the thymus to react with every conceivable antigen, why should some not become programmed to react with the protein macromolecules of the body in which they form? Apparently, either such T lymphocytes do not form or, if they do, there must be some mechanism in the thymus whereby they are destroyed before they can gain entrance to the blood circulation and kill the body cells that possess antigens against which they are programmed to react. The evidence that suggests that such lymphocytes are actually formed will now be described. As was explained in discussing immunological tolerance in Chapter 9, whether any macromolecule is regarded as foreign or not in a particular body depends on whether that macromolecule was present in the body and exposed to body fluids before, roughly, the time of birth. As will be mentioned in later chapters, some protein macromolecules produced in the body before birth are in such secluded environments that they do not come into contact with any body fluids. However, if the organ in which they were formed (and were protected from body fluids) is affected, for example, by a disease process that causes such a protein to become exposed to body fluids after birth, it is found that these proteins are regarded as foreign. When this happens it is called autoimmune disease (*auto,* self) because a person's own immunological mechanisms are reacting against his own cells. So the existence of autoimmune disease, occurring under the conditions described above, show that the normal macromolecules that are formed and exist in a person's own body are not automatically excluded from acting as antigens in that body, as might be expected because of their having been derived from the same cell —the fertilized ovum—that also gives rise to the same body's T and B lymphocytes. It is of interest in this connection that there are certain cells in the body that are not produced until puberty, for example the germ cells of the male. Moreover, when these are normally produced after puberty, their formation occurs in an environment that is more or less sealed off from body fluids. But if they are removed from this environment and injected, say, into loose connective tissue of the body in which they were produced, they are regarded by that body as foreign antigens.

The above evidence indicates that, whatever the reason for a body not possessing lymphocytes programmed to react against its own cells, it is not because of inherited genetic limitations being placed on the kind of immunological specificities that can be coded for in that body. So if we grant that the body attempts to produce cells of the lymphocyte series that would react against the body cells of the individual in which they are produced, we must seek some explanation as to why such cells do not appear in the circulation and destroy body cells.

A very plausible hypothesis (and it is only a hypothesis) has been put forward which explains why the T lymphocytes of a particular body do not react against any cells or macromolecules which were present in, or had contact with, a body fluid in embryonic and fetal life: If a cell of the lymphocyte series that is being formed and programmed to react with macromolecules of cells in the body in which it is being formed has *premature contact* with these macromolecules, it is destroyed by this contact. Thus, it may be that any developing T lymphocyte that would find body proteins antigenic is not permitted to mature into a functioning cell but is killed by premature contact. It might be suggested that this premature contact with body macromolecules that destroys cells of the lymphocyte series that are being programmed to react with them occurs in the thymus at the level of the lymphoblast or possibly at the level of the cells of the next smaller size which still have potentiality to reproduce, because any programming that occurs in lymphocytes occurs at a cell level which permits clones of lymphocytes with identical programming to be produced. However, as produced in the thymic cortex, T lymphocytes do not seem to be as yet immunologically competent; so it may be at this stage that they are destroyed by antigens they are programmed to react with. It has been suggested that the high rate of lymphocyte death in the thymus may be accounted for by the destruction of T lymphocytes that are programmed to react to body macromolecules which they encounter before they are mature. Experiments have shown that an animal can be made tolerant to a foreign antigen by injecting it into its thymus but only if this is done before the thymus has had time to seed the other parts of the lymphatic system with programmed T lymphocytes. Presumably, if the thymus is injected with an antigen under these circumstances, no T lymphocytes programmed to react against that antigen would emerge from the thymus; they would be destroyed by premature contact with the antigen. It therefore seems clear that in some manner the thymus is chiefly responsible for the phenomenon of tolerance.

The Thymic Barrier. The next interesting question that should engage our attention is why T lymphocytes that are programmed to react with various foreign antigens are not all weeded out as they are being formed by having premature contact with these antigens in the thymus. The reason seems to be that the thymic cortex in which T lymphocytes are formed is protected from antigens that may gain entrance to a body by a *thymic barrier*. This barrier is a leaky one in fetal life, as has been shown by Horivchi, Gery and Waksman, but the fetus is not normally exposed to foreign antigens; otherwise, tolerance to them would be induced, because they would gain entrance to the thymic cortex, like the macromolecules of the fetal body that circulate in its bloodstream and to which tolerance is induced.

There are several factors that prevent foreign antigens from gaining entrance to the thymic cortex where T lymphocytes are being programmed.

First, in contrast to the lymph nodes—into which the lymphatics drain lymph that originates from various parts of the body which are often sites of infection —and which are constructed so as to give any antigen present in lymph wide exposure within the node to both T and B lymphocytes, the thymus has no lymphatics that empty into it. Second, unlike the spleen which, as we shall see, is designed to give wide exposure of any antigen in blood to both T and B lymphocytes, the site of production of T lymphocytes in the thymus is separated by a barrier from both antigens and B lymphocytes that might be present in blood circulating through it. To explain the barrier between blood and the sites of developing lymphocytes in the cortex, we must first describe the blood supply of the cortex.

The Blood Supply of the Cortex. The cortex of the thymus is supplied *only with capillaries*. In an extensive study in the mouse, Raviola and Karnovsky have shown by injecting the vascular bed of the thymus that the capillaries originate from arterioles that are located at the cortico-medullary junction and that from these they ascend into the cortex where they form anastomosing capillary arcades from which capillaries return to the cortico-medullary junction where they drain into the postcapillary venules of the medulla.

The Components of the Blood-Thymus Barrier in the Cortex. Clark, with the EM in 1963, found evidence of a continuous epithelium surrounding the capillaries of the cortex (Fig. 13-4, EP). Thus the reticular epithelial cells form a lining for narrow channels in the cortex in which individual capillaries are conducted on their course. Between the capillaries and such pericytes as are associated with them and the epithelial membrane, a space may be seen; this is labeled SPACE in Figure 13-4. There is basement membrane material associated with both the epithelial reticular cells and the endothelium of the capillaries. The space between a capillary and the epithelial lining of the channel in which it lies may contain lymphocytes and macrophages. There are thus three components of

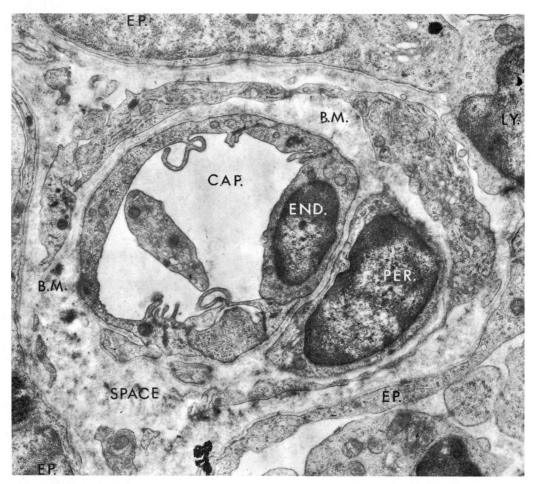

Fig. 13-4. Electron micrograph ($\times$ 12,000) of section of cortex of thymus of mouse. A capillary (CAP.) is cut in cross section. It is surrounded by a connective tissue space (SPACE), which contains a pericyte (PER.) and its processes. Surrounding this space is an epithelial membrane composed of cells (EP.) joined together by desmosomes. At the upper right a lymphocyte (LY.) has been caught in the act of migrating between two epithelial cells of the barrier, presumably to enter the connective tissue space. (Clark, S. L., Jr.: Am. J. Anat., *112*:1, labeling added)

the blood-thymic barrier through which antigens in a capillary would have to pass in order to reach lymphocytes that were forming in the cortical substance. An antigen would first have to penetrate the wall of the capillary and its basement membrane. Second, macromolecules would then enter a perivascular space (Fig. 13-4, SPACE), which presumably would contain tissue fluid and macrophages. It might be thought that the flow in this extravascular space would be toward the medulla which would wash an antigen to the medulla. Moreover, macrophages in the space could take up antigen that gained access to the space. Third, such macromolecules as crossed the tissue-fluid-filled space and reached the epithelial barrier would then have to

penetrate it to enter the area where lymphocytes are forming.

There has been controversy as to whether the blood-thymic barrier is effective in postnatal life with regard to shielding forming lymphocytes from antigens. In considering this matter it should be realized that when foreign antigens gain entrance to the bloodstream, they become greatly diluted; this is in contrast to the concentration of antigens that can occur in the lymph that drains into a lymph node. Recently, however, Raviola and Karnovsky have shown in a most extensive study with different antigens which they could trace that some confusion about the effectiveness of the barrier stems from not limiting the barrier concept to the cortex. They found the barrier was effective in preventing antigens from reaching the parenchyma of the cortex but that the blood-thymic barrier in the medulla was not effective in this respect. Their work should be read for details.

How T Lymphocytes Formed in the Cortex Leave the Thymus

The thymic cortex is a very active site of lymphocyte production, particularly in fetal and early postnatal life. There are more lymphocytes in the blood that leaves the thymus than in the blood that enters it, as was shown by Sainte-Marie and Kostuik (*The Thymus and Immunobiology*, p. 221). There has been much investigation and speculation with regard to the extent to which the excess of cells leaving the thymus over those that enter it can account for all the lymphocytes that are produced in the thymus; in other words, it is difficult to ascertain what percentage of the lymphocytes produced in the thymus die in the thymus. The concept outlined previously, to the effect that T lymphocytes that are programmed so as to recognize macromolecules of the body in which they were formed as antigenic would all die in the thymus, may account for much cell death in the thymus. Furthermore if the variability of the programming of lymphocytes in the thymus is due to there being a high rate of mutation occurring in them the total cell death that occurs could be explained by some of the mutants not being viable. In any event those lymphocytes that are viable because of cell proliferation behind them are pushed along through the interstices of the epithelial reticulum of the thymus to emerge into the medulla from which they enter the bloodstream, as will next be described. Some may enter the medulla by way of the perivascular spaces of the cortex which lead to those of the medulla.

On reaching the medulla, the lymphocytes formed in the cortex enter the blood circulation by migrating through the walls of postcapillary venules. In order to reach the wall of the venule they have to pass between the epithelial reticular cells that line the canals that contain the postcapillary venules. The endothelium of the venules is surrounded by a basement membrane which is of substantial thickness and associated with scattered pericytes. As can be seen in Figure 13-5 two lymphocytes (indicated by asterisks on their nuclei) have migrated through the epithelial reticular network that lines the canal in which the venule lies and have broken through the basement membrane to bulge inward into the venules, pushing a thin layer of endo-

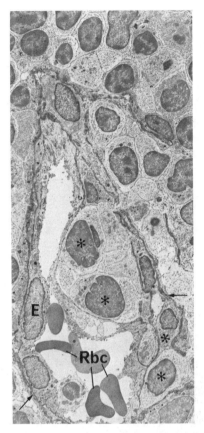

Fig. 13-5. Electron micrograph ($\times$ 1,800) of thymic medulla showing lymphocytes (marked by asterisks) migrating through the wall of a postcapillary venule so as to enter the lumen of the venule. The lumen of the venule contains some red blood cells (Rbc). The endothelium that lines the venule is labeled E and the basement membrane is indicated by arrows. The lymphocytes marked by asterisks have broken through the basement membrane but have still to pass between endothelial cells to gain entrance to the lumen of the venule. (From W. S. Hwang and G. T. Simon)

thelium ahead of them which thus separates them from the lumen of the venule which contains some red blood cells (Rbc). From this position lymphocytes enter the lumen by passing through the sites of junctions of endothelial cells (other explanations of how they pass through endothelium have also been suggested).

The blood drains from the thymic medulla by way of veins that are associated with some perivascular connective tissue in which there are some lymphatics which drain away such lymph as is formed in association with the capillaries and which probably reaches these lymphatics by connections with perivascular spaces.

Plasma cells are not normal constituents of the thymus for two reasons: (1) T lymphocytes cannot develop into plasma cells, and (2) if any B lymphocyte should penetrate a capillary and enter the thymic cortex, it would be in an environment in which it would be most unlikely that it could encounter an antigen. However, some blood-borne B lymphocytes may emerge in the thymus in its medulla and here there is no blood-thymic barrier to prevent blood-borne antigens from escaping into the perivascular tissue, so an occasional B lymphocyte may here form a few plasma cells. Furthermore, if the thymus is injured in such a way that parts of it are vascularized from the adjacent connective tissue, B lymphocytes and antigens could both have access to the injured area, in which plasma cells could subsequently form.

Before beginning the study of lymph nodes it should be mentioned that the germinal centers, to be described in connection with lymph nodes, do not develop in the thymus; the reasons for this will become apparent.

Sites To Which T Lymphocytes Migrate. T lymphocytes enter the other lymphatic tissues (lymph nodules, lymph nodes and spleen) and will be described as these tissues are dealt with. The T lymphocytes take up certain positions in the latter two organs which are termed thymus-dependent zones or areas. T lymphocytes, moreover, constitute most of the lymphocytes that recirculate from lymph nodes to thoracic duct to blood and then from the blood back again into the lymph in lymph nodes in which they are carried again to the thoracic duct.

DOES THE THYMUS PRODUCE AN INTERNAL SECRETION?

Development of Knowledge. A time-tested way for determining whether any given organ produces an internal secretion (a hormone) is to remove that organ from an experimental animal and see what happens. Until 1961 the thymus had been removed from animals without its removal seeming to exert any serious or remarkable effect (it is now known there is some effect). In 1961, however, both Archer and Pierce and Miller reported that removal of the thymus from a *newborn* animal resulted in an impaired development of its immunological capacities.

As this discovery was followed up, it became established that animals that were thymectomized at birth had fewer lymphocytes in their blood and lymphatic tissues than normal animals of the same age. It was shown that their ability to reject skin grafts from homologous animals was impaired, and also that they were unable to produce some of the immunoglobulins

that can be produced by normal animals. Furthermore, the members of several strains of mice that were thymectomized at birth were found to sicken in the first few months of life with a wasting type of disease.

In seeking the explanation for the defective immunologic mechanisms resulting from thymectomy at birth, consideration was given to the view that it was caused by the lymphatic tissue of the body being cut off from the supply of lymphocytes it would ordinarily receive from the thymus in early postnatal life. (At that time it was not known that there were two kinds of lymphocytes, T and B, with different functions.) It was also assumed that if the thymus is not removed until a week or two after birth, enough time would have elapsed during the first week or two of life for the thymus to have built up the lymphocyte population of the other lymphatic organs sufficiently for them to carry on independently thereafter, and that this explained why thymectomy performed later did not seem to be nearly as serious. However, evidence for another theory was soon forthcoming. It was found that if a thymus is transplanted from another animal (even another newborn animal) into an animal that has been thymectomized at birth, the thymectomized animal with the transplanted thymus recovers most of its immunologic competence. It might be thought that this is due to the transplanted thymus immediately producing lymphocytes (of donor origin) and feeding them to the other lymphatic organs of the host. But when a thymus gland is transplanted, it takes several days for the capillaries of the host to connect with the blood vessels of the transplant and to re-establish a circulation in transplanted syngeneic tissue. Since lymphocytes are sensitive cells, the lymphocytes of a thymic transplant that stay in the transplant (for some migrate from it) mostly undergo pyknosis before a circulation is established in the transplant, and, as a result, the cells that survive in the transplant are at least mostly the hardier epithelial reticular cells.

Evidence from transplantation experiments thus began to raise the possibility that the thymus is necessary for animals to become immunologically competent in the first week or so of life because of some humoral factor (such as a hormone) that is secreted into the blood by the epithelial cells of the thymus. To test this hypothesis, bits of thymus tissue were placed in little millipore chambers before they were transplanted into animals that were thymectomized at birth. The pores of the chambers were believed to be too small to permit any cells to leave the chambers, but fluid could, of course, enter and leave through the pores. Numerous experiments of this kind by Osoba and Miller and others have shown that thymic tissue in chambers transplanted into newborn thymectomized animals at least partially prevent the usual effects of thymectomy. Sections taken from the thymic tissue contained in chambers of this sort that have been transplanted and left in place for some time show that all that remains of the lymphatic tissue that was placed in the chamber is a mass of cells of the epithelial reticular type. Accordingly, it seemed reasonable to conclude that the epithelial reticular cells of the thymus, through the medium of a soluble product—a humoral factor—exert some influence on lymphocytes far away from the thymus, an influence which in the first week or so of life is necessary for lymphocytes in the other lymphatic organs to proliferate, develop and function immunologically in a normal way.

Perhaps because the postulated humoral factor seemed to elude attempts to obtain extracts of it that would prevent the effects of thymectomy, doubts arose about its existence. Hence increasing attention began to be paid to the importance of the long recognized function of the thymus in serving as a source of lymphocytes for the blood and other lymphatic tissues. In due course it was shown that the thymus produced T lymphocytes, which as already explained, perform a particular role. It was shown that if animals are thymectomized at birth, the number of lymphocytes obtained from the thoracic duct is profoundly reduced. If animals several months old are thymectomized, the number of lymphocytes that can be obtained from the thoracic duct is, with time, substantially reduced. So with the development of knowledge that T lymphocytes can originate in the thymus only and, hence, if the thymus is removed at birth the other lymphatic tissues do not become properly seeded with them, it became generally considered that the effects of thymectomy at birth could be explained by a lack of production of T lymphocytes. After a few weeks of life, the effect of thymectomy in a mouse would not be so severe because by then the other lymphatic organs could have been seeded with T lymphocytes. It is now generally thought that whereas a humoral factor that has some effect on the immunological system may indeed be produced by the thymic epithelium, the main effects of thymectomy at birth can be explained by the lack of formation of T lymphocytes.

EFFECTS OF CERTAIN HORMONES ON THE THYMUS

The growth hormone of the pars anterior of the pituitary gland and the thyroid hormone (Chap. 25) both stimulate the growth of the thymus gland. Most steroid hormones (Chap. 25) on the other hand—if sufficient quantities of them are present in the blood-

stream—tend to bring about the involution of the gland. Hence, the appearance of substantial quantities of sex hormone in the circulation at the time of puberty is probably an important factor in causing the thymus gland to begin to involute at this time. Selye, from his many studies on the effects of stress, believes that the premature involution of the gland observed in children who suffer from serious diseases or other forms of stress is caused by the oversecretion of adrenal cortical steroid hormones that occur as a result of the disease or stress condition. A deficiency of either adrenal cortical hormone or sex hormone in an animal, brought about by removing the endocrine glands responsible for these hormones, is associated with the hypertrophy of the thymus gland.

Distinguishing a Section of Thymus From One of a Lymph Node or Other Lymphatic Tissue. There are many ways to do this; however, since Hassal's corpuscles are seen only in the medulla of the thymus and not in other lymphatic tissues, their presence denotes a section of the thymus. EM studies have shown that the epithelial cells involved in forming Hassal's corpuscles pass through the same changes that are seen in the formation of keratinized epithelium and described in Chapter 7.

Lymph Nodules and Lymph Nodes

In contrast to the lymphatic component of the thymus, which is relatively protected from contact with foreign antigens, the cells of the lymphocyte series in the other lymphatic tissue of the body, (1) the non-encapsulated lymphatic nodules of loose connective tissue, (2) the lymph nodes, and (3) the spleen, are all placed so as to be exposed as extensively as possible to foreign antigens that enter (1) loose connective tissue, (2) lymph, and (3) blood respectively.

THE NONENCAPSULATED LYMPHATIC NODULES OF LOOSE CONNECTIVE TISSUE

Antigens in a variety of forms—such as pollens, viruses or bacteria—may penetrate the wet epithelial membranes that line various tubes in the body that have contact with the outside world—in particular, those membranes that line the respiratory and digestive tract and even the genitourinary tract. To provide a line of defense behind such wet epithelial membranes, little depots of lymphatic tissue called *lymphatic nodules* are variously scattered about in the loose connective tissue that lies beneath and supports the wet epithelial membranes that line these tracts. The association between lymphatic tissue in loose connective tissue and wet epithelium is particularly intimate in what are termed *tonsils,* which are paired structures disposed in 3 different sites (tongue, pharynx and nasopharynx), where they more or less stand on guard at the entrance of the respiratory and digestive tracts; these will be described in connection with the respiratory system because they have a special structure. Although most prevalent beneath wet epithelial membranes, lymphatic nodules occasionally are seen in other sites.

Histologic Features. Most nonencapsulated lymphatic nodules in loose connective tissue are single but in some sites—for example, in tonsils or in the ileum—they become confluent. In the lower part of the small intestine, the confluent nodules form structures called *Peyer's patches* which are large enough to be seen with the naked eye. An isolated nodule in loose connective tissue is roughly spherical and from a few hundred microns to a millimeter or more in diameter (Fig. 13-6). In an H and E section it appears under low power as a dark blue area. Under higher magnification the blue appearance is seen to be due to the nodule's being packed with cells of the lymphocyte series; since these cells have little cytoplasm, there is a great concentration of nuclei in the nodule; and since the densely packed nuclei are all colored blue, the whole nodule stands out as a rounded blue area. Most of the lymphocytes are of the small variety but larger cells of the series are also seen.

The periphery of a nodule is not very sharply defined (Fig. 13-6, *left side*). Lymphocytes produced in the nodule may be pushed out from its periphery so that at this site the appearance gradually changes from a dense concentration of lymphocytes to a decreasing concentration in the adjacent tissue. Lymphatic nodules are *not* encapsulated; they lie naked in whatever tissue they are in. To avoid misunderstanding, it should be noted that the *lymph nodes* and the *spleen* are enclosed by connective tissue capsules.

The Development of Lymphatic Nodules in Loose Connective Tissue. Lymphatic nodules are not as common in loose connective tissue before birth as after birth. Furthermore, they do not develop nearly as extensively in germ-free animals after birth as they do in ordinary animals. It seems, therefore, that the presence and recognition of antigens have much to do

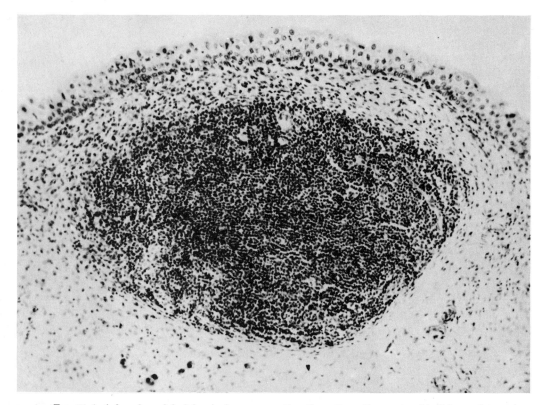

Fig. 13-6. A lymph nodule lying in loose connective tissue beneath a wet epithelial membrane. Specifically this figure illustrates a section cut from the wall of the urinary bladder of a dog. The epithelium that is above the lymphatic nodule is of the transitional type.

with their development. It seems probable that their development in postnatal life depends on three factors; (1) the trapping of antigen on the surface of a reticular cell or macrophage as shown in Figure 13-14 at the site where a nodule develops; (2) the arrival of some B and T lymphocytes from the bloodstream to the area, whereupon (3) blast cells would develop and give rise to the lymphocytes of the nodule.

Lymphatic nodules in loose connective tissue sometimes acquire what are termed *germinal centers*. The morphology of these will be described in more detail in connection with lymph nodes in the next section of this chapter. Here it is enough to say that they are rounded areas that appear in the central parts of lymphatic nodules; they stain differently from the remainder of the nodule, usually, but not always, by appearing lighter, and sometimes they exhibit many mitotic figures. Germinal centers therefore seem to be related to the presence of antigens. Possible functions will be discussed in connection with lymph nodes.

Functions of Lymphatic Nodules in Loose Connective Tissue. Their precise functions are not very clearly established; they probably serve much the same purpose as the lymphatic nodules of lymph nodes soon to be described. Certainly they produce lymphocytes. Since plasma cells often form in association with them—as, for example, in tonsils or in the alimentary tract—both B and T lymphocytes must enter into their composition. The fact that some of the nonencapsulated nodules in the intestine have some resemblance to the bursa of Fabricius of birds (which produces the B lymphocytes of birds) has raised the question as to whether some of the depots of confluent nodules that are in close association with the epithelium that lines the intestine—as, for example, in the tonsil, appendix or Peyer's patches—are a normal source of some B lymphocytes in mammals.

Difference Between Nonencapsulated Nodules and Lymphatic Infiltrations. In tissues that have been the site of some disease process, commonly of an inflammatory nature, there may be a considerable infiltration of lymphocytes in and around the site of the injured tissue. These diffuse infiltrations are regarded as inflammatory reactions and differ from nodules because they are not round as are isolated nodules but of an irregular shape, and they differ also from sites of confluent nodules because in the latter the outlines of the individual nodules that have fused are apparent on close scrutiny. Furthermore, lymphocytic infiltrations do not have any germinal centers as both discrete or confluent nodules may have. Tissue infiltrations of cells of the lymphocyte series may be seen in homograft reactions and also in what are

termed delayed hypersensitivity reactions which will be mentioned later in this chapter. Some other types of leukocytes are generally present along with lymphocytes in lymphocytic infiltrations.

Lymph Nodes

Most of the lymph collected by the lymphatic capillaries of the body, before being returned to the blood circulatory system by the thoracic or the right lymphatic duct, passes through one or more little round, oval or bean-shaped structures called *lymph nodes*. (They are sometimes called lymph glands, but since they are not designed for secretion, *node* is the preferable term. However, a physician may sometimes say a patient has swollen glands when the swollen structures are lymph nodes.) The student in using the term *node* must be careful to distinguish between nodes and nodules; the latter have already been briefly described.

Distribution. Many lymph nodes are situated in the axilla and in the groin. A great many are distributed along the great vessels of the neck and a considerable number in the thorax and the abdomen, particularly in association with the great vessels and the mesentery. A few are associated with the popliteal vessels, and a few are at the elbow. In general, then, lymph nodes are distributed, not where the lymph originated (like lymphatic nodules) but rather along the course of the main tributaries that flow into the thoracic and the right lymphatic ducts.

THE MICROSCOPIC STRUCTURE OF LYMPH NODES

Some Preliminary Consideration. An H and E section of a lymph node bears some resemblance to a section of thymus because much of the section is colored a deep blue (Fig. 13-7, *bottom*) for the same reason that a section of thymus is colored blue which is that the tissue is densely packed with lymphocytes which have deep blue nuclei. Furthermore, a lymph node, like the thymus, has a cortex and a medulla, with lymphocytes moving generally from the cortex to the medulla. The cortex of a lymph node, however, differs from that of the thymus because it is made up to a great extent of lymphatic nodules (Fig. 13-7, *bottom*). Another point of difference is that there is no epithelial component in lymph nodes.

It is a mistake to approach the study of the microscopic structure of a lymph node with the impression that it is a static structure. Lymph nodes are actually the site of great activity. As noted, lymph

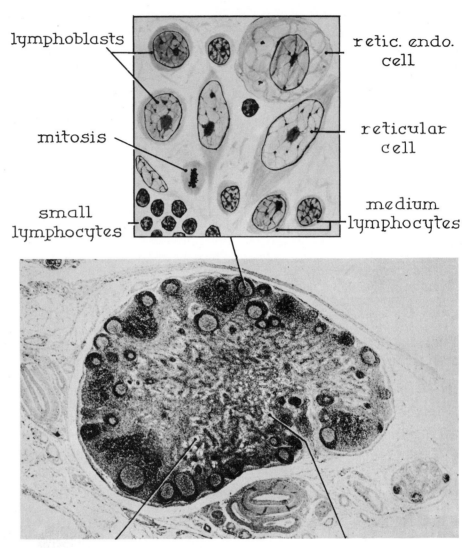

FIG. 13-7. (*Bottom*) Low-power photomicrograph of a lymph node. (*Top*) High-power drawing
of cells in germinal center. The two bottom leaders point to medullary sinuses.

drains through them and much phagocytosis by macrophages occurs in connection with any particulate matter that may be in lymph. Lymphocytes, both those produced in the node and those that are constantly being added to those of the node from the bloodstream, pass into the lymph that drains through the node. Killer cells and plasma cells that secrete antibodies are being formed in nodes as needed from activated T and B lymphocytes respectively. Structures called germinal centers come and go, depending on demands for immunological function. In other words, the study of a section of a lymph node suffers from the same limitations as a snapshot of a very active and ever changing scene. Frequent reference to Figs. 13-8 and

13-7 in the following descriptions should help to sort out the sites where various activities occur.

Size and Shape. Lymph nodes range in size from as small as seeds to as large as (shelled) almonds. Each has (1) a thick outer part called its cortex (bark), and (2) an inner part called its medulla. Bean-shaped nodes are common and facilitate description because they possess convex and concave surfaces, so we shall describe the minute structure of a node of this shape.

Capsule and Afferent and Efferent Lymphatics. A lymph node is surrounded by a connective tissue capsule (Fig. 13-8) which overlies its cortex. Since nodes commonly lie in fat tissue, some fat usually adheres to the outer aspect of the capsule when nodes are removed for sectioning. This may help the student distinguish a section of a lymph node from one of spleen which has a smooth peritoneal surface. Lymphatic vessels penetrate the capsule covering the convex aspect of the node (Fig. 13-8) and others leave from the deepest part of the indentation which is called the *hilus*. The lymphatic vessels that bring lymph *to* the node through the capsule are called *afferent lymphatics,* and those that *carry it away* from the hilus of the node are called *efferent lymphatics* (Fig. 13-8). Both kinds are provided with valves of the flap type so that the lymph in them cannot pass backward toward its point of origin (Fig. 13-8).

The capsule (black in Fig. 13-8) is thicker at the hilus where it gives off trabeculae (little beams) of connective tissue that extend into the substance of the node to provide support and carry blood vessels (Fig. 13-8). Trabeculae also extend inward from the capsule that covers the convex aspect of the node (Fig. 13-8).

The Stroma of a Node. Like bone marrow, the substance of the node consists of a stroma in which free cells are held, generally loosely, in place. The stroma consists of cells and intercellular substance. The latter is mostly in the form of networks of reticular fibers associated often with basement membrane material; these fibers connect with the capsule (Fig. 13-8, *left*) and also with the connective tissue (collagenic) trabeculae that extend into the node from both the capsule and the hilus to provide internal support (Fig. 13-8, *left*). The cells of the stroma are generally believed to be reticular cells (Fig. 13-7, *top right,* reticular cell) and to produce the reticular fibers (and possibly to perform other functions to be described presently).

The reticular net in a node varies from being fairly closely woven to fairly open. In the cortex there are rounded areas where the net is almost nonexistent (Fig. 13-8, *germinal center*). These rounded areas lie in more or less pyramidal areas of a looser mesh (shaded in Fig. 13-8). The bases of these pyramidal areas face, but do not abut on, the capsule; they are however, connected to it by a few reticular or collagenic fibers. The spaces between adjacent pyramidal areas are crossed by a more open reticular net. Many such spaces contain a trabecula derived from the capsule (black in Fig. 13-8). The network of reticular fibers of the pyramidal areas (shaded in Fig. 13-8) continue into the medulla where the narrow ends of the pyramidal areas merge into structures called medullary cords

LYMPH NODE

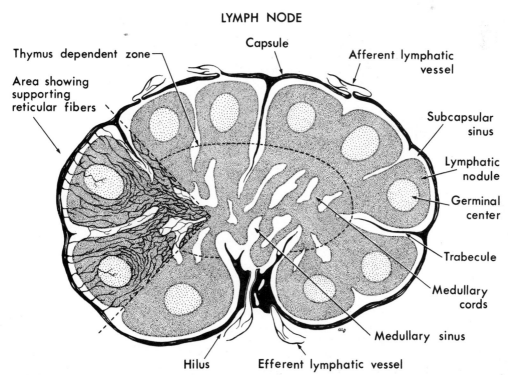

Fig. 13-8. Diagram of a lymph node. The thymus-dependent zone extends for a variable distance to each side of the dotted line.

(Fig. 13-8). The net in these often contains more plasma cells than lymphocytes. The medullary cords commonly branch and anastomose with one another as well as connecting with the pyramidal areas. The number of connective tissue trabeculae and the distribution of the mesh of reticular fibers seem to vary somewhat in different species. The density of the reticular mesh is generally greater around blood vessels, which structures it supports. The sites where free cells, which are mostly lymphocytes, are held in the stroma of a lymph node are shaded in Figure 13-8.

Nature of Sinuses. As already mentioned, some reticular or collagenic fibers extend between the broad bases of the pyramidal areas and the capsule which

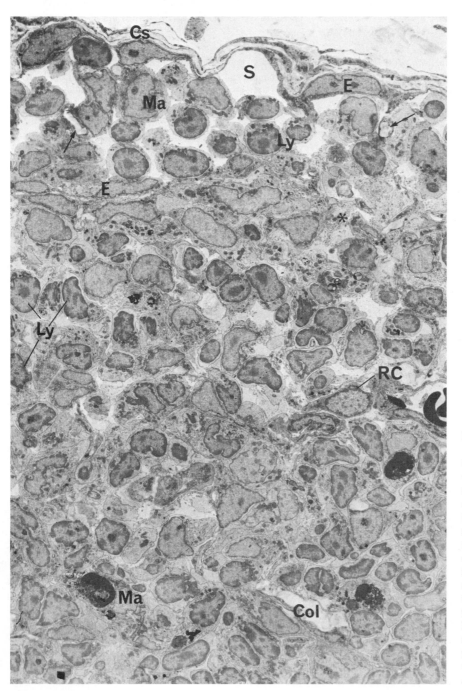

Fig. 13-9. Electron micrograph (× 2,100) of the cortex of a lymph node. The thin capsule (Cs) is seen at the top. Below this is the subcapsular sinus (S) which contains lymphocytes (Ly) and macrophages (Ma). The subcapsular sinus is lined with endothelial cells (E) and traversed by some fine trabeculae of collagenic fibers which are covered with endothelium (see also the next illustration). An asterisk indicates a gap in the endothelial lining of the sinus. In the lymphatic nodule that lies below the sinus some lymphocytes are labeled Ly, a reticular cell, RC, and a macrophage, Ma. (From Nopajaroonsri, C., Luk, S. C. and Simon, G. T.: Am. J. Path., *65:*1, 1971)

they face. A similar arrangement exists between the sides of adjacent pyramidal areas, in which space a trabecula may or may not be present (Fig. 13-8), and in the spaces between medullary cords (Fig. 13-8). These spaces that are crossed by a few reticular or/and collagenic fibers constitute what are called the *sinuses* of the node as will now be described.

THE FLOW OF LYMPH THROUGH A NODE

The Lymphatic Sinuses

Afferent lymphatics empty lymph through the capsule of a node into a space that exists between the capsule and the bases of the pyramidal areas and is called the subcapsular sinus (Figs. 13-8 and 13-9, S). In the past this space, from studies with the LM, was generally described as containing branching reticulo-endothelial phagocytic cells whose cytoplasmic processes connected with one another so that they formed a type of network reminiscent of a cobweb through which lymph passed and was strained of particulate matter by the phagocytic action of the reticulo-endothelial cells of the cobweb.

The study of rat lymph nodes with the EM by Nopajaroonsri, Luk and Simon, at relatively low magnifications, indicates a different type of structure. The subcapsular sinus (Fig. 13-9, S) proves to be a space but one that contains many *free cells,* mostly lymphocytes and macrophages. It is lined by what they term *lymphatic endothelium* (Fig. 13-9, E), which consists of flattened cells not significantly different from the ordinary endothelium that lines lymphatic and blood vessels in general. They found, however, that while the endothelium lining the capsule was continuous, that which lined the deeper side of the sinus was discontinuous. Neither had a basement membrane. They found that occasional collagenic or reticular trabeculae cross the subcapsular sinus (Fig. 13-10) and that these are covered with endothelium. The sinus contains a great many free cells most of which are macrophages and lymphocytes (Fig. 13-9, M and Ly). Their findings therefore differ from the older views held about the structure of lymph sinuses but, since both concepts indicate the existence of many phagocytic cells in the sinuses, both support the concept of filtration occurring in sinusoids. According to the newer view both macrophages and lymphocytes in the pyramidal areas already described would have easy access to the sinuses via the discontinuous endothelium at this side of the sinus.

From the subcapsular sinus lymph continues through the node by way of the *cortical* and *subcortical sinuses* which exist between the sides of the pyramidal areas

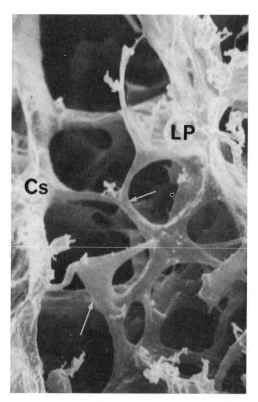

FIG. 13-10. Scanning electron micrograph ($\times$ 1,900) of a subcapsular lymphatic sinus showing the meshwork of trabeculae (arrows) joining the capsule (Cs) to the lymphoid parenchyma (LP). These trabeculae correspond to the collagen bundles seen traversing the sinus with transmission electron microscopy. (Illustration courtesy of S. C. Luk and G. T. Simon)

previously described. Here further lymphocytes are added to the lymph. These channels in turn connect with the *medullary sinuses* which exist between the medullary cords (Fig. 13-8) and deliver lymph to the efferent lymphatics that leave the node. All these sinuses were found, in the EM study mentioned above, to have the same type of structure as the subcapsular sinus in that they are lined with lymphatic endothelial cells but these are all discontinuous. Furthermore, as in the subcapsular sinus there is no definite basement membrane. Here also gaps between the lining cells would permit the free entry or exit of cells from the pyramidal areas or the medullary cords. In all of these other sinuses lymphocytes and macrophages were the common types of cells seen.

THE LYMPHATIC NODULES OF A NODE

The areas of fine reticular mesh described above which provide a framework for the pyramidal areas

and join with medullary cords are packed, except in
their central parts (when germinal centers are present)
with cells of the lymphocyte series; these are mostly
small lymphocytes but larger progenitor cells are also
present. The mesh of the medullary cords is likewise
packed with free cells which vary from lymphocytes
to blast cells and cells in various stages of development
into plasma cells. Next, the roughly pyramidal areas
packed with cells of the lymphocyte series have enough
of a rounded appearance to be termed lymphatic
nodules and, indeed, if they contain germinal centers,
as they do in Figure 13-7, the appearance of more or
less rounded nodules is accentuated by the fact that
densely packed lymphocytes form a sort of ring around
each germinal center (Fig. 13-7). These nodules, however, have tails that continue into medullary cords;
this does not necessarily show in every section. It is
therefore common to speak of the cortex of a lymph
node such as is illustrated in Figure 13-7, *bottom,* as
containing lymphatic nodules (instead of pyramidal
areas) which are often separated from one another
or often confluent as so many are in Figure 13-7.

The Thymus-Dependent Zone of Lymph Nodes.
Thymectomy performed at birth has a very characteristic and specific effect on the structure of an animal's
lymph nodes. In the normal adult mouse the cortex
consists of lymphatic nodules that are often confluent
and may or may not have germinal centers. The zones
of the node between the level of germinal centers and
the medullary cords are termed the mid- and deep-
cortical zones; these are not as densely packed with
lymphocytes as the more superficial part of the cortex.
Most postcapillary venules with walls of more or
less cuboidal endothelium through which lymphocytes
commonly migrate from blood to lymph (Figs. 13-18,
13-19 and 13-20) are present in these zones.

As described by Parrott the effects of thymectomy
at birth are manifested chiefly in the mid- and deep-
cortex which become depleted of lymphocytes, and the
postcapillary venules nomally present become thin
walled. This region was termed by Parrott, de Sousa
and East the *thymus-dependent* zone of a lymph node.
In Figure 13-8 this zone extends for a variable distance
to either side of the line labeled thymus dependent
zone. It is now believed that the lymphocytes of this
area are chiefly T lymphocytes and that this zone
must be seeded from the thymus to develop and, to a
lesser extent, be maintained.

The thymus-dependent zone of lymph nodes is the
zone primarily involved when homografts are placed
in normal animals in regions that drain into the nodes.
Parrott showed that clusters of large free cells with

basophilic cytoplasm appear in this area in a few days.
The clusters are often associated with postcapillary
venules. However, in homografts made in mice thymectomized at birth, no early changes of this kind
were seen in the lymph nodes along drainage routes.
Later a few free cells with basophilic cytoplasm
appeared. It has been shown, moreover, that if transplants of thymic tissue are made into mice thymectomized at birth, lymphocytes from the transplant
migrate into the bloodstream and eventually take up
a position in the thymus-dependent areas of lymph
nodes.

It therefore seems that the inability of thymectomized mice to reject homografts is due to the fact
that they lack T lymphocytes in the parts of their
lymph nodes that are primarily concerned with producing lymphocytes of the nature of killer cells.

Location of B Lymphocytes in a Node. In the
diagram in Figure 13-8 the thymus-dependent zone
of the node would be a zone that extends for a short
distance to either side of the dotted line labeled
thymus-dependent zone. Extending from somewhat
above this line to the broad base of a pyramidal
area, the lymphocytes would be primarily of the B
type. There is, of course, much movement of lymphocytes of both types so there is a good deal of mixing
of the two types. B lymphocytes are also present in
the tip region of the pyramidal areas and along their
sides and also in the medullary cords, for the latter
are the chief site where plasma cells are formed and
these are derived from B lymphocytes.

SOURCES AND TYPES OF PROGENITOR CELLS
OF SMALL LYMPHOCYTES IN LYMPH NODES

What was long believed to be the progenitor cell of
cells of the lymphocyte series in lymph nodes has long
been termed a lymphoblast. In H and E sections this
cell is generally described as having a large nucleus
and a rim of basophilic cytoplasm that is thicker on
one side than on the other (Fig. 13-11, C). With
the EM the cytoplasmic basophilia of cells of this type
is seen to be due to very numerous free ribosomes.
The cytoplasm also contains some rER, a Golgi apparatus, centrioles and a few mitochondria and microtubules.

Blast Cells. A usual view in the past was that the
reticular cells of lymph nodes which are described as
having large pale nuclei (Fig. 13-7, reticular cells, and
Fig. 13-11, B, arrow) gave rise to the lymphoblasts
of lymph nodes, that these formed lymphocytes by
dividing into daughter cells, which have somewhat

Fɪɢ. 13-11. High-power photomicrographs of somewhat different magnifications of different parts of a mediastinal lymph node of a rat.

A. An active germinal center. Arrows indicate cells in mitosis.

B. A germinal center. Arrow indicates the nucleus of a reticular cell. Note that its cytoplasm is very indistinct.

C. Edge of a germinal center. Arrow indicates a large cell with a ring of basophilic cytoplasm that has a sharp edge. This is a free, rounded cell, either a lymphoblast or a plasmoblast.

D. A medullary cord. Arrows indicate some of the plasma cells that are present. Note the negative Golgi areas in their cytoplasm.

E. A medullary sinusoid. Arrows indicate reticuloendothelial cells (macrophages).

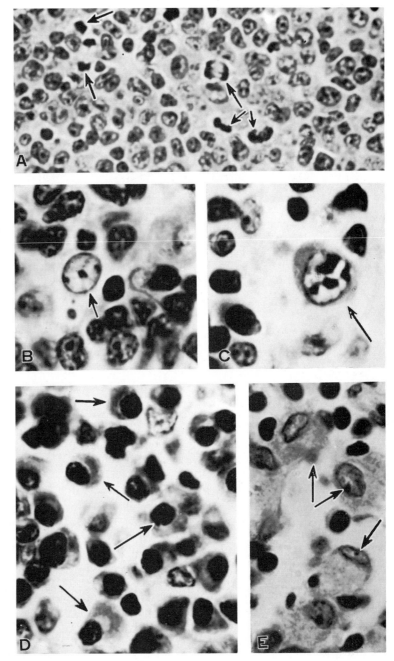

smaller nuclei plus basophilic cytoplasm and which were variously called medium-sized lymphocytes or prolymphocytes, and that these could, in turn, divide to give rise to the small lymphocytes that were formed in the node. Parts of this sequence have been changed with the knowledge that lymph nodes are seeded by T and B lymphocytes formed in the thymus and bone marrow respectively and that either type of lymphocyte in a node can be activated by suitable antigenic stimulation to grow larger and become a blast cell that is somewhat smaller than the classic description of lymphoblasts. So the term blast cell is now used for cells that do not necessarily fit the classic description of lymphoblasts in that blast cells can also be of medium size. Each of course has a rim of basophilic cytoplasm as does the classic lymphoblast.

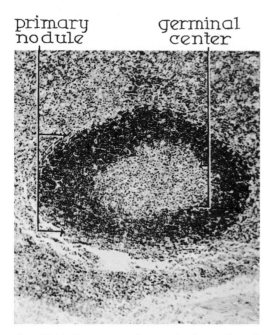

FIG. 13-12. Low-power photograph of a section of a lymph node of a dog, showing a primary nodule. The central part of this contains a pale germinal center.

How T and B Lymphocytes Form Lymphocytes of Nodules. It is generally conceded that small lymphocytes as such do not divide. How then are lymphocytes formed from them when they seed lymph nodes? As mentioned above, this is because both kinds of lymphocytes under the proper stimulus can develop into blast cells which can divide and form more small lymphocytes. To explain the nature of the stimulus that induces the lymphocytes that seed lymph nodes from the thymus and bone marrow to become blast cells it should be pointed out that, unlike all other body cells, they, when they arrive at lymph nodes, are variously programmed to be able to respond specifically to particular antigens. It is mostly in lymph nodes and spleen that lymphocytes meet these different kinds of antigens. As was described in connection with lymphocytes in Chapter 10, it is probably generally necessary for two lymphocytes, a T and a B, to cooperate in order for a B lymphocyte to be stimulated to develop into a blast cell that will give rise to a plasmablast that will form plasma cells that will produce (in quantity) the particular antibody for which the lymphocyte was programmed. However, T lymphocytes in a node can be stimulated to become blast cells that will form killer cells specific for some foreign antigen that induces a cell-mediated type of response without having to have help from B lymphocytes.

GERMINAL CENTERS

Germinal centers are often, even commonly, involved in B lymphocytes becoming blast cells. Germinal centers are rounded areas commonly seen in the central parts of the lymphatic nodules (often termed primary nodules) of the cortex; their position in relation to the pyramidal cortical areas is shown in Figure 13-8 and their appearance in a very low-power view of a section of a lymph node is shown in Figure 13-7, *bottom*. Individual germinal centers are also shown at slightly higher magnifications in Figures 13-12 and 13-13.

We shall first discuss briefly some things that are known about their significance.

Germinal centers do not develop in lymph nodules before birth, nor do they develop in postnatal animals raised in germ-free environments. Other evidence also indicates that they develop in the nodules of a lymph node only because the node has been exposed to an antigen which in all probability has reached it via the lymph that is brought to it from some body site where a foreign antigen is present. Commonly this occurs as a result of a bacterial infection in the part of the body from which the lymph that drains through the node was derived.

Next, although it has been shown that antibody can be produced in lymph nodes in which the nodules have not developed germinal centers, they commonly develop during the course of a sufficiently prolonged

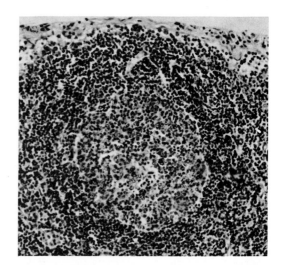

FIG. 13-13. Low-power photomicrograph of a primary nodule that contains a germinal center which is not pale but basophilic. On close inspection it would be seen to contain many mitotic figures (see Fig. 13-11 for higher-power views of this type of germinal center).

exposure of a lymph node to an antigen. Moreover, what is of great interest is that they make their appearance much more rapidly when a lymph node, in the course of time, is exposed a second time to some antigen with which it had a previous contact. These facts indicate that germinal centers represent tissue responses designed to facilitate the production of humoral antibody.

The formation of germinal centers could therefore be visualized as occurring when enough of some antigen drains through a lymph node in which there are B lymphocytes that are programmed to react with that antigen and particularly when the antigen has been there before. With the direct help of T lymphocytes (see top of Figure 13-14) (or indirect, as will be described presently), the B lymphocytes are activated to become blast cells and multiply. The multiplication, if extensive, causes a group of blast cells to form which create a rounded mass of cells with basophilic cytoplasm in the central part of the nodule (Fig. 13-13). The cells, however, mostly migrate down into medullary cords before becoming plasmablasts and forming plasma cells.

Indirect Interaction of T and B Lymphocytes. This concept hinges on the interaction between B and T lymphocytes being indirectly mediated through the agency of reticular cells or macrophages as follows:

In the sites where germinal centers develop in nodules there are cells, called reticular cells, that have large pale nuclei (Fig. 13-11, B, arrow) and cytoplasm that is relatively indistinct and often extends in various directions in the form of processes; hence these cells have an extensive surface. The way these cells attach antigens or antigen-antibody complexes to their surfaces is believed to be as follows. T lymphocytes have on their surface a low concentration of receptors which, though they do not have all the characteristics of a complete immunoglobulin, nevertheless can interact with antigen (see Fig. 13-14) and, when this happens, a complex consisting of the antigen and the receptor is released from the T lymphocyte. Reticular cells and macrophages have, on their surface, receptors to which the free complex can become attached in such a way as to leave the attached antigen exposed so that it can react specifically with a B lymphocyte for which it is programmed (Fig. 13-14). Thus the B lymphocytes make contact with the antigen in an indirect manner, whereupon they are activated and become the blast cells (Fig. 13-11) of a germinal center and in due course they or their progeny tend to migrate toward medullary cords as plasmablasts.

Investigation of Primary and Secondary Responses by the Immunofluorescence Technic. The

TENTATIVE SCHEMES OF B-LYMPHOCYTE-T-LYMPHOCYTE INTERACTION *

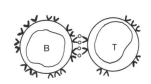

The antigen may be brought into contact with a B lymphocyte receptor by an encounter between a B and a T lymphocyte; the antigen is attached to the surface of the T lymphocyte through the latter's own specific immunoglobin receptor molecules.

- or -

INDIRECT INTERACTION

The immunoglobin receptor molecule may be set free from the surface of a T lymphocyte after the antigen has become attached to it.

The free T cell immunoglobin molecule bearing the antigen may then become attached to the surface of a reticular cell. When a B lymphocyte encounters a reticular cell, B lymphocyte receptors can come into contact with the antigen.
Either type of interaction would serve to present the antigen to the B lymphocyte receptors in an optimal configuration, thus increasing the chance of "triggering" the B lymphocyte.

* after Mitchison and Feldmann & Nossal

FIGURE 13-14.

sequence of events that occur in a node on its first exposure to an antigen is described as a *primary response*. If some time after a primary response an animal is again given an injection of the same antigen, it (except in the instance of certain antigens) responds much more quickly, producing antibody in what is termed a *secondary response* and it produces more antibody in the secondary response than it did in the primary response.

Coons in 1958 used the immunofluorescence sandwich technic which he devised (Fig. 9-19) to study these responses in lymph nodes. He found that by the fourth day in a primary response there were about 50 cells in a section cut from a node that revealed antibody, and that their numbers did not increase to any extent over the next 4 days. However, in a secondary response he found that by the second day after the antigen was injected there were hundreds of cells demonstrating some antibody in an area that was comparable to the one in which a primary response showed only 50 cells. Furthermore he found these cells to be distributed irregularly enough (Fig. 13-15) to indicate that they did not belong to a single clone but instead had arisen independently (Fig. 13-15).

In the light of what is now known about lymphocytes and blast cells, the differences between a primary and a secondary response and the relation of these responses to the formation of germinal centers could be explained as follows: On first exposure to an antigen, the B lymphocytes that are preprogrammed to react with that antigen are present at low frequency —in the order of 50 per million cells. These become activated and proliferate and either differentiate to plasma cells or return to the state of small lymphocytes which tend to remain in the lymph node. Thus there are now many more B lymphocytes (perhaps 100 times as many), all of which are identical with the first one that became activated and each is programmed exactly in the same way as the first. Since there are now many more of them reacting on second exposure

to the same antigen, more antibody is now produced per unit time and thus high levels are reached in a shorter time. Similarly, the visible effects of their activation—e.g., the formation of a germinal center, which requires the participation of a number of activated B lymphocytes—will also appear sooner.

The Cells of Germinal Centers. In addition to blast cells, germinal centers contain both reticular cells and macrophages (Fig. 13-7, *top*); the two latter cells may merely represent different forms of the same cell type and heritage. Reticular cells are generally described as having large pale nuclei (Fig. 13-7, *top*) and indistinct cytoplasm. Macrophages have more clearly defined cytoplasm (Fig. 13-7, *top*, labeled reticendo cell) and their phagocytic properties are readily shown by vital staining. As already noted, the blast cells that appear in primary and secondary responses do not all necessarily possess the morphology of the classic lymphoblast, primarily because many of them are smaller. A blast cell typically has a nucleus that is

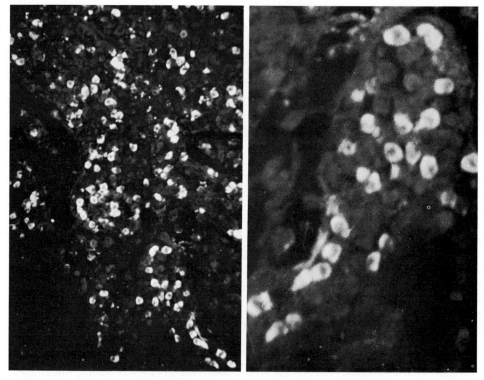

FIG. 13-15. Low-power and high-power photomicrographs of sections of a portion of a popliteal lymph node of a rabbit after it had received a second injection of diphtheria toxoid. The photomicrographs were taken from paraffin sections prepared by a new method devised by G. Sainte-Marie. The photomicrographs were taken using an ultraviolet source of light, and sites where antibody was present appear in the photomicrographs as bright areas. Careful inspection of the picture on the right will show that antibody is present in the cytoplasm of cells which have the characteristic structure of young plasma cells. (Preparation by G. Sainte-Marie)

larger than that of a small lymphocyte and in which the chromatin is not so condensed. It has a rim of basophilic cytoplasm as seen in sections with the LM. With the EM the nucleus of a blast cell is relatively pale (Fig. 13-16, *left*). The cytoplasm of a blast cell is characterized by an abundance of free ribosomes and polyribosomes (Fig. 13-16, *left*). Blast cells of the B lymphocyte type that differentiate into plasma cells are sometimes called immunoblasts; part of the one illustrated on the left side of Figure 13-16 is so labeled (they are also called plasmablasts). When such a cell becomes a plasma cell it develops large cisternae of rER in its cytoplasm and a larger Golgi so as to become a secretory cell that elaborates antibody as is shown on the right side of Figure 13-16. Blast cells customarily migrate to medullary cords where they complete their development into plasma cells. In a light microscope study of the formation of plasma cells in the medullary cords of the mediastinal lymph nodes of rats, Leblond and Sainte-Marie distinguished three stages in their formation; plasmablasts, proplasmacytes and plasmacytes (plasma cells). These are indicated by arrows and numbers in Figure 13-17. Note that as differentiation occurs the nucleus becomes smaller and the cytoplasm more abundant.

Although the greatest numbers of plasma cells are seen in medullary cords of lymph nodes, some may also develop in germinal centers in secondary responses and produce antibody in that location. As an infection that induced a secondary response is overcome by the defenses of the body, the activity in the germinal centers that were involved slows down and the germinal center gradually assumes a different appearance. While it is active not only is it very cellular, as can be seen in Figure 13-13, but in addition most of these cells (immunoblasts and plasma cells) have basophilic cytoplasm and so the germinal center appears dark. When the center becomes relatively inactive, the cells of the plasma cell series which have basophilic cytoplasm have mostly disappeared and so the germinal center appears lighter than the lymphatic nodule in which it lies (Fig. 13-12).

The Different Classes of Immunoglobulins. As was mentioned in Chapter 9 in connection with mast cells and allergy, there are different kinds of antibodies. We have since then discussed the immune response and where it occurs in more detail and to round out the account for those who would like, at this time, more information, we shall describe, very briefly, the different immunoglobulins.

Based on their molecular size and composition, 5 classes of immunoglobulins are now recognized. As more is learned about them, it appears that those of different classes perform different functions in the body and are synthesized in different locations.

IgG (also known as γG) is the immunoglobulin that is present in highest concentration in normal serum and it is the one that is usually thought of when one is considering antibodies that circulate after prolonged immunization. It is of the size class referred to as 7S, with a molecular weight of 160,000 daltons.

IgG is produced by plasma cells and by cells that have the appearance of activated lymphocytes and have, or are acquiring, cytoplasmic rER. These are found free in loose connective tissues, in lymphatic nodules under wet epithelial surfaces, in the medulla of lymph nodes, and in the red pulp of the spleen. IgG is the only class of immunoglobulins that can cross the placenta; this allows a baby to be provided with antibodies from its mother which help it after it is born until it has time to make its own.

IgM is much larger than IgG, having a molecular weight of nearly a million daltons, and has a sedimentation coefficient of 19S. It is in fact composed of 5 subunits, each of which is like an IgG molecule, all held together in a ring by hydrogen bonds. This is the immunoglobulin that is characteristically produced, early in the humoral antibody response to an antigen, by the same kinds of cells that produce IgG and at the same sites. There is still some doubt as to whether one cell can produce both kinds of antibody. IgM is more efficient than IgG in fixing complement and therefore in reactions of cytoxicity. IgM is less efficient than IgG in reactions of neutralization where the activity of a functional molecule such as an enzyme or a molecule at the surface of a virus is inactivated as a result of combination with antibody. On interacting with an antigen, IgM is more likely than IgG to produce an antigen-antibody complex that precipitates.

IgA is another major class of immunoglobulins. It is characteristic of bodily secretions. It also occurs in serum, where its concentration is usually greater than that of IgM. It occurs in tears and milk but predominantly in the mucous secretions of the respiratory and gastrointestinal tracts. These molecules have the general character of immunoglobulins but they are composed of one or more immunoglobulin subunits (as IgM is composed of 5). The IgA that appears in secretions is mainly in the form of a dimer held together by a polypeptide component known as the secretory piece. The precursor molecules for IgA are synthesized in plasma cells; the secretory piece seems to be synthesized in epithelial cells, and both components combine before the secretory IgE is secreted. Since they have antibody activity and are secreted

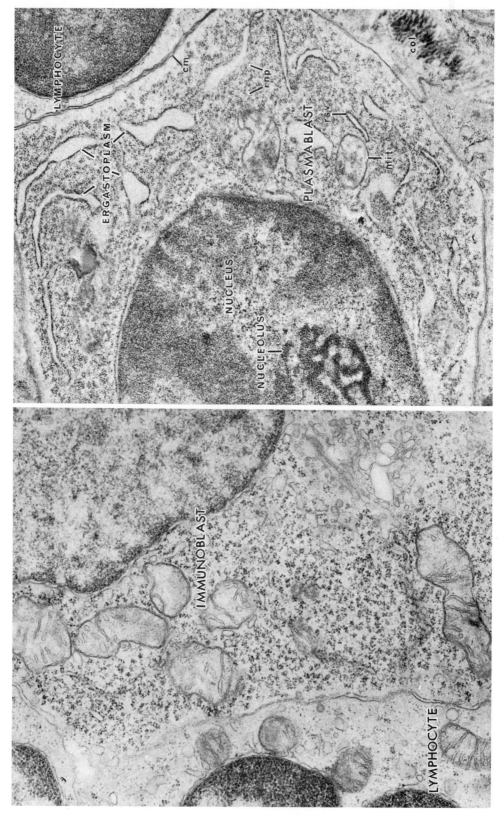

FIGURE 13-16. (*Caption on facing page*)

onto wet epithelial surfaces, secretory IgA immunoglobulins provide a first line of defense against
potential invaders before the latter actually enter the
body. IgA is believed to be especially active against
viruses.

IgD is a minor immunoglobulin class that differs
from IgC only in the detail of structure of its molecules. Its function is unknown.

IgE, as mentioned in connection with mast cells in
Chapter 9, represents a minor class of immunoglobulins
that have a special affinity for mast cells and mediate
allergic reactions. These molecules whose production
is stimulated by antigens like pollens, dusts, etc. become attached to the surface of mast cells at their
Fc end, leaving their antigen-combining sites free to
interact with these antigens. The result is sudden
release of mast cell granules, with the pharmacological
consequences attendant upon exposure of blood vessels
to histamine and the other vasoactive substances contained in mast cell granules. IgE is produced in plasma
cells that are situated under wet epithelial surfaces,
i.e., in the same regions as IgA but different from those
of IgG. IgE is of about the same molecular size as IgG,
but the amino acid structure of its light chains is
slightly different.

On exposure to any antigen, the production of
immunoglobulins of all 5 classes is stimulated but complex regulatory mechanisms soon come into play so
that, under different conditions, one or other of the
immunoglobulins eventually predominates.

The Blood Supply of Lymph Nodes

A lymph node is supplied entirely or almost entirely
from arteries that enter it at the hilus.

Arterioles from these arteries ascend into the substance of the node. They have been described as
ascending within the substance of both the trabeculae
and the medullary cords. The arterioles reach as far as
the cortex, but, according to Menzies, the arterioles end
in capillaries before germinal centers are approached.
The germinal center and the area of cortex imme-

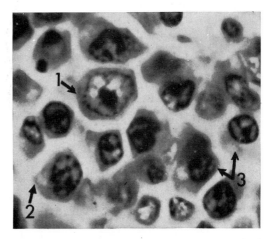

Fig. 13-17. Photomicrograph of a medullary cord of a
thoracic lymph node of a rat showing (1) a plasmablast,
(2) a proplasmacyte, and (3) mature plasmacytes
(plasma cells). (Leblond, C. P., and Sainte-Marie, G.: *In
Ciba* Symposium on Haemopoiesis. p. 152. London,
Churchill, 1960)

diately surrounding it are thus supplied only with
capillaries.

Many capillaries which descend in the cortex
(toward the medulla) become postcapillary venules
which in many instances are relatively long and lined
with cuboidal (or even taller) endothelium (Fig. 13-
18). These venules are most numerous in the cortical
area indicated roughly in Figure 13-8 as the thymus-
dependent zone of the node. It is through the walls of
these curious venules that lymphocytes chiefly migrate
from blood to lymph in their recirculation. Different
views have arisen about how lymphocytes pass through
the endothelium of these vessels because of the problems of interpreting from a two-dimensional thin slice
of tissue what was really happening in three dimensions. The situation has recently been studied and
analyzed by Schoefl who presents convincing evidence
to the effect that the lymphocytes migrate through the
endothelium by passing between contiguous endothelial

Fig. 13-16. These two electron micrographs were taken from a lymph node a few days after an
antigen was injected into a site which drained into it. These micrographs are thought to show the
changes that occur in the cytoplasm of a properly programmed lymphocyte as it develops into a
plasma cell. (*Left*) At the very left some cytoplasm of inactive lymphocyte (labeled lymphocyte)
is shown to contain only a few ribosomes and a few mitochondria. It abuts, on its right, on a
lymphocyte that presumably has been activated by the antigen. It is labeled immunoblast and its
cytoplasm shows abundant ribosomes. (*Right*) This picture shows the cytoplasm of a cell (labeled
plasmablast) which would represent a further development of the immunoblast: as well as having
an abundant content of free ribosomes it now has also a considerable content of rER, which indicates its differentiation into a cell of the plasma cell series. (Electron micrographs courtesy of H. Z.
Movat)

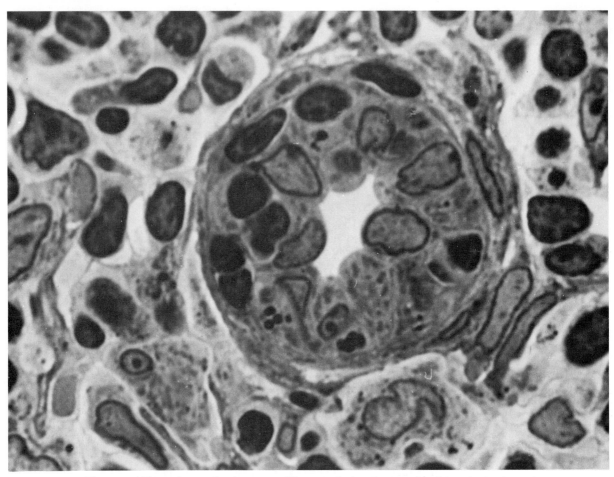

Fɪɢ. 13-18. Photomicrograph of a postcapillary venule in nonencapsulated lymphatic tissue. It exhibits the same features as the postcapillary venules in lymph nodes, in that it is lined by thick endothelium the cells of which are cuboidal or even columnar in shape. Lymphocytes can be seen migrating through the endothelium to enter the substance of the node. The endothelium is ringed by flattened perivascular cells and some intercellular substance through which the lymphocytes have to pass to enter the substance of the node. The way lymphocytes migrate through the endothelium is shown in the following illustration. (Provided by G. I. Schoefl)

cells. He points out that because the endothelial cells are tall in these postcapillary vessels the endothelium remains as a seal as a lymphocyte passes between two cells, because by the time a lymphocyte reaches the basement membrane the two cells between which it has passed have closed over the opening between them on the lumen side (Fig. 13-19). Figure 13-20 shows two lymphocytes migrating through the endothelium which has closed over on their lumen side. The lower lymphocyte has broken through the basement membrane in order to enter the substance of the node, from which it will probably be carried away in the lymph to eventually enter the thoracic duct and from there return to the bloodstream again. The recirculation of

lymphocytes is dealt with in connection with lymphocytes in Chapter 10.

Differences Between Various Nodes. There is some difference between the microscopic appearances of lymph nodes taken from different parts of the body. In some the lymph nodules of the cortex are highly developed and little medulla is apparent. In a section of a node of this type, the student will have difficulty finding medullary cords and sinuses. In nodes taken from other parts of the body the medulla rather than the cortex is well developed. These should be used for the study of medullary cords. It should always be remembered that a single slice cut through a node may not be representative of its microscopic structure.

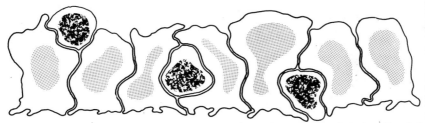

Fɪɢ. 13-19. Diagram showing how lymphocytes can migrate between the relatively tall endothelial cells that line the venules in such a manner that the endothelial cells can remain sealed to one another at some level and so prevent undue fluid loss. (From Schoefl, G. I.: J. Exp. Med., *136:*568, 1972)

HEMAL LYMPH NODES AND HEMAL NODES

Most mammals have, in addition to lymph nodes, a much smaller number of structures that are similar except that they are yellow or red instead of gray in color. On section, these structures resemble lymph nodes except that they have somewhat better defined channels in their coarse mesh, and either some of these channels or all of them are filled with blood instead of lymph. If only some are filled with blood and others with lymph, the structure is called a *hemal lymph node.* If all the channels are filled with blood, it is called a *hemal node.*

There is some question as to whether hemal lymph nodes or hemal nodes are constant structures in man, but they have often been described as commonly occur-ring in the prevertebral peritoneal tissue, in the root of the mesentery, near the rim of the pelvis and occasionally in other sites. There are not enough of them in man to filter very much blood, but it is important to know of them, lest, on being discovered at operation or at autopsy, they can be mistaken for pathologically altered tissue.

SUMMARY OF THE IMMUNOLOGICAL RESPONSES THAT OCCUR IN LYMPH NODES

When an antigen or antigens make their appearance in some part of the body the lymph nodes through which the lymph formed in this part of the body is drained (and these nodes are termed the regional lymph nodes) can manifest two different types of

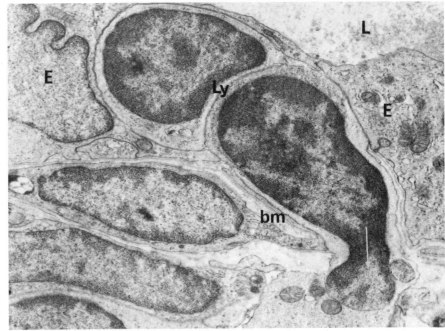

Fɪɢ. 13-20. Electron micrograph showing two lymphocytes migrating through the wall of this postcapillary venule. On the luminal side the endothelial cells (E) have sealed over their point of entry. Part of the lower lymphocyte (arrow) has created a gap in the basement membrane (bm) of the venule through which it would escape into the adjacent parenchyma. Lumen of postcapillary venule (L). (From Nopajaroonsri, C., Luk, S., and Simon, G. T.: Am. J. Path., *65:*1, 1971)

immunological response to the antigen or antigens present in the lymph. The two immune responses are termed (1) the cell-mediated type, and (2) the humoral antibody type.

(1) **The Cell-Mediated Response.** If the antigen or antigens involved are components of foreign cells, such as would occur if skin were transplanted from one animal to another (except in pure strains), although both types of response occurs, the cell-mediated response is more effective than the humoral antibody response in destroying the cells of the transplant. Antigens from the foreign cells, on being conveyed by lymph to a lymph node, encounter T lymphocytes which are programmed to react with them and are located in the thymus-dependent zone of the node. The T lymphocytes thereupon are activated to become blast cells and proliferate to produce many blast cells that are programmed in the same way. Many of these enter the circulation but soon leave it to enter the connective tissue at the site where the foreign cells are present; these cells aggregate on the foreign cells, and adhere specifically to the antigens on them. By a direct action which is cytotoxic and which gives them the name killer cells, they destroy the foreign cells. The blast cells which developed as a result of activation by antigens of T lymphocytes in the thymus-dependent zone of the lymph node do not all leave the node in the form of blast cells. Many once more take on the appearance of small lymphocytes and then leave the node. These are committed with regard to the antigen that induced their formation and there are now many more of them than there were at first. They circulate and are long-lived and, since they are available when the body has a second experience with the same antigen, they have been called memory cells. This is manifested by the fact that the first time some foreign tissue is transplanted to an animal it takes about two weeks for it to be completely rejected, whereas the second time the same type of foreign tissue is transplanted to the animal it takes less than one week to complete the rejection. Moreover, the reaction is more violent. The shortened time and increased violence of the reaction are due to the fact that many more cells are now available to supply specific killer cells than there were at the time of first exposure to the foreign cells.

As was described in connection with lymphocytes in Chapter 10, foreign cells also initiate a humoral antibody response, but antibodies do not react lethally with cells unless they cause complement to be fixed and this occurs only in the instance of certain cells that have a high concentration of antigen on their surfaces. Hence antibody may interfere to some extent with the

activity of killer cells by covering up the antigens on the foreign cells so that they are not recognized by the killer cells, or by inhibiting the induction of a cell-mediated immune response in other ways.

The cell-mediated response may be very important in connection with the destruction of body cells that undergo a malignant transformation to become cancer cells. Since the malignant transformation is due to some genetic change in the cell, it may result in the affected cells having sufficiently different antigens from normal cells to induce the formation of specific killer cells that destroy the cancer cells before they have become too numerous to be destroyed by this mechanism.

It should be mentioned here that the cell-mediated response is also principally responsible for a phenomenon termed the *delayed hypersensitivity reaction*. This concerns a type of lesion that develops at the site of a second exposure to some antigen which generally is of a type that, on first exposure, did not induce, or induced very little of, a humoral antibody response. The first exposure nevertheless causes T lymphocytes to form memory cells (in other language, lymphocytes are said to become sensitized to the antigen). So at a later, second encounter with this antigen the memory cells capable of reacting with it become blast cells so more cells capable of reacting with the antigen are formed. These elaborate biologically active materials that cause enough damage to the tissue at the site of the antigen to cause an inflammatory lesion in which other leukocytes, chiefly monocytes and macrophages, participate. This type of recation can be of importance in many diseases. It has been much studied in tuberculosis. It is also the cause of what is known as *contact sensitivity* to certain chemicals.

(2) **The Humoral Antibody Response.** Lymph draining from a body site where there is, for example, a bacterial infection passes to the regional lymph nodes where the antigen or antigens it contains triggers B lymphocytes that are programmed to react with the antigen or antigens to become blast cells and form cells of the plasma cell series which produce antibody specific for the antigen that triggered the B cells. However, as already explained, for the B cell that was programmed for this antibody to be triggered it generally needs help from a T cell. This help may be given either directly or indirectly via a reticular cell as shown in Figure 13-14. In prolonged primary, or in secondary, responses the blast cell proliferation that occurs in this type of reaction can bring about the formation of germinal centers.

The Spleen

The nonencapsulated lymph nodules, the lymph nodes and the spleen are the important sites in the body in which lymphocytes become activated to form cells that either produce antibodies or are responsible for the cell-mediated type of immunological reaction. However, there is a division of labor among these three types of lymphatic tissue so that there can be a suitable response to antigens present in any of the three main types of body fluids—tissue fluid, lymph, and blood. The nonencapsulated lymphatic nodules are exposed to antigens that may be present in the tissue fluid in which the nodules are bathed. Lymph nodes are arranged along lymphatic vessels and constructed in such a way that lymphocytes are exposed to the lymph that drains through them. Finally, the spleen is an organ that is isolated from the above-mentioned two types of body fluids but is designed to give antigens present in blood wide and reasonably prolonged exposure to variously programmed immunologically competent cells as the blood circulates through it. The reasons for its exposure to antigens being limited to those in blood will become evident when its gross structure and location are examined.

Gross Characteristics. The spleen is an organ that is roughly the size and shape of a clenched fist. It lies in the abdomen in the shelter of the left 9th, 10th and 11th ribs, with its long axis parallel with them. Its purple color is due to its great content of blood. It is soft in consistency and more friable than most organs. (The possibility of it being ruptured from severe crushing type injuries must be taken into account.) Most of its surface is smooth and not attached by fat or loose connective tissue to the organs or structures with which it is in contact. A long fissure may be seen close to its medial border; this is termed the hilus. On approaching this, the splenic artery divides into several branches that enter the substance of the spleen separately at different points along the elongated hilus. Veins and lymphatics leave the spleen in association with the arteries that enter it. The veins later unite to form the splenic vein.

No afferent lymphatics enter the free surface of the spleen as occurs in lymph nodes, the surfaces of which are of course attached to the tissue in which they lie. Such lymphatics as exist in the spleen are of the efferent type and they are confined to the connective tissue sheaths of the blood vessels, as will be described presently. As noted, they leave the hilus.

FUNCTIONS OF THE SPLEEN

First, as already noted, the spleen serves as the site where antigens in the blood can activate suitably programmed lymphocytes to develop into immunologically functioning cells.

Second, in many animals the spleen in postnatal life is a hemopoietic organ producing not only the cells of the lymphocyte series but also cells of the erythrocyte and granulocyte series as well as megakaryocytes and platelets. In man it serves this function under normal conditions only in fetal life; however, the spleen retains the potentiality for blood cell formation even in adult life. Under certain pathological conditions it may again become a hemopoietic organ producing the cells ordinarily formed in bone marrow. This phenomenon, when it occurs, is called extramedullary hemopoiesis.

Third, the spleen abounds in macrophages which have access to the blood that circulates through it. The chief matter they phagocytose in filtering the blood to which they are exposed are old, worn-out erythrocytes but they also participate in the phagocytosis of worn-out leukocytes and platelets. Most of the iron they liberate from the hemoglobin of old, worn-out erythrocytes that they phagocytose they restore to the circulation where it is used over again in the formation of new erythrocytes in the bone marrow. The macrophages of the spleen also produce the pigment bilirubin from the breakdown of hemoglobin; this circulates to the liver where it becomes a constituent of bile.

Fourth, the spleen can serve a mechanical function. In normal life it is more or less distended with blood that is circulating through it and in this sense it is more or less of a storehouse for blood. Particularly in animals that are sometimes called upon for great bursts of activity it can liberate much of its stored blood into the circulation so as to provide for a more efficient pumping action of the heart; in this sense the spleen can act as an automatic transfusion bank. The fact that it is normally somewhat distended with blood in life is apparent if the size of the spleen seen at a surgical operation is compared to that which is seen at an autopsy, because after death the spleen contracts and squeezes much of its blood into the splenic vein as the pressure within it falls.

Finally, it is believed the spleen permits blood cells to become concentrated by separating them from the plasma in which they are suspended. The concentrated cells may be retained in the spleen for varying periods and then released into the circulation. In addition to cells, platelets may be held in the spleen, for a considerable proportion of the body's platelets are normally found in it.

The Internal Structure of the Spleen

Much can be learned about the internal structure of the spleen by examining, with the naked eye or a magnifying glass, a slice cut through a spleen (this is commonly done at postmortem examinations). It will be seen to be surrounded by a connective tissue capsule (Figs. 13-21 and 13-22). The capsule has some smooth muscle fibers in it but these cannot be seen with the naked eye. The capsule is smooth because it is covered with a continuous layer of mesothelium. Trabeculae of connective tissue (Figs. 13-21 and 13-22) extend into the substance of the organ both from the hilus and to a lesser extent from the capsule. The remainder of the interior of the spleen is filled with what is called

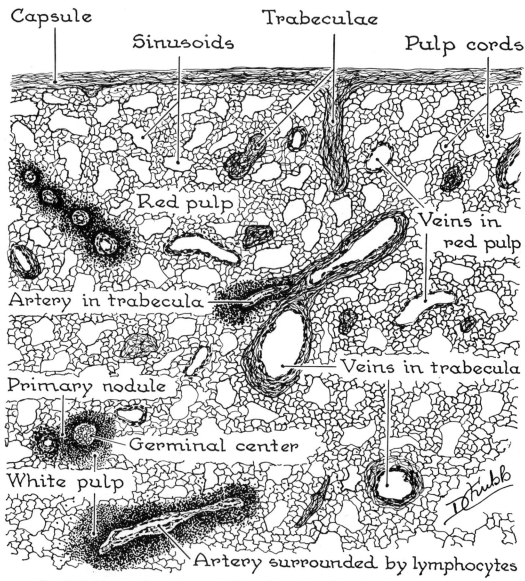

Fig. 13-21. Diagram of a section cut at right angles to the surface of a distended human spleen. Notice that the white pulp (*left lower corner*) consists of nodules and aggregations of lymphocytes, and that the red pulp is an open mesh with sinusoids running through it. A trabecula with veins may be seen in the central part of the illustration.

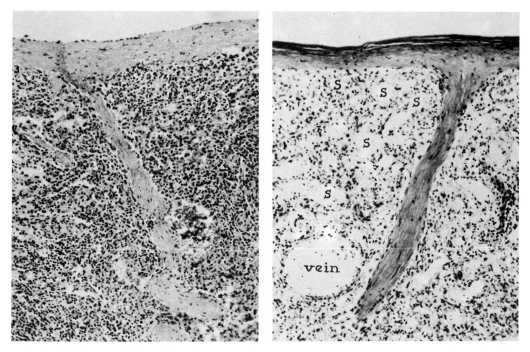

FIG. 13-22. Low-power photomicrographs of 2 sections cut at right angles to the capsule of the spleen. (*Left*) Picture taken from a section of collapsed spleen. The capsule and also a trabecula extending in from the capsule may be seen. (*Right*) Picture taken from a spleen that was distended with fixative through its veins. Notice that the red pulp has been opened up by this procedure, and that the sinusoids (S) are apparent.

splenic pulp. Two kinds of pulp can be seen with the naked eye: *white,* and *red*. The white pulp is distributed as tiny little firm gray islands (dark in Fig. 13-21) somewhat less than 1 mm in diameter, among the soft red pulp that fills all the remaining space. The basic framework of the pulp is a network of reticular fibers (Fig. 13-21).

General Microscopic Structure. If sections cut at right angles to the capsule are examined with the LM, it will be obvious that the little nodules of gray pulp observed on the cut surface of the spleen with the naked eye are lymphatic nodules (Fig. 13-23). These, then, are the chief sites of lymphocyte production in the spleen. Moreover, it will be seen that the red pulp that surrounds the lymphatic nodules contains vast numbers of red blood cells in its mesh (these are not shown in Fig. 13-21) and so the red pulp represents the part of the spleen that is designed to filter blood.

THE MICROSCOPIC STRUCTURE OF THE HUMAN SPLEEN

Some Problems Associated With the Study of the Spleen. While the spleens of many laboratory animals

serve the functions performed by the spleen of man, in postnatal life they perform the additional functions of producing erythrocytes, granular leukocytes and platelets, which functions are not performed by the spleen of man after birth. Accordingly, it is much simpler in many respects to limit our discussion of the microscopic structure and function of the spleen in postnatal life to the spleen of man. However, since the spleens of laboratory animals possess many of the features of spleens of man it is possible to obtain certain photo and electron micrographs from them to illustrate certain features of the spleen that are related to its function in man, so selected illustrations of mouse spleen will be used in addition to those of human spleen in the following section.

Another factor is that so far as possible a histological description of any organ should relate to its structure as it is during life. Special measures must be taken if sections of the spleen are to serve this purpose, because the splenic vein drains into the portal vein in which blood, instead of being under very slight pressure, as it is in the vena cava, is under a pressure of around 10 mm. This pressure is transmitted back along the

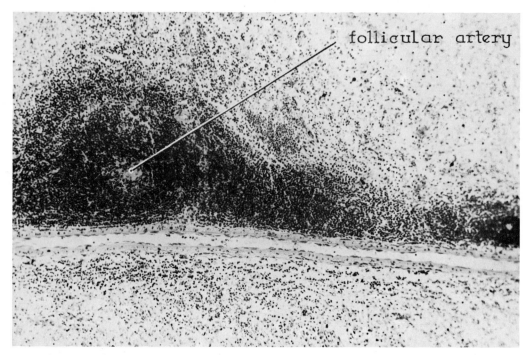

FIG. 13-23. Low-power photomicrograph of a section of a distended human spleen. In this particular section an artery that has left a trabecula and is passing through red pulp is cut longitudinally. Many lymphocytes, disposed in a fine reticular mesh, are to be seen above the artery. Toward the left-hand side of the picture, the lymphatic tissue accompanying the artery is expanded into a primary nodule. The artery at the site of the primary nodule has given off a branch which has entered the nodule as a follicular artery (labeled as such). The border area between the white and red pulp is sometimes referred to as the transitional zone.

splenic vein to its tributaries within the spleen and from them into the large passageways called sinusoids within the red pulp of the spleen. Because of the venous pressure these are normally mostly congested and expanded with blood. A spleen removed at operation, as they sometimes are, will contract as soon as a clamp is taken from the splenic vein which allows the blood that was in the sinusoids and veins under pressure to escape from the opened vein. Likewise, after death, pressure in the vascular system, including that in the portal system, ceases, so that the spleen then contracts and forces its blood out through its vein into a site of lower pressure. Accordingly, unless special measures are taken, sections of spleen reveal the microscopic structure of a collapsed spleen and not the microscopic structure of the spleen as it was during life. Since it is venous pressure that is responsible for the size and structure of the spleen during life, the logical procedure to obtain sections of spleen that represent its structure as it is during life would be to perfuse the veins of collapsed spleen with a fixative under sufficient pressure to restore it to its normal size.

Robinson studied human spleens obtained from operation by this method years ago and the author was fortunate in obtaining some of his material to section and photograph; some of these sections are used here.

The Capsule and Trabeculae. The capsule (Fig. 13-22) consists of collagenic and elastic fibers in which fibroblasts and perhaps some smooth muscle cells are distributed. Some animals have enough smooth muscle cells in the capsule for them to be demonstrated more readily than they can be in man, and its contraction can materially assist the smooth muscle of the trabeculae in contracting the spleen and so forcing blood into the circulatory system in times of emergency. It is doubtful whether there is enough smooth muscle in the capsule of the spleen of man to function very efficiently in this respect.

The plentiful elastin content of the capsule allows it to be stretched under life conditions; hence, in the collapsed spleens so commonly used for preparing sections the capsule is thicker than it is during life.

The capsule is covered with a serous (peritoneal) coat of mesothelium; this consists of a single layer of squamous cells. Their cytoplasm is too scant to be seen in ordinary sections but their flat nuclei may be noticed.

Trabeculae. These are scattered through the substance of the spleen (Figs. 13-21, 13-22 and 13-24). They extend in from the hilus like a branching tree, and branches pass in various directions to connect often with trabeculae that extend in from the capsule. In any section trabeculae will be cut in almost every plane. Most, of course, will be cut obliquely. Like the capsule, they consist of dense connective tissue in which there is a fairly high percentage of elastin. They also contain a few smooth muscle cells, but, as is true of the capsule, the amount of smooth muscle in them is not as great in man as in certain other animals.

The trabeculae from the hilus convey both the arteries and veins and the nerves that supply the spleen. In general, the largest trabeculae are seen near the hilus, and these contain the largest vessels. The detailed microscopic structure of arteries and veins will not be considered until a later chapter, but if the student will glance at Figure 19-16 he will see that arteries are ringed with a much thicker layer of smooth muscle cells than are veins. By using these criteria the student should readily distinguish an artery from a vein in most trabeculae (Fig. 13-24). In Figure 13-24 the artery is on the left and the vein on the right. The wall of the vein here is thin, but the vein here lies in a thick trabecula.

Microscopic Structure and Function of the White and the Red Pulp. Perhaps the easiest order to follow in describing the microscopic structure and functions of the various parts of the spleen is to take these parts up in the order in which they are supplied with blood. So we shall follow the blood from the arteries of the trabeculae out into the splenic pulp and back to the veins of the trabeculae because in taking this journey through the spleen all its significant components will be encountered.

The Relation of Arteries to the White Pulp. The arteries that travel in from the hilus in the larger trabeculae branch into small branches *that leave the trabeculae* (the smaller trabeculae, therefore, contain only veins) to enter the pulp. To support the arteries, the reticular fibers of the stroma of the splenic pulp become condensed chiefly along one side of them but to some extent around them, to provide them with fairly substantial reticular sheaths. The reticular fibers in these hold lymphocytes in their meshes, and as a result the sheaths are heavily infiltrated with lymphocytes (Fig. 13-23). Although these sheaths, infiltrated with lymphocytes, are not true lymphatic nodules along most of their course, they become expanded (usually at one side) from time to time to form lymphatic

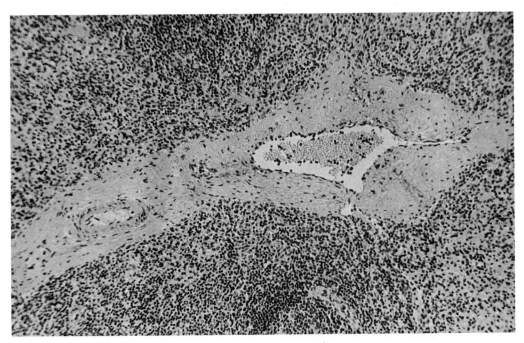

Fig. 13-24. Low-power photomicrograph of a section of collapsed spleen cut near its center. The picture shows a large trabecula containing an artery on the left and a vein on the right.

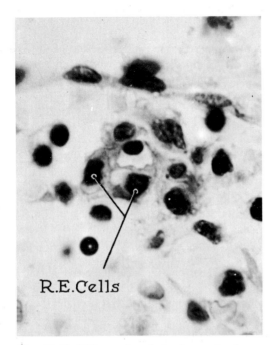

Fig. 13-25. Oil-immersion photomicrograph of a section of distended human spleen. An ellipsoid, cut in cross section, may be seen in the center of the illustration. It consists of an arrangement of reticuloendothelial cells surrounding a capillary. The lumen of the capillary may be seen immediately above the labeled reticuloendothelial cells. A lymphocyte is present in the lumen of the capillary.

nodules (Fig. 13-21, *lower left;* Fig. 13-23, *left*), which may contain germinal centers. The white pulp of the spleen, then, is distributed along the arteries that leave the trabeculae.

In each site where a sheath is expanded into a lymphatic nodule the artery gives off a branch to supply the nodule (Fig. 13-23, *left*). This is termed a follicular artery (in the spleen lymphatic nodules are often termed lymphatic follicles). A follicular artery gives off branches to supply the capillary beds of the lymphatic nodule and then emerges from the follicle into the surrounding red pulp as described below.

The Arterial Supply of Red Pulp. A follicular artery, on leaving white pulp and entering the adjacent red pulp, according to Solnitzky divides into 2 to 6 branches which radiate in different directions from their point of origin. Since these arterial branches are straight, they are called *penicillar arteries* or penicilli. Each of these, according to Solnitzky, divides into 2 or 3 arterioles, most of which soon enter curious little structures called ellipsoids (Fig. 13-25), whereupon they lose all their arteriolar characteristics (muscular

and elastic walls) to become capillaries. Before considering the further course of the blood through the red pulp of the spleen, we should briefly discuss the role of the white pulp in immunological responses.

Immunological Responses in the Spleen. In considering the immunological responses in the spleen it may help to compare its structure and function with those of lymph nodes.

First, the spleen is concerned with antigens that are present in the bloodstream and, except in the relatively rare instances of septicemia (a generalized infection of the blood), the concentration of antigens in the blood could not be expected to be nearly as great as that which might occur in lymph draining to a lymph node from a site of infection. Next, it seems much more likely that lymph nodes would be concerned with cell-mediated reactions (because of antigens draining directly from, say, sites of foreign transplants via lymph to regional nodes), rather than the spleen which, because of its receiving blood from all over the body, would receive low concentrations of such antigens. There is therefore reason to think that the spleen is concerned mostly with the formation of antibodies and we shall now discuss where the cells develop that form them.

Movat and Fernando studied the spleens of rabbits after the latter were given an antigen intravenously. They found that the first indication of an immunological response was the development among lymphocytes of blast cells. These appeared between the second and the fourth day in the lymphocyte sheaths of the arteries and the arterioles that run from trabeculae to primary nodules. They also were seen at this time in the peripheral parts of primary nodules. By the sixth day both immature and mature plasma cells were seen in these same sites. Moreover, some plasma cells by this time had spilled over from the white pulp into the red pulp.

Nine days after antigenic stimulation, Movat and Fernando found that the penicillar arteries radiating from the lymphatic nodules of the white pulp to deliver blood into the red pulp, which are normally ensheathed with lymphocytes, became ensheathed mostly with plasma cells. Accordingly, it seems that certain B lymphocytes of the white pulp of the spleen under the influence of antigenic stimulation become blast cells of the same type as those that appear in the lymphatic follicles of lymph nodes that are stimulated antigenically: cells which in the EM are characterized by a great abundance of free ribosomes in their cytoplasm. Cells of this type that form in the spleen migrate toward the red pulp and, according to the present concepts, serve as a source of plasmablasts which divide and differentiate to form the plasma cells seen in the red pulp.

Respective Sites of T and B Lymphocytes and Interactions Between Them. The above described studies gave information about the sites at which blast cells of the plasma cell series develop after intravenously administered antigen. When this study was made it was not known that there were two kinds of lymphocytes, T and B, and that interaction had to occur between them, either directly or indirectly, as shown in Figure 13-14, for blast cells of the plasma cell series to develop. Since this has become known it has become of interest to know the respective locations of T and B lymphocytes in the spleen and where they interact with one another. It should, of course, be appreciated that the lymphocyte population in the spleen is by no means static; it changes from hour to hour and from day to day, so determining where different kinds of lymphocytes are located is not as simple a matter as determining where different cells are located in organs in which there is a stable population.

One approach to the problem has been that of removing the thymus at birth and then determining which sites in the spleen are thereafter not properly populated. Experiments along this line indicate that the population of lymphocytes in the perivascular lymphatic sheaths of the arteries and arterioles that extend from trabeculae to lymphatic nodules is greatly reduced from normal, so it is assumed that the lymphocytes in these sheaths are mostly of the T type. Likewise, there is a considerable reduction of the lymphocyte population of the lymphatic follicles, so many of the lymphocytes that are normally present in these are also thought to be T lymphocytes.

Other experiments give some information about the source of these lymphocytes. It seems that the T lymphocytes of the sheaths and those of follicles are not derived directly from the arterial vessels that they surround but instead the T lymphocytes take up their positions after the blood in which they were being carried has been emptied from the terminations of these vessels into what is called the marginal zone between the white and red pulp.

The Marginal Zone. To explain this it may help to consult Figure 13-23 which shows that the border between the white pulp and the red pulp is not sharp. Instead there is a zone around the lymphatic follicle at the left and also around the periarterial lymphatic sheath of the artery that is shown where there are more lymphocytes than there are in the red pulp but fewer lymphocytes than are in the white pulp. This zone of transition between white and red pulp is called the

marginal zone and that which surrounds the periarterial sheaths is continuous with the marginal zones around the follicles to which the arteries lead.

It is mostly into this marginal zone that the terminations of the blood vessels that enter the nodule, branch within it and leave at various points around its periphery, empty their blood. Whether this blood is emptied into the splenic pulp itself or into the sinusoids of the pulp will be discussed later in connection with the circulation through the red pulp. However, it is around the periphery of the nodules that the T lymphocytes that are contained in the blood are delivered. From the marginal zone they move or are carried into the nodules where they mix with B lymphocytes. They also migrate from the marginal zone into the periarterial sheaths of the arteries of the pulp and penetrate deeply into the sheaths to account for at least most of the lymphocyte population of the sheaths. Hence the marginal zone is the site where T lymphocytes arrive from the circulation and have their first opportunity to encounter the B lymphocytes of the spleen so that they can interact with them. Those that migrate into the nodule can also, of course, encounter reticular cells and by this means have indirect interaction with B lymphocytes. The marginal zone therefore is a site where blast cells of the plasma cell lineage commonly appear. Another place can be the site where a germinal center has appeared or will appear. The basic cells of germinal centers are activated B lymphocytes but the rim of lymphocytes that immediately surrounds a germinal center is composed most probably of T lymphocytes. From either position where blast cells of the plasma cell series appear they could move readily into the red pulp where as plasma cells they could elaborate antibodies.

Since the topics discussed in the preceding paragraphs are the subject of much current research with new findings becoming available more or less constantly, further information on this subject, if desired, should be sought from the recent and current literature.

The Sinusoids of the Red Pulp. The nonliving framework of red pulp consists basically of a mesh of reticular fibers which are continuous with the collagenic fibers of the trabeculae and the capsule (Fig. 13-21). Next, the reticular mesh of red pulp, though of an open type itself, is permeated by clear passageways that measure from 12 to 40 microns in width. Since these passageways drain into veins, they are termed the *venous sinusoids* of the red pulp (Fig. 13-21). The walls of many (if not all) of these sinusoids are made of long, narrow endothelial cells that run longitudinally along the sinusoid wall (Fig. 13-26). Whereas the cells bulge into the lumen slightly where their nuclei are

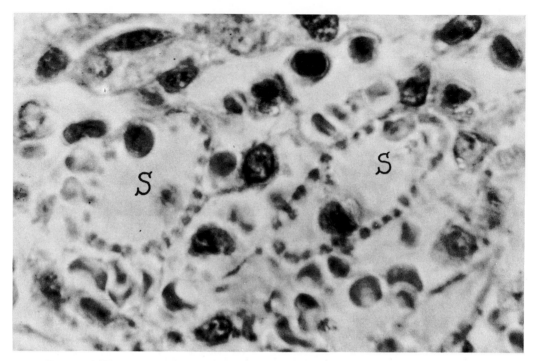

Fɪɢ. 13-26. Oil-immersion photomicrograph of a section of distended spleen taken with the phase microscope. In this picture 2 sinusoids are cut in cross section. These are marked S. The cytoplasm of their longitudinally disposed narrow stavelike lining cells is cut in cross section. The cells can be seen to be slightly separated from one another.

located, their cytoplasm which extends along a sinusoid in each direction from their nuclei, is, in a distended spleen, not very bulky. Cross sections of the sinusoids across these cytoplasmic processes, which are separated from each other in a distended spleen, are seen in Figure 13-26. Hence it is said there are longitudinal slits between the long endothelial cells that line sinusoids.

A sinusoid in life is therefore something like an old leaky barrel whose longitudinal staves have shrunken away from one another to leave slits between them. Like barrels that are supported by surrounding iron hoops the endothelial staves of the venous sinusoids are somewhat similarly surrounded and supported by hoops of basement membrane material as will be described presently.

The So-called Pulp Cords. From the appearance seen in a single section, the red pulp between two adjacent sinusoids often resembles a cord; indeed these areas have been termed *Billroth* or *pulp cords* (Fig. 13-21, *right*). However, the student who thinks in three dimensions will quickly realize that this name is misleading. For anything to be a cord it should be surrounded on all sides by a material different from itself

—for example a fishing line dangling in water is a cord and is surrounded on all sides by water. A so-called pulp cord, although in a particular section it may have a sinusoidal space on each side of it, is not surrounded by a space, for sections taken below and above the section under view would show the substance of the so-called cord to be continuous with the substance of the red pulp in general. Sinusoids are tubular-like spaces in a spongework of red pulp, and just as the substance between the two holes in a single slice of Swiss cheese is not a cord, as cutting further slices shows, the pulp between two sinusoids is not in the form of cords.

Robinson, in his studies on distended human spleens, included some of thick sections which he examined with a binocular microscope arranged to give stereoscopic vision. He described the pulp between the sinusoids as consisting of a vast, delicate network of starlike cells having long, irregular protoplasmic processes running in all directions and uniting one cell with another. He visualized interstices of this cellular network as a vast cavernous system of intercellular spaces that were in free communication with the venous sinusoids through the longitudinal slits in the walls of the latter (Fig. 13-26). Moreover, Robinson described blood from the follicular arteries as being emptied into the substance of the red pulp (and not directly into the sinusoids, as will be described presently) and red blood cells, leukocytes and platelets from the pulp between sinusoids entering sinusoids through the slits between their endothelial cells.

In a random section cut from a distended spleen, sinusoids and the so-called pulp cords are cut in various planes. In many of the planes in which sinusoids are cut they are not as distinct as when cut in cross section. As is shown in Figure 13-27, it is sometimes difficult to distinguish between sinusoids and the pulp between them, because both the sinusoids and pulp contain erythrocytes and nucleated cells which, in the instance of sinusoids, are mostly leukocytes. Macrophages are numerous in the pulp between sinusoids; two are seen in the center of Figure 13-27; one has phagocytosed a red blood cell (labeled R.B.C.). Other phagocytic

cells are labeled R.E. cells; these too are macrophages. The endothelium of the sinusoids where it is cut more or less longitudinally in this section is thin.

Fine Structure of the Red Pulp. In interpreting observations made with the EM it is of course important to know whether a given study was made on the spleens of man or laboratory animals and whether or not the spleens were collapsed or distended to life size. In general, the EM has confirmed that the basic structural framework of the red pulp consists of a network of reticular fibers that are continuous with the collagenic fibers of the trabeculae. Chen and Weiss in their EM studies of human spleen, have shown that, at the edges of sinusoids, the reticular fibers are associated with basement membrane material and that the latter forms rings around the sinusoids (Fig. 13-28). Among other things, they have also described two types and arrangements of filaments in the endothelial cells of sinusoids, which they believe may be

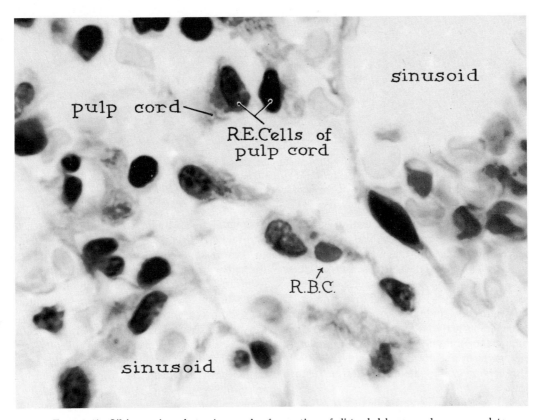

FIG. 13-27. Oil-immersion photomicrograph of a section of distended human spleen removed to alleviate excessive red blood cell destruction. Sinusoids may be seen at the lower left and the upper right; between them is a pulp cord. In this, several reticuloendothelial cells (macrophages) may be seen. One near the center has phagocytosed a red blood corpuscle (labeled R.B.C.), which is lying in its cytoplasm. The spotty appearance of the cytoplasm of the cell immediately below it is due to granules of pigment formed as a result of the breakdown of hemoglobin in its cytoplasm.

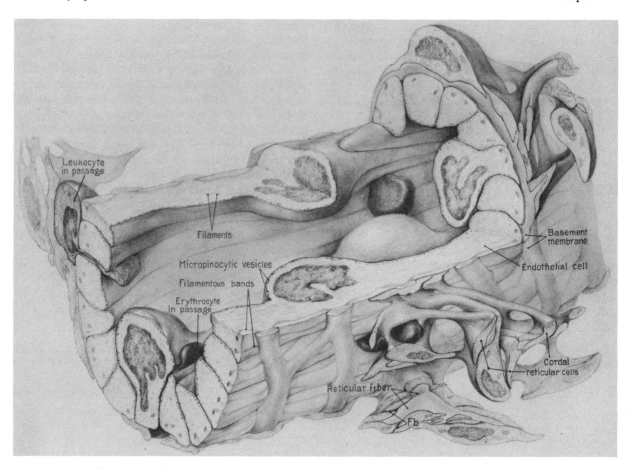

FIG. 13-28. A diagram representing the structure of a sinus of the red pulp based on studies made with the EM. (This illustration was provided by Dr. Leon Weiss; Chen, L-T., and Weiss, L.: Electron microscopy of the red pulp of the human spleen. Am. J. Anat., *134:425,* 1972.)

contractile (and play a role in the removal of damaged blood cells), as well as the presence of many pinocytotic vesicles just beneath the membranes of the endothelial cells on their lateral sides and on their sides that face the lumen of the sinusoids. They also describe adventitial cells which border the endothelial cells of the sinusoids and are associated with the basement membrane material that comprises the rings that surround the sinusoids and also incompletely covers other parts of their walls (Fig. 13-28). Their study, and others by Weiss, should be read for further information.

What seem to be the indigenous cells of the red pulp are termed reticular cells and they are believed to be responsible for forming the reticular fibers. They have relatively large nuclei with little condensed chromatin. Their cytoplasm has a most irregular shape and tends to extend from the cell body in an irregular fashion. It contains a Golgi apparatus, some rER, lysosomes,

and bundles of filaments as well as some free ribosomes and mitochondria. It is believed the reticular cells are to some extent phagocytic but not as phagocytic as the great many macrophages with which they are associated in the red pulp. In addition to reticular cells and macrophages the red pulp in life contains blood cells, both red and white, in relatively large numbers as well as many plasma cells. It is believed that erythrocytes are strained through the slits between the endothelial cells that line the sinusoids at sites not occluded by basement membrane. It is probable that worn-out erythrocytes (or imperfect, fragile erythrocytes) are not sufficiently elastic to pass undamaged through the slits and so are phagocytosed by macrophages in the substance of the pulp. Leukocytes, being mobile and labile, can pass through the slits fairly readily.

What we have termed the macrophages of the pulp and the endothelial cells lining the sinusoids were once believed to be very similar with regard to their phagocytic properties and were both spoken of as being reticuloendothelial cells. As is shown from the study of Burke and Simon, the endothelial cells of the sinusoids, when tested with colloidal carbon, evidence little phagocytic capacity as compared with macrophages within the pulp; so here, as in bone marrow, the cells lining sinusoids are not primarily phagocytic, as was once postulated. The extensive phagocytosis that seems, with the LM, to occur along sinusoidal walls could be due to macrophages which Burke and Simon show often protrude into the sinusoidal lumen between endothelial cells.

Summary of the Functions of the Red Pulp. In postnatal life in man the two most important functions of the red pulp are to dispose of worn-out erythrocytes and other cellular material that might otherwise clutter up the bloodstream, and to provide antibodies. The first function is performed by the macrophages of the red pulp and the second by the plasma cells which are also present in it and whose origin can be traced to the white pulp. A third but less important function of the red pulp is to act as a storage reservoir for blood. Finally, in a sense it could be said that the spleen produces both iron and a bile pigment; these are formed by the breakdown of hemoglobin in macrophages that have phagocytosed erythrocytes.

Fate of Macrophages That Enter the Sinusoids. The splenic vein drains into the hepatic portal system and so the large number of macrophages that enter the sinusoids and leave the spleen via the splenic vein go into the liver. This problem will be discussed again in relation to the liver, from which phagocytic cells of the same general type may be released into the circulation. It seems probable that these, being large cells, are unable to pass through the capillaries of the lungs. They make their way into the air spaces and are ultimately coughed up or swallowed and disintegrate in the stomach.

THEORIES OF CIRCULATION OF BLOOD THROUGH THE RED PULP

Studies of sections of spleen have in the past given rise to two main theories about the circulation through the red pulp. According to one—the open circulation theory—arterial blood from the ellipsoids is delivered directly into the substance of red pulp (Fig. 13-29) and only gains entrance to the sinusoids by percolating through the slits in sinusoidal walls. According to the other—the closed circulation theory—arterial blood is delivered via capillaries directly into sinusoids (Fig. 13-29), and the great content of erythrocytes in the

red pulp between sinusoids is explained by the erythrocytes passing back and forth between the pulp and the sinusoids via the slits in the walls of the latter.

In evaluating these two theories we encounter again the problem of whether studies are made on human spleens or on the spleens of other animals. Different animals reveal differences, for example, in the structure and size of ellipsoids; these, for example, are highly developed in cats. The spleens of mice and rats, as already noted are hemopoietic. Then again, the question arises as to whether studies made on distended spleens would support the same theory as studies made on collapsed spleens. Indeed, there is a third theory to the effect that the circulation in a collapsed spleen is closed but in a distended spleen, open.

Robinson in his studies of human spleens which he distended through the veins concluded that blood from the ellipsoids empties into the substance of the red pulp and therefore has to pass from there through sinusoidal walls to gain entrance to their lumens. Chen and Weiss in their recent study with the EM on human spleens noted that all terminal arterial vessels that were observed opened into red pulp between sinusoids. There is therefore substantial evidence for the open circulation theory in human spleens.

In studies on the spleens of rabbits with the EM Burke and Simon place emphasis on the existence of zones between areas of white pulp and red pulp, which they term transitional zones, and where there is a large marginal sinus from which they believe the majority of other sinusoids arise, but they were unable to show any direct connection between capillaries and sinusoids or the substance of red pulp. In another study, however, they found that carbon injected intravenously appeared so quickly in the sinusoids that it suggested that they have direct connections with capillaries.

Perhaps in trying to decide whether the splenic circulation is open or closed it is often assumed that the beginning of a sinusoid is as definite a structure as it becomes farther along its course. In a distended spleen, as is shown in Figure 13-27, there are many areas where it is difficult, if not impossible, to distinguish sinusoids from interstices between cells of pulp cords and it would probably be a matter of opinion as to whether the terminations of capillaries were in pulp or sinusoids. This could be the basis for the theory that the circulation can be *either closed or open,* depending on circumstances. According to this view, the beginnings of the venous sinusoids which appear as tubular structures in a contracted spleen may exhibit in a distended spleen so many openings between the cells of their walls that they cease to be structures and become no more than fairly open passageways

CIRCULATION OF BLOOD THROUGH THE SPLEEN

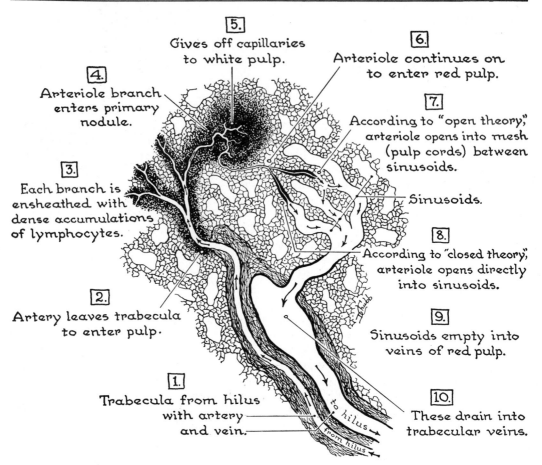

5. Gives off capillaries to white pulp.

6. Arteriole continues on to enter red pulp.

4. Arteriole branch enters primary nodule.

7. According to "open theory," arteriole opens into mesh (pulp cords) between sinusoids.

Sinusoids.

3. Each branch is ensheathed with dense accumulations of lymphocytes.

8. According to "closed theory," arteriole opens directly into sinusoids.

2. Artery leaves trabecula to enter pulp.

9. Sinusoids empty into veins of red pulp.

1. Trabecula from hilus with artery and vein.

to hilus
from hilus

10. These drain into trabecular veins.

FIG. 13-29. Diagram to show the course of blood taken through the spleen according to the open and the closed theories of circulation. The legends on the figure should be read in a clockwise fashion.

through a reticular mesh that abounds with communicating spaces. In other words, some consider that the first parts of the venous sinusoids, when they are distended, are so leaky that they should not here be considered as structures and hence that the circulation under these conditions is open. But when the spleen is contracted, the cells of the walls of the sinusoids come close enough together to justify the view that they are tubular structures; under these conditions, the circulation is closed.

Another approach to the problem was made by Knisely when he utilized the quartz-rod illuminator to study the passageways by which blood circulates between the arteries and the veins in the exposed spleen of a living animal. Knisely found that the arterial capillaries branch after passing through the region of ellipsoids, and that some of the branches pass directly to the veins. These capillaries (Fig. 13-30, capillary shunts), which are controlled by sphincters, provide a *bypass* or *shunt* circulation so that blood can pass through the spleen without being emptied into either the red pulp or the sinusoids. Knisely found that the other set of capillary branches empty into the sinusoids; in this respect Knisely's findings seem to support the closed circulation theory. Knisely found, moreover, that there were sphincters at each end of the sinusoids, and that, depending on the contraction or the relaxation of these sphincters, sinusoids exhibit different states of form and function which he termed phases (Fig. 13-30). With both sphincters open, a sinusoid would be relatively narrow; in this state it would be said to be in a conducting phase. With the efferent sphincter contracted and the afferent one open, a sinusoid is said to be in a *filtration-filling* phase, with its walls retaining erythrocytes but allowing plasma to escape into the pulp cords. When the sinusoid becomes filled with erythrocytes, the afferent sphincter closes, and the sinusoid enters the *storage phase*. Then, when both sphincters open, it enters the *emptying phase,* and the red blood cells that are packed in it are washed into the circulation.

The study of the circulation of the living spleen by the quartz-rod illuminator is a difficult technic to employ and cannot be expected to reveal the kind of tissue or cellular detail obtainable in sections studied with either the LM or the EM. In their use of this method, MacKenzie, Whipple and Wintersteiner were unable to confirm many of Knisely's findings. However Peck and Hoerr made a further study of both the method and the problem. Their work emphasized the necessity for very exacting precautions if the method is to yield information of value, and they found, when these precautions were taken, that the intermediary circulation in the spleen is essentially as Knisely described it. However, while these studies on living spleen elicited physiological information that would not be obtainable from studying sections, such as capillary bypasses and the same sinusoid existing in different phases, they could be scarcely expected to prove that there was always unbroken endothelial continuity between capillaries and the beginnings of sinusoids and hence settle the open versus closed circulation controversy.

References and Other Reading

THE THYMUS

General References

Defendi, V., and Metcalf, D. (eds.): The thymus. *In* A. Wistar Institute Symposium Monograph No. 2. Philadelphia, Wistar Inst. Press, 1964.

Good, R. A., and Gabrielsen, A. E. (eds.): The Thymus in Immunobiology. New York, Hoeber, 1964.

Hess, M. W.: Experimental Thymectomy. New York, Springer, 1968.

Metcalf, D., and Moore, M. A. S.: Haemopoietic Cells. Amsterdam, North-Holland, 1971.

Miller, J. F. A. P.: The thymus, yesterday, today and tomorrow. Lancet, *2:*1299, December 16, 1967.

Osoba, D.: Thymic function, immunologic deficiency and autoimmunity. Med. Clin. N. Am., *56:*319, 1972.

Special References

Alapper, C.: Morphogenesis of the thymus. Am. J. Anat., *78:* 139, 1946.

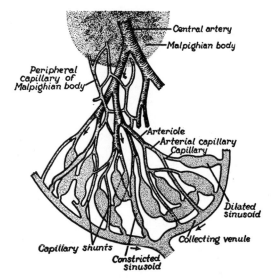

Fig. 13-30. Diagram of splenic circulation, according to Knisely. (Peck, H. M., and Hoerr, N. L.: Anat. Rec., *109:*447)

Archer, O. K., and Pierce, J. C.: Role of the thymus in development of the immune response. Fed. Proc., *20:*26, 1961.

Auerbach, R.: Experimental analysis of the origin of cell types in the development of the mouse thymus. Develop. Biol., *3:* 336, 1961.

Clark, S. L., Jr.: The thymus in mice of strain 129/J studied with the electron microscope. Am. J. Anat., *112:*1, 1963.

————: The penetration of proteins and colloidal materials into the thymus from the bloodstream. *In* Defendi, V., and Metcalf, D. (eds.): A Wistar Institute Symposium Monograph No. 2, p. 9. Philadelphia, Wistar Inst. Press, 1964.

Horiuchi, A., Gery, I., and Waksman, B. H.: Role of the thymus in tolerance. VII. Diatribution of nonaggregated and heat aggregated bovine globulin in lymphoid organs of normal newborn and adult rats. Yale J. Biol. Med., *41:*13, 1968.

Ito, T., and Hoshino, T.: Fine structure of the epithelial reticular cells of the medulla of the thymus of the golden hamster. Z. Zellforsch., *69:*311, 1966.

Jerne, N. K.: Waiting for the end (summary of symposium on antibodies). Symp. Quant. Biol. (Cold Spring Harbor), *32:* 591, 1967.

Law, L. W., Trainin, N., Levey, R. H., and Barth, W. F.: Humoral thymic factor in mice: Further evidence. Science, *143:*1049, 1964.

Metcalf, D.: The thymic lymphocytosis stimulating factor and its relation to lymphatic leukemia. Ann. N.Y. Acad. Sci., *73:* 113, 1958.

Miller, J. F. A. P.: Role of the thymus in immunity. Brit. Med. J., *2:*459, 1963.

————: Functions of the thymus. *In* Scientific Basis of Medicine, Annual Reviews. p. 218. London, Athlone Press, 1964.

————: The thymus and the development of immunologic responsiveness. Science, *144:*1544, 1964.

Mitchell, G. F., and Miller, J. F. A. P.: Immunological activity of thymus and thoracic-duct lymphocytes. Proc. Nat. Acad. Sci., *59:*296, 1968.

Osoba, D.: Immune reactivity in mice thymectomized soon after birth. Normal response after pregnancy. Science, *147:* 298, 1965.

Raviola, E., and Karnovsky, M. J.: Evidence for a blood-thymus barrier using electron-opaque tracers. J. Exp. Med., *136:* 466, 1972.

Sainte-Marie, G.: Lymphocyte formation in the thymus of the rat, Proc. Canad. Cancer Conf. vol. 3, p. 337. New York, Academic Press, 1958.

Sainte-Marie, G., and Leblond, C. P.: Thymus-cell population dynamics. *In* Good, R. A., and Gabrielsen, A. E. (eds.): The Thymus in Immunobiology. p. 207. Harper and Row, New York, 1964.

Sainte-Marie, G., and Messier, B.: Thymus and node labelling by intramediastinal injection of tritiated tracers and its bearing on present concepts of lymphocyte cytokinetics. Scand. J. Haematol., *7:*163, 1970.

Sainte-Marie, G., and Peng, Fuh-Shiong: Emigration of thymocytes from the thymus. A review and study of the problem. Rev. Canad. Biol., *30:*51, 1971.

Smith, C.: Studies on the thymus of the mammal. VIII. Intrathymic lymphatic vessels. Anat. Rec., *122:*173, 1955.

Smith, C., and Parkhurst, H. T.: A comparison with the staining of Hassall's corpuscles and the thick skin of the guinea pig. Anat. Rec., *103:*649, 1949.

LYMPHATIC NODULES AND NODES

Ada, G. L.: Antigen, Lymphoid Cells and the Immune Response. New York, Academic Press, 1971.

Andreasen, E., and Christensen, S.: The rate of mitotic activity in the lymphoid organs of the rat. Anat. Rec., *103:*401, 1949.

Brahim, F., and Osmond, D. C.: The migration of lymphocytes from bone marrow to popliteal lymph nodes demonstrated by selective bone marrow labeling with ^{3}H thymidine in vivo. Anat. Rec., *175:*737, 1973.

Clark, S. L., Jr.: The reticulum of lymph nodes in mice studied with the electron microscope. Am. J. Anat., *110:*217, 1962.

Conway, E. A.: Cyclic changes in lymphatic nodules. Anat. Rec., *68:*487, 1937.

Coons, A. H.: Fluorescent antibody methods. *In* Danielli, J. F. (ed.): General Cytochemical Methods. pp. 399–422, New York, Academic Press, 1958.

———: The cytology of antibody formation. J. Cell. Comp. Physiol., *52* (Suppl. 1):55, 1958.

Coons, A. H., Leduc, E. H., and Connolly, J. M.: Leukocytes involved in antibody formation. Ann. N.Y. Acad. Sci., *59:* 951, 1955.

———: Studies on antibody production: I. A method for the histochemical demonstration of specific antibody and its application to a study of the hyperimmune rabbit. J. Exp. Med., *102:*49, 1955.

Dumonde, D. C.: The role of the macrophage in transplantation immunity. Symposium on Tissue and Organ Transplantation. J. Clin. Path. (Suppl.), p. 430, May 1967.

Everett, N. B., and Tyler (Caffrey), R. W.: Lymphopoiesis in the thymus and other tissues: functional implications. Int. Rev. Cytol., *22:*205, 1967.

Krumbhaar, E. B.: Lymphatic tissue. *In* Cowdry, E. V. (ed.): Problems of Ageing. p. 149. Baltimore, Williams & Wilkins, 1939.

Leduc, E. H., Coons, A. H., and Connolly, J. M.: Studies on antibody production. II. The primary and secondary responses in the popliteal lymph node of the rabbit. J. Exp. Med., *102:*61, 1955.

Menzies, D. W.: The blood supply of the para-aortic lymph node of the rat. *In* Further Studies in Pathology. p. 176. Melbourne, Australia, University Press, 1965.

Micklem, H. S., Ford, C. E., Evans, E. P., and Gray, J. G.: Interrelationships of myeloid and lymphoid cells. Studies with chromosome-marked cells transfused into lethally irradiated mice. Proc. Roy. Soc. (Biol.), *165:*78, 1966.

Movat, H. Z., and Fernando, N. V. P.: The fine structure of lymphoid tissue. Exp. Molec. Path., *3:*546, 1964.

———: The fine structure of lymphoid tissue during antibody formation. Exp. Molec. Path., *4:*155, 1965.

Messier, P., and Sainte-Marie, G.: Location of lymphocytes in endothelium of postcapillary venules of rat lymph nodes. Rev. Canad. Biol., *31:*231, 1972.

Nopajaroosri, C., Luk, S. C., and Simon, G. T.: Ultrastructure of the normal lymph node. Am. J. Path., *65:*1, 1971.

Nopajaroosri, C., and Simon, G. T.: Phagocytosis of colloidal carbon in a lymph node. Am. J. Path., *65:*25, 1971.

Nossal, G. J. W.: Genetic control of lymphopoiesis, plasma cell formation, and antibody production. Int. Rev. Exp. Path., *1:*1, 1962.

———: How cells make antibodies. Sci. Am., *211:*106, 1964.

Parrott, D. M. V.: The response of draining lymph nodes to immunological stimulation in intact and thymectomized animals. J. Clin. Path., 20 (Symp. Tissue Org. Transplant., Suppl.):456, 1967.

Rebuck, J. E. (ed.): The Lymphocyte and Lymphocytic Tissue. New York, Hoeber, 1960.

Sainte-Marie, G.: Study on plasmocytopoiesis. 1. Description of plasmocytes and of their mitoses in the mediastinal lymph nodes of ten-week-old rats. Am. J. Anat., *114:*207, 1964.

Sainte-Marie, G., and Coons, A. H.: Studies on antibody production. X. Mode of formation of plasmocytes in cell transfer experiments. J. Exp. Med., *119:*743, 1964.

Sainte-Marie, G., and Sin, Y. M.: Structures of the lymph node and their possible function during the immune response. Rev. Canad. Biol., *27:*191, 1968.

Sainte-Marie, G.: Labelling of lymphoid organs by repeated injections of ^{3}H-thymidine. Rev. Canad. Biol., *32:*251, 1973.

Schoefl, G. I.: The migration of lymphocytes across the vascular endothelium in lymphoid tissue, a reexamination. J. Exp. Med., *132:*568, 1972.

Weller, C. V.: The hemolymph nodes. *In* Downey's Handbook of Hematology. p. 1759. New York, Hoeber, 1938.

Yoffey, J. M., and Courtice, F. C.: Lymphatics, Lymph and the Lymphomyeloid Complex. New York, Academic Press, 1971.

SPLEEN

Bradfield, J. W., and Born, G. V. R.: The migration of rat thoracic duct lymphocytes through the spleen in vivo. Brit. J. Exp. Path., *54:*509, 1973.

Burke, J. S., and Simon, G. T.: Electron microscopy of the spleen. I. Anatomy and microcirculation. Am. J. Path., *58:* 127, 1970.

———: Electron microscopy of the spleen. II. Phagocytosis of colloidal carbon. Am. J. Path., *58:*157, 1970.

Chen, L.-T., and Weiss, L.: Electron microscopy of the red pulp of human spleen. Am. J. Anat., *134:*425, 1972.

Doggett, T. H.: The capillary system of the dog's spleen. Anat. Rec., *110*:65, 1951.

Foot, N. C.: The reticulum of the human spleen. Anat. Rec., *36*:79, 1927.

Ford, W. L.: The kinetics of lymphocyte recirculation within the rat spleen. Cell Tissue Kinet., *2*:171, 1969.

Knisley, M. H.: Spleen studies: I. Microscopic observations of the circulatory system of living unstimulated mammalian spleens. Anat. Rec., *65*:23, 1936.

———: Spleen studies: II. Microscopic observations of the circulatory system of living traumatized, and of drying spleens. Anat. Rec., *65*:131, 1936.

Krumbhaar, E. B.: Function of the spleen. Physiol. Rev., *6*: 160, 1926.

Lewis, O. J.: The blood vessels of the adult mammalian spleen. J. Anat., *91*:245, 1957.

———: The development of the circulation in the spleen of the foetal rabbit. J. Anat., *90*:282, 1956.

MacKenzie, D. W., Jr., Whipple, A. O., and Wintersteiner, M. P.: Studies on the microscopic anatomy and physiology of living transilluminating mammalian spleens. Am. J. Anat., *68*:397, 1941.

MacNeal, W. J.: The circulation of blood through the spleen pulp. Arch. Path., *7*:215, 1929.

McNee, J. W.: The spleen: its structure, functions and diseases (Lettsomian Lectures). Lancet, *1*:951, 1009, 1063, 1931.

Mall, F. P.: On the circulation through the pulp of the dog's spleen. Am. J. Anat., *2*:315, 1903.

Movat, H. Z., and Fernando, N. V. P.: The fine structure of the lymphoid tissue during antibody formation. Exp. Molec. Path., *4*:155, 1965.

Peck, H. M., and Hoerr, N. L.: The effect of environmental temperature changes in the circulation of the mouse spleen. Anat. Rec., *109*:479, 1951.

———: The intermediary circulation in the red pulp of the mouse spleen. Anat. Rec., *109*:447, 1951.

Robinson, W. L.: Some points on the mechanism of filtration by the spleen. Am. J. Path., *4*:309, 1928.

———: The vascular mechanism of the spleen. Am. J. Path., *2*:341, 1926.

———: The venous drainage of the cat spleen. Am. J. Path., *6*:19, 1930.

Solnitzky, O.: The Schweigger-Seidel sheath (ellipsoid) of the spleen. Anat. Rec., *69*:55, 1937.

Waksman, B. H., Arnason, B. G., and Jankovie, B. D.: The role of the thymus in immune reactions in rats. III. Changes in the lymphoid organs of thymectomized rats. J. Exp. Med., *116*:187, 1962.

Weiss, L.: A study of the structure of splenic sinuses in man and in the albino rat, with the light microscope and the electron microscope. J. Biophys. Biochem. Cytol., *3*:599, 1957.

———: An experimental study of the organization of the reticuloendothelial system in the red pulp of the spleen. J. Anat., *93*:465, 1959.

———: The Cells and Tissues of the Immune System. Englewood Cliffs, N.J., Prentice-Hall, 1972.

14 Dense Ordinary Connective Tissue and Cartilage

Perspective. In describing the connective tissue we first considered the loose kind which represents a judicious mixture of cells and intercellular substances. We next described the hemopoietic tissues which represent types of connective tissue that consist almost entirely of cells. We shall now consider the connective tissues that consist chiefly of intercellular substances. There are three of these: one ordinary kind called Dense Ordinary Connective Tissue and two special kinds called Cartilage and Bone respectively.

Dense Ordinary Connective Tissue. Dense ordinary connective tissue consists mostly of collagenic fibers except in a few places where it contains a good deal of elastin. Such cells as it contains are mostly those that are concerned with producing intercellular substance.

Since dense ordinary connective tissue consists mostly of collagen, which is a nonliving material, dense ordinary connective tissue does not require many capillaries to be distributed throughout its substance in relation to its bulk and indeed it is sparingly supplied with only enough capillaries to nourish its few cells. Such capillaries as are present are generally invested in a little loose connective tissue.

There is not always a sharp line of demarcation in the body between loose and dense ordinary connective tissue. Often one type merges into the other. In sites where they merge ordinary connective tissue may be neither very dense nor very loose, and hence impossible to classify in a clear-cut way.

Classification. Dense ordinary connective tissue is commonly classified into 2 main types, the regularly arranged, and the irregularly arranged. In the regularly arranged kind, the collagenic fibers all run more or less in the same plane and more or less in the same direction. Hence structures built of it have great tensile strength and can withstand tremendous pulls exerted in the plane and the direction of their fibers without stretching. Obviously, dense regularly arranged connective tissue is ideal for tendons and ligaments which join muscles to bones and bones to bones and for sites where pull is exerted in one general direction (Fig. 14-1). The cells in the dense regularly arranged kind are nearly all fibrocytes and are located between the parallel bundles of collagenic fibers (Fig. 14-1).

In the irregularly arranged type, the collagenic fibers run either in different directions but in the same plane or in every direction. In the sheets of dense, irregularly arranged connective tissue that comprise aponeuroses and sheaths of various sorts, the fibers are more or less in the same plane but may run in different directions. Such sheets can withstand stretching in those directions in which their fibers run. In other body sites, however, such as in the reticular layer of the dermis of the skin (which comprises most of the substance of the skin—to be studied later), the collagenic fibers run both in different directions and in different planes, and hence dermis can withstand stretching in any direction.

The capsules of many organs—for example, lymph nodes and spleen—are composed of thin dense, irregularly arranged connective tissue, and this type of connective tissue often extends from the capsule into organs as septa or trabeculae. Dense connective tissue is often seen as an outer wrapping for tubes of various sorts in the body, as well as for muscles and nerves. It forms a sheath in which the central nervous system (brain and spinal cord) is enclosed. In short, it is a very common tissue and will be seen in many of the sections that will be studied in the laboratory. Here we shall study only one example of it—the dense, regularly arranged connective tissue of tendons.

Tendons

Development. Tendons appear in the embryo as dense bundles of fibroblasts that are oriented in the same plane and packed closely together. The fibroblasts proliferate to permit the growth of the tendon. But, as development proceeds, the fibroblasts become arranged in rows and secrete more and more collagen between the rows to form what is shown in Figure 14-1. The

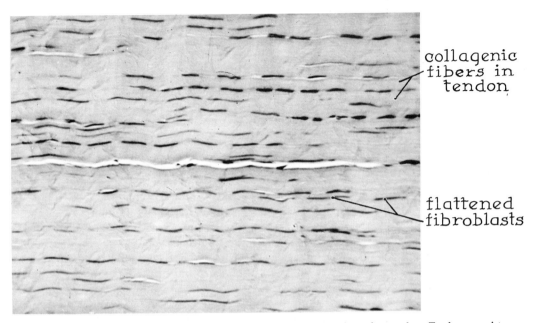

collagenic fibers in tendon

flattened fibroblasts

FIG. 14-1. Low-power photomicrograph of a longitudinal section of a tendon. Tendons consist chiefly of collagenic fibers and bundles of collagenic fibers which run in one direction, with rows of flattened fibroblasts between them. Notice that this tissue is chiefly intercellular substance.

character of the structure thus changes from being primarily cellular to being primarily intercellular substance.

Blood Supply. During development, when tendons are cellular, they have a reasonably good blood supply which is necessary for the collagen to be synthesized and secreted. But when the fiber bundles of collagen become built up, the capillary blood supply within the tendon bundles almost entirely disappears.

Tendon Sheaths. Some tendons in certain sites where they otherwise might rub against bone or other friction-generating surfaces are enclosed in sheaths. Actually a tendon sheath consists of 2 sheaths. The outer one is a connective tissue tube, and its exterior is attached to the structures that surround it. The inner sheath directly encloses the tendon and is firmly attached to it. There is a space between the inner and the outer sheath, and this is filled with a slippery solution of mucopolysaccharide similar to *synovial fluid,* which will be described in connection with joints in Chapter 16.

The inner surface of the outer tendon sheath and the outer surface of the inner sheath do not possess a continuous lining of cells, so the surfaces that glide over one another are mostly surfaces of intercellular substances, chiefly collagen, along which, however, some cells are scattered as in the synovial membranes

of joints (Fig. 16-10). The synovial fluid between the two sheaths is an excellent lubricant.

Regeneration of Tendons. Tendons may be severed in accidents. With proper surgical treatment they heal excellently and in due course become as strong as before. Repair is effected by fibroblasts from the inner tendon sheath or, if the tendon has no proper sheath, from the loose connective tissue around its periphery growing into the site where the cut ends are apposed, proliferating all the while. Gradually the fibroblasts become oriented in the axis of the tendon. Here they re-enact the same scene that is to be witnessed when a tendon develops. At first the fibroblasts have a good capillary blood supply and produce much collagen, which becomes deposited in bundles between them and so arranged in the long axis of the tendon. Some of the cells grow into the cut ends of the tendon where the new collagen that is being formed unites with the old. As more and more collagen is deposited' between the fibroblasts, the capillary blood supply diminishes, and the site of the repair eventually becomes almost free of capillaries. It is not generally believed that the old fibrocytes between the fiber bundles of the original tendon contribute very much, if anything, to the repair process; these old fibroblasts (fibrocytes) have probably lost their reproductive powers.

An interesting factor in regard to the repair of

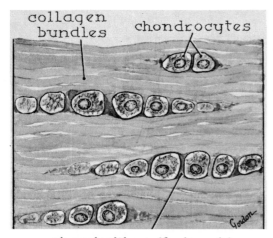

chondroitin sulfuric acid

FIG. 14-2. High-power drawing of an H and E section of fibrocartilage that was taken from a tendon close to its point of insertion. The mucopolysaccharide of cartilage is labeled chondroitin sulfuric acid.

tendons is described by Peacock and Van Winkle, who should be read for details by students inclined toward surgical careers. They point out that the problem of achieving successful repair of a severed tendon more or less hinges on the same factors that could cause adhesions of the tendon so that its subsequent gliding functions might suffer. Isolating the connected ends of a severed tendon from adjacent connective tissue, so that adhesions between the healing tendon and adjacent connective tissue will not occur, prevents the tendon ends from becoming united, because repair of the severed ends depends on connective tissue cells and blood vessels reaching the severed ends from outside the tendon. However here, as in bone, natural remodeling of the healing structure can be extraordinarily efficient in aiding the restoration of function. In addition to pointing out the best ways to obtain good functional results they describe the differences in procedures that should be used for repairing extensor and flexor tendons so as to obtain the best results.

Grafts of Tendons. It was once thought that grafts of dense connective tissue structures such as tendons and fascia continue to live on autologous transplantation. Indeed sutures of fascia were sometimes used in repairing wounds and were termed *living sutures*. It seems probable that the basis for this belief was an uncritical attitude that viewed everything in the body as being alive. Actually most of the substance of dense connective tissue is nonliving material. The relatively

few cells in these dense tissues that are transplanted probably all die, but the intercellular substances of which the transplants mostly consist, and which are of course nonliving materials, persist long enough for new cells to invade and replace those of the transplant and in due course replace also at least much of its intercellular substance with newly formed tissue. Such autologous grafts are useful, not because their cells live, but because their intercellular substance persists long enough to provide a suitable model for replacement by new cells which invade the transplant from host tissue, and produce new intercellular substance as needed.

Tendon Insertions. Tendons can be inserted into either cartilage or bone.

The word insertion is somewhat misleading because it infers that the collagenic bundles of a tendon burrow their way into cartilage or bone and become cemented in place. Actually what happens is that a tendon joined to cartilage develops as such. Where tendon develops the fibroblasts make collagen. Where the cartilage develops closely related cells called chondroblasts make collagen and the mucopolysaccharides of cartilage intercellular substance. Between the tendon and the cartilage the cells make bundles of collagen continuous with the tendon but also some of the mucopolysaccharides of cartilage; such a tissue is termed fibrocartilage (Fig. 14-2).

The way that tendons are inserted into bones by means of *Sharpey's fibers* will be described later in connection with bone.

Elastic Ligaments. It should be noted that there are some ligaments that are composed primarily of elastin, for example, *ligamenta flava* and *ligamentum nuchae*. In these structures the elastin is formed by fibroblasts. The formation of elastin will be dealt with in more detail in connection with the elastic laminae of elastic arteries in Chapter 19.

Cartilage

Cartilage is one of the two kinds of *special* dense connective tissue, bone is the other. Both cartilage and bone consist chiefly of intercellular substance in which their respective cells are housed in little individual cavities called *lacunae* (see chondrocyte in lacuna in Fig. 14-3). The intercellular substance of cartilage differs from that of a tendon (which, although it will not stretch, will bend easily) because in cartilage the collagen fibers are embedded in a mucopolysaccharide which physically has some of the attributes of a plastic; for the intercellular substance of cartilage is firm enough to bear a certain amount of weight.

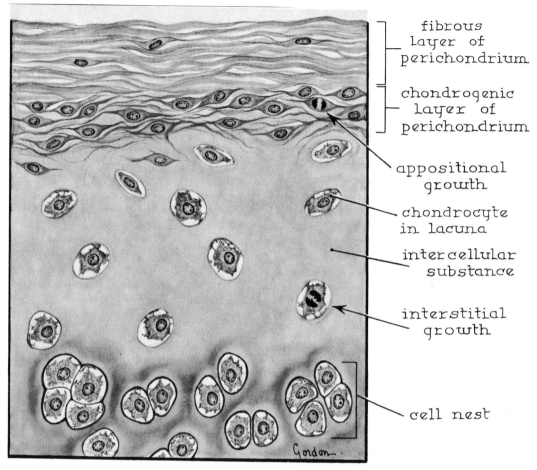

fibrous layer of perichondrium

chondrogenic layer of perichondrium

appositional growth

chondrocyte in lacuna

intercellular substance

interstitial growth

cell nest

Fig. 14-3. Semidiagrammatic drawing of a section of uncalcified hyaline cartilage covered with perichondrium. It illustrates the processes of both appositional and interstitial growth.

Furthermore, a free cartilage surface can be very smooth and with proper lubrication, as it has in freely movable joints, it can be very slippery, which allows the two or more cartilaginous surfaces to glide over each other with a minimum of friction or wear.

Importance of Cartilage in the Body. There is so little cartilage in relation to other tissues in the adult body that a student might think its study is not very important. This would be a real mistake. If it were not for cartilage and its unique properties we would, of course, have no freely movable joints such as knees, elbows and so on. But what is not readily apparent is that without cartilage we would have no long bones to move, because the growth in length of the long bones of our arms and legs is absolutely dependent on the unique properties (to be described soon) of cartilage. Cartilage plays much of its role in permitting bones to grow in length in prenatal life but it also continues to serve this function in postnatal life until the longitudinal growth of bones is over. Afterward cartilage persists in only a few sites in the human body as will next be described.

There are 3 types of cartilage:

$$\text{Cartilage} \begin{cases} \text{hyaline} \\ \text{elastic} \\ \text{fibro} \end{cases}$$

Of the 3 types, hyaline is the most common, so we shall describe it here in detail.

HYALINE CARTILAGE

Hyaline cartilage was given this name because seen with the naked eye fresh hyaline cartilage has a pearly white, glassy (*hyalos,* glass), translucent appearance which is a familiar sight to anyone who has bought soup bones. This appearance is due entirely to the special character of its intercellular substance.

Hyaline cartilage persists in adult life not only in the articular surfaces of joints but also in parts of the ear, and it plays a prominent role in providing support in the nose, the larynx, the trachea and the bronchi and in the walls of the upper respiratory passages. The ring-like cartilages of the trachea are commonly studied in the laboratory to illustrate persisting hyaline cartilage (Figs. 23-5 and 23-6). However, by far the most informative way to study hyaline cartilage is to study it in prenatal life where it plays such an important role. In prenatal life models of most of the bones-to-be in the body are first formed from cartilage and these are later replaced by bone. In fetal tissues there is, therefore, an abundance of hyaline cartilage to study. Since some of this cartilage persists into postnatal life in the long bones in what are termed epiphyseal plates or disks (but only until the longitudinal growth of bones is completed), hyaline cartilage can be studied here also if tissue is obtained from animals that have not yet finished their growth.

Development. Cartilage develops from mesenchyme. To form cartilage, mesenchymal cells first come closer together and lose the processes that, up to this time, have extended off from their cytoplasm. Soon the area in which cartilage is to form becomes composed of rounded mesenchymal cells which are packed closely together (Fig. 14-4, a; only the nuclei show up well at this stage). The next change to be observed is that these cells gradually become separated from one another again. This is due to their beginning to form the intercellular substance of cartilage which, as it is laid down in increasing amounts between the cells, gradually pushes them apart (Fig. 14-4, b). Since the mesenchymal cells have now differentiated and lie in lacunae in intercellular substance, they could be called chondrocytes (cartilage cells), or since they can still divide (Fig. 14-3, interstitial growth) and form more intercellular substance, they could at this stage still be called chondroblasts.

The Development and Structure of the Perichondrium. The mesenchyme surrounding the area in which cartilage develops remains closely applied to the forming cartilage and becomes its perichondrium. In the outer part of this mesenchyme, the mesenchyme cells tend to differentiate into fibroblasts and to form collagenic fibers (Fig. 14-3, fibrous layer of the perichondrium). In the deeper part of the perichondrium, that is, the part applied closely to the cartilage tissue, the mesenchymal cells of the perichondrium do not differentiate into fibroblasts but remain in a relatively undifferentiated state, retaining their capac-

ity to form chondroblasts and chondrocytes. This layer of cells could be called the chondrogenic layer of the perichondrium as it is in Figure 14-3. This layer of the perichondrium is a feature of young cartilage. In adult life the perichondrium of—for example—the cartilage rings in the trachea seems to be reduced to its fibrous layer.

Microscopic Structure. The cells of cartilage are called *chondrocytes* and reside in little spaces in the intercellular substances called *lacunae* (Fig. 14-3). In some instances, a lacuna contains but a single chondrocyte. In others, pairs or even larger numbers of chondrocytes may be present. When many chondrocytes are present in a single lacuna, it is said to constitute a *cell nest*. Often when several cells are present in a single large lacuna, very fine partitions of intercellular substance may exist between the individual cells so that a large primary lacuna, which is still called a cell nest, is thereby broken up into a number of smaller secondary ones (Fig. 14-3). Typically, chondrocytes have a rounded nucleus with one or more nucleoli. In life their cytoplasm fills the lacunae in which the cells reside. However, in stained sections the cytoplasm is commonly seen to be shrunken away from the sides of the lacunae because of shrinkage artifact. Glycogen and fat may be demonstrated in the cytoplasm of large chondrocytes. Chondrocytes vary considerably in size and shape. Young chondrocytes, which could be called chondroblasts, like the lacunae that contain them, instead of being spherical are often flattened (Fig. 14-3). Old or, more precisely, fully differentiated cartilage cells tend to be large and rounded (Fig. 14-3). Size, then, is an important indication of the degree to which any given chondrocyte has differentiated. Small, more or less flattened chondrocytes are to be regarded as not nearly so well differentiated as the large hypertrophied rounded ones.

The *intercellular substance* of hyaline cartilage is a firm gel. Although it appears to be homogeneous both in the gross and in most ordinary kinds of microscopic preparations, it contains considerable quantities of both fibrous and amorphous kinds of intercellular substance. The fibrous kind is represented by collagenic fibrils and fibers, and a considerable quantity of these are present. However, they are immersed in a relatively large quantity of amorphous intercellular substance. Most of this is one of the mucopolysaccharides described in Chapter 8 and known as *chondroitin sulfuric acid*. The amorphous intercellular substance of cartilage is of approximately the same refractive index as the collagen fibrils and fibers which lie in it;

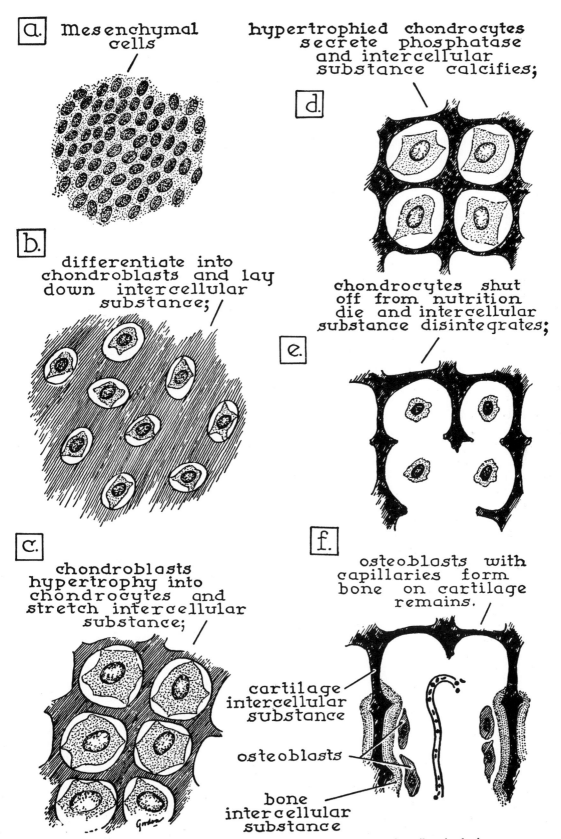

a. Mesenchymal cells

b. differentiate into chondroblasts and lay down intercellular substance;

c. chondroblasts hypertrophy into chondrocytes and stretch intercellular substance;

d. hypertrophied chondrocytes secrete phosphatase and intercellular substance calcifies;

e. chondrocytes shut off from nutrition die and intercellular substance disintegrates;

f. osteoblasts with capillaries form bone on cartilage remains.

cartilage intercellular substance

osteoblasts

bone intercellular substance

FIG. 14-4. Diagrams to show the development, life history and usual fate of cartilage in the body.

hence the collagen fibers cannot be seen at all distinctly unless the amorphous intercellular substance is dissolved away. The lining of each lacuna seems to consist of an intercellular substance somewhat different in consistency from that present throughout most of the substance of cartilage (Fig. 14-3). If cartilage is stained with toluidine blue, strong metachromasia is evidenced by the thin layer of intercellular substances that lines each lacuna. This suggests that it is largely chondroitin sulfuric acid because this substance stains metachromatically with toluidine blue. Frequently, this lining layer of the lacuna is sometimes referred to as the *capsule* of the cartilage cell.

Fine Structure. The fine structure of hyaline cartilage is described later in connection with articular cartilage in Chapter 16.

Growth of Cartilage

Unlike bone, which as we shall see can grow by only one method, young cartilage can grow by two different methods a fact of the greatest importance, as we shall see when we study bone. These two methods are (1) interstitial growth, and (2) appositional growth. They are both illustrated in Figure 14-3.

Interstitial Growth. Since *interstitium* means a small hole in the substance of a tissue, the word *interstitial* refers to the cells in the lacunae in the substance of the cartilage. These cells (the chondrocytes), until they become mature, retain their ability to divide; hence more chondrocytes can form within the substance of cartilage. The new cells that are formed by this growth mechanism can give rise to new and more intercellular substance. The formation of new cells with their subsequent formation of intercellular substance within the substance of cartilage causes the cartilage to expand from within (Fig. 14-3, interstitial growth). A piece of cartilage growing by the mechanism of interstitial growth increases in size in much the same way as dough "rises" when bread is made. For this type of growth to occur in cartilage, the intercellular substance must be sufficiently malleable to allow the cartilage to expand from within when internal cells divide and make new intercellular substance. Obviously, cartilage in which the amount of intercellular substance is not yet great permits interstitial growth to occur much more readily than cartilage that has become older, and in which the intercellular substance has become great in amount and of a stiffer consistency. Interstitial growth, then, is limited to moderately young cartilage.

Appositional Growth. The second mechanism by which any piece of cartilage can increase in size is

known as *appositional growth*. As the name implies, this means a mechanism whereby new layers of cartilage are apposed to one of its surfaces. Appositional growth depends on activity in the inner chondrogenic layer of the perichondrium. In this, the deeper cells of the perichondrium divide, which increases their numbers. Some of the cells so formed then differentiate into chondroblasts and then into chondrocytes and, as they do, they surround themselves with intercellular substance, which is applied to the surface of the cartilage. By this mechanism a new layer of cartilage is laid down under the perichondrium on the surface of the cartilage and this causes the cartilage to grow in width. Furthermore, since the deeper cells of the perichondrium divide before differentiation occurs, their numbers are not depleted by the process, and so there are plenty more, should additional growth by this mechanism be necessary. (Fig. 14-3 illustrates the appositional growth of cartilage.)

The free surfaces of freely movable joints are not covered with perichondrium, so such growth as can occur in articular cartilage is possible by the interstitial method only and, as we shall see when we later study joints, this appears to be limited to the period of growth of the skeleton.

The Nutrition of Cartilage. It might be expected that any tissue that develops from mesenchyme would be abundantly supplied with capillaries. Cartilage in this respect is also unique, because it contains no capillaries within it to nourish its cells. The capillaries that supply cartilage with nourishment lie outside its substance (Fig. 14-5). Consequently, chondrocytes are nourished by means of dissolved substances, because of diffusion gradients, diffusing through the wet gelled intercellular substance that surrounds them as is shown in Figure 14-5. The fact that the only way that chondrocytes can receive nutrients from the blood in capillaries is for the nutrients to diffuse from capillaries outside the cartilage through the intercellular substance, often for long distances, has profound implications with regard to understanding the weight-bearing tissues, as will next be described.

Calcification of Cartilage. Bone, as will be described in the next chapter, can bear great amounts of weight because its organic intercellular substance becomes thoroughly impregnated with calcium salts which makes it something like reinforced concrete. Even though they are surrounded by this calcified intercellular substance, the cells of bone can remain alive because there are tiny little passageways through the intercellular substance by which they can receive nutrients. However, there are no such passageways in the intercellular substance of cartilage, so if its intercellular substance becomes impregnated with calcium salts it is no longer able to serve as a means for the diffusion of nutrients, because what was previously a water-containing gel becomes changed to a dense impermeable stonelike calcified material. As a result, as is shown in Figure 14-5, the chondrocytes of cartilage are shut off from nutrition and die when the intercellular substance around them becomes calcified.

The mechanism of calcification of cartilage or bone is complicated and is still not thoroughly understood. However, under normal conditions there are enough Ca and PO_4 ions in the tissue fluid that permeates cartilage intercellular substance for us to visualize that local increases in one or the other ion or increased alkalinity could cause the relatively insoluble $Ca_3(PO_4)_2$ to precipitate into the organic intercellular substance. As we shall see when we study bone, it is normal for the intercellular substance of cartilage that precedes the formation of bone in prenatal life to become calcified and die. It is also normal for cartilage that persists in the growing sites of long bone to become calcified and die. Indeed, calcification and death is the normal fate for most of the cartilage that forms in the body, as is illustrated on the right side of Figure 14-4. If cartilage does not become calcified at its regular rate in a growing child, the child suffers from a condition called rickets, which condition arises when the product obtained by multiplying the levels of calcium and phosporus in the blood together falls below a certain level, below which calcium phosphate does not precipitate or is not precipitated from tissue fluid into intercellular substance. Another point is that the calcification of the intercellular substance of cartilage is almost always normally associated with the chondrocytes attaining such a large size they are said to be hypertrophied (Fig. 14-4, c and d). It was shown long ago that when they become this large they secrete an enzyme, *alkaline phosphatase,* which it is known can split certain phosphate-containing compounds to liberate free phosphate ions. However, it is not certain that there are compounds of this nature available at the site where calcification occurs so that enough extra PO_4 ions would become available to induce precipitation. Nevertheless, there is such a general association between alkaline phosphatase and normal calcification in the body it seems that this enzyme must play some role in the calcification of intercellular substance which normally follows its secretion by hypertrophied chondrocytes.

The phenomenon of calcification will be considered further in the next chapter. How the interstitial growth of cartilage and the calcification and death of cartilage are indispensable for the development and longitudinal

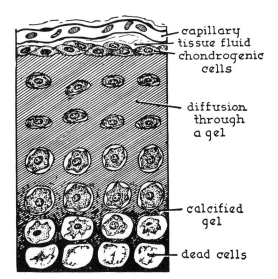

FIG. 14-5. Diagram of a section of hyaline cartilage. A capillary which forms tissue fluid is shown outside the limits of the cartilage. For the cells of the cartilage to be nourished, substances dissolved in tissue fluid must diffuse through the gelled intercellular substances of the cartilage to deeply buried cells. If the intercellular substance becomes calcified, as is indicated in the lower part of the diagram (black), diffusion cannot occur, and the cells die. (Ham, A. W.: J. Bone Joint Surg., *34-A:* *701*)

growth of bones will also be explained in the next chapter.

ELASTIC CARTILAGE

Although hyaline cartilage is elastic to some degree, it is not as elastic as cartilage that contains considerable numbers of elastic fibers in its intercellular substance. Some sites—for example, the external ear and epiglottis—require a tissue that is at once stiff and yet elastic, and in these elastic cartilage is found. While similar to hyaline cartilage, its intercellular substance, in addition to collagen fibers and chondroitin sulfate, contains elastic fibers scattered throughout it (Fig. 14-6).

FIBROCARTILAGE

This has already been mentioned and illustrated in Figure 14-2.

The Grafting of Cartilage—Absence of the Homograft Reaction

Two tissues commonly transplanted by plastic surgeons are skin and cartilage. Skin transplanted from

elastic fibers
in intercellular subst.

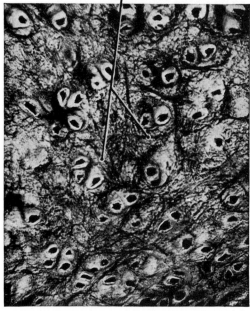

Fig. 14-6. Low-power photomicrograph of a section cut through the external ear. Elastic fibers may be seen as dark fine lines in the intercellular substance.

out its being gradually absorbed, *its cells must continue to live.* Grafts of dead cartilage eventually become resorbed. Even autografts of cartilage sometimes become resorbed in part; it is now thought that this is due to the fact that the graft bed at the sites where resorption occurs does not furnish enough nutrient that can diffuse through the intercellular substance to keep the chondrocytes of the graft alive. Cartilage grafts must be placed in beds that will provide nutrients for the chondrocytes of the graft. If this is done, it has been found that as a general rule homografts will survive for long periods of time.

The unique feature of cartilage that permits homografts to survive is that its cells live by diffusion through intercellular substance that probably prevents any antigenic features of the cells being known to the body and, furthermore, would keep any antibodies or killer cells from coming in contact with its constituent cells.

The repair of cartilage is considered in Chapter 16.

References and Other Reading

CARTILAGE REFERENCES OTHER THAN THOSE ON CALCIFICATION

Amprino, R.: Uptake of S^{35} in the differentiation and growth of cartilage and bone. *In* Wolstenholme, G. E. W., and O'Connor, C. M. (eds.): Ciba Foundation Symposium on Bone Structure and Metabolism. p. 89. London, J. & A. Churchill, 1956.

Bélanger, L. F.: Autoradiographic studies of the formation of the organic matrix of cartilage, bone and the tissues of teeth. *In* Wolstenholme, G. E. W., and O'Connor, C. M. (eds.): Ciba Foundation Symposium on Bone Structure and Metabolism. p. 75. London, J. & A. Churchill, 1956.

Benninghoff, A.: Form und Bau der Gelenkknorpel in ihren Beziehungen zur Funktion, Z. Zellforsch., 2:783, 1925.

Fell, H. B.: Skeletal development in tissue culture. *In* Bourne, G. H. (ed.): The Biochemistry and Physiology of Bone. p. 401. New York, Academic Press, 1956.

Gibson, Thomas: The transplantation of cartilage. *In* Porter, K. A. (ed.): The College of Pathologists Symposium on Tissue and Organ Transplantation. Tavistock Square, London, British Medical Association, 1967.

Laskin, D. M., Sarnat, B. G., and Bain, J. A.: Respiration and anaerobic glycolysis of transplanted cartilage. Proc. Soc. Exp. Biol. Med., 79:474, 1952.

Martin, A. V. W.: Fine structure of cartilage matrix. *In* Randall, J. T., and Jackson, S. F. (eds.): Nature and Structure of Collagen. p. 129. New York, Academic Press, 1953.

Pritchard, J. J.: A cytological and histochemical study of bone and cartilage formation in the rat. J. Anat., 86:259, 1952.

Robinson, R. A., and Cameron, D. A.: Electron microscopy of cartilage and bone matrix at the distal epiphyseal line of the femur in the newborn infant. J. Biophys. Biochem. Cytol. (Suppl.), 2:253, 1956.

Scott, B. L., and Pease, D. C.: Electron microscopy of the epiphyseal apparatus. Anat. Rec., 126:465, 1956.

See also References and Other Reading for Chapter 16.

one person to another (a homograft or allograft) is almost invariably rejected, and so for skin to be transplanted with any hope of a permanent take, it is necessary to use autografts. Fortunately this can be done in such a way that an individual ends up with skin in the site from which the graft was removed and also has skin in the site to which it was transplanted, as will be described when we deal with skin in Chapter 20.

The grafting of cartilage is different from the grafting of skin in two main ways. A person has a good deal of skin that can be used for grafts, but a person does not have much cartilage. So if a nose or an ear has to be reconstructed using cartilage as the supporting tissue, there is not much material to be drawn on for autografts. This led, many years ago, to attempts to use cartilage obtained from people who had just died for grafts in people who needed reconstructive surgery. It might be thought that such grafts, being homografts, would be destroyed by the homograft reaction. However, it was found that the cartilage in some homografts survived. This is the other way grafts of cartilage differ from those of skin.

Before considering why homografts of cartilage, in contrast to skin grafts, can survive, we should point out that for any kind of cartilage graft to persist with-

CALCIFICATION OF CARTILAGE

Bélanger, L. F.: The entry of CA^{45} into the skin and other soft tissues of the rat: An autoradiographic and spodographic study. J. Histochem. Cytochem., *5:*65, 1957.

Bourne, G. H.: Phosphatase and calcification. *In* The Biochemistry and Physiology of Bone. ed. 2, vol. 2. New York, Academic Press, 1972.

Dixon, T. F., and Perkins, H. R.: The chemistry of calcification. *In* Bourne, G. H. (ed.): The Biochemistry and Physiology of Bone. p. 287. New York, Academic Press, 1956.

Gutman, A. B., and Yu, T. F.: Concept of the role of enzymes in endochondral calcification. *In* Reifenstein, E. C., Jr. (ed.): Trans. of the Second Conference on Metabolic Interrelations. p. 167. New York, Macy, 1950.

————: A further consideration of the effects of beryllium salts on in vitro calcification of cartilage. *In* Reifenstein, E. C., Jr. (ed.): Trans. of the Third Conference on Metabolic Interrelations. p. 90. New York, Macy, 1951.

————: Further studies of the relation between glycogenolysis and calcification in cartilage. *In* Reifenstein, E. C., Jr. (ed.): Trans. of the First Conference on Metabolic Interrelations. p. 11. New York, Macy, 1949.

Hass, G. M.: Pathological calcification. *In* Bourne, G. H. (ed.): The Biochemistry and Physiology of Bone. p. 767. New York, Academic Press, 1956.

Rathbun, J. C.: Hypophosphatasia, a new developmental anomaly. Am. J. Dis. Child., *75:*822, 1948.

Robison, R.: The Significance of Phosphoric Esters in Metabolism. New York, New York University Press, 1932.

Wells, H. G.: Chemical Pathology. ed. 5. Philadelphia, W. B. Saunders, 1925.

See also References for Chapter 16.

15 Bone

In order to take advantage in the study of bone of what has been learned about cartilage in the previous chapter, we shall first compare and contrast certain features of these two tissues.

Some Similarities Between Cartilage and Bone

Bone resembles cartilage in the respect that it consists chiefly of intercellular substance and its constituent cells, like the chondrocytes of cartilage, live in little lacunae (OS in LAC in Fig. 15-1) within the intercellular substance (I.S. in Fig. 15-1) where they are termed osteocytes (Fig. 15-1). Compare Figures 15-1 and 14-3.

Bone also resembles cartilage (except articular car-tilage) in that the outer free surface of a bone is covered with a membrane that is the counterpart of the perichondrium that covers cartilage. In bone the membrane is called *periosteum* (Fig. 15-1). Like the perichondrium (Fig. 14-3) it has two main layers, an outer and an inner. The outer is not very thick and consists of dense, irregularly arranged connective tissue which contains some fibroblasts; this layer is termed the fibrous layer (Fig. L. in Fig. 15-1), and, just as the deeper layer of the perichondrium contains chondrogenic cells, the deeper layer of the periosteum contains osteogenic cells; the layer containing them is termed the osteogenic layer (OS.L. in Fig. 15-1). Osteogenic cells are flattened, spindle-shaped cells with

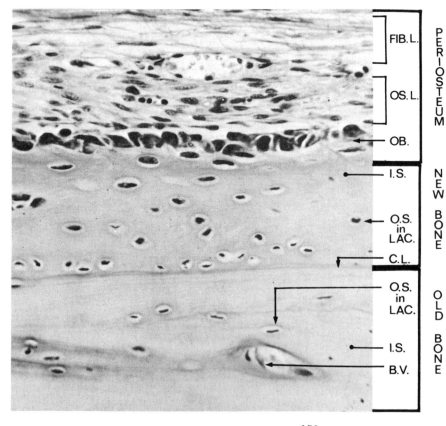

FIG. 15-1. Photomicrograph of a longitudinal section of a rabbit's rib close to a fracture that had been healing for a short time. During this time the osteogenic cells of the periosteum have proliferated and some have differentiated into osteoblasts which have laid down a layer of new bone on the original bone that was fractured. Three layers are labeled at the right: periosteum, new bone and old bone. Within the periosteum the fibrous layer is labeled FIB.L., the osteogenic layer, OS.L., and the layer of osteoblasts, OB. Within the layer of new bone the intercellular substance is labeled I.S., an osteocyte in a lacuna is labeled O.S. in LAC., and the cementing line between the new bone and the old is labeled C.L. Within the old bone intercellular substance is labeled I.S., an osteocyte in a lacuna, O.S. in LAC., and a blood vessel in a canal is labeled B.V.

no distinctive morphology but, as we shall see, with considerable potentiality (OS.L. in Fig. 15-1).

Like cartilage, bone can grow by the appositional growth mechanism. In cartilage this mechanism depends on chondrogenic cells of the perichondrium multiplying, with some of their numbers differentiating into cartilage cells, in which process they surround themselves with intercellular substance which thus adds to the bulk of the cartilage (Fig. 14-3). In bone the process is similar in most respects but somewhat different in others. First, for bone to grow by the appositional mechanism the osteogenic cells of the deep layer of the periosteum must proliferate (this is shown very diagrammatically in Fig. 15-2, A and B). Next, those closer to the bone surface differentiate into what are termed *osteoblasts* (OB in Fig. 15-1). With the LM these appear as relatively large cells characterized by an abundance of cytoplasm that is colored a deep blue in H and E sections (Fig. 15-1); this staining reaction is due to the cytoplasm of osteoblasts containing a great deal of rER which is responsible for the osteoblasts being able to synthesize and secrete the organic intercellular substance of bone around themselves. When they finish this they are entombed in the lacunae in intercellular substance they have produced (Fig. 15-2, C) at which stage of development they have become *osteocytes*. By this appositional growth mechanism new layers of bone are added to bone surfaces; this is how the new bone formed in Figure 15-1 (NEW BONE). A line called a water mark or cementing line can usually be detected between a new layer and the bone that was formed previously (C.L. in Fig. 15-1).

Some Differences Between Cartilage and Bone

Unlike cartilage, which can grow by an interstitial growth mechanism (see Fig. 14-3) as well as by the appositional mechanism, bone is limited to growing by only the appositional mechanism. Note that in Figure 15-2 the nails never become farther apart. It is only by means of new bone being added to pre-existing surfaces that the bony skeleton of a fetus becomes the skeleton of an adult.

A second and very important difference between cartilage and bone is that under normal conditions the organic intercellular substance of bone begins to become calcified as soon as it is formed. The intercellular substance of cartilage, it will be recalled, does not become calcified unless chondrocytes become hypertrophied and begin to secrete alkaline phosphatase. The fact that the intercellular substance of bone normally begins to calcify as soon as it is formed has

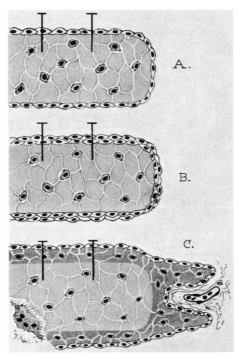

Fig. 15-2. Diagrams showing that bone cannot grow by the interstitial mechanism, but only by appositional growth, which requires new layers of bone to be deposited on surfaces. (A) This shows that a trabecula of bone is covered on all surfaces with a layer of osteogenic cells. (B) This shows that the surface cells can proliferate so as to increase their numbers. (C) This shows that the innermost layer of surface cells can form a new layer of bone by secreting organic intercellular substance about them, and that the surface still remains covered by a continuous layer of osteogenic cells except as sites of resorption where osteoclasts are present. One is shown at the lower left corner. At the right end, the diagram illustrates how new bone can be laid down on surfaces, extending the length of a trabecula to surround a capillary, so that the cells of the newly formed bone will have a source of nutrition. (Ham, A. W.: J. Bone Joint Surg., *34-A:*701)

some very important consequences which will now be described.

1. Unlike the hypertrophied cartilage cells that are shut off from nutrients when the intercellular substances surrounding them become calcified, the osteocytes of calcified bone continue to live when the intercellular substance about them is rendered impermeable by its becoming impregnated with calcium salts. The osteocytes survive because the intercellular substance of bone is permeated with tiny little canals, called canaliculi (light in Fig. 15-2), which contain the deli-

cate cytoplasmic processes of the osteocytes together with a certain amount of tissue fluid. The canaliculi that radiate from one lacunae in bone join with those that radiate from others and the canaliculi from lacunae that are close to a free surface of bone where there are capillaries, extend to and open out on that surface (Fig. 15-2, C, *right*). Hence tissue fluid formed from the capillaries close to bone surfaces is in communication with that in canaliculi. Accordingly, the canalicular mechanism provides a means whereby nutrients can diffuse from capillaries to osteocytes that are otherwise surrounded by calcified intercellular substance. Likewise, waste products can diffuse from osteocytes to bone surfaces in the other direction (Fig. 15-2, C, *right*).

2. The distance, however, over which osteocytes can be kept alive by the canalicular mechanism is limited and hence even what appears in the gross to be solid (compact) bone will be seen under the microscope to be a relatively vascular tissue containing enough capillaries so that no osteocyte (according to measurements made by the author on the radius of a dog) is generally more than from one tenth to one fifth of a millimeter away from a capillary. Since capillaries do not bore holes into dense bone, this means that dense bone must be formed around pre-existing capillaries. One way this could occur is shown at the right side of Fig. 15-2, C. The usual way it occurs in growing bones will be described shortly.

3. The next point to make in the present context is that if bone intercellular substance begins to calcify as soon as it is formed, it is obvious, that unlike cartilage, bone cannot grow by means of the interstitial mechanism, for it would be impossible for a stone-like intercellular substance to be expanded from within. But even if its intercellular substance did not become properly calcified, as sometimes happens under conditions of an abnormal mineral metabolism, bone cannot grow by the interstitial mechanism because osteocytes cannot divide. Even osteoblasts are so highly specialized for function that they, too, have lost their ability to divide, as Pritchard's work showed so long ago; this has been more recently verified, for it was shown using labeled thymidine that when osteogenic cells become osteoblasts their DNA is rarely duplicated.

The fact that solid bone substance cannot be expanded from within by an interstitial growth mechanism was shown over a century ago by driving two metallic pins into the shaft of the bone of a growing animal and finding that after the bone had attained full growth the distance between the pins had not changed; this is shown in the diagram (Fig. 15-2). Somewhat later we shall describe how it is possible

for a long bone with a joint at each, or even one end, to increase in length by only the appositional method of growth. But first some more details about bone.

How Canaliculi Are Formed. For bone to form anywhere osteoblasts must be present. As will be explained later, the origin of osteoblasts can be traced in the embryo to mesenchymal cells. Perhaps the easiest place to see where this happens is where certain bones of the skull will later appear. In a central point in an area where a bone will develop, certain mesenchymal cells develop connecting cytoplasmic processes as is shown at the top of Figure 15-3, and as these former mesenchymal cells differentiate into osteoblasts in this little area they begin to synthesize and secrete the intercellular substance of bone around their cell bodies and their processes so that they become surrounded by the organic intercellular substance of bone. In this procedure the cytoplasmic processes of the osteoblasts serve the same purpose as molds serve when metals are cast; for when the organic intercellular substance "sets" and becomes calcified (Fig. 15-3, *middle* and *bottom*) the intercellular substance is riddled with tiny canals (canaliculi) which connect the lacunae, in which the osteoblasts (which have now become osteocytes) reside, with each other and with the surface of the bone.

As was shown in Figures 15-1 and 15-2, most bone is formed, layer by layer, on surfaces by osteoblasts which on that surface bury themselves by the intercellular substance they secrete. The canaliculi that form around their processes and extend to the surface of each new layer of bone that forms permit tissue fluid from capillaries at that surface to permeate the canaliculi and this allows nutrients to reach the cells that lie within the calcified intercellular substance of bone.

Canaliculi cannot be seen in the usual H and E section of bone that is studied in the laboratory such as the one illustrated in Figure 15-1, for reasons that will become apparent in the following.

Special Types of Preparations Are Required for a Rounded-out Study of Bone

Since bone is calcified, it is difficult to slice it into thin sections. Accordingly, for routine work, pieces of bone are decalcified before they are dehydrated and embedded in paraffin for sectioning.

Pieces of bone are commonly decalcified in solutions of acids, such as nitric or formic or chelating agents. For details see books on histologic technic.

Decalcified bone contains both its cells and most of the organic intercellular substance that its cells had

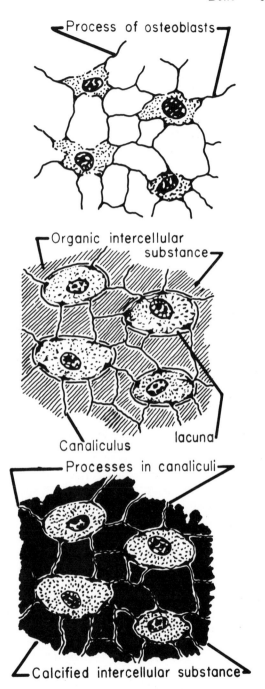

Fɪɢ. 15-3. Diagrams to show how bone forms. As shown in the top picture, special cells called osteoblasts, must be present before bone is made. The osteoblasts always have cytoplasmic arms that contact or connect with one another. The osteoblasts secrete the organic intercellular substance of bone both around their cell bodies and around the cytoplasmic arms that extend from the cell bodies. During the time when the intercellular substance is being secreted, the cytoplasmic arms serve as molds for tiny passageways called canaliculi; these passageways remain to provide communication between adjacent osteoblasts and the surface on which the bone is forming. When the osteoblasts are completely surrounded by the intercellular substance they have secreted, they are termed osteocytes. The organic intercellular substance then becomes impregnated with calcium salts and so rendered stonelike. However, the osteocytes entombed in the stonelike intercellular substance are not cut off from oxygen and nutrition, because the canaliculi provide a means whereby materials can be transported between surfaces and the cells buried in the calcified intercellular substance, provided that the distance over which transport has to be effected is not very great.

secreted around themselves, but the mineral that formerly permeated the organic intercellular substance is dissolved away. Hence a decalcified bone (and it is possible to decalcify a whole bone) has the same form as a normal calcified bone (Fig. 15-4, *bottom*). The great difference between a decalcified bone and a calcified bone is not in its gross appearance but in the fact that the decalcified bone cannot bear weight; indeed, a decalcified bone is so flexible it can be tied into a knot, as is shown in Figure 15-4.

Paraffin sections of decalcified bone can be cut and stained with H and E like ordinary tissues. Such sections permit the study of the cells and at least most of the organic intercellular substance of bone. However, the lumens of canaliculi are by no means readily apparent in such sections (see Fig. 15-1). Possibly the decalcifying solution causes the collagen of the intercellular substance to swell enough to obliterate their lumens to such an extent they become too narrow to be resolved with the LM. Their sites, however, can at least sometimes be indicated in decalcified sections by special staining, possibly because their immediate lining contains enough chondroitin sulfate to bind certain basic stains (such as those in blood stains). However, to see canaliculi in bone with the LM it is usual to study sections of undecalcified bone. There are two main ways by which sections can be prepared from undecalcified bone.

The older way is to cut thin slices of calcified bone with a fine saw and then grind them down on a stone until they are thin enough to transmit light. Such sections are termed *ground bone sections*. Ground bone sections are not suited for study of cell detail but since mineral is still present in them, the intercellular substance remains rigid. As a result, the canaliculi remain open and stand out as dark lines and appear as in

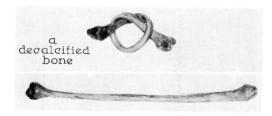

Fig. 15-4. This illustration shows that although a decalcified bone closely resembles a calcified bone, it may be tied into knots, as is illustrated in the upper picture.

Figure 15-5. Furthermore, the lacunae which contain the osteocytes can also be seen as dark ovoid cavities (Fig. 15-5). The layered nature of bone can also be seen in such sections.

By using special hard embedding media and special kinds of microtomes adapted for heavy work, it is possible to cut sections of bone without the material having been decalcified. This technic has permitted many kinds of studies to be made that were not previously possible. Several will be described later in this chapter. It is even possible to cut sections of undecalcified bone that are thin enough to study with the EM as will be apparent shortly.

The Intercellular Substance of Bone

The intercellular substance of bone consists of two fundamentally different components. One is organic and the other inorganic. The intercellular substance is often referred to as *bone matrix*. Strictly speaking, this word should be used to denote the organic component because it means roughly a basic material to which something else can be added, with the something else in this instance being mineral. However, matrix is often used to denote the complex of organic and inorganic material that surrounds osteocytes.

The term *ossification* refers to osteoblasts evolving in some part of the body and secreting the unique organic intercellular substance of bone. The term *calcification* refers to the deposition of calcium salts in a tissue which, however, is not necessarily bone or cartilage. It is normal for the organic matrix of bone to become calcified but it is abnormal if the wall of an artery becomes calcified; thus there is such a thing as normal calcification and pathological calcification. Ossification can occur under conditions of an abnormal calcium metabolism without its being accompanied by calcification; thus there is such a thing as *uncalcified bone* or, as it is often termed, *osteoid tissue*. Uncalcified bone is of course different from decalcified bone.

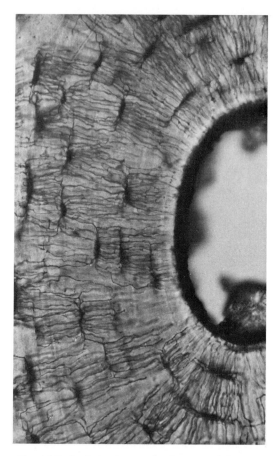

Fig. 15-5. A photomicrograph of a ground bone section. The lacunae in which the osteocytes reside are dark flattened oval structures. The fine lines connecting these are canaliculi. The canaliculi extend to the empty canal on the right. In life this contained blood vessels that supplied tissue fluid to the canaliculi. (Preparation by H. Whittaker)

Uncalcified bone can develop in the body as described above but decalcified bone can only be produced in the laboratory by using decalcifying agents on bone that is being prepared for sectioning. The reason for this is that after bone has become thoroughly calcified, the only mechanism whereby the body can remove the calcium from it removes the organic intercellular substance as well. The process by which this is done is known as *bone resorption* and this is almost as common a phenomenon in the body as bone formation. Bone resorption occurs on the surfaces of bony structures and is brought about through the agency of large multinucleated cells called *osteoclasts* (Fig. 15-10) as will be described in detail in due course.

Chemical Composition of Intercellular Substance. Studies on calcified bone have shown that by dry weight around 76 to 77 percent of bone substance is inorganic and the balance organic. The organic material in turn is 88 to 89 percent collagen. Various studies on the collagen of bone generally, but not always, seem to indicate that it is no different from the collagen of ordinary connective tissue which is formed by fibroblasts. The collagen of bone is formed by osteoblasts by the same mechanism described in connection with fibroblasts in Chapter 9. The organic intercellular substance of bone contains in addition to collagen some sulfated mucopolysaccharide and some glycoprotein as well as some other materials. Weinstock has described in detail the recent knowledge on the carbohydrates of matrix and their relation to protein (*see* Other Reading). Since bone contains cells and blood vessels, there are problems associated with attempting to procure pure intercellular substance for analysis. For those wishing detailed information about the composition of the organic intercellular substance, an extensive review by E. M. Herring is available (*see* Other Reading).

Osteoblasts and Osteocytes. The Formation and Calcification of the Organic Intercellular Substance

The organic intercellular substance of bone is synthesized and secreted by osteoblasts. Seen with the LM in routine H and E sections, osteoblasts commonly appear as large blue cells in which it may be difficult to distinguish nucleus from cytoplasm (Fig. 15-1, OB) because both are basophilic and also because it is difficult to obtain perfect fixation of calcified bone and the decalcification procedures may cause some distortion and affect their staining. Hence, in routine H and E sections of bone, cellular detail is often not all that could be desired (as in Fig. 15-1). However, in good preparations the nucleus of an osteoblast can be seen to be eccentrically situated (Fig. 5-30) and the cytoplasm is extensive. Its basophilia is due to its substantial content of rER. A large negative Golgi can often be demonstrated close to the nucleus (Fig. 5-30). Osteoblasts are generally irregularly rounded in shape but they are sometimes drawn out in one direction so as to appear roughly fusiform.

Fine Structure of Osteoblasts. Since osteoblasts are secretory cells, their cytoplasm, as might be expected, is characterized by an extensive development of rER and Golgi stacks (Fig. 15-6). Their fine structure does not therefore differ materially from that of young fibroblasts. Indeed Weinstock and Leblond have recently shown that the pathway described for the synthesis and secretion of procollagen in the osteoblasts of the alveolar bone of the rat (Fig. 15-6) is much the same as was described in detail in connection with fibroblasts in Chapter 9 and illustrated in Figure 9-6.

As already noted, it is possible to prepare sections of undecalcified bone for study with the EM. Osteoblasts in such a section are shown in Figure 15-7. It is of course somewhat more difficult to demonstrate fine structure in such sections than in sections of decalcified bone such as Figure 15-6. However, it can be seen in Figure 15-7 that some osteoblasts are relatively elongated and that in such cells the nuclei tend to be at one end, the rER toward the other end and the Golgi in the middle. Sections of undecalcified bone have, however, the advantage of showing where material is deposited in the organic intercellular substance that the osteoblasts are secreting. The mineral is black and it is seen that it is not as dense close to the osteoblast as it is farther away. The organic intercellular substance farther away would have been formed sooner than that closer to the osteoblast and so it would have had more time to become thoroughly calcified. It is to be noted that the mineral as it is being deposited appears in the form of scattered granular-appearing deposits.

Osteocytes. When an osteoblast has surrounded itself with organic intercellular substance it becomes an osteocyte. In routine H and E sections little, if anything, more than their nuclei are seen in the ovoid lacunae in which they lie (Fig. 15-1, OS in LAC). The osteocytes and the lacunae in which they lie are larger in new bone than in older bone (Fig. 15-1), which suggests that young osteocytes add some intercellular substance to the walls of their lacunae for at least a brief period.

Fine Structure. This can be studied with the EM in thin sections of decalcified or calcified bone. Figure 15-8 is a low-power electron micrograph of an osteocyte in a decalcified section and it shows to advantage the processes of the osteocyte extending into canaliculi. It also shows two canaliculi cut in cross section in the intercellular substance; each contains a process.

Figure 15-9 shows an osteocyte in a section of undecalcified bone. Some rER and a few mitochondria can be seen in its cytoplasm.

In both types of preparation the osteocyte does not completely fill the lacuna in which it lies. Even if shrinkage accounts for the space between the cell body of the osteocyte and the lacuna, and the space between the walls of a canaliculus and the process it contains, the existence of a space of any extent indicates the existence of accommodation for tissue fluid at this site.

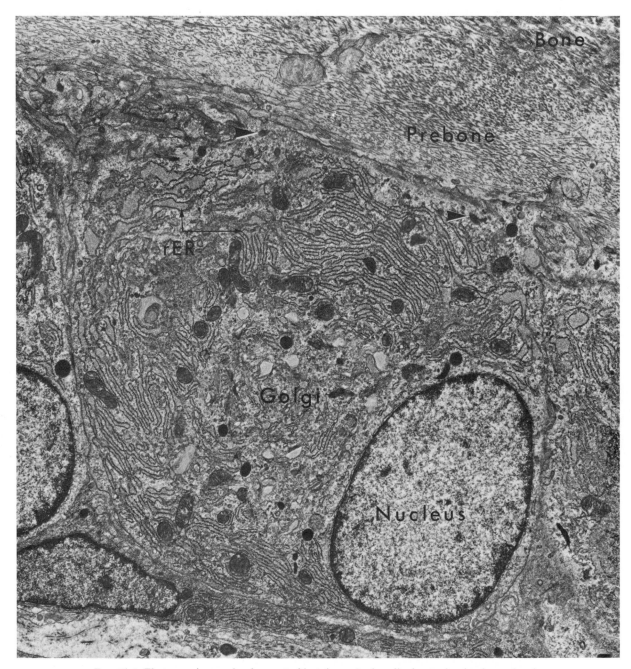

Fig. 15-6. Electron micrograph of an osteoblast from demineralized rat alveolar bone showing the arrangement of the organelles ($\times$ 12,000). Numerous collagen fibrils which these cells secrete are present in the adjacent prebone and bone (*upper right*). The procollagen, which is the precursor of the collagen fibrils, is carried within secretory granules (arrowheads) originating from the Golgi saccules. Procollagen is released into the prebone by fusion of the secretory granule with the apical plasma membrane of the cell. A portion of a cell of the type that gives rise to osteoblasts is seen at lower left. (Illustration courtesy of Melvyn Weinstock)

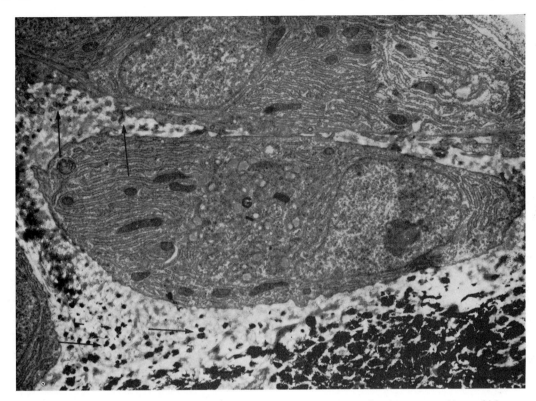

FIG. 15-7. Electron micrograph ($\times$ 7,600) of undecalcified bone showing an osteoblast which extends across the middle of the picture, and part of another above it. In the lower one a nucleus can be seen near its right end, a Golgi apparatus (G) in its central region, and many flattened rough-surfaced vesicles of endoplasmic reticulum at its left end. The vertical arrows point to cytoplasmic processes that extend off from the cell body and are cut in cross and oblique section. The horizontal arrows point to mineral deposits that are just forming. At the lower right the mineral is more dense. In the intercellular substance just below the nucleus some collagenic microfibrils with cross banding can be seen. (Preparation by B. Boothroyd and N. M. Hancox)

The Mechanism of Calcification of Bone

All aspects of this very complex subject are not as yet understood. The following account will be limited to what seems suitable for a student reader who will doubtless hear more about the subject in physiology, biochemistry and pathology courses. For those wishing more advanced reading some recent reviews are listed under "References and Other Reading."

The mineral with which bone matrix is impregnated in mature, fully calcified bone is believed to be at least mostly in the form of crystals of hydroxyapatite $(Ca_{10}(PO_4)_6(OH)_2)$. Their form has been described as needle-shaped, rodlike or tubular, around 30 to 50 Å in diameter and up to 600 Å long. There has been a great deal of study of the relation of the crystals to the collagen. It has been suggested that they lie linearly along the collagenic fibrils or even that crystals may form and lie within collagenic fibrils. If so, the most probable site would be in the gap regions (often called "holes") between the ends of the tropocollagen molecules that do not meet end-to-end in the dark segments of collagenic fibrils (see Gap region, Fig. 9-8).

In order to consider theories about how and why crystals of hydroxyapatite form in bone matrix, we must first discuss calcium and phosphorus metabolism briefly.

The mineral that is deposited in bone must be transported there by the bloodstream and then pass from capillaries into the tissue fluid so that the mineral dissolved in tissue fluid can be deposited in bone. Long ago it was believed that osteoblasts took up mineral salts and secreted these somehow in the form of particulate matter into the organic matrix. Actually with the development of modern methods there has been some further exploration of this possibility, but a recent radioautographic study of calcification in dentin

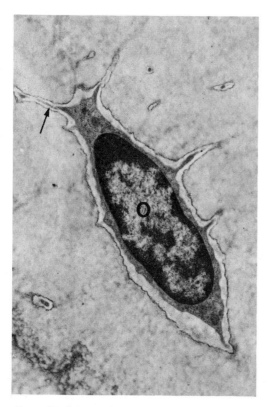

FIG. 15-8. Low-power electron micrograph of an osteocyte and its processes in a section of decalcified bone. The nucleus is indicated by O and an arrow points to a process in a canaliculus. Two processes in canaliculi cut in cross section can be seen, one near the upper right corner and the other toward the lower left corner. (From S. C. Luk and G. T. Simon)

by Munhoz and Leblond, in which they used semithin sections and radioactive calcium, revealed no label in odontoblasts but it did almost immediately reveal labeled calcium phosphate in the dentinal matrix. It therefore seems conclusive that insoluble calcium salts are not secreted as particulate matter into an organic matrix.

There is, moreover, long-standing evidence that osteoblasts or osteocytes are not essential for matrix to become calcified. The organic matrix of bone has in itself a physical or chemical proclivity for becoming calcified under conditions where other tissue components would remain uncalcified. Long ago Wells showed that dead uncalcified cartilage would become calcified if it was transplanted to some part of a body where it had access to tissue fluid. More particularly, Robison and his colleagues performed some very interesting experiments to show that calcification would proceed in the absence of living cells. They showed that if

slices of the growing zone of a long bone (to be described in detail presently), where calcification is normally occurring, were treated with an agent to kill its cells, the intercellular substance would not continue to calcify in suitable solutions of calcium salts. However, they found that the dead bone and cartilage would continue to calcify if the enzyme alkaline phosphatase was added to the solutions.

As already noted, chondrocytes secrete alkaline phosphatase when they become hypertrophied and this is when the organic intercellular substance around them becomes calcified. Osteoblasts produce abundant alkaline phosphatase. Indeed when a fractured bone is being repaired by the activity of many new osteo-

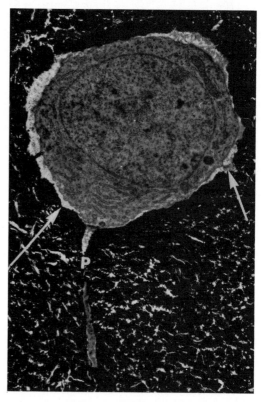

FIG. 15-9. Electron micrograph ($\times$ 7,500) of undecalcified section of bone, showing an osteocyte in its lacuna, which is surrounded by heavily calcified intercellular substance. The osteocyte has less cytoplasm than an osteoblast and fewer rough-surfaced vesicles. The arrows point to sites where cytoplasmic processes probably extend off from the main cell body but disappear from the substance of the section. However, one process is cut in longitudinal section for some little distance; this is labeled P. (Preparation by B. Boothroyd and N. M. Hancox)

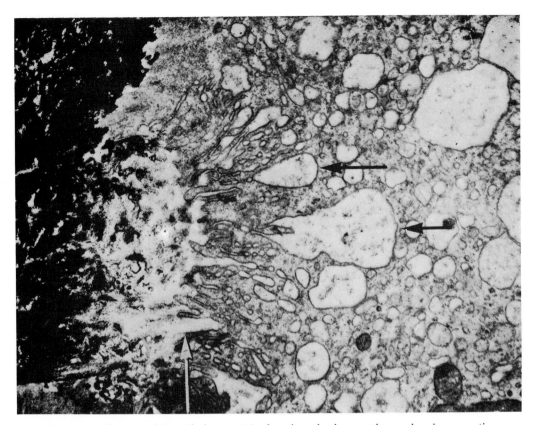

FIG. 15-14. Electron micrograph ($\times$ 20,000) of section of a bone surface undergoing resorption. Calcified bone appears black at the left. The main part of the picture is occupied by the cytoplasm of an osteoclast. Extending from the top to the bottom, in the middle of the picure, is the ruffled border of the osteoclast; this consists of complex folds and projections which abut on the bone at the left. Between the ruffled border of the osteoclast and the heavily calcified bone is an area where the calcium content is much less, which suggests that the osteoclast is dissolving or otherwise removing mineral from this area. Black granules of mineral can be seen in some of the large vesicles which are indicated by horizontal arrows, and which probably form because of the bottom of crypts being pinched off. In the original print a collagenic microfibril showing typical periodicity could be seen at the site indicated by the vertical arrow. (Preparation by B. Boothroyd and N. M. Hancox)

seen with the LM. The appearance of a fluffy border in a thicker section viewed with the LM would in our opinion be no more than a fuzzy fringe, and indeed that is the way the borders that most osteoclasts present to bone surfaces appear with the LM.

Theories of Mechanism of Resorption by Osteoclasts

In considering this matter it must be remembered that the resorption of bone involves the removal of both its mineral and its organic intercellular substance which, as already described, is mostly collagen.

There seem to be three possibilities (1) that osteoclasts act primarily by dissolving the mineral and secondarily by depolymerizing the organic constitu-

ents; (2) that they depolymerize the mucopolysaccharides and/or glycoproteins and that these are concerned in binding the mineral so that their dissolution leads to the freeing of mineral, and (3) that they act primarily on the collagen. In connection with these possibilities Hancox discussed several observations that have been made under various experimental conditions and show that osteoclasts are found not in association with osteoid tissue (uncalcified bone) but always in association with calcified bone and that for osteoid tissue to be resorbed it must first become calcified, whereupon osteoclasts do the work. Accordingly it seems most probable that the primary action of osteoclasts is on the mineral.

Obviously, the easiest way for osteoclasts to remove

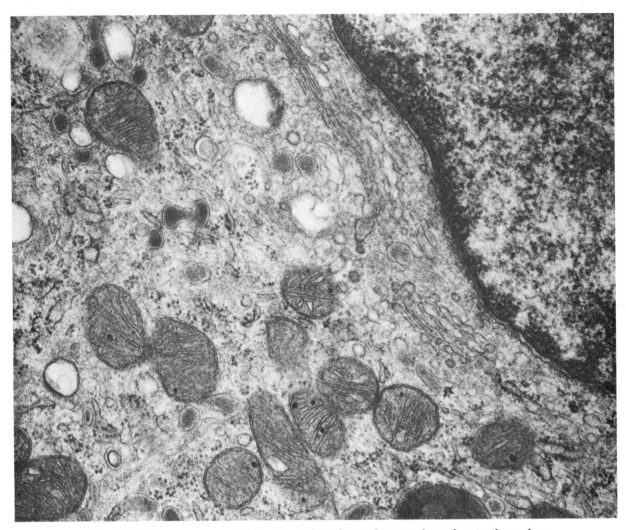

Fɪɢ. 15-15. Electron micrograph showing portion of osteoclast cytoplasm close to the nucleus, part of which is seen at the upper right. To the left of its envelope there is a good deal of Golgi material from which vesicles are leaving; most or at least many of these are probably primary lysosomes. Some free ribosomes are scattered about in little groups and a little rER is evident. The mitochondria are abundant in this region. (From Cameron, D. A.: The Ultrastructure of Bone. *In* Bourne, G. H. (ed.): The Physiology and Biochemistry of Bone. ed. 2, vol. 1. New York, Academic Press, 1972)

mineral would be to provide a sufficiently local acid environment at the surface of the fluffy border to cause the bone salts to act as a buffer does. In buffering an acid a calcium phosphate would become a much more soluble salt than it was before; for example, $CaHPO_4$ is many times more soluble than $Ca_3(PO_4)_2$. It has been suggested that precipitate observed between the villous folds or in the underlying vesicles (Fig. 15-14) in undecalcified sections could be explained not as phagocytosed insoluble salts but as

precipitates of a soluble salt caused by the action of the phosphate buffers used preparing the material for sectioning. How an osteoclast could provide a relatively acid environment at its surface is unsolved. Hancox has pointed out an interesting association in that both the cytoplasm of the parietal cells of the stomach (which secrete hydrochloric acid) and osteoclasts are commonly acidophilic. The former (Fig. 21-26) have a very complicated set of invaginations of the surface membrane which are concerned in the phenomenon of acid secretion, but whether or not the invaginations of the fluffy border of the osteoclasts could serve a similar purpose is not known.

Several enzymes have been shown to be present in the lysosomes of osteoclasts. Hancox observed a long time ago that osteoclasts in cultures liquefied fibrin clots, which suggested the presence of proteolytic enzymes in them. It is established that β glucuronidase is one of the enzymes; this enzyme could conceivably play a role in resorption by affecting the mucopolysaccharides of the organic matrix.

As will be described at a more appropriate time, the hormone produced by the parathyroid gland exerts a profound effect on osteoclasts, activating those already in existence and stimulating the formation of more. To discuss this matter further we must next consider the problems of the origin of osteoclasts and to do this we must describe the type of cell that covers and lines the surfaces of bones.

Osteogenic Cells. The exterior of a bone is covered with a connective tissue membrane called the periosteum (Fig. 15-1) and the interior of the bone is lined with a primarily cellular membrane called the *endosteum*. The cells which we wish to discuss here are what we term osteogenic cells and other authors often term *osteoprogenitor cells*. Osteogenic cells are normally found apposed to the bone surface in the deep layer of resting periosteum, and they also comprise the endosteum where they are also apposed to the bone surface. During the growing period the osteogenic cells of the periosteum proliferate and the deepest ones give rise to osteoblasts (Fig. 15-1) which add new bone to the surface, which accounts for growth in width. In the endosteum the appearances suggest that the osteogenic lining cells give rise to the osteoclasts which erode the inner surface of a shaft so as to enlarge the marrow cavity. In sites of erosion the membrane of osteogenic cells that lines the bone surface is thus interrupted by osteoclasts taking the place here and there of the osteogenic cells previously at these sites. The endosteal membrane may also give rise to osteoblasts because some bone is sometimes formed on this surface as well, although resorption is the rule.

In attempting to describe the morphology of an osteogenic cell we encounter the same problem as was encountered in connection with attempts to describe the morphology of the stem cell of blood cells (the CFU); for we cannot expect the cytoplasm of a stem cell that can give rise to different lines of cells to display any particular complement of organelles that would denote which line of cells it was going to form. All that we know about its morphology is that on a resting bone surface there are thin flattened cells that

abut directly on the surface of the underlying bone. What we know about the potentiality of at least some of these cells is learned by finding out what they do during growth, in the repair of fractures and in their transplantation. Information on these matters is gained by following their behavior under these conditions.

Behavior of Osteogenic Cells of Periosteum During Growth. As bones grow in width it is comparatively easy to find mitotic figures in the deeper part of the periosteum at the site where growth is occurring. However, when a cell is in mitosis, it is difficult to decide whether it is—for example—an osteogenic cell or an osteoblast. As was described in Chapter 3, it is easy to settle a question such as this by using labeled thymidine and making radioautographs. By using single doses of labeled thymidine several investigators [Kember (1960), Hunt and Poynter (1961), Tonna and Cronkite (1961, 1962) and Owen (1963)] showed that it was the osteogenic cells (sometimes called by other names such as osteoprogenitor cells or preosteoblasts) in growing bones that took up label and that only later (in almost all instances) did label appear in osteoblasts, so that the general conclusion was that for all practical purposes osteoblasts themselves do not duplicate their DNA and undergo mitosis. Osteoblasts (with possibly a few exceptions) become labeled only because a *labeled* osteogenic cell differentiates into an osteoblast. When the labeled osteoblast becomes an osteocyte, the osteocyte is labeled.

Behavior of Osteogenic Cells of Periosteum After a Fracture. An informative way to study what happens when resting periosteum becomes active is to examine sections taken from, for example, a rabbit's rib 24 hours or so after the rib is fractured. As is shown in Figure 15-16, there is a great proliferation of the cells in the deeper (osteogenic) layer of the periosteum close to the site of the fracture. Many mitotic figures can be seen among them (arrows). What is particularly informative about the study of osteogenic cells in the repair of a fracture, however, is that a few days later the cells that have proliferated, in addition to differentiating into osteoblasts and bone cells, also differentiate into chondroblasts and chondrocytes (Fig. 15-17). This was pointed out by the author in 1930 who then suggested that whether osteogenic cells differentiated to form bone or cartilage depended on whether their environment was vascular or nonvascular. In other words, close to the capillaries they differentiate into osteoblasts but away from capillaries they differentiate into chondrocytes. Tissue culture experiments by Bassett and Hermann in 1961 showed that oxygen tension was the determining factor with

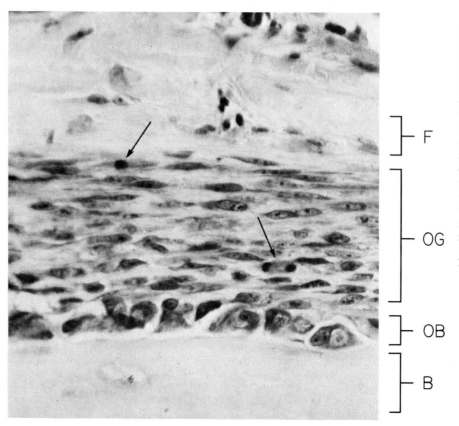

Fig. 15-16. Photomicrograph showing what happens in the periosteum shortly after and close to a fracture. The fibrous layer (F) is lifted away from the bone (B) by the greatly thickened osteogenic layer (OG) in which osteogenic cells are proliferating. Mitotic figures are indicated by arrows. At the bone surface the osteogenic cells have differentiated into osteoblasts which will soon form a new layer of bone on the surface on which they lie. (Ham, A. W., and Harris, W. R.: *In* Bourne's Biochemistry and Physiology of Bone. ed. 2, vol. 3. New York, Academic Press, 1971)

regard to whether certain cells with which they were working formed bone or cartilage.

The fact that osteogenic cells can differentiate so as to form both cartilage and bone has recently been confirmed by Tonna and Pentel who labeled the osteogenic cells of 30-week-old mice by giving them 4 injections of tritiated thymidine. They then fractured one femur of each animal and found that 7 days later the label was present in both the cartilage cells and the osteoblasts and new bone cells that had developed in the new callus tissue that had formed around the site of the fracture from the labeled cells.

Are Osteoclasts Derived from Osteogenic Cells? The foregoing indicates the osteogenic cells of the periosteum to be a type of stem cell which has proliferative capacity and whose differentiation can be directed by an environmental factor to form either bone or cartilage. The questions now arise (1) whether or not osteogenic cells have the potentiality to also form osteoclasts, and (2) if there is any environmental factor that induces their differentiation along the latter line.

Since mitosis does not occur in osteoclasts, the question of their origin boils down to the kind or kinds of cells that fuse to become osteoclasts. Since they make their appearance on bone surfaces previously covered with osteogenic cells and/or osteoblasts, it has been commonly assumed through the years that osteogenic cells and/or osteoblasts fuse together to form them, at the sites where they are seen. As a result of their eroding bone at these sites, osteocytes (previously in the bone that is eroded) may be released from their lacunae, and it is thought that these would melt into the osteoclast responsible for their liberation, with their nuclei adding to those of their liberator.

That osteogenic and osteoblasts are at least the usual source of osteoblasts seems to be supported by numerous experiments that have been performed using labeled thymidine to trace their origin. After an animal is given tritiated thymidine, osteogenic cells are the first to become labeled. Subsequently, after there has been time for some to differentiate into osteoblasts, label appears in osteoblasts and later still in the osteocytes of the new bone that forms. But particularly on the inner surfaces of a bone where osteoclasts are prone to form, at about the same time that label would begin to show up in osteoblasts, some osteoclasts will show the occasional labeled nucleus among their other unlabeled nuclei. Tonna and Cronkite have shown, however, that after the continuous administration of labeled thymidine over a sufficiently long period, all of the nuclei seen in the osteoclasts then seen may be labeled.

All of the above would fit with the concept that, since thymidine labels the cells of bone surfaces that have proliferative capacity, it labels osteogenic cells. Since label is found later in the nuclei of both osteo-blasts and osteoclasts (neither of which can undergo mitosis), the label that appears in their nuclei must have been incorporated into those nuclei when they were the nuclei of osteogenic cells. It would, therefore, follow that labeled nuclei of osteoclasts must be de-rived from those of labeled osteogenic cells. Since, however, osteoclasts form as a result of cell fusions and since, by the time labeled nuclei appear in osteo-clasts in an animal given tritiated thymidine, osteo-blast nuclei have also become labeled, some of the labeled nuclei in an osteoclast could be derived from labeled osteoblasts that participated in the cell fusions that produced the osteoclast.

Monocytes and Macrophages As a Possible Source of Osteoclasts. There is, however, some evi-dence that osteogenic cells and/or osteoblasts are not the only cells that can fuse to form osteoclasts. For example, we have found what appear with the LM to be typical osteoclasts forming around dead bone chips that were transplanted to muscle. Since pieces of dead bone in muscle would be foreign bodies, it is not sur-prising that foreign body giant cells originating from monocytes and/or macrophages would develop beside them. The surprising feature about them is, however, that what would be termed foreign body giant cells in association with any other kind of foreign body, in association with bone develop a typical striated border (Figs. 15-12 and 15-13), a fact that suggests strongly that the striated borders seen with the EM on osteo-clasts is a feature of the bone and not of the osteo-clast, as has already been emphasized.

The facts that cells having, at the level of the LM, the morphology of osteoclasts can arise in association with dead bone transplanted to muscle and that such cells must arise from monocytes or macrophages, to-gether with the fact that monocytes are produced in bone marrow, might seem to suggest the possibility of osteoclasts in living bone developing from the mono-cytes of marrow instead of from the osteogenic cells and osteoblasts that normally cover and line bone sur-faces. Reasons will be given shortly that detract from this view. But to explain these reasons we must first comment on how certain hormones affect the cells con-cerned with the formation and resorption of bone.

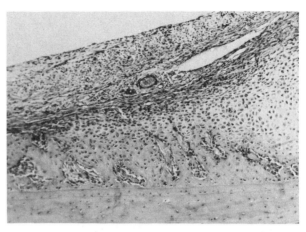

Fig. 15-17. Photomicrograph of a longitudinal section of a rabbit's rib close to a fracture (that is to the right) and after healing for 5 days. Over a period of a few days the osteogenic cell proliferation shown in Figure 15-16 has continued and toward the left the osteogenic cells have differentiated into osteocytes to form bony trabeculae that are cemented to the bone of the rib. This area is vascular—see blood vessels between the trabeculae. Toward the right the osteogenic cells have differentiated into chondrocytes, thus forming a mass of cartilage which has no blood vessels in it. (Ham, A. W., and Harris, W. R.: *In* Bourne's Biochemistry and Physi-ology of Bone. ed. 2, vol. 3. New York, Academic Press, 1971)

EFFECTS OF PARATHYROID HORMONE AND CALCITONIN ON BONE

The Parathyroid Hormone. As knowledge devel-oped about hormones, it was learned that if the hormone of the parathyroid gland was administered in sufficient amounts to an experimental animal, it would cause a great increase in the number and activity of osteo-clasts as well as an increase in the calcium level of the blood. In due course it became accepted that the increase in the level of the blood calcium was to be attributed largely to the increased resorption of bone by osteoclasts that was taking place which process caused increased amounts of bone calcium to be lib-erated into the blood so that its level was raised.

As mentioned above, administration of parathyroid to an animal does much more than stimulate such osteoclasts as are already in existence into greater activity; it also causes a great increase in the numbers of osteoclasts. The photomicrographs shown in Figure 15-18 were taken from a site in a growing bone in which processes are occurring that will be explained in detail a few pages further on. It is enough at this time to say that in the lower half of the section of

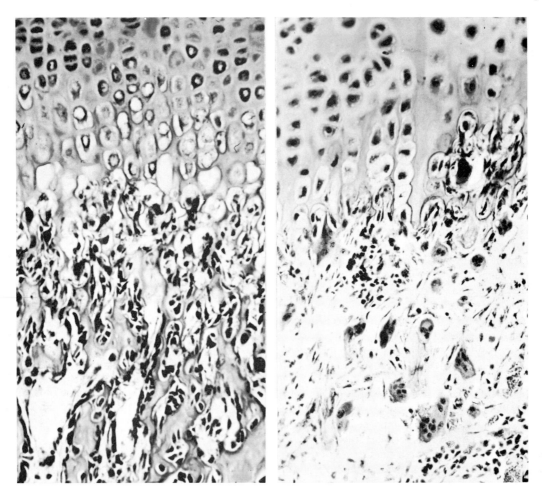

Fɪɢ. 15-18. (*Left*) Low-power photomicrograph of a small portion of a longitudinal section of the metaphysis of a long bone of a young, normal guinea pig. (*Right*) A similar preparation from a littermate who was given a very large injection of parathyroid hormone 48 hours before. Note that the trabeculae on the diaphyseal side of the epiphyseal disk have melted away and that osteoclasts are left in their place.

bone on the left, bone formation is occurring at a rapid rate and a large number of osteogenic cells and osteoblasts are present and responsible for this activity. The bone shown on the right shows what happens to the same site 48 hours after a large dose of parathyroid hormone. The abundant osteogenic cells and osteoblasts and new bone have almost all disappeared and in their place there are a great many osteoclasts.

Parathyroid hormone, as is shown by administering large doses to animals, or as occurs in man in instances of tumors of the parathyroid gland which secrete excessive amounts of hormone, acts on the cells that normally cover and line bone surfaces to cause more and more of them to differentiate so as to form osteoclasts which actively resorb bone. At the same time

the formation and function of bone-forming cells is impaired, because excessive parathyroid hormone prevents the cells that are not directed into becoming osteoclasts from forming more new bone to compensate for that which is being lost. There is even evidence to the effect that in long-continued hyperparathyroidism the lacunae in which the osteocytes within bone substance reside become somewhat larger which indicates that the effects of the hormone affect even the most highly differentiated cells of the bone cell series (Meunier, P., Bernard, J. and Vignon, G.).

It therefore seems that all the cells of the bone cell series—osteogenic cells, osteoblasts, osteoclasts and even osteocytes—are affected to different degrees by the hormone; hence, the cells of this particular lineage seem to have some special characteristic that allows them to specifically react to changes in the concentration of this hormone in the bloodstream and tissue fluid.

Calcitonin. As will be described in Chapter 25, Copp and his associates in 1961 discovered a new hormone, calcitonin, which is now known to be formed in man by certain cells in the thyroid gland. Whereas the secretion of parathyroid hormone is normally increased when the level of calcium in the blood falls below its normal level, whereupon the hormone stimulates the formation and activity of osteoclasts so that calcium is released from bone to raise its level in the blood, the hormone calcitonin is secreted when the level of the calcium in the blood increases, for one reason or another, over its normal level. Calcitonin acts to lower the level of calcium in the blood. It does this in a way that is more or less the reverse of the way parathyroid hormone acts, by diminishing resorptive processes in bone and perhaps also by stimulating osteoblastic activity so there is more new bone formed to absorb calcium from the blood. The net result is that it brings about a lowering of the level of calcium in the blood.

As already mentioned, the growth of width of any given bone from birth to adulthood is dependent on bone being formed on its exterior and being resorbed from its interior. If a high blood calcium level is maintained in an animal so as to cause calcitonin to be secreted or if excessive amounts of calcitonin are being secreted for any other reason the process of resorption does not keep up with the process of formation; hence a given bone comes to contain more bone substance than it should, as will be discussed somewhat further when we consider calcitonin as a hormone in Chapter 25.

Kallio, Garant and Minken have recently described an effect that calcitonin exerts on osteoclasts in cell cultures. They have made EM studies of preparations of osteoclasts in cultures with and without calcitonin being present and have shown that the effect that it has on osteoclasts is manifested chiefly by the virtual disappearance of their ruffled borders. A good many experiments by others have indicated that calcitonin also actually increased the rate of formation of new bone in an animal as well as decreasing the formation and activity of osteoclasts. Apparently, calcitonin, like parathyroid hormone, affects all the cells of the bone cell lineage, and not just osteoclasts.

Conclusions Regarding the Osteogenic Cell. From all the foregoing it seems reasonable to conclude that there is a "bone cell lineage" (Fig. 15-19) of cells that are responsive to two different hormones. Furthermore, the stem cell of this lineage is the osteogenic cell (called by some authors the osteoprogenitor cell) which can differentiate along three sub-lines as is indicated in Figure 15-19 to form osteoblasts, osteoclasts or chondroblasts. In growth processes, whether osteogenic cells form cartilage or bone seems to depend on the oxygen content (low or high) of the environment in which they differentiate. Differentiation in this cell lineage apparently is determined also by the concentration of two hormones in the blood. Parathyroid hormone seems to direct differentiation into osteoclasts whereas calcitonin seems to direct differentiation away from osteoclasts and into the formation of osteoblasts.

So far as the morphology of the osteogenic cell is concerned, about all that can be said is that it could be expected that a resting osteogenic cell is a flattened cell that lies along or close to the surface of a bone and that because it is of the nature of a stem cell its cytoplasm would reveal no particular distinguishing organelles; indeed, it could not be expected that it would contain in noticeable amounts anything more than free ribosomes and some mitochondria. However, when osteogenic cells are stimulated to go into cycle, as for example when a bone is fractured, it could be expected that they would assume more of a fusiform shape, like many of the cells shown in Figure 15-16, and that as any in the G_1 phase differentiated into either chondroblasts and osteoblasts, their cytoplasm would reveal well developed rER and Golgi stacks as well. In other words, the existence of resting osteogenic cells in the deep layer of the periosteum, in endosteum or in bone marrow is not to be established by morphological means but by what they do when they are stimulated to proliferate and differentiate, whereupon they give rise to cells and tissues that can be identified by morphological means.

The Prenatal Development of Bone

Endochondral and Intramembranous Ossification. The term ossification refers to the formation of bone. The terms endochondral and intramembranous refer to the sites or environments in which ossification (the formation of bone) occurs. Endochondral means "in cartilage" and intramembranous means "within membrane." In both instances, bone forms because osteoblasts evolve and secrete the organic intercellular substance of bone. It is important to emphasize this because a great deal of confusion has been caused by the bones that form as a result of endochondral ossification sometimes being called cartilage bones and those that develop as a result of intramembranous os-

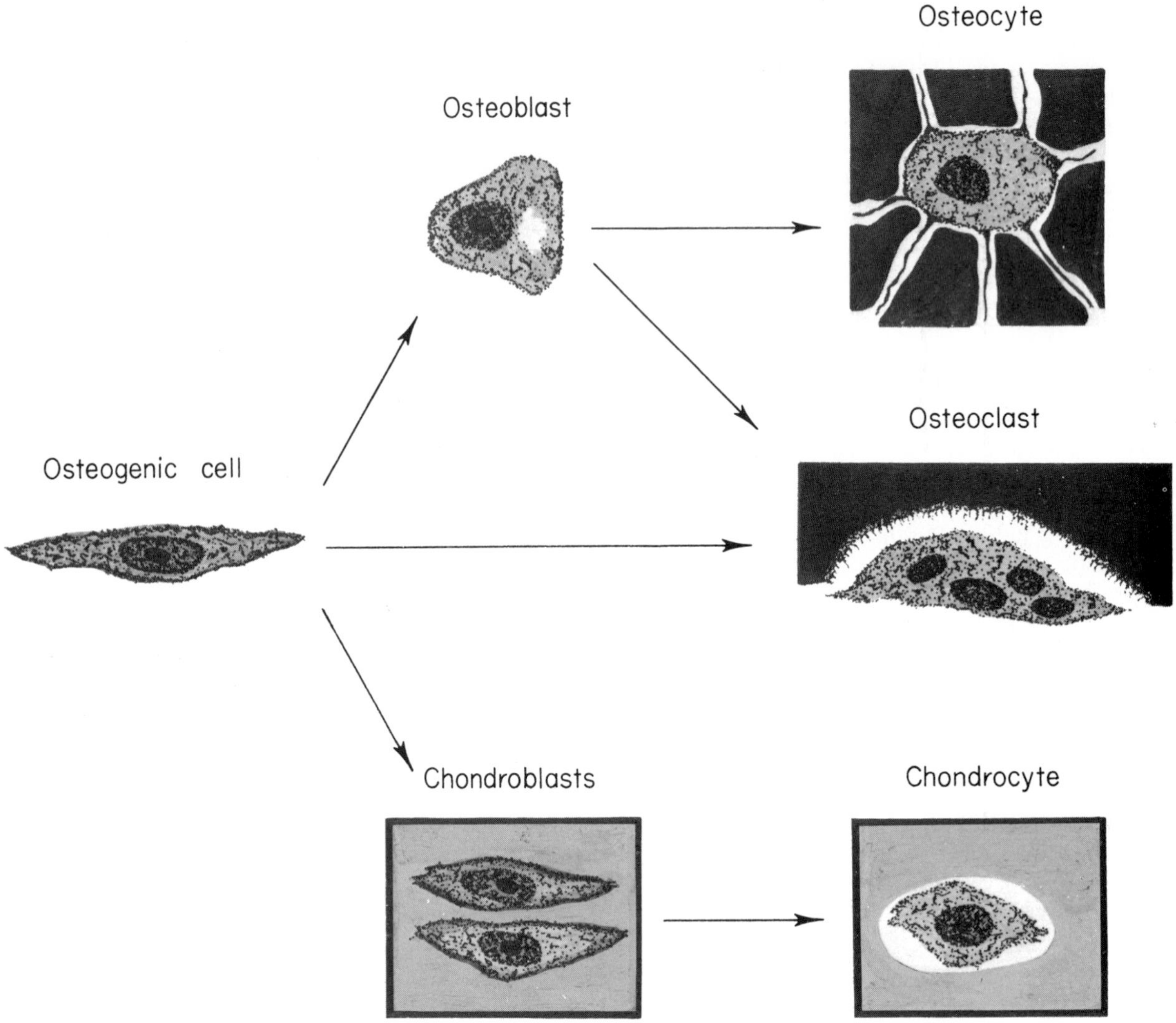

FIG. 15-19. This illustration is not intended to depict the microscopic structure of the cells concerned with exactitude; they are only represented diagrammatically to show their relationships. The osteogenic cell at the left does not represent a resting cell but one of the type seen when a growth process has been set in motion as in the repair of a fracture where, as shown at the top, it gives rise to osteoblasts and osteocytes in sites where capillaries are present. Under conditions of parathyroid stimulation it is believed it is induced to follow the middle pathway of differentiation to fuse with others and even with previous osteoblasts to form osteoclasts. If the osteogenic cell differentiates in a nonvascular environment, it follows the pathway into cartilage as is shown below. It should be noted that this diagram is not intended to rule out the fact that osteoclasts may also arise from some form of blood cell; it merely depicts what is believed to be their usual normal source. (Ham, A. W., and Harris, W. R.: *In* Bourne's Biochemistry and Physiology of Bone. ed. 2, vol. 3. New York, Academic Press, 1971)

sification being called membrane bones. This practice can lead to students making two false assumptions: (1) that in endochondral ossification, membrane turns into bone and in endochondral ossification cartilage turns into bone, and (2) that there are two different kinds of bone. The bone that forms in cartilage is the same as bone that forms in membranous areas.

We shall consider endochondral ossification first because an understanding of this process opens the door to easily understanding how bones grow in length and in width, how fractures are repaired and how many kinds of joints are formed. Most of the skeleton develops as a result of endochondral ossification.

ENDOCHONDRAL OSSIFICATION

The process of endochondral ossification can be followed to advantage in observing the histological changes that successively occur as limb buds develop in the embryo as will now be described.

As the embryo of what will become a four-legged mammal develops, four little appendages push out from its trunk at the sites where its four legs will later appear. These are called *limb buds* and they are essentially mesodermal outgrowths covered with ectoderm. In man, two of the limb buds develop into arms and two into legs, and at their ends they branch to form fingers and toes respectively. A longitudinal section of a developing toe of a rabbit embryo is shown in Figure 15-20.

The first indication of the formation of bones in a limb bud appears in the mesenchyme that occupies part of a bud (or a branch of a bud that is to become a toe) where a bone will eventually develop. The mesenchymal cells at this site become very numerous so that a very rough outline of the bone-to-be is indicated

by mesenchyme becoming so cellular it appears condensed (Fig. 15-20). However, in the central core of this otherwise condensed mesenchyme the cells soon begin to become increasingly separated from one another, owing to their beginning to differentiate into chondrocytes and secrete cartilage intercellular substance which of course separates them from one another. Soon clearly recognized cartilaginous models of the bones-to-be make their appearance (Fig. 15-21), as a result of the continuing differentiation of mesenchymal cells.

The Formation of Perichondrium. The mesenchyme immediately adjacent to the sides of each developing cartilage model becomes arranged into a surrounding membrane for it; this membrane is called *perichondrium* (Fig. 15-21). It has two ill-defined layers. The cells in its outer part in due course differentiate into fibroblasts, and these form collagen. The outer part of the perichondral membrane thus becomes a connective tissue sheath. The mesenchymal cells in its inner part (between its fibrous layer and the cartilage of the model) do not differentiate to any great extent. Instead, they remain relatively undifferentiated and so possess almost all the potentiality of the mesenchymal cells from which they are derived. They

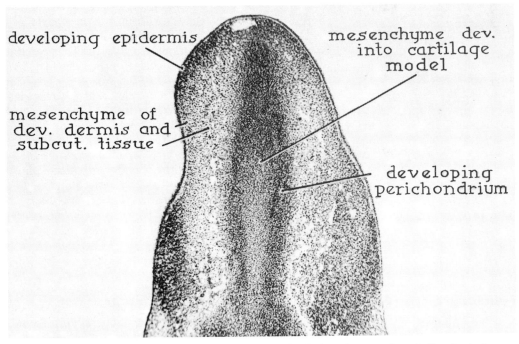

FIG. 15-20. Low-power photomicrograph of a longitudinal section cut through the developing toe of an embryonic rabbit. In the central part of the developing toe the mesenchyme is becoming condensed and is beginning to differentiate into the cartilage model of the terminal phalanx.

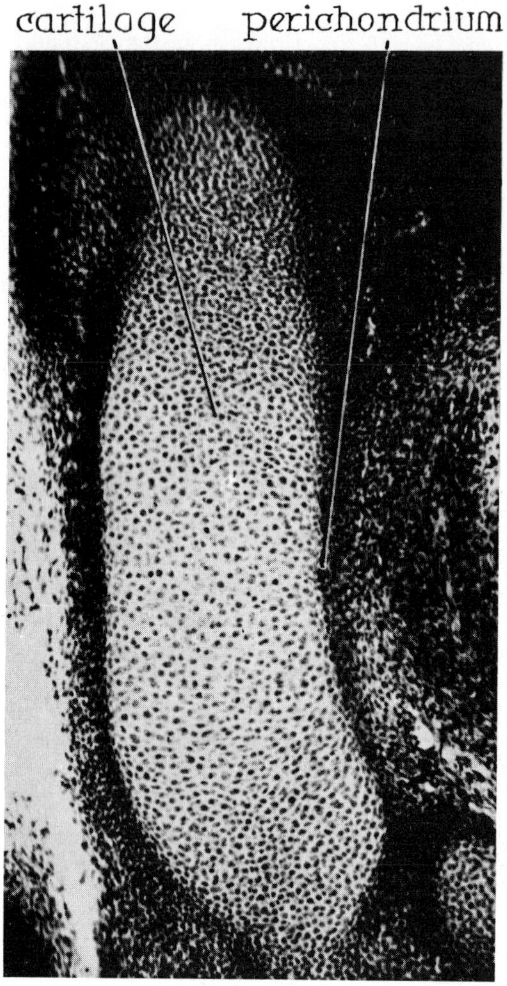

cartilage   perichondrium

Fig. 15-21. Low-power photomicrograph of a longitudinal section of a developing leg (rabbit). In the middle of this picture a cartilage model is differentiating from the mesenchyme. In its more central part, the cartilage is fairly well developed. The mesenchyme along the side of the cartilage model forms a sheath for it; this is called the perichondrium.

constitute the inner or chondrogenic layer of the perichondrium (see Fig. 14-3).

THE GROWTH OF THE MODEL

Cartilage models increase in length by interstitial growth (described in the previous chapter). This requires division and enlargement of chondrocytes within the substance of the cartilage and the formation of additional intercellular substance by them. The models also grow in width. Although interstitial growth may be a factor in this, it is likely that most growth

in width is accomplished by the appositional mechanism; that is, new layers of cartilage are added to the surface of the sides of the model by the proliferation and the differentiation of the cells of the chondrogenic layer of the perichondrium.

The cell division responsible for the interstitial growth of any model tends to occur more near its ends than in its midsection. Hence, as growth continues, the chondrocytes left in the midsection of the model have time to mature. As they become larger, the intercellular substance about them becomes somewhat thinned out (Fig. 15-22), and when the chondrocytes have become sufficiently hypertrophied to secrete phosphatase, the intercellular substance becomes calcified (Fig. 15-23). This prevents the intercellular substance from any longer serving as a means for the diffusion of nutrients to the chondrocytes so they die. With the death of the hypertrophied chondrocytes, the intercellular substance, particularly in the central part of the midsection of the model, begins to break up, and some of it dissolves away to leave cavities within the substance of the model (Fig. 15-23).

During the period in which the changes described above are taking place in the midsection of a cartilage model, the progressive development of the vascular system of the embryo is responsible for the perichondrium of the model being invaded by capillaries. Before their appearance, the relatively undifferentiated cells of the inner (chondrogenic) layer of the perichondrium, by proliferation and differentiation into chondroblasts and cartilage cells, have been adding new layers of cartilage to the sides of the model (appositional growth). The appearance of capillaries in the perichondrium is associated with a changing differentiation pattern on the part of the relatively undifferentiated cells of what we have termed previously the chondrogenic layer of the perichondrium. For, instead of continuing to differentiate into chondroblasts and chondrocytes, they, in the presence of capillaries, begin to differentiate into osteoblasts and osteocytes, with the result that a thin layer or shell of bone is soon laid down around the shaft of the model (this has already happened in Fig. 15-23). Since the membrane that was previously termed perichondrium because it surrounded cartilage now covers a shell of bone (see details in Fig. 15-24) that has been laid down around the cartilage model, the name of the membrane is changed from perichondrium to *periosteum*.

The fact that the proliferating cells in the deep layer of the perichondrium now begin to turn into osteoblasts instead of chondroblasts should not be interpreted as indicating a change in the nature of these cells; rather, a change in their environment has

hypertrophied
chondrocytes

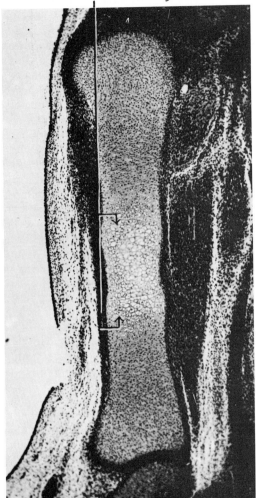

FIG. 15-22. Low-power photomicrograph of a longitudinal section of a developing leg (rabbit). This shows a cartilage model in a somewhat more advanced stage than that shown in Figure 15-21. The form of the bone-to-be is well outlined. Furthermore, the cartilage cells in the central part of the model have become hypertrophied and are about to secrete phosphatase.

occurred which is probably that more oxygen is brought to them by the invading capillaries. That the cells of the inner layer of the periosteum retain their ability to differentiate into chondroblasts and form cartilage even into adult life is easily demonstrated in the repair of broken bones; for, when bones are fractured, the cells of the inner layer of the periosteum situated close to the break proliferate vigorously and, in sites where capillaries are unable to keep up with

spaces in breaking-
down calcified
cartilage

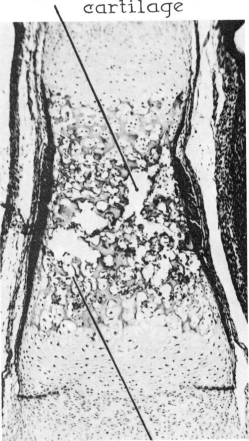

being invaded by
blood vessels and
osteoblasts of
periosteal bud

FIG. 15-23. Low-power photomicrograph of a longitudinal section cut through a developing human phalanx. At this stage of development the calcified cartilage in the central part of the model has broken down, and this has resulted in the formation of spaces in this area. Subperiosteal bone has formed along the sides of the model; this stains more darkly than the cartilage which it covers. Furthermore, osteogenic cells and blood vessels from the periosteum have grown into the spaces in the breaking-down cartilage, and the osteogenic cells in this area are beginning to differentiate into osteoblasts and lay down bone on what is left of the old calcified cartilage matrix.

their rapid growth, differentiate into chondroblasts and so form cartilage (Fig. 15-17). However, in other sites, where capillaries are able to keep up with their growth, they differentiate into osteoblasts and so form bone (Fig. 15-17).

THE FURTHER DEVELOPMENT OF THE MODEL

At this stage of development, then, the calcified cartilage in the midsection of the model is beginning to break down (Fig. 15-23) and the shaft of the model has gained a surrounding shell of bone which has been laid down by the recently vascularized perichondrium, which is now termed the periosteum (Fig. 15-24). The inner layer of the periosteum at this time consists of osteogenic cells and osteoblasts which have formed from them (Fig. 15-24, *right*). It also contains capillaries. As the calcified cartilage in the midsection of the model begins to disintegrate, osteogenic cells and osteoblasts, together with capillaries, at an appropriate site along the model, begin to move from the inner

layer of the periosteum into the breaking-down midsection of the cartilage model (Fig. 15-23). The invading osteogenic cells, osteoblasts and capillaries constitute what is called the *periosteal bud*.

When the osteogenic cells, the osteoblasts and the capillaries of the periosteal bud reach the interior of the midsection of the cartilage model, they are said to constitute a *center of ossification;* this means that bone formation that begins here will spread out to soon replace most of the cartilage model. In this process proliferating osteogenic cells gather round such remnants of calcified cartilage as still remain and form osteoblasts which lay down bone intercellular substance on the remnants of calcified cartilage. The calcified cartilaginous intercellular substance that still remains at this time is, in this part of the model, in the form of an irregular network riddled with spaces. The first bone that is formed in this area is deposited on these cartilage remnants. Hence it is cancellous bone (cancellous means in the form of a lattice) in type, with its individual trabeculae (trabeculae means

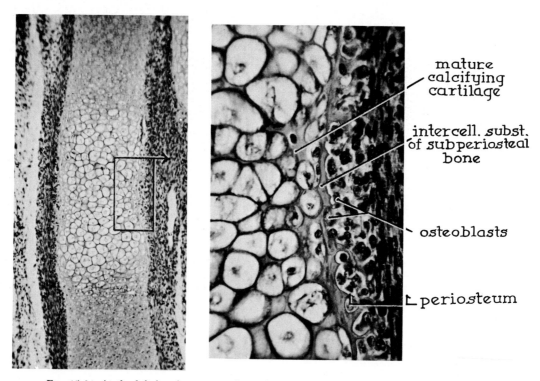

mature
calcifying
cartilage

intercell. subst.
of subperiosteal
bone

osteoblasts

periosteum

FIG. 15-24. At the left is a low-power photomicrograph of a longitudinal section of the developing leg of a rabbit. The cartilage cells in the central part of the model are seen to be hypertrophied and are presumably secreting phosphatase, which is bringing about the calcification of the intercellular substance about them. Furthermore, as may be seen in the picture at the right, which is a high-power photomicrograph of the area indicated by a rectangle in the picture on the left, the osteogenic cells of the perichondrium have differentiated into osteoblasts and have laid down a thin layer of bone intercellular substance (subperiosteal bone) on the side of the model.

little beams which may be isolated from one another or connected together to form a lattice-work) having cores of calcified cartilage. In a good H and E section, this makes a very pretty picture because the cores of cartilage intercellular substance are blue, while the bone covering them is pink or red. The osteoblasts applied to the surface of the trabeculae are blue. Trabeculae of bone with cores of cartilage are illustrated on the right side of Figure 15-27 and also in the drawing Figure 15-30.

Up to this time the only cartilage in the model that has matured, become calcified and died in that part which was situated in its midsection and whose remnants by this time are covered with bone. The young cartilage at each end of the model continues to grow by means of the interstitial growth mechanism, thus increasing the length of the model. However, a time soon arrives when the interstitial growth of the younger cartilage at the ends of the model, while it increases the length of the model, no longer increases the amount of cartilage in the model. The reason for this is that those cartilage cells next to the bone that has formed from the ossification center continue to mature, and the intercellular substance about them becomes calcified. This brings about their death. When this occurs, the calcified cartilage intercellular substance breaks up into cavities, and these are rapidly invaded by capillaries, osteogenic cells and osteoblasts that are migrating up and down the model from the center of ossification and form bone on such cartilage remnants as are left. Thus cartilage is destroyed at the edge of the ossification front as fast as it grows by interstitial growth at the ends of the model. The net result is that the model grows longer by more and more of it becoming bone.

The spread of ossification in the middle of the bone soon results in the formation of a marrow cavity (Fig. 15-25). This is possible because the model continues to grow in width by means of the osteogenic cells of the periosteum continuing to add further bone to the sides of the model. As the periphery of the model thus becomes stronger, the cancellous bone in its central part is no longer necessary for support, so it is mostly resorbed so as to leave a cavity that is called the marrow cavity (Fig. 15-25). This soon becomes filled with myeloid tissue. However, during the postnatal growing period, the marrow cavity never extends quite all the way to the cartilaginous ends of the model but instead is always separated from each cartilaginous end by a region of longitudinally disposed trabeculae of bone which have cartilaginous cores. The nature of these will be described in detail presently after we have described epiphyseal centers of ossification.

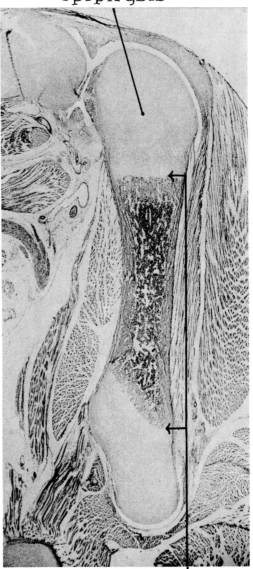

cartilaginous epiphysis

bony diaphysis

FIG. 15-25. A very low-power photomicrograph of a longitudinal section of the developing thigh of a rabbit. At this stage the cartilage of the model is replaced by bone except at its ends. The bone that has formed from the periosteum and periosteal bud constitutes the diaphysis. The cartilage left at each end constitutes the epiphyses.

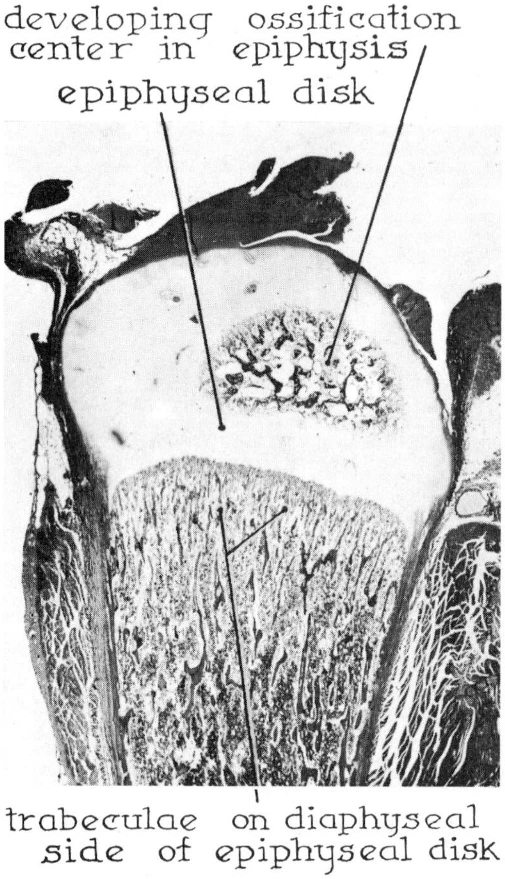

developing ossification
center in epiphysis
epiphyseal disk

trabeculae on diaphyseal
side of epiphyseal disk

Fig. 15-26. Low-power photomicrograph of a longitudinal section of the upper part of the tibia of a kitten. This shows the stage of development shortly after the appearance of a center of ossification in an epiphysis. The cartilage that remains between the bone that forms from the epiphyseal center of ossification and that from the diaphyseal center constitutes an epiphyseal disk.

Epiphyseal Centers of Ossification. An ossification center that arises in the midsection of a cartilage model, as has been described, is spoken of as a *diaphyseal center* of ossification, since it gives rise to the diaphysis (diaphysis means shaft) of the bone concerned. However, the development of the larger long bones of the body is complicated by the development of further centers of ossification in their cartilage models. These further centers of ossification appear in the growing cartilaginous ends of the models and are termed *epiphyseal centers* of ossification (Fig. 15-26) (epiphysis means roughly something on an end of something which in this instance is a shaft (diaphysis)). The centers of ossification that develop in the

cartilaginous ends of the bone give rise to the bony epiphyses that form later.

The development of an epiphyseal center of ossification is heralded by the maturation of the cartilage cells situated in and near the central part of the cartilaginous end of a model. These hypertrophy and the intercellular substance about them becomes thinned out and calcified and they die. Cavities soon form and are invaded by capillaries and osteogenic cells which form osteoblasts which lay down bone on the remnants of the cartilage intercellular substance just as occurs in a diaphyseal center. Meanwhile, the living chondrocytes immediately surrounding this area also begin to mature and die; hence the process of ossification is able to spread out from the epiphyseal center in all directions. However, ossification stops short of replacing all the cartilage in the end of a model. Enough is left at each articulating end of a model to constitute an articular cartilage (Fig. 15-27, *left, artic. cart.*). Furthermore, a transverse disk or plate of cartilage that extends across from one side of the bone to the other is left between the bone derived from the epiphyseal center of ossification and that from the diaphyseal center. This transverse disk or plate of cartilage that separates epiphyseal bone from diaphyseal bone is termed the *epiphyseal disk* or *plate* (Figs. 15-26 and 15-27, *left*), and it persists until the postnatal longitudinal growth of bones is completed; only then is it replaced by bone. It is of tremendous importance, for, as we shall soon describe, it is responsible for allowing long bones to grow in length until full growth is obtained.

The route by which capillaries and osteogenic cells gain entrance to the central part of an epiphysis probably is indicated later by the course of the larger blood vessels that supply that epiphysis. The blood supply of epiphyses will be described later in connection with the blood supply of bones.

THE GROWTH OF MODELS IN WHICH
EPIPHYSEAL CENTERS HAVE APPEARED

The further longitudinal growth of the shaft of a long bone is accounted for by the continuance of the interstitial growth of cartilage cells in the epiphyseal disk. Since epiphyseal disks separate bone-containing epiphyses from bony diaphyses, interstitial growth occurring in the cartilage of the epiphyseal plate which separates the bone of the epiphysis from the bone of the diaphysis (Fig. 15-30) constantly tends to thicken the plate and hence move the bone of the epiphysis

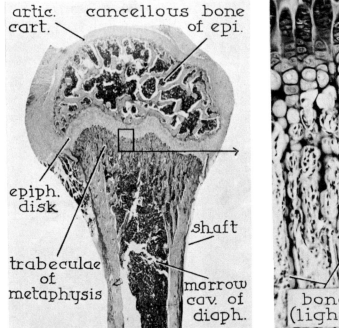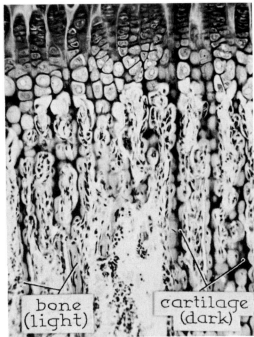

Fɪɢ. 15-27. At the left is a low-power photomicrograph of a longitudinal section cut through the end of a long bone of a growing rat. At this stage of development osteogenesis has spread out from the epiphyseal center of ossification so that only the articular cartilage above and the epiphyseal disk below remain cartilaginous. On the diaphyseal side of the epiphyseal plate are the metaphyseal trabeculae, which, as may be seen from the high-power picture on the right, consist of cartilage cores on which bone has been deposited. The cartilage cores of the trabeculae formerly were partitions between columns of cartilage cells in the epiphyseal disk.

away from the bone of the diaphysis. (Remember bone cannot grow by the interstitial mechanism.) The result is that the total length of the model becomes increased by this interstitial growth in epiphyseal plates. However, the thickness of the epiphyseal disks does not become increased because of the interstitial growth that occurs in them. This is because another process that tends to reduce the thickness of the disk is at work simultaneously, namely, the continuing maturation, death and replacement of cartilage on the diaphyseal side of the disk. Hence, in an epiphyseal disk there is a persistent race between two processes: (1) interstitial growth, which tends to thicken it, and (2) the calcification and death of cartilage on the diaphyseal side of the plate where it is continuously replaced by the appositional growth of bone. The latter process continues to increase the length of the bony shaft. The race is not won by the latter process until full growth has been obtained, for at this time interstitial growth ceases in the plate and it is all replaced with bone from the diaphysis.

An epiphyseal disk and that part of the diaphysis adjacent to it constitute what is termed a *growing zone* of a long bone. (The term *zone* is used in this connection in the same way that it is commonly used, for example, in zoning bylaws—to indicate a region and not necessarily an encircling band which is its precise meaning.) In a child this zone is the site of tremendous cellular activity. Many different processes (the interstitial growth, maturation, calcification, death and disintegration of cartilage, and the formation, calcification and destruction of bone) are at work in this area simultaneously. Any interference with any one of these different processes, while the others continue, is quickly reflected by an alteration in the normal histological picture of the part.

Since different abnormal states (for example, dietary deficiencies and endocrine gland imbalances) affect different processes at work in this region and so produce different kinds of alteration in the histological picture in the part, we shall consider the growing zone of long bones in some detail.

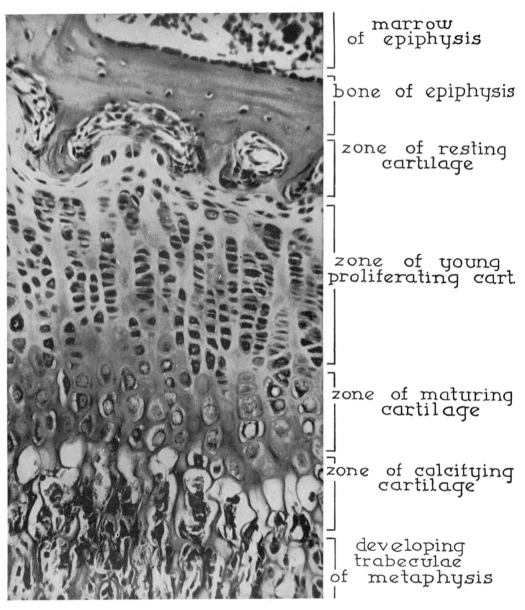

marrow
of epiphysis

bone of epiphysis

zone of resting
cartilage

zone of young
proliferating cart.

zone of maturing
cartilage

zone of calcifying
cartilage

developing
trabeculae
of metaphysis

Fig. 15-28. High-power photomicrograph of a longitudinal section cut through the upper end of the tibia of a guinea pig. This picture illustrates the different zones of cells in the epiphyseal plate.

Microscopic Structure of an Epiphyseal Plate. If a longitudinal section of a growing bone is placed under the microscope and examined so as to allow the eye to sweep across the thickness of the epiphyseal disk from its epiphyseal to its diaphyseal aspect (Fig. 15-28), the cartilage of the disk will be seen to present four successively different appearances. Accordingly, the epiphyseal disk is divided into 4 different parts. From the epiphysis to the diaphysis these regions, com-

monly called zones, are: (1) the zone of resting cartilage, (2) the zone of proliferating young cartilage, (3) the zone of maturing cartilage and (4) the zone of calcified cartilage. These 4 zones imperceptibly merge into one another. Their special characteristics and functions will now be described.

(1) The layer of resting cartilage is immediately adjacent to the bone of the epiphysis. Chondrocytes of moderate size are scattered irregularly throughout its

intercellular substance. In some sites the cartilage of this zone is separated from the bone of the epiphyses by spaces which contain blood vessels (Fig. 15-28). This zone of cartilage does not participate in the growth of the epiphyseal plate. It serves, first, to anchor the plate to the bone of the epiphysis; second, the capillaries in the spaces between it and the bone (Fig. 15-21) have been shown to be the source of the nutrients that by diffusion nourish the cells in the other zones of the plate.

(2) The second zone is composed of young proliferating cartilage cells. These are commonly thin, and many of them are wedge-shaped. The cells in this zone are more or less piled on top of one another like stacks of coins so that they form columns whose axes are parallel with that of the bone (Fig. 15-28). In a growing bone, mitotic figures can be found among these cells. The plane in which mitosis occurs exhibits considerable variability. It seems likely that the column arrangement is maintained because the bundles of collagenic fibrils in the partitions of intercellular substance between the columns run longitudinally. The function of this zone is cell proliferation. This is the site where a sufficient number of new cells must be produced to replace those that hypertrophy and die at the diaphyseal surface of the disk, as will be described.

(3) The third zone or layer contains cartilage cells that are in various stages of maturation. These, too, are arranged in columns. Those nearest the zone of proliferating cartilage are the least mature, and those nearest the diaphysis are the oldest and most mature (Fig. 15-28).

The cells of this zone were originally in the proliferating zone but were left behind as their neighbors on their epiphyseal side continued to proliferate and so drew away from them. The cells left behind in this zone gradually mature. In this process they become larger and accumulate glycogen in their cytoplasm. In becoming larger they take up more space and hence expand the epiphyseal disk longitudinally. The epiphyseal plate is then expanded in the long axis of the bone by the proliferation of cells in the second zone and by the maturation of cells in the third zone. Moreover, the cells of this zone produce alkaline phosphatase, as may be demonstrated in sections by histochemical methods (Fig. 15-29). As this zone merges into the next the intercellular substance around the cartilage cells becomes increasingly calcified. This causes their death. When this happens, the third zone has turned into the fourth zone.

(4) The fourth zone is very thin, being only one or a few cartilage cells thick. This zone abuts directly on the bone of the diaphysis. Most of the cells in this zone

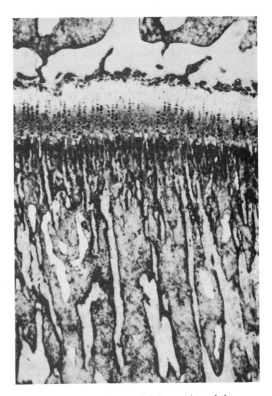

Fig. 15-29. Photomicrograph of a section of the growing bone of a tibia of a normal rat. The section was prepared so that the darkened areas are due to the presence of alkaline phosphatase. Notice that there is a dark band of phosphatase activity in the region of the hypertrophied cartilage cells in the plate and another in the region of the osteoblasts that are invading the diaphyseal side of the plate. Notice that the zone of calcified cartilage is relatively free from phosphatase (it contains few living cells). (Morse, A., and Greep, R. O.: Anat. Rec., *111*:193)

have died because the intercellular substance about them became calcified (Fig. 15-28). The calcified intercellular substance then begins to break up in a special way, next to be described, and the breaking-down cartilage is invaded from the diaphysis by osteogenic cells and capillaries. The osteogenic cells give rise to osteoblasts that lay down bone on the calcified cartilage that persists.

Osteogenesis is very active at the diaphyseal border of the epiphyseal disk and results in bone being formed in such intimate contact with the cartilage of the disk (Figs. 15-27 and 15-30) that the cartilaginous disk is normally always firmly cemented to the bone of the diaphysis that is forming in association with the calcified intercellular substance of the dying cartilage. It is important to understand exactly where this bone is formed. As is shown in Figure 15-30, as the cartilage cells in the zone of calcification die and the intercellular substance about them begins to disintegrate, the horizontal partitions between the cells in any given column and some of the vertical partitions between adjacent columns melt away. However, some (probably the stouter) vertical partitions between columns remain, and these are immediately utilized as sites for bone deposition (Figs. 15-30 and 15-27). Osteoblasts form on these partitions from osteogenic cells that grow up into the area from the adjacent diaphysis. Capillary loops are formed to accompany them. The osteoblasts that form line up on the partitions of calcified cartilage that remain and lay down bone inter-

cellular substance on them. This results, on the diaphyseal side of the epiphyseal disk (the metaphysis), in the formation of what appear in longitudinal sections as longitudinally disposed bony trabeculae with cartilaginous cores, the cartilage cores of which are continuous with as yet only partly calcified cartilaginous intercellular substance of the disk (partitions between columns), and by this means the newly formed bony trabeculae are united firmly with the substance of the cartilaginous disk. By this arrangement the metaphysis of a bone is joined firmly to the epiphyseal disk (Figs. 15-30 and 15-27).

The osteoblasts also produce phosphatase which may assist in bringing about the calcification of the

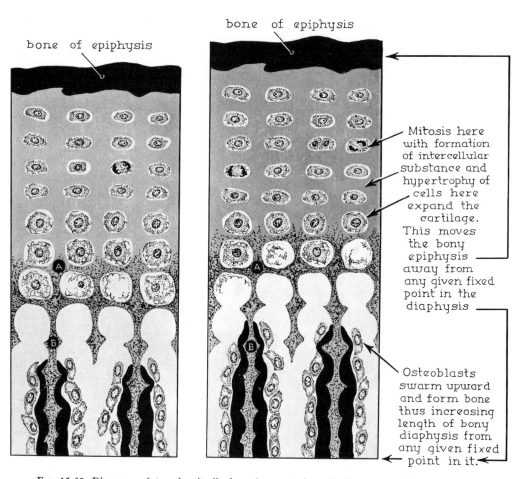

Fɪɢ. 15-30. Diagrams of two longitudinal sections cut through the same epiphyseal plate and part of the diaphysis of growing long bone. The diagram on the right illustrates the changes that occur in what is represented in the left over a short space of time. Cartilage is gray, calcified cartilage is stippled, and bone is black. The sites labeled A and B are fixed points and remain at the same level in both diagrams. Note, however, that the "bone of epiphysis" has moved upward in the diagram on the right, and that the level of calcified cartilage and bone is also higher in the diagram on the right. (Ham, A. W.: J. Bone Joint Surg., *34-A:*701)

organic intercellular substance of bone that they form. (See Fig. 15-29, which is a photomicrograph of a section on which a histochemical test for phosphatase has been performed. It shows dark bands both where hypertrophied chondrocytes and active osteoblasts are present.)

The growth mechanism described above is the only mechanism by which the diaphysis can become lengthened. Bone cannot grow by interstitial growth. It can grow only by appositional growth, and, as is shown in Figure 15-30, the new bone that is "apposed" and accounts for the growth in length of the diaphysis is added *to the ends of the prolongations of bone that extend into the cartilage;* this increases the penetration of the cartilage and makes the metaphysis longer (Fig. 15-30).

Resorption at the Diaphyseal Ends of Trabeculae. Since the (epiphyseal) ends of the bony trabeculae in this zone are constantly being elongated by the mechanism described above, it might be thought that the zone of trabeculated bone in the metaphysis would become increasingly elongated. Instead, however, except at its periphery, this zone of trabeculated bone does not become elongated during the growing period; it stays about the same length (Fig. 15-27, *left*). This can only mean, then, that as rapidly as bone is added to the (epiphyseal) ends of the metaphyseal trabeculae in the zone of calcification, bone is resorbed from their free (diaphyseal) ends that project toward the marrow cavity of the diaphysis. Osteoclasts commonly are seen here; often they are wrapped around the free ends of the trabeculae at which sites the free ends of the trabeculae are resorbed at roughly the same rate the epiphyseal ends are being elongated.

That the trabeculae that are present under the more central part of an epiphyseal disk of a growing animal at any given time are not the same ones that are present several days later is illustrated beautifully by means of radioautographs. As is shown in Figure 15-31, *top,* a single dose of radioactive phosphorus labels the newly forming and calcifying bone in this area in 5 minutes. However, the bone continues to grow in length, and so new bone is added continuously to the (epiphyseal) ends of the trabeculae—the ends that extend into the epiphyseal disk—and this new bone is not labeled by radiophosphorus because now there is not enough in the circulation to mark it. A considerable band of new unlabeled bone is already present 2 days after the administration of the radiophosphorus (Fig. 15-31, *center*). Meanwhile, the labeled bone of the trabeculae has been dissolving from the free (diaphyseal) ends of the trabeculae, so that the average

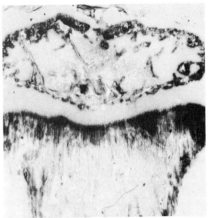

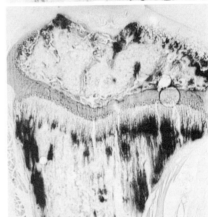

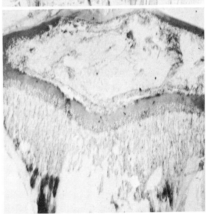

Fig. 15-31. (*Top*) Coated radioautograph of a safranin-stained section of the end of a tibia of a 50-gm. rat sacrificed 5 minutes after injection of radiophosphorus. (*Center*) Similar preparation from rat sacrificed 2 days after the injection. (*Bottom*) Similar preparation from rat sacrificed 8 days after the injection. (All 3 preparations from Leblond, C. P., Wilkinson, G. W., Bélanger, L. F., and Robichon, J.: Am. J. Anat., *86:* 289)

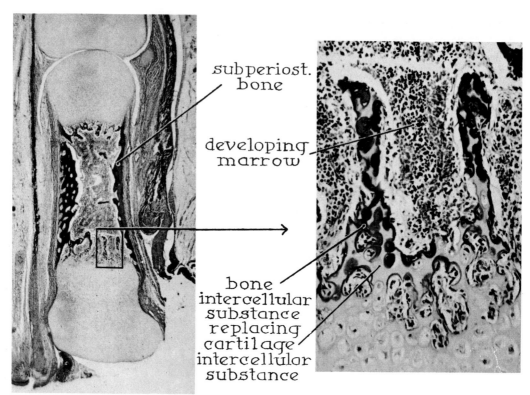

subperiost. bone

developing marrow

bone intercellular substance replacing cartilage intercellular substance

Fig. 15-32. (*Left*) A low-power photomicrograph of a longitudinal section of a developing human phalanx. The amount of subperiosteal bone is increased, and the cartilage of the entire central part of the model has disappeared. Marrow now occupies the central part of the model. Bone formation is advancing toward each end. (*Right*) The photograph shows the characteristic picture of bone being deposited on cartilage remnants. The bone intercellular substance is dark, that of the cartilage is light in this particular illustration.

total length of labeled bone in the trabeculae is shorter than it was 2 days previously. After 8 days all the labeled bone has been eroded from the trabeculae under the central part of the disk (Fig. 15-31, *bottom*); hence, the trabeculae that are present at this time (8 days after the radiophosphorus was administered) are composed of bone that has formed and calcified during the 8 days; therefore they are not the same trabeculae that were present 8 days before. However, it is to be noted that Figure 15-31, *bottom,* shows the persistence of some of the labeled bone in the developing shaft, some distance below the epiphyseal disk; why some of the bone that formed 8 days before under the periphery of the epiphyseal disk has persisted and has now become part of the shaft will be explained in the next section.

Under the *periphery* of the epiphyseal disk, the fate of the metaphyseal trabeculae is different from that described for the trabeculae under its more central part. However, an explanation of what happens to

these involves a discussion of how a long bone *as a whole* changes during the growing period, and so we shall discuss this matter first.

The Growth of a Bone As a Whole

Speaking generally, the growth in length ot bones that develop in cartilage is fundamentally dependent on the ability of the cartilage that persists in them as epiphyseal disks or at their ends to grow by the interstitial mechanism while at one of its surfaces it is replaced by bone growing by the appositional mechanism at the same rate.

1. Short bones such as a phalanx do not develop epiphyseal centers of ossification and hence they depend for longitudinal growth on the interstitial growth of cartilage at their ends. This is replaced by bone from the diaphyseal center of ossification in the same way that cartilage is replaced on the diaphyseal side of an epiphyseal plate (Fig. 15-32). What is left of it

when growth in length is over becomes the articular cartilage of a joint.

2. In long bones in which epiphyseal centers of ossification develop and hence which have epiphyseal disks, the interstitial growth of the cartilage of the part of the epiphyses that becomes the articular cartilages provides only for the growth in size of the epiphyses and not for the growth of the diaphysis. Articular cartilage may provide for growth in width of the epiphysis as well as for its growth in length, as will be described in the next chapter.

3. In long bones that have epiphyseal disks, the interstitial growth of the cartilage in the disks does not assist in the growth of the epiphysis after the bony epiphyses are reasonably well developed. After an epiphysis is well developed, the cartilage of an epiphyseal disk is no longer replaced with bone on its epiphyseal side but only on its diaphyseal side (Fig. 15-28). Hence, the interstitial growth of cartilage in epiphyseal disks accounts only for the growth in length of diaphyses during all but the early stages of the growing period (Fig. 15-33).

With these facts established we can now consider some further points about the growth of a long bone as a whole.

The diaphyses of many long bones funnel outward as they approach their epiphyses (Fig. 15-33); hence, many bones are of a much greater diameter in their metaphyseal regions (the metaphysis is the part of the shaft that in a growing bone is composed of bony trabeculae that have cores of cartilage and is directly adjacent to a diaphyseal side of the epiphyseal disk) than in their midsections (Fig. 15-33). As may be seen by comparing the left and the right sides of Figure 15-33, the site, along the longitudinal axis of a bone, that is occupied by the flared metaphyseal portion of the diaphysis will, as the bone continues to elongate, be occupied later by the tubular and considerably narrower portion of the shaft. This means that as growth in length continues, the diameter of the portion of the shaft that is flared at any given time subsequently must become decreased. This requires that bone be resorbed continuously from the exterior of the flared portion (and osteoclasts are numerous here) and built up continuously on its inner aspect so that it can become a narrower shaft. We shall now consider how bone is built up on the inner aspect of the flared portion so that bone can be resorbed safely from its outer aspect.

Why What Appear as Isolated Trabeculae Are Really the Walls of Tunnels. It is easy to get the impression from longitudinal sections of growing bone that the trabeculae of the metaphysis are like stalac-

tites, hanging down from the diaphyseal side of the plate. However, if cross sections are cut of the metaphyses of larger mammals close to the plate, it will be found that only the free ends of the trabeculae are stalactite-like. Closer to the plate the structures that in longitudinal sections appear as stalactite-like trabeculae are revealed in cross sections to be connected together to constitute a network that is honeycombed with spaces which are the lumens of tunnels (Fig. 15-34). Why the newly formed bony trabeculae (which have cartilaginous cores) appear to be isolated from one another in longitudinal sections and should appear, when they are seen in cross section, to comprise a cancellous network will now be explained.

In the zone of maturing cartilage the cartilage cells are arranged in longitudinal rows that are separated from one another by partitions of intercellular substance. If this area is visualized in 3 dimensions, it will be obvious that the rows of cells are contained in longitudinal tunnels, and that the partitions of intercellular substance between the rows of cells are the walls of these longitudinally disposed tunnels. As the cartilage cells in a tunnel mature and die at its diaphyseal end, the thinner partitions between tunnels tend to dissolve, and by this means tunnels only one cartilage-cell wide fuse with others of the same size to become relatively large tunnels as shown in longitudinal section in Figure 15-30. These are invaded from the diaphysis by osteogenic cells, osteoblasts and capillaries. The osteoblasts line up along the sides of the tunnels and deposit bone on the tunnel surfaces (Fig. 15-30). Hence, in a longitudinal section, the wall between 2 adjacent tunnels will appear as a trabecula with a cartilage core that is covered on each side by a layer of bone (Fig. 15-34, *left* and *middle*). In other words, the bone seen covering the cartilaginous cores of the trabeculae in longitudinal sections is the bone that in cross section is seen to line the tunnels in cartilage (Fig. 15-34, *middle*). The osteoblasts that cover the trabeculae of longitudinal sections similarly are the osteoblasts that line the insides of the tunnels that are seen in cross sections. And the capillaries and the osteogenic tissue that fill the spaces between the trabeculae of longitudinal sections are the contents of the tunnels seen in cross section.

How a Shaft of Compact Bone With Haversian Systems Forms Under the Periphery of the Plate. On the diaphyseal side of the more central part of the epiphyseal disk only a single layer of bone is commonly deposited inside the cartilaginous tunnels. Hence, the trabeculae seen in a longitudinal section of this area are narrow. However, at the periphery of the disk successive layers of bone are deposited inside the larger tunnels that have formed by the coalescence of a few smaller tunnels (Fig. 15-33). This narrows the lumens of these larger tunnels and the several layers of bone that are laid down in them and imparts a *lamellar* appearance to their thickened walls. The successive layers of bone deposited inside the tunnels are the result of successive waves of appositional growth. The osteogenic cells in the tunnel proliferate by mitosis

to increase their numbers. Simultaneously some of them differentiate into osteoblasts and then into osteocytes which surround themselves with intercellular substance. This results in a layer or lamella of bone being deposited inside the tunnel. The osteogenic cells that remain to line the tunnel then repeat the full procedure, so a second layer of bone is deposited. Finally, after several layers have been deposited, the tunnel is

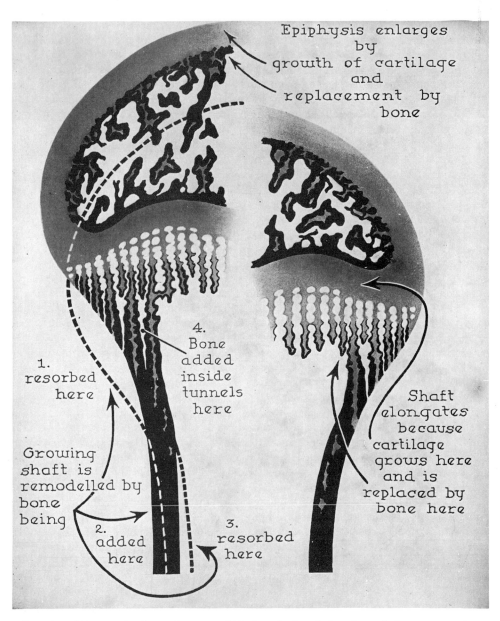

FIG. 15-33. Diagram showing surfaces on which bone is deposited and resorbed to account for the remodeling that takes place at the ends of growing long bones that have flared extremities. (Ham, A. W.: J. Bone Joint Surg., *34-A*:701)

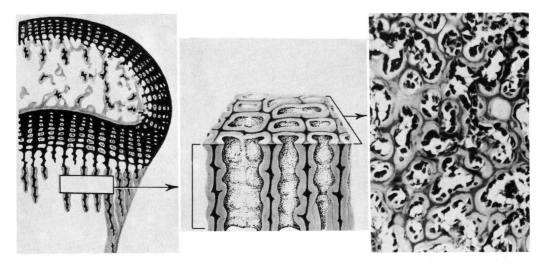

Fɪɢ. 15-34. The diagram at the left illustrates the appearance seen in a longitudinal section of the end of a growing long bone. The trabeculae appear stalactite-like in such a preparation. However, if they could be seen in 3 dimensions, as illustrated in the drawing in the middle, it would be seen that, close to the plate, the structures that appear as trabeculae in a longitudinal section are slices that have been cut through walls that surround spaces; they are slices cut through the walls of tunnels. The photomicrograph at the right represents what is seen in a cross section cut through the metaphysis of a growing long bone of a rabbit, close to the epiphyseal disk. In it the trabeculae of bone have cartilaginous cores, and they surround spaces. These spaces under the periphery of the disk become filled in to form haversian systems, and such compact bone as is present in the flared extremities of bone is built by spaces such as these becoming filled in.

reduced to a narrow canal, which contains a blood vessel, some osteoblasts or osteogenic cells and perhaps a lymphatic. This arrangement of a canal with concentric layers of bone surrounding it is called a *haversian system* or an *osteon* (Fig. 15-37). Haversian systems, in a sense, are units of structure of what is called compact or dense bone. Each has one or two blood vessels in its canal, and this provides tissue fluid to nourish the osteocytes in the surrounding lamellae. Haversian systems are limited in the number of lamellae they can contain by the distance over which the canalicular mechanism can nourish osteocytes. This, of course is not very great; hence, commonly a haversian canal is surrounded by less than half a dozen concentric lamellae (Fig. 15-37).

A haversian system (osteon) can develop only by means of a tunnel being filled in from its inside with concentric layers of bone. A haversian system, then, is in the nature of a bony tube with thick walls and a very narrow lumen. However, if ordinary tubes are bundled together side by side, crevices are left between them. Compact bone, though generally composed of longitudinally disposed tubular haversian systems, does not exhibit such crevices. With what are they filled?

Since the first compact bone that forms under the periphery of a disk is the result of a cartilaginous tunnel being filled in with bone, the crevices between the haversian systems that form in this manner are filled with cartilage (Fig. 15-34, *middle* and *right*). Hence, in the shaft of a very young growing bone, irregular bits of cartilage commonly will be seen (Fig. 15-33). It should be kept in mind by any student who wishes to understand bone growth well, that each of these bits of cartilage seen incorporated into the shaft of bone and situated between haversian systems was once part of a partition between rows of cartilage cells in the epiphyseal plate and somewhat later was the cartilaginous core of a metaphyseal trabecula under the periphery of the plate. In the shafts of older bones, the crevices between adjacent haversian systems are filled with what are termed interstitial lamellae of bone. Why there is no cartilage between haversian systems in older bone (Fig. 15-37) will be made clear when we study how shafts of bones grow in width—our next subject.

How Shafts of Bones Grow in Width

A long bone grows in width by new layers of bone being added to the outer aspect of the shaft while at

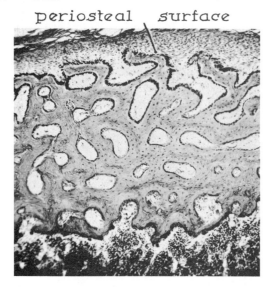

periosteal surface

FIG. 15-35. Low-power photomicrograph of a cross section of the radius of a growing puppy. It is to be noted that the periosteal surface is not smooth but consists of longitudinally disposed ridges and grooves. The ridges are covered by osteoblasts, and the grooves are lined by them. Developing haversian systems can be seen throughout the substance of the shaft.

the same time bone is dissolved away from the inner aspect of the shaft. The result of these two processes proceeding simultaneously is that, although the shaft as a whole becomes wider, its walls do not become unduly thick, and the width of the marrow cavity gradually increases. It also means that the bone of the shaft of an adult is not the same bone that made up the shaft of that bone when he was a young child. The latter has all been resorbed as new bone was added to the exterior of the shaft during the growing period.

The shaft of a bone grows in width by the appositional mechanism (Fig. 15-2). New bone is laid down beneath the periosteum by the osteogenic layer of that membrane. However, if a cross section through the shaft of a young bone that is growing in width is examined, it will be seen that much of the new bone of which it is composed is in the form of haversian systems. It has been explained that haversian systems always are formed as a result of tunnels (not necessarily cartilaginous ones) being filled in from the inside. How, then, can bony tunnels, to be subsequently filled in from the inside, be formed under the periosteum of a young growing bone?

A brief study of the periphery of a cross section of an actively growing shaft of a young animal will reveal how this occurs. The surface of such a shaft is not

smooth; instead, it demonstrates a series of longitudinal ridges with grooves between them (Figs. 15-35 and 15-36). The osteogenic cells and the osteoblasts of the periosteum cover the tops of ridges and extend down to the bottoms of the grooves between them. The periosteum here also contains blood vessels (Fig. 15-36, 1). Longitudinal tunnels form from this arrangement as follows: the osteogenic cells of the periosteum covering the ridges proliferate, and some differentiate into osteoblasts which lay down bone so as gradually to extend the ridges over toward one another (Fig. 15-36, 2) till they meet (Fig. 15-36, 3). This converts the groove that formerly existed between 2 ridges into a tunnel. Since the groove was lined with periosteum containing osteogenic cells, osteoblasts and blood vessels, the tunnel now contains a lining of osteogenic cells and osteoblasts with a blood vessel somewhere in its lumen. As is shown in Figure 15-36 (4, 5 and 6), the continued proliferation of the osteogenic cells lining the tunnel, with their subsequent differentiation into osteoblasts and osteocytes, results in the tunnel being converted into a haversian system. It is in this manner that new haversian systems are added beneath the periosteum to the periphery of a young actively growing shaft.

As the growth in width of a bone slows down, the surface of the shaft becomes smoother. Appositional growth occurring under the periosteum, then, tends to add smooth, even layers to the surface of the shaft (Fig. 15-37). These are called *circumferential lamellae* because they tend to surround the whole shaft. However, if growth in width continues after they have formed, haversian systems can replace them by means of longitudinal troughs being eroded on the surface of the shaft by osteoclasts. When a longitudinal trough becomes sufficiently deep, the osteogenic cells and the osteoblasts of the periosteum line it and those at the surface roof over the trough and convert it into a tunnel which thereupon is filled up from its interior by osteogenic cells and osteoblasts laying down successive lamellae of bone. By this means, bone consisting originally of circumferential lamellae or bone in almost any kind of arrangement can be replaced by bone consisting of haversian systems. In this instance, the crevices between the haversian systems filled with what are called interstitial lamellae would be the remains of the former circumferential lamellae.

The Incorporation of Periosteal-derived Blood Vessels Into Growing Shafts of Bone—The Nature of Volkmann's Canals. As the two processes of bone deposition and bone resorption, on the outer and inner surfaces of a shaft, respectively, continue through the growth period, it comes to pass that the bone of the

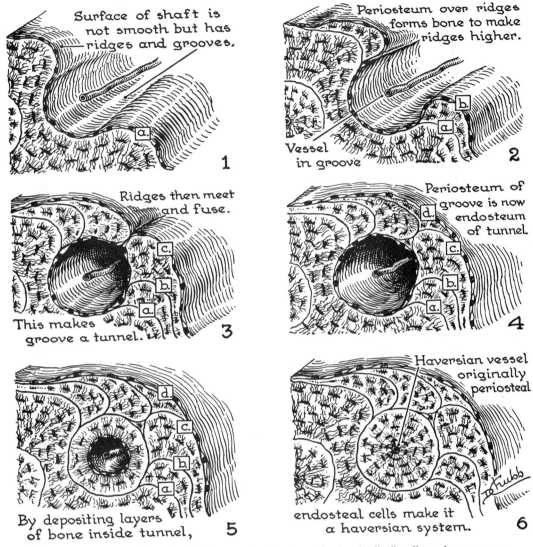

FIG. 15-36. Three-dimensional diagrams showing how the longitudinally disposed grooves on the exterior of a growing shaft become roofed over to form tunnels and how these become filled in to form haversian systems which thereupon are added to the exterior of the shaft. These diagrams also show how the blood supply of a shaft of a long bone comes to be derived, when it is fully grown, to a great extent from the periosteum by means of vessels having been buried in its substance.

original shaft is all resorbed, and that the shaft comes to be composed entirely of bone that has been deposited under the periosteum during the growing period. Since each haversian system that forms under the periosteum is built around a periosteal vessel (Fig. 15-36), the blood vessels of the shaft, as growth in width continues, would seem to be vessels that were once in the periosteum and became incorporated into bone as the troughs that they were in became roofed over. However, the roof that forms over each trough is not quite complete. A hole is left in it at the site at which the periosteal vessel descends into the trough. As the successive haversian systems are added to the surface, the first-formed ones become more deeply buried, and so what were originally only holes in the roofs of troughs become elongated to constitute canals which run at right angles to the haversian systems between them and the periosteum. These canals that thus come to convey periosteal vessels into the haversian canals of the compact bone shaft are called Volkmann's canals (Fig. 15-37). Because of the way they are formed, they, unlike haversian canals, are not surrounded by concentric lamellae.

From the foregoing account of how a bone grows in width, it may seem that most of the blood supply of the cortex of the diaphysis of a fully grown bone would be derived from the periosteum. However, the circulation is more complicated than it seems, as will be described presently.

Circumferential, Haversian and Interstitial Lamellae. As a bone attains its full width, it is usual for the osteoblasts covering its outer surface and lining its inner surface to smooth these by adding a few more or less final circumferential lamellae. These are called the outer and the inner circumferential lamellae (Fig. 15-37). In a sense, they are like the finishing coats that a plasterer applies to the walls of a room as he completes his work. Between the outer and the inner circumferential lamellae, the shaft of a bone consists of haversian systems made of haversian lamellae (Fig. 15-37). The crevices between these (interstitial lamellae) are either the remaining parts of old outer circumferential lamellae or old haversian systems (Fig. 15-37). There would be, of course, infinitely more haversian systems in the wall of a shaft than is shown in the simplified diagram that is Figure 15-37.

The Remodeling of Bone

The remodeling of bone can only be achieved by bone being resorbed from surfaces and added to surfaces.

Remodeling occurs under different circumstances. We have already described one kind that occurs as long bones grow in length and width. This kind ends up with a bone having its adult form and size. As has been described, it is not the same bone tissue that is in the bone of an adult as that that was present in the bone of the child because during growth the latter is all resorbed. This type of remodeling is sometimes called "structural remodeling."

Structural remodeling also occurs in connection with the increased use or a changed use of a particular bone. The formation of new extra bone, or a changed alignment of the trabeculae of cancellous bone or even of the cortex of cortical bone can occur so as to improve the ability of the bony structure to bear weight or stand up better to some new type of stress. Why the need for increased or altered function can bring about resorption in some areas and new bone formation in others is not understood. What is known, however, is

that the function of a bone has a great deal to do with determining its microscopic structure. For example, if a bone that is much used is put to rest, the amount of bone tissue in it becomes considerably reduced; this is termed "atrophy of disuse."

In addition to structural remodeling there is another type sometimes termed "internal remodeling." Internal remodeling is required because the haversian systems in compact bone or the trabeculae of cancellous bone do not last throughout the life of an adult. Some systems or parts of systems are always being resorbed with new ones being built in the tunnels caused by the resorption. Internal remodeling occurs because bone does not last throughout life; it, like so many other tissues, must be constantly renewed but not nearly so rapidly as others.

There are many reasons for bone tissue not lasting as long as might be expected from its gross appearance. First, the canalicular mechanism by which the cells of compact bone are nourished is not a very efficient system. Anyone who understands the histology of bone and how osteocytes are nourished would expect that parts of haversian systems, particularly those parts that are farthest from haversian canals, might suffer nutritional deficiencies and hence the osteocytes in these more remote parts of systems would die. This brings up the problem of what happens to *dead bone,* that is, calcified bone in which the lacunae are empty because the osteocytes they formerly contained have died and dissolved or in which lacunae contain only the pyknotic remains of dead osteocytes.

Parts of haversian systems in which the osteocytes have died may persist for a long time if they are completely surrounded by haversian systems in which the bone is still alive. Hence it is not unusual in compact bone to see empty lacunae, particularly in interstitial lamellae. The probable reason for the persistence of dead bone in such locations is that any mechanisms that could bring about its resorption have no access to it. But if dead bone is exposed to the contents of a haversian canal—that is, capillaries and osteogenic cells—the osteogenic cells form osteoclasts and the dead bone is resorbed. By this means what is termed a *resorption cavity* (Fig. 15-38) is formed within bone substance. These are generally elongated tubular cavities and the normal fate for them in a healthy adult is that after they have been tidied up by osteoclasts in much the same way that a dentist tidies up a cavity in a tooth before he fills it (Fig. 15-38), the osteogenic cells line up around the inner surface of the cavity and form osteoblasts. The way a resorption cavity appears in an H and E section as it is being filled in by successive new layers of bone is shown in Figure 15-39.

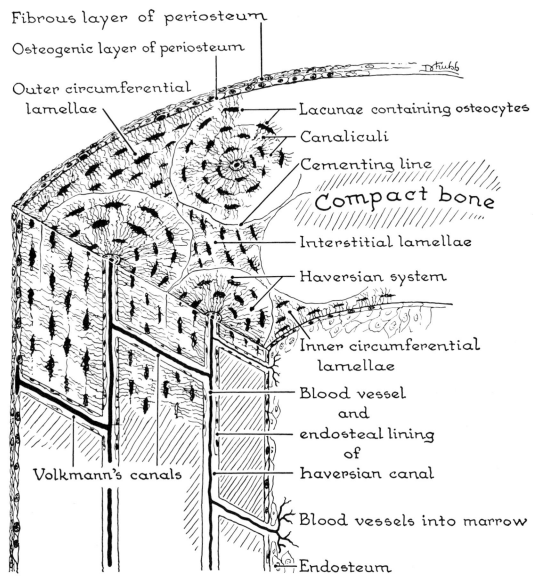

Fibrous layer of periosteum

Osteogenic layer of periosteum

Outer circumferential lamellae

Lacunae containing osteocytes

Canaliculi

Cementing line

Compact bone

Interstitial lamellae

Haversian system

Inner circumferential lamellae

Blood vessel and endosteal lining of haversian canal

Volkmann's canals

Blood vessels into marrow

Endosteum

Fig. 15-37. A 3-dimensional diagram showing the appearance of both a cross and a longitudinal section of the various components that enter into the structure of the cortex of the shaft of a long bone. It should be kept in mind, of course, that there would be many more haversian systems in the cortex than are shown here. The diagram shows the different kinds of lamellae that are present and the relation between the blood vessels of the periosteum, Volkmann's canals, haversian canals and the marrow cavity.

The border between the edge of a resorption cavity that thus becomes a new haversian system and the new bone of the system can be distinguished in most ordinary sections as what is called a cementing line (Fig. 15-40). There is moreover another line that can be detected which is called a frontier line or calcification front (Fig. 15-40, not labeled); this line is seen between what appears to be the last layer of organic

intercellular substance that has been formed in the new haversian system and the layer that was formed previously and has become calcified. The reason for this line is that, in forming a haversian system, it takes some time for each layer of organic intercellular substance that is deposited to become calcified; in a new system the last layer to be formed, which is the layer that abuts on the lumen of the system, remains for a

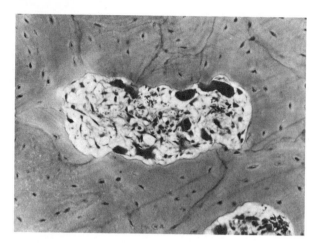

Fig. 15-38. Photomicrograph of a cross section of the shaft of a bone showing a resorption cavity in cross or somewhat oblique section. The large dark cells are osteoclasts; their activity explains the etched-out borders of the cavity. (Preparation courtesy of C. P. Leblond)

time in an uncalcified state and so during this period it is referred to as *osteoid tissue* or *prebone*. Leblond and Weinstock have shown by radioautography that the collagen of prebone is not associated with as much glycoprotein as that in the bone beyond the frontier line.

The last layers of bone that are being deposited in the various sites where bone is being laid down in the body are believed to be of metabolic significance in that the calcium of the calcium salts that are gradually being deposited in it remains more or less in equilibrium with the ionized calcium of the blood. Hence, if some condition arises that causes the level of the calcium in the blood to fall, the calcium in this newly forming bone shifts quickly into the blood to help maintain its proper calcium level. Thus the tissue that is newly formed and just in the process of becoming calcified is sometimes referred to as metabolic or labile bone because of its reservoir function. This is in contrast to structural bone which is thoroughly and permanently calcified and from which calcium can be removed only by means of the calcified matrix being eroded by cellular activity.

Although it is easily possible from studying cross sections of bone to see resorption cavities developing and new haversian systems being formed, it is difficult to gain any appreciation of how long systems last or how long it takes for new ones to form; in other words, ordinary studies give little information about the rate of turnover of haversian systems. There are, however, vital staining methods available that allow new bone

to be labeled as it is formed and calcified, and these can be used to determine how much new bone is formed over the time they are available in the circulation.

A vital staining method for following the deposition and calcification of new bone so that the amount that formed over a given time could be calculated was first discovered in 1736 by a young surgeon who instead of having to work at nights in a laboratory to make his discovery did so under the pleasant circumstances of having dinner at a friend's house where he noticed, as his host carved the joint, that the bone in it was red. Being interested in this phenomenon he inquired into the origin of the meat and found that his host, who was a dye merchant, raised his own pigs and also that he fed his pigs some of the leftover materials from which he extracted dyes, from one of which (a vegetable substance called madder) he extracted a dye now known as alizarin. The young surgeon found that if he fed this dye to an animal it colored red such bone as was being formed and becoming calcified while it was being fed. Although much of interest was elicited about bone growth and repair by feeding or injecting animals with alizarin, the method has been superseded by radioautography and the use of radioactive calcium or phosphorus for labeling newly forming calcium deposits or a labeled amino acid (for example, proline)

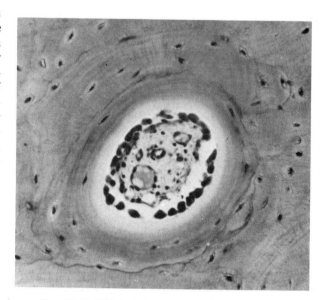

Fig. 15-39. This is the way a former resorption cavity that is being filled in to make a new haversian system appears in an H and E cross section of compact bone. The dark cells that ring the cavity are osteoblasts. For details see next illustration. (Photomicrograph courtesy of C. P. Leblond)

Fig. 15-40. In Figure 15-39 the osteoblasts are seen to be separated from the bone by a pale material. As is shown on the right side of this figure the material of that layer is called Prebone. It consists of organic matrix which is not as yet calcified. At its periphery a line called the frontier line (not labeled) marks the site where mineral begins to be deposited. Farther out *cementing lines* indicate the borders between new layers of bone that have been formed on older layers. The left side of the picture illustrates a fully formed osteon. (Illustration courtesy of C. P. Leblond)

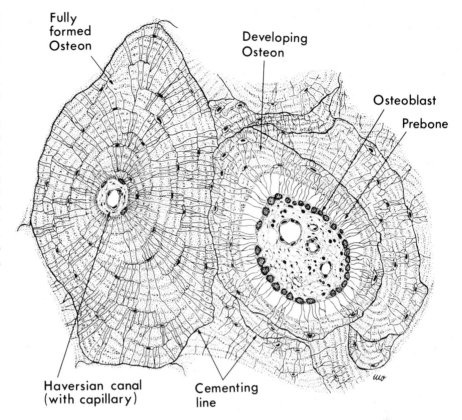

to label newly forming organic matrix. It was also found that certain fluorescent substances could be injected into animals to label sites where calcification was occurring; tetracyclines have been much used for this purpose. These latter methods require examining the sections that are obtained by means of fluorescence microscopy. The various results obtained by these methods indicate that remodeling occurs to different extents in different bones and also to different extents in the same bone. From studies on dogs made by the newer methods, it appears that the annual rate at which the bone of the cortex of a long bone is replaced is somewhere between 5 and 10 percent a year. (For details of this matter see Lacroix and Harris and Heaney.)

How Certain Nutritional and Metabolic Factors Can Affect Growing Bones and the Structure of Bones in the Adult

One of the meanings of meta is "between," so a metaphysis of a long bone is the region between its epiphysis and its diaphysis. This region could be thought of as encompassing the zone of the epiphyseal plate that is being replaced by bone and the region of

trabeculae that are forming beneath the plate and which have cores of calcified cartilage. The metaphyses of growing bones are the site of great *anabolic* activity. The proliferation of osteogenic cells, their differentiation into osteoblasts and the synthesis of the organic matrix of bone at this site all involve a great deal of collagen synthesis as well as the synthesis of mucopolysaccharides and glycoproteins. With all this anabolic activity taking place, it should be obvious that any nutritional deficiencies or metabolic alterations that affect protein or even carbohydrate synthesis may quickly be reflected is some alteration of the growth pattern in this region.

Second, the metaphyseal region of a growing bone is a site where calcium salts are being deposited into newly formed organic matrix at a very rapid rate. The normal growth of bone in the metaphyseal region depends on calcification occurring normally, just as it depends on protein synthesis occurring normally. In the normal the two processes, (1) the synthesis of organic materials and (2) the calcification of organic intercellular substance, are synchronized. It is important to realize that the normal growth of bone depends on *two different processes* that generally operate in harmony with one another and that the factors that affect the anabolic synthetic processes are not the same factors that affect the calcification process, and vice versa. Next, because the metaphysis is the site of such great activity it is a very sensitive one to any metabolic disturbance that may develop in a growing individual and as a result of a metabolic disturbance its histological picture is soon altered. If a disturbance of the normal growth pattern is seen in the metaphysis of a growing bone, perhaps the first question to ask is, which process is primarily affected, the synthesis of the organic components of bone or the calcification of the organic intercellular substance?

To illustrate that interference with each of these processes is reflected in a different kind of histological picture in the metaphysis, we shall describe briefly one example each of an interference with (1) the synthesis of the organic components of bone, and (2) the calcification of the organic intercellular substance of bone.

(1) **Scurvy.** Perhaps the most dramatic interference with the synthesis of organic materials in a metaphysis is seen in scurvy, a disease that can affect adults as well as growing children, although in adults, in whom growth is no longer occurring in metaphyses, its manifestations in bone appear more slowly and in relation to bone maintenance and in the maintenance of other structures, for example, capillaries. It was once the greatest threat to the life and welfare of sailors who were on long voyages (where it was noted that the disease often appeared after they ran out of potatoes). The possibility of an outbreak of scurvy always hung heavily over the heads of those who engaged in polar exploration, and, indeed, in the early days of the settlement of the northern part of North America scurvy became so widespread and serious in the long winters that it is a wonder anyone stayed here unless he had to.

In due course it became fairly well established that scurvy did not develop in children and adults whose diets contained a supply of fresh fruits and vegetables and that a dietary supplement of lemon juice would prevent the disease from occurring. However, for a long time it was believed that the disease was caused by a *positive agent* of some sort, for example, poor air or tainted food and therefore it was assumed that fresh fruits and vegetables somehow prevented this elusive unknown agent from exerting its evil effects. It was not until the present century that it became clear that diseases could be caused by a *lack of something*—for example, the essential food factors that we now term vitamins—and that scurvy was caused by a lack of vitamin C.

Although a vitamin C deficiency affects the metabolism of types of various cells in the body, its effects are particularly noticeable in the metaphysis of a growing bone. The proper multiplication of both chondroblasts and osteogenic cells is affected and in particular osteoblasts are unable to synthesize and secrete the organic constituents of normal bone matrix. The net result is that on a diet inadequate but not completely deficient in vitamin C, the metaphysis of, for example, the upper end of the tibia of a guinea pig (guinea pigs, like man, are sensitive to dietary deficiencies of vitamin C; many animals can make their own), shows very little anabolic activity (Fig. 15-41). Growth in the epiphyseal plate is slowed, and almost no new bone formation occurs on the diaphyseal plate (Fig. 15-41). The almost complete cessation of the formation of bone results in the shaft of the bone being very thin (Fig. 15-41). As a consequence, both the epiphyseal plate, lacking support by bony trabeculae beneath it, and the shaft are easily fractured.

The process of calcification, however, is *not* interfered with by scurvy. The little organic matrix that is formed becomes heavily calcified. Scurvy, therefore, represents a condition in which the defect lies in anabolic activities that are concerned with the multiplication of cells and their synthesis of organic intercellular substances. There are other metabolic defects which act in a different way to interfere with normal growth and the formation of organic intercellular substances; for example, we shall see, when we consider the endocrine glands, that the synthesis of protein can be affected by several of the hormones.

(2) **Rickets.** The mechanism of calcification is probably dependent on a concentration of calcium and phosphate ions being achieved in the vicinity of calcifying bone or cartilage that approaches their solubility product and so permits a local mechanism to operate and cause a local precipitation of calcium salts into the organic matrix. It has been shown that calcification does not proceed normally in the growing zone of the bones of an infant if the product obtained by multiplying the number of milligrams of calcium per 100 ml of serum by the number of milligrams of phosphorus per 100 ml of blood is below a certain figure. It is to be noted that a reduced level of calcium *or* phosphorus in the blood does not necessarily interfere with calcification; it is the concentration of the product of the two that determines whether calcification will continue.

In a baby the growing skeleton normally absorbs large amounts of calcium phosphate which necessitates that the infant's diet contain an adequate amount of calcium and phosphorus. Further, for these minerals to be absorbed into the bloodstream, the infant also requires an adequate supply of vitamin D. If an infant's diet is deficient in these essentials, the CaP product of

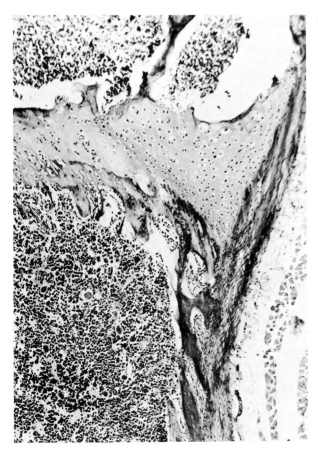

normally, but continue to live. The result is that, since growth continues in the growing zone of the disks, the epiphyseal disks become thicker than normal (Fig. 15-42). Inasmuch as calcification is not entirely arrested but occurs in a few sites on the diaphyseal sides of the disk, the thickening of the disks tends to be irregular (Fig. 15-42). In the meantime, osteoblasts continue to lay down the organic intercellular substance of bone in the metaphysis, but this also does not become calcified because of the low CaP product. Instead, it exists in an uncalcified state until the diet is remedied. This new bone, during the time it remains uncalcified, is termed *osteoid tissue* (Fig. 15-42). Fur-

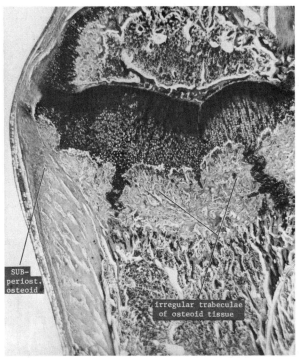

Fig. 15-41. A low-power photomicrograph of a longitudinal section of the upper end of the tibia of a guinea pig that for some weeks had been fed a diet containing an inadequate amount of vitamin C. Under conditions of prolonged vitamin C deficiency, bone building almost ceases on the diaphyseal side of the disk, and, as a result, the epiphyseal plate is not supported by a proper number of trabeculae. Furthermore, bone building almost ceases in the shaft, and, as a result, it becomes fragile and breaks easily. (Ham, A. W., and Elliott, H. C.: Am. J. Path., *14:323*)

Fig. 15-42. Low-power photomicrograph of a longitudinal section of the upper end of the tibia of a young rat that had been fed a Steenbock diet with calcium carbonate added to produce a blood-calcium level of 10 mg. and a blood-phosphorus level of 2 mg. per 100 ml. Since the product of calcium and phosphorus was only 20, proper calcification did not ensue on the diaphyseal side of the epiphyseal plate. This had resulted in the cartilage cells living much longer than they should, and as a result the epiphyseal disk has become thicker than normal and in some sites very thick. Furthermore, such trabeculae as have formed on the diaphyseal side of the disk are irregular and poorly calcified (osteoid tissue). Osteoid tissue also may be seen to have formed under the periosteum at the left side of the picture. This is an example of severe low-phosphorus rickets.

the blood may fall below the level at which calcification would occur in the growing zone, with the result that a condition known as *rickets* develops. The earliest change noted is that although growth continues and organic matrix continues to be synthesized, the calcification of cartilage almost ceases in the epiphyseal disks. If the intercellular substance surrounding the mature cells in this zone fails to become impregnated with mineral, the cells of this zone are not shut off from nutrition. Hence, they do not die, as they do

thermore, it seems as if the osteoblasts of the periosteum in the region of metaphysis realized that calcification was not proceeding normally, for they increase their activities and lay down large amounts of osteoid tissue in the metaphyseal region just beneath the periosteum (Fig. 15-42, subperiost. osteid). This makes the metaphyseal regions knobby. The knobs so produced at the growing ends of the ribs are responsible in a rachitic child's chest for what is termed the "rachitic rosary."

It is to be kept in mind that the changes that occur in the growing zones of bone in rickets are the result of growth continuing while calcification fails. For this reason, a disturbed mineral metabolism will cause more severe rickets in a child who is actively growing than in one who is not. The poorly calcified intercellular substance of bone seen in rickets bends with weightbearing. Hence, rachitic children may be bowlegged.

A deficiency of vitamin D in the diet is the usual cause of rickets. The condition is more common in cold countries and where there is little sunshine and exposure to it. In humans vitamin D is made by the effects of sunshine on their skin, as will be explained in the chapter on skin.

Effects of Disturbances of Mineral Metabolism on the Bones of Adults

Nutritional and metabolic defects show up in the metaphyses of growing bones much more quickly than they do in the bones of adults. However, as has been described, there is a turnover of both cancellous and compact bone throughout life. As has already been described, parts of old haversian systems die, resorption tunnels develop, and new haversian systems form in the tunnels. As people become older, it seems that the rate of resorption becomes greater, and as a result the compact bone of skeleton becomes more porous than it is in middle life (compare middle and right in Fig. 15-43). Not uncommonly, particularly in women who have passed the menopause, the resorptive processes exceed the building processes to a point beyond what can be considered normal, and bone becomes unduly porous and hence fragile; this condition is termed *osteoporosis*. The cause of this condition is not entirely clear, and at the moment osteoporosis is the subject of much research. One of the tools used to investigate this and allied problems is microradiography. For those interested, Jowsey's papers will be found both informative and a guide to the literature.

Microradiography. Determining the extent to which different lamellae in a given haversian system are calcified and different, and the extent to which different haversian systems in the same section of bone are calcified, has been made possible by the development of the technic of microradiography. Undecalcified sections must, of course, be employed; these have been variously prepared by grinding or by special embedding of calcified bone and cutting it into sections with special heavy microtomes. Even more elaborate methods can be employed. Sections are placed over and in direct contact with a film or plate covered with fine-grain emulsion. The preparation is then exposed (section side up) to very soft x-rays from a special source. The soft x-rays penetrate the section in relation to the amount of calcium present in its different parts. The developed film or plate constitutes a microradiograph of the section and shows the extent to which its different parts are calcified. The microradiograph can be compared with the actual section under the microscope. By this means histological appearances can be correlated with the sites of different densities indicated in the microradioautograph. Three microradiographs of cross sections of cortical bone from people of different ages and kindly supplied by Jennifer Jowsey are seen in Figure 15-43. The interpretation is explained in the caption, which should be read carefully.

The Skeleton As the Calcium Reservoir of the Body. The calcium of the blood exists in different forms; roughly half of it is ionized and the remainder is combined with protein. The proper operation of nerve tissue is dependent on the concentration of calcium ions being maintained at a certain level and if the concentration falls below it, a condition called tetany develops which is manifested by spasms of certain muscles and even convulsions. It is therefore of paramount importance that a proper level of calcium ions be maintained in the blood. There are two factors involved in this: the amount of calcium in the blood, and the pH of the blood. The significance of the latter factor is probably due to the fact that the salts that calcium ions form at a high pH are less soluble (and so provide fewer calcium ions in solutions) than those they form at a lower pH. However, given a normal pH, the concentration of calcium ions is related to the total calcium content of the blood and this in turn depends primarily on the balance between calcium intake in the diet and calcium excretion and on the functioning of the parathyroid glands. The calcium content of the diet may be less than it should be, or there may be factors that operate to somewhat inhibit its absorption from the intestine into the blood. In any event, if the excretion of calcium from the body exceeds calcium absorption, the blood calcium level

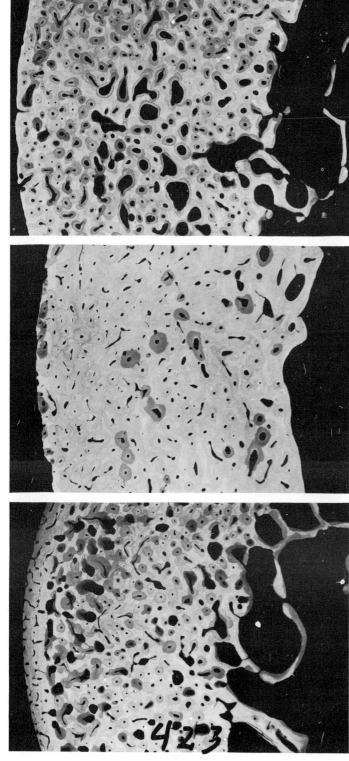

Fɪɢ. 15-43. Microradiographs of undecalcified sections from the midshaft of the femur of people of different ages. (*Left*) This section was from a 7-year-old, and it indicates the relatively rapid turnover of bone normal for this age in that it shows many resorption tunnels and many newly formed haversian systems (the bone of which shows darker than that of the older and hence more heavily calcified systems, which, being denser, are whiter in the illustration). (*Center*) This section was from a 25-year-old person. There is little indication here of the turnover of systems, for there are almost no resorption tunnels, and most of the systems are well calcified and of the same density. (*Right*) This section was from an 85-year-old person. It shows two features characteristic of bone of people this age in that (1) there are many resorption tunnels, which indicate an increased rate of resorption, and (2) the new layers of bone which are beginning to fill in some of the tunnels are poorly calcified (darker than well-calcified bone), and hence bones of the old have a higher content of bone of low density than the bone of young adults (Microradiographs by Jennifer Jowsey)

tends to fall but, as it does, the parathyroid glands are stimulated to secrete more parathyroid hormone. This, by its action on the cells of the bone cell lineage, causes the liberation of calcium from the bones so that a proper level of calcium is maintained in the blood. But this is at the expense of the skeleton.

It is believed that the calcium most easily obtainable in bones is that which has been described as being in the labile calcium of bone which is in turn believed to be that which has just been deposited in prebone where it may not as yet have become firmly bound to organic intercellular substance and hence can pass back into the tissue fluid and blood without the organic matrix, with which it was as yet loosely associated, having to be destroyed by cellular activity. However, if the demand for calcium for the blood is not satisfied by the limited amount of labile calcium available, the parathyroid gland secretes enough hormone to stimulate the formation and activities of osteoclasts. Probably the easiest place for them to provide more calcium is from cancellous bone but they also are stimulated to form in compact bone and this in due course leads to the formation of more resorption tunnels.

It should perhaps be kept in mind that a reasonably normal blood calcium level does not necessarily mean that the skeleton is not being drawn upon for calcium, because the parathyroids, in order to maintain a reasonably normal blood calcium level in a person whose diet or absorption of calcium is deficient, would be drawing upon the bone.

Osteolysis. In addition to absorption of bone by osteoclasts it has been suggested by Belanger and his associates (see references) that calcium may be removed from the bony walls of the lacunae in which osteocytes reside. They have described changes in the nature and amounts of organic intercellular substance in the intercellular substance surrounding lacunae as well as alterations in its mineral content under conditions where resorption was occurring. They have termed the phenomenon *osteolysis* and they point out that the lacunar surfaces with which osteocytes are in contact and the canalicular surfaces with which their processes are in contact represent a vast area from which mineral could be removed when the calcium metabolism was unfavorable. However, the lacunae and their osteocytes in haversian systems are not nearly as accessible to the bloodstream as the external surfaces of cancellous and compact bone or the internal surfaces of haversian canals, all of which are close to capillaries, and whose covering or lining cells could be expected to react promptly to increased parathyroid hormone in the blood by forming osteo-

clasts which are specialized for resorption. It might, therefore, be thought that resorption at the level of osteocytes would only be substantial in long continued drains on the bone calcium and after resorption from surfaces, where there are capillaries, had been thoroughly exploited.

The Blood Supply of a Long Bone

We shall first consider a long bone whose growth is over. In such a bone the epiphyseal plates have finished their work in connection with its growth in length and have been resorbed, so there is no barrier between the marrow cavity of the diaphysis and that of the epiphyses.

How Do 3 Sets of Blood Vessels Become Incorporated Into a Bone? Our study of the development of a long bone makes it easy to understand there are three ways that blood vessels can and do become incorporated into a long bone as it develops.

1. *The Nutrient Artery and Vein.* First, it will be recalled that the cartilage in the midsection of a cartilage model of a bone begins to calcify and develop cavities within its substance just as the osteogenic cells along the side of the model are beginning to form a shell of bone around the model (Figs. 15-23 and 15-24). Then, at some site around the circumference of the model, some osteogenic cells and capillaries break through into the substance of the cartilage to enter it at the site where it is cavitating. This ingrowth of osteogenic cells and capillaries into the cartilage model is called a periosteal bud, and the blood vessels within it become increasingly larger as the bone continues to grow, to become the nutrient artery and vein of that particular bone. In some bones (for example, the femur) nutrient arteries form at different sites in this manner but in other bones (for example, the tibia) there is only one.

As was described in connection with myeloid tissue, the nutrient artery (or arteries) provide the blood supply for bone marrow. The branches of the artery however, besides serving the marrow, supply also much of the shaft of the bone. When the growth of a long bone is over, and the epiphyseal plates have been resorbed, there is no cartilaginous barrier between the marrow of the diaphysis and the epiphyses of a long bone and so the blood vessels of the diaphysis can anastomose with those of the marrow of the epiphysis, the origin of which will next be described.

2. *The Metaphyseal Vessels.* To understand how these vessels obtain access to the marrow cavity of a bone it will be helpful to glance again at Figure 15-33. It is to be noted here that around the flared end of

the bone the spaces between the trabeculae that are just below the periphery of the epiphyseal plate extend out to the periosteum that covers the flared portion of the diaphysis. Blood vessels from the periosteum are present in these canals and they extend to the epiphyseal plate. But when growth is over and the epiphyseal plate is resorbed, these blood vessels can pass directly into the marrow cavity of the epiphysis which is now in free communication with the marrow cavity of the diaphysis and so they are able to anastomose with vessels from the nutrient vessels, which they do.

3. *The Periosteal Vessels.* In connection with our description of how the shaft of a bone grows in width, we pointed out that capillaries from the periosteum become successively buried in each new haversian system that is added to the exterior of a shaft and that, as successive systems are buried, their vessels retain their connection with periosteal vessels by way of Volkmann's canals (Figs. 15-36 and 15-37). From the way these vessels are incorporated into the shaft of a bone it might be assumed that these vessels would provide the chief blood supply for the cortex of the shaft. But this does not seem to be what happens. Suspicion that the compact bone of a shaft is not supplied with blood primarily from the periosteal vessels might be aroused from the fact noted by De Haas and Macnab that a nutrient vein is generally smaller than its companion nutrient artery, which leads to the thought that much of the blood that enters a bone by way of the nutrient artery must leave by some route other than the nutrient vein. The studies of Brooks indicate that, instead of the blood flowing inward from the periosteum through the cortex of a bone, the circulation is in the other direction—that is, that blood from the nutrient artery is fed by means of anastomoses into the system of vessels that lie in the haversian canals of the cortex of a long bone and that the blood flows out through these vessels to be drained away from the bone by way of periosteal vessels. It now seems generally accepted that under normal conditions at least the inner two thirds of the cortex receives its blood supply from the nutrient artery and that only in some sites do the periosteal vessels contribute significant amounts of blood to the haversian systems of the cortex. However, should the medullary supply be injured, as might occur in some fractures or in operative procedures as when some of the marrow cavity is reamed out, it seems probable that periosteal vessels can then supply more of the cortex than they do under ordinary circumstances.

It should be very clear, from the above discussion, that a thorough knowledge about the blood supply of a long bone is a matter of profound importance to those who propose specializing in orthopedic or reconstructive surgery and that further investigation as to what happens under different types of injury or operative procedures is indicated. The problem has recently been extensively studied and reviewed by Rhinelander (*see* "Other Reading").

The Blood Supply of the Epiphyses of Long Bones

The blood supply of epiphyses and the epiphyseal plate is of great interest with regard to certain problems in connection with growing children.

Blood Supply of Epiphyses. Dale and Harris point out that in growing bones there are two kinds of epiphyses, in the sense that, in one kind, the articular cartilage is continuous with that of the epiphyseal plate, as is shown in the picture on the right in Figure 15-44, and, in the other kind, the articular cartilage is not continuous with the epiphyseal plate, as is shown in the left-hand picture in Figure 15-44. In the first kind the blood vessels that supply the epiphysis have to travel through the site where the cartilage of the epiphyseal plate is continuous with articular cartilage in order to reach the marrow cavity of the epiphysis (right side, in Fig. 15-44). In the second kind of arrangement, shown on the left in Figure 15-44, the blood vessels that enter the epiphysis do not have to pass through articular or epiphyseal plate cartilage to enter the epiphysis; instead they pierce the perichondrial-like tissue that covers one side of the epiphysis. These two types of epiphysis behave differently if a separation due to an accident occurs across the epiphyseal plate, as will now be described.

Epiphyseal separations sometimes occur in children. If some shearing or other force operates to cause an epiphyseal separation, the separation, as has been shown by both Haas and Harris, generally occurs in the zone of hypertrophied cartilage cells of the plate, as is shown in Figure 15-45, for this is the weakest part of the plate. If this happens in an epiphysis of the type illustrated on the right side of Figure 15-44, the blood vessels that are conducted through the cartilage at the edge of the plate are likely to be ruptured. On the other hand, if a separation occurs in the type illustrated on the left in Figure 15-44, the epiphysis still retains its blood supply. Harris and Hobson showed that the upper femoral epiphysis is of the type illustrated on the right in Figure 15-44, and that separation of an epiphysis of this type, by experimental means, leads to the death of the detached fragment. Dale and Harris, however, have shown that the epiphysis of the type illustrated on the left in Figure

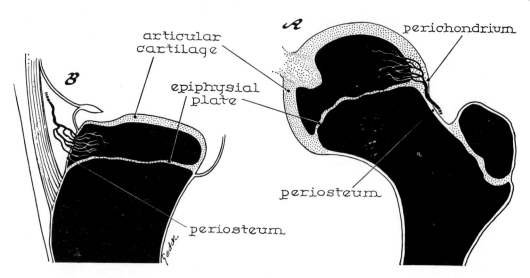

FIG. 15-44. Diagram to demonstrate that when an epiphysis is entirely covered by articular cartilage (*A*) (*right side*), its blood vessels must enter it by traversing the perichondrium at the periphery of the epiphyseal plate. This makes them vulnerable to rupture after epiphyseal displacement. By contrast, when an epiphysis is only partly covered by articular cartilage (*B*) (*left side*), its blood vessels enter it in such a way that separation could occur without serious damage to them. (Dale, G. G., and Harris, W. R.: J. Bone Joint Surg., *40-B*:116)

15-44 may be detached without death of the fragment occurring (Fig. 15-45). Furthermore, the experimental detachment of this type of epiphysis gave valuable information in regard to the source from which the proliferating cells of an epiphyseal plate receive their nourishment, as will next be described.

The Nutrition of the Epiphyseal Plate. Since the diaphyseal side of an epiphyseal plate abounds in capillary loops which are disposed between the forming trabeculae of bone in that region, and which penetrate into the zone of calcifying cartilage of the plate, it might be assumed that these capillaries of diaphyseal (nutrient artery) origin provided the nourishment necessary for the cell division that occurs toward the epiphyseal side of the plate and for the synthesis of such intercellular substance as occurs in association with the chondrocytes in a growing plate. However, as has been stressed by the author, the calcification of the intercellular substance of cartilage makes it much less able to serve as a medium for diffusion, and hence nourishment might have difficulty in penetrating from diaphyseal capillaries through the zone of calcified cartilage to reach the zone of proliferating cells. Moreover, inspection of Figure 15-28 will show that there are on the diaphyseal side of the layer of epiphyseal bone that abuts on the epiphyseal plate, in the zone labeled *resting cartilage,* canals that contain capil-

laries. These have been studied by injection methods by Salter and Harris, one of whose preparations is seen in Figure 15-46; this shows branches from epiphyseal vessels penetrating the bone of the epiphysis to supply the zone of "resting" cartilage cells of the plate. That nourishment from these capillaries diffuses through the remainder of the plate to nourish the cells of its various living layers was shown by Dale and Harris; for they found that if the blood supply of the epiphysis remained intact, epiphyseal plates could be separated from the metaphysis (and hence from metaphyseal blood vessels), and yet the separated plates would continue to grow in thickness (Fig. 15-45). These experiments and others show clearly that the cartilage of the epiphyseal plate obtains the nutriment it requires for growth from its epiphyseal side and probably principally from the small vessels seen in the canals immediately on the diaphyseal side of the bone of the epiphysis illustrated in Figures 15-28 and 15-46. Some nourishment may also diffuse in from the periphery of the plate.

The Blood Vessels of Haversian Systems (Osteons) of Compact Bone. The arrangement of haversian systems in compact bone is very complex as new ones are substituted for old ones in the slow remodeling of compact bone that takes place during life. Jonathan Cohen and William H. Harris have made a 3-

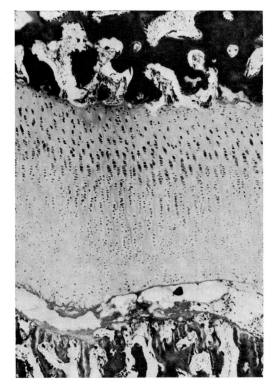

FIG. 15-45. Photomicrograph of section of radial epiphyseal plate of a rabbit 10 days after the epiphysis with the epiphyseal plate was separated from the diaphysis. Note that the line of separation occurs across the zone of hypertrophied cells. During the 10 days that followed the separation, the plate has grown greatly in thickness, which shows that its source of nutrition was provided from the epiphysis by the vessels illustrated in Figure 15-46. (Dale, G. G., and Harris, W. R.: J. Bone Joint Surg., *40-B*:118)

some site where they anastomose. Between this site and the fracture the osteocytes in the compact bone have no source of nutrition so they die. This means there is dead bone on either side of a fracture back to where haversian vessels anastomose with one another, as will be mentioned further as we discuss fractures.

Intramembranous Ossification

Having discussed endochondral ossification and how bones that develop in cartilage grow and are remodeled, we should now briefly discuss intramembranous ossification which is responsible particularly for forming most of the bone of the skull. Since bone that forms in membrane has no cartilage in it to provide for interstitial growth, we shall find that the way that bones of the skull grow in extent is different from the way those that form in cartilage do. Intramembranous ossification is easily studied by studying sections of the developing vault of the skull. Areas in which these bones develop are occupied first by mesenchyme. Intramembranous ossification begins when a cluster of

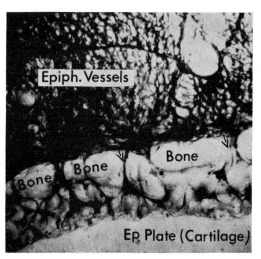

FIG. 15-46. Photomicrograph of longitudinal section that passes through epiphyseal plate and part of an epiphysis of a growing long bone of a rabbit. The arteries supplying the epiphysis were injected with an opaque material, and the illustration shows that arterial vessels from the epiphysis penetrate the bone that lies between the marrow of the epiphysis and the epiphyseal plate of cartilage to supply nutriment to the epiphyseal border of the epiphyseal plate. These vessels can support the life and growth of the plate if it is separated from the diaphysis. (Salter, R. M., and Harris, W. R.: J. Bone Joint Surg., *45-A*:587)

dimensional study of haversian systems and their anastomoses in compact bone, and their report should be read for details about their sizes and the courses they pursue.

In completed haversian systems there may be only a single vessel, as is shown on the left in Figure 15-47, or two vessels, as shown on the right in Figure 15-47. The vessel on the left is of the order of a large capillary, while those on the right are a precapillary arteriole and a beginning venule.

Since vessels in haversian systems run more or less parallel with the shaft of a long bone, their severance, when a fracture occurs, leads to their open ends becoming sealed off and so circulation in them ceases back to

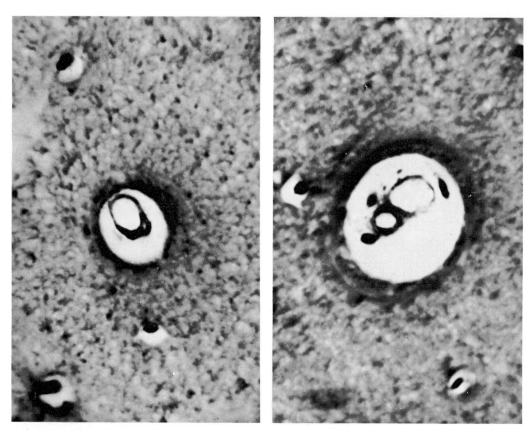

Fig. 15-47.   Photomicrographs ($\times$ 800) of blood vessels in haversian canals as they appear in cross sections of the radius of a dog. (*Left*) The canal in the center contains a single vessel which is a large capillary. (*Right*) The canal in the center contains 2 vessels, a very small arteriole and a very small venule. The stippled appearance of the bone intercellular substance is due to the presence of canaliculi that are cut in cross section and obliquely. A few bone cells in lacunae may be seen. (Ham, A. W.: J. Bone Joint Surg., *34-A*:701)

mesenchymal cells differentiate into osteoblasts as shown in Figures 15-3 and 15-48.

Sites where clusters of osteoblasts first appear are spoken of as centers of ossification. There are usually two centers for each of the bones of the vault of the skull.

Soon after osteoblasts appear they begin to secrete the organic matrix of bone. Those that completely surround themselves with this become osteocytes residing in lacunae (Fig. 15-49). However, not all the cells of the osteoblast-osteocyte family that arise from mesenchyme differentiate immediately into functioning secretory osteoblasts. In due course the least differentiated cells of the bone cell lineage that arise from the mesenchyme cells (osteogenic cells) set up a self-maintaining population of stem cells that proliferate to supply new osteoblasts in the region. Both osteogenic cells and osteoblasts remain fairly closely applied to the margin of the bone already formed, with some of the osteogenic cells continuing to proliferate and others differentiating and secreting intercellular substance about themselves to become osteocytes to form a beam of bone called a spicule. Spicules are covered with osteogenic cells and osteoblasts. Figure 15-49 is probably a cross section of a spicule.

Well developed spicules that radiate out from the ossification center are also termed *trabeculae* (*trabs*, a beam). This term is apt because individual trabeculae (beams) of bone are commonly joined together to form a scaffolding (Fig. 15-50). Bone that consists of a scaffolding of trabeculae joined together is termed *cancellous* bone.

The Nourishment of the Cells of Cancellous (Trabeculated) Bone. The trabeculae of cancellous bone are bathed in tissue fluid which is derived from the blood vessels in spaces between the trabeculae.

Within each trabecula, canaliculi extend out from each lacuna and anastomose with canaliculi from all adjacent lacunae (Fig. 15-2). Moreover, canaliculi from more superficial lacunae extend to the exterior of the trabecula and so permit tissue fluid or substances dissolved in tissue fluid to enter the anastomosing canalicular system of the trabecula. Consequently, nutrients, to reach the bone cells in the middle of a trabecula that is one fifth of a millimeter in thickness, must pass along the canalicular system for one tenth of a millimeter. In the experience of the author, trabeculae of more than one fifth of a millimeter in thickness generally have blood vessels disposed in canals near their middles to provide the more deeply disposed bone cells with nourishment. Accordingly, the thickness of solid trabeculae is limited. If too many layers are deposited on the surface of one, the osteocytes that are disposed deep within it are too far from capillaries to survive.

How the Cancellous Bone Is Converted to Compact Bone in the Skull. In order to understand this, it is necessary to realize that a section such as the one shown in Figure 15-50 is only a slice cut through what is really a 3-dimensional network of bone trabeculae and hence the spaces in such a section are more or less

of the nature of tunnels that have bony walls even though the latter are not always continuous. So if new lamellae are added to the sides of trabeculae in a cancellous network, the spaces between the trabeculae are correspondingly narrowed, exactly in the same way that a tunnel becomes narrowed if workers inside the tunnel continue to apply further layers of stone or reinforced concrete to the inside of its walls. Accordingly, the continued deposition of fresh bone lamellae on trabeculae that enclose spaces soon changes the character of the bone in that it changes from a structure consisting of large spaces with little bone (Fig. 15-50) to one of narrow spaces with much bone (Fig. 15-51). *When bone substance (instead of spaces) becomes the predominant feature of the tissue, it is said to be compact or dense bone.*

Growth of Bones of the Skull. At birth ossification has advanced far enough for the bones of the skull to have approached one another so closely that they are separated from one another only by narrow seams of relatively undifferentiated connective tissue. An arrangement whereby adjacent bones are joined by connective tissue is termed a *suture* (Fig. 16-1). However, at points where more than 2 bones meet, the sutures

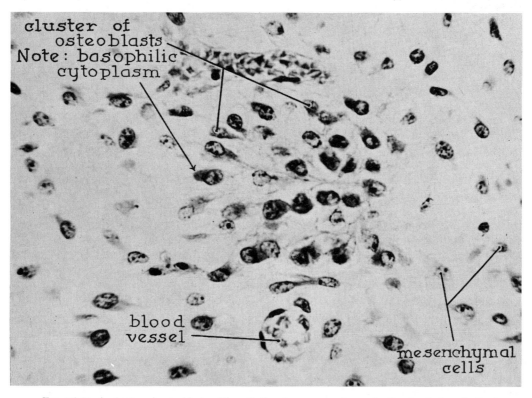

FIG. 15-48. A cluster of osteoblasts differentiating from mesenchyme in the developing skull of a pig embryo.

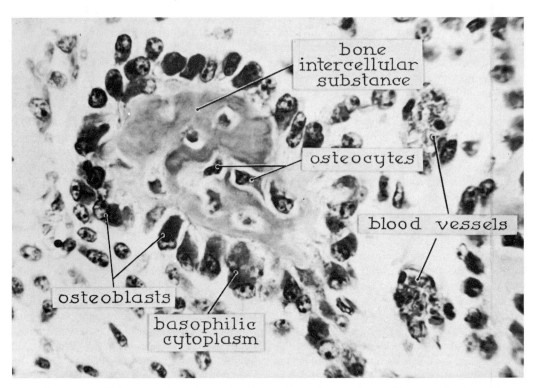

Fig. 15-49. High-power photomicrograph of a section cut through a newly formed spicule of bone in the developing skull of a pig embryo. Observe that some of the osteoblasts have differentiated into osteocytes and have surrounded themselves with intercellular substance so that they have come to reside in lacunae. Note that osteoblasts are arranged around the periphery of the spicule, where they are engaged in increasing its extent.

are wide, and such areas are termed *fontanelles*. There are 6 of these membranous areas in the skull of the newborn infant. The most prominent one, the anterior or frontal fontanelle, is situated at the point where the 2 parietal bones and the bone advancing from 2 centers of ossification of the frontal bone meet. Its inspection, in an infant, can give valuable information as to whether ossification is proceeding normally.

The vault of the skull enlarges in postnatal life by appositional growth. However, there are somewhat different views as to whether the appositional growth that is primarily responsible occurs in the sutures (Fig. 15-52) or on the convex surfaces of the bones that comprise the vault. As Figure 15-52 illustrates, appositional growth on the convex surfaces alone could account for the individual bones becoming larger (resorption on their inner surfaces would keep them from getting much thicker) without bone actually being deposited *in* the sutures. Weinmann and Sicher favor sutural growth and say that in some sutures more bone is added to one bone than the other. Brash, however, favored the second view.

How the Curvature of Bones Changes as the Skull Enlarges. As the cranium enlarges, the curvature of its bones must decrease. This requires that the bones of the skull be remodeled continuously as they grow, and this involves the deposition of bone on some surfaces and resorption of bone from others. Figure 15-52, shows how deposition and resorption, at different sites, could change the curvature of a skull bone. The bones that are remodeled in this fashion are, for some time after birth, composed of only a single plate of bone which, however, contains some spaces filled with mesenchyme and thin-walled veins (Fig. 15-51). As the growth of the skull continues, the remodeling process gradually converts these single plates of bone, over most of the skull, into double plates of compact bone, with cancellous bone and a considerable amount of marrow between them.

The layer of cancellous bone and marrow between the two plates of compact bone is termed the *diploë*, and it comes to contain many large, thin-walled veins called the *diploic veins*. The double-plate arrangement over most of the skull is attained in childhood (around

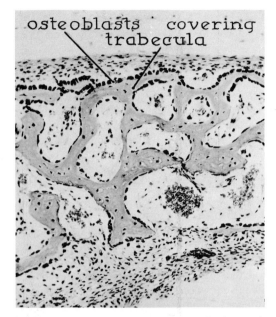

Fig. 15-50. Low-power photomicrograph of a section cut from the skull of a pig embryo somewhat more developed than that in Figure 15-49. This picture illustrates trabeculated (cancellous) bone, with the trabeculae arranged so as to enclose spaces. Observe the osteoblasts, with their dark-staining cytoplasm, arranged along the surface of the trabeculae.

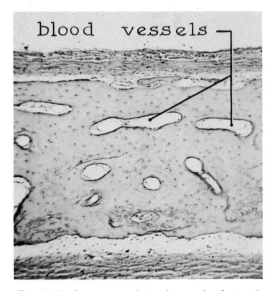

Fig. 15-51. Low-power photomicrograph of a section cut through the skull of a child. The trabeculated bone shown in Figure 15-50 has become filled in to constitute a plate of compact bone, as is shown here. The former spaces in the trabeculated area are reduced to canals which transmit the blood vessels.

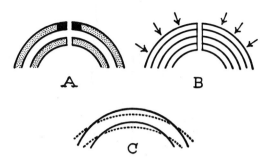

Fig. 15-52. (A) Diagram to show how appositional growth in sutures could enlarge the vault of the cranium. The new bone is black. (B) Diagram to show how appositional growth on the convex surfaces of the bones could enlarge the cranium without new bone being deposited in the sutures. It is to be understood that resorption would occur from the concave surfaces as new bone is laid down on convex surfaces. (C) Diagram to show how apposition at some sites and resorption from others could change the curvature of a skull bone.

the age of 8). Later on in adult life the bones meeting at the various sutures become fused, and it becomes possible for diploic veins to pass from one bone to another.

Immature and Mature Bone

We have dealt with both endochondral and intramembranous ossification and have seen that the bone that develops in one is the same as that which develops in the other and hence that there is no such entity as cartilage bone or membrane bone. There are, however, different kinds of bone that are distinguished from one another because of the arrangement and relative amounts of the various components of their intercellular substance and also by the relative numbers of osteocytes that they possess in relation to their content of intercellular substance. By these morphological criteriae Pritchard describes three types: (1) bundle bone, (2) woven bone, and (3) fine-fibered bone.

Bone can also be classified as immature and mature bone. The reason for this is that bundle bone and woven bone are for the most part the types of bone that are the first to develop in embryonic life—for example the bone in Figure 15-49 is immature. Later the fine-fibered type of bone is the kind that is formed and so it is referred to as mature bone. For the most part the immature types of bone have only a temporary existence in the body, being replaced as growth continues with mature bone.

Immature Bone. Immature bone (Fig. 15-53) has proportionately more cells than mature bone. Imma-

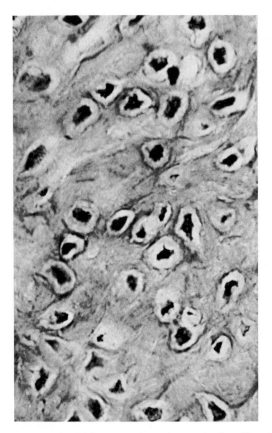

FIG. 15-53. High-power photomicrograph of an H and E section of decalcified immature bone.

ture bone is of two types, *woven bone* or *coarsely bundled* bone. In the former the bundles of collagen fibers of its matrix run in various directions; this accounts for the term woven. The intercellular substance, moreover, appears to have a greater percentage of mucopolysaccharide and/or glycoprotein than mature bone because it is colored blue in H and E sections. It is reported as having a greater calcium content than other types of bone. Bundle bone differs from woven by having thick bundles of collagen fibers which may parallel each other with osteocytes between them.

Although the matrix of immature bone stains very unevenly it so often demonstrates basophilia that areas of immature bone that have become surrounded by mature bone may be spotted easily on low-power examination (Fig. 15-54). *Unless it is appreciated that bits of immature bone can become surrounded by, and hence incorporated into, dense mature bone as seen in Figure 15-54, its presence might mistakenly be interpreted as being due to some degenerative change having occurred in mature bone.*

Almost all the immature bone that forms during embryonic life is in due course replaced with mature bone, which will be described next. Pritchard, who gives an excellent and comprehensive account of types of bone, states that some immature bone persists in tooth sockets, near cranial sutures, in the osseous labyrinth and near tendon and ligament attachments, but that in these sites it usually is mixed with mature bone. It should be mentioned also that immature bone often makes its appearance in postnatal life in the repair of fractures. It is also seen in postnatal life in rapidly growing tumors of bone that arise from osteogenic cells.

Mature Bone. The formation and growth of mature (also called lamellar) bone is characterized by new layers being added to bony surfaces in an orderly way. Each layer, according to Weinmann and Sicher, is from 4 to 12 μ thick. The osteoblasts responsible for producing the successive layers of lamellated bone become incorporated as osteocytes within or between the layers of bone matrix that they form. In general, the direction of the collagenic fibrils in any given layer is usually at an angle to that of the fibrils in immediately adjacent layers. Sometimes the direction of the fibrils in one layer is at right angles to the direction of those in the next. Since the direction of the fibrils in immediately adjacent layers is not the same, adjacent layers may appear to be optically different.

Mature bone is to be distinguished from immature bone because its matrix stains evenly and lightly (Fig. 15-54), by the regularity of its lamellae, by the fact that the direction of fibrils in immediately adjacent lamellae is different and by its fewer cells, which are more regularly arranged and in flatter lacunae than they are in immature bone (Fig. 15-54).

The Healing of a Simple Fracture of a Long Bone

In the usual fracture a single bone is broken into two parts, each of which is termed a *fragment*. Further, in the usual fracture the periosteum is torn, and the fragments are displaced, so that their ends are not in perfect apposition to one another. Hence it is usually necessary for fractures to be reduced; that is, the fragments are led back, usually by manipulation so that their broken ends are in apposition to one another, and the line of the bone is restored. The bone is then immobilized to keep things in place, usually by a cast.

For one reason or another a fracture may be reduced at an open operation and the two fragments joined by a metallic device. Under these conditions

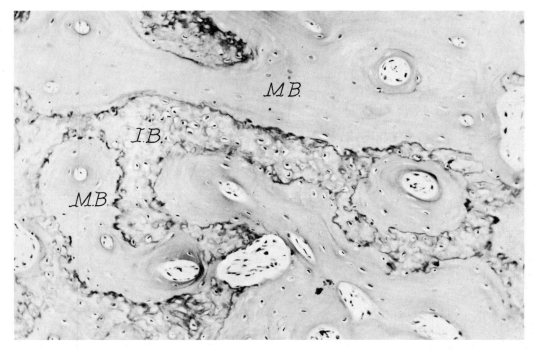

Fig. 15-54. Low-power photomicrograph of an H and E section of decalcified bone, showing areas of immature bone (I.B.) that have been surrounded or otherwise encroached upon by mature bone (M.B.) that formed later.

the healing process, as will be described later, may be different from that which we shall first describe.

Immediate Effects of the Injury. There is both direct and indirect injury to tissue. The trauma itself causes direct injury; it breaks the bone and tears the soft tissues associated with the bone (Fig. 15-55). Both the blood vessels that cross the line of the fracture and those of the adjacent soft tissue are torn. The more displacement there is the more blood vessels are torn and bleed into and around the fracture area. This blood soon coagulates to form a clot in and about the site of the fracture (Fig. 15-55). The next and second type of injury caused by a fracture is indirect; it depends on the fact that when the ends of the torn blood vessels are sealed off by hemostatic mechanisms, circulation stops in all these vessels back to sites where they anastomose with still functioning vessels. Since haversian blood vessels run more or less longitudinally in bone, the vessels in haversian systems are all torn at the fracture line, and circulation in them stops back to sites where they anastomose with other haversian vessels. Since anastomoses between vessels of adjacent haversian systems are probably not overly abundant, this means that circulation ceases in haversian vessels for some distance each side of the fracture line. This results in *the death of the osteocytes of the haversian systems for a certain distance from each side of the fracture line;* this is shown by empty lacunae (Fig. 15-55, dead bone).

Injury to blood vessels also accounts for the death of both some periosteal and some marrow tissue on each side of the fracture line. However, since both of these tissues have a better blood supply than the bone itself, the periosteal tissue and the marrow tissue do not die for as great a distance from each side of the fracture line as does the bone (Fig. 15-55).

Dead bone is generally recognized because dead osteocytes undergo lysis; hence, in most dead bone the lacunae, at least after some days, appear to be empty (Figs. 15-55, 15-56 and 15-57). However, the osteocytes, before dissolving, sometimes become pyknotic (dark and rounded). After 48 hours, the irregular line of demarcation between the dead bone (with empty lacunae), which extends from both sides of the fracture line, and living bone (the lacunae of which contain normal osteocytes), farther away from the fracture line, generally can be recognized, as in Figures 15-55, 15-56 and 15-57. The distance from a fracture line over which bone dies as a result of its blood supply being interrupted differs, depending on the site of the fracture in the bone and the particular bone that is fractured.

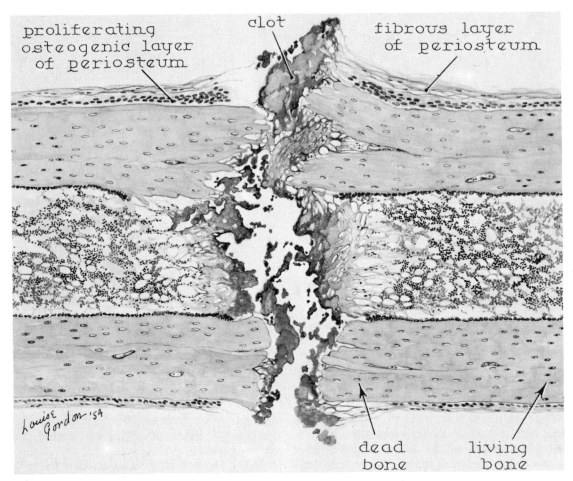

FIG. 15-55. A drawing of a longitudinal H and E section of a rabbit's rib in which a fracture had been healing for 48 hours. The territory encompassed by the drawing was that which could be seen with a very low-power objective, but the detail has been depicted at higher magnification to obviate the necessity of making several drawings at different magnifications. (Ham, A. W., and Harris, W. R.: *In* Bourne, G. H. (ed.): The Biochemistry and Physiology of Bone. ed. 2, vol. 3, p. 338. New York, Academic Press, 1971)

Early Stages of Repair

The Term Callus. A fracture is repaired by a growth of new tissue that develops around and between the ends of the fragments; this new tissue, which soon or late forms a bridge between the fragments so that they are united (Figs. 15-55, 15-56 and 15-57), is termed a *callus*. Some accounts of fracture healing are unnecessarily complicated by using names such as *provisional callus, temporary callus, bridging callus* and *permanent callus*. These terms suggest that different calluses exist at different times, each being replaced by another. Actually, what happens is that only one callus develops and, like any bony structure, it is remodeled as it grows. However, there is one clas-

sification that is helpful in describing callus formation; that is to speak of the callus that forms *around* the opposing ends of the bone fragments as the *external callus* and that which forms *between* the 2 ends of the bone fragments and between the 2 marrow cavities as the *internal callus* (Fig. 15-58).

The Cellular Origin of Callus. The least complicated and most informative method for investigating the cellular origin of callus tissue is to study sections of healing fractures in rabbits' ribs. A rib can be fractured in an anesthetized rabbit with the fingers without any incision being necessary and during healing the adjacent ribs act as a splint for the one that is fractured. By using a group of rabbits and preparing sections of a fractured rib each day over a period of a couple of weeks what happens day by day is readily apparent.

Sections taken over the first two days following the fracture show that the cells responsible for bringing about the eventual bony repair of the fracture have already begun to proliferate. The greatest proliferation seen this early is in the deep layer of the periosteum which is close to, but not directly at, the site of the fracture. This layer becomes thicker (Fig. 15-55) because of active cell proliferation occurring among the osteogenic cells (Fig. 15-16). The thickening of the osteogenic cells lifts the fibrous layer of the periosteum farther away from the bone. Over the first few days the osteogenic cells that line the marrow cavity also begin to proliferate but the thickening of this layer is not as great as that of the osteogenic layer of the periosteum (Fig. 15-55).

Over the next few days the proliferation of osteogenic cells continues in both periosteal and endosteal regions, but those cells in the deep layer of the periosteum show the greater activity. They proliferate so rapidly that they soon form a distinct collar around each fragment close to the line of the fracture (Figs. 15-56, *top* and 15-57). In addition to proliferating, these cells now begin to manifest signs of differentiation. When the osteogenic cells begin to proliferate after a fracture, the capillaries among them also proliferate, but they do not seem to grow as quickly as the osteogenic cells. As a result, the osteogenic cells that are more deeply disposed in the collars (those closest to the bone) differentiate in the presence of a blood supply; consequently, they become osteoblasts and form bony trabeculae in this region (Figs. 15-17, 15-56 and 15-57). The new trabeculae that develop are

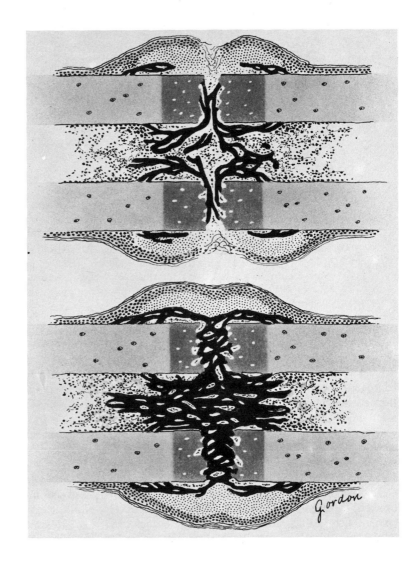

FIG. 15-56. Drawings to show the periosteal collars that form, approach each other and fuse in the repair of a fracture. The drawings also show the formation of internal callus and how the trabeculae become cemented to the original fragments. Living bone of the original fragments is light gray, dead portions of the original fragments are dark gray, and new bone in the external and the internal callus is black. In the external callus, cartilage is stippled lightly, and proliferating osteogenic cells are stippled darkly.

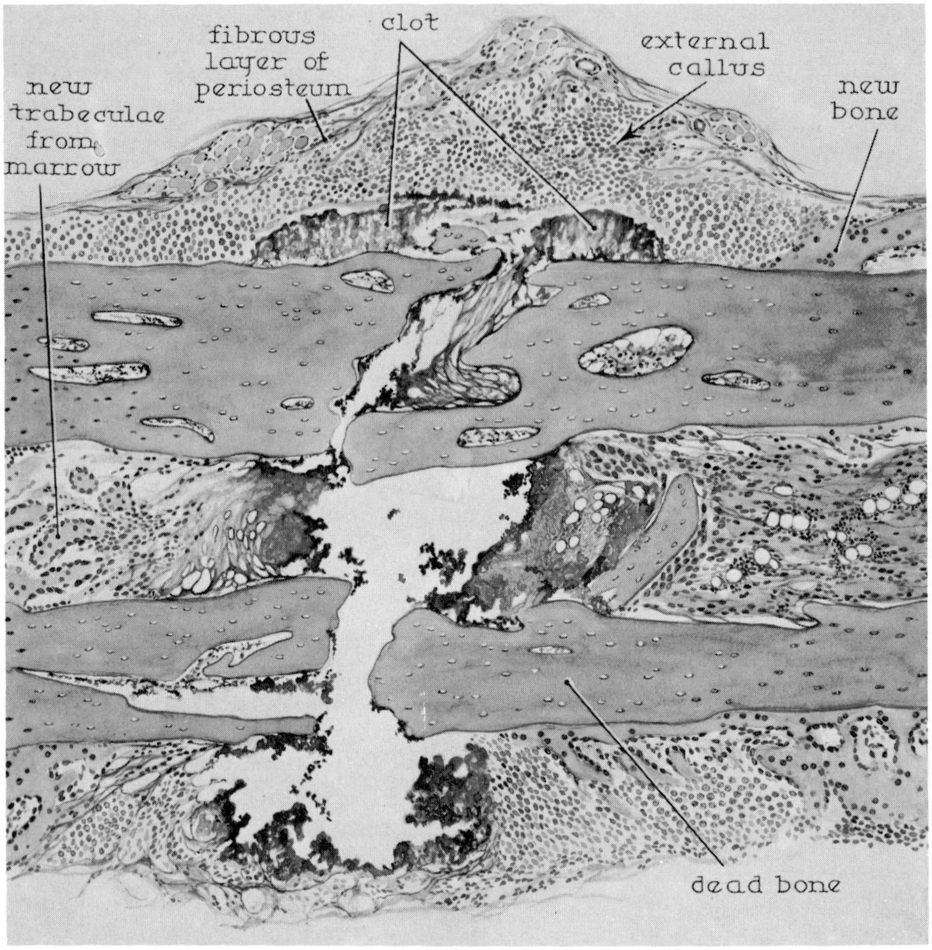

Fig. 15-57. A drawing of a longitudinal H and E section of a rabbit's rib in which a fracture had been healing for 1 week. The territory encompassed by the drawing was that which could be seen with a very low-power objective, but the detail has been filled in at higher magnification to obviate the necessity of making several drawings at different magnifications. (Ham, A. W., and Harris, W. R.: *In* Bourne, G. H. (ed.): The Biochemistry and Physiology of Bone. ed. 2, vol. 3, p. 338. New York, Academic Press, 1971)

cemented firmly to the bone matrix of the fragment, even though the bone of the fragment may be dead (Fig. 15-56). Those osteogenic cells in the more superficial parts of a collar (those farther away from the bone) seem to grow so quickly that the capillaries from the periosteum cannot keep up with them. When these osteogenic cells differentiate, they must do so in a nonvascular environment, so they tend to differentiate into chondroblasts and chondrocytes, and as a result cartilage develops in the outer parts of the collars (Figs. 15-17, 15-56 and 15-57).

Two comments should be made about the significance of cartilage in the external callus: (1) Its development here should not be unexpected, because the osteogenic cells that cover bone surfaces and prolif-

erate to repair a fracture are direct descendants of the cells of the perichondrium of embryonic bones, where they of course once formed cartilage. (2) The amount of cartilage that forms in a callus is, we think, dependent to a great extent on how quickly the callus tissue grows; if it grows very rapidly, capillaries seem unable to keep up with it, so its outer parts become nonvascular and cartilaginous. However, if callus tissue develops more slowly, new capillaries can keep pace with the osteogenic cells, so the osteogenic cells in such a callus differentiate in a vascular environment and so form bone. There also may be other factors that influence the amount of cartilage that forms—for example, species and movement.

When the collars resulting from the growth and the

differentiation of the osteogenic cells of the deep layer of the periosteum are well developed, they generally exhibit 3 layers that merge into one another (Figs. 15-56 and 15-57). The layer closest to the fragment consists of bony trabeculae that are cemented to the bone; the next and intermediate layer consists of cartilage which merges imperceptibly into the outer parts of the bony trabeculae on one side and into the third and outer layer of the callus on the other. The third and outer layer consists of proliferating osteogenic cells. The merging of these layers into one another is shown to advantage in Figure 15-17.

The collars continue to grow chiefly because of the proliferation of osteogenic cells in their outer layer and to a lesser extent because of the interstitial growth of cartilage in their middle layers. Such growth as occurs in the collars makes them thicker and makes them bulge toward each other. Sooner or later the collars from the two fragments meet and fuse (Figs. 15-56 and 15-57); when this occurs, union of the fragments has been achieved. Union is also achieved in the marrow cavity by developing trabeculae there forming a bridge (Fig. 15-56, *bottom*). Soon the histological picture of the healing fracture comes to resemble that illustrated in Figure 15-58.

The Fate of the Cartilage. The cartilage that develops in a callus normally has a temporary existence only; like that which develops in embryonic bones, it is eventually replaced with bone. Those cartilage cells that are closest to the newly formed bone mature and the intercellular substance around them becomes calcified, and this causes their death. The region in which this occurs is seen as a V-shaped line in a longitudinal section of a fracture at this stage of healing (Fig. 15-58). As the cartilage becomes progressively calcified it is replaced progressively with bone; this makes the

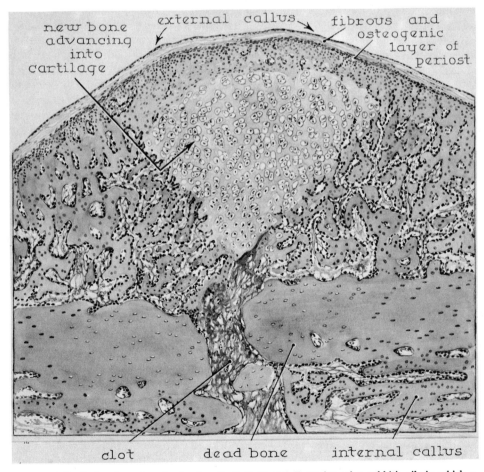

Fig. 15-58. A drawing of part of a longitudinal H and E section of a rabbit's rib in which a fracture had been healing for 2 weeks. (Ham, A. W., and Harris, W. R.: *In* Bourne, G. H. (ed.): The Biochemistry and Physiology of Bone. ed. 2, vol. 3, p. 338. New York, Academic Press, 1971)

angle of the V become increasingly acute. Finally the cartilage is all replaced with bone; this is of the cancellous type. It is to be observed that the trabeculae of this cancellous bone that replace the calcified cartilage have cores of cartilage as do those that replace calcified cartilage on the diaphyseal side of an epiphyseal plate.

The Remodeling of the Callus. To understand the remodeling process it is important to realize that those trabeculae of bone that form close to the original fragments are firmly cemented to the fragments. Since they also connect with one another, the two fragments are bridged by a cancellous network (Fig. 15-56, *bottom*). Moreover, it is important to realize that osteoblasts in building new trabeculae can lay down their matrix on dead portions of the fragments (as well as on living portions of them), so that by this means new trabeculae of bone become firmly cemented here and there to dead bone. However, between these trabeculae there are capillary-containing spaces, and the matrix of the dead bone is slowly etched away by osteoclasts (except where new trabeculae fasten onto it). Next, osteoblasts move into the spaces that have been deepened into the matrix of the dead bone by this process and lay down new living bone in them. By this means the matrix of the dead bone eventually is almost all replaced with new living bone.

At this stage the external callus constitutes a fusiform mass of cancellous bone around the two fragments from which much of the dead bone has been resorbed. By this time an internal callus has also been developed (Fig. 15-56). This has two parts that are continuous with one another. First in the marrow of each fragment new trabeculae of bone develop from both the endosteum that lines the marrow cavity and the osteogenic cells of the marrow itself. As is shown in Figure 15-56 trabeculae from one fragment connect with those of the other. Second, internal callus forms also between the ends of the fragments. In a rabbit's rib, which has a very thin cortex, this originates from osteogenic cells from the external surfaces of the bone growing down into the space between the two fragments and also from endosteal cells from the marrow growing outward in the space between the two ends of the bone, to form some cancellous bone between the ends of the broken bone (Fig. 15-56, *top* and *bottom*).

Remodeling. As the cartilage of the callus is being replaced with bone, and continuing afterward, when the callus consists of cancellous bone, the callus is gradually remodeled. We have already described how cancellous bone can be converted into compact bone, and this phenomenon occurs in the cancellous bone

that is directly between the two fragments and around their immediate periphery. This makes the bone strong in this site, and, as a consequence, the trabeculae in the periphery of the callus are no longer necessary to provide strength, so they are gradually resorbed. Eventually, the original line of the bone may be so well restored by this process that the site of the fracture can no longer be felt as a bony thickening.

It should be remembered that these various steps in the remodeling procedure merge into one another and proceed more or less simultaneously.

The Healing of Fractures of Bone With Thick Cortices. While the study of the healing of fractures in rabbits' ribs provides superb material for observing the nature of the osteogenic cells that repair a fracture, the cortex of a rabbit's rib is so thin that it does not disclose properly the participation of the osteogenic cells of the haversian canals (Fig. 15-59) that occurs in the healing of thick bones which contain large numbers of haversian systems. Hence to appreciate what happens in the healing of fractures of the larger long bones of man, studies must be made in the healing of fractures of these bones in man or in bones of larger experimental animals. If these are treated by the usual method without operation and by means of a cast an external callus develops and healing is much the same as in a rabbit's rib except that in due course osteogenic cells and capillaries grow out into the gap between the fractured bones from the exposed ends of the fragments from the haversian canals and they make a contribution to the part of the internal callus that develops between the cortices of the fragments. However, with rigid fixation of a fracture obtained by fixing the fragments firmly together at open operation the haversian canals become a more important source of callus tissue, as will next be described.

The So-Called Primary Healing of Bone. The terms primary and secondary healing or their counterparts, healing by first or second intention, originated a long time ago in connection with the healing of wounds, particularly the healing of incisions made through the skin and underlying tissues. It was then believed that if the edges of a wound were carefully brought together and sutured and there was no infection, the respective layers that had been cut would grow together with a minimum, or absence, of scar tissue. On the other hand, if the edges of the wound were not in direct apposition with one another, or if infection supervened, healing would require that for the space between the edges of the wound to be closed it must be filled first with a growth of fibroblasts and capillaries, called granulation tissue, and that in due course the collagen formed by the fibroblasts result in the gap being filled with a sizeable scar. This was referred to as secondary healing or healing by second intention.

As will be explained and illustrated in Chapter 20, modern studies on the healing of wounds show that the old view of primary healing was erroneous, for an incision does not heal by the respective layers that the surgeon believes are closely apposed to one another immediately growing together layer by layer. In fact, primary healing as it was conceived of, and still taught to some extent, is a myth.

The term primary healing seems to have been introduced with regard to the healing of fractures to designate those that heal without the development of an external callus. Through the years it was noticed that if fractures were treated by an open operation at which the two fragments were joined firmly together by some form of metallic plate that would hold the fragments rigidly in place until the fracture healed, no, or very little, external callus would form in the repair process. Repair would, therefore, depend almost entirely on the formation of internal callus. This finding seems to have led to an external callus being visualized as the counterpart of the scar tissue that forms in wounds in so-called secondary healing. The healing of a fracture without the formation of an external callus was therefore visualized as an example of healing by first intention and dependent on the ends of the two fragments being directly united with one another as various layers were believed to become united with one another in the old concept of primary healing. In due course, advances were made in connection with apparatus that would keep the two ends of the fragments in close apposition and rigidly immobilized in that position to facilitate this kind of healing.

Experimental studies made on dogs or even larger animals in which the shaft of a bone with a substantial cortex was cut across by a fine saw or by some other method that would permit the ends of the two fragments to be smooth and even enough to be brought into direct apposition with one another over much of their cut surfaces, and held rigidly in close apposition through the healing period, were made. It was shown that when the edges of the bone fragments were in direct apposition to one another healing between the ends occurred as follows: As already described, the osteogenic cells and endothelial cells of capillaries all die for some distance back from the fracture line because circulation in the capillaries is interrupted by the fracture back to the site where the capillaries in the canals anastomose with functioning vessels. Likewise, the osteocytes in the bone surrounding the haversian canals close to the fracture line also die, so that the

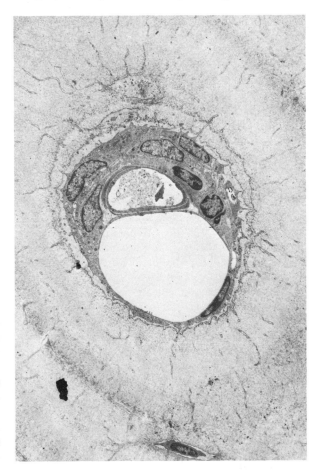

Fig. 15-59. This electron micrograph of a cross section of a haversian canal shows to advantage that the canal is lined by cells of the bone cell series. The outermost of these have cytoplasmic processes extending into canaliculi. Osteogenic cells would be scattered along the canal between these cells which are differentiating into osteoblasts and the cells of the walls of the blood vessels. (From S. C. Luk and G. T. Simon)

fracture line is faced on both its sides by dead bone. But on both sides of the fracture line, back at the sites where osteogenic cells and capillaries are still alive in the haversian canals, there is proliferation and, as a result, osteogenic cells and capillaries grow toward the fracture line. The osteogenic cells differentiate into osteoclasts which ream out the canals to make them larger; further, the osteogenic cells, which continue to proliferate, also differentiate into osteoblasts and begin to rebuild new haversian systems within the widening canals. This dual process advances to the fracture line and under the best of circumstances newly forming osteons from one fragment may cross the line and extend into the fragment on the other side of the line so that a new osteon that crosses the fracture line is formed. The process is much the same as that which occurs in the ordinary remodeling that takes place in the shaft of a bone and by which old osteons which have died are replaced by new ones that form to take their place. The process, however, is believed to be much more rapid than occurs in ordinary remodeling, because of its being stimulated by the injury. For a detailed account of what happens in experiments of this nature, the reader is referred to the study by Schenk and Willengger.

Fractures, however, as they occur in man, do not often lead to the ends of the fragments being smooth and even so that they can be fitted together so as to be in close apposition over their whole extents. Indeed, in a recent study made by Grant in which fractures were produced by the same kind of forces that would operate say in an accident, the two ends of the fragments were not sufficiently smooth or even for them to be fitted to achieve direct contact with one another except at a few sites. Hence, when they were joined together by mechanical means so as to approach each other as closely as possible, a space was found to exist between their ends over much of the areas of the latter. In the healing process Grant observed that although haversian canals on each side of the fracture line became reamed out by osteoclasts, and osteogenic cells and capillaries grew along these to reach the fracture site, before there could be any attempt to cross the line they first had to fill the spaces between the fragments with bone, which they did. The bone formed here was commonly of the immature type. Thus the first union achieved between the two fragments is that the two fragments are merely glued together as it were by immature bone and, at this time, are not joined by osteons crossing from one fragment to the other to provide pegs of living bone (new osteons) that are inserted into each fragment as may occur later. Moreover, at this time the fracture line previously seen in an x-ray picture may no longer be apparent, and thus give an impression that substantial healing of the so-called primary type has been achieved. Substantial union does not occur under these conditions until the whole area of bone encompassing the fracture area is remodeled, in which process new haversian systems are built which extend across the fracture line to peg one fragment directly into the other. Grant found that this takes a long time, not being complete even by the end of a year.

Grant found, moreover, that in fractures treated with less stable fixation, so that an external callus developed, the external callus had mostly disappeared after about 18 weeks and that the histological changes

that occurred between the two fragments from that point on were much the same as those observed in the animals in which rigid fixation had been obtained. It is obvious therefore that the so-called primary healing of a fracture is not the result of a different or novel type of healing, and that rigid fixation by plating merely substitutes, as it were, for an external callus, which under ordinary circumstances forms quickly to provide the support required for the extensive remodeling of bone that must occur in the area encompassing the ends of the two fragments. In both instances an internal callus from the endosteum and marrow helps in providing some new bone for the remodeling process.

An immensely interesting problem relates to why an external callus does not develop when rigid fixation is instituted. The formation of one must be inspired by movement. Perhaps this is just another example of the still mysterious quality of bone that is responsible for its growing where it is needed.

(For those wishing an extensive account of the healing of fractures together with some clinical implications, a recent review of the subject by the author and W. R. Harris is available in the Physiology and Biochemistry of Bone, ed. 2, vol. III, 1971. *See* References and Further Reading.)

THE TRANSPLANTATION OF BONE

Bone transplants are often used when fractured bones fail to heal by the ordinary method. They are also used when substantial parts of a bone are destroyed by accident or disease. They are useful in permitting certain reconstructions of the face to be made by plastic surgeons. They are sometimes employed to bring about bony union between two bones separated by a joint that has become diseased. Indeed, the transplantation of bone is a common surgical operation.

The transplanting of bone is also referred to as bone grafting although, as we shall see, this is not a very accurate term to use with regard to the transplantation of bone.

Bone transplants can be classified into two types in two ways. First, there are autologous transplants, in which bone is transplanted from one site to another in the same individual, and homologous transplants, in which bone is transplanted from one individual to another. Second, transplants may be made of either compact or cancellous bone.

Transplants of Autologous Bone. In depicting the problems associated with successfully transplanting bone it is best to begin with describing what happens when a piece of compact bone is cut from one bone and transplanted into a bed cut for it at some other bony site in the same individual.

Decades ago it was believed by many surgeons that transplanted compact bone continued to live in its new site. Now it is known that the osteocytes of a piece of compact bone that is transplanted die, and that sooner or later the dead transplanted bone is replaced by new bone.

When a graft of compact bone is cut, it is, of course, severed from its blood supply (Fig. 15-60). When it is fitted into its new position, its osteocytes, if they were to live, would have to obtain all their oxygen and nourishment through canaliculi. Hence, the only osteocytes that survive after a piece of compact bone is transplanted are the very few that are close enough to functioning capillaries in the bed of the host bone to permit the canalicular mechanism to function. This means that at best only a few osteocytes very close to a surface where there is tissue fluid can survive in transplanted bone.

However, the osteogenic cells of the periosteum and such endosteal cells as are present on a transplant, being situated at surfaces, are more likely to be sufficiently well bathed in tissue fluid to survive than are the osteocytes within the transplant. Indeed, some of the covering and lining cells of compact bone do survive and grow if they are in a suitable environment, and they may contribute a little toward osteogenesis, which, however, comes mostly from the covering and lining cells of the bone into which the transplant is inserted (Fig. 15-60).

If most of the osteocytes of transplanted compact bone die, it might be thought that a transplant of compact bone would be of little use; but a transplant can be of the greatest use even if most of its constituent cells do die. Bone transplants are placed so that each of their ends extends well into living bone tissue of the two fragments they bridge. Cells from the osteogenic layer of the periosteum, the endosteum and the marrow of the host bone proliferate and, together with capillaries, push out toward the transplant, forming new trabeculae of bone (Fig. 15-60). After a time the bony trabeculae, increasing in length and breadth by new bone being deposited on their surfaces, reach the transplant and unite with it (Fig. 15-60). It is to be understood that new bone deposited on dead bone becomes firmly cemented to it, just as the new bone that is deposited on the calcified cartilage on the diaphyseal side of the epiphyseal plate becomes firmly cemented to the cartilage. This step in the history of a compact bone transplant is illustrated in Figure 15-60 and shows that new trabeculae from the host have firmly united with the dead bone of the transplant.

It is also evident in this illustration that the osteogenic cells and the osteoblasts from which these new trabeculae arose came from some little distance behind the dead edge of the graft bed.

After the transplant is united to its host, it must be resorbed slowly and replaced with new bone. Resorption occurs in two general sites: (1) on the outer surfaces of the transplant in between areas where trabeculae of new bone have become cemented to it, and (2) on the inner surface of haversian canals (Fig. 15-60, *bottom*).

It is to be understood that functioning blood vessels are as necessary for the resorption of bone as for the deposition and the maintenance of the life of bone. Accordingly, little resorption can occur from the inner surfaces of the haversian canals of a transplant until there are functioning blood vessels in these haversian canals. Commonly it takes many weeks for new blood vessels to grow into the haversian canals of a compact bone graft.

The growth of new blood vessels and osteogenic cells into the haversian canals of the transplant is associated both with the resorption of dead bone from the canals by osteoclasts, which widens them (Fig. 15-60), and also with the deposition of new bone on the sides of the canals, which narrows them again (Fig. 15-60). The same two processes operate simultaneously on the exterior of the transplant and also at the dead edges of the graft bed, so before long the transplant and the edge of the bed both become a conglomerate of living, host-derived, bone and dead bone (Fig. 15-60, *bottom*). Eventually, nearly all, if not all, of the dead bone is resorbed, with new bone being substituted for it, but this takes time.

THE TRANSPLANTATION OF HOMOLOGOUS COMPACT BONE

As was pointed out in connection with the fate of transplanted autologous bone, the value of a transplant of compact bone does not depend upon the survival of any of its cells but upon the ability of its calcified intercellular substance to somehow stimulate osteogenesis from the bed of the host into which it is placed. The osteogenesis that it incites will in due course replace the bone of the transplant (Fig. 15-60). It might, therefore, seem that homologous transplants of compact bone would serve this purpose as well as autologous bone.

In Chapter 10 the homograft reaction was described. The question therefore arises here as to whether or not homologous bone would incite a homograft reaction that would prevent its serving the purpose out-

HISTORY OF A COMPACT BONE GRAFT

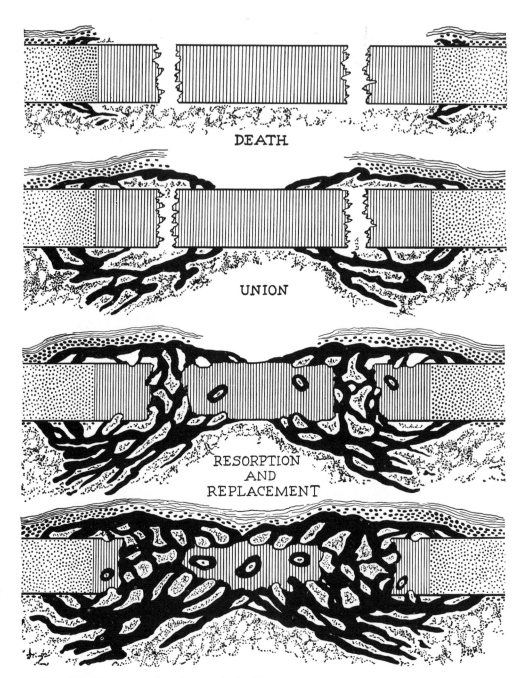

Fig. 15-60. Diagrams to show the steps in the history of a block of cortex of a bone which is cut free from its blood supply and placed back into the defect its removal caused. The periosteal surface is above and the marrow surface is below in each of the 4 pictures. Preexisting bone still alive is shown in medium stipple, dead bone is lined, and new bone is black. (Ham, A. W.: J. Bone Joint Surg., *34-A*:701)

lined in the above paragraph. In considering the possibilities of a homologous transplant of compact bone inciting a homograft reaction we have to think of both its cells and its intercellular substance. We shall consider the latter first.

The intercellular substance of bone is nonliving. Moreover it seems probable that the calcified intercellular substance of the bone of one individual is not sufficiently antigenic in another individual to incite enough of a homograft reaction to cause enough inflammation around a transplant to interfere with its being replaced by new bone from the host into which it is transplanted; otherwise homografts of compact bone would never be successful. However, any living cells associated with a freshly obtained homograft of compact bone would be sufficiently antigenic to incite a serious homograft reaction, as will be shown when we discuss the transplantation of cancellous bone. Even dead cells associated with a homologous transplant of compact bone could incite a temporary homograft reaction. So theoretically a homograft of compact bone should serve its purpose to best advantage if it has no living cells associated with it and if all the dead cells that can possibly be removed from it are removed before it is transplanted. Even so in treating a patient an autologous transplant is the first choice but if this is not feasible it is generally considered that a transplant of homologous bone will not usually be antigenic enough to prevent its being replaced by host bone in due course. However, in any situation where successive bone transplants have to be made in a patient, consideration should be given to the possibility of the dangers of a homograft reaction increasing with each transplant if homologous bone is used.

THE TRANSPLANTATION OF FRAGMENTS OF CANCELLOUS BONE

Autologous Transplants. Cancellous fragments or, as they are often termed cancellous chips, of autologous bones can be obtained, for example, from the crest of the ileum. They are transplanted for an entirely different purpose from that for which compact bone is used.

Early observations made on the transplantation of cancellous chips led to the concept that the osteocytes of the small chips received enough nutrient in their new location to survive. But more critical studies showed that when cancellous chips were transplanted, for example, into muscle, the osteocytes of the chips died. However, the osteogenic cells that covered and/or lined the cancellous bone from which the chips were obtained continued to live and quickly gave rise to

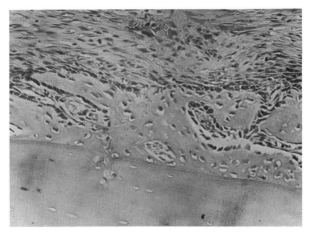

FIG. 15-61. Photomicrograph of autologous cancellous bone chip transplanted to muscle 10 days previously. The bone of the original transplant lies below and the new bone (of the immature type) above has formed during the 10 days from the osteogenic cells that covered its surface. (From Chalmers, J.: J. Bone Joint Surg. Brit., *41*:160, 1959)

new bone on some surface of the otherwise dead fragment of cancellous bone that had been transplanted, as is shown in Figure 15-61. From experiments such as this it became evident that autologous cancellous fragments could be used to set up little centers of osteogenesis in sites where new bone formation was required and they are now much used for this purpose.

Some confusion about their effects arose because the possibility was raised that they acted by virtue of their being able to induce bone formation from some type of cell such as fibroblasts or undifferentiated mesenchymal cells in the site to which they were transplanted. This idea led to the concept that chips of compact bone might serve the same purpose as cancellous chips. However, Gordon and the author showed that if autologous chips of cancellous bone were frozen and thawed three times to kill all their cells and then transplanted into muscle no new bone formed on any of their surfaces. Similar cancellous chips not frozen and thawed, and similarly transplanted, showed new bone forming on their surfaces. They concluded from their work that the bone seen in association with transplanted cancellous chips was not induced bone but bone that formed from the osteogenic cells that covered or lined the chips.

Cancellous bone has a high percentage of covering and lining cells (osteogenic cells) in relation to its bulk. Chips of compact bone would almost never have covering or lining cells on their surfaces. Hence since the bone that forms in association with transplanted

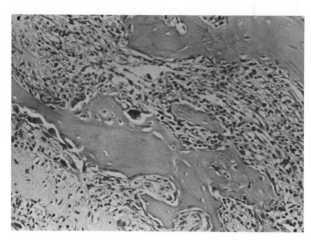

Fig. 15-62. Photomicrograph of homologous cancellous bone chip transplanted to muscle 10 days previously. The transplanted bone was lamellar and it can be seen that some immature bone has formed at its periphery in some sites from its osteogenic covering cells. By day ten, however, there is a well-developed homograft reaction which is resulting in the death of the cells of, and cells associated with, the new bone that had formed. The homograft reaction is indicated here by the large number of free nucleated cells that have infiltrated between the two main fragments of cancellous bone. The types of cells involved in the homograft reaction were described in Chapter 10. For illustrations of earlier stages in the process see Chalmers. (From Chalmers, J.: J. Bone Joint Surg. Brit., *41*:160, 1959)

cancellous bone chips is not induced bone but arises from their covering or lining osteogenic cells, transplants of autologous cancellous bone, and not chips of compact bone, should be used to set up centers of osteogenesis when these are needed to encourage bone formation.

Transplants of Homologous Chips of Cancellous Bone. Chambers has shown that chips of homologous cancellous bone, for the first few days, act similarly to transplanted autologous chips in that the covering or lining cells of the chips proliferate and begin forming new bone on the surface of the bone of the chip that was transplanted. But, as shown in Figure 15-62, by 10 days a homograft reaction has set in which is destroying the living cells of the new bone that formed, and many osteoclasts have appeared to resorb both the bone of the transplanted chips and the new bone that at first formed from the covering and lining cells.

Since the new bone that begins to form in association with transplanted homologous chips is by 10 days being destroyed by a homograft reaction it is obvious that the new bone must have developed from the osteogenic cells of the transplanted homologous bone. If it was induced bone of host origin it would not incite a homograft reaction. (It should, however, be mentioned that very occasionally homologous bone chips left in position for months may reveal a little bone formation beside them; this, it is believed, is an example of transplanted bone inducing bone formation from some type of host cell; for details, see Chambers, 1959.)

References and Other Reading

A Comprehensive General Reference

Bone is such an interesting and important subject it has been the subject of an enormous number of articles and other publications, and to list all those relevant to this chapter would require far more space than is available. Fortunately for those who wish to indulge in further reading there is a recent and most informative general reference in which various aspects of bone are dealt with at some length by authors having a particular interest in the aspect of bone on which they write. The great many chapters by different individuals are accompanied by extensive bibliographies. This comprehensive general reference is:

Bourne, G. H. (ed.): The Biochemistry and Physiology of Bone. ed. 2, vols. 1, 2 and 3. New York, Academic Press, 1971 and 1972.

In the following, to save space, articles by various authors in this general reference will be referred to by name and the topic they deal with and give only the page number and volume in which their chapter appears in the General Reference.

In addition, further references and suggestions for further reading will be listed under suitable headings for a variety of reasons.

Some Further Books on Bone

Hancox, N. M.: Biology of Bone. New York, Cambridge University Press, 1972.
Lacroix, P.: L'Organisation des Os. Liège, Desoer, 1950.
McLean, F. C., and Urist, M. R.: Bone: An Introduction to the Physiology of Skeletal Tissue. ed. 3. Chicago, University of Chicago Press, 1967.
Vaughan, J. M.: The Physiology of Bone. Oxford, Clarendon Press, 1970.
Weinmann, J. P., and Sicher, H.: Bone and Bones: Fundamentals of Bone Biology. ed. 2. St. Louis, C. V. Mosby, 1955.
Wolstenholme, G. E. W., and O'Connor, C. M. (eds.): Ciba Foundation Symposium on Bone Structure and Metabolism. London, J. & A. Churchill, 1956.

The following references are arranged in an order which so far as possible follows that in which various aspects of bone are dealt with in the text.

Mechanism of Nutrition in Bone

Ham, A. W.: Some histophysiological problems peculiar to calcified tissues. J. Bone Joint Surg., *34-A:*701, 1952.

Harris, W. R., and Ham, A. W.: The mechanism of nutrition in bone and how it affects its structure, repair and transplantation. *In* Ciba Foundation Symposium on Bone Structure and Metabolism. p. 135. London, J. & A. Churchill, 1956.

The Organic Intercellular Substance of Bone

Eanes, E. D., and Posner, A. S.: Structure and chemistry of bone collagen. *In* Schraer, H. (ed.): Biological Calcification. Cellular and Molecular Aspects. pp. 1-26. 1970.

Eastoe, J. E.: Chemical aspects of the matrix concept in calcified tissue organisation. Calc. Tiss. Res., *2:*1, 1968.

Engström, Arne: Aspects of the Molecular Structure of Bone. General Reference, vol. 1, p. 237.

Fernandez-Madrid, F.: Collagen biosynthesis. A review. Clin. Orthop., *68:*103, 1970.

Herring, G. M.: Chemistry of the bone matrix. Clin. Orthop., *36:*169, 1964.

————: The Organic Matrix of Bone. General Reference, vol. 1, p. 128.

Leblond, C. P., and Weinstock, M.: Radiographic Studies of Bone Formation. General Reference, vol. 3, page 181.

Weinstock, A.: Elaboration of Enamel and Dentin Matrix Glycoproteins. General Reference, vol. 2, p. 121.

Osteoblasts and Osteocytes

Cameron, D. A.: The Ultrastructure of Bone. General Reference, vol. 1, page 191.

Carniero, J., and Leblond, C. P.: Role of osteoblasts and odontoblasts in secreting the collagen of bone and dentin as shown by radioautography in mice given tritium-labeled glycine. Exp. Cell Res., *18:*291, 1950.

Pritchard, J. J.: General Histology of Bone. General Reference, vol. 1, page 1.

————: The Osteoblast. General Reference, vol. 1, page 21.

The Mechanism of Calcification

Bourne, G. H.: Phosphatase and Calcification. General Reference, vol. 2, page 79.

Bowness, J. M.: Present concepts of the role of ground substance in calcification. Clin. Orthop., *59:*233, 1968.

Munhoz, C., and Leblond, C. P.: Deposition of calcium phosphate into dentin and enamel as shown by radioautography of semithin sections of incisor teeth following injection of ^{45}calcium into rats. Calc. Tissue Res. In Press, 1974.

Robison, R.: The Significance of Phosphoric Esters in Metabolism. New York, New York University Press, 1932.

Tanes, D. R.: Mechanisms of calcification. Clin. Orthop., *42:*207, 1965.

Osteoclasts

Cameron, D. A.: The Ultrastructure of Bone. General Reference, vol. 1, page 191.

Fischman, D. A., and Hay, E. D.: Origin of osteoclasts from mononuclear leukocytes in regenerating newt limbs. Anat. Rec., *143:*329, 1962.

Gonzales, F.: Electron microscopy of osteoclasts. Anat. Rec., *139:*330, 1961.

Gonzales, F., and Karnovsky, M. J.: Electron microscopy of osteoclasts in healing fractures of rat bone. J. Biophys. Biochem. Cytol., *9:*299, 1961.

Ham, A. W., and Gordon, S. D.: Nature of the so-called striated border of osteoclasts. Anat. Rec., *112:*147, 1952.

Hancox, N. M.: The osteoclast. Biol. Rev., *24:*448, 1949.

————: The osteoclast. *In* The Biochemistry and Physiology of Bone. ed. 1. New York, Academic Press, 1956.

————: Motion picture studies of osteoclasts. *In* Rose, G. G. (ed.): Cinemicrography in Cell Biology. pp. 141-190. New York, Academic Press, 1963.

————: The Osteoclast. General Reference, vol. 1, p. 45.

Hancox, N. M., and Boothroyd, B.: Structure-function relationships in the osteoclast. *In* Sognnaes, R. F. (ed.): Mechanisms of Hard Tissue Destruction. Am. Assoc. Adv. Science, Washington, D.C., 1963.

Kallio, D. M., Garant, P. R., and Minkin, C.: Ultrastructural effects of calcitonin on osteoclasts in tissue culture. J. Ultrastruct. Res., *39:*205, 1972.

Owen, M.: The Origin of Bone Cells. Int. Rev. Cytol., *28:*213, 1970.

Scott, B. L.: Thymidine ^{3}H electron microscope radioautography of osteogenic cells in the fetal rat. J. Cell Biol., *35:*115, 1967.

Tonna, E. A., and Cronkite, E. P.: Skeletal cell labeling following continuous infusion with tritiated thymidine. Lab. Invest., *19:*310, 1968.

The Stem Cell of Bone: The Bone Cell Lineage

Ham, A. W.: A histological study of the early phases of bone repair. J. Bone Joint Surg., *12:*827, 1930.

————: Cartilage and Bone. *In* Cowdry's Special Cytology. ed. 2. vol. 2, p. 979. New York, Hoeber, 1932.

Ham, A. W., and Gordon, S. D.: The origin of bone that forms in association with cancellous chips transplanted into muscle. Brit. J. Plast. Surg., *5:*154, 1952.

Owen, M.: Cell population kinetics of an osteogenic tissue. J. Cell Biol., *19:*19, 1963.

————: Uptake of ^{3}H uridine into precursor pools and RNA in osteogenic cells. J. Cell Sci., *2:*39, 1967.

————: The origin of bone cells. Int. Rev. Cytol., *28:*213, 1970.

————: Cellular Dynamics of Bone. General Reference, vol. 3, page 271.

Tonna, E. A., and Cronkite, E. P.: Autoradiographic studies of cell proliferation in the periosteum of intact and fractured femora of mice utilizing DNA labeling with H^3-thymidine. Proc. Soc. Exp. Biol. Med., *107:*719, 1961.

————: An autoradiographic study of periosteal cell proliferation with tritiated thymidine. Lab. Invest., *11:*455, 1962.

————: The periosteum: autoradiographic studies on cellular proliferation and transformation, utilizing tritiated thymidine. Clin. Orthop., *30:*218, 1963.

————: The effects of extraperiosteal injection of blood components on periosteal cell proliferation. J. Cell Biol., *23:*79, 1964.

Tonna, E. A., and Pentel, L.: Chondrogenic cell formation via osteogenic cell progeny transformation. Lab. Invest., *27:*418, 1972.

Young, R. W.: Cell proliferation and specialization during endochondral osteogenesis in young rats. J. Cell Biol., *14:357*, 1962.

Parathyroid Hormone and Calcitonin

See also References and Other Reading in Chapter 25.

Arnaud, C. D., Jr., Tenenhouse, A. M., and Rasmussen, H.: Parathyroid hormone. Ann. Rev. Physiol., *29:349*, 1967.

Bingham, P. J., and Owen, M.: Effects of PTE on bone metabolism in vivo. Can. Tiss. Res. *2*(Suppl.):46, 1968.

Copp, D. H.: Calcitonin. General Reference, vol. 2, page 337.

Gaillard, P., Talmage, R. V., and Budy, A. M.: The Parathyroid Glands. Chicago, University of Chicago Press, 1965.

Prenatal Development of Bone

Ascenzi, A., and Benedetti, L.: An electron microscope study of the foetal membranous ossification. Acta Anat. (Basel), *37:370*, 1962.

Bassett, A. L.: Current concepts of bone formation. J. Bone Joint Surg., *44-A:1217*, 1962.

Bernard, G. W., and Pease, D. C.: An electron microscope study of initial intramembranous osteogenesis. Am. J. Anat., *125:271*, 1969.

Bertelson, A.: Experimental investigation into postfoetal osteogenesis. Acto Orthop. Scand., *15:139*, 1944.

Bevelander, G., and Johnson, P. L.: An histochemical study of the development of membrane bone. Anat. Rec., *108:1*, 1950.

Decker, J. D.: An electron microscope investigation of osteogenesis in the embryonic chick. Am. J. Anat., *118:591*, 1966.

Fell, H. B.: Skeletal development in tissue culture. *In* The Biochemistry and Physiology of Bone. ed. 1. New York, Academic Press, 1956.

Gardner, Ernest: Osteogenesis in the Human Embryo and Fetus. General Reference, vol. 3, p. 77.

The Fine Structure of Bone

Anderson, C. E., and Parker, J.: Electron microscopy of the epiphyseal cartilage plate. Clin. Orthop., *58:225*, 1968.

Ascenzi, A., Bonucci, E., and Boccia-Relli, S.: An electron microscope study on primary periosteal bone. J. Ultrastruct. Res., *18:605*, 1967.

Baud, C. A.: Submicroscopic structure and functional aspect of the osteocyte. Clin. Orthop., *56:227*, 1968.

Boyde, A., and Hobdell, M.: Scanning electron microscopy of lamellar bone. Z. Zellforsch. Mikrosk. Anat., *93:213*, 1969.

———: Scanning electron microscopy of bone. Calcif. Tissue Res. *2*(Suppl.):4-4B, 1968.

Cameron, D. A.: The fine structure of bone and calcified cartilage. Clin. Orthop., *26:199*, 1967.

———: The Ultrastructure of Bone. General Reference. vol. 1, p. 191.

Jande, S. S.: Fine structural study of osteocytes and their surrounding bone matrix with respect to their age in young chicks. J. Ultrastruct. Res., *37:279*, 1971.

Luk, S. C., Nopjaroonsri, C., and Simon, G. T.: The ultrastructure of endosteum—a topographic study in young adult rabbits. J. Ultrastruc. Res., 1974. In Press.

———: The ultrastructure of cortical bone in young adult rabbits, J. Ultrastruct., Res., 1974. In Press.

Scott, B. L.: Electron microscopy of the epiphyseal apparatus. Anat. Rec., *124:470*, 1956.

Scott, B. L., and Pease, D. C.: Electron microscopy of the epiphyseal apparatus. Anat. Rec., *126:465*, 1956.

Growth and Remodeling of Bone

Amprino, R.: On the growth of cortical bone and the mechanism of osteon formation. Acta Anat., *52:177*, 1963.

Cohen, J., and Harris, W. H.: The three dimensional anatomy of haversian systems. J. Bone Joint Surg., *40-A:419*, 1958.

Lacroix, P.: The Internal Remodelling of Bones. General Reference, vol. 3, page 119.

Leblond, C. P., Wilkinson, G. W., Belanger, L. F., and Robichon, J.: Radioautographic visualization of bone formation in the rat. Am. J. Anat., *86:289*, 1950.

Sissons, H. A.: The Growth of Bone. General Reference, vol. 3, page 145.

Effects of Nutritional and Metabolic Disturbances on Bone Growth and Remodeling

Amprino, R.: Bone histophysiology. Guy's Hosp. Rep., *116:51*, 1967.

Amprino, R., and Marotti, G. A.: Topographic Quantitative Study of Bone Formation and Reconstruction. *In* Blackwood, H. J. J. (ed.): Bone and Tooth. p. 21. London, Pergamon Press, 1964.

Bailie, J. M., and Irving, J. T.: Changes in the metaphysis of the long bones during the development of rickets. Brit. J. Exp. Path., *29:539*, 1948.

Barer, M., and Jowsey, J.: Bone formation and resorption in normal human ribs. Clin. Orthop., *52:241*, 1967.

Burkhart, J. M., and Jowsey, J.: Parathyroid and thyroid hormones in the development of immobilization osteoporosis. Endocrinology, *81:1053*, 1967.

Campo, R. D., and Dziewiatkowski, D. D.: Turnover of the organic matrix of cartilage and bone as visualized by autoradiography. J. Cell Biol., *18:19*, 1963.

Frost, H. M.: Tetracycline-based histological analysis of bone remodelling. Calcif. Tissue Res., *3:211*, 1969.

Hall, Kathleen: Changes in the bone and cartilage of the symphysis pubis of the mouse during pregnancy and after parturition, as revealed by metachromatic staining and the periodic acid-Schiff technique. J. Endocr., *11:210*, 1954.

Ham, A. W., and Elliott, H. C.: The bone and cartilage lesions of protracted moderate scurvy. Am. J. Path., *14:323*, 1938.

Ham, A. W., and Lewis, M.: Hypervitaminosis D rickets. Brit. J. Exp. Path., *15:228*, 1934.

Harris, W. H., and Heaney, R. P.: Skeletal renewal and metabolic bone disease. New Eng. J. Med., *280:193-253*, 303, 1969.

Hess, A. F.: Collected Writings. Springfield, Ill., Charles C Thomas, 1936.

———: Rickets, Including Osteomalacia and Tetany. Philadelphia, Lea & Febiger, 1929.

Jowsey, J.: The structure of normal and osteoporotic bone. J. Bone Joint Surg., *44-A:1255*, 1962.

Jowsey, J., and Gershon-Cohen, J.: Clinical and experimental osteoporosis. *In* Blackwood, H. J. J. (ed.): Bone and Tooth: Proceedings of the First European Symposium held at Somerville College, Oxford, April 1963. pp. 35-48, New York, Symposium Publication Division, Pergamon Press, 1964.

Jowsey, J., and Gordan, G.: Bone Turnover and Osteoporosis. General Reference, vol. 3, page 202.

Jowsey, J., and Riggs, B. L.: Assessment of bone turnover by microradiography and autoradiography. Seminars Nuclear Med., *2:*3, 1972.

Murray, P. D. F., and Kodicek, E.: Bones, muscles and vitamin C: I. The effect of a partial deficiency of vitamin C on the repair of bone and muscle in guinea pigs. J. Anat., *83:*158, 1949.

———: Bones, muscles and vitamin C: II. Partial deficiencies of vitamin C and mid-diaphyseal thickenings of the tibia and fibula in guinea pigs. J. Anat., *83:*205, 1949.

———: Bones, muscles and vitamin C: III. Repair of the effects of total deprivation of vitamin C at the proximal ends of the tibia and fibula in guinea pigs. J. Anat., *83:*285, 1949.

Silberberg, M., and Silberberg, R.: Steroid Hormones and Bone. General Reference, vol. 3, p. 401.

Osteolysis

Baud, C. A.: The Fine Structure of Normal and Parathormone Treated Bone. Proc. 4th Europ. Symp. on Calcified Tissues. Excerpta med. (Leiden), *120:*4, 1966.

Belanger, L. F., Migicovsky, B. B., Copp, D. H., and Vincent, J.: Resorption without osteoclasts (osteolysis). *In* Sognnaes, R. F. (ed.): Mechanisms of Hard Tissue Destruction. p. 531. Washington, Am. Assoc. Adv. Sci., 1965.

Belanger, L. F., and Robichon, J.: Parathormone-induced osteolysis in dogs. J. Bone Joint Surg., *46-A:*1008, 1964.

Belanger, L. F., Semba, T., Tolnai, S., Copp, D. H., Krook, L., and Gries, C.: The two faces of resorption. Third European Symposium on Calcified Tissues. New York, Springer-Verlag, New York, 1966.

Belanger, L. F.: Osteocytic osteolysis. Calcif. Tissue Res., *4:*1, 1969.

———: Osteocytic Resorption. General Reference, vol. 3, p. 240.

Cameron, D. A., Parshall, H. A., and Robinson, R. A.: Changes in the fine structure of bone cells after the administration of parathyroid extract. J. Cell Biol., *33:*1, 1967.

The Blood Supply of Bones

Brookes, M.: Femoral growth after occlusion of the principal nutrient canal in day-old rabbits. J. Bone Joint Surg., *39:*563, 1957.

———: Sequelae of experimental parietal ischemia in long bones of the rabbit. J. Anat., 94:552, 1960.

Brookes, M., and Harrison, R. G.: The vascularization of the rabbit femur and tibiofibula. J. Anat., *91:*61, 1957.

Dale, G. G., and Harris, W. R.: Prognosis of epiphyseal separation. J. Bone Joint Surg., *40-B:*116, 1958.

Harris, W. R., and Bobechko, W. P.: The radiographic density of avascular bone. J. Bone Joint Surg., *42-B:*626, 1960.

Harris, W. R., and Ham, A. W.: The mechanism of nutrition in bone and how it affects its structure, repair and transplanta-

tion. *In* Ciba Foundation Symposium on Bone Structure and Metabolism. p. 135. London, J. & A. Churchill, 1956.

Harrison, R. C., and Gámez, F. N.: Hormonal effects on the vascularization of bone. Symp. Zool. Soc. London, *II:*I, 1964.

Irving, M. H.: The blood supply of the growth cartilage in young rats. J. Anat., *98:*631, 1964.

Johnson, R. W.: A physiological study of the blood supply of the diaphysis. J. Bone Joint Surg., *9:*153, 1927.

Rhinelander, F. W.: Circulation of Bone. General Reference, vol. 2, p. 1.

Salter, R. B., and Harris, W. R.: Injuries involving the epiphyseal plate. J. Bone Joint Surg., *45-A:*587, 1963.

Trueta, J., and Harrison, M. H. M.: The normal vascular anatomy of the femoral head in adult man. J. Bone Joint Surg., *35:*442, 1953.

The Repair and Transplantation of Bone

Chalmers, J.: Bone transplantation. Symp. on Tissue and Organ Transplantation. J. Clin. Path., *20*(Suppl.):540, 1967.

Gordon, S., and Ham, A. W.: The fate of transplanted cancellous bone. *In* The Gallie Addresses. p. 296. Toronto, University of Toronto Press, 1950.

Grant, C. G.: An investigation of the mechanical aspects of long-term fracture healing following rigid fixation. Ph.D. Thesis, Institute of Medical Science, University of Toronto, 1973.

Haas, S. L.: The importance of the periosteum and the endosteum in the repair of transplanted bone. Arch. Surg., *8:*535, 1924.

Ham, A. W.: An histological study of the early phases of bone repair. J. Bone Joint Surg., *12:*827, 1930.

Ham, A. W., and Harris, W. R.: Repair and transplantation of bone. General Reference, vol. 3, pp. 338 and 379.

Ham, A. W., Tisdall, F. F., and Drake, T. G. H.: Experimental noncalcification of callus simulating nonunion. J. Bone Joint Surg., *20:*345, 1938.

Pritchard, J. J.: Repair of fractures of the parietal bone in rats. J. Anat., *80:*55, 1946.

Pritchard, J. J., and Ruzicka, A. J.: Comparison of fracture repair in the frog, lizard and rat. J. Anat., *84:*236, 1950.

Schenk, R., and Willenegger, H.: Morphological findings in primary fracture healing. Symp. Biol. Hung., *7:*75, 1964.

Urist, M. R., and Johnson, R. W.: Calcification and ossification: IV. The healing of fractures in man under clinical conditions. J. Bone Joint Surg., *25:*375, 1943.

Urist, M. R., and McLean, F. C.: Calcification and ossification: II. Calcification in the callus in healing fractures in normal rats. J. Bone Joint Surg., *23:*1, 1941.

———: Calcification and ossification: II. Control of calcification in the fracture callus in rachitic rats. J. Bone Joint Surg., *23:*283, 1941.

Wilkinson, G. W., and Leblond, C. P.: The deposition of radiophosphorus in fractured bones in rats. Surg. Gynec. Obstet., *97:*143, 1953.

16 Joints

Introduction

Diseases of joints are said to constitute the greatest single cause of disability encountered by the medical profession which is a good reason for the medical and paramedical student trying to learn as much as possible about them.

Definition and Function. The words *articulation* (*articulare,* to connect) and *joint* (*jungere,* to join) are used synonymously to refer to those structural arrangements that connect two or more bones together at their site of meeting. Although many joints permit movement between the two or more bones that they connect, the permitting of movement is not essential for a connecting structure to be termed a joint; indeed some joints become as solid as the bones they connect. Another function of some joints is that they make it possible for the structures they connect to grow in extent.

Classification. Joints may be classified in several ways: according to how they develop (on an embryologic basis), according to their structure (on a morphologic basis), or according to the kind of movement they permit (on a physiologic basis). Classified on a morphologic basis there are 5 kinds of joints:

1. Syndesmoses
2. Synchondroses
3. Synostoses
4. Symphyses
5. Synovial

The prefix *syn* is used with joints because it means *together.* The term *desmosis* refers to a *band* or a *bond,* but in connection with joints the term has become restricted to imply bands or bonds of dense connective tissue. Syndesmoses, then, are joints wherein bones, at their site of meeting, are held together by bands of dense fibrous tissue. It is important to understand that in a syndesmosis the bands of dense connective tissue extend from one *bare* bony surface to another; if the bones that are connected with dense fibrous tissue are capped with cartilage, another term, as we shall see, is

employed to describe them. *Synchondroses,* as might be supposed, are joints wherein two bones are connected with cartilage. Likewise, since *osteon* means *bone, synostoses* are joints wherein two bones are cemented together with bone. A synostosis, in effect, makes two bones into one, but synostoses are thought of as joints because they connect bones that developed separately and remained individual through the growing period, during which time they were connected by some other tissue (cartilage or fibrous tissue). The term *symphysis* means literally a *growing together;* actually the term is used with reference to joints wherein bones that are capped with cartilage at the joint site are held together (through the medium of their cartilage caps) by dense fibrous tissue or fibrocartilage. In one sense, then, a symphysis is a type of syndesmosis, but it is easier to think of it as a different type of joint, the difference lying in the fact that the dense fibrous tissue of the joint, in a syndesmosis, is inserted into bone tissue, and in a symphysis, into the cartilage that caps the bones of the joint at their site of meeting. The term *synovial* is derived from *syn* and *ovum.* Ovum, as used here, refers to the egg of the domesticated bird, and in particular, to the "white" of the egg, which is a glairy fluid. Synovial joints, then, are joints wherein a glairy fluid is present (in a closed cavity, called a synovial cavity) between the ends of the bones that participate in the joint. The glairy fluid, as we shall see, is of the nature of a lubricant to allow the smooth surfaces of the cartilage-capped bones that meet in the joints to slide freely on one another. Synovial joints, then, represent a specialized type of joint for free movement. Synovial joints, moreover, are sometimes termed *diarthroses* (*di,* apart; *arthron,* joint) because the two bones entering into one are, in a sense, kept *apart* by the synovial cavity. Furthermore, any of the first 4 types given in our classification can be termed a *synarthrosis* because in this type 2 bones are not kept apart, but *together,* by the joint.

The particular features of the various types of joints will now be described.

448

Syndesmoses

The sutures of the skull provide good examples. The flat bones of the skull develop from separate centers of ossification and thereafter grow in extent because new bone is continuously added to their edges in sutures by appositional growth. As a result the young connective tissue that at first exists between the edges of two adjacent bones becomes reduced eventually to a narrow band (Fig. 16-1) which joins the edges of the two bones together; hence, a suture is a syndesmosis. Osteogenic cells between the two bones in the suture can still proliferate and differentiate into bone cells. By this means layers of new bone can be added to the edges of the bones in the suture, and this permits the two bones that meet at the suture to grow in extent as the skull increases in size. Thus a syndesmosis permits bones to increase in extent by the appositional growth mechanism. When growth is over, the connective tissue in a suture may be replaced by bone; thus the syndesmosis becomes converted into a synostosis. When this occurs, the two bones that meet at the joint can no longer grow in extent.

Suture lines are commonly irregular; the edges of the bones concerned may be serrated, or they may interlock by means of toothlike processes. When a suture is cut in cross section, the suture line is usually seen to be oblique (Fig. 16-1). Not uncommonly an isolated ossicle, called a Wormian bone, may be seen in the connective tissue of a suture; such a bone forms as a result of the detachment of a little group of osteo-

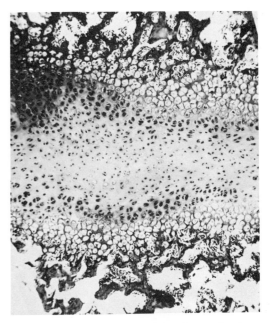

FIG. 16-2. Low-power photomicrograph of a section cut through the basisphenoid joint of an adult rat. Notice that the cartilage is being replaced by bone on both its sides.

blasts or a little spicule from the edge of one of the bones that meet in the suture.

Synchondroses

During the growing period epiphyseal disks are examples of synchondroses because they consist of hyaline cartilage and connect the bony epiphyses that arise from epiphyseal centers of ossification with bony diaphyses which arise from diaphyseal centers of ossification. It is to be understood that in most epiphyseal plates any substantial growth of bone occurs only on the diaphyseal side of the plate. However, the synchondrosis between the basioccipital and the basisphenoid bones is unlike an epiphyseal plate in this respect, for it provides for the growth of both of the bones that meet at this joint; in sections, then, it appears as a "doublesided" epiphyseal disk (Fig. 16-2).

Synostoses

When growth is over, most syndesmoses and synchondroses become synostoses. This is emphatic evidence to the effect that the chief function of the first two described types of joint is to permit growth rather than movement. It is of interest that operative procedures (including the use of bone transplants) are often

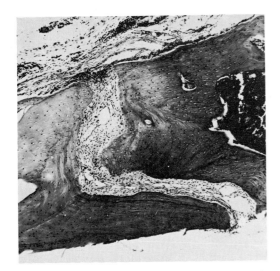

FIG. 16-1. Low-power photomicrograph of a section cut through the parietotemporal joint of an adult rat. This is an example of a suture and a syndesmosis.

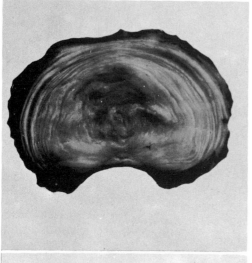

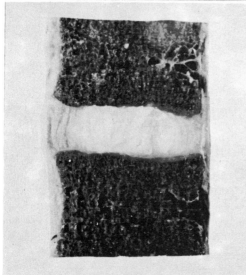

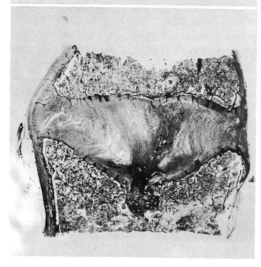

employed to convert symphyses and synovial joints into synostoses when pathologic conditions arise which make movement undesirable.

Symphyses

In a symphysis, the ends of the bones meeting in the joint are each capped with hyaline cartilage, and in turn the cartilage caps are joined by strong fibrous tissue which blends with the hyaline cartilages through a transitional zone of fibrocartilage. This arrangement provides great strength with a limited amount of movement.

In the *symphysis pubis* the tissue between the cartilage caps of the bones concerned consists almost entirely of fibrocartilage. A tiny slitlike space exists in the fibrocartilage, and in women during pregnancy this becomes larger, thus allowing for greater movement between the pubic bones during the passage of the fetus through the birth canal. In some lower animals the pubic bones actually become separated during pregnancy. Hall and her associates have studied the process in pregnant mice and have investigated the effects of hormones on the process (see references).

The *intervertebral joint* or, as it is often called, the *intervertebral disk* is a specialized type of symphysis. In each of these joints the flat bony surfaces of the bodies of the vertebrae concerned are capped with a layer of hyaline cartilage; the cartilage of one is joined to that of the other by fibrocartilage and dense fibrous tissue that is disposed so as to form a ring around the periphery of the joint (Figs. 16-3 and 16-4). This ring, called the annulus fibrosus, surrounds a central space that is filled with a pulpy semifluid material; this central space, so filled, is termed the nucleus pulposus (Figs. 16-3 and 16-4). The nucleus pulposus is believed to represent a remnant of the notochord. It contains cells (at least in the young) and intercellular substance, and under normal conditions it is under pressure; this, since the annulus fibro-

Fig. 16-3. (*Top*) Very low-power photomicrograph of a horizontal section cut through an intervertebral disk. The circularly disposed fibers in the annulus fibrosus may be seen in the periphery of the picture. The central dark area is the nucleus pulposus. (*Center*) Very low-power photomicrograph of a vertical section cut through the bodies of two vertebrae and the disk between them. The fibers of the annulus fibrosus may be seen near the edges of the disk; the paler material in the more central part of the disk is the nucleus pulposus. (*Bottom*) Very low-power photomicrograph of a vertical section cut through two vertebrae and the disk between them. The nucleus pulposus has ruptured into the substance of the body of the vertebra below. (Dr. William Donohue)

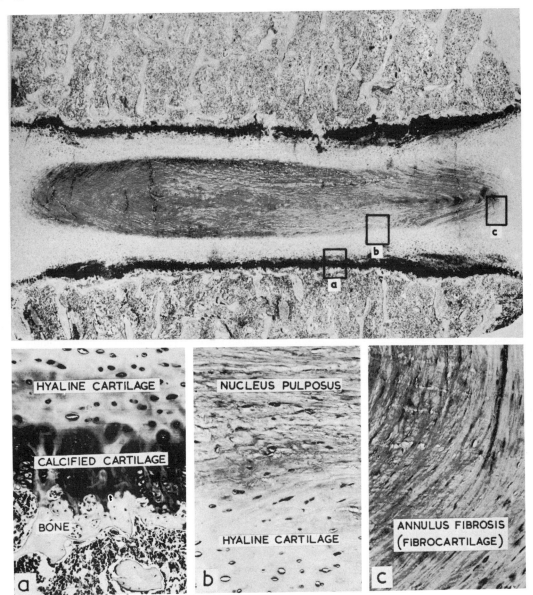

FIG. 16-4. Very low- and medium-power photomicrographs of an H and E section of an intervertebral disk of a young child. The areas marked a, b and c in the upper picture are shown in higher magnifications in the lower pictures.

sus is slightly elastic, makes the spine more resilient than it would be otherwise. In the aged, the nucleus pulposus loses some of the water content and so becomes smaller. This change is partly responsible for the spine becoming shorter and less resilient in old age.

The nucleus pulposus may herniate through the annulus fibrosus into the spinal canal, where it may press on the roots of the spinal nerves. These herniations or extrusions of the nucleus pulposus commonly occur between the 4th and the 5th lumbar vertebrae or between the 5th lumbar and the 1st sacral vertebrae. Pressure on the roots of the 5th lumbar or the 1st sacral nerve as a result of this condition is a common cause of a painful condition known as sciatica. Extrusions of the nucleus pulposus through the annulus fibrosus may also occur in the cervical region, where the extrusion may compress the entire spinal cord or the roots of the nerves of the brachial plexus. Some-

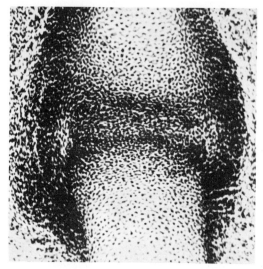

FIG. 16-5. Low-power photomicrograph of a longitudinal section cut through the developing interphalangeal joint in a 20-mm. human embryo. The developing cartilaginous ends of the two bones-to-be are pale. The dark-staining material that extends across the middle of the picture is the condensed mesenchyme that makes up the articular disk. The dark-staining stripes that run up and down each side of the ends of the developing cartilage models represent the condensed mesenchyme that is destined to form the capsule of the joint. The little clear areas seen in the dark-staining, otherwise condensed mesenchyme of the disk represent the beginnings of the synovial cavity.

times the nucleus pulposus herniates through the hyaline cartilage covering the body of a vertebra into the cancellous bone of its substance; this causes a characteristic lesion called a Schmorl's nodule (Fig. 16-3, *bottom*).

Synovial Joints

Development. It has been explained (Chapter 15) that the central mesenchyme in the limb buds of embryos gradually differentiates into cartilage in such a way that cartilage models of the bones-to-be are formed. It has also been said that the mesenchyme immediately surrounding the shaft of a cartilage model becomes arranged into an indistinctly 2-layered membrane, the perichondrium, that the outer layer of this membrane assumed a fibrous nature, and that the inner remains cellular and chondrogenic so that by the appositional growth mechanism it can add further layers of cartilage to the sides of the shaft, thus causing the shaft to grow in width. We shall now consider the series of events that occur in regions where the

ends of cartilage models approach one another (Fig. 16-5) and where a synovial joint develops.

The mesenchyme between the ill-defined ends of two developing models becomes condensed; this is called the *articular disk of mesenchyme* or the primitive joint plate (Fig. 16-5). And, in a fashion similar to that in which the perichondrium forms around the shafts of the cartilage models, the mesenchyme that surrounds the whole area in which the two ends of the cartilage models are developing also becomes condensed to form the counterpart of the perichondrium in this region (Fig. 16-5); this is the forerunner of what is called the *capsule* of the joint. This fits like a sleeve over the end of each of the cartilage models that enters into the joint and extends along the sides of terminal parts of the cartilage models for a sufficient distance to become continuous with the perichondrium that covers and is adherent to the sides of the shafts of the models.

As development proceeds, the jellylike amorphous intercellular substance and tissue fluid disposed between the mesenchymal cells of the articular disk begin to increase, and as a result, the cells in the disk become widely separated from one another in at least certain areas in the disk. The continuance of this process soon leads to the appearance of fluid-filled clefts in the substance of the disk; these gradually fuse with one another so that soon a continuous cavity, the *synovial cavity,* comes to occupy the site formerly occupied by the bulk of the disk. This permits the ends of the two cartilage models to come into contact and articulate with each other.

The process which accounts for the formation of a synovial cavity is not confined to the area between the two ends of the models; the same process operates to cause the cavity to extend along the sides of the terminal portions of the two models for some distance. The condensed mesenchyme which surrounds the joint area, and which is the counterpart of the perichondrium of the shafts of the models, thereby becomes separated from the sides of the ends of the models as it develops into a joint capsule. However, the developing joint capsule remains continuous with the tightly attached perichondrium (or periosteum, as the case may be) that covers the shaft of the models some little distance back from the end of each model.

As development continues, differentiation occurs in the forming joint capsule. The mesenchyme comprising its outer and thicker layer tends to differentiate into dense fibrous tissue which becomes the joint capsule while that of its inner layer becomes more or less specialized to constitute its synovial layer, or, as it is often called, the *synovial membrane* of the joint. Its microscopic structure will be described presently.

General Structure. The appearance of a longitudinal section of a synovial joint—the knee joint of a man—is illustrated in Figure 16-6. This figure shows the various structures that are involved in a complex synovial joint and their relations to one another. This figure should be consulted frequently as the microscopic structure of various components of a synovial joint are considered in the following section.

Articular Cartilage

This is a typical example of hyaline cartilage (Fig. 16-7). It has no blood vessels, nerves or lymphatics within it; the blood vessels seen near the bottom of Figure 16-7 are in the underlying bone. Near the surface the chondrocytes are flattened and small and disposed with their long axes running parallel with the articular surface. In the deeper layer the chondrocytes are larger and more nearly round and are disposed in

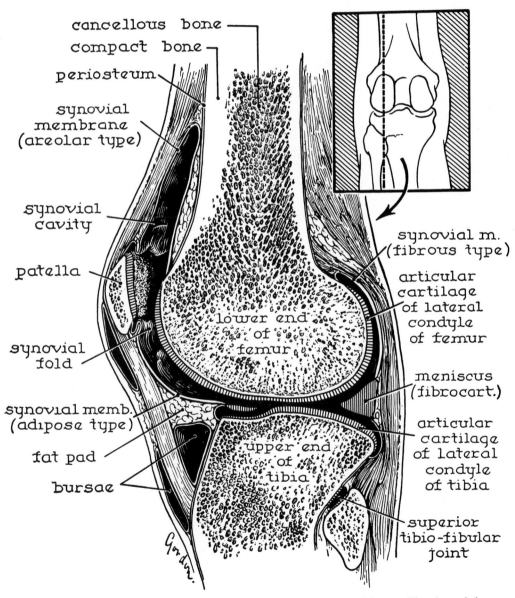

FIG. 16-6. A drawing of a longitudinal section of a knee joint of an adult man. The plane of the section that is illustrated in the main drawing is indicated in the inset (*upper right*).

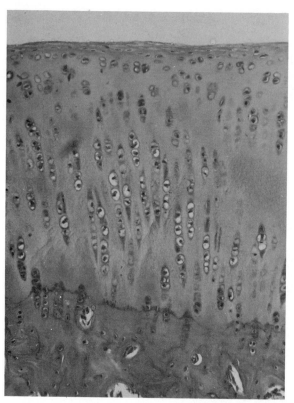

FIG. 16-7. Photomicrograph of an H and E section from the femur of a nearly full grown rabbit. The section is cut at right angles through the articular cartilage and its supporting bone. Note that the chondrocytes near the articular surface are thin, with flattened nuclei the long axes of which are more or less parallel to the articular surface. Deep to these the chondrocytes are arranged in columns. Near the bottom of the picture a dark line is seen crossing from one side to the other; this indicates the line between calcified and noncalcified intercellular substance. Deep to the line of calcification the calcified cartilage has mostly been replaced with bone which contains some canals with blood vessels in them. (Illustration courtesy of R. B. Salter, D. F. Simmonds, B. W. Malcolm and E. J. Rumble)

columns that run at right angles to the surface. In the deepest part of this layer the intercellular substance is calcified and stains more deeply even in decalcified H and E sections than does the intercellular substance that surrounds the cells in the outer part of this layer (Fig. 16-7). During the period of growth this layer is more or less constantly being replaced by bone while the cartilage cells in the more (but not most) superficial layers proliferate by mitosis which enables the epiphysis of a bone to become larger.

The intercellular substance of articular cartilage

consists of collagenic fibers embedded in a sulfated amorphous type of intercellular substance (chondroitin sulfuric acid). In sections cut from the articular cartilages of young animals the fibers are effectively masked by the amorphous intercellular substance. But in older animals the fibers are demonstrated more readily and can be seen (Fig. 16-8) to form coarse bundles that, deep in the cartilage, run at right angles to the surface between the rows of cells. As the fibers approach the surface, however, they become separated into smaller bundles which eventually spread out in a fountainlike fashion to run parallel with the surface (Fig. 16-8). This creates a densely tangled network of fibers immediately under the surface; this network probably is suited to bear the constantly altered stresses to which a joint surface is subjected.

Fine Structure. Figure 16-9 shows a large chondrocyte in a lacuna in articular cartilage surrounded by intercellular substance. See also Figure 4-3.

During the time a young animal is growing, the chondrocytes of the articular cartilage are synthesizing and secreting both the protein (tropocollagen) and the mucopolysaccharide components of the intercellular substance. As might be expected, chondrocytes engaged in this activity demonstrate the usual components of a cell that is synthesizing protein and carbohydrate for export; their cytoplasm reveals well-developed rough-surfaced vesicles of endoplasmic reticulum and a well-developed Golgi apparatus (Fig. 16-9). The borders of chondrocytes are very ragged; this appearance is caused by their cytoplasm extending off for short distances into the intercellular substance in the

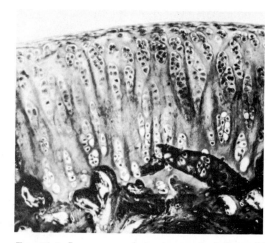

FIG. 16-8. Low-power photomicrograph (taken with the phase microscope) of a section cut through the upper end of the tibia of an aged rat. The direction of the collagenic fibers in the articular cartilage may be seen.

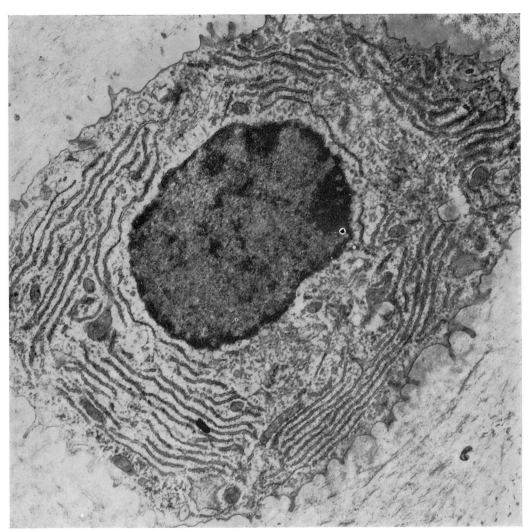

Fig. 16-9. Electron micrograph ($\times$ 19,500) of chondrocyte of articular cartilage. Note well-developed rough-surfaced vesicles, Golgi material, cytoplasmic footlets and fibrillar material lying in an amorphous intercellular substance. (Preparation by Ruth and Martin Silberberg)

form of processes which are much like microvilli but which are generally termed cytoplasmic footlets. The intercellular substance, best seen in the lower part of Figure 16-9, consists of interlacing fibrillar material, which is collagen, and an amorphous material, which appears structureless in the EM and is of the order of a sulfated mucopolysaccharide.

As chondrocytes become older, the organelles associated with protein synthesis and secretion, the rough-surfaced vesicles and the Golgi apparatus, become less prominent, and glycogen and lipid material accumulates in the cytoplasm. Silberberg and Silberberg think that chondrocytes that die in the substance of the

cartilage and are not immediately replaced by bone are replaced by fibrillar scars.

Nourishment and Metabolism. Since articular cartilage is nonvascular, nourishment must diffuse into its cells from outside its substance. The calcification of its intercellular substance in its deeper layers probably shuts off nutriment from the capillaries of the cancellous bone that underlies it; it is said, however, that there are certain sites where some nourishment may percolate through to it by this route. Around its periphery articular cartilage probably obtains some nourishment from the vessels of the synovial membrane in a manner to be described presently. But the greater part of the articular cartilage obtains its nourishment from the synovial fluid. It has been demonstrated repeatedly that fragments of cartilage, detached by injury or disease and floating freely in the synovial fluid, not only can survive but also in many instances can grow and increase greatly in size. Furthermore, in experimentally produced fractures of the necks of the femurs of dogs, in which the heads are separated completely from all blood supply and then pinned in place, and which the author was privileged to study, the articular cartilages of the heads over the succeeding months, as seen in sections, seemed generally to survive. When good results are obtained in such fractures, the dead bone and marrow of the head is all replaced, as has been described in connection with the healing of a fracture, and new bone develops to support the living articular cartilage which has survived through the whole procedure. Since a head has no blood supply until it is revascularized, and since the region directly beneath the articular cartilage is the last part of the head to be revascularized, it seems evident that the synovial fluid is capable of supporting the life of the chondrocytes of articular cartilage. This suggests that synovial fluid, under normal circumstances, provides the chief source of nourishment for most of the cells of articular cartilage.

Chondrocytes probably have a low metabolic rate. There is some evidence indicating that their metabolism is primarily of the anaerobic type, for their oxygen consumption ·is almost negligible (Bywaters). Moreover, their oxygen consumption diminishes with advancing age (Rosenthal).

Growth and Maintenance. As has been noted before, the articular cartilage provides for the growth of a bony epiphysis in the same way that an epiphyseal disk provides for the growth in length of a bony diaphysis; indeed, in short bones in which there are no epiphyseal disks, the articular cartilages serve as the sites wherein the bones as a whole grow in length. During the growing period, mitotic figures are to be observed among the chondrocytes of articular cartilage, not in the most superficial layer of flat cells (which might otherwise be assumed to be the youngest cells in the cartilage), but somewhat deeper, in about the third or fourth layer of cells below the surface. Deep to this layer the chondrocytes of articular cartilage are more mature, and still deeper, next to the bone, they are hypertrophied, and the intercellular substance surrounding them is calcified. During the period of active growth this zone of calcified cartilage is continuously being replaced by bone, which forms from the osteogenic cells and osteoblasts that invade this layer of cartilage from the bone below.

However, when the epiphysis has grown to its full size these two processes—the growth of the cartilage and its replacement by bone—appear to cease. It is the author's experience that mitotic figures can no longer be found in the articular cartilage after growth is over. Elliott could not find mitotic figures in the articular cartilages of adult animals even if they were specially exercised.

If there is no mitosis in adult articular cartilage it must be assumed that its chondrocytes, for the most part, have a very long life span and that they compensate for any wear that occurs by producing intercellular substance throughout life. Indeed Rosenthal and his associates have shown that the number of cells in articular cartilage decreases in relation to the amount of intercellular substance throughout life. Since articular cartilage persists, this suggests that some wear and tear is compensated for by such cells as persist continuing to produce more intercellular substance.

The Healing of Wounds of Articular Cartilage. Since the chondrocytes of adult articular cartilage seem unable to divide, it might be thought that wounds of articular cartilage would not be repaired. However, this is not necessarily true as will now be described.

Two classes of wounds that can affect articular cartilage must be considered: (1) those that are limited to the cartilage, and (2) those that extend through both the cartilage and the supporting bone that lies deep to the cartilage.

1. Wounds limited to cartilage that are close enough to the attachments of the synovial membrane for its cells to become involved in the repair can undergo at least some healing by means of the synovial cells proliferating and producing, generally, fibrocartilage. However, wounds limited to the cartilage anywhere except around its periphery where there is synovial membrane do not heal, because of the inability of the chondrocytes of adult articular cartilage to undergo mitosis. It seems probable, however, that there could be some slight molding of the edges of such a wound because of nearby chondrocytes producing some intercellular substance and also because the edges of the wound have no support.

2. Healing occurs in wounds of adult articular cartilage if they extend through both the cartilage and the underlying bone; this has been known for a long time but experience showed that this type of healing did not result in the articular cartilage being restored so as to possess a smooth cartilaginous slippery surface. As will be described presently, it has now been shown in some very recent experiments by R. B. Salter, D. F. Simmonds, B. W. Malcolm and E. J. Rumble that,

under conditions of continuous passive motion of the joint in which the wound has been made, there can be a restoration of the articular cartilage. But before attempting to explain how this occurs, we shall describe the healing of a wound such as a drill hole made through the articular cartilage and underlying bone as occurs when an experimental animal is kept under ordinary cage conditions (Fig. 16-10).

The first point to make is that the cells that attempt to repair a wound through both articular cartilage and bone, even though cartilage forms in the repair process, are not derived from the articular cartilage. The cells that respond to the injury are the osteogenic cells that cover the surfaces of the trabeculae of cancellous bone which supports the cartilage and the connective tissue cells of the marrow that lies between the bony trabeculae of the epiphysis. Cells from the latter source include both the osteogenic cells of marrow and pericytes associated with the blood vessels. As a result of the injury to the cancellous bone the osteogenic cells that cover it and osteogenic cells of the marrow respond as they would in an ordinary fracture by multiplying and differentiating, and by doing so they begin to fill the defect with what might be regarded as a callus which contains both new bony trabeculae and masses of cartilage. In addition the pericytes associated with the blood vessels of the marrow also proliferate and, depending on circumstances, the defect that extends through the cartilage and its underlying bone becomes more or less filled with what is often a mixture of bony trabeculae, masses of cartilage and fibrous tissue (Fig. 16-10). In due course the bone intercellular substance becomes calcified and that of at least some of the cartilage also becomes calcified; hence in most instances the reparative tissue that reaches the articular surface is not a suitable substitute for articular cartilage and this can lead to an arthritic condition. In Figure 16-10, the repair tissue is mostly of a fibrous character and contains several blood vessels.

As mentioned above, however, Salter et al. have found that if by means of suitable apparatus the joint in which a defect has been created in and through the articular cartilage is maintained under conditions of continuous passive motion the repair process which begins as described above ends with the defect, at the level of the articular cartilage, becoming filled with cartilage that resembles that seen in normal articular cartilage, as is shown in Figures 16-11 and 16-12. It is of interest to inquire how and why this kind of a result could be achieved.

First, it must be understood that the new articular cartilage does not arise from the edges of the pre-

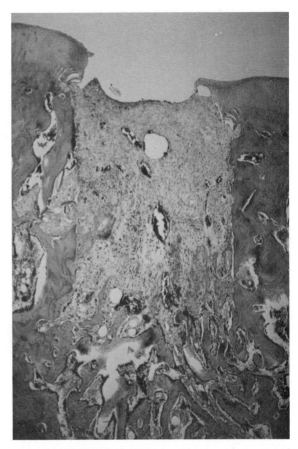

FIG. 16-10. Low-power photomicrograph showing the degree and character of healing of a drill hole through the articular cartilage and underlying bone of a femoral condyle of a nearly full grown New Zealand rabbit. After the operation the rabbit had been kept under ordinary cage conditions for a period of 3 weeks when the specimen was taken. There has been a good deal of new bone formation at the site of the injury to the cancellous bone and, as can be seen above this area, there has been some formation of cartilage as well. But most of the reparative tissue that is closer to the surface is what might be termed a primitive type of ordinary connective tissue which contains several blood vessels. (Illustration courtesy of R. B. Salter, D. F. Simmonds, B. W. Malcolm and E. J. Rumble)

existing articular cartilage but is derived from below. This fact is clearly apparent in Figures 16-11 and 16-12.

Second, as the author pointed out in 1930 (his first paper), when the osteogenic cells that cover and line bone surfaces proliferate in the repair of a fracture, they can differentiate so as to form either cartilage or bone (see Figs. 15-17 and 15-19), and which course

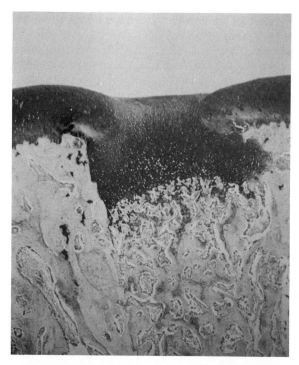

Fig. 16-11. The procedure and the time of healing of the rabbit from which this specimen was recovered were the same as those in the one illustrated in Figure 16-10, but the knee joint in this rabbit was subjected to continuous passive motion over the healing period. The section was stained with toluidine blue which colors the intercellular substance of cartilage deeply. It is to be noted that while new bony trabeculae have formed, deep to the defect most of the reparative tissue is cartilaginous and a great deal of it has formed so that it has bulged upward and restored a cartilaginous articular surface. For higher powers see Figure 16-12. (Illustration courtesy of R. B. Salter, D. F. Simmonds, B. W. Malcolm and E. J. Rumble)

they take seems to depend on whether or not they differentiate in a nonvascular or vascular environment. That is to say that if differentiation occurs in the absence of capillaries they differentiate into chondroblasts but if differentiation occurs in the presence of capillaries they differentiate into osteoblasts and form bone. As was described in Chapter 15, the actual determinant seems to be oxygen.

It is therefore of interest to inquire into two matters: why the growth of the reparative tissue should be so extensive under the conditions of continuous passive motion and why, as the new tissue grew up from below into the defect, the environment should become increasingly nonvascular, so as to lead to differentiation into, and continued growth of, cartilage.

First, as Salter et al. have pointed out to the author, continuous passive motion would prevent the development of adhesions and would also maintain the normal lengths of associated ligaments and muscle. It would also improve the return circulation of blood from the affected limb and prevent the disuse osteoporosis that follows immobilization. Continuous passive motion would moreover stimulate the healing process. It could therefore be expected that the reparative growth induced by the injury would be more vigorous than would occur if the joints were kept relatively immobilized.

The next question is why the reparative tissue as it ascends from below up into the wound becomes increasingly cartilaginous. It seems to the author that this could be explained if the environment became increasingly nonvascular and more anoxic as the growth of reparative tissue neared the articular surface. In this connection it should be recalled that articular cartilage itself is nourished from the synovial fluid so that most of it is a long way from capillaries. It might also be pointed out that under conditions of continuous passive motion the circulation of synovial fluid would be greatly enhanced, which would bring more nutrients to the wound area. It might also be supposed that, as the reparative growth reached the level of the base of the articular cartilage, it would increasingly derive its nutrients from synovial fluid; in particular the young cartilage in the reparative tissue would be nourished by it because of the excellent diffusion mechanism that exists in the intercellular substance of cartilage. It could therefore be thought that the growth of such young cartilage that formed in the reparative growth would be increasingly favored as the reparative tissue neared the articular surface and that, as it became increasingly nourished from the synovial fluid, it would become subjected to the same physical conditions as those that apply to normal articular cartilage so that it would increasingly assume the appearance of normal articular cartilage, which it does (Fig. 16-12).

It seemed to the author that it is of such interest both to orthopaedics and to the biology of differentiation, that defects in articular cartilage have been shown to be repaired by the formation of new articular cartilage, it should be described briefly here even though the reports of Drs. Salter, Simmonds, Malcolm and Rumble on this work are not in print at the time of this writing. The author is grateful to these investigators for allowing him to have access to this work and to describe it briefly here.

Effects of Compression on Articular Cartilage. Salter, having observed that degenerative changes were sometimes associated with joints that had been

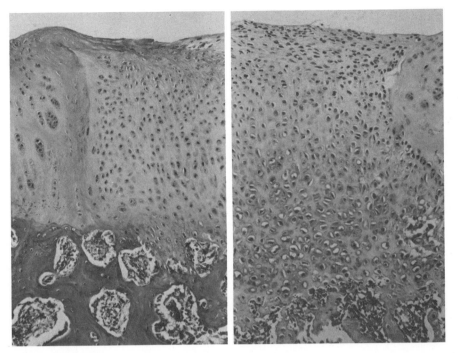

FIG. 16-12. High-power photomicrographs of an H and E section showing the cartilaginous repair of the articular cartilage in a rabbit after a defect was created as described in the legend for Figure 16-10. The knee joint of this animal was subjected to continuous passive motion for the 3 weeks after the defect was created. Note that in the region of the articular cartilage the reparative tissue which originated from the bone below is entirely cartilaginous in character and that the intercellular substance of the reparative tissue for the most part seems to be fusing with the edges of the original articular cartilage with which it is in apposition. The cell nests visible in and close to the edges of the original cartilage are probably to be explained by the fact that the rabbits used were not quite full grown and hence a few mitoses could have occurred in chondrocytes of the articular cartilage close to the site of the injury. (Illustration courtesy of R. B. Salter, D. F. Simmonds, B. W. Malcolm and E. J. Rumble)

immobilized in forced positions, has made an experimental study with Field and shown that artificially induced compression on joint cartilages will lead to their degeneration. Moreover, they have shown experimentally that if joints are immobilized in forced positions, degeneration will occur. Degenerative changes may appear as soon as 6 days after the compression has been applied. They think that the effects of compression interfere with the nutrition of the cells of the articular cartilage, which, as has been explained, is probably dependent on diffusion through the synovial fluid and then through the intercellular substances of the cartilage. It seems logical to assume that the maintenance of a joint in one position with a compression of the cartilage would interfere with this mechanism of nutrition, which, it might be thought, would ordinarily be facilitated by movement, which

would result in surfaces being more or less continuously coated with fresh synovial fluid.

The Joint Capsule and the Synovial Membrane

As already mentioned, the joint capsule consists of two layers: an outer fibrous layer which is commonly called the fibrous capsule of the joint and an inner layer which commonly is called the synovial membrane of the joint (Fig. 16-6).

The fibrous capsule of a joint is continuous with the fibrous layer of the periosteum of the bones that meet at the joint (Fig. 16-6). It is composed of sheets of collagenic fibers that run from the periosteum of one bone to that of the other. It is relatively inelastic and hence makes a contribution to the stability of the joint.

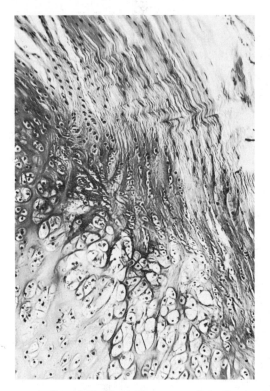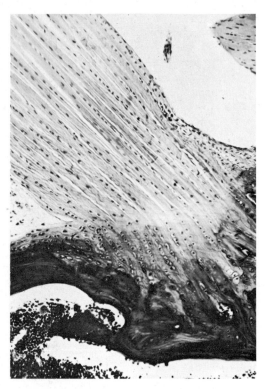

Fig. 16-13. (*Left*) Low-power photomicrograph of a section cut through the site of the insertion of the patellar tendon of an adult rat. (*Right*) Low-power photomicrograph of a section cut through the site of the insertion of the anterior cruciate ligament of an adult rat. Observe the bundles of collagenic fibers in bone (Sharpley's fibers).

Occasionally, gaps are present in fibrous capsules; if so, the synovial membrane rests on muscles or such other structures as surround the joint. The ligaments of a joint represent cordlike thickenings of the capsule. These may be incorporated in the capsule or may be separated from it by bursae that are formed by outpouchings of the synovial lining (Fig. 16-6, bursae). Near their attachments the structure of ligaments undergoes a transition into fibrocartilage (Fig. 16-13). The collagenic fibers become associated with increased amounts of amorphous intercellular substance, and the fibroblasts become encapsulated and resemble chondrocytes (Fig. 16-13).

Sharpey's Fibers. The collagenic fibers extend into the substance of the bone to which they are attached as typical Sharpey's fibers (Fig. 16-13, *right*). It is to be remembered that bundles of collagenic fibers can become buried in bone as Sharpey's fibers to serve as an anchorage for tendons, muscles or the periodontal membrane only when the fibers are formed before, or as, bone intercellular substance is deposited around them and onto the surface of the bone (appositional

growth mechanism) by the osteoblasts which lie between the fiber bundles close to the bone. In this sense, a tendon serves as the periosteum of a bone at the site of its insertion (see Sharpey's fibers, Fig. 16-13, *right*).

Synovial Membrane. The synovial membrane, the inner layer of the joint capsule, lines the joint everywhere except over the articular cartilages (Fig. 16-6). The inner surface of the synovial membrane is usually smooth and glistening, and it may be thrown into numerous processes; some of these are termed *villi*. It is abundantly supplied with blood vessels, nerves and lymphatics, as will be described presently.

The cells in this membrane are called synovial cells. They are of a relatively undifferentiated type and tend to be concentrated along the inner border of the membrane; indeed, in some instances they may be so concentrated as to give the appearance of forming a continuous cellular membrane. However, the careful microscopic study of such a membrane will show that the cells disposed along its inner surface lie *in among* rather than *on* the collagenic fibers which also partici-

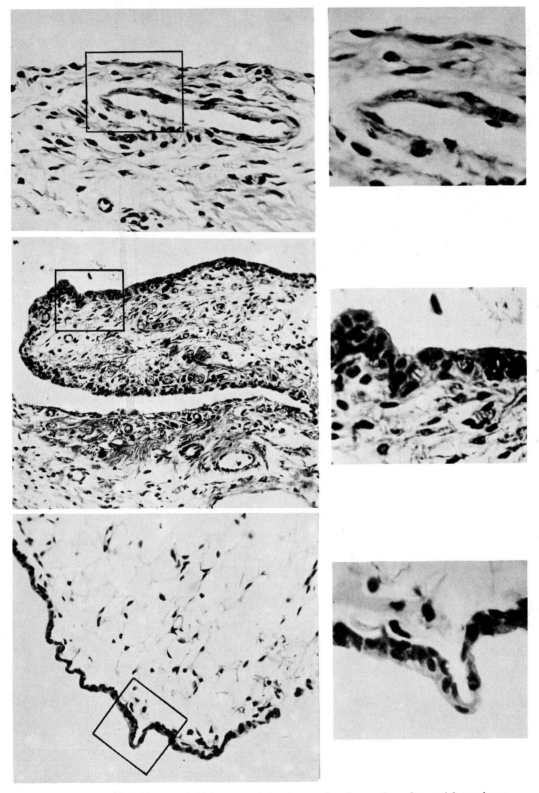

FIG. 16-14. (*Top*) Low- and high-power photomicrographs of a section of synovial membrane of the fibrous type. (*Center*) Low- and high-power photomicrographs of a section of synovial membrane of the areolar type. (*Bottom*) Low- and high-power photomicrographs of a section of a synovial membrane of the adipose type. All of the sections are of rat tissue.

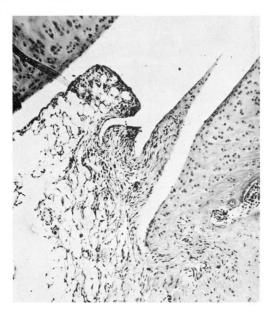

Fig. 16-15. Low-power photomicrograph of a section cut through the border of the patella of a rat. The synovial fold is wedge-shaped in this section.

pate in forming the inner lining of the membrane.

The inner lining of the joint capsule, which contains the synovial cells, may lie directly on the fibrous capsule of the joint or may be separated from the fibrous capsule by a layer of areolar tissue or a layer of adipose tissue (Fig. 16-6). Accordingly, Key distinguishes three morphologic types of synovial membrane: (1) fibrous, (2) areolar and (3) adipose. These are illustrated in Figures 16-6 and 16-14 and will now be described.

The fibrous type is found over ligaments and tendons and in other areas where the synovial lining is subjected to pressure (Fig. 16-6). The surface cells are characteristically widely separated from one another (Fig. 16-14, *top*), and although they are slightly larger and more numerous that the fibroblasts that are farther removed from the surface, it is often difficult to distinguish them from ordinary fibroblasts in sections. Since intercellular substance, rather than cells, comprises most of the lining of this type of synovial membrane, this type of membrane provides strong evidence in favor of the concept that synovial cavities are of the nature of connective tissue spaces.

The areolar type of synovial membrane is found where the membrane is required to move freely over the fibrous capsule of the joint, as, for example, in the suprapatellar pouch of the knee joint (Fig. 16-6). The surface cells are grouped fairly closely together in this type of lining (Fig. 16-14, *center*), usually in 3 or 4

rows, and are embedded in a layer of collagenic fibers which blend smoothly into those of the areolar tissue. Usually many elastic fibers are present in this type of lining; these usually are arranged in a lamina, and this probably serves to keep synovial projections from being nipped between the articular cartilages (Davies).

The adipose type of synovial lining covers the intra-articular fat pads (Fig. 16-6) and most closely resembles a true cellular lining membrane in appearance. The surface cells are usually formed into a single layer which appears to rest on the adipose tissue (Fig. 16-14, *bottom*). However, careful inspection will reveal that the surface cells are more or less embedded in a thin layer of collagenic fibers, as are the surface cells in the other two types of lining membrane.

Synovial cells vary quite a bit in appearance, as might be expected if they represented a mesenchymal-derived family of cells, the members of which were in different stages of differentiation. Asboe-Hansen has observed that there are numerous mast cells in synovial membranes.

Transition Zone. At the site of attachment of the synovial membrane to the periphery of the articular cartilage, the synovial cells undergo a transition into chondrocytes. This region is known as the *transition zone*. In this site a fold or fringe of synovial tissue may be seen to overlie the articular cartilage for a short distance. This fold, which is cut in cross section in a longitudinal section of a joint, appears wedge-shaped (Fig. 16-15). The tip of the wedge is relatively non-cellular, and the base is cellular. The areolar tissue that underlies the base of the wedge undergoes an abrupt change into fibrous tissue as it nears the articular cartilage, and this tissue, in turn, merges with the articular cartilage.

Since the synovial cells are relatively undifferentiated, synovial tissues are capable of rapid and complete repair. It is helpful to know this fact because synovial tissues must be removed in certain types of operations on joints. Key found that following the removal of a portion of the synovial lining from the knee joints of rabbits, there was a rapid deposition of fibrin in the wounded area, and that this quickly became organized by young connective tissue cells which grew in from the fibrous capsule. These soon differentiated into synovial cells, so that within 60 days the newly formed synovial lining could not be distinguished from that of undamaged adjacent areas.

Intra-articular Menisci. These structures (Fig. 16-6) develop from portions of the articular disk of mesenchyme (Fig. 16-5) which once occupied the space between the developing articular cartilages of the joint concerned. In these, the mesenchyme tends to differentiate into fibrocartilage. They may have a free inner border, as they have in the knee joint, or they may traverse the joint, dividing it into two separate synovial cavities, as in the sternoclavicular joint.

The menisci of the knee joint may be torn as the result of an injury, and it is common practice to excise an affected meniscus. Following the removal of a meniscus, a new one sometimes forms, growing in from the fibrous capsule of the joint. The new structure that forms in this fashion is an almost complete duplicate of the former meniscus but it consists of dense fibrous tissue rather than of fibrocartilage. New menisci that form in this fashion may themselves become injured and require removal; indeed, it was because of this that it was found that intra-articular menisci can regenerate (Smillie).

Blood Vessels and Lymphatics. Synovial joints have a relatively rich blood supply. The branches of arteries that approach a joint commonly supply three structures: one goes to the epiphyses, a second to the joint capsule and a third to the synovial membrane. In these sites they supply capillary beds. There are arteriovenous anastomoses in joints; the significance of these has not yet been determined.

The synovial membrane has a very rich supply of capillaries, and in many sites these approach the inner surface of the membrane very closely. As a result blood may escape into the synovial fluid from a relatively minor injury to the joint.

Blood vessels are arranged in a circular network at the periphery of the articular cartilage in the transition zone; this arrangement constitutes the circulus articuli vasculosus of Hunter.

Gardner's paper should be consulted for details regarding the blood supply of joints.

The lymphatic plexus lies somewhat more deeply from the synovial surface than do the blood capillaries. The lymphatic capillaries begin as blind tubes; these are often enlarged at their blind ends. After piercing the elastic lamina of the synovial lining they converge into larger vessels which pass in the general direction of the flexor aspect of the joint. Here they anastomose freely with the periosteal lymphatics and then empty into the main lymphatic vessels of the limb (see Davies).

Nerve Supply. The student will find it easier to understand the following section if he returns to it after reading the section on nervous tissue. Hilton's law, first enunciated by John Hilton in 1863, continues to be the fundamental statement about the nerve supply of joints: "The same trunks of nerves whose branches supply the muscles moving a joint also furnish a distribution of nerves to the skin over the insertions of the same muscles, and . . . the interior of the joint receives its nerves from the same source." Articular cartilage contains no nerve endings. The capsular structures contain different types of endings, as will now be described.

Joints are supplied with both myelinated and nonmyelinated fibers.

The larger myelinated fibers that reach joints are those of afferent neurons. These terminate for the most part in the joint capsule. The nerve endings on these fibers, according to Gardner, are mostly of the Ruffini type (described in Chapter 28), and these in this site are sensitive to changes in pressure and probably other types of stimuli concerned in providing a proprioceptive function. The endings are aggregated chiefly in sites in the capsule that are most likely to be compressed by joint movements.

Small myelinated fibers pass to the joint capsule and to the ligaments of the joint, where they end in free endings. These fibers are concerned with the sense of pain. There are very few of these free endings in the connective tissue of the synovial membranes; hence it would not seem to be very sensitive to pain. That the synovial membrane is not very sensitive to pain has been confirmed at operations in which joints have been opened under local anesthesia. The free endings in the capsule and ligaments of joints seem to be stimulated most easily by stretching or twisting these structures. Small myelinated fibers also form free endings in the adventitia of blood vessels; these are probably vasosensory, and at least some probably are concerned with the sense of pain. Endings of this type in the adventitia of blood vessels are probably the only kind of free afferent endings in synovial membranes.

Nonmyelinated sympathetic fibers, which, of course, are efferent, end in the smooth muscle of the blood vessels of joints to regulate flow through them.

Fibers reach larger joints from many spinal nerves, and any given nerve may supply more than one joint. Joint pain is generally poorly localized.

Gardner has made extensive studies on the nerve supply of joints, and his papers should be read to obtain detailed information on this subject.

Synovial Fluid. Since the synovial cavity develops as a connective tissue space, it should contain a ground substance and be perfused with tissue fluid. This concept of the cavity and its contents has been supported by the investigations of Bauer and his colleagues, who showed that synovial fluid was an ultrafiltrate or dialysate of blood (as is tissue fluid) plus what they termed mucin. Meyer identified the so-called mucin of synovial fluid as hyaluronic acid. In synovial fluid, in contrast to the aqueous humor, hyaluronic acid is highly polymerized; this accounts for the viscous quality of synovial fluid and doubtless adds to its lubricating qualities.

The various projections of the synovial membrane that extend into the synovial cavity and the closeness of the capillaries to the surface of the cavity make it easy to understand how tissue fluid readily could gain access to the cavity. The presence of hyaluronic acid in synovial fluid is to be explained by the fact that synovial cells produce it, and that which is produced constitutes the ground substance of the synovial membrane and also gains entrance to the synovial fluid.

The cell content of synovial fluid appears to vary considerably from joint to joint and from species to species. Key points out that it tends to become increased after death. Counts of from 80 to several thousand cells per cubic millimeter have been found by different investigators. Key found a typical differential count to yield 58 percent monocytes, 15 percent macrophages, 14 percent ill-defined types of phagocytes, 1 percent primitive cells, 3 percent synovial cells and 5 percent of other types of blood leukocytes.

The passage of substances into and out of the synovial fluid depends upon their size. Crystalloids diffuse readily in both directions. This is of importance in the treatment of joint diseases, for soluble drugs given an individual can quickly enter the synovial fluid. Gases also diffuse readily in both directions. Hence, in caisson disease (the bends), nitrogen bubbles frequently appear in joint cavities. This disease occurs when divers or other people working under high atmospheric pressure return too quickly to normal atmospheric pressure. The sudden decompression of the individual as a whole causes a too sudden release of gases dissolved in the bloodstream and other fluids, just as carbon dioxide bubbles from soda water when the cap is removed from a bottle.

Proteins, with their large colloidal molecules, leave synovial fluid by way of lymphatics. Particulate matter must be removed from synovial fluid by phagocytosis. Although synovial cells have some phagocytic powers, most of the phagocytosis of particulate matter introduced into synovial fluid is brought about by macrophages. The removal of particulate matter from joints is a slow process, and phagocytes containing hemosiderin may be seen in the synovial tissues of joints months after blood has escaped into the synovial fluid.

Age Changes. A condition called *osteoarthritis* tends to develop in joints as individuals age. This condition is so common that its development to some degree is considered, by some investigators, to be a normal consequence of the aging process. As has already been described, the cells of articular cartilage seem unable to divide and so maintain articular cartilage in the same way that many other body tissues are maintained. Should the condition develop prematurely or in a severe form, it is, of course, considered to be pathologic. It consists essentially of a curious combination of degenerative and proliferative phenomena.

The degenerative changes that occur are seen to best advantage in the more central parts of articular cartilages (rather than at the periphery of articular cartilages). The cement substance of the cartilage (chondroitin-sulfuric acid) appears to be involved and to change in character. As a result, the collagenic fibers and even the fibrils of the intercellular substance of the cartilage become unmasked and visible in sections. As the condition progresses, the collagenic fibers become freely exposed on the articular surface; this gives the surface an appearance like the "pile" of a carpet, and the condition is termed fibrillation of the cartilage.

The proliferative changes occur around the edges of the articular cartilage, particularly in the transition zone and at the sites of attachment of tendons and ligaments. Cartilage proliferates in these regions and is replaced by bone in such a fashion that bony spurs, termed *osteophytes,* grow so as to form lips around the joint. It may be that these outgrowths represent an attempt to restrain movement to the joint.

This combination of degenerative and proliferative changes, although it occurs commonly in the aged, may occur in younger individuals, particularly if the direction of a stress borne by a joint has been altered by some kind of injury. Hence the condition to some extent appears to be the consequence of joints having to perform too much or the wrong kind of work.

References and Other Reading

GENERAL

Barnett, C. H., Davies, D. V., and MacConaill, M. A.: Synovial Joints. London, Longmans, Green & Co., 1961.
Davies, D. V.: The anatomy and physiology of joints. *In* Copeman's Textbook of the Rheumatic Diseases. ed. 2, p. 40. Edinburgh, E. & S. Livingstone, 1955.
Silberberg, Ruth: Ultrastructure of articular cartilage in health and disease. Clin. Orthop., *57:*233, 1968.

SPECIAL

Bauer, W., Ropes, M. W., and Waine, H.: The physiology of articular structures. Physiol. Rev., *20:*272, 1940.
Benninghoff, A.: Form und Bau der Gelenkknorpel in ihren Beziehungen zun Funktion (II). Z. Zellforsch., *2:*783, 1925.

Bradford, F. K., and Spurling, R. G.: The Intervertebral Disc. Springfield, Ill., Charles C Thomas, 1941.

Crelin, E. S., and Koch, W. E.: Development of mouse pubic joint in vivo following initial differentiation in vitro. Anat. Rec., 153:161, 1965.

Crelin, E. S., and Southwick, W. O.: Changes induced by sustained pressure in the knee joint articular cartilage of adult rabbits. Anat. Rec., 149:113, 1964.

Davies, D. V.: Anatomy and physiology of diarthrodial joints. Ann. Rheum. Dis., 5:29, 1945.

Elliott, H. C.: Studies on articular cartilages. I. Growth mechanisms. Am. J. Anat., 58:127, 1936.

Gardner, E.: The anatomy of the joints. Instruc. Lect. Am. Acad. Orthop. Surg. vol. 9. Ann Arbor, Edwards, 1952.

———: Blood and nerve supply of joints. Stanford Med. Bull., 11:203, 1953.

———: The innervation of the elbow joint. Anat. Rec., 102:161, 1948.

———: The innervation of the hip joint. Anat. Rec., 101:353, 1948.

———: The innervation of the knee joint. Anat. Rec., 101:109, 1948.

———: The innervation of the shoulder joint. Anat. Rec., 102:1, 1948.

———: The nerve supply of diarthrodial joints. Stanford Med. Bull., 6:367, 1948.

———: Physiology of movable joints. Physiol. Rev., 30:127, 1950.

Gardner, E., and Gray, D. J.: Prenatal development of the human hip joint. Am. J. Anat., 87:163, 1950.

Grant, J. C. B.: Interarticular synovial folds. Brit. J. Surg., 18:636, 1931.

Haines, R. W.: The development of joints. J. Anat., 81:33, 1947.

Hall, Kathleen: The effect of hysterectomy on the action of oestrone on the symphysis pubis of ovariectomized mice. J. Endocrinol., 7:299, 1951.

———: The effect of oestrone and progesterone on the histologic structure of the symphysis pubis of the castrated female mouse. J. Endocrinol., 7:54, 1950.

Hall, Kathleen, and Newton, W. H.: The action of "Relaxin" in the mouse. Lancet, 1:54, 1946.

———: The effect of oestrone and relaxin on the x-ray appearance of the pelvis of the mouse. J. Physiol., 106:18, 1947.

———: The normal course of separation of the pubes in pregnant mice. J. Physiol., 104:346, 1946.

Ham, A. W.: *See* reference in previous chapter for 1930.

Key, J. A.: The reformation of synovial membrane in the knees of rabbits after synovectomy. J. Bone Joint Surg. (N.S.), 7:793, 1925.

———: The synovial membrane of joints and bursae. *In* Cowdry's Special Cytology. ed. 2, p. 1053. New York, Hoeber, 1932.

Lanier, R. R.: The effects of exercise on the knee-joints of inbred mice. Anat. Rec., 94:311, 1946.

Lever, J. D., and Ford, E. H. R.: Histological, histochemical and electron microscopic observations on synovial membrane. Anat. Rec., 132:525, 1958.

Paulson, S., Sylvén, B., Hirsch, C., and Snellman, O.: Biophysical and physiological investigations on cartilage and other mesenchymal tissues. III. The diffusion rate of various substances in normal bovine nucleus pulposus. Biochim. Biophys. Acta, 7:207, 1951.

Ropes, M. W., and Bauer, W.: Synovial Fluid Changes in Joint Disease. Cambridge, Mass., Commonwealth Fund, Harvard University Press, 1953.

Rosenthal, O., Bowie, M. A., and Wagoner, G.: Studies in the metabolism of articular cartilage. I. Respiration and glycolysis of cartilage in relation to its age. J. Cell. Comp. Physiol., 17:221, 1941.

Ruth, E. B.: Metamorphosis of the pubic symphysis. I. The white rat (Mus norvegicus albinus). Anat. Rec., 64:1, 1935.

———: Metamorphosis of the pubic symphysis. III. Histological changes in the symphysis of the pregnant guinea pig. Anat. Rec., 67:409, 1937.

———: A note on the fibrillar structure of hyaline cartilage. Anat. Rec., 96:93, 1946.

Salter, R. B., and Field, P.: The effects of continuous compression on living articular cartilage. J. Bone Joint Surg., 42-A:31, 1960.

Salter, R. B., Simmonds, D. F., Malcolm, B. W., and Rumble, E. J.: Personal Communication. 1973.

Silberberg, M., Silberberg, R., and Hasler, M.: Ultrastructure of articular cartilage of mice treated with somatotrophin. J. Bone Joint Surg., 46-A:766, 1964.

Silberberg, R., Silberberg, M., and Feir, D.: Life cycle of articular cartilage cells: An electron microscope study of the hip joint of the mouse. Am. J. Anat., 114:17, 1964.

Walmsley, R., and Bruce, J.: The early stages of replacement of the semilunar cartilages of the knee joint in rabbits after operative excision. J. Anat., 72:260, 1938.

Whillis, J.: The development of synovial joints. J. Anat., 74:277, 1940.

17 Nervous Tissue

Nervous tissue is the third of the four basic tissues to engage our attention. The fourth, muscle tissue, the functions of which are controlled by nervous tissue will be considered in the next chapter.

The Term System. The nervous tissue of the body is organized into what is termed the *nervous system.* A system is a group of organs or structures that work together to carry out some special function for the body. Presently we shall try to explain the nature of the special functions that are carried out by the nervous system. These functions are carried out by the nervous tissue of what are termed the two divisions of the system which will now be described.

The Two Divisions of the System. The first division is called the Central Nervous System or, for short, the C.N.S. This division is surrounded and protected by bone. It consists of the brain (black in Fig. 17-1) which is contained within the skull, and the *spinal cord* (black in Figure 17-1) which is continuous with the brain above and is contained in the canal of the vertebral column where it extends to the level of between the first and second lumbar vertebrae (Fig. 17-1).

The second division is called the Peripheral Nervous System or, for short, the P.N.S. It consists of cordlike structures called *nerves* (black in Fig. 17-1) which lead off from the brain and spinal cord. These nerves are in pairs, with one of each pair going toward one side of the body and the other to the other side. Those that emerge from the brain are called *cranial nerves* and to reach their destinations they have to pass out through small canals that exist in the bones of the skull and are called *foramina.* Those nerves that pass out from each side of the spinal cord into the body are called *spinal nerves;* they pass through canals that are located between contiguous vertebrae and are called intervertebral foramina, as will be described in more detail later.

Perspective. For those readers who may not have had any previous introductory instruction about nervous tissue it may be helpful for purposes of perspective about its role in the body to here use an analogy.

Nervous tissue serves the same general role in the body as the telegraph and telephone systems of communities of people. It provides the means whereby instantaneous communication is possible between the cells of its different parts as well as between epithelial, connective and muscle tissue. Messages are sent in the nervous system over threadlike structures called nerve fibers which are very much like telephone wires; for, like them, they are wrapped with insulation, which is necessary because the passage of a nervous impulse along a nerve fiber is associated with a wave of changing electrical potential as it travels along the fibers at an almost incredible speed.

The core of a nerve fiber, however, instead of being a metallic conductor, is a delicate strand of living cytoplasm. A nerve fiber is a strand of cytoplasm that extends off from what is termed the *cell body* of a nerve cell which is the part of it that contains its nucleus and around which there is a substantial amount of cytoplasm to house its organelles (Fig. 17-2). It is because of the organelles in the cell body that the cytoplasmic threads which are nerve fibers are constantly renewed and kept alive.

Neurons. A nerve cell including all the nerve fibers that extend from it is called a *neuron.* As is shown in Figure 17-2, a neuron is classified as a unipolar if it has a single process (a nerve fiber) extending off from its cell body (Fig. 17-2, *left*), or bipolar if it has two processes (Fig. 17-2, *middle*) or multipolar if it has more than two (Fig. 17-2, *right*).

Axons and Dendrites. Nerve impulses in the body customarily travel one way over neurons. All three types—unipolar, bipolar and multipolar—have a single fiber that conducts impulses away from the cell body; this single fiber is termed an *axon* (Fig. 17-2). This is the only kind of process possessed by a unipolar neuron so in these the nervous impulse has to originate at the surface of its cell body (Fig. 17-2, *left*). A bipolar neuron has an axon but also another process which is called a *dendrite* (Fig. 17-2, *middle*). Impulses initiated at the free end or at any other part of a dendrite are conducted to the cell body and from there along the axon to its termination. Multipolar neurons, which are the most common kind in the body

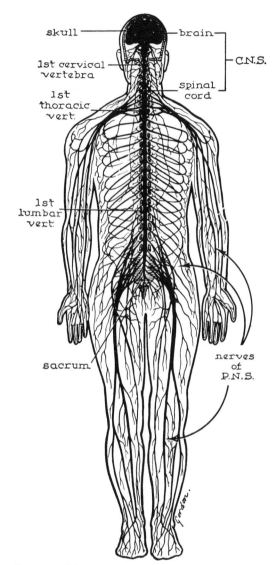

skull

brain

1st cervical vertebra

C.N.S.

spinal cord

1st thoracic vert.

1st lumbar vert.

sacrum

nerves of P.N.S.

Fig. 17-1. Diagrammatic drawing showing the C.N.S. and the P.N.S. and how they are continuous with one another.

neuron to another much in the same way as relays are used in long-distance telegraph and telephone transmission. The counterparts of relays used in the nervous system are termed *synapses* and, as will be explained later, a synapse (from the Greek *to clasp*) is an arrangement whereby the axon of one neuron ends in a special structure on some part of a second neuron. The arrival of enough nervous impulses at the synapse of one neuron on another can trigger the initiation of a nervous impulse in the second neuron which travels along it to the termination of its axon which, of course, may end in another synapse on still another neuron.

Nerve fibers from many different neurons may end in synapses on a single neuron where they appear as little bodies called end-feet (Fig. 17-3). However, as will be described later, not all synapses are of the excitatory type described above. Some synapses are inhibitory and thus impulses arriving at them tend to prevent initiation of impulses in their immediate vicinity in the second neuron. The fine structure of synapses and a description of how they function will be given later.

The Organization of Nervous Tissue Within the Nervous System

The way the nervous tissue of the body is organized is most easily understood by considering briefly the way it evolved.

The Evolution of Neurons. An organism consisting of a single cell cannot have either nerve tissue or a nervous system. It was not until the multicellular organism evolved that it became possible for cells to become specialized so that one kind would do one kind of work, and other kinds, other kinds of work in a body. Muscle cells—specialized for contractility— probably appeared in the animal kingdom before nerve cells, because certain of the sponges, though vegetable-like, possess some cells specialized for contractility around their pores. These are in direct contact with sea water, and, should it contain a noxious substance, these musclelike cells are directly stimulated to contract and close the pores.

As multicellular organisms evolved further and became composed of more and more different kinds of cells, muscle cells came to be more deeply located in the multicellular body. This development required that some sufficiently irritable cells of the organisms be exposed to surface stimulation and arranged so that they could conduct waves of excitation to the deeply situated muscle cells. One of the first arrangements of this sort to evolve is illustrated in Figure 17-4; this shows that one of the ectodermal cells (the black one)

have several dendrites (*dendron,* tree) which may emerge from the cell body like the branches of a tree from its trunk (Fig. 17-2, *right*). This gives them wide exposure to sites of possible stimulation.

Neurons Are Individual Units but Connect With One Another. There seems to be a limit as to how long a nerve fiber can be if it is to be adequately maintained by a cell body. Many nerve fibers are quite short while the longest are around two or three feet long. So for a nervous impulse to be conducted over long distances in the body it must be relayed from one

TYPES OF NEURONS

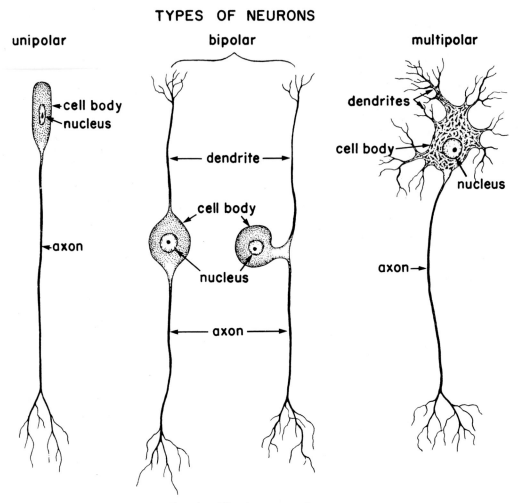

Fig. 17-2. The three types of neurons.

has differentiated into a neuron (labeled *sensory cell*), and although its cell body, which contains the nucleus of the cell, remains at the surface, its cytoplasm has extended in the form of a long threadlike process (a *nerve fiber*) to a deeply disposed muscle cell; thus this represented the development of a unipolar neuron. In this arrangement the cell body of the neuron is exposed to environmental stimuli, and, when stimulated, a nervous impulse is set up in it which travels along the nerve fiber (which would be an axon) to the muscle cell, making it contract.

The Evolution of the Reflex Arc. The further evolution of nervous tissue hinged on the development of nervous pathways consisting of two or more neurons. In these pathways the process of one neuron comes into contact with either the cell body or a process of another by means of a synapse. An arrangement of

two or more neurons is required if a stimulus, received anywhere by a higher animal, is to evoke a response in a muscle or gland. A simple example of a working arrangement of two neurons is to be seen in each segment of an earthworm (Fig. 17-5); this illustrates the simplest kind of a reflex arc as will be described below.

The Afferent and Efferent Neurons of Reflex Arcs. The first neuron, which in the earthworm (but not in man) has its cell body at the surface (Fig. 17-5, cell body etc.), sends a nerve fiber into the substance of the segment where the fiber terminates in synaptic connection with the fiber of a second neuron (labeled synapse in Fig. 17-5). The first neuron, because it carries a nervous impulse toward the more central part of the earthworm, is said to be an *afferent (affere,* to carry on) neuron (labeled in Fig. 17-5). The second neuron, in turn, carries the impulse away from the

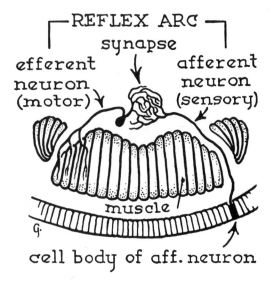

FIG. 17-5. Diagram of an afferent and efferent neuron arranged to constitute a reflex arc in the earthworm. (Redrawn from Parker, G. H.: The Elementary Nervous System. Philadelphia, J. B. Lippincott)

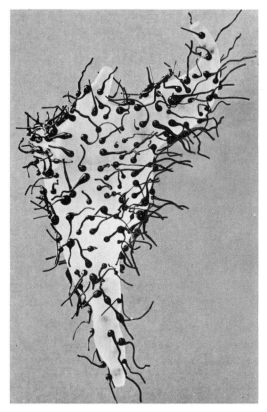

FIG. 17-3. Photograph of a model of the body of a nerve cell in the dorsal horn of the cat's spinal cord. The model as a whole was made by fitting together individual models made from serial sections, and it shows the enormous number of nerve fibers that terminate as end-bulbs (end-feet) on the body of the nerve cell to effect synaptic relations with it. (Haggar, R. A., and Barr, M. L.: J. Comp. Neurol., *93*:17)

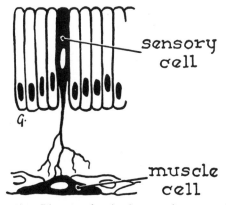

FIG. 17-4. Diagram of a simple type of receptor-effector system such as is seen in the tentacles of sea anemones. (Redrawn from Parker, G. H.: The Elementary Nervous System. Philadelphia, J. B. Lippincott)

deeper part of the organism to the muscle and is said to be an *efferent* (*effere,* to carry away) neuron (labeled in Fig. 17-5). The two neurons together constitute the very simplest form of a *reflex arc.* This term (*reflectere,* to bend back; *arcus,* a bow or a curved line) aptly describes the arrangement, because the nervous impulse brought into the organism by means of the afferent neuron is reflected outward again by means of the efferent neuron.

The Evolution of Segmented Animals and Connector Neurons. Most of the larger animals that evolved became elongated, generally by basic units of body structure, called segments, becoming duplicated and reduplicated in the longitudinal axis of an animal. In lowly segmented organisms, such as the earthworm, the boundaries between segments are easily seen, and each segment retains a considerable amount of autonomy. Of particular interest to us is the fact that each segment contains an afferent and an efferent neuron and an individual unit of muscle to which the efferent neuron leads; hence, reflex activity is possible within each segment. It is most important to realize that man, too, is a segmented organism, and each segment has its afferent and efferent neurons, as we shall see.

The evolution of the elongated segmented organism was associated with a new type of neuron which could provide nervous connections between segments and so permit their activities to be regulated in the interests of the animal as a whole. Hence, segmented organisms have, in addition to the afferent and efferent neurons

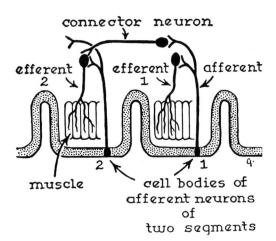

FIG. 17-6. Diagram of a portion of a hypothetical segmented organism, showing how connector neurons permit correlation between segments.

of each segment, *intersegmental connector neurons*. In the diagram of a hypothetical segmented animal (Fig. 17-6) it may be seen that these intersegmental connector neurons permit a stimulus received in one segment to cause a response in another. Intersegmental connector neurons *broaden the base of reflex arcs from one segment to many segments*.

Emergence of a Spinal Cord and a Brain. As evolution proceeded, there came to be more and more of these connector neurons, with some running for only short distances and others for long distances. Furthermore, they tended to become bundled together in the longitudinal axis of an animal in a more or less central position to account eventually for the structure called a *spinal cord*. In the head region the counterpart of the spinal cord became expanded, as it were, to become the brain; this expansion, as will be explained presently, is due in part to a still more greatly increased number of connector neurons being present in this region and also to the great input of afferent impulses from the special receptors in the nose, eyes, ears and taste buds, all of which are located in this area.

From the foregoing it is obvious that all connector neurons are contained in the C.N.S. However, in addition to these, the C.N.S. contains parts of both the afferent and the efferent neurons of each body segment. The remaining parts of the afferent and the efferent neurons—and these, of course, are outside the C.N.S. in peripheral nerves—constitute the P.N.S. To explain which parts of the segmental afferent and efferent neurons are contained in the P.N.S. requires that we discuss the changes in position that took place in the cell bodies of these neurons as evolution continued.

The Evolution of Posterior Root Ganglia. It is very important to understand the nature of what are termed the posterior root ganglia, two of which are present in each body segment, one on each side of the vertebral column.

The first sensory cells to evolve had their cell bodies at the surface of the organism (Fig. 17-4), and the cell bodies remained there in a few lower animals—for example, the earthworm—that have neurons, synapses and reflex arcs (Fig. 17-5). But the surface of an animal is not a suitable place for the cell bodies of afferent neurons, for in this position they are too easily injured and destroyed. The destruction of the *body* of a nerve cell is a very serious matter, because nerve cells seem to be too highly specialized to divide; hence, if one is destroyed, another cannot divide to provide a replacement for it. However, as can be shown in connection with the nerves of the P.N.S., the bodies of nerve cells can, under suitable circumstances, regenerate new fibers. So a much better arrangement is for the cell bodies of afferent neurons to be located more deeply, out of harm's way, with a long dendrite going to the surface to pick up stimuli. If the fiber is injured at the surface, it can be regenerated from the uninjured cell body. This is the kind of arrangement found in connection with almost all the afferent sensory neurons in higher animals. In these the nerve cell bodies of afferent neurons seem to have come as close to the C.N.S. as they could without actually getting into the C.N.S. In this position the cell bodies are housed in little nodules of nervous tissue called *ganglia* (a ganglion is a lump) (Fig. 17-7, body of ganglion cell). The particular ganglia that house the cell bodies of those afferent neurons that enter the spinal cord from each side of the body in each segment of the body are called *spinal, dorsal* or *posterior root ganglia*. There are two of these for each segment of the body, one on each side. The segments of the body in man are indicated by the vertebrae in the vertebral column, but each segment is not indicated by a particular individual vertebra but by adjacent halves of each of two contiguous vertebrae. An intervertebral foramen extends out from the vertebral canal on each side between contiguous vertebrae; this marks, as it were, the middle of the segment, and the spinal ganglion of each side is located in the intervertebral foramen of that side. (At this time the left side of Figure 17-34 should be briefly examined to see a spinal ganglion in position.)

Some afferent neurons enter the brain by way of certain cranial nerves. The cell bodies of these afferent neurons are also situated in ganglia that are close to, but not actually inside, the brain. These are termed cranial ganglia. The term *cerebrospinal* ganglia refers to both groups. All the cell bodies of the afferent neurons that enter the C.N.S. from the body segments are therefore housed in spinal or cranial ganglia.

The afferent neurons are fundamentally bipolar cells. They began, as it were, by having a dendrite that passed out to the surface and brought impulses into the cell body from which an axon which passed inward to conduct the impulse away from the cell body to a synapse in the spinal cord. This first type of bipolar afferent neuron is shown on the left of the middle illustration in Figure 17-2. However, as evolution proceeded further, the dendrite leading into the cell body and the axon leaving it seem to have swung around like the hands of a clock, until they came together and then fused. As a result the bipolar cells become seemingly unipolar (Fig. 17-2, right side of middle illustration). The single process of each, however, is short and soon branches into two, one of which extends to a sensory ending and the other into the spinal cord. Functionally, the peripheral branch is a dendrite, and the other an axon, but since both processes have the histologic structure of axons (to be described in detail in due course), both are commonly called axons, which is somewhat confusing.

The axons that enter the spinal cord from afferent neurons do so at the posterior-lateral aspects of the cord (Fig. 17-7). One entering the cord they may synapse directly with efferent neurons, as is shown in Figure 17-7 or with connector neurons, or they may pass for short distances down the cord, or for longer distances up the cord, before synapsing with efferent neurons of other segments or with connector neurons.

Efferent Neurons. The cell bodies of all efferent neurons, with the exception of certain of those of the autonomic nervous system, which will be described later, are all confined to the C.N.S. The axons from the cell bodies of efferent neurons of the spinal cord may pass directly out from the segment in which they lie as nerve fibers of a peripheral nerve as shown in Figure 17-7.

Most Actions of Man Involve Reflex Arcs. The medical or paramedical student reader will soon be testing the reflexes of patients to learn if various parts of their nervous system are functioning properly. A common and important reflex tested is the knee jerk. This is done as follows, first having the patient cross his knees and relax; then the upper knee is given a sharp tap just below the patella, as is shown in Figure 17-7. The indentation of the tendon occasioned by the tap pulls on the muscle and stretches little spindle-shaped structures within it called *neuromuscular spindles* (to be described later), which thereupon generate afferent impulses that flow toward the cell body of the afferent neuron which is contained in a posterior root ganglion of the segment (Fig. 17-7, posterior root ganglion). From it an axon extends into the spinal cord where it synapses with the cell body of an efferent neuron, which sends an axon by means of the same peripheral nerve to the muscle fibers of the quadriceps femoris, as is shown in Figure 17-7. The contraction of the muscle causes the foot to kick forward smartly.

Notice, as is shown in Figure 17-7, that both afferent and efferent fibers travel in the same peripheral nerve.

A SIMPLE REFLEX ARC (Knee Jerk)

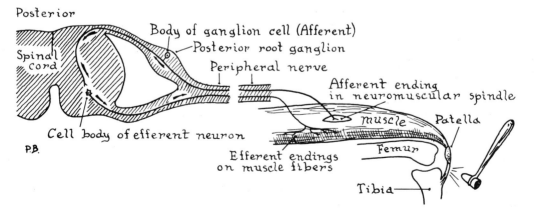

FIG. 17-7. Diagram illustrating a simple two-neuron reflex in man, the knee jerk or stretch reflex. Note that the cell body of the afferent neuron is in a posterior root ganglion, outside the central nervous system.

The knee jerk is the simplest kind of reflex found in the body, involving only two neurons. Most reflexes involve many neurons.

Segmental Nerve Supply in Man. In understanding the nerve supply in any part of the body and the reflexes that can be elicited in man, it is of the greatest importance to remember that man is a segmented organism. The spinal cord contains the intersegmental connector neurons. The peripheral nerves that pass out from the spinal cord, one on each side, through the foramen between individual vertebrae (Fig. 17-34) in man contain the fibers of the afferent and efferent neurons of that body segment. The spinal nerves that extend from each foramen into the body contain the fibers of both its afferent and the efferent neurons. Moreover, the afferent (sensory) fibers in these nerves will be found to extend only to sites in the skin and other tissues that develop from that same segment. Likewise, the efferent fibers in each nerve will be found to pass only to muscle fibers that develop from that same segment. During development, the muscle fibers that develop from any given segment only sometimes remain independent of those from other segments, as occurs, for example, in the intercostal muscles; more commonly, muscle fibers that develop from a particular segment meet with muscle fibers from other segments to become parts of larger muscles that traverse many segments. Nevertheless, the fibers that develop from any segment retain their efferent innervation from that same segment; hence, large muscles may have innervation from several segments.

The importance of the foregoing becomes obvious in determining the site of an injury or lesion of the spinal cord; for if the lesion or injury destroys the afferent or efferent neurons in a segment, the site of the lesion can be determined by locating the skin in which sensation is lost or the muscles which lose their function.

To Sum Up. The cell bodies of all afferent neurons are in spinal or cerebral ganglia just outside the C.N.S. The cell bodies of all connector neurons, and all efferent neurons, except certain of those of the autonomic nervous system (to be described later), are in the C.N.S. The skin and muscles that develop from any body segment are innervated by nerves from that segment.

Afferent Nerve Endings and the Basis for Sensations

Man has many senses: touch, pressure, heat, cold, pain, sight, hearing, taste, position and movement. These sensations are experienced in the brain. However, the stimuli that give rise to these sensations do not reach the brain; only nervous impulses reach the brain. These impulses are initiated at the endings of afferent neurons in various body segments and are conducted into the spinal cord and from there via connector neurons to certain parts of the brain. So we shall next inquire briefly into how nervous impulses from different afferent neurons give rise to different sensations and permit the site of the cause of the sensation—for example, cold—to be located, say, in a finger.

The Nature of Afferent (Sensory) Nerve Endings. The passage of a nervous impulse along a nerve fiber is not precisely the same as the passage of an electric current along a wire, but is somewhat similar to it. Any amateur electrician could wire up a battery and an induction coil so that he can give himself a shock when he closes a switch. Furthermore, switches can be obtained or made which could be said to be specialized with regard to different kinds of stimuli. For example, a telegraph key (Fig. 17-8) completes a circuit if it is touched or pressed; it is either a *touch* or a *pressure* receptor, depending on how tightly its spring is adjusted. Contrivances can also be built, some of which would complete a circuit if they were heated, others if they were cooled (Fig. 17-8). Indeed, it is possible to build or obtain electrical contrivances that will complete a circuit when they are exposed to any of the different kinds of stimuli that can stimulate the afferent neurons of man (Fig. 17-8).

Much the same kind of phenomena occur in the afferent nerve endings in man. For example, the different afferent nerve fibers that end in the skin terminate at different kinds of nerve endings. Some initiate a nervous impulse when they are lightly touched. Others do so when they are firmly pressed, others when they are warmed and others when they are cooled and so on. They will be described in Chapter 28. The impulses generated by any one ending being stimulated travel by way of a special separate neuron chain to a particular part of the brain and the proper sensation is aroused when this part of the brain is stimulated.

Locating the Site of a Stimulus. A blindfolded person can tell whether he is touched on a finger or foot and furthermore if he is touched on a particular finger. The mechanism here is somewhat similar to that of a person who lives in a house with a front door, a side door and a back door, and has a touch receptor (a push button) on each door, each of which is wired to one of three lights in a call box. If the light connected to the push button at the back door flashes on he knows his house was touched in that region. Similarly the neuron pathways that reach the brain from afferent touch receptors located at innumerable body sites are wired to somewhat different sites in the same general area of the brain so as to also give the precise location of the particular part of a body that is touched.

Since it is difficult to describe the microscopic structure of afferent nerve endings in various body parts until we have studied the microscopic structure of those body parts, we shall postpone their description until the last chapter when we will have covered the histology of all parts of the body.

Efferent Nerve Endings. There are two main types, those that end in muscle to control its function and those that end in association with secretory cells. The structure of those that terminate in muscle will be described in the next chapter. Those that end in association with secretory cells will be described later in this chapter.

Inherited and Conditioned Reflex Responses

Reflexes are basic to human behavior. However, reflex behavior can be modified by conditioning so that people do not all react in the same way to the same stimulus.

A common analogy that helps to explain how this happens is to liken the brain to a giant switchboard. Afferent pathways from all parts of the body lead to it, and efferent pathways lead from it to all parts of the body. Although connections exist between afferent and efferent neurons in the spinal cord, most afferent impulses that are set up in the body pass to the brain by means of afferent pathways before they activate efferent systems. The number of different circuits available between afferent and efferent systems in this organ is enormous, so the possibility exists for different afferent impulses to "set off" different efferent systems. Higher animals inherit some preferred circuits between afferent and efferent systems which seem to account for instinctive reflex responses. For example, if food is placed in a puppy's mouth, a reflex action occurs which results in efferent impulses causing his salivary glands to secrete. Pavlov, the famous Russian psychologist, showed first that the *only* stimulus that would evoke salivation in a newborn puppy was the actual presence of food in its mouth. The afferent pathway activated in this instance would be a pathway leading from receptors in the mouth itself. In its brain the puppy had inherited a preferred connection, as it were, between this afferent pathway and the efferent pathway that controls the salivary glands. But then Pavlov showed that the puppy, after being fed a few times, would salivate as soon as he smelled the food that was

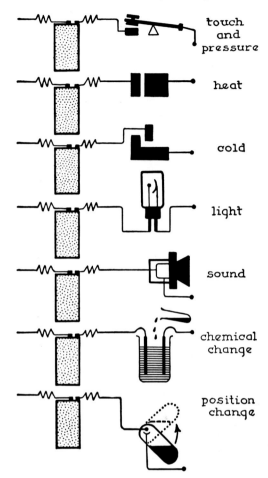

FIG. 17-8. Diagrams of pieces of apparatus which could be employed to complete an electrical circuit when subjected to the different kinds of stimuli listed on the right side.

put before him. Obviously, this would require the use of a different afferent pathway from the first one employed—one from the nose rather than from the mouth. So there must be some connection in the brain between afferent pathways from the nose and the afferent pathways from the mouth. The neurons by which such connections are made are termed *association neurons.* These permit the puppy to associate the taste of food with the smell of food, and once this association is built up, the proper stimulus applied to the nose brings about the same reflex responses as does food in the mouth. This next reflex response, which involves a different afferent pathway, and association neurons, Pavlov termed a *conditioned response.* He showed that the possibilities in conditioned responses are very considerable. A pup, for example, soon learns to salivate at the sight of food and can even be trained to salivate at the ringing of a bell, if a bell is rung every time it is fed. Then, by further conditioning procedures which need not be described here, the conditioned response to the ringing of the bell can be inhibited. Therefore, conditioning procedures are effective in broadening not only the base of our possible responses to stimuli but also the base of our inhibitions. All in all, we are exposed to so many different associations in our lives that it is not strange that a particular stimulus does not evoke the same response in all men, or that what may attract one may repel another.

Development of the Nervous System

In order to understand very much about the histology of the nervous system, it is essential to know something about how it develops. A brief and simple account of this matter follows.

The early development of the neural tube and neural crests from ectoderm was described in Chapter 6 and illustrated in Figure 6-3. This illustration shows how the tube develops into a spinal cord and brain. The neural crests give rise to the posterior root ganglia (spinal ganglia).

The cells of the neural tube and crests constitute the *neuroectoderm*. We shall now consider its further history and learn how the neuroectodermal cells of the neural tube develop into the C.N.S. and then, several pages further on, how the neuroectodermal cells of the neural crests give rise to much of the P.N.S.

THE DEVELOPMENT OF THE GROSS STRUCTURE OF THE SPINAL CORD AND BRAIN

Spinal Cord. As a result of cell proliferation within its wall, a neural tube becomes longer and wider and, at the same time, the lumen of the tube is encroached upon because of its wall becoming thickened. In due course the lumen of the tube is reduced to a tiny size (Fig. 6-3, *bottom left*). As the cord continues to develop, its appearance in cross section, although remaining oval, becomes somewhat flattened in front.

Results of a Disproportionate Growth of Cord and Vertebral Column. As already described, man is a segmented organism. The afferent neurons that extend into the cord from any given body segment pass through the intervertebral foramen belonging to that segment and into the vertebral canal (Fig. 17-34), where they extend to and enter the posterior part of the segment of the spinal cord that belongs to that body segment (Fig. 17-7). Likewise, the efferent fibers that extend out from that same segment of the cord

pass through the same intervertebral foramen to reach and innervate, by way of a peripheral nerve, the muscles that belong to that particular body segment (Fig. 17-7). However, during development the vertebral column elongates to a much greater extent than the spinal cord that is contained in its canal. This has two important effects. First, since the cord must remain connected to the brain, the lower end of the cord in the adult does not reach nearly to the lower end of the vertebral canal but only to the level of the 1st or the 2nd lumbar vertebra (Fig. 17-1). Second, the various segother courses and here should learn something of the general structure of this organ.

It seems almost incredible to anyone who examines a brain for the first time that an organ of such a complex appearance (Fig. 17-9) could have developed from something as simple as one end of the neural tube. Probably two general mechanisms are involved in its development: (1) the dissimilar growth rates in different parts of the wall of the neural tube, which results in the wall of the tube becoming thick and even forming protrusions in some sites while remaining thin in other sites, and (2) the vast amount of longitudinal growth that occurs in the wall of the neural tube in the site where the brain develops results in the growing neural tube becoming too long to fit into the long diameter of the space it occupies. As a result it can be accommodated only if it becomes more or less kinked (flexed), as a rubber tube might become kinked or flexed if it was pushed into a space shorter than it was.

The first change seen as the anterior end of the tube begins to form a brain is that it develops three swellments of the cord, which originally are in line with the body segments to which their afferent and efferent fibers are connected, gradually assume higher levels than their respective body segments; hence the afferent and the efferent fibers that pass out from each segment of the cord to reach their respective body segments must pass down along the sides of the cord to reach their intervertebral foramina. This condition, of course, becomes increasingly prominent as the caudal end of the cord is approached and accounts for the fact that although the caudal division of the vertebral canal does not contain any spinal cord, it does contain afferent and efferent fibers that are extending down from the lower segments of the cord to reach their proper intervertebral foramina.

The Development of the Neural Tube Into the Brain. Since it is essential for the reader to have some concept of the gross structure of the brain in order to describe its microscopic components, the following account is presented for purposes of reference for students who have not yet learned about the brain from

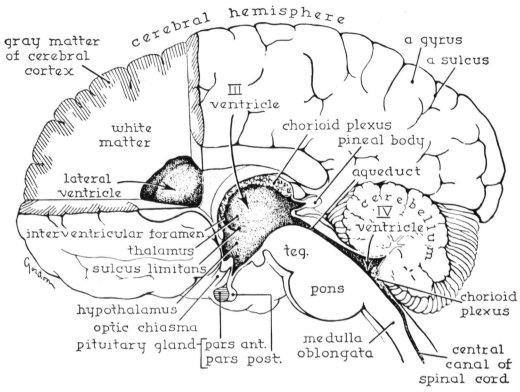

Fig. 17-9. A median sagittal section of the brain of man. A portion of the frontal lobe has been cut out (*upper left*) so as to disclose that lateral ventricle. What was originally the lumen of the neural tube is shown in dark stipple. In reading the text the student should begin at the right lower corner and follow the central canal of the cord into the various ventricles of the brain and visualize how the main parts of the brain have developed from the parts of the wall of the neural tube that originally surrounded the divisions of its lumen that later became ventricles.

ings separated by two constrictions. The swellings are called *vesicles* and are named the forebrain, the midbrain and the hindbrain, respectively. Various important parts of the brain represent *thickenings* or *bulgings* of the wall of these vesicles. It is hoped that it should be easily possible, from the following description, to obtain a general idea of how some of the more important parts of the brain that are illustrated in Figure 17-9 developed from the three vesicles. In order to help the reader's orientation, the lumen of the tube which becomes the ventricles (a ventricle is a cavity in a hollow organ) of the brain, is shown in dark stipple in Figure 17-9.

In the following description we shall begin with the hindbrain (which is the part of the brain that is continuous with the spinal cord) and work forward.

The Hindbrain. This is divided into two parts by the *pontine flexure*. If a rubber tube is kinked or bent upon itself, the region of the kink is no longer tubular but broad and flattened, and the lumen is distorted to a transverse slit. Thus, when the neural tube is bent at the pontine flexure, the lateral walls diverge, and the form described for the rubber tube is assumed. However, the thin roof stretches more than the floor of the tube, so the roof of the tube becomes a thin cover over the shallow, widened cavity of the neural tube at this site. The floor of the lumen of the tube becomes *very thick* in the hindbrain (Fig. 17-9). The hindpart of the flexed tube is called the medulla oblongata (Fig. 17-9) because of its oblong cavity and is distinguishable from the cord, with which it is continuous, by its greater width, thicker floor and thinner roof.

The forepart of the hindbrain at first resembles the hindpart, but further development alters its appearance. The floor here, which becomes very thick, is called the *pons* (*pons*, bridge) (Fig. 17-9). However, apart from this, the sides of the developing neural tube undergo rapid development and form two large lateral swellings; these eventually meet and fuse to constitute a large mass, the cerebellum (Fig. 17-9), which forms the roof over the lumen at this site. These two lateral swellings which fuse medially are termed the *cerebellar hemispheres* (Fig. 17-9).

The lumen of the neural tube persists in the hindbrain as a flattened cavity called the *fourth ventricle* (Fig. 17-9). As will be explained in due course, this ventricle contains cerebrospinal fluid, and it communicates with other ventricles, as will be described. The thin roof plate, which roofs over the fourth ventricle behind the cerebellum, is called the *posterior medullary velum* (*velum*, veil).

The Midbrain. Of the three divisions of the primitive brain, the midbrain alone retains a frank tubular structure, for the growth rate of the different parts of the wall of the tube is more nearly equal here than elsewhere. In it the lumen of the neural tube is reduced to a small ductlike passage in the dorsal part of the midbrain. This passage, called the aqueduct (Fig. 17-9), connects the cavities (ventricles) of the forebrain and the hindbrain.

The medulla, the pons and the midbrain contain many important groups of cell bodies of neurons. The areas of frank gray matter that contain many bodies of neurons are termed *nuclei*. Fiber tracts of white matter containing either ascending or descending fibers may synapse in these regions or pass through them uninterruptedly. The nature of gray and white matter will soon be described.

The Forebrain. The cephalic flexure that develops between midbrain and forebrain does not produce the rubber-tube effect that occurs in the instance of the pontine flexure. Here the neural tube conforms more readily to bending, without its lumen becoming flattened.

The forebrain undergoes so many changes, particularly in its forepart, that it is helpful to regard it as consisting of two portions. The hindpart of the forebrain gives rise to thickenings of the wall of the tube called the *thalamus*, the *hypothalamus* and the *subthalamus*, and the forepart to two huge thickened bulges, the *cerebral hemispheres* (Fig. 17-9).

In the hindpart of the forebrain the growth rate is less than in the forepart. The thalamus is concerned primarily with relaying afferent (particularly sensory) impulses from the lower levels of the brain and the cord to the higher centers of the cerebral hemispheres. The hypothalamus is concerned essentially with the automatic innervations of smooth muscles and glands; this matter will be described when the autonomic nervous system is considered. It is also involved in producing neurosecretions, as will be described in connec-

tion with endocrine glands in Chapter 25. The lumen of the neural tube persists here to become a vertical slit and is known as the *third ventricle* (Fig. 17-9).

In the forepart of the forebrain the more dorsal parts of the lateral walls of the neural tube undergo enormous development and form two huge evaginations called the *cerebral hemispheres* (Fig. 17-9). The cavities of these become the *lateral ventricles* (Fig. 17-9), which connect with the third ventricle through the interventricular foramina (Fig. 17-9). In man the surface of the brain becomes greatly corrugated. The deeper grooves are termed *fissures*, and the shallower ones *sulci*. The latter separate *gyri* (Fig. 17-9).

Basic Histology of the Nervous Tissue of the C.N.S.

Cellular Development. The nervous tissue of the C.N.S. develops from the cells of the wall of the neural tube. As shown in Figure 17-10 the neuroectodermal cells of the cellular wall of the tube differentiate along three separate pathways to form (1) neurons, (2) the supporting cells of the nervous tissue of the C.N.S. which are of two kinds, termed astrocytes and oligodendrocytes respectively, and (3) ependymal cells which originally form a lining for the lumen of the tube. The latter become of importance later to form a lining for ventricles of the brain.

The pathways of differentiation are illustrated in Figure 17-10 which also illustrates more or less diagrammatically the appearance of the cells involved as differentiation proceeds along the three main lines.

The first step in learning about the microscopic structure of the nervous tissue of the C.N.S. is to understand the difference between the gray matter and white matter of which it is composed.

Gray and White Matter of the C.N.S.

The C.N.S. consists of two kinds of what was long ago called *gray,* and *white matter* from their gross appearance. As we shall learn, there is nothing special to make gray matter gray but there is something special to make some of the nervous tissue of the C.N.S. white.

Gray Matter. As a result of mitosis in the inner part of the neural tube (Fig. 17-10), the cells that are formed are pushed into the middle layer of the tube. Here most of them become neuroblasts and eventually nerve cells (Fig. 17-10). A minority becomes *neuroglia* (*neuro,* nerve; *glia,* glue) which is a comprehensive term for the supporting cells of the nervous tissue of the C.N.S. The combination of the cell bodies of

HISTOGENESIS
OF
CELLS OF C.N.S.

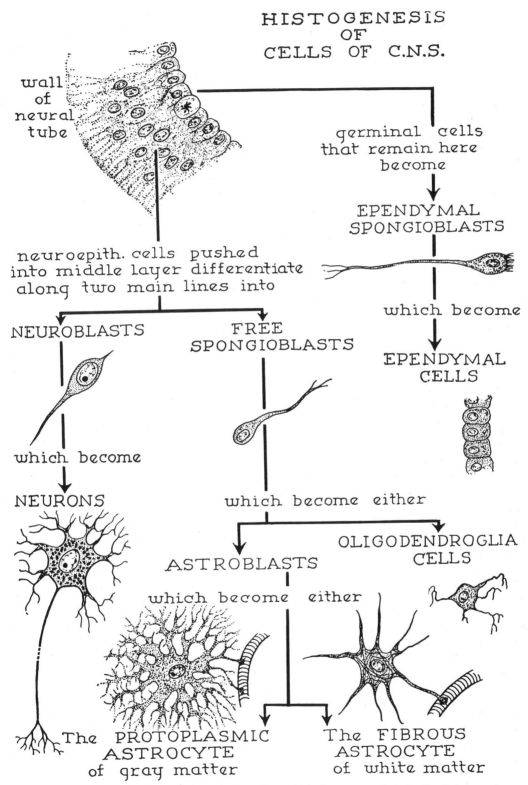

wall of neural tube

germinal cells that remain here become

EPENDYMAL SPONGIOBLASTS

neuroepith. cells pushed into middle layer differentiate along two main lines into

which become

NEUROBLASTS   FREE SPONGIOBLASTS

EPENDYMAL CELLS

which become

NEURONS

which become either

OLIGODENDROGLIA CELLS

ASTROBLASTS

which become either

The PROTOPLASMIC ASTROCYTE of gray matter

The FIBROUS ASTROCYTE of white matter

Fɪɢ. 17-10. Diagrams showing the main lines along which the neuroectodermal cells of the neural tube differentiate.

neurons with some supporting neuroglia cells constitutes the bulk of what, from its appearance in the
gross, was called *gray matter*.

The gray matter becomes arranged in the form of a
structure which roughly resembles an "H" when the
spinal cord is seen in cross section (Fig. 17-11). From
its appearance in a single cross section, this H-shaped
mass of gray matter is said to have two dorsal or posterior *horns* and two ventral or anterior horns (Fig.
17-11). Actually, the horns are continuous columns
that extend up and down the cord. In some parts of
the cord there is a lateral horn or column on each side
as well. Cell bodies of neurons are seen to best advantage in the horns, and in particular in the anterior
horns (Fig. 17-11, *lower left*).

A more detailed account of the cells of gray matter

GRAY AND WHITE MATTER OF SPINAL CORD

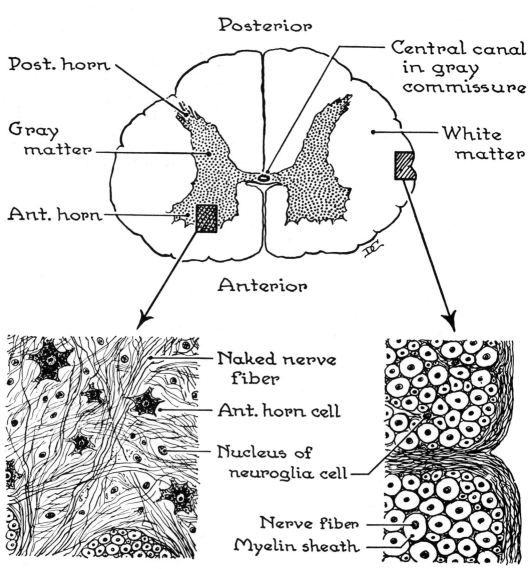

Fig. 17-11. (*Top*) Diagram of a cross section of the spinal cord (low-power), showing the distribution of gray and white matter in it. (*Bottom*) Two diagrams (high-power), showing the contents of the gray and the white matter, respectively.

will be given in due course. Gray matter is gray because it contains a lot of cells and because it does not contain the material which makes white matter white.

White Matter. The white matter of the spinal cord surrounds the H of gray matter (Fig. 17-11). The white matter contains the vast number of axons that extend up and down the cord. It is white because so many of these axons are ensheathed with a white fatty material called *myelin*. Myelin makes up most of the substance of white matter.

White matter does not contain any cell bodies of neurons. The axons it contains originate from cell bodies that are in the gray matter of the brain or spinal cord together with some from spinal ganglia.

As will be learned in other courses, the axons in the white matter are organized, with bundles or tracts which contain axons of neurons engaged in the same function. For example, there are motor tracts and sensory tracts. In the latter the fibers that, for example, lead to the brain center where pain is experienced are in the same tracts. Likewise, those responsible for certain aspects of the sense of position of arms and legs in space are segregated in another pair of tracts, and so on.

Although white matter contains no cell bodies of neurons it contains many cells of the neuroglia type. As shown in Figure 17-10, the outer layer of the part of the neural tube destined to become the spinal cord is invaded not only by axons but also by some free spongioblasts (from the developing middle layer), which differentiate into *astrocytes* and *oligodendrocytes*. These two types of neuroglia cells (chiefly oligodendrocytes) fit into the crevices between the axons and send their processes out among them (Fig. 17-11, *right*). The oligodendrocytes are commonly arranged in rows between adjacent myelinated axons.

Myelination. Myelin is a nonliving fatty material. It contains cholesterol, phospholipids, proteins and other components; its chemical composition is dealt with in biochemistry courses and textbooks. Myelination usually begins near the cell body and advances along the axon toward its termination. Myelination begins early in the 4th month and is not complete at birth; some fiber tracts become myelinated afterward. The total amount of myelin in the C.N.S. increases from birth to maturity; individual fibers become more heavily myelinated during the growth period. Myelin is not necessary for fibers to conduct nervous impulses but is necessary for fibers to conduct nervous impulses sufficiently well to permit muscles to make delicate and precise movements; the functions of myelin in this respect will be considered later in connection with peripheral nerves.

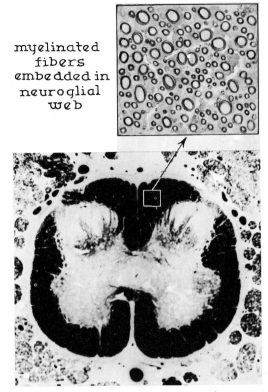

myelinated fibers embedded in neuroglial web

FIG. 17-12. (*Bottom*) Low-power photomicrograph of a cross section of spinal cord (sacral region) fixed in osmic acid. The white matter appears black. (*Top*) High-power drawing of a small area of white matter showing that the black material seen in the low-power illustration is the myelin of the sheaths of the nerve fibers. Observe that the fibers are of different calibers.

Myelin is soluble in fat solvents; hence, when ordinary paraffin sections of the spinal cord are prepared, most of the myelin of the white matter dissolves away in the dehydrating and clearing agents. When such sections are stained, the sites where myelin was present appear as round spaces that would be empty except that each contains a little round dot which represents a cross section of the axon that in life is surrounded by myelin (Fig. 17-11, *lower right*). The occasional nuclei that are seen in white matter between the empty round spaces are the nuclei of neuroglia cells.

By the use of fixatives that make myelin insoluble it is possible to demonstrate it in H and E paraffin sections. *Osmic acid* fixes myelin so that it does not dissolve away in paraffin sections. Osmic acid, in itself, colors myelin black, so that if a cross section of spinal cord fixed in osmic acid is examined under very low power, the white matter of the cord appears black (Fig. 17-12, *bottom*). If the white matter is examined

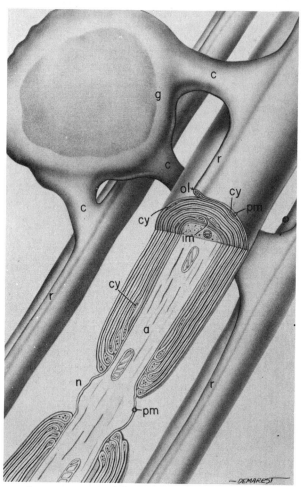

FIG. 17-13. Diagrammatic drawing illustrating the concept of how oligodendrocytes are related to the nerve fibers in white matter and how myelin is formed around the fibers by means of widened, thinned and flattened processes wrapping fibers with successive layers of themselves and, since these processes consist of little more than cell membrane material, the wrappings become converted to myelin. Note that an oligodendrocyte (o) sends processes (c) to more than one nerve fiber so oligodendrocytes can be involved in myelinating parts of more than one nerve fiber. The junction between the part of a fiber myelinated by the process of one oligodendrocyte and the part myelinated by the next oligodendrocyte is indicated by a node of Ranvier (n). (From Bunge, M. L., Bunge, R. P., and Ris, H.: J. Biophys. Biochem. Cytol., *10*:67, 1961)

under high power, the blackened myelin will be seen to be arranged in little rings around each nerve fiber (Fig. 17-12, *top*).

The Formation of Myelin in the C.N.S. As was described in Chapter 5, the cell membrane contains

much lipid material. Myelin is formed in the C.N.S. by the oligodendrocytes that lie between the nerve fibers in the white matter; these fibers run up and down in the outer part of the cord. The way an oligodendrocyte makes myelin is essentially that of wrapping a nerve fiber with successive layers of one of its processes which becomes widened and flattened, with almost all the cytoplasm that was in the process being squeezed back to the cell body, so the wrapping material consists of little more than a double layer of cell membrane (Fig. 17-13). The process of myelination here is similar to that which occurs in the myelination of nerve fibers in the P.N.S. and which will be explained in more detail shortly, so if the above is not understood it should become clear later. In peripheral nerves, however, myelination is of course not performed by oligodendrocytes but by another type of cell, as will be described.

To Sum Up Some of the Foregoing. Gray matter contains the cell bodies of all the nerve cells that are present in the spinal cord. Gray matter also contains neuroglia cells that provide support and protection of the nerve cells. Gray matter also contains the beginnings and endings of nerve fibers that lead from or to its nerve cells; myelin is not prominent on these parts of the fibers. The white matter of the cord consists of myelinated fibers that run up and down the cord. They are separated from each other, supported and protected by neuroglia, which are oligodendrocytes and astrocytes.

White matter is white because of the myelin it contains. White matter contains no cell bodies of nerve cells, only those of neuroglia. The oligodendrocytes wrap the nerve fibers with many layers of cell membrane which is what becomes myelin. Gray matter appears gray in the gross because it contains so many cells and only a trace of myelin, which is on some of the fibers entering or leaving it.

In due course we shall describe the cells mentioned above in more detail. But before doing so we must briefly describe the distribution of the white matter and gray matter in the brain.

THE GENERAL DISTRIBUTION OF GRAY AND WHITE MATTER IN THE BRAIN

Up to a point the formation of the gray and the white matter of the brain follows a similar pattern to that seen in the development of the spinal cord where gray matter forms from the cells of the middle layer of the tube, and white matter forms in the outer layer of the neural tube. In the medulla, the pons, the midbrain and in parts of the forebrain, gray matter develops in positions that are roughly comparable with those in which it develops in the spinal cord, and it becomes covered by the white matter that develops in the outer layer of the tube as it does in the cord. But in certain parts of the developing brain, neuroblasts from the middle layer of the neural tube migrate out through the outer layer of the wall of the tube, where white matter will later develop, to take up a position on the outside of the tube. *Because of this phenomenon the cerebral and the cerebellar hemispheres come to possess a thin covering or cortex of gray matter (Fig. 17-9).* Hence in these two parts of the brain gray matter exists not only deep to the white matter but also superficial to it.

It should now be clear why the surface of the spinal cord is white and that of the cerebral and cerebellar hemispheres is gray. Furthermore, the reason for the tissue of the C.N.S. being so soft, delicate and easily injured should also be understood: unlike the other tissues of the body, which are supported by connective tissue possessing strong intercellular substances, the tissue of the C.N.S. is supported internally only by ectodermal-derived neuroglia cells. In other words, the absence of strong intercellular substances within the substance of the tissue of the C.N.S. accounts for its softness and fragility.

Having considered the formation of the nervous tissue of the C.N.S. and having learned something about the different parts of the brain and spinal cord, we shall now describe the cells and certain other features of the C.N.S. in more detail.

The Cells of the Nervous Tissue of the C.N.S. As Seen With the L.M. and the E.M.

Most neurons of the C.N.S. are multipolar; they have 2 or more dendrites (Fig. 17-2, *right*). However, the single axon may branch. The branches come off an axon more or less at right angles and are termed *collaterals*. The terminations of axons break up into treelike branches.

Cell Bodies. The cell body is sometimes designated by the longer term, the *perikaryon (peri,* around; *karyon,* nut or nucleus). The cell bodies of neurons vary from small to large. The larger ones are among the largest cells in the body. The cell bodies of different kinds of neurons vary in shape; they may be round, oval, flattened, ovoid or pyramidal, as is shown in Figure 17-2. As noted, the cell bodies of the neurons of the C.N.S. are all located in gray matter.

Nuclei. The nucleus commonly has a central position in the cell body, but in at least one type of neuron it is eccentrically disposed. Nuclei are generally large

and spherical (Figs. 17-14 and 17-15). In small neurons the nucleus, although actually smaller, is larger in relation to the size of the cell body than it is in larger neurons. The chromatin of the nuclei of many kinds of neurons is almost entirely of the extended type (Fig. 17-15); hence chromatin granules either are very fine or are not seen. As a result the nucleolus of a neuron is generally prominent, often appearing as an island in what appears as nuclear sap (Fig. 17-15). In electron micrographs a little peripheral chromatin can be seen on the inner aspect of the nuclear envelope (Fig. 17-14).

Polyploidy in Neurons. Microspectrophotometric technics have indicated that the DNA content of certain types of neurons with large cell bodies are characteristically tetraploid; that is, they have double the DNA content of diploid cells (Lapham and Herman and Lapham).

Neurofibrils. With the light microscope and certain technics it is possible to demonstrate what seem to be fibrils in the cytoplasm of nerve cell bodies and also in nerve fibers. With the EM what are termed *neurofilaments* are demonstrable in the cytoplasm (Fig. 17-14). The latter, of course, are much too fine to be seen with the LM, but they are often arranged in bundles, which are the fibrils seen with the LM. Microtubules are also present in neurons; they are similar to those seen in other kinds of cells. Neurofilaments can be seen in electron micrographs. In Figure 17-14 neurofilaments are labeled "F." Microtubules are labeled "MT."

Nissl Bodies (Clumps of Basophilic Material in the Cytoplasm). With the LM clumps of basophilic material are commonly seen in the cytoplasm of nerve cells (Fig. 17-15). These are often termed Nissl bodies in honor of Franz Nissl, who described them in the last century.

Seen with the EM a Nissl body consists of an aggregation of flattened membranous cisternae of rER with numerous ribosomes and polysomes scattered between the adjacent cisternae (Fig. 17-16). The rRNA is, of course, responsible for the basophilia seen with the LM. The arrangement of the flattened vesicles in Nissl bodies differs in different kinds of nerve cells. In large motor neurons the Nissl bodies are large, and the flattened cisternae in each are arranged more or less parallel with one another (Fig. 17-16). In other types of nerve cells the arrangement of the flattened vesicles is not so regular and, in some the rough-surfaced vesicles, are disposed in an irregular fashion in the cytoplasm.

As will be described when axons are considered in detail, the free ribosomes in the cell bodies of nerve cells are responsible for continuously synthesizing new

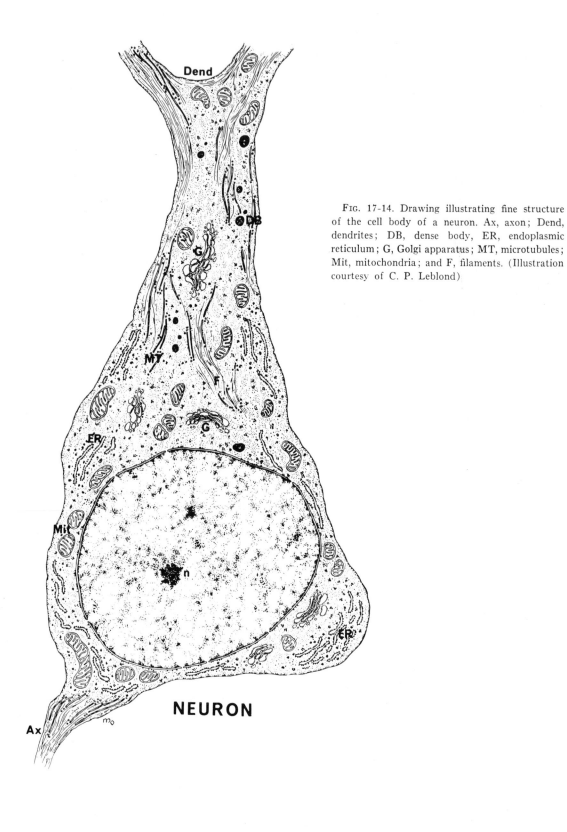

NEURON

Fig. 17-14. Drawing illustrating fine structure of the cell body of a neuron. Ax, axon; Dend, dendrites; DB, dense body, ER, endoplasmic reticulum; G, Golgi apparatus; MT, microtubules; Mit, mitochondria; and F, filaments. (Illustration courtesy of C. P. Leblond)

cytoplasmic substance which flows down the axon to replace that which is metabolized.

Axon Reaction. If the axon of a neuron is severed, what is known as an axon reaction occurs; the basophilic material of the cytoplasm tends to melt away temporarily (chromatolysis), and the nucleus moves to one side (Fig. 17-17).

Mitochondria. The mitochondria show no unusual features and are disposed haphazardly in the cytoplasm (Fig. 17-14).

Golgi Apparatus. It was in the cell bodies of neurons that Golgi first demonstrated the network that bears his name. Its location varies in different kinds of nerve cells; in some, elements of the apparatus are scattered so as to seem (with the LM) to surround the nucleus. The common distribution in a nerve cell is shown in Figure 17-14, G.

Pigments. Two kinds of pigments may appear in nerve cells. The first, *lipofuscin* (Fig. 5-64), appears during postnatal life, first in ganglion cells and later in cells of the C.N.S. Its amount increases with age. Its significance is not known. *Melanin* occurs in nerve cells in a few parts of the C.N.S., perhaps most notably in what is termed the *substantia nigra* (*niger,* black), a landmark in the midbrain that will be seen by the student when the brain is dissected. The significance of the presence of melanin in the bodies of some nerve cells of the C.N.S. is not known.

Dendrites extend from the various surfaces of multipolar neurons like branches from the trunk of a tree (Fig. 17-2). The dendrites themselves branch; hence, several different orders of branches that become smaller with branching are common. In their stouter parts, close to the cell body, the cytoplasm of dendrites contains both Nissl bodies and mitochondria (Fig. 17-2, *right*). Neurofibrils probably extend into their finest branches. Their surface provides a most extensive site on which synapses could be located and by which axons of many different neurons could terminate.

Axons. In contrast with dendrites, only one axon extends from the cell body of even a multipolar neuron. It arises from a special part of the periphery of the cell body termed the *axon hillock* (Fig. 17-14, lower left). Axons carry impulses away from the cell body. They vary from being part of a millimeter to several feet in length. The axons of different neurons vary in diameter from less than a micron to several microns. The larger ones conduct impulses more rapidly than the smaller ones. Axons may give off branches; these are termed *collaterals* because they come off the axon at right angles (laterally). They may then make a right-angle turn and proceed in the same direction as the axon from which they branch.

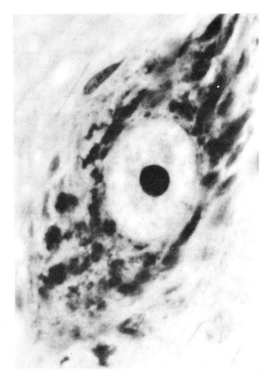

Fig. 17-15. Oil-immersion photomicrograph of anterior horn cell in section of the spinal cord of a male cat. Cresyl violet stain. Nissl bodies are seen to advantage. (Barr, M. L., Bertram, L. F., and Lindsay, H. A.: Anat. Rec., *107:283*)

The axons that pass up and down the white matter of the cord, in the different afferent and efferent pathways, and those that extend through the white matter of the brain are myelinated. However, outside of their myelin sheaths they have no covering except that provided by the processes of oligodendrocytes and astrocytes.

The Fine Structure of Axons. An axon, being a fiberlike extension of the cytoplasm of a nerve cell, must of course be covered with the cell membrane of the nerve cell to which it belongs. The cell membrane that surrounds an axon is called the *axolemma.* It is labeled in Figure 17-18 which is a cross section of an axon in which the following organelles can be seen: (1) Mitochondria; these are arranged generally with their long axes parallel with the axon; three can be seen in Figure 17-18. (2) Axoplasmic vesicles; these are the representatives in the nerve fibers of smooth-surfaced endoplasmic reticulum; several are labeled in Figure 17-18. (3) Neurofilaments; these appear as small dots in a cross section seen in the EM (Fig. 17-18). They are probably seen best in longitudinal sections at structures termed nodes of Ranvier which

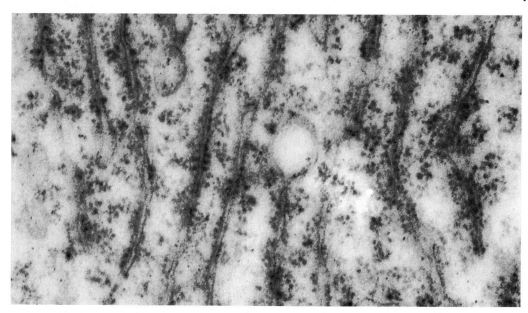

FIG. 17-16. Electron micrograph (× 85,000) of a section cut through the nucleus abducens of a rat. The field illustrated here is that of a Nissl body in a motor neuron. The illustration shows ribosomes to advantage; they are arranged along the flattened membranous vesicles (which appear in the illustration as double lines) and between adjacent flattened vesicles. The seemingly empty ovoid area in the center of the picture is the expanded end of a vesicle. (Palay, S., and Palade, G.: J. Biophys. Biochem. Cytol., *1*:69)

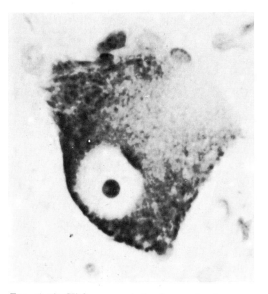

FIG. 17-17. High-power photomicrograph of a nerve cell, showing severe chromatolysis during axon reaction. The axon hillock of this cell is at the upper right, and the chromatolysis is typically most severe between the nucleus and the axon hillock. The nucleus has taken up an eccentric position, and a good "nuclear cap" is shown. (Barr, M. L., and Hamilton, J. D.: J. Comp. Neurol., *89*:93)

will be described when we describe the P.N.S. where they are more crowded together. (4) Neurotubules; the microtubules of nerve cells are very delicate, being only slightly larger than neurofilaments. Most of them seem to run longitudinally and so appear in cross section in Figure 17-18, but some run in other directions and hence are cut at various angles in this illustration. Unlike dendrites, few or no ribosomes or rough-surfaced vesicles of endoplasmic reticulum are to be seen in axons. Elements of the Golgi apparatus are likewise not seen. The absence of the cytoplasmic components that are concerned in protein synthesis and secretion in axons is perhaps to be expected because protein synthesis is active in the cell bodies of neurons, and the protein formed in the cell bodies travels down the axon at a fairly regular rate as will next be described.

Axonal Flow. Free ribosomes are even more abundant than membrane-attached ribosomes in Nissl bodies. Free ribosomes are involved in the synthesis of proteins which are used within the cell body and its dendrites and axon to replace those proteins used up in the course of metabolism. Although, in sections, axons appear rather small in comparison to cell bodies, they may be very long; hence their volume may be several hundred times that of the cell bodies from which they originate. Since little or no protein synthesis occurs within axons, most of their required protein must flow down the axon from the cell body. Decisive evidence for the existence of this axoplasmic flow was first provided by the radioautographic studies of Droz and Leblond. They gave animals labeled amino acids required for the synthesis of protein in the cell bodies of nerve cells and found that, within minutes, the label appeared in the cytoplasm. Shortly afterward, the label was seen to migrate into axon hillocks and later still into the axons. They found the labeled proteins to travel down the axon at a rate of about 1.5 mm. per day. The proteins migrating at this rate constitute

what is now known as the *slow flowing component,* and it may be that the whole axoplasm flows down the axon at this rate.

More recently it has been found that a *fast flowing component* also exists in axonal flow. In this the proteins migrate along the axon with a velocity ranging between 100 and 500 mm. per day. Different cell organelles appear to be carried in the different flows, i.e., neurofilaments and neurotubules in the slow flow and vesicles and mitochondria in the fast flow.

Using the dark field microscope, Dr. R. S. Smith, of the Department of Surgery at the University of Alberta, observed the motion of spherical organelles

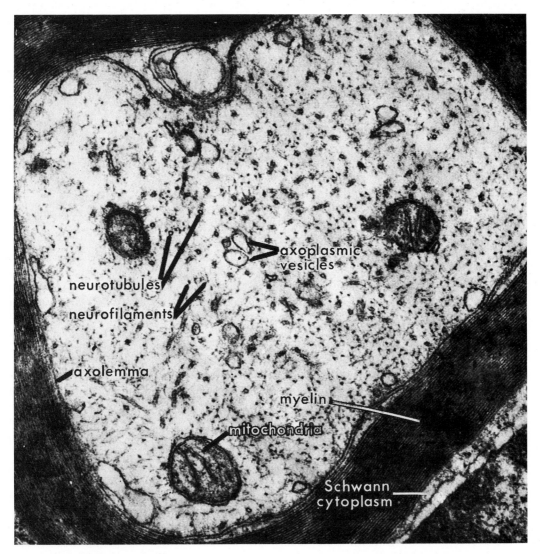

FIG. 17-18. Electron micrograph of a cross section of a single myelinated nerve fiber (an axon) showing mitochondria, axoplasmic vesicles, neurofilaments and neurotubules, all of which are labeled. (Preparation by B. Droz)

of the size of mitochondria in the axoplasm of isolated nerves. In the amphibian *Xenopus laevis,* this migration was very rapid (1 mm. in 16 minutes) in the sciatic nerve and ventral roots of the spinal cord whereas there was little motion in the portion of the dorsal roots central to the spinal ganglia. In the first case, he counted a mean of 18 microtubules per cross section of axon, whereas in the central portion of dorsal roots he counted only two. He concluded that microtubules were responsible for the fast flow of mitochondria.

Finally, substances other than simple proteins also appear to be axonally transported. Recent studies with labeled sugars have provided evidence that glycoproteins are also transported down the axon; these are almost completely carried in the fast flow, and may be involved in the renewal of components of synaptic vesicles (to be described shortly) and the cell surface coat (Bennett and Droz). Other substances for which axonal transport has been demonstrated in some axons include norepinephrine, dopamine glutamate, neurosecretory granules, and other substances (e.g., phospholipids).

The Nervous Impulse

Since this topic will be dealt with in detail in courses and textbooks that deal with neurophysiology, it will be given only introductory treatment here. In Chapter 5 it was pointed out that under ordinary conditions the cell membrane does not permit the ready diffusion of sodium ions through it. It was also mentioned that a mechanism termed the *sodium pump* has been postulated which, with an expenditure of energy, is able to transport sodium ions (which, of course, carry positive charges) from the inner surface of a cell membrane to its outer surface, and that the operation of the sodium pump accounts under normal conditions for there being an excess of sodium ions on the outer surface of a cell membrane, and that the positive charges on these ions is a very important factor in causing the outer surface of the cell membrane to be positively charged in relation to its inner surface. An axon is, of course, part of the cytoplasm of a cell. It is encased in a cell membrane (the axolemma), and under conditions of rest the outer surface of its membrane has an excess of sodium ions and is positively charged in relation to the inner (cytoplasmic) side of its covering membrane. The difference in electrical potential is around 85 millivolts and this is called its resting potential.

The stimulus that institutes a nervous impulse can be physical (as in some nerve endings), electrical

(as in a physiology laboratory) or chemical (as in synapse). If any site along an axon is effectively stimulated, the stimulus acts by making the cell membrane of the fiber at the site where the stimulus is applied, and for an infinitesimal fraction of a second, permeable to sodium ions, and at this site the excess of the latter on the outer surface of the membrane instantaneously diffuse through the membrane to its inner surface; as a result the outer surface of the membrane is no longer positively charged in relation to its inner surface—indeed, the inner surface of the membrane may even develop a positive charge. In any event, the membrane at this site is therefore said to have become *depolarized.* However, it just as quickly becomes polarized again. The rapid change in the electrical potential of the membrane that occurs when it becomes depolarized and repolarized is described as the *action potential.*

The almost instantaneous repolarization of the membrane at the site where it had become depolarized is also to be explained by a change in the permeability of the membrane to the diffusion of positively charged ions but in this instance those involved are potassium ions. Before the activation of the membrane by a stimulus there are far more potassium ions in the axon, on the inner aspect of the axolemma than on its outer aspect. So the diffusion of sodium ions from the outer to the inner side of the membrane that occurs when the membrane becomes permeable due to its activation by a stimulus is immediately followed by the diffusion of potassium ions outward through the membrane, and the positive charges in these are sufficient to cause the exterior of the membrane to become positively charged again in relation to its inner surface. Subsequently, the action of the sodium and potassium pumps move sodium ions back to the outside and potassium ions from the outside to the inside. For ions to be shifted by the two pumps, however, takes longer than it takes for them to diffuse through a membrane that has its permeability altered because of its activation by a stimulus; hence the almost instantaneous repolarization of a membrane is not to be accounted for by sodium ions being pumped out to the exterior of the membrane but by potassium ions diffusing through it from its inner to outer aspects.

Propagation of the Nervous Impulse Along Nerve Fibers. In order to make the following account as simple as possible we shall first describe what happens in connection with the propagation of a nervous impulse along a fiber that is not ensheathed with myelin.

If a stimulus is applied say, close to the end of an

unmyelinated nerve fiber, the axolemma at this site is activated and becomes depolarized, thus losing the positive charge on its outer surface. However, the axolemma just beyond the site where it becomes depolarized is still polarized, with its outer surface still being positively charged. So a current instantaneously flows from the positive charge on the outer side of the polarized membrane to the site where its outer surface has become depolarized. Similarly, a current flows along the inner surface of the membrane between the depolarized and the as yet polarized site in an opposite direction. These events somehow cause the membrane immediately adjacent to the site where it became depolarized by a suitable stimulus to become permeable to sodium and so it becomes depolarized in turn. This in turn causes the polarized membrane next to it to become depolarized and so on. The net result is that a wave of depolarization sweeps along the axolemma at incredible speed from the end of the axon that received the stimulus to its other end.

The wave of depolarization and repolarization (the nervous impulse) that sweeps along the fiber is referred to as the *action potential.*

Conduction Along Myelinated Fibers. The Role of Nodes of Ranvier. The myelin of myelinated fibers is not continuous; it is interrupted periodically by constrictions (also called nodes) of Ranvier (one is labeled n in Figure 17-13). Nodes of Ranvier are present along the myelinated fibers of both the C.N.S. and the P.N.S. At these nodes there is no myelin. In these sites, as has been shown by the EM studies of Robertson, the nerve fiber is therefore at least partially uncovered. In the P.N.S. there is one sheath of Schwann cell (these cells will be described later) between each two nodes, and in the C.N.S. there is one oligodendrocyte between two nodes (Fig. 17-13). The distance between adjacent nodes of Ranvier in the same fiber varies; it may be up to one millimeter.

Between nodes of Ranvier the outer surface of the cell membrane of the axon is closely invested with a relatively thick coat of myelin, which is an excellent insulator. There is, furthermore, neither tissue fluid on the outer aspect of the membrane in this region nor cytoplasm to serve as a means of keeping electrolytes in solution available. Indeed, the myelin sheath of the nerve fiber between nodes of Ranvier is in effect a great impervious thickening of cell membrane material. Accordingly, along myelinated fibers there is not the same electrolyte medium that is present on the outer surface of unmyelinated fibers for conducting a nervous impulse smoothly. However, at nodes of Ranvier, the membrane of the axon of a myelinated fiber is freely exposed to tissue fluid, and hence there

are electrolytes present at these sites that can be involved in depolarization of the membrane. Here sodium ions that have previously accumulated on the outer surface of a membrane can enter the axon through the membrane to cause it to become depolarized.

When a node of Ranvier becomes depolarized because of a nervous impulse reaching it, the inner surface of the membrane of the axon at that node of Ranvier has a greater positive charge than the inner surface of the axon at the next node of Ranvier, so a current flows in that direction. The current, on reaching the unpolarized node of Ranvier, causes a partial depolarization of the membrane of the axon at the node, and when this partial depolarization reaches the firing level, the membrane at this site becomes permeable to sodium ions and depolarized. This in turn sets up a current between it and the next node, which in turn becomes depolarized and so on.

So in myelinated fibers, the wave of depolarization jumps, as it were, along the nerve fibers from one node to the next; this is the reason that conduction is so fast in myelinated fibers. It seems that the potential differences that generate the current between adjacent nodes of Ranvier would not be great enough for one that becomes depolarized to cause the depolarization of the next if nodes were very far apart. Nodes of Ranvier are not more than a millimeter apart.

The speed of the nerve impulse along a fiber varies with the diameter of the fiber; the larger it is, the faster it conducts.

How Nerve Impulses Arriving at Nerve Endings on Cells Exert an Effect on the Cells That They Contact

The axons of efferent neurons end in four general sites. First, within the nervous system an axon can terminate on some part of another nerve cell in a synapse. Second, an efferent axon in the body can terminate on, or close to, secretory cells such as those of glands or close to cells which are not, strictly speaking, secretory cells but carry out metabolic functions such as fat cells. Third, they can terminate on muscle cells. Fourth, some terminate at perivascular spaces into which they discharge secretory granules as will be described in Chapter 25. The question arises as to how the arrival at a nervous impulse at any of these sites elicits a response in the cell at which the nerve fiber terminates.

Development of Knowledge. As nerves were studied in physiological laboratories it became evident that if a nerve that led to a muscle was stimulated

by an electric current, or even if it was pinched, it
would cause the muscle on which its fibers terminated
to contract. It was also found that if a muscle was
directly stimulated by an electric current it would
contract. So it is not surprising that with no other
explanation available it was more or less assumed that
a nervous impulse arriving at a nerve ending induced
a response in the cell that it innervated by giving them
something of the nature of a minute electric shock.

To describe the next development, we must explain
briefly here something that will be described in more
detail shortly in connection with the P.N.S. Among
the afferent neurons of the P.N.S. there is a division
of labor between those whose activities are under the
control of the conscious mind and those that function
automatically outside the control of the conscious
mind. The latter group of efferent neurons constitute
what is termed the *autonomic nervous system*. The
efferent neurons of the autonomic system control the
activities of the kind of muscle cells that are found,
for example, in the viscera (for example, the muscle
cells in the wall of the intestine) and the walls of
blood vessels and they also affect the secretory functions of many glands and the metabolic activities
of certain other cells. There are two parts to the
autonomic system (glance at Fig. 17-48) which will
be described in detail later, one is called its *sympathetic* division and the other its *parasympathetic*
division. In general, efferent nerve fibers from both
reach each type of cell that is innervated by the
system and in general the impulses from one system
arriving at any given target cell have opposite effects—
for example, the fibers from one system may stimulate
a muscle cell to contract while the impulses from the
other system will cause it to relax.

The next development depended on the discovery
that the inner part of the adrenal gland produced the
hormone called epinephrine which was described in
Chapter 6. Giving an animal epinephrine was found
to produce most of the effects that were produced by
stimulating the sympathetic division of the autonomic
nervous system. It was only natural that at first it
was assumed that epinephrine must act by stimulating
the nerves or nerve endings of the sympathetic division
of the autonomic nervous system. But then in 1904
Elliott performed a most interesting experiment in
which he found that administration of epinephrine to
an animal would produce the effects attributed to
stimulation of the sympathetic nerves in some part
of the body even though the sympathetic nerves to
that part of the body were severed. This finding raised
problems and in due course it came to be realized that
epinephrine (actually it turned out to be a companion

chemical norepinephrine) brought about a response
in the cells innervated by efferent fibers of the sympathetic system not by stimulating the nerve endings
but by actually itself causing the response by its effect
on the membrane of the cell that responded. In
the meantime another substance—acetylcholine—was
found to act this way in connection with the other
(parasympathetic) division of the autonomic nervous
system. The net result of all this work led to the
concept that the arrival of a nervous impulse at a
nerve ending causes the nerve ending to liberate a
chemical substance such as norepinephrine or acetylcholine that is actually the agent that incites the
response in the cell on which the nerve ending ends;
it does this by affecting the cell membrane of the cell
that is capable of responding. This phenomenon is
termed the *chemical mediation of the nervous impulse.*

Establishing that there were two chemical mediators
of the nervous impulses in connection with the nerve
endings in the autonomic nervous system raised the
question as to whether this was the way that nerve
impulses brought about responses in the muscles that
are under the control of the conscious mind, and also
whether or not the same sort of mechanism was
involved in the transmission of nervous impulses from
one neuron to another at synapses. It is now considered
that this is the universal way nerve impulses cause
effects at their terminations, including those at
synapses. However, as research has continued it has
been found that there are several kinds of chemical
substances that act as chemical mediators in various
synapses, as will be learned about in courses and
books that specialize in this area. We shall now
describe the fine structure of synapses and discuss how
the chemical mediators are formed and liberated.

Synapses and Their Fine Structure

Long before it was known that chemical mediation
was involved in nervous impulses being conducted over
synapses, it had been shown that the propagation of
an impulse over a synapse was always a one-way
phenomenon. Knowledge of chemical mediation explained why synapse can transmit impulses in only
one direction, as will become apparent in the following.

Types of Synapses and Terminology. The neuron
that delivers nervous impulses to a given synapse is
termed the presynaptic neuron. At its termination it
is usually expanded into a bulblike structure; this is
called an end bulb or end foot (shown but not labeled
in Figure 17-19). The end bulb, being the termination
of an axon, is of course, surrounded by the axolemma
(cell membrane) of the axon. The part of the axolemma

that closely approaches the cell membrane of some part of the postsynaptic neuron is called the *presynaptic membrane,* and that part of the cell membrane of the postsynaptic neuron that is slightly separated from the presynaptic membrane is called the postsynaptic membrane. Between the pre- and post-synaptic membranes there is a space of around 200-Å wide; this is termed the *synaptic cleft* which is shown but not labeled in Figure 17-19. It is labeled in Figure 17-20.

One way synapses are classified is with regard to where they are located on the postsynaptic neuron. The terminations of axons on dendrites are termed *axondendritic synapses* (Fig. 17-19). In some of these the dendrite involved possesses little protrusions called dendritic spines on and around which the terminal end bulbs of the axon fits (Fig. 17-19). Axon endings that terminate on the cell bodies of neurons are termed *axosomatic synapses.* Those that terminate on other axons are termed *axoaxonic synapses.* An axon can end on another axon to form a synapse only on a part of that axon that is not myelinated, and this situation is encountered only on the very first part of an axon, close to its origin at the axon hillock, for at this point an axon remains naked because myelination does not begin immediately at the hillock but a short distance away from it.

Physiologically, synapses are classed as being either excitatory or inhibitory. The arrival of a nervous impulse at the end of the presynaptic neuron has the effect of slightly lowering the electrical potential between the inner and the outer surfaces of that part of the axolemma of the postsynaptic neuron that participates in the synapse. The arrival of an impulse at the end of a presynaptic neuron in an inhibitory type of synapse tends to raise the potential between the inner and the outer surfaces of the axolemma of the postsynaptic neuron at the site of the synapse. Thus the arrival of impulses at excitory synapses act to make the postsynaptic neuron more excitable and the arrival of impulses at the inhibitory synapses tend to make the postsynaptic neuron less excitable. If there are considerably more impulses arriving at excitatory synapses than at inhibitory synapses, the potential between the inner and the outer surfaces of the axolemma of the postsynaptic neuron at the synapse can be reduced sufficiently to trigger the initiation of a nervous impulse in the postsynaptic neuron. Data on just how much the potential between the outer and the inner layers of the axolemma of a postsynaptic neuron must be reduced in terms of millivolts before it is triggered are to be found in texts that deal with neurophysiology, as will information of how excitatory impulses that

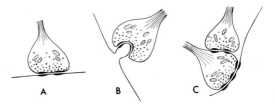

Fig. 17-19. Ultrastructure of synapses. A. Axodendritic or axosomatic synapse. B. Axodendritic synapse, in which an end-bulb is in synaptic relation with a dendritic spine. C. Axoaxonic synapse of the end-bulb to end-bulb type. See text for details. (From Barr, M. L.: The Human Nervous System. New York, Harper and Row, 1972)

come quickly enough in succession can become more or less cumulative.

The Fine Structure of Synapses. The end bulb (end foot) is of course covered with the axolemma of the presynaptic neuron and is filled with cytoplasm. The latter generally contains some mitochondria which indicates that metabolic activity occurs in the end foot. Another and distinctive component of the cytoplasm of an end foot is that it contains very numerous membranous vesicles that range in diameter from around 200 to 650 Å (20 to 65 nm.) but are probably mostly around 500 Å (50 nm.) in diameter. These are believed to contain the chemical mediator (also called the neurotransmitter substance). The vesicles tend to accumulate close to the surface of the axolemma at the site where it participates directly in the synapse (the presynaptic membrane). At this site the axolemma appears to be somewhat irregularly thickened. It is separated from the axolemma of the postsynaptic neuron by a space of around 200 Å (20 nm.), which as noted, is termed the *synaptic cleft.* On the postsynaptic side of the cleft the axolemma of the postsynaptic neuron (the postsynaptic membrane) also shows the irregular thickenings that are observed in association with the axolemma of the presynaptic axon.

It is believed that the arrival of a nervous impulse at a synapse somehow causes the membranous walls of the vesicles containing the chemical mediator to fuse with the presynaptic membrane of the synapse, layer by layer, as they break open so that their contents are discharged into the synaptic cleft. The mechanism of fusion of the membrane of the vesicle with that of the presynaptic membrane appears to be the same as that which occurs when a Golgi-derived vesicle fuses with the cell membrane of a cell and empties its contents of cell coat material on the surface. This was illustrated in Figure 5-37 which figure should

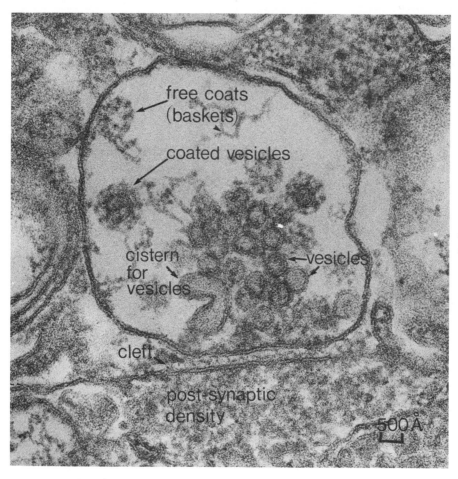

FIG. 17-20. Electron micrograph of a synapse in the cerebral cortex of the rat. The 500-Å wide vesicles fuse with the presynaptic membrane and release their contents of neurotransmitter. Coated vesicles subsequently arise from the presynaptic membrane by endocytosis (the free coats may be contractile, initiating the endocytosis). The free coats or baskets fall off, leaving the smooth vesicle which fuses with the collecting cistern. The vesicles later bud off from the cistern, becoming reloaded with neurotransmitter. The postsynaptic region is a dendrite. (Courtesy of P. Seeman)

be consulted at this time. It will be recalled that the fusion of Golgi-derived membranous vesicles with the cell membrane of a cell not only provides for more cell coat material; it also, because its membranous wall fuses with that of the cell membrane, with the membrane being "right-side-up" as it were, provides new and extra membrane for the cell itself, as is shown in Figure 5-37. Likewise, the fusion of membranous synaptic vesicles with the presynaptic membrane adds more membrane to it, which, of course, would expand it if the process continued. However, the studies of Heuser and Reese indicates that this extra membrane is recycled, because it is used for the formation of new vesicles, as will now be described.

These investigators have shown that new vesicles form from the axolemma covering the parts of the end bulbs (other than the presynaptic membrane) by the same sort of mechanism as occurs in phagocytosis or pinocytosis shown in Figure 5-7, or in endocytosis shown in Figure 5-39. Actually, the vesicles that form from the axolemma were shown to be of the coated variety, the formation of which, in another site, is illustrated in Figure 5-43. The coats of the vesicles that form from the axolemma are termed baskets (Fig. 17-20). As the coated vesicles move inward they lose their baskets, so their membranous walls are naked. In this state they fuse with a membranous cistern (Fig. 17-20) into which they presumably empty their contents. However, new vesicles bud off from the cistern, just as vesicles bud off from the Golgi in Figure 5-37; these then accumulate and hence are ready to fuse with the presynaptic membrane and empty their contents into the synaptic cleft when enough nervous impulses arrive at the end bulb.

Thus, according to Heuser and Reese, the axolemma membrane of the end foot is constantly recycled. That which is "used up" in forming coated vesicles is added back to the axolemma when the vesicles fuse with the presynaptic membrane.

Exactly where the neurotransmitter substance (chemical mediator) is synthesized and how it comes to be contained in the cisternae from which synaptic vesicles bud off, does not seem as yet to have been clearly established.

Having now considered neurons in some detail we can describe the other cellular components of the C.N.S., including their fine structure. But first we shall comment briefly on the general microscopic structure of gray matter and how it was determined.

How the Microscopic Structure of Gray Matter Was Elucidated

Before describing some of what has been learned about the microscopic structure of gray matter from the use of metallic impregnation methods we should first comment on how relatively little could have been learned about its complex structure from the study of paraffin sections and ordinary stains alone.

The left side of Figure 17-21 illustrates a low-power view of a paraffin section of human cerebral cortex stained with H and E. Four components can be identified in it.

(1) The cell bodies of neurons. These are shown to better advantage on the right side of the figure which was taken at higher magnification.

(2) Nuclei, which are scattered about and do not reveal enough cytoplasm for the identification of the cells in which they reside. Some of these are the nuclei of small neurons but most are the nuclei of the supporting cells of the central nervous system which are called neuroglia, to be described shortly.

(3) Capillaries. These can be seen winding through the substance of the gray matter; one can be identified in each of the two pictures.

(4) The *neuropil* (*neuro*, nerve; *pilus*, felt). The neuropil is a pale blue-gray seemingly structureless background seen in an H and E section in which the first three components mentioned above are contained. About all that can be seen in an H and E section is that it seems to have a feltlike texture. It constitutes the bulk of gray matter. What it consists of has been shown as a result of the development, first of metallic impregnation methods and secondly, and more recently, by electron microscopy as will be described in the following pages.

Evolution of Silver-Impregnation Methods. In 1872 a discovery was made which was a great advance toward elucidating the microscopic structure of the C.N.S. At this time an Italian anatomist, Camillo Golgi, was forced by economic circumstances to terminate temporarily his association with a proper

laboratory and take a position as chief resident physician and surgeon in a hospital for incurable patients. Such was his zeal for anatomic research that he attempted to set up a histologic laboratory in the kitchen of his house, where he could work at night. He had little more than a microscope and a few simple instruments, and with these he made the discovery that revolutionized the study of nervous tissue.

Golgi had fixed some tissue of the C.N.S. in a solution of potassium bichromate and had left the tissue in this solution for a long time. He then soaked the tissue in silver nitrate and, probably to his surprise, silver was deposited as a dark precipitate on *only some* of the cells in the tissue but not on most of them. Furthermore, the ones that were impregnated stood out against a clear background as if they had been mounted in a relatively clear plastic. By this means it is possible to demonstrate whole neurons (both their cell bodies and their processes) in thick sections (for example, as shown in Fig. 17-22) and it also shows that supporting cells of the C.N.S. have innumerable processes (Fig. 17-23).

Subsequently, a young man in Spain who was destined to become the greatest neurohistologist of the time, Santiago Ramon y Cajal, saw the possibilities of Golgi's method, made improvements in it and, with his pupils, devised still further metallic impregnation methods with which he systematically investigated the histology of nervous tissue. Among other things he provided evidence for the individuality of neurons. Cajal published nearly 300 papers and many books on neurohistology, and much of what is known today about neurohistology can be traced to him. In 1906 he was awarded, jointly with Golgi, the Nobel prize in Physiology and Medicine. Students will find inspiration and enjoyment in reading his *Recollections of My Life* (this has been translated into English by E. Horne Craigie).

With the development of metallic impregnation methods and the use of relatively thick sections it became possible to demonstrate the processes of neurons over considerable distances as well as to show the different sizes and shapes of the nerve cell bodies from which they arise. It therefore is possible to portray the arrangement in which they exist in, for example, the cerebral cortex as is shown in Figure 17-22.

Microscopic Structure of Cerebral Cortex

The gray matter that constitutes the cerebral cortex varies from about 1.5 to 4 mm. in thickness and covers the white matter of the cerebral hemispheres (Fig.

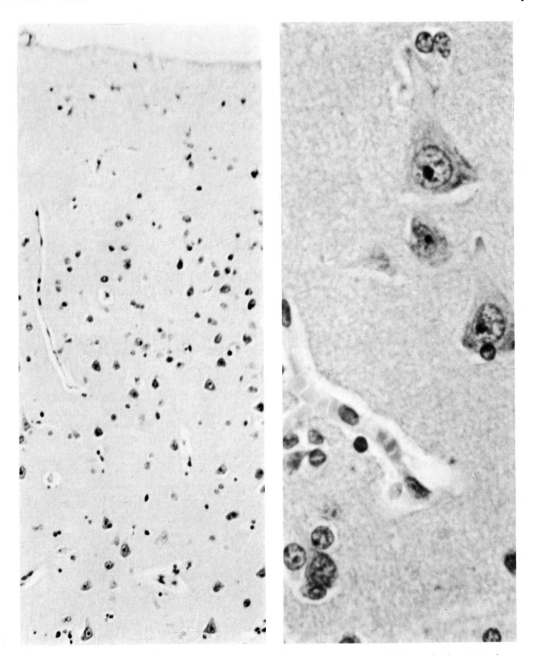

FIG. 17-21. Low- and high-power views of H and E section of parts of the cerebral cortex of man. Note the capillaries separated from the neuropil (the gray background) by a shrinkage space. The bodies of nerve cells and the nuclei of neuroglia cells can be seen on the left. One nerve cell body in the right picture has an oligodendrocyte as a satellite. (Photomicrograph by H. Whittaker)

17-9). The extensively convoluted surface of the hemispheres of man (Fig. 17-9) permits the gray matter to be much more extensive than it would be if the surfaces of the hemispheres were smooth, as they are in some animals. Preparations made from different parts of the hemisphere show the same general plan of microscopic structure, but also that the general plan is sufficiently modified in different cortical areas to imply that different areas of the cortex perform somewhat different functions. The cortex, speaking generally, exhibits 6 layers (Fig. 17-22). The extent to which each of these 6 layers is developed differs in

LAYERS OF CEREBRAL CORTEX

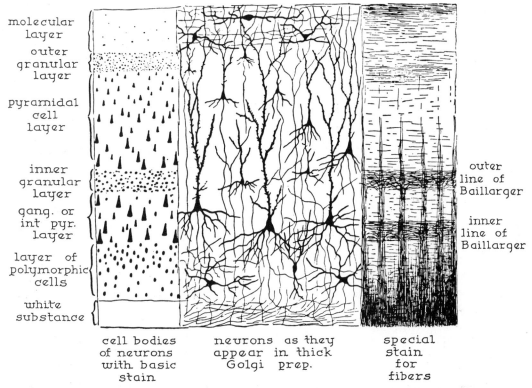

molecular layer

outer granular layer

pyramidal cell layer

inner granular layer

gang. or int. pyr. layer

layer of polymorphic cells

white substance

outer line of Baillarger

inner line of Baillarger

cell bodies of neurons with basic stain

neurons as they appear in thick Golgi prep.

special stain for fibers

FIG. 17-22. Schematic representation of the structure of the cerebral cortex. (Modified from Villiger, E.: Brain and Spinal Cord. Philadelphia, J. B. Lippincott)

various areas; the significance of this is a matter for consideration in neuroanatomy textbooks. Here we shall describe only some of the characteristics of the 6 layers.

The most superficial is called the *molecular layer* (Fig. 17-22). It contains relatively few cells and consists chiefly of fibers of underlying cells which run in many directions but generally parallel with the surface (Fig. 17-22). The 2nd layer is called the *outer granular layer* because it contains many small nerve cells which give it a granular appearance when it is examined under low power (Fig. 17-22). The 3rd layer is called the *pyramidal cell layer* because of its content of pyramid-shaped cell bodies of neurons (Fig. 17-22). The 4th layer is termed the *inner granular layer* because it is "granulated" with small nerve cells (Fig. 17-22). The 5th layer is termed the *internal pyramidal layer* because its most prominent feature is its content of pyramidal cell bodies. In one part of the cortex, called the *motor area,* the pyramidal cells of this layer are huge; they are called *Betz cells.* The 6th and final layer is named the layer of *polymorphous cells* because the cells of this layer have

many shapes. It will be noticed in Figure 17-21, *left,* that the size of the cell bodies of the neurons in the deeper parts of the cortex are larger than those in the more superficial parts, hence the existence of the layers

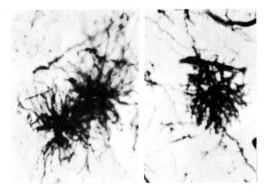

FIG. 17-23. Medium-power photomicrographs of two protoplasmic astrocytes in a Golgi preparation of the cerebral cortex of a dog. The heavy black line obliquely crossing the top of the picture on the right is a blood vessel, and the feet of the processes of the astrocyte are attached to it.

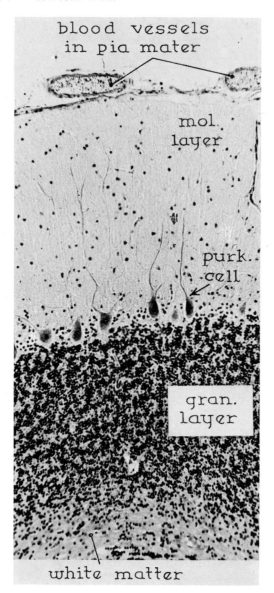

FIG. 17-24. Low-power photomicrograph of an H and E section of the cerebellum.

fibers), a layer of huge flask-shaped (Purkinje) nerve cells and an inner granular (small nerve cell) layer.

The Supporting Cells of the Nervous Tissue of the C.N.S. (Neuroglia)

Since living cells are jellylike, they must be supported both individually and collectively in the body. In most body parts support is provided by various kinds of intercellular substance (reticular, collagenic and elastic fibers and mucopolysaccharide jellies) that are produced by connective tissue cells all of which develop from the mesoderm. But the substance of gray and white matter of the brain and spinal cord develops from ectoderm and hence it does not contain connective tissue cells throughout its substance that produce intercellular substance. Accordingly, the substance of the brain and cord is soft and delicate; indeed, a brain removed at autopsy is so soft it cannot be cut into slices to investigate sites of internal disease until it has been hardened by placing it whole in a solution of fixative for an appropriate period of time. An important reason for the soft brain and cord not being injured more commonly is that in life they are more or less suspended in a bath of fluid (the cerebrospinal fluid), as will be described shortly. Nevertheless, the neurons of the C.N.S. are provided with an intimate type of support by cells of a type termed *neuroglia* (*neuron*, nerve; *glia*, glue); these cells are essential for permitting the cell bodies and processes of neurons to be arranged and maintained in a proper spacial arrangement with one another and they serve other purposes as well.

An understanding of the form and supporting function of neuroglia cells in the C.N.S. awaited the development of metallic impregnation methods. *Ordinary stains such as H and E give no intimation that these cells possess innumerable processes that permeate the substance of the nervous tissue of the C.N.S. and so bind it together and to the blood vessels that course through it.* Even an ordinary Golgi preparation shows that a cell of which only the nucleus could be seen in an H and E section possesses innumerable processes which connect various parts of neurons to capillaries as is shown in Figure 17-23. Furthermore, the use of more refined impregnation methods and more particularly modern studies with the EM has shown that the neuropil—the pale gray background of gray matter —is a vast conglomerate of the cell bodies and processes of neuroglia and the processes of neurons which in the neuropil are mostly unmyelinated. But before

described from impregnation methods can be correlated roughly with what is seen in an H and E section.

It has been estimated that there are close to 10,000 million neurons in the cerebral cortex, and since one neuron may effect synaptic connection with a great many others, the possibilities with regard to the number of pathways that are available here are indeed overwhelming.

The gray cerebellar cortex (Fig. 17-24) has an outer molecular layer (a few cells and many unmyelinated

considering the neuropil further, we shall describe the 3 types of neuroglial cells.

The use of silver and gold impregnation methods by Cajal and del Rio-Hortega (one of his pupils) permitted neuroglia cells to be classified into three groups: (1) oligodendrocytes (Fig. 17-10, *bottom*), so-named because they were small and had treelike processes (*oligo*, little; *dendron*, tree); (2) astrocytes (Figure 17-10, *bottom*), so-named because they were cells with starlike cytoplasmic processes (*astron*, star), and (3) microglia (Fig. 17-28).

We shall now consider their fine structure.

OLIGODENDROCYTES

There are metallic impregnation methods which are fairly reliable for identifying astrocytes and microglia but oligodendrocytes cannot be identified with any assurance by any of these methods. Hence Mori and Leblond, in order to study oligodendrocytes with the EM in the large bundle of axons that join the two cerebral hemispheres (the corpus callosum), used the reasonably specific metallic stains to mark the astrocytes and the microglia and assumed that the cells that did not stain by these methods were oligodendrocytes. These were studied with the EM and also in semithin sections with the LM.

Three classes of oligodendrocytes were identified—light, medium and dark; all three classes revealed certain features in common—for example, their cytoplasm possessed a considerable content of free ribosomes and contained a substantial content of microtubules. They all revealed fine nonbranching processes extending from their cell bodies but the number of processes varied from cell to cell.

1. The light oligodendrocyte (Fig. 17-25) has a relatively large pale nucleus with a large nucleolus. The cytoplasm is abundant and its most striking characteristic is a large content of evenly spread free ribosomes. The large oligodendrocytes were found to constitute about 6 percent of all the neuroglial cells in the corpus callosum. Radioautographic studies showed that the large oligodendrocytes were the ones that underwent mitosis.

2. The medium-shade types of oligodendrocytes were found to make up about 25 percent of the neuroglia of the tissue studied. They too were found to undergo mitosis but not as extensively as the light ones. They are in general smaller and denser than the light cells.

3. The dark oligodendrocytes (Fig. 17-25) constitute about 40 percent of the neuroglia of the tissue

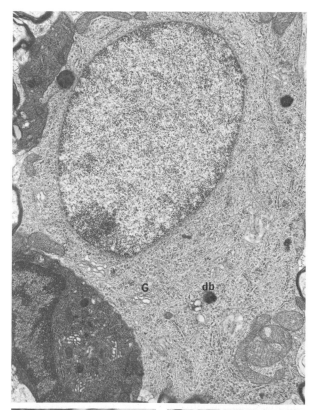

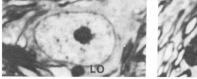 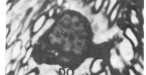

FIG. 17-25. (*Top*) Electron micrograph ($\times$ 15,000) of a *light oligodendrocyte* occupying most of the picture and a *dark oligodendrocyte* (at lower left), from adult rat brain. The light oligodendrocyte has a large nucleus and cytoplasm, the latter rich in ribosomes and microtubules. A Golgi (G) and a dense body (db) are indicated. The dark oligodendrocyte is small, shows densely staining cytoplasm and nucleoplasm, and has coarse chromatin in the nucleus. The Golgi saccules stand out in the cytoplasm. (At upper left, part of another dark oligodendrocyte is seen as well as parts of axons in cross section.) (*Bottom*) These are photomicrographs, not electron micrographs. At left is a light oligodendrocyte ($\times$ 3,000) and at right a dark oligodendrocyte ($\times$ 3,000) as seen in a 0.5-μ Epon section stained with toluidine blue. The light oligodendrocyte (LO) has a light nucleus with grainy chromatin and prominent nucleolus; its ample cytoplasm is less pale. The dark oligodendrocyte (DO) shows large dense chromatin patches in the nucleus, and the cytoplasm stains very deeply. (From E. A. Ling, J. Paterson and C. P. Leblond)

investigated. They were found to be smaller and denser than the medium-shade cells. No evidence was found that they undergo mitosis. They apparently develop from medium-shade types of cells.

It seems that the light cell is the progenitor cell of the series and that the dark cell is the most highly differentiated. It seems logical, therefore, that free ribosomes would characterize the cytoplasm of the progenitor cell and that as the cells become smaller and darker, the rER and the Golgi become more prominent in their cytoplasm.

It has been noticed for decades that neuroglia cells with small dark nuclei are commonly seen in gray matter in close association with the bodies of nerve cells where they are often referred to as satellites. One can be seen at the middle of the right side of Figure 17-21.

Myelin-Forming Function. The metallic staining methods had suggested that oligodendrocytes were commonly disposed in rows between myelinated fibers in white matter (Fig. 17-27). As has already been mentioned it is believed that in this position they are able to wrap nerve fibers with extensions of their cell membrane from which the cytoplasm is mostly squeezed out (Fig. 17-13). By this means they can cover the nerve fibers with layer after layer of double cell membrane which becomes the myelin coat of the nerve fiber. Thus it is believed that oligodendrocytes, as well as providing support, serve the same myelin-forming function attributed to the sheath of Schwann cells that we shall describe shortly in connection with myelinated nerve fibers of the P.N.S.

Turnover. Radioautography after thymidine labeling reveals that after growth is over there is a low degree of proliferation of oligodendrocytes in the adult. As noted, the larger oligodendrocytes are those which have the most ability to divide. Division, therefore, seems to continue beyond the age when a myelin sheath has been provided for all myelinated axons. Whether it is for the purpose of increasing the degree of myelination or for the replacement of oligodendrocytes is not known.

ASTROCYTES

Astrocytes are stained in a reasonably specific manner by Cajal's gold chloride-sublimate method. On a yellow background the astrocytes appear as dark stars, due to the staining of processes that extend in various directions. Some are also stained in Golgi preparations (Fig. 17-23). Some of the processes go to blood vessels (Fig. 17-23); others go to the surface of neurons. In either case, as will be described in detail later, they

widen at the end and spread out over the surface with which they are in contact—capillary or neuron—to cover as much as they can, thus making up a sheath of astrocyte feet. An astrocyte foot spreads until it comes close to and partly in contact with another astrocyte foot. Hence, astrocytic feet make up a complete sheath around capillaries, with only the odd microglia interrupting it. They do the same around many neurons. Astrocyte feet also end on the basement membrane that underlies the pia mater (to be described shortly).

Examination of gold-stained astrocytes in the light and electron microscopes reveal that only two structures are stained in their cytoplasm: dense bodies (referred to by Cajal as gliosomes and now presumed to be lysosomes), and bundles of fine filaments (Fig. 17-26); these are the structures responsible for the dark staining of astrocytic processes shown in Figure 17-27. In fact, a filament bundle arising in an astrocytic foot runs along in a process and reaches the perinuclear region of the cell but does not stop there and instead continues into another process up to its end. The cytoplasm is disposed irregularly around the bundles of filaments as these follow a straight or gently curving path. These bundles are responsible for the rigidity of astrocytic processes; thus the bundles in astrocytic processes extending from one capillary to the next provide a fairly rigid link between them.

Gold-stained astrocytes may be divided into two categories. *Fibrous astrocytes* are characterized by particularly long and straight processes which branch little or not at all (Fig. 17-27, *right*). These astrocytes are observed in the white matter. Gliosomes are found in the cytoplasm that surrounds the bundles of filaments present in the processes and even in the end-feet. It was long held that fibrous astrocytes were the only ones to contain fibers, that is, bundles of filaments, but the EM showed that the protoplasmic type, next to be described, also contain such bundles.

Protoplasmic astrocytes have branching cytoplasmic processes extending from all aspects of their cell bodies so that they resemble bushy shrubs after metallic staining (Figs. 17-10 and 17-23). Their processes are shorter and branch more extensively than in fibrous astrocytes, but, as noted, the EM shows that they are also made rigid by the presence of short bundles of filaments.

Examination of astrocytes of either type in the EM shows a light, rather large nucleus (Fig. 17-26). Often the nucleus is somewhat indented, a fact that may be noted even in the LM. These indentations are presumed to be caused by pressure from the adjacent

Fɪɢ. 17-26. (*Top*) Electron micrograph (× 13,800) of the nucleus and cytoplasm of an astrocyte from the corpus callosum of an adult rat. Note the homogeneous paleness of nucleoplasm and cytoplasm. Bundles of filaments (f) may be seen in the cytoplasm. Two of the sectioned neighboring axons are indicated (ax). (*Bottom*) Photomicrograph (× 3,000) of two astrocytes (A) near a capillary lumen (L) bounded by an endothelial cell whose nucleus is evident. This is an Epon section, cut 0.5 μ thick, and stained with toluidine blue. The ovoid astrocytic nucleus is homogeneously pale and a continuous fine rim of chromatin lies along the nuclear envelope. A pale cytoplasmic process extends at left, between the dark myelinated axons. (From E. A. Ling, J. Paterson and C. P. Leblond)

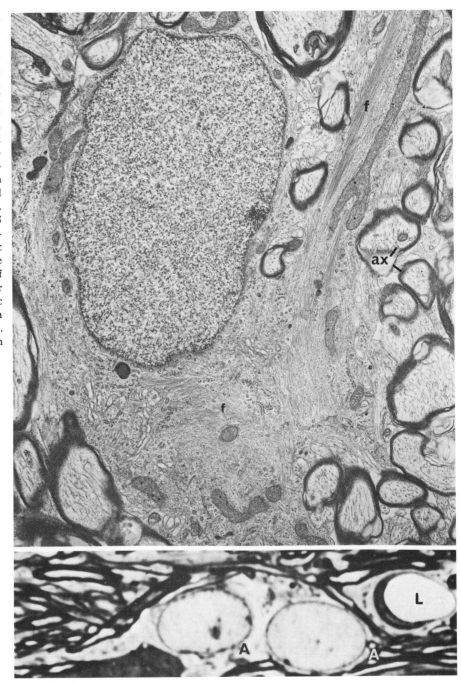

bundles of filaments. The cytoplasm is rather light because of its low content of ribosomes and rER. As shown in Figure 17-26, axons (dark rims) are commonly enveloped by astrocyte cytoplasm. Astrocytes are fairly numerous; in the corpus callosum they make up one quarter of the glial population. A few astrocytes, which contain sparse filaments, are able to divide, as shown by radioautography after ^{3}H-thymidine. These cells, which might be considered as "spongioblasts" (Fig. 17-10) would slowly produce astrocytes. An occasional degenerating astrocyte may be encountered. Some degeneration would balance the production of new astrocytes, thus ensuring turnover of the astrocyte population.

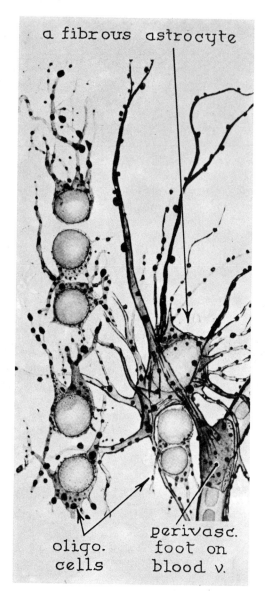

FIG. 17-27. White matter of the brain of a rabbit stained by del Rio-Hortega's method for gliosomes. It shows a row of oligodendroglia cells on the left and a fibrous astrocyte on the right. (Modified from Penfield, W.: Brain, *47*:430)

The Association Between Astrocytes and Capillaries: How Nutrients Reach the Cell Bodies of Neurons in Gray Matter

The capillaries that supply nutrients to the cells within the substance of the gray matter that covers the surface of the cerebral and cerebellar hemispheres, and the capillaries that supply the gray matter of the

cord, are derived from arterial vessels that are close to the surface of the brain and cord and carried in the deeper layers of a connective tissue wrapping that surrounds the brain and cord, collectively called the *meninges* which will be described shortly. What concerns us here, however, is the fact that small vessels, derived from the deepest layer of the meninges which is called the *pia mater,* penetrate brain substance and terminate in capillaries that supply nutrients to neurons and neuroglia as follows.

The Blood Vessels of Pia and Perivascular Spaces. The blood vessels that penetrate the substance of the brain are at their beginnings covered with a thin layer of pia mater. Furthermore, the pia mater dips into the little tunnels which contain the vessels so as to line the tunnels with pia mater. Between this and the pia that covers the vessels there is a true *perivascular space* (Fig. 17-28, perivascular space). This is found only in connection with the larger vessels; it does not extend as far as the capillaries, as was believed formerly. This true perivascular space com-

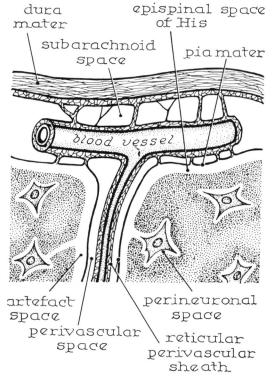

FIG. 17-28. Diagram to illustrate the relations of the perivascular space. Note that the epispinal and perineural spaces seen in ordinary paraffin sections are not true spaces but artifacts. (Redrawn from Woollam, D. H. M., and Millen, J. W.: J. Anat., *89*:193)

municates with the subarachnoid space (to be described presently) and contains cerebrospinal fluid.

From the study of ordinary H and E sections of brain, two false impressions were given by artefacts over the years. First, as a result of shrinkage a space could be seen between the pia that lines the tunnels and brain substance; this is labeled "artefact space" at the left of Figure 17-28. Second, a space was also seen between the cell bodies of neurons and brain substance; this was termed the perineural space (Fig. 17-28, *right*). This so-called perineural space was believed to communicate with the space that was supposed to exist between the pia and brain substance but all these spaces, with the exception of the perivascular space found around the larger vessels have been proven, particularly by the EM and excellent fixation, to be artefacts.

As noted above, the true perivascular space, recognizable with the LM and seen around larger vessels, disappears by the time capillaries are reached, so there are no continuous spaces around capillaries as there may appear to be in H and E sections—for example, in Figure 17-21, *right*, below the middle of the figure; as noted, this space is an artefact.

The Formation and Absorption of Tissue Fluid and the Diffusion of Nutrients in Gray Matter and the Blood-Brain Barrier. As was described in connection with loose connective tissue in most body sites, tissue fluid is found at the arterial ends of capillaries and reabsorbed from their venous ends (Fig. 8-6). Any excess that is formed is drained away by lymphatic capillaries (Fig. 8-6). Furthermore, in sites where the production of tissue fluid is substantial, the capillaries may be of the fenestrated type (Fig. 8-7, *right*). Furthermore, the barrier between blood and tissue fluid normally permits the escape of some of the macromolecules of blood protein; these do not accumulate because they are drained away by the more porous lymphatic capillaries.

The situation in gray matter is very different from that in loose connective tissue. First, there are no lymphatic capillaries to drain away tissue fluid, a situation that in other parts of the body would result in edema (Fig. 8-8, *top right*). Next, the capillaries are of the continuous type—they have no fenestration and furthermore the endothelial cells are joined together by what appear to be almost continuous tight (occludens type) junctions (described in Chapter 5). It is, therefore, apparent that little tissue fluid would be produced by these capillaries. Next, the capillaries of gray matter are all surrounded by a substantial basement membrane (Fig. 17-29, BM); this is often split to house a pericyte.

There has been a difference of opinion as to whether or not the basement membrane of a capillary is completely surrounded by astrocyte feet or whether this covering is discontinuous. In a recent study, Robertson (personal communication) has shown that at least 88 percent of the basement membrane is covered with astrocytic processes (Fig. 17-29). The cytoplasm of oligodendrocytes, moreover, accounted for covering 4 percent of the basement membrane surface and the remaining 8 percent was covered by very small cell processes, either neuronal or neuroglial, the nature of which could not be determined precisely.

Nature of the Neuropil. As already described, between the capillaries and the cell bodies and processes of neurons, an H and E section reveals only a pale blue finely mottled, seemingly structureless substance called the neuropil (Fig. 17-21) that contained some nuclei. The EM, however, shows this seemingly structureless substance is a conglomerate of the cell bodies and processes of astrocytes and the processes of neurons; only a few of the latter reveal myelin (Fig. 17-29). Between the cell bodies and processes of the astrocytes there is a network of intercellular spaces; it has been suggested that these may be up to 200 Å (20 nm.) wide. Unlike loose connective tissue or even cartilage, there is no mucopolysaccharide or fibrous intercellular material to fill these interstices between cells which are connected together only by spot-type junctions. It seems, therefore, that these intercellular spaces must contain tissue fluid which permits diffusion to occur between capillaries and neurons; the latter are, of course, very sensitive to a lack of oxygen and also to low blood sugar levels.

The Blood-Brain Barrier. Clinical and experimental findings probably suggested the existence of a *blood-brain barrier* before studies with the EM were made to determine its basis. It was found, for example, that if transplants of foreign tissue were made into the brains of animals, they were not rejected nearly as quickly as if they were transplanted into connective tissue. This could perhaps be explained by the absence of any lymphatic capillaries in the brain substance that would convey antigen to regional lymph nodes where T lymphocytes could be activated. However, it was also noted that certain substances that would have therapeutic value if given intravenously did not enter the brain from the blood, as would occur in other body parts. Moreover, certain dyes that would gain entrance from the blood to other parts of the body were found to not pass into gray matter, so there is no doubt about the existence of there being some kind of a blood-brain barrier.

Its components seem to be (1) the continuous capil-

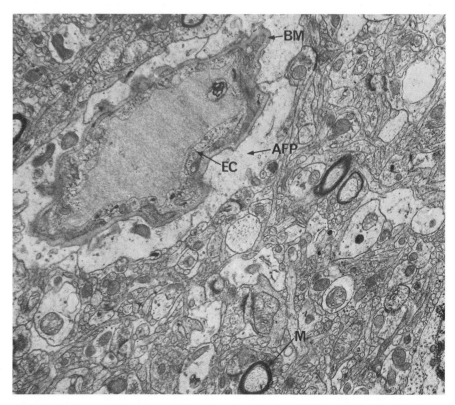

FIG. 17-29. Electron micrograph ($\times$ 12,000) of a capillary in the neuropil of the cerebral cortex. An endothelial lining cell of the capillary is labeled EC and the basement membrane around the capillary, BM. Just outside the basement membrane there is a light zone around the capillary, AFP, composed of the expanded astrocyte feet which are presumably attached to the basement membrane. The cell bodies of the astrocytes lie farther away from the capillary. Except for the capillary, most of the area seen in the micrograph is neuropil which consists of a conglomerate of astrocyte processes intertwined with nerve fibers most of which are unmyelinated; however an occasional myelinated fiber is encountered in the neuropil (labeled M). In the lower right corner a small portion of the cell body of a neuron can be seen; its cytoplasm is light and its nucleus dark. (Illustration courtesy of Ian Robertson)

laries with extensive tight junctions between contiguous endothelial cells, and (2) a very substantial basement membrane. However, the diffusion of gases and at least many of the components of simple solutions essential for the nutrition of neurons must occur through the barrier with relative ease.

MICROGLIA AS BRAIN MACROPHAGES

As their name implies, microglia are small cells originally believed to make up part of the gluelike glial tissue that held nerve tissue together. They are evenly scattered in white and gray matter. They make up about 5 percent of the glial cells in the white matter of the corpus callosum. They are stained reasonably specifically by the so-called weak silver carbonate method of del Rio-Hortega. This technic stains both

nucleus and cytoplasm, as well as long angular processes (Fig. 17-30). With the EM the cytoplasm of the cell bodies and processes is shown to contain a little rER and a fair number of dense bodies. Microglia normally do not divide (and do not take up ^{3}H-thymidine), and they show little indication of mobility and phagocytosis. However, whenever there is a local emergency, such as a stab wound or inflammation, dramatic changes occur; they acquire the ability to divide, both nucleus and cytoplasm enlarge, and they become mobile and fill up with phagocytosed material.

Origin. The origin of microglia has been the subject of much discussion. The majority opinion is that they come from the blood, probably by transformation of monocytes. However, there is some interference to their entry into brain substance because they have to

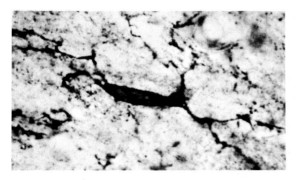

Fig. 17-30. A photomicrograph ($\times$ 1,100) of a microglia stained by del Rio-Hortega's weak silver carbonate method. The nucleus and cytoplasm are deeply stained. A number of long dark cytoplasmic processes extend to the edge of the figure. (Illustration courtesy of C. P. Leblond)

pass through the capillary basement membrane; what seems to happen is that after they have passed from the blood through the endothelium of a capillary they become enclosed by an expansion of its basement membrane, thus becoming a "perithelial cell." These stain like microglia by the del Rio-Hortega method, but their cytoplasm and processes are minimal. Eventually they break out of their basement membrane enclosure, especially in emergencies, and enter brain tissue.

It would probably have been less complicated if they had never been classed as part of the nerve glue (neuroglia) because they do not develop, as do the other cells of brain tissue, from neuroepithelium and their function is not primarily to play a supporting or adhesive role.

Appearances of Nuclei in the Three Types of Glial Cells. Since the nuclei of neuroglia are all that

can generally be seen in H and E sections, the question arises as to whether or not the different kinds can be identified by their nuclei. In general there are some differences between the nuclei of the three types, as is shown in Figure 17-31, but particularly if there are any small nerve cells in the same general area whose cytoplasm is indistinct, attempts to classify the cells of the gray matter by nuclear appearances alone is not recommended, at least for the inexperienced.

EPENDYMAL CELLS

It is not unusual to classify these also as a type of neuroglia cell. The ependymal cells that line the lumen of the neural tube perform three more or less consecutive functions. At first their function is proliferative (Fig. 17-10). Their second is supportive. As the wall of the neural tube thickens, the lining cells send out long processes that for a time reach the exterior of the tube and help to form the external limiting membrane that surrounds the tube. Still later they gradually relinquish their supporting role and function chiefly in forming a continuous epithelial lining, known as the ependyma, for the ventricles of the brain (Fig. 17-32). They also persist in the central canal of the spinal cord. In certain sites in the ventricles the ependyma is pushed inward by the vascular tufts to form choroid plexuses, as will be explained presently. The ependyma that comes to cover the capillaries of the choroid plexuses is termed *choroid plexus epithelium*.

The Meninges

The spinal cord and brain are protected not only by a bony encasement (the cranium and the vertebral column) but also by 3 connective tissue wrappings

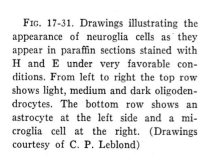

Fig. 17-31. Drawings illustrating the appearance of neuroglia cells as they appear in paraffin sections stained with H and E under very favorable conditions. From left to right the top row shows light, medium and dark oligodendrocytes. The bottom row shows an astrocyte at the left side and a microglia cell at the right. (Drawings courtesy of C. P. Leblond)

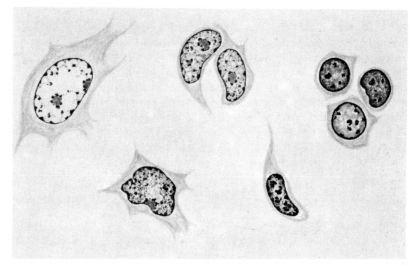

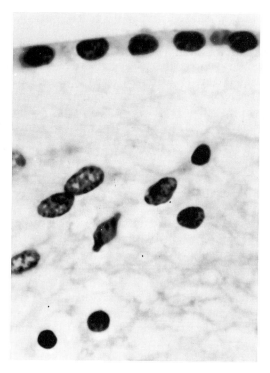

FIG. 17-32. High-power photomicrograph of an H and E section of brain, showing the ependyma lining of lateral ventricle.

called the *meninges* (*menix*, membrane) (Fig. 17-28). The innermost of these is applied directly to the surface of the brain and the cord and is called the pia mater (Fig. 17-28). The 2nd and middle one is called the arachnoid (Fig. 17-28) and the 3rd and outermost one is called the *dura mater* (Fig. 17-28). The structure of these three membranes will now be considered in turn.

Pia Mater. As its name implies (*pia*, tender; *mater*, mother), this membrane is delicate. It consists of interlacing bundles of collagenic fibers but has some fine elastic networks in it as well. It is covered with a continuous membrane of flattened squamous cells which are morphologically similar to those of the mesothelial membranes of the great body cavities. The substance of the membrane contains a few fibroblasts and macrophages and many blood vessels; these blood vessels are distributed by the pia mater over the surface of the brain (Fig. 17-28).

The Arachnoid. The middle membrane of the meninges is called the arachnoid because it is separated from—and, at the same time, joined to—the pia by a cobwebby (*arachnoid*, cobweb) network of trabeculae (Fig. 17-28). The term *arachnoid* includes both the

continuous roof over the pia and the network of pillars which extend from the pia to the roof.

The pia and the arachnoid are sometimes described as a single membrane, the *piarachnoid*.

Both the membrane and the trabeculae are composed chiefly of delicate collagenic fibers together with some elastic fibers. Both the outer and inner surfaces of the membranous roof and the trabeculae, are covered with a continuous lining of thin, flat lining cells that are similar to those that cover the pia. The space between the membranous roof of the arachnoid and the pia mater, through which the delicate arachnoid trabeculae extend, is filled with *cerebrospinal fluid* (soon to be described).

The surface of the brain is extraordinarily convoluted (Fig. 17-9). Whereas the pia extends down into the sulci and the fissures to cover the surface of the brain intimately, the membranous part of the arachnoid, except in the instance of some of the larger fissures, does not. Hence, over grooves there is more accommodation for cerebrospinal fluid than there is in other sites. Indeed, there are some sites where the brain surface is a considerable distance from the covering arachnoid, and in these there is accommodation for considerable amounts of cerebrospinal fluid. The precise location and nature of these will be learned in neuroanatomy; they are termed *cisternae*.

Dura Mater. As its name implies (*dura*, hard; *mater*, mother), this outermost membrane is of a tough consistency and is made up chiefly of dense connective tissue (Fig. 17-33). The collagenic fibers tend to run

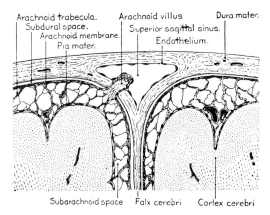

FIG. 17-33. Schematic diagram to illustrate the meninges, the sagittal sinus and an arachnoid villus. The potential subdural space is shown of greater size than is normal. The subarachnoid space over the convolutions also is increased so as to illustrate the character of the subarachnoid mesh. (Weed, L. H.: Am. J. Anat., *31:* 203)

longitudinally in the spinal dura but somewhat irregularly in the cranial dura. Some elastic fibers are mixed with the collagenic. There are certain differences between the dura of the vertebral canal and that of the cranium. In the vertebral canal the dura consists of a relatively free dense connective tissue sheath. The potential space between its inner surface and the outer surface of the arachnoid is called the *subdural space* (Fig. 17-34), and it normally contains a slight amount of fluid which is *not* cerebrospinal fluid. The outer surface of the spinal dura abuts on the *epidural space* (Fig. 17-34), which is filled with loose areolar tissue containing a certain amount of fat and many veins. The internal periosteum of the vertebrae, which lines the vertebral canal, forms the outer limit of the epidural space. The space between the arachnoid and pia is, of course, called the subarachnoid space (Fig. 17-34).

In the cranium there is no potential epidural space

because here the dura is fused with the internal periosteum of the cranial bones.

The cranial dura is therefore often described as having 2 layers, its inner being the counterpart of what has been termed *dura* in the vertebral canal, and its outer being the internal periosteum of the bones of the cranium. However, since these 2 layers adhere to one another, the dura of the cranium is adherent to the bones of the skull. Furthermore, since its outer layer serves as the inner periosteum of the bones, it contains blood vessels. The inner layer is much less vascular than the outer layer. Next, although the outer and the inner layers of the cranial dura are continuous with one another over most of the brain, they are separated in a few specific sites. In these sites the inner layer of the dura extends deep into fissures in the brain to form large partitions (Fig. 17-33). Along the line from which a partition extends into the fissure a cavity may exist between the 2 layers of the dura. This is roughly tri-

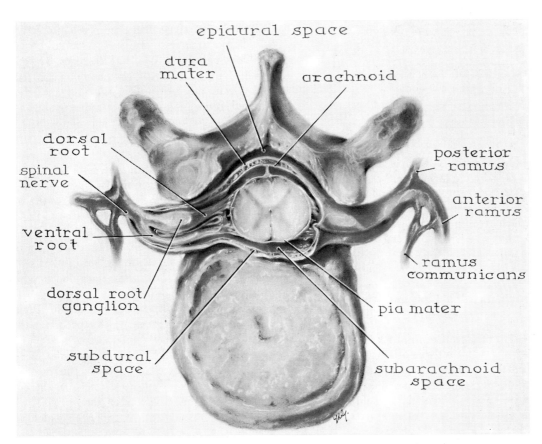

Fig. 17-34. Semidiagrammatic drawing of a cross section of the vertebral column at the level of an intervertebral foramen. It shows the relations of the meninges to the spinal cord and the way the central nervous system is connected to the peripheral nervous system. Note the spinal (dorsal root) ganglion.

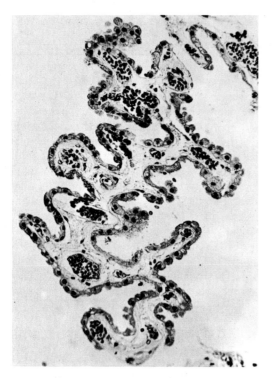

Fɪɢ. 17-35. High-power photomicrograph of a portion of a section cut from a human choroid plexus. (Section from Professor E. A. Linell)

angular on cross section (Fig. 17-33) and is bordered on its base above by the outer layer of the dura and on the other 2 sides by the inner layer, which sweeps from both sides of the fissure into it to form a partition there (Fig. 17-33). These spaces between the layers of the dura which are disposed along the lines from which partitions originate are lined by endothelium and contain venous blood; they constitute the *sinuses of the dura mater* (Fig. 17-33).

Formation, Circulation and Absorption of Cerebrospinal Fluid

Distribution of Cerebrospinal Fluid. Protection is provided for the delicate tissue of the C.N.S., first, by its being contained in bony cavities and, second, by its being more or less suspended in a fluid cushion. This cushion is contained in the piarachnoid, for all the interstices of its cobwebby structure are filled with a modified tissue fluid called *cerebrospinal fluid* (Fig. 17-33). The fluid-filled piarachnoid completely surrounds the brain and the cord and functions as a hydraulic shock absorber.

The ventricles of the brain, which form a continuous passageway (Fig. 17-9), also are filled with cerebrospinal fluid which is in communication with that outside the brain in the piarachnoid through the medium of 3 openings in the roof of the 4th ventricle. Normally, fluid flows through these openings from the interior of the brain to the exterior.

Sites of Formation of Cerebrospinal Fluid. Some is formed on the exterior of the brain, but most of it is formed in the ventricles by structures called *choroid plexuses,* which are little tufted structures, rich in capillaries, that project into the lumens of certain of the ventricles (Fig. 17-35). Like the glomeruli of the kidney, the choroid plexuses are structures specialized to produce tissue fluid. The capillaries are close to the free surfaces that are exposed to the fluid-filled lumens of the ventricles (Fig. 17-35). The free surfaces of the plexuses are, however, covered with a cuboidal type of epithelium (Fig. 17-35) through which the tissue fluid must pass before it enters the lumen of a ventricle to become cerebrospinal fluid; for this and other reasons it is more difficult for some substances, particularly those of macromolecular size, to get into cerebrospinal fluid than to get into ordinary tissue fluid.

Development of Choroid Plexuses. The part of the wall of the neural tube that becomes the roof of the third and the fourth ventricles becomes very thin; indeed, it comes to consist of no more than the single layer of cuboidal cells that compromise the ependyma plus the vascular piarachnoid which covers it. In these sites the piarachnoid, pushing the ependyma ahead of it, pushes into the ventricles to form the tufted *choroid plexuses* (Fig. 17-35). A similar phenomenon occurs in the medial wall of the cerebral hemisphere along the line of attachment of the hemispheres to the hindpart (thalamus) of the forebrain; this accounts for the development of the choroid plexuses of the lateral ventricles. Thus, there are 4 choroid plexuses formed: one in the fourth, one in the third and one in each of the lateral ventricles of the brain.

Microscopic Structure of Choroid Plexuses. A choroid plexus has many leaflike processes that hang, as it were, from the counterpart of a stem. A leaf is supplied with blood by a small artery or an arteriole; this supplies a capillary plexus. The capillaries, becoming tortuous, produce elevations in the epithelium called *villi,* as may be seen in Figure 17-35, which is a section cut through a leaf and from which villi, containing large capillaries, project on either side.

The epithelium that covers the leaves and the villi of the choroid plexuses develops from the ependyma. It is of the cuboidal type and is termed choroid plexus epithelium (Fig. 17-35). It rests on delicate connective tissue derived from the little piarachnoid that is pushed in behind it but ahead of the blood vessels.

With the EM the free surfaces of the epithelial cells of the choroid plexus are seen to be studded with microvilli, the free ends of which are often somewhat bulbous.

The choroid plexuses of the lateral ventricles, as described by Hudson and Smith, go through many changes during development which modify their vascular pattern considerably. They point out that degenerative changes may be seen in these plexuses relatively early in life. The degenerative changes are manifested by calcium deposits (termed *concentric bodies*), which may be scattered or concentrated in masses and/or by cysts.

Circulation of Cerebrospinal Fluid—Internal Hydrocephalus. The cerebrospinal fluid produced in the lateral ventricles must circulate through the interventricular foramina and, with that produced in the third ventricle, pass through the cerebral aqueduct of the midbrain to the fourth ventricle and out through its roof into the subarachnoid space. Most of the cerebrospinal fluid in the piarachnoid spaces surrounding the brain and the cord is formed inside the brain. If the outflow through the roof of the fourth ventricle is blocked, cerebrospinal fluid accumulates in the ventricles and causes them to expand, which stretches the brain from within. Such a condition can occur as a result of disease or deformity and is called *internal hydrocephalus.*

A minor amount of cerebrospinal fluid is formed by the smaller blood vessels which penetrate the brain surface, producing some tissue fluid; this makes its way back to the surface of the brain via the piarachnoid that ensheaths these vessels. At the brain surface it mixes with and becomes part of the cerebrospinal fluid.

Since cerebrospinal fluid is formed more or less continuously, it must be absorbed continuously, or a great increase in intracranial pressure would result. The little structures that function to absorb cerebrospinal fluid into the bloodstream at the same rate as that at which cerebrospinal fluid is produced are known as *arachnoid villi;* these are buttonlike projections of the arachnoid into certain of the venous sinuses of the dura mater (Fig. 17-33). The more or less hollow cores of these arachnoid villi are filled with cerebrospinal fluid, which is separated from the blood in the sinuses only by the thin cellular caps of the villi (Fig. 17-33). Cerebrospinal fluid seeps through these thin caps to enter the venous blood of the sinus.

Relation of the Formation and Absorption of Cerebrospinal Fluid to the Formation and Absorption of Tissue Fluid Elsewhere. The whole arrangement for the formation and the absorption of tissue fluid reminds one of the mechanisms by which tissue fluid is formed and absorbed in most parts of the body (Chapter 8). Presumably, the hydrostatic pressure in the capillaries of the choroid plexuses is fairly high (for capillaries); this could be inferred from the congested state that many of them exhibit. Tissue fluid, then, would be produced readily in choroid plexuses. On the other hand, the hydrostatic pressure in the venous sinus, into which the arachnoid villi project, is low, and in this site it might be expected that the greater osmotic pressure of the blood, imparted to it by its protein content, would draw cerebrospinal fluid (which is normally of a low protein or colloid content) back into the blood through the cells of the arachnoid villi. However, this arrangement differs from that ordinarily concerned in the absorption of tissue fluid because lymphatics are not provided in the C.N.S. to draw off excess fluid. Some cerebrospinal fluid may be drained away by passing along spaces in the nerves that leave the C.N.S. to go to various parts of the body (see Steer and Horney).

Composition. Cerebrospinal fluid is clear and limpid. It contains inorganic salts but very little protein. In its normal state it contains only a very few cells, and these are mostly lymphocytes. Its examination in suspected injuries or diseases of the C.N.S. is of the greatest help in diagnosis. For example, the finding of blood in the cerebrospinal fluid may provide confirmation of a skull fracture involving a rupture of vessels from which blood has escaped. Or an increase in the number of cells in the cerebrospinal fluid may be of assistance in diagnosing certain inflammatory diseases of the nervous system or the meninges. Even the pressure under which the cerebrospinal fluid exists is often a great help in distinguishing between different types of pathologic conditions of the brain or the cord. However, a complete study of the cerebrospinal fluid is reserved for the later and clinical years of the medical course.

The Nervous Tissue of the Peripheral Nervous System

The P.N.S. consists of:

(1) **Nerves.** These are branching cordlike structures that extend out from the brain as cranial nerves and from the spinal cord as spinal nerves to reach almost every part of the body (Fig. 17-1). Nerves each contain many nerve fibers, commonly both afferent and efferent. By means of nerves, nerve fibers are distributed to almost every part of the body. Nerves are sometimes termed nerve trunks.

(2) **Ganglia.** These little nodules contain the cell bodies of neurons. There are two general kinds of ganglia in the P.N.S.: first, cerebrospinal ganglia, which contain the cell bodies of the afferent neurons of the body segments (Figs. 17-7 and 17-34), and, second, ganglia of the autonomic nervous system (soon to be described), which contain the cell bodies of efferent neurons of the autonomic system.

(3) **Nerve Endings and Organs of Special Sense.** A description of the various kind of endings of afferent nerve fibers as well as the organs of special sense is given in a separate chapter at the end of this book because these structures can be studied to better advantage after the organs and the structures in which many of them are distributed have been described. Efferent nerve endings among the secretory cells of exocrine glands will be described later in this chapter and efferent nerve endings in muscle will be described in the next chapter.

The following outline of the components of the P.N.S. provides a basis for completing our classification of nervous tissue:

Nervous Tissue

$$\text{The tissue of the C.N.S.} \begin{cases} \text{Gray matter} \\ \text{White matter} \end{cases}$$

$$\text{The tissue of the P.N.S.} \begin{cases} \text{Nerves} \\ \text{Ganglia} \\ \text{Nerve Endings} \end{cases}$$

The Development of the P.N.S.

The afferent and efferent components of the P.N.S. are developed from different sources. The afferent components will be considered first.

Afferent. The neural plate gives rise to two neural crests (Fig. 6-3) as well as to the neural tube. Soon each neural crest breaks up into a chain of nodules, and these are the forerunners of the posterior (dorsal) root ganglia of the spinal cord and their cranial counterparts. Each segment of the cord has two ganglia: one on each side in a posterolateral position (Figs. 17-34 and 17-36). As these develop, the neuroectodermal cells differentiate along two main lines, as they do in the neural tube. Along one line they form neuroblasts. These are at first bipolar cells, but as they turn into neurons, their two processes, like the hands of a clock, move around their circumference toward each other until they meet and fuse; by this maneuver the bipolar neurons become unipolar neurons (Fig. 17-2). However, their single process branches, with one branch (the functional) axon growing centrally along

the line indicated with an arrow in Figure 17-36 to the dorsal root of the spinal cord; the other process, though functionally a dendrite, is morphologically an axon, and it grows peripherally and becomes enclosed with other fibers in a nerve trunk through which it extends to reach the tissue in which it is to provide a sensory ending (Fig. 17-36).

Neuroectodermal cells in a developing spinal ganglia differentiate along a second pathway to form supporting cells; these are not neuroglia but their P.N.S. counterparts. These cells are of two main types: *capsule cells,* which form capsules around the cell bodies of the ganglion cells (Fig. 17-37), and *neurolemma* or *sheath of Schwann cells* (to be described later), which form sheaths for the nerve fibers.

Efferent. The efferent components of the P.N.S. arise, not from neural crests but from the middle layer of the neural tube (Fig. 17-36). Here neuroblasts become neurons and sprout axons that extend out from the anterolateral surface of the spinal cord to account for the efferent nerve fibers of peripheral nerves. The efferent fibers of cranial nerves originate in the same way. The axons escape the confines of the C.N.S. by passing out through foramina (Fig. 17-34), from there passing into nerve trunks, along the line indicated by arrows in Figure 17-36, by which they are distributed to the structures that they innervate.

When we deal with the autonomic nervous system, we shall find that it consists only of efferent neurons, and that the cell bodies of some of these are in the brain and the cord, but the cell bodies of many others are scattered in autonomic (not posterior root) ganglia in various parts of the body. Therefore the cell bodies that are in these ganglia represent the cell bodies of efferent neurons that are outside the confines of the C.N.S. They develop from neuroectodermal cells of the neural tube, but they leave the tube and migrate outward into the body early in development. Where they go and what they do will be described shortly.

Microscopic Structure of Spinal Ganglia

The bodies of the nerve cells here are unusually rounded. Many of them are large (Fig. 17-37), but some are small. Their nuclei are large and pale and contain prominent nucleoli (Fig. 17-37). Their cytoplasm contains neurofibrils and basophilic material; the latter is characteristically more dispersed than that in anterior horn cells. Accumulations of the yellow-brown pigment, lipofuscin, may be present in the cytoplasm (Fig. 5-64). The rounded cell bodies of ganglion cells are each separated from the connective tissue framework of a ganglion by a single layer of

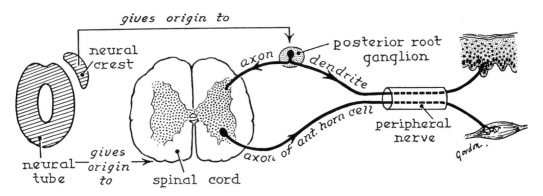

FIG. 17-36. Diagram illustrating the origin of the P.N.S. The neural crest gives rise to posterior root ganglion cells. Processes from these grow both outward and inward; hence the neural crests give rise to the afferent components of the P.N.S. The efferent components of the P.N.S. develop from the neural tube by means of axons from anterior horn cells growing out from the developing spinal cord.

special flattened cells called *capsule* cells or *amphicytes* (Fig. 17-37), which are derived from neuroectoderm; as noted, these are the P.N.S. counterparts of the neuroglia of the C.N.S.

The single process of each ganglion cell extends from its cell body to approach the mainstream of fibers in the dorsal root, and in doing so the process divides into two branches. One passes into the spinal nerve, which conducts it out to a receptor ending (Fig. 17-36). The other branches pass inward via the dorsal root to reach the posterior column of gray matter on that side of the cord (Fig. 17-36). Structurally, both processes have the appearance of axons, and most of them are myelinated. The connective tissue in which the ganglion cells and their processes lie is the counterpart of the connective tissue sheaths of nerves; it will be described shortly.

Microscopic Structure of Peripheral Nerves

The Connective Tissue Components of Peripheral Nerves. The peripheral nerves encountered ·in gross dissection are cordlike and relatively strong. This is due to peripheral nerves having a fairly extensive connective tissue component which is more or less arranged to form tubes of three different orders. In cross section of a large peripheral nerve, there is more or less of a tubelike arrangement of connective tissue that encases the whole nerve; this is called the epineurium of the nerve (Figs. 17-38 and 17-39). Its wall is not very thick or strong—not nearly as strong as the walls of the next size of tubes of connective tissue in its interior. The smaller (next order of) tubes have walls of relatively dense connective tissue; this is called

perineurium (Figs. 17-38 and 17-39.) Each tube of perineurium contains a great many nerve fibers, each of which is itself encased in a delicate tube of connective tissue termed *endoneurium*. Shanthaveerappa and Bourne have studied the perineurium of nerves of many species and describe the existence of an epithelial sheath made of flattened cells that forms a lining for the connective tissue perineurial sheath. They suggest that this perineurial epithelium has its origin from the leptomeninges, and that it extends to the terminations

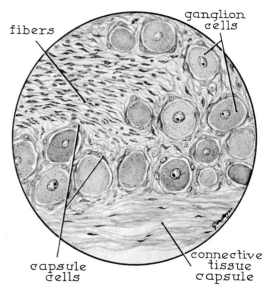

FIG. 17-37. Drawing of a portion of a section cut from a human spinal ganglion (high-power).

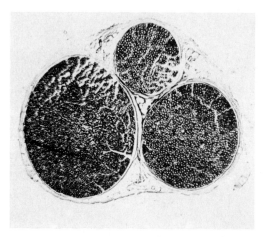

FIG. 17-38. A low-power photomicrograph of a cross section of the sciatic nerve of a dog; this was cut from material fixed in osmic acid.

of nerve fibers (see pacinian corpuscles in Chapter 28).

Smaller nerves lack epineurium. A small nerve consists of a tube of perineurium within which are endoneurial tubes, each containing a nerve fiber.

The Nerve Fibers of Peripheral Nerves. The fine structure of nerve fibers (axons) was described in connection with Figure 17-18. Each nerve fiber in the P.N.S. is covered with a thin delicate cytoplasmic

sheath termed the *neurolemma* (also spelled *neurilemma*) or *sheath of Schwann* (Fig. 17-41). The cells that comprise this sheath are derived from neuroectodermal cells that grow out along with the nerve fibers as they push out from the neural crests or the neural tube. In one kind of nerve fiber there is a sheath of myelin between the nerve fiber and the sheath of Schwann that is of substantial thickness (Figs. 17-39 and 17-41); such fibers are termed *myelinated fibers*. In the other kind of fiber—and these tend to be smaller—the myelin covering is very thin, so these are termed *nonmyelinated fibers,* and anywhere up to a dozen or more of these are enclosed by the cytoplasm of the same sheath of Schwann cell (Fig. 17-40).

Nodes of Ranvier. The myelin of myelinated fibers is not continuous; it is interrupted periodically by constrictions (also called nodes) of Ranvier (Figs. 17-39 and 17-41). At these nodes there is no myelin and the sheath of Schwann of the nerve fiber dips down toward the nerve fiber but does not completely cover it. In these sites, as has been shown by the EM studies of Robertson, the nerve fiber is therefore partially uncovered. There is one sheath of Schwann cell between each two nodes. The distance between adjacent nodes of Ranvier in the same fiber varies; it may be up to one millimeter. Nodes of Ranvier are also present in the C.N.S. (Fig. 17-13) but there, of course, there are no sheath of Schwann cells for there myelin is produced by oligodendrocytes.

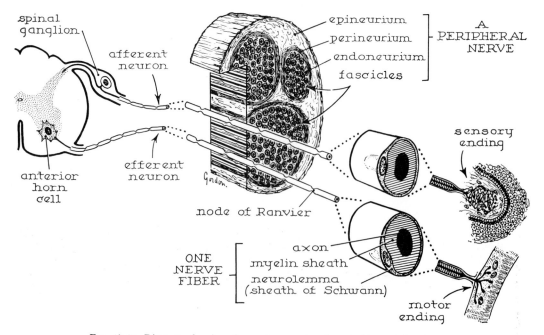

FIG. 17-39. Diagram showing the various parts of a sizable peripheral nerve.

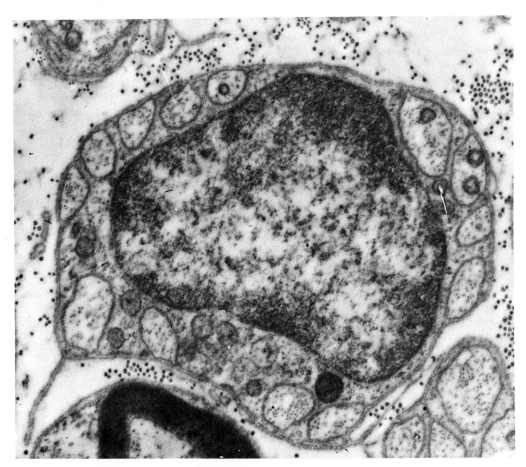

FIG. 17-40. Electron micrograph ($\times$ 26,000) of a Schwann cell, the cytoplasm of which houses over a dozen unmyelinated axons. The latter are cut in cross section and appear as the lighter, generally ovoid areas. The dots seen in them are neurofilaments. The darker bodies seen in the cytoplasm of the Schwann cell are mitochondria. An occasional mitochondrion, much smaller, can be seen in the axoplasm of a few of the unmyelinated fibers. Each unmyelinated fiber is surrounded by two cell membranes—its own and, peripheral to its own, the cell membrane of the Schwann cell, the cytoplasm of which closed over the fiber as it was engulfed by the Schwann cell. (Illustration courtesy of E. J. H. Nathaniel and D. C. Pease)

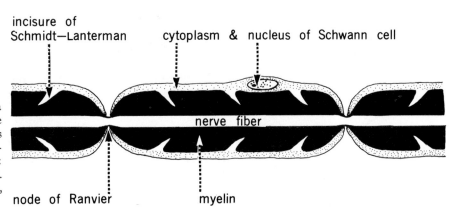

FIG. 17-41. Diagram showing a portion of a mylelinated nerve fiber of the peripheral nervous system and two nodes of Ranvier. (Redrawn from Barr, M. L.: The Human Nervous System. New York, Harper and Row, 1972. Labeling added)

The role of nodes of Ranvier in connection with the transmission of the nervous impulse was described previously in connection with these nodes in the C.N.S. As already mentioned, unmyelinated nerve fibers, with minimal myelin sheaths and no nodes of Ranvier, do not conduct nervous impulses as quickly as myelinated fibers.

In peripheral nerves fixed with osmic acid, the myelin between constrictions of Ranvier is broken up by little incisures or clefts that extend down into it from the surface; these are termed the *clefts of Schmidt-Lanterman* and the segments between them are termed *Schmidt-Lanterman segments*. The clefts have been studied by histochemical methods by Shanklin and Azzam.

The Formation and the Fine Structure of Myelin Sheaths. According to the hypothesis now generally accepted, a myelin sheath in the P.N.S. is formed as follows: The cytoplasm of a Schwann cell surrounds an axon (Fig. 17-42, *left*). The axon then lies in a long trough in the Schwann cell. The Schwann cell (or part of it) then begins to rotate around the axon (Fig. 17-42, *left, center,* and *right*). It should be noted here that the cell membrane of the Schwann cell is represented in this simple diagram (Fig. 17-42), designed to illustrate a particular point, as a single line; later, for the EM appearance, it will be shown as a double line. When Schwann cell cytoplasm begins to wind around the axon, the cell membrane lining one side of the groove in which the axon lies comes into contact with the cell membrane that lines the other side of the groove (Fig. 17-42, *middle,* and *right*). These two membranes that come and stay together are seen, as the cell continues to wind around the axon, as a series

of rings made of double lines; each of these lines represents a cell membrane (Fig. 17-42, *right*). Between these adjacent double rings there is at first cytoplasm (stippled in Fig. 17-42). As the winding continues, the cytoplasm is squeezed back toward the cell body of the Schwann cell or lost in some other way. Accordingly, the myelin sheath evolves from 2-layered rings of cell membrane. To understand how a sheath made up of these rings of membrane becomes myelin, we no longer have to consider cytoplasm, for this is all squeezed out or lost; all that we have to consider is how a structure consisting of concentric rings, with each ring consisting of 2 cell membranes, takes on the appearance of myelin.

Under high resolution a fully formed myelin sheath reveals concentric dark rings termed major dense lines (Fig. 17-43, *bottom*) that are about 25 Å thick. These are separated from each other by a layer of a lighter material about 100 Å thick (Fig. 17-43, *bottom*). With special fixation and excellent resolution, a thinner dark line can be seen in the middle of each of the lighter layers; these fine lines that are halfway between the major dense lines are termed *intraperiod lines* (Fig. 17-43, *bottom*). We shall now consider how this appearance can evolve from concentric layers of cell membranes.

As was explained in Chapter 7, a cell membrane under appropriate conditions appears in the EM as 2 dark lines with a light space between them (Figs. 5-3 and 5-4), the whole membrane being about 95 Å thick. Evidence suggests that the middle layer of the cell membrane (the light layer) contains much lipid, whereas the 2 dark layers, which bound the membrane on each of its sides, contain protein. To follow the

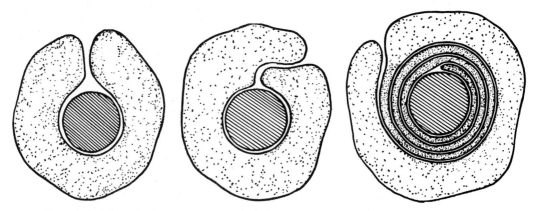

FIG. 17-42. Diagram illustrating the earlier stages of the formation of a myelin sheath according to the jelly-roll hypothesis. (Diagrams based on those of Green, B. B., and Schmitt, F. O.: Symposium on the Fine Structure of Cells. p. 251. Groningen, Holland, Noordhoff, and diagrams supplied by Schmitt in a personal communication)

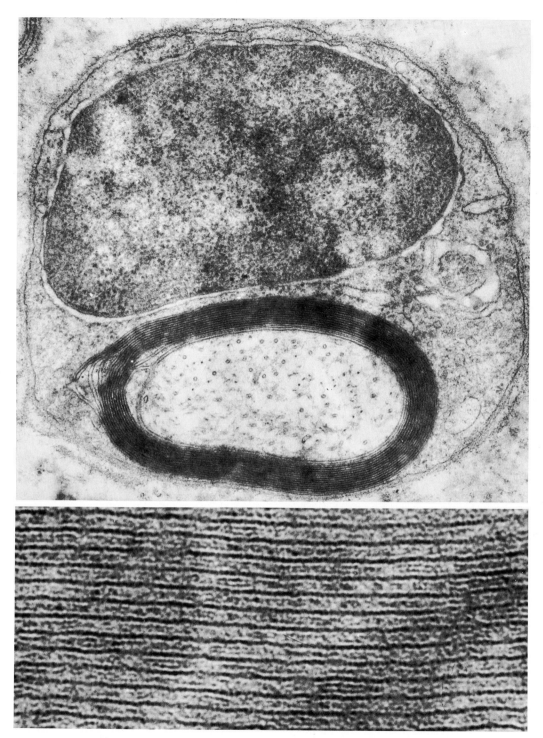

FIG. 17-43. Electron micrographs (*top*, × 70,000; *bottom*, × 360,000) of cross sections of sciatic nerve of rat. (*Top*) This is a cross section of a single myelinated nerve fiber surrounded by a sheath of Schwann. The upper part is occupied by the nucleus of a sheath of Schwann cells. Below the nucleus, lying in the cytoplasm of the Schwann cell, is a myelin sheath surrounding a nerve fiber. Details of a fiber are shown at higher magnification in Figure 17-18. (*Bottom*) This shows the major dense lines of the myelin sheath. Between the major dense lines, the intraperiod lines (the formation of which is illustrated in Fig. 17-44) can be seen; these are often double. (Preparation by Martha Nagai and A. F. Howatson)

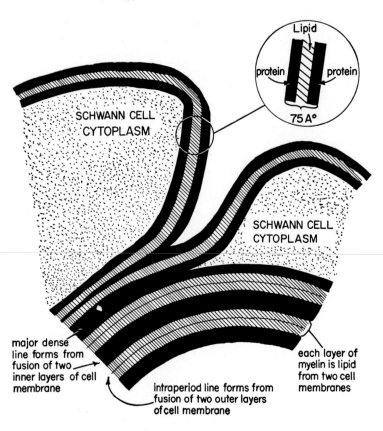

formation of myelin in Figure 17-44, we must think of the 2 cell membranes that come together as the Schwann cell rotates, not as each being represented by a single line, as in Figure 17-42, but as *each* being a double line with light material between; they are represented this way in Figure 17-44.

As the Schwann cell cytoplasm continues to encircle the nerve fiber, the outer lamellae of 2 cell membranes continue to come into contact with each other and fuse (Fig. 17-44). The dark line so formed becomes compressed to form the fine intraperiod line (Fig. 17-44). Next, as cytoplasm is squeezed away, the inner lamellae of the cell membranes that previously bordered this cytoplasm come together and fuse, and this forms the major dense line (Fig. 17-44). Therefore, the myelin that fills the space between 2 major dense lines is derived chiefly from the lipid that existed in the middle layers of the 2 cell membranes that fuse. Why the fusion of the outer lamellae of 2 cell membranes should result in only a thin dark (intraperiod) line and the fusion of 2 inner lamellae of cell membrane in a heavy major dense line, is not entirely clear. Both lines can be seen in Figure 17-43, *bottom.*

The fine structure of nonmyelinated fibers is illustrated in Figure 17-40; this shows that several such fibers lie in the cytoplasm of a single Schwann cell where the axolemma of each fiber is covered with at least one layer of cell membrane of the Schwann cell.

How Nerves Appear in Sections Studied With the LM

In preparing an ordinary paraffin section, the myelin surrounding the individual nerve fibers, unless it is treated with special mordants, will, because of its fatty nature, dissolve away in the dehydrating and clearing agents. This allows the nerve fiber to slip to one side of the tubular space that is left by the myelin dissolving away. Hence ordinary H and E cross sections of nerves show the site previously occupied by the myelin sheaths as little rounded spaces, mostly empty except for the nerve fiber, and this may be situated toward one side rather than in the center of the space (Fig. 17-45, *right*). At the exterior of the space, or bulging somewhat into it, the faint-staining sheath of Schwann may be seen. The nuclei seen in the substance of a nerve bundle in an H and E preparation are those of the sheath of Schwann cells and those of the fibroblasts and macrophages of the endoneurium, together with the nuclei of the cells of the blood vessels which lie in the endoneurium. However, in an osmic acid preparation the myelin surrounding the nerve fibers is not dissolved away but is preserved and blackened. Hence the myelin sheaths of nerve fibers appear as blackened rings in this type of preparation (Fig. 17-45, *left*). However, the other elements of the nerve do not show up very well in the usual osmic acid preparation. Osmic acid preparations show very clearly that the fibers in a nerve are of different sizes.

In routine H and E preparations, nerves cut obliquely, or in planes approaching the longitudinal, have an appearance which is often substantially different from that which might be expected from their cross-section appearance. Instead of seeing rings, where myelin has dissolved away, one sees streaks. Moreover, the streaky appearance of obliquely and longitudinally sectioned nerves is accentuated by the long, thin, flat nuclei seen between fibers; those are the nuclei of the sheath of Schwan cells and the cells of the endoneurium (Fig. 17-46). The streaks do not run directly longitudinally but in a wavy snake-fence manner along it (Fig. 17-46).

Most peripheral nerves are of the mixed variety; they contain both afferent and efferent fibers (Fig. 17-39).

Some Histological Features of Nerves of Clinical Interest

Variability of Fascicles. A large nerve contains several fascicles of fibers each surrounded with a dense sheath of perineurium (Fig. 17-39). Sunderland has shown that there is much communication between fascicles, in that nerve fibers pass from one to another. Consequently, the relative sizes and content of fibers of the fascicles in a nerve changes continually along its course. Hence if a small section of a nerve is, for example, destroyed and an attempt is made to join the two stumps together the fascicles in the two stumps may not match each other.

In order to join the two stumps of a nerve, a portion of which has been lost, recourse may be taken to stretching the two parts of the nerve that are to be joined. Nerves can be stretched to some extent without damage to them (see Sunderland). This is probably due at least in part to the fact that nerve fibers

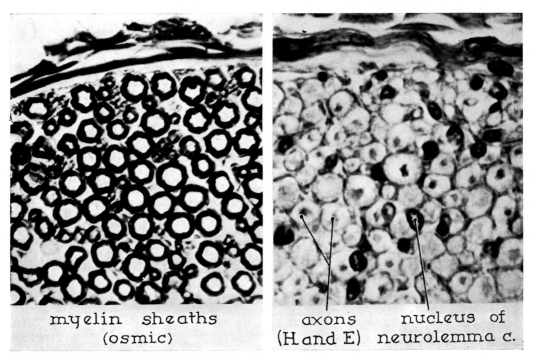

myelin sheaths
(osmic)

axons   nucleus of
(H and E) neurolemma c.

Fig. 17-45. (*Left*) High-power photomicrograph of a portion of a cross section of a peripheral nerve fixed in osmic acid. (*Right*) A similar preparation of a nerve fixed in formalin and stained with H and E.

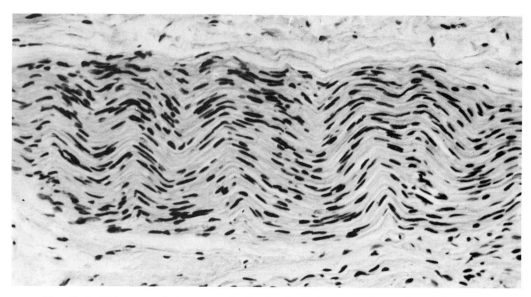

Fɪɢ. 17-46. High-power photomicrograph of a longitudinal section of a small peripheral nerve, showing the snake-fence appearance which is typical in longitudinal sections of nerves in sections.

do not pursue a straight course along a nerve but instead follow a zigzag course (Fig. 17-46). Stretching a nerve (up to a point) merely straightens out the fibers and does not stretch them. The strong perineurial sheaths provide a limiting factor in stretching a nerve (for details see Sunderland).

Small nerves are composed of only a single fascicle. This is surrounded by a perineurial sheath (Fig. 17-46).

The number of nerve fibers within a fascicle varies greatly, as does the diameter of the nerve fibers in the fascicle. Sunderland, Lavarack and Ray found, for example, that the lateral cutaneous nerve on the right side of one subject consisted of only 1 fascicle, and that it contained 3,160 fibers. The same nerve on the left side consisted of 7 fascicles that contained a total of 10,178 fibers. They measured the diameters of the fibers (including their myelin sheaths) in 1 fascicle that contained 1,242 fibers and found that about 60 percent of these were less than 8 μ wide, 15 percent were between 8 and 15 μ wide, 23 percent were between 16 and 23 μ wide and 0.5 percent were wider than 23 μ.

Laverack, Sunderland and Ray have counted the number of fibers in nerves at different levels and have found more fibers in the distal parts of some nerves than at more proximal levels. The increased number of fibers is attributed to the branching of fibers within nerves.

The Blood Supply of Nerves. In surgical procedures, nerves must sometimes be freed of their attachments for certain distances, and it is important to know whether or not this will interfere sufficiently with their blood supply to cause serious damage within them. Fortunately, nerves are supplied by a profusion of vessels that anastomose freely. The vessels are of several orders. There are longitudinally disposed epineurial interfascicular, perineurial and intrafascicular arteries and arterioles. The endoneurium contains a capillary network. Nutrient arteries from vessels outside the nerve, and from longitudinally disposed vessels accompanying the nerve, penetrate the nerve frequently along its course to communicate with the neural vessels. The number of anastomoses between all these vessels is so great that nerves can be freed for considerable distances from their surrounding attachments. Sunderland, who should be read for details about blood supply, stresses the importance of preserving the superficial vessels that run along nerves when the nerves are being freed from adjacent structures, for these superficial vessels are important links in the system that provides such efficient anastomoses.

The Degeneration and the Regeneration of Peripheral Nerves

Nerve injuries are of different orders of severity.

First-degree Injuries. These are common and generally are caused by pressure being applied to a nerve at a particular site for a limited time; this may act by squeezing the blood vessels in the nerve to cause local anoxia of the axons sufficient to interfere with their function. Sensory fibers are affected more readily by pressure than motor fibers, and different kinds of sensory fibers vary in their susceptibility. After the pressure is released, recovery of sensation or motor function may occur in a matter of minutes, hours or weeks, depending on the severity of the injury. If recovery does not occur in a *few weeks,* the injury must be regarded as more severe than a first-degree type, as will now be described.

Second-degree Injuries. This kind is generally caused by prolonged and/or severe pressure being exerted on some part of the nerve—enough to destroy the axon at the point where it is subjected to pressure. Nerves sometimes are injured purposefully in this fashion to bring about the temporary paralysis of some muscle or muscles whose actions are interfering with the rest and recovery of some part of the body (for example, the nerves to one side of the diaphragm sometimes are squeezed hard enough to put the lung on that side to rest).

The severe pressure required to bring about second-degree injuries to nerves causes the *death of the axons* of the nerve at the site where the pressure is applied. In this respect the second-degree type of injury has *fundamentally different* consequences from the first-degree type. When even a small segment of an axon dies, the part of the axon distal to the injury also dies because it is separated from the cell body on which it depends for its existence. Accordingly, nerve function in a second-degree type of injury can be restored only by all parts of axons distal to the injury being regenerated.

When the cell body recovers from the axon reaction (Fig. 17-17), it begins again to synthesize new axoplasm. This results in new axoplasm pushing into and through the site where the axon was crushed. To discuss its further fate we must consider certain other changes that result from the injury.

When the axons distal to the site of the injury die, the myelin sheaths surrounding them also degenerate. Since the degeneration of the axon and its myelin sheath was first described by Waller, the process often is termed Wallerian degeneration. Macrophages from the endoneurium phagocytose the degenerating material. It has been suggested that Schwann cells also become phagocytic and help rid the area of debris.

A second-degree type of injury, however, *is not believed to interrupt the continuity of the endoneurial tubes at the site of injury.* Accordingly, when the cell bodies supplying the axons in the nerve begin to send axoplasm into and through the site of the injury, the new axoplasm from each neuron pushes into the same endoneurial tube that formerly was occupied by the axon from that same neuron. Axoplasm generally extends down the endoneurial tubes at a rate of about 2 to 3 mm. per day, but the rate is said to become slower as the new axoplasm approaches the terminations of the fibers. When it reaches the terminations of the fibers, function is restored. The way in which the new axoplasm becomes myelinated and covered with a sheath of Schwann is similar to that in severed and reunited nerves, as will now be described.

Regeneration in Severed Nerves That Are Rejoined Surgically. If a peripheral nerve is cut, the muscular action in the part of the body it supplies and the reception of sensation from that part need not be lost forever. If two cut ends of the nerve are brought together and fastened in place by sutures through their connective tissue wrappings, or held together by some other means, at least partial function, after a considerable period of time, may be restored to the part affected.

In the part of the nerve distal to the cut, the nerve fibers of afferent and efferent neurons are, of course, severed from their cell bodies, so they die and become necrotic. The disintegration of the axons takes only a short time, and in a few days only a little debris is left in the space that the living axon formerly occupied (Fig. 17-47). The myelin sheaths of these axons that are severed from their cell bodies also decompose (Fig. 17-47). The myelin breaks down rather more slowly than the material of the axon, but soon it becomes reduced to droplets (Fig. 17-47). The cells of the sheaths of Schwann proliferate and are believed to form cords that lie in the endoneurial tubes (Fig. 17-47). Macrophages from endoneurium phagocytose and digest the droplets of broken-down myelin and the remnants of the dead axons. After they phagocytose this debris, they move away. Fibroblasts, particularly those close to the place where the nerve is cut, proliferate, but unless the site of the cut has become infected, they do not usually proliferate as rapidly as the cells of the sheath of Schwann, which at this site bulge from the cut ends of the endoneurial tubes of the distal stump, and also, but not so rapidly, from the endoneurial tubes of the proximal stump. The slitlike spaces between the proliferating sheath of Schwann cells offer a means for nerve fibers to push across the gap from the proximal into the distal stump (Fig. 17-47).

While all these changes are taking place in the portion of the nerve distal to the cut, changes also take place in the proximal stump. Near the cut the axons at first degenerate. As has been mentioned already, the sheath of Schwann cells proliferate and grow out into the gap and meet those from the distal stump.

DEGENERATION AND REGENERATION OF A SEVERED NERVE

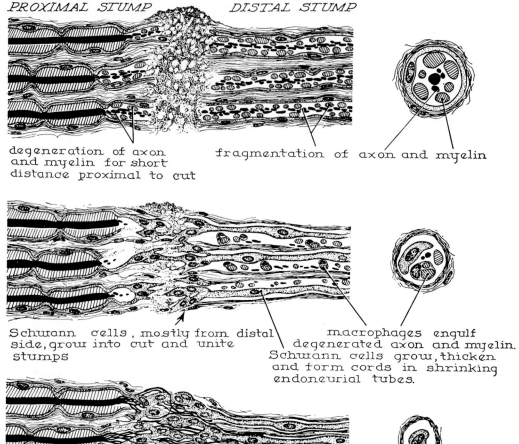

PROXIMAL STUMP   DISTAL STUMP

degeneration of axon
and myelin for short
distance proximal to cut

fragmentation of axon and myelin

Schwann cells, mostly from distal
side, grow into cut and unite
stumps

macrophages engulf
degenerated axon and myelin.
Schwann cells grow, thicken
and form cords in shrinking
endoneurial tubes.

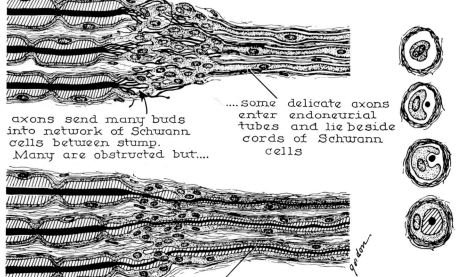

axons send many buds
into network of Schwann
cells between stump.
Many are obstructed but....

....some delicate axons
enter endoneurial
tubes and lie beside
cords of Schwann
cells

axons continue to push along
endoneurial tubes of distal stump and are
enfolded by Schwann cells after which new myelin is formed

FIG. 17-47. Diagram showing the changes that occur in a nerve when it is severed and regenerates.

Thus continuity is established across the cut by the sheath of Schwann cells, and, as noted before, these cells have longitudinally disposed slits between them. The axons from the proximal portion of the severed nerve now start to push forward a little each day, and after a few days they reach the space where union has occurred between the two outgrowths of the sheath of Schwann cells. The axons on growing into this maze-like arrangement often branch into many branches (Fig. 17-47), and the various branches push their way through such slits and spaces as are available; before long, many may manage to traverse the region of the cut and from then on grow along the tiny passageways that exist in the syncytium provided by the sheath of Schwann cells into the open ends of the endoneurial tubes of the distal stump: these, while they have become smaller, are still open. Under good conditions, the fibers grow down these tubes at a rate that has been variously estimated at from 1 to 4 mm. a day (Fig. 17-47). As they near the termination of the nerve, they grow somewhat more slowly.

It is to be observed that no matter how carefully severed nerves are joined together, it could scarcely be expected that the majority of axons that grow down it would ever find their proper paths. It seems almost incredible under the circumstances that efficient motor function and reasonably good sensation should ever return to a part of the body after the nerve supplying it has been severed. Nevertheless, good results often are obtained by the joining of cut nerves. Perhaps one thing that helps is that the axons, on reaching the sheath of Schwann syncytium that forms at the site of the cut, branch into many branches. Hence, more axons actually may try to grow down the severed nerve than were present in the first place. Sometimes several enter one endoneurial tube; perhaps only the one that should be there survives.

In an endoneurial tube the new axon lies against a cord of Schwann cells (Fig. 17-47). The latter gradually enfold the axon, probably much as occurs in normal development (Fig. 17-47). New myelin then forms, probably as it does during development, and the cordlike Schwann cells once more assume their mature appearance.

Nerve Transplantation. In certain types of injuries a whole section of a nerve may be destroyed. Under these conditions the two cut ends cannot be approximated; hence recourse may be taken to what is called *nerve grafting.* In this procedure a piece of some superficial nerve that is not essential is removed, and this is placed and sutured so as to fill the gap. On transplantation, the sheath of Schwann cells in an autogenous nerve graft appear to survive and proliferate. In this respect the graft acts very much like the distal fragment. However, even though its sheath of Schwann cells proliferate at both of its cut ends, to join with the distal and the proximal fragments, respectively, of the injured nerve, it is obvious that the use of a graft necessitates axons finding their way through two mazes rather than one. It is understandable, then, that the results from nerve grafting are not nearly so satisfactory as those that are obtained by joining the two cut ends of a nerve directly.

The Autonomic Nervous System

To recapitulate: nervous tissue is structurally specialized to be excited selectively by different kinds of stimuli, originating both within and without the body, and to conduct nervous impulses rapidly to (1) the gland cells of the exocrine type, and (2) the cells of muscle tissue. These are the kinds of cells that account for *responses.*

It is to be observed further that only some of these responses are under the direct control of the conscious mind—that is, those that occur in striated muscle (this is the kind attached to the bones of the skeleton and which we can control; see next chapter for details). The control of all heart muscle and smooth muscle (the latter is the kind that, for example, controls the diameter of blood vessels and the intestine and other tubes in the body; see next chapter for details) and all exocrine glands is outside the direct influence of the conscious mind. However, these activities are controlled by reflex phenomena. Some of the afferent impulses concerned in these reflexes make their way into consciousness; for example, stimulation of the nerve endings in the taste buds of the mouth give rise to the sensation of taste as well as initiating the response of salivation. But other afferent impulses (for example, those arising from the stimulation of nerve endings in the viscera) do not ordinarily appear even dimly in consciousness. Hence, we say that the function of smooth and cardiac muscle and glands is automatically controlled in the body.

The *efferent* neurons concerned in the automatic innervation of the smooth and cardiac muscle and the exocrine glands of the body constitute the *autonomic nervous system.*

Next, cardiac muscle and most of the smooth muscle and glandular structures of the viscera are doubly innervated by this system. This is accomplished by its having two divisions, with each division sending efferent neurons to most bits of muscle or gland that the autonomic nervous system innervates (Fig. 17-48) so that each has a double supply. Further, the efferent

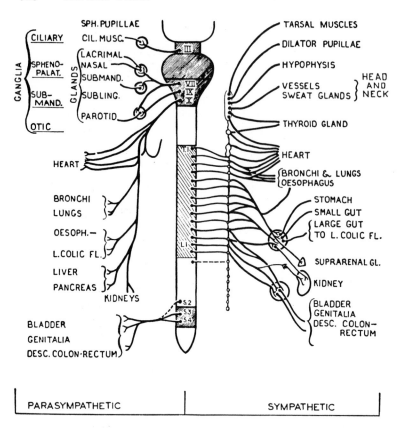

Fig. 17-48. Diagram of the autonomic nervous system. The parasympathetic division is shown on the left, and the sympathetic division on the right. (After Stopford. In Grant, J. C. Boileau, and Basmajian, J. V.: Grant's Method of Anatomy. ed. 7, p. 47. Baltimore, Williams & Wilkins, 1965)

PARASYMPATHETIC   SYMPATHETIC

impulses arriving at muscle or gland by neurons of the two divisions tend to cause different physiologic effects. For example, the impulses arriving by way of the neurons of one division may lead to the contraction of a certain bit of smooth muscle, while those arriving at the same muscle by way of neurons of the other division cause it to relax. The two divisions of the autonomic system are thus, in the viscera, functionally antagonistic to each other, with the responses in the muscle and the glands controlled by the system being more or less the result of a balance struck between the activities of the two divisions of the system. However, outside the viscera—for example, in the skin—smooth muscle or secretory cells involved may be innervated by only one or the other of the two divisions of the system. Hence, although the two divisions of the autonomic nervous system may be said to be functionally antagonistic to one another, it does not mean that every structure innervated by the system has innervation from both divisions.

The two divisions of the autonomic nervous systems are termed the *sympathetic* and the *parasympathetic* division, respectively. Both divisions of the system arise in the C.N.S. but from different parts of it (Fig. 17-48). Hence, the neurons by which muscle and

glands are innervated by the two systems travel along different routes. Moreover, *in each system two efferent neurons are always required to join the C.N.S. with each gland or muscle innervated* (Fig. 17-48). The cell body of the first neuron in each efferent chain in each system is situated in the C.N.S. but the cell body of the second is out somewhere in the body in a ganglion of the autonomic system. The two neurons involved in each instance are called preganglionic and postganglionic, respectively. We shall now consider briefly the microscopic structure of the ganglia of the autonomic nervous system and then consider the two systems in more detail, and where the ganglia are located.

Autonomic Ganglia. The ganglia of the autonomic nervous system are generally similar to cerebrospinal ganglia in that both have connective tissue framework and contain ganglion nerve cells. However, there are certain differences. The nerve cells of cerebrospinal ganglia are multipolar and, since they give off many dendrites, they have somewhat more irregular contours than those of cerebrospinal ganglia cells (Fig. 17-49). In general, the nerve cells of autonomic ganglia are smaller than those of cerebrospinal ganglia, and not all of them are surrounded by capsules. Moreover, the nuclei are disposed eccentrically more often than are

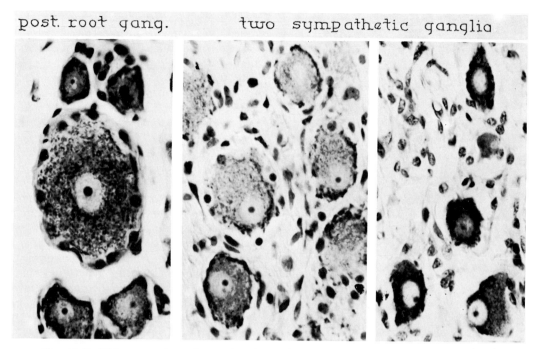

post. root gang.   two sympathetic ganglia

FIG. 17-49. High-power photomicrographs of ganglion cells as they appear in sections stained with cresyl blue. Observe the larger size of the dorsal root ganglion cell on the left and the eccentric distribution of the nuclei in some of the sympathetic ganglion cells.

those of cerebrospinal ganglia cells (Fig. 17-49). The terminal ganglia of the parasympathetic system may be very small; indeed, sometimes a single ganglion cell may be concerned.

The Sympathetic Division. In the thoracic and upper part of the lumbar portion of the spinal cord, a lateral as well as an anterior and a posterior column of gray matter is present. The nerve cell bodies in these lateral columns of gray matter differ somewhat from those in the ventral columns; they are smaller, have fewer Nissl bodies and peripherally rather than centrally disposed nuclei. These cell bodies give rise to thin, lightly myelinated axons which leave the cord by way of the ventral roots to reach the spinal nerves (Figs. 17-50, 17-51 and 17-52), along which they extend to enter the ventral branches of the spinal nerves for only a short distance, whereupon they leave them by way of little nerve trunks (Fig. 17-50) called *white rami communicantes* (*ramus,* branch; *communicans,* communicating; and *white* because the axons are myelinated. Before considering the course of these axons further, it is necessary first to describe the ganglia of the sympathetic division of the autonomic nervous system. According to their position these are called *paravertebral* or *prevertebral* ganglia.

The paravertebral ganglia are disposed in the form

of chains, one on each side of the vertebral column, and are said to constitute two sympathetic *trunks* (Fig. 17-51). In the cervical region there are 3 ganglia in each: the superior, the middle and the inferior cervical ganglia. The middle cervical ganglia are not al-

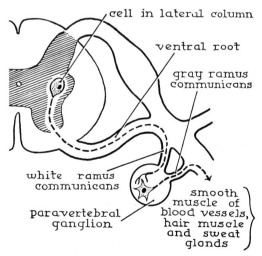

cell in lateral column

ventral root

gray ramus communicans

white ramus communicans

paravertebral ganglion

smooth muscle of blood vessels, hair muscle and sweat glands

FIG. 17-50. Diagram showing one course taken by preganglionic and postganglionic fibers of the sympathetic division of the autonomic nervous system.

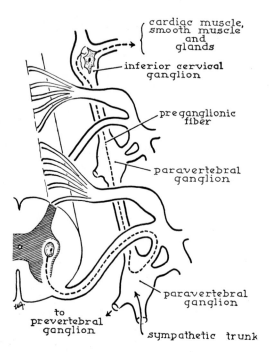

FIG. 17-51. Diagram showing a second course taken by preganglionic and postganglionic fibers of the sympathetic division of the autonomic nervous system.

ways present. In the thoracic region 10 or 11 ganglia are distributed along each side of the vertebral column (Fig. 17-48). In some instances the first thoracic ganglion is fused with the inferior cervical; if so, the fused mass is termed the stellate ganglion. In the lumbar region 4 ganglia are present on each side, and in the sacral region 4 also are present on each side of the vertebral column. Nerve fibers extend between the ganglia in each chain. Since the position and the connections of these ganglia will be presented in detail in other courses, the student should not attempt to obtain anything but a general knowledge of them at this time (see Fig. 17-48, *right*).

The prevertebral ganglia constitute a group of ganglia that lie in front of the vertebral column and in closer association with the viscera than do the paravertebral ganglia. There are 3 of them—the celiac ganglion, the superior mesenteric and the inferior mesenteric. An extension of the last may be present in the pelvis. These, too, will be learned about in detail in other courses, so the names need not be memorized here.

The axons from the bodies of nerve cells in the lateral column of the spinal cord, which we have traced to the white rami communicantes, end either in the paravertebral (Figs. 17-50 and 17-51) or the preverte-

bral (Fig. 17-52) ganglia. Therefore they are all called preganglionic fibers. They reach one or the other of these ganglia by 3 different routes, a description of which is rather the prerogative of gross anatomy and neuroanatomy than histology. However, for the convenience of the interested student, the 3 routes are illustrated in Figures 17-50, 17-51 and 17-52.

The number of postganglionic fibers that emerge from a sympathetic ganglion is considerably greater than the number of preganglionic fibers that enter it. Preganglionic fibers, then, in ganglia must enter into synaptic relation with many different neurons whose cell bodies are situated in that ganglion. This arrangement allows ganglia to serve as instruments for broadening the stream of nervous impulses that enter them.

The Parasympathetic Division. Nerve fibers belonging to the parasympathetic division of the system also innervate most of the glands and muscles innervated by the sympathetic division, and, as noted before, the two systems are to some extent antagonistic to each other. Between each structure innervated by the parasympathetic division and the C.N.S., from which the parasympathetic division arises, a chain of two efferent neurons is always to be found.

The parasympathetic division has its origin from two widely separated parts of the C.N.S. The bodies of the nerve cells that give rise to one group of its preganglionic fibers are situated in nuclei of gray matter in the medulla and the midbrain, and the pregangli-

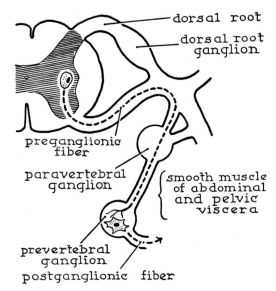

FIG. 17-52. Diagram showing a third course taken by preganglionic and postganglionic fibers of the sympathetic division of the autonomic nervous system.

onic fibers arising from these cell bodies make their way out of the C.N.S. by way of the 3rd, 7th, 9th and 10th cranial nerves (Fig. 17-48, *left*). The cell bodies from which the remainder of its preganglionic fibers arise are found in the lateral column of the sacral portion of the spinal cord, and they make their way out of the C.N.S. by way of the 2nd, 3rd and 4th sacral spinal nerves, which they soon leave by way of the visceral rami of these nerves (Fig. 17-48, *bottom, left*).

Since the preganglionic fibers of the parasympathetic division of the autonomic system emerge by way of cranial and sacral nerves from the C.N.S., the parasympathetic division is also termed the craniosacral division of the autonomic system (in contrast to the thoracolumbar division).

The preganglionic fibers of the parasympathetic division are, in general, longer than those in the sympathetic division, and with certain exceptions, they proceed all the way to the muscle or the gland with whose innervation they are concerned. When they approach the gland or the muscle, they generally end in small ganglia that are closely associated, particularly in the viscera, with the gland or the muscle innervated. These are sometimes called *terminal ganglia*, and in them the preganglionic fibers come into synaptic relation with the second neurons, whose cell bodies are situated in the terminal ganglia, and send axons, the postganglionic fibers, to the nerve endings in muscle or gland. The postganglionic axons are, then, generally short.

However, in the head region the ganglia of the parasympathetic division of the system are not within, or on the surface of, the gland or the muscle innervated, and in these instances the postganglionic fibers are correspondingly longer (Fig. 17-48, *top, left*).

NERVE ENDINGS IN THE AUTONOMIC NERVOUS SYSTEM

The endings of the postganglionic fibers of the sympathetic and the parasympathetic systems in smooth or cardiac muscle or glands cannot be seen in H and E sections, although the terminal ganglia of the parasympathetic system show to advantage (Fig. 21-43). The ways that nerve endings on muscle cells are demonstrated, and their fine structure, are described in the next chapter. However, the endings of the efferent fibers of the autonomic system are essentially like the termination of a presynaptic neuron at a synapse and the stimulation of a muscle or gland cell is effected by the nervous impulse causing a release of the contents of vesicles containing a chemical mediator (as shown in Figure 17-20) which induces a response in a smooth

muscle or glandular secretory cell. For the demonstration of the nerve endings of the fibers of the autonomic system in muscle or glands, special technics are necessary. Silver impregnation methods or the treatment of fresh tissue by methylene blue are commonly employed to reveal them. Even with these special technics it is difficult to establish definitely how and where the fibers end. However, the EM has disclosed that nerve endings on smooth muscle cells are somewhat similar to the motor end plates on striated muscle fibers which are described in the next chapter. The nerve endings of the autonomic system at secretory cells will now be described.

HOW NERVOUS IMPULSES FROM THE AUTONOMIC NERVOUS SYSTEM AFFECT THE SECRETORY PROCESS OF THE CELLS OF EXOCRINE GLANDS

The chemical mediation of the nervous impulse was described at some length in connection with synapses. In the development of knowledge about the autonomic system it was at first concluded that parasympathetic endings elaborated acetylcholine and endings of the sympathetic system elaborated norepinephrine. However, it was found later that some sympathetic fibers could elaborate acetylcholine, for it was shown that although the innervation of the sweat glands of the skin is provided by sympathetic fibers the chemical transmitter at their endings at sweat glands is acetylcholine. Accordingly, it became usual to class the fibers of the autonomic system, not necessarily as to whether they were parasympathetic fibers or sympathetic fibers but as to whether they were adrenergic (which means the chemical mediator they elaborate is norepinephrine), or cholinergic (which means their endings elaborate acetylcholine). In the instance of the sweat glands of the skin this means, for example, that cholinergic fibers are controlled by activities of the sympathetic division of the autonomic nervous system. Both adrenergic and cholinergic fibers are found to innervate secretory cells of many glands—for example, the parotid gland of rats as will be described shortly. It should perhaps be pointed out, however, that there seems to be a considerable variation with regard to the innervation of the parotid and other salivary glands in other species.

As Hand, from whose studies Figures 17-53 and 17-54 were provided, points out, the term nerve ending is not appropriate for describing the innervation of the secretory cells of glands. The reason for this is that the axons responsible for the innervation do not necessarily possess a single terminal bulb that is applied

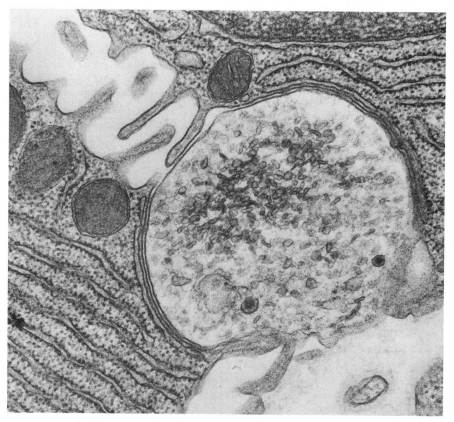

FIG. 17-53. Electron micrograph ($\times$ 65,750) showing a bulb of an axon lying between the sides of the basal parts of two acinar cells of a secretory unit of the parotid gland of a rat. The bulb contains vesicles which presumably contain the neurotransmitter. Note that the bulb is not separated from the acinar cells by basement membrane. The acinar cells in contact with the bulb have cytoplasm that is rich in both free ribosomes and rER. Note that the cisterna of ER that closely approaches the bulb and runs parallel with it has no ribosomes on its outer surface but that its inner surface that faces the cytoplasm of the acinar cells has ribosomes on it. (From Hand, A. R.: J. Cell Biol., *47:* 540, 1970)

closely to the particular cells it will affect by elaborating a chemical mediator as appears to be the case in Figure 17-53. Instead, an axon may possess several swellings along its terminal part (Fig. 17-54) each of which can elaborate a chemical mediator, and so the influence of a single axon is not limited to one particular site as a single end bulb at an axon termination would be.

In order for nerve fibers to serve acinar cells they must first be conducted in the connective tissue that lies between acini. Here the fibers are covered by sheath of Schwann cells (Fig. 17-54) and sometimes more than one fiber is enclosed by the same Schwann cell. Usually the axon sheds its Schwann cell covering as, or before, it penetrates the basal lamina of an acinar cell so that a bulb can come into very close contact with the cell membrane of the acinar cell as is seen in Figure 17-53. However, this does not always happen, for sometimes relatively close contact is achieved with the bulbs along axons not having lost their Schwann cell covering as in Figure 17-54.

Hand describes two types of bulbs that serve as the source of a chemical mediator in the rat parotid. About two thirds of them contain granular vesicles that are from 300 to 700 Å in diameter and have dense cores from 130 to 300 Å in diameter. The evidence indicates that these are adrenergic. The remaining one third of the bulbs contain mostly small agranular vesicles but they also contain a few much larger vesicles. These bulbs are considered to be cholinergic.

The way in which the release of a chemical mediator affects the function of a secretory cell is not understood. Hand, however, notes that a cisterna of endoplasmic reticulum can often be seen close to, and parallel with, the cell membrane of the acinar cell at the site where an axon bulb is present; this occurs with both adrenergic and cholinergic types of bulb. The side of the cistern that faces the bulb is devoid of ribosomes but the other side of the cistern is covered with ribosomes. These structures which may be found to have something to do with how the chemical mediator affects secretion are to be seen in Figures 17-53 and 17-54.

The number of bulbs associated with an acinus varies. Hand discusses the possibility that gap (nexus) type junctions between acinar cells may be instru-

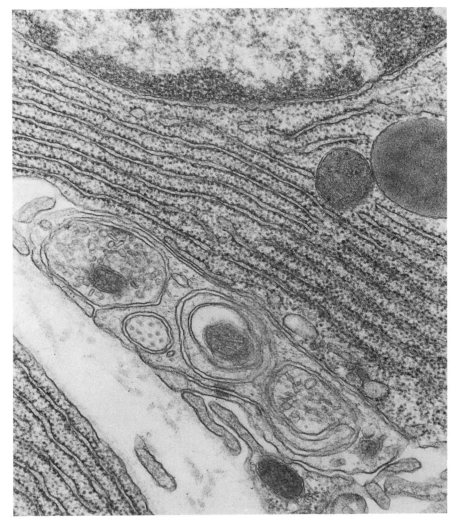

FIG. 17-54. Electron micrograph showing 4 axons within the cytoplasm of a Schwann cell at the base of an acinar cell of the rat parotid gland. Here as well as in Figure 17-53 there is a cisterna of ER lying close to, and parallel with, the area where it might be expected that chemical mediation would occur; note that this cisterna has no ribosomes on the surface that is closest to the axon bulbs. (Illustration courtesy of Arthur R. Hand)

mental in transmitting stimulation from one or more cells throughout a whole secretory unit.

References and Other Reading

See also Textbooks on the Nervous Systems, Neuroanatomy, Gross Anatomy, Neurophysiology and Neurology.

GENERAL

Bourne, G. H. (ed.): Structure and Function of Nervous Tissue. New York, Academic Press, vol. 1, 1968; vols. 2 and 3, 1969; vols. 4 and 5, 1972.

Penfield, W.: Cytology and Cellular Pathology of the Nervous System. vols. 1. 2 and 3. New York, Hoeber, 1932.

Peters, A., Palay, S. L., and Webster, H. de F.: The Fine Structure of the Nervous System: The Cells and Their Processes. New York, Harper and Row, 1970.

SPECIAL

Central Nervous System

Barr, M. L., and Hamilton, J. D.: A quantitative study of certain morphological changes in motor neurons during axon reaction. J. Comp. Neurol., *89:*93, 1948.

Bodian, D.: A note on the nodes of Ranvier in the central nervous system. J. Comp. Neurol., *94:*475, 1951.

———: The generalized vertebrate neuron. Science, *137:*323, 1962.

———: An electron microscope study of the monkey spinal cord. I. Fine structure of normal motor column; II. Effects of retrograde chromatolysis; III. Cytological effects of mild and virulent poiio virus infection. Bull. Johns Hopkins Hosp., *114:*13, 1964.

Brightman, M. W.: The distribution within the brain of ferritin injected into cerebrospinal fluid compartments. II. Parenchymal distribution. Am. J. Anat., *117:*193, 1965.

Brightman, M. W., and Reese, T. S.: Junctions between intimately apposed cell membranes in the vertebrate brain. J. Cell Biol., *40:*648, 1969.

Bunge, R. P.: Glial cells and the central myelin sheath. Physiol. Rev., *48:*197, 1968.

Bunge, R. P., Bunge, M. B., and Ris, H.: Ultrastructural study of remyelination in an experimental lesion in adult cat spinal cord. J. Biophys. Biochem. Cytol., *10:*67, 1961.

Caley, D. W., and Maxwell, D. S.: Development of the blood vessels and extracellular spaces during postnatal maturation of rat cerebral cortex. J. Comp. Neurol., *138:*31, 1970.

———: An electron microscopic study of neurons during postnatal development of the rat cerebral cortex. J. Comp. Neurol., *133:*17, 1968.

Cameron, G.: Secretory activity on the choroid plexus in tissue Culture. Anat. Rec., *117:*115, 1953.

Causey, G.: The cell of Schwann. Edinburgh, E. & S. Livingstone, 1960.

Finean, J. B.: The nature and stability of nerve myelin. Int. Rev. Cytol., *12:*303, 1961.

Gabe, M.: Neurosecretion. Oxford, Pergamon Press, 1966.

Gray, E. G., and Guillery, R. W.: Synaptic morphology in the normal and degenerating nervous system. Int. Rev. Cytol., *19:*111, 1966.

Haggar, R. A., and Barr, M. L.: Quantitative data on the size of synaptic end-bulbs in the cat's spinal cord; with a note on the preparation of cell models. J. Comp. Neurol., *93:*17, 1950.

Hess, A., and Young, J. Z.: Nodes of Ranvier in the central nervous system. J. Physiol., *108:*52P, 1949.

Heuser, J. E., and Reese, T. S.: Evidence for recycling of synaptic vesicle membrane during transmitter release of the frog neuro-muscular junction. J. Cell Biol., *57:*315, 1973.

Hudson, A. J., and Smith, C. G.: The vascular pattern of the choroid plexus of the lateral ventricle. Anat. Rec., *112:*43, 1952.

King, J. S.: A light and electron microscopic study of perineuronal glial cells and processes in the rabbit neocortex. Anat. Rec., *161:*111, 1968.

Kruger, L., and Maxwell, D. S.: Electron microscopy of oligodendrocytes in normal rat cerebrum. Am. J. Anat., *118:*411, 1966.

Kuffler, S. W., Nicholls, J. G., and Orkand, R. K.: Physiological properties of glial cells in the central nervous system of amphibia. J. Neurophysiol., *29:*768, 1966.

Ling, E. A., Patterson, J. A., Privat, A., Mori, S., and Leblond, C. P.: Identification of glial cells in the brain of young rats. J. Comp. Neurol., *149:*43, 1973.

McEwen, B. S., and Graftsein, B.: Fast and slow components in axonal transport of protein. J. Cell Biol., *38:*494, 1968.

Maxwell, D. S., and Pease, D. C.: Electron microscopy of the choroid plexus. Anat. Rec., *123:*331, 1956.

Mori, S., and Leblond, C. P.: Identification of microglia in light and electron microscopy. J. Comp. Neurol., *155:*57, 1969.

———: Electron microscopic features and proliferation of astrocytes in the corpus callosum of the rat. J. Comp. Neurol., *157:*197, 1969.

———: Electron microscopic identification of three classes of oligodendrocytes and a study of their proliferative activity in the corpus callosum of young rats. J. Comp. Neurol., *139:*1, 1970.

Orkland, R. K., Nicholls, J. G., and Kuffler, S. W.: Effects of nerve impulses on the membrane potential of glial cells in the central nervous system of amphibia. J. Neurophysiol., *29:*788, 1966.

Palay, S. L.: Structure and function in the neuron. *In* Korey, S. R., and Nurnberger, J. I. (eds.): Trends in Neurochemistry and Allied Fields. vol. 1. New York, Hoeber, 1955.

———: Synapses in the central nervous system. J. Biophys. Biochem. Cytol., (Suppl.) *2:*193, 1956.

———: The structural basis for neural action. *In* Brazier, M. A. B. (ed.): Brain Function. vol. 2, p. 69. Berkeley, University of California Press, 1963.

Palay, S. L., and Palade, G. E.: The fine structure of neurons. J. Biophys. Biochem. Cytol., *1:*69, 1955.

Patterson, J. A., Privat, A., Ling, E. A., and Leblond, C. P.: Transformation of subependymal cells into glial cells as shown by radioautography after ³H thymidine injection into the lateral ventricles of the brain of young rats. J. Comp. Neurol., *149:*73, 1973.

Pease, D. C., and Schultz, R. L.: Electron microscopy of rat cranial meninges. Am. J. Anat., *102:*301, 1958.

Weed, L. H.: The cerebrospinal fluid. Physiol. Rev., *2:*171, 1922.

———: Certain anatomical and physiological aspects of the meninges and cerebrospinal fluid. Brain, *58:*383, 1935.

———: Meninges and cerebrospinal fluid. J. Anat., *72:*181, 1938.

Wislocki, G. B.: The cytology of the cerebrospinal pathways. *In* Cowdry's Special Cytology. ed. 2, p. 1485. New York, Hoeber, 1932.

Woollam, D. H. M., and Millen, J. W.: The perivascular spaces of the mammalian central nervous system and their relation to the perineuronal and subarachnoid spaces. J. Anat., *89:*193, 1955.

Peripheral Nervous System

Droz, B., and Leblond, C. P.: Axonal migration of proteins in the central nervous system and peripheral nerves as shown by radioautography. J. Comp. Neurol., *121:*325, 1963.

Fernand, V. S. V., and Young, J. Z.: The sizes of the nerve fibers of muscle nerves. Proc. Roy. Soc. (Biol.), *139:*38, 1951.

Geren, B. B., and Raskind, J.: Development of the fine structure of the myelin sheath in sciatic nerves of chick embryos. Proc. Nat. Acad. Sci., *39:*880, 1953.

———: The formation from the Schwann cell surface of myelin in the peripheral nerves of chick embryos. Exp. Cell Res., *7:*558, 1954.

———: Structural studies on the formation of the myelin sheath in peripheral nerve fibers. *In* Cellular Mechanisms in Differentiation and Growth. Princeton, N.J., Princeton University Press, 1956.

Geren, B. B., and Schmitt, F. O.: Electron microscope studies of the Schwann cell and its constituents with particular reference to their relation to the axon. *In* Fine Structure of Cells. p. 251. Groningen, Holland, Noordhoff, 1955.

Hess, A.: The fine structure of young and old spinal ganglia. Anat. Rec., *123:*399, 1955.

Hess, A., and Lansing, A. I.: The fine structure of peripheral nerve fibers. Anat. Rec., *117:*175, 1953.

Lavarack, J. O., Sunderland, S., and Ray, L. J.: The branching of nerve fibers in human cutaneous nerves. J. Comp. Neurol., *94:*293, 1949.

Nathaniel, E. S. H., and Nathaniel, D.: The ultrastructural features of the synapses in the posterior horn of the spinal cord in the rat. J. Ultrastruct. Res., *14:*540, 1966.

Peterson, E. R., and Murray, M. R.: Myelin sheath formation in cultures of avian spinal ganglia. Am. J. Anat., *96*:319, 1955.

Robertson, J. D.: The unit membrane of cells and mechanism of myelin formation. *In* Ultrastructure and Metabolism of the Nervous System. p. 94. Proc. Assoc. Res. Nerv. Ment. Dis. Baltimore, Williams & Wilkins, 1962.

Shanklin, W. M., and Azzam, N. A.: Histological and histochemical studies on the incisures of Schmidt-Lanterman. J. Comp. Neurol., *123*:5, 1964.

Shanthaveerappa, T. R., and Bourne, G. H.: The "perineural epithelium," a metabolically active, continuous, protoplasmic cell barrier surrounding peripheral nerve fasciculi. J. Anat., *96*:527, 1962.

Steer, J. C., and Horney, F. D.: Evidence for passage of cerebrospinal fluid along spinal nerves. Canad. Med. Assoc. J., *98*:71, 1968.

Weiss, P., and Hiscoe, H. B.: Experiments on the mechanism of nerve growth. J. Exp. Zool., *107*:315, 1948.

Nerve Regeneration

Bacsich, P., and Wyburn, G. M.: The effect of interference with the blood supply on the regeneration of peripheral nerves. J. Anat., *79*:74, 1945.

Bueker, D., and Meyers, E.: The maturity of peripheral nerves at the time of injury as a factor in nerve regeneration. Anat. Rec., *109*:723, 1951.

Clark, E. R., and Clark, E. L.: Microscopic studies on regeneration of medullated nerves in living mammal. Am. J. Anat., *81*:233, 1947.

Guth, L.: Regeneration in the mammalian peripheral nervous system. Physiol. Rev., *36*:441, 1956.

Gutmann, E., and Guttmann, L.: Factors affecting recovery of sensory function after nerve lesions. J. Neurol. Psychiat., *5*:117, 1942.

Gutmann, E., Guttmann, L., Medawar, P. B., and Young, J. Z.: The rate of regeneration of nerve. J. Exp. Biol., *19*:14, 1942.

Gutmann, E., and Sanders, F. K.: Functional recovery following nerve grafts and other types of nerve bridge. Brain, *65*:373, 1942.

———: Recovery of fiber numbers and diameters in the regeneration of peripheral nerves. J. Physiol., *101*:489, 1943.

Highet, W. B., and Sanders, F. K.: The effects of stretching nerves after suture. Brit. J. Surg., *30*:355, 1943.

Holmes, W., and Young, J. Z.: Nerve regeneration after immediate and delayed suture. J. Anat., *77*:63, 1942.

Ramon y Cajal, S.: Degeneration and Regeneration of the Nervous System. London, Oxford, 1928.

Sanders, F. K.: The repair of large gaps in the peripheral nerves. Brain, *65*:281, 1942.

Sanders, F. K., and Young, J. Z.: The degeneration and reinnervation of grafted nerves. J. Anat., *76*:143, 1941.

Seddon, H. J.: Three types of nerve injury. Brain, *66*:237, 1943.

———: War injuries of peripheral nerves. Brit. J. Surg. (War Surg., Suppl. No. 2), p. 325, 1948.

Seddon, H. J., Medawar, P. B., and Smith, H.: Rate of regeneration of peripheral nerves in man. J. Physiol., *102*:191, 1943.

Sunderland, S.: The capacity of regenerating axons to bridge long gaps in nerves. J. Comp. Neurol., *99*:481, 1953.

———: Capacity of reinnervated muscles to funtion efficiently after prolonged denervation. Arch. Neurol. Psychiat., *64*:755, 1950.

———: A classification of peripheral nerve injuries producing loss of function. Brain, *74*:491, 1951.

———: Factors influencing the course of regeneration and the quality of the recovery after nerve suture. Brain, *75*:19, 1952.

———: Rate of regeneration in human peripheral nerves. Arch. Neurol. Psychiat., *58*:251, 1947.

Windle, W. F.: Regeneration of axons in the vertebrate central nervous system. Physiol. Rev., *36*:427, 1956.

Young, J. Z.: The effect of delay on the success of nerve suture. Proc. Roy. Soc. Med., *37*:551, 1944.

———: Effects of use and disuse on nerve and muscle. Lancet, *2*:109, 1946.

———: Factors influencing the regeneration of nerves. Advances Surg., *1*:165, 1949.

———: Histology of peripheral nerve injuries. *In* Cope, Z. (ed.): Medical History of the Second World War: Surgery. p. 534. London, Her Majesty's Stat. Off., 1953.

———: Structure, degeneration and repair of nerve fibers. Nature, *156*:132, 1945.

Young, J. Z., Holmes, W., and Sanders, F. K.: Nerve regeneration—importance of the peripheral stump and the value of nerve grafts. Lancet, *2*:128, 1940.

Blood Supply of Nerves

Adams, W. E.: The blood supply of nerves. J. Anat., *76*:323, 1942.

Sunderland, S.: Blood supply of the nerves of the upper limb in man. Arch. Neurol. Psychiat., *53*:91, 1945.

———: Blood supply of peripheral nerves. Arch. Neurol. Psychiat., *54*:280, 1945.

———: Blood supply of the sciatic nerve and its popliteal divisions in man. Arch. Neurol. Psychiat., *54*:283, 1945.

Nerve Endings

For Afferent Endings *see* Chapter 28.
For Efferent Endings in Muscle *see* next chapter.
For the Fine Structure of Nerve Endings in Secretory Organs, *see below*.

Hand, A. R.: Nerve-acinar relationships in the rat parotid gland. J. Cell Biol., *47*:540, 1970.

———: Adrenergic and cholinergic nerve terminals in the rat parotid gland. Electron microscopic observations on permanganate-fixed glands. Anat. Rec., *173*:131, 1972.

18 Muscle Tissue

Introduction. Muscle tissue, the fourth basic tissue, is highly specialized for contractility. The early anatomists by dissection found that muscles are composed of elongated structures which they called *fibers*. With the advent of the LM and the cell theory, each muscle fiber was shown to be a cell. Some kinds, however, are so large they have many nuclei. Despite the realization that muscle fibers are living structures they are still usually called fibers—which at first may be confusing to a beginner who has just learned about collagenic fibers which, of course, are composed of a nonliving material.

The most impressive feature of a muscle fiber is that on stimulation it shortens in its long axis, thus pulling the attachments of its two ends closer together. In performing this work muscle fibers in effect act as tiny engines that perform work by burning (metabolizing) fuel (food) at a relatively low temperature with an efficiency that is probably only equaled by excellent diesel engines. Their operation causes no pollution—indeed, the CO_2 they produce, and which the animal body exhales, is used for the growth of plants—and, finally, they operate noiselessly. How they could perform the mechanical function of contracting posed a problem for decades. The advent of the EM permitted studies to be made which disclosed that the mechanical function was performed at the level of longitudinally disposed protein filaments within the fiber which were so fine they could not be seen with the LM. The filaments were found to be of two types; one kind, the thicker, was found to contain the protein myosin and the other, thinner kind, the protein actin. In a relaxed fiber these two types of filaments were found to interdigitate but only over part of their lengths. But when a fiber was stimulated, the attraction between them became so great they slid along each other until their interdigitation was complete. As will be described in detail later, the attachments of the filaments within the fiber are such that the complete interdigitation of the filaments can only be achieved by their pulling the two ends of the fiber closer together. With this introductory information we shall now describe the types of muscle tissue.

Three Kinds of Muscle Tissue. They are all composed of muscle fibers but differ from one another in microscopic structure, distribution, innervation and the particular kind of function they perform. The most typical and most thoroughly investigated is called *striated muscle* for reasons soon to be explained. This is the kind that is connected to the bones of the skeleton and is the most abundant kind in the body. The second type is microscopically similar; it is found in the walls of the heart and pulmonary veins and is known as the *cardiac muscle*. Both striated and cardiac muscle fibers contain similar filaments, whose actin and myosin have been thoroughly investigated. The third kind, referred to as *smooth muscle*, appears to be somewhat different from the other two; it is found in the walls of viscera and blood vessels. The contraction of smooth muscle differs in several ways from that of other muscles, particularly in being rather slow. Although smooth muscle contains actin and myosin components, they are somewhat different from the corresponding proteins in striated and cardiac muscle, and resemble those found in the other cell types endowed with some contractility or in cell derivatives such as blood platelets.

Because striated muscle may serve as a model, it will be described first and in greater detail than the other two types.

Striated Muscle

This is the kind that makes up what people call their muscles. With striated muscle man performs voluntary actions; these may require a rapid, powerful contraction (for example, throwing a baseball) or maintaining a prolonged state of partial contraction (for example, holding the head erect; this is called tonus).

Striated muscle fibers may be of considerable length, so much so that they possess many nuclei, the number of which is proportional to their volume (Moss). The name striated (or striped) was given this kind of muscle because, with the LM, the fibers reveal cross striations (Figs. 18-1 and 18-3). It is also referred

Fig. 18-1. Striated muscle fibers cut longitudinally. Cross striations are evident in all fibers but show subtle variabilities due to fixation and contractile state. All muscle nuclei are peripherally placed, but sometimes appear to be in the center of the fibers due to the plane of section. Two nuclei of connective tissue cells between muscle fibers are labeled. (Illustration by E. Schultz and C. P. Leblond)

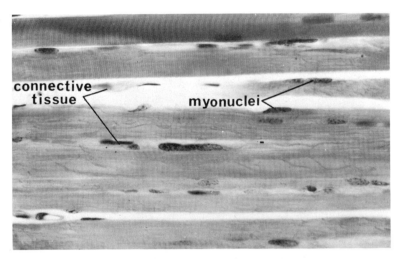

to as *skeletal muscle* because it is generally attached to the skeleton and responsible for moving bones or as *voluntary muscle* because it is usually under the control of the conscious mind.

Striated muscle fibers are cylindrical in form, measuring from 1 to 40 mm. in length and from 10 to 40 μ in width. They are multinucleated cells. The nuclei are elongated ovoids and, in the striated muscles of man and most, but not all, animals they are situated in the peripheral cytoplasm of the cylindrically shaped fibers. This fact helps the student distinguish striated from smooth and cardiac muscle, for in the latter two the nuclei have a more central position in the fiber. The peripheral distribution of striated muscle fiber nuclei is seen to advantage in cross sections (Fig. 18-2). In longitudinal sections, there may be some ambiguity, since a peripheral nucleus viewed in a longitudinal section grazing the top or bottom of a fiber may seem to be in its middle (Fig. 18-1). Furthermore, individual striated muscle fibers are each enclosed in a delicate connective tissue network containing nuclei of fibroblasts, which are often elongated like those of muscle fibers. In a longitudinal section these may seem, if they are above or beneath the part of the fiber that is present in the section, to be within the fiber. The thinner the section used, the easier will it be to see nuclei at the periphery of longitudinally cut fibers.

Sarcolemma and Basement Membrane. Each striated fiber has, and is enclosed by, a cell (plasma) membrane called the *sarcolemma*. The sarcolemma is part of the muscle fiber but cannot be seen in ordinary sections with the LM because it is very thin, stains poorly, and remains tightly adherent to the sides of the fiber. It is best studied with the EM. The sarcolemma is covered with a layer of PA-Schiff-

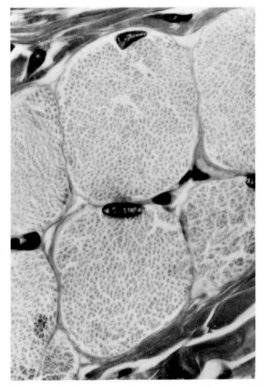

Fig. 18-2. Photomicrograph of cross section of striated muscle fibers. Note myofibrils and peripheral nuclei.

positive material which is of the nature of a basement membrane and, when stained, can be seen with the LM.

Cross Striations. Because of the unevenness of fixation, every longitudinally cut striated muscle fiber seen in an H and E section does not necessarily exhibit cross striations. But a search of different fields in a

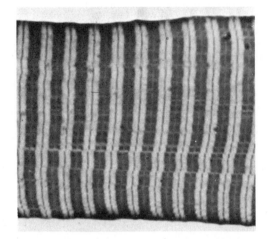

FIG. 18-3. A high magnification (× 2,000) LM photomicrograph of a longitudinal section of a striated muscle fiber, stained with toluidine blue. The thick dark vertical stripes are composed of the A bands of juxtaposed myofibrils, while the light stripes are the I bands (centered by the Z lines). The tiny faint lines running horizontally across the dark A bands are areas of sarcoplasm which slightly separate the myofibrils. The bands of most myofibrils are in exact register with one another to produce continuous striations across the fiber. A sarcomere is the portion of one myofibril between two Z lines. (Courtesy of Dr. E. Schultz)

section, or of other sections, should reveal some fibers that show them (Fig. 18-1).

The cross-striated appearance is due to the cytoplasm of the fiber seeming to consist of alternating bands (sometimes called disks) of light and dark material (Fig. 18-3). With polarized light the bands that seem darker with the ordinary light microscope are anisotropic (birefringent), whereas those that are lighter are isotropic. Accordingly, the darker bands are called A bands (A for anisotropic) and the lighter ones are called I bands (I for isotropic).

In good preparations each I band can be seen to be bisected by a thin dark line; this is called the Z line (Z for the German *Zwischenscheibe*, which means intermediate disk) (Fig. 18-3).

In the usual preparation seen in the LM (Fig. 18-3) the cross striations seem to be continuous from one side of a fiber to the other. But they are not, because a striated muscle fiber consists of two main components: (1) longitudinally disposed myofibrils which are slightly separated from one another, as can be seen to advantage in cross sections of fibers (Fig. 18-2) and which are cross striated, and (2) cytoplasm between the myofibrils which is termed sarcoplasm. The sarcoplasm shows no cross striations but does

contain certain organelles, for example, mitochondria and smooth-surfaced endoplasmic reticulum, as will be described presently. Cross striations are features exclusively found in the myofibrils. The chief reason for cross striation *seeming* to extend from one side of a fiber to the other is that the myofibrils are close together and their cross striations *are approximately, but not perfectly, in register with one another* (Fig. 18-3). In this figure, the A band of one myofibril is separated from the A band of the next one by tiny pale lines of sarcoplasm; yet the A bands remain in register; likewise, the I bands and Z lines are beside their counterparts in adjacent myofibrils. Therefore with the LM, it *seems* that the A and I bands extend as continuous stripes from one side of a fiber to the other.

The portion of one myofibril between two Z lines is termed a *sarcomere*, but before describing it in detail, the differences between the two main types of striated muscle must be examined.

Fiber Types. Nearly all skeletal muscles are an admixture of fibers which belong to two main types: (a) one type characterized by a small diameter and

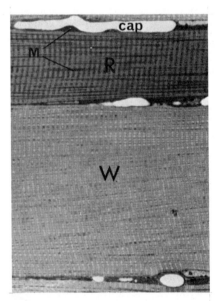

FIG. 18-4. A photomicrograph (× 720) of a longitudinal section of striated skeletal muscle (stained with toluidine blue) which shows the two basic fiber types. The small diameter red fiber (R) contains large numbers of intensely stained mitochondria (M) packed between the myofibrils or in accumulations at the fiber periphery, especially in association with apposed capillaries (cap). The large diameter white fiber (W) contains relatively few mitochondria. (Courtesy of Dr. E. Schultz)

abundance of a reddish protein, myoglobin; a fiber of this type is known as *red fiber* (Fig. 18-4), and (b) one type characterized by a large diameter and a relatively low content of myoglobin, a fiber of this type is known as a *white fiber* (Fig. 18-4). Fibers *intermediate* between these two types are also encountered. Red fibers and, hence, muscles composed predominantly of red fibers are capable of carrying on sustained activity over prolonged periods of time (as required of postural muscles). White fibers, on the other hand, are more suited to short bursts of brisk activity and, with continued demand, will show relatively rapid fatigue. The efficient use of these fiber types in nature can be seen by comparing domestic and wild birds. The domestic fowl, which do little or no flying, have dark meat (that is, red muscle) in the constantly used leg and thigh musculature, while the little-used wing and breast musculature is white. Wild fowl, on the other hand, have red muscle in wing and breast, since flight for long distances requires muscle composed of the fiber types most resistant to fatigue. Certain wing muscles, however, do contain large portions of white muscle which probably aid during the strenuous demands of take-off.

Because of the need for a lasting source of energy, red fibers are richly supplied with capillaries and their sarcoplasm is heavily populated with mitochondria. Characteristic aggregations of the latter are found along the periphery of the fibers. Mitochondria are also packed between myofibrils and run longitudinally behind one another (Fig. 18-4), whereas white fibers have relatively few mitochondria. Histochemical reactions confirm that the enzymes associated with mitochondria (e.g., succinoxidase) are more abundant in red than in white fibers.

The Fine Structure of Sarcomeres

Light microscopy established the presence of A and I bands and also that the I band is bisected by a Z line, all these structures being visible in longitudinal sections (Fig. 18-3). In addition, good preparations of relaxed muscle fibers sometimes show the A band bisected by a relatively narrow light area, the H zone.

In the EM, the myofibrils are seen to be separated by cytoplasm containing mitochondria. In Figure 18-5, the myofibrils at *top right,* are associated with few mitochondria, which are restricted to a region corresponding to the I bands on either side of the Z line; the Z line itself is rather thin (Z_3); such myofibrils belong to a white fiber. In contrast, the lower micrograph in Figure 18-5 shows two red fibers with large accumulations of mitochondria and a rather thick Z line (Z_1).

Each myofibril shows a number of Z lines separated by a constant distance, about 2.4 μm (Fig. 18-6). The material between two Z lines constitutes a sarcomere. Thus a myofibril is composed of successive sarcomeres juxtaposed longitudinally.

As after H and E staining in the LM, the routine lead-uranyl staining in the EM shows the I bands light and the A bands dark (Fig. 18-5). While the I bands contain Z lines, the A bands are bisected by the H zone, in the middle of which a slightly darker line may be distinguished, the M line (Fig. 18-6).

These aspects result from the relative arrangement of the thick myosin-containing filaments and the thin actin-containing filaments. The thick filaments have a diameter of 140 Å and a length of the order of 1.6 micron, whereas the thin filaments have a diameter of 80 Å and extend for 1 micron on either side of the Z line to which they are attached.

The thick filaments characterize the A band and *the thin filaments, the I band,* as seen in Figure 18-7. While the thin filaments are alone in making up the I band, one of their extremities extends into the A band where they interdigitate with the thick filaments, so that both contribute to make the A band stain dark. However, the thin filaments terminate in free ends before reaching the middle of the sarcomere. The gap between the free ends of the thin filaments accounts for the portion of the A band referred to as the H zone. Hence, in this region only the thick filaments are present; the absence of thin filaments here accounts for the H zones being relatively pale. Finally, in the middle, the M line results from the presence of fine threads connecting the central portions of the thick filaments.

Appearance of Bands in Cross Section. Cross sections cut through the I band of a relaxed fiber will reveal only the thin filaments (Fig. 18-6, *lower left*). Of course, cross sections through much of the A band will reveal both thick and thin filaments (Fig. 18-6; second of the four lower pictures). In this case, the thin filaments are seen in a cross section to be arranged so as to form hexagons, with a thick filament in the center of each hexagon. The thick filaments are arranged so as to form triangles, each of which has a thin filament in its center. Cross sections through the H zone show only the thick filaments (Fig. 18-6; third of lower pictures). Finally, cross sections through the M line show the thick filaments, with fine connections holding them together (last of lower pictures).

Composition. The building block of the *thin filaments* is a molecule with a weight of 42,000 daltons,

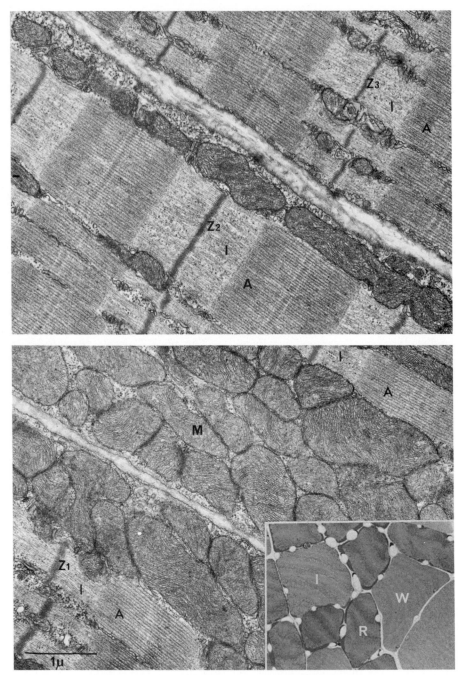

FIG. 18-5. Electron micrographs ($\times$ 33,000) and a photomicrograph (inset, lower right) showing differences between red and white muscle fibers. At the upper right of the top micrograph a white fiber is cut in longitudinal section. It shows small numbers of mitochondria arranged in pairs in the sarcoplasm on each side of the narrow Z line (Z3). The lower micrograph illustrates a red fiber with a large number of mitochondria many of which are arranged in subsarcolemmal aggregations. The Z line here (Z1) is approximately twice the thickness of the one in the white fiber. The lower fiber shown in the top micrograph is of an intermediate type. The thickness of the Z line (Z2) is intermediate between that in red and white fibers.

The inset (lower right) shows the appearances of red, white and intermediate fibers (R, W and I) in cross section as seen with the LM. (Illustration courtesy of Dr. J. P. Dadoune)

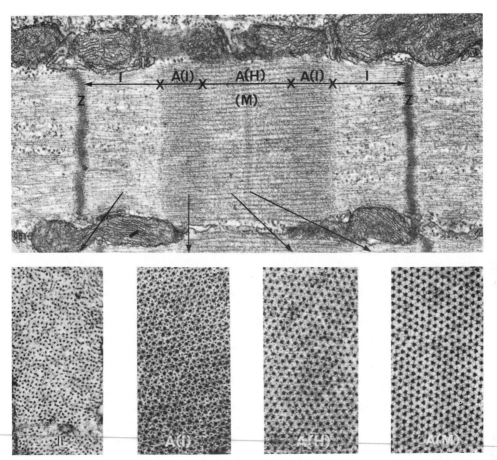

Fig. 18-6. The upper electron micrograph shows a sarcomere, that is, the portion of a myofibril between two Z lines, cut in longitudinal section. On either side of the Z lines are the lightly stained I bands composed entirely of thin actin filaments. The thin filaments extend from the Z line to interdigitate with the darkly stained thick myosin filaments which make up the A band. The region where both thick and thin filaments are present in the A band ✕—A(I)—✕ is darker than the area where only thick filaments are present, that is, the H zone ✕—A(H)—✕. The H zone is bisected by the darker M line of the A band (M), the region where the thick filaments are linked by delicate interconnections.

The appearance of these portions of the sarcomere in cross section is shown in the lower 4 figures. The first one represents cross sections of thin filaments (I); the second shows cross sections of the thick filaments, each one of which is surrounded by 6 thin ones ✕—A(I)—✕; the third shows cross sections of the thick filaments at the beginning of the H zone ✕—A(H)—✕, with a few thin filaments still visible at left, but only thick filaments at center right; the last figure represents cross sections of the thick filaments with fine connections as seen at the M line, A(M). ✕ 33,000. (Illustration provided by E. Schultz and C. P. Leblond)

known as G-actin. Seen in the electron microscope, the molecule is spherical or globular (hence the name G-actin) with a diameter of 56 Å. The G-actin molecules line up in two rows which coil around each other into a long helix (Fig. 18-8) to form the main component of the thin filament. In association with this coil, two additional proteins are found. Tropomyosin is a fibrous, narrow molecule about 400 Å long which runs between the two helicoidal rows of G-actin and is represented as two continuous thin rods in Figure 18-8. Troponin is a complex protein occurring at regular intervals of about 400 Å along the helix (dark in Fig. 18-8). These two proteins play a regulatory role in muscle contraction as will be discussed later. Finally, another protein found in muscle, α actinin, is believed to be a component of the Z line.

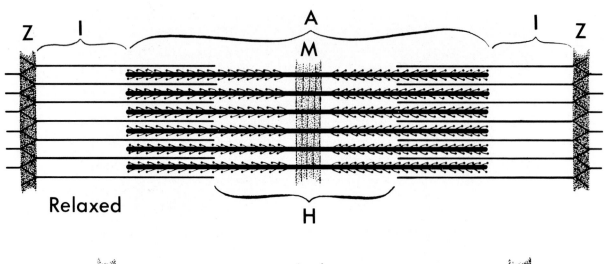

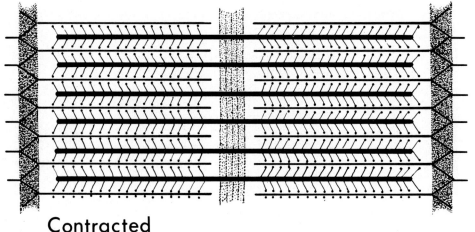

Fig. 18-7. Diagram of a sarcomere in the relaxed state (*above*) and the contracted state (*below*). The sarcomere is the portion of a myofibril between two Z lines. The relaxed sarcomere is composed of two portions of I band (composed of thin actin filaments) located on either side of the darker A band (containing thick myosin filaments). The A band includes a lighter central portion, the H zone, which is centered by the M line. In the relaxed sarcomere the interdigitation of the thick and the thin filaments is at a minimum. As a result the I band and H zone are relatively large. The heads of the myosin molecules projecting from the surface of the thick filaments do not reach the thin filaments. During contraction the tiny processes along the thick filaments, known as myosin heads, interact with the thin filaments and pull them toward the M line, thus causing the Z lines to move toward the free ends of the thick filaments, thereby decreasing the width of the I band and H zone. As another consequence, the distance between the filaments increases, since the filament lattice reflects the increase that occurs in the girth of the muscle belly. The type of movement thought to occur at the molecular level is seen in detail in Figure 18-8. (Illustration provided by E. Schultz and C. P. Leblond)

The *thick filaments* are built from the large (500,000 daltons) myosin molecules. These molecules have an over-all length of about 1,500 Å. Using proteolytic enzymes they can be broken down into two subunits: one is rodlike and measures about 800 Å in length; the other has a rodlike portion which is continuous with the first and is about 600 Å long, but it terminates in a globular double structure referred to as the myosin head (Fig. 18-8). At the point of junction between the two subunits the myosin molecule is flexible, thus allowing the subunits to move in relation to each other.

The myosin molecules are packed together to form

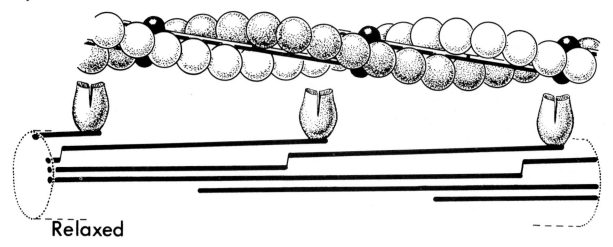

Relaxed

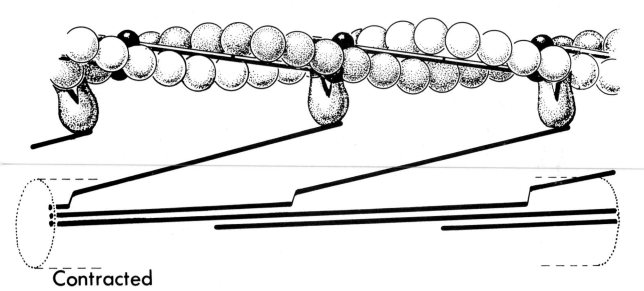

Contracted

FIG. 18-8. A diagram showing the relation between an actin thin filament and a myosin thick filament during relaxation and contraction. The actin filament is made up of globular G-actin monomers aggregated in a manner that forms a helix. Bound to the actin monomers along the length of the helix are long narrow tropomyosin molecules. At regular intervals, globular troponin molecules (dark spheres) are bound to the tropomyosin. These latter two proteins play a regulatory role in the interaction of actin and myosin (after Ebashi et al., 1969). The thick filament is composed of myosin molecules, which consist of two rodlike portions hinged together; one of the portions carries the globular myosin head.

During relaxation the interaction of actin and myosin is inhibited by tropomyosin (under troponin influence) and the myosin heads do not make contact with G-actin monomers. With initiation of contraction, troponin causes tropomyosin to remove the inhibition of the actin-myosin interaction, so that the myosin heads repeatedly couple with active sites on the G-actin monomers.

Because of the increase in the distance between the filaments resulting from the increase in girth of the muscle belly, the swing of the myosin head away from the body of the thick filament must increase to allow continued actin-myosin interactions in prolonged contraction. (Illustration provided by E. Schultz and C. P. Leblond)

the thick filament. The straight portions of the molecules lie parallel to the long axis of the filament, and are oriented so that the head is always on the end of the molecule that is away from the M line (Fig. 18-7). The myosin head is seen in the EM as a tiny projection, which is capable of interacting with G-actin and forming cross bridges during contraction (Fig. 18-7).

The myosin heads are arranged in pairs on either side of thick filaments; the pairs are at intervals of 143 Å along the length of these filaments (Fig. 18-9). The x-ray diffraction studies of Hugh Huxley indicate that each pair of myosin heads is rotated 120° relative to the next pair. Such an arrangement results in 6 rows of myosin heads on the surface of the thick filament, with each row having a myosin head every 429 Å (3 × 143 Å) (Fig. 18-9). Each myosin head approaches the nearest thin filament to form a cross bridge during contraction (Fig. 18-7). There are about 180 to 200 of them per thick filament, which interact with the 6 adjacent thin filaments.

The Changes That Occur as Myofibrils Contract. From the studies of Hugh Huxley it became apparent that the contraction of a sarcomere (and hence of a muscle fiber) does not entail any significant shortening of either the thick or the thin filaments. Contraction of the sarcomere is due to the thin filaments (which extend from each end of the sarcomere toward but, in a relaxed muscle, not reaching its middle) sliding farther and farther into the interstices between the thick filaments (with which they interdigitate). This pulls the Z lines to which they are attached with them, until the free ends of the thin filaments meet in the middle region of the sarcomere. Of course, as the Z lines are pulled closer together, the sarcomere shortens (Fig. 18-7).

Since the relative lack of density of the H zone of the A band in a relaxed myofibril is due to its containing only thick filaments, it is obvious that in a contracted myofibril, in which the thin filaments slide into this area to meet one another, this area will then have both types of filaments and so will be as dense as the rest of the A band (and will no longer be visible). On the other hand, the sliding of the thin filaments between the thick ones pulls the Z line close to the free ends of the thick filaments, so that the I band becomes very small. In cases of extreme contraction, the I band may no longer be visible. In such cases, the extremities of the thin filaments not only meet in the middle of the sarcomere but even pass each other.

From the foregoing it would seem that contraction is due to the thin and the thick filaments suddenly coming to possess an increased attraction for each other, an attraction that results in one kind of filament sliding along the other so that the maximum attachment between their respective surface areas can be obtained.

Molecular Biology of Contraction. The thin filaments are composed of two helicoidal rows of G-actin molecules, with two strands of tropomyosin between the rows and, at 400-Å intervals, the troponin complex (Fig. 18-8). The troponin complex is known to combine with the tropomyosin which, in turn, combines with the G-actin molecules. At a distance of 135 Å from the thin filaments are the thick filaments which are composed exclusively of myosin molecules. The space is bridged, but only partly, by the protruding heads of the myosin molecules which approach but do not make contact with G-actin molecules. This is the situation in the relaxed fiber. The interpretation at the molecular level will be that of Ebashi and his co-workers. In the

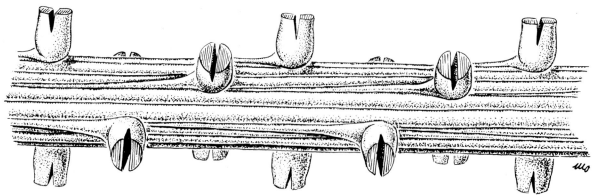

FIG. 18-9. A diagram showing the arrangement of myosin heads that project from the surface of the thick filament. The heads are arranged in pairs, one on each side of the filament, at 143-Å intervals. Each pair is rotated 120 degrees, so that heads appear in the same row every 429 Å (3 × 143 Å). Viewed on end the thick filament exhibits 6 rows of myosin heads. (Illustration provided by E. Schultz and C. P. Leblond)

relaxed myofibril calcium ions are absent, and troponin appears to be combined with tropomyosin, which under these conditions prevents G-actin from interacting with the myosin heads. The mechanism of this inhibition is not clear. Perhaps tropomyosin is located in such a way as to block the reactive sites of G-actin.

When contraction is initiated, the first step is the appearance of calcium ions within the myofibril. It will be shown below how calcium ions are stored nearby and may be released. These ions react with troponin, which then frees the tropomyosin to which it is combined. Perhaps, as a result, tropomyosin moves away from the active sites of G-actin. In any case, the myosin heads combine with G-actin molecules (Fig. 18-8).

Hugh Huxley has observed that, when a muscle contracts, the extent of the sliding of the actin filaments along the myosin filaments is much greater than the distance between any two successive myosin heads on the thick filaments. It has therefore been suggested that, during contraction, the myosin heads alternately disconnect and reconnect to new sites along the actin filament. At each reconnection, there would be a gain of a distance equal to that of the diameter of a G-actin molecule (56 Å) for each sarcomere of a myofibril. The summation of these gains would account for the amplitude of a given muscle contraction. Thus, as contraction occurs, the cross bridges from the myosin filaments probably resemble the feet of a caterpillar in motion, walking along the active parts of actin filaments. The relative displacement of thick and thin filaments in this manner is known as the "sliding filament mechanism" of contraction.

Source of Energy for Muscular Contraction. As calcium ions release the inhibitory effect exerted by troponin through tropomyosin, actin and myosin combine and thus trigger contraction. The energy required is provided by the breakdown of adenosine triphosphate (ATP) to adenosine diphosphate (ADP) and free phosphate ions, a reaction that releases large amounts of energy. However, there is no appreciable store of ATP in the muscle, only about enough for less than 10 brief contractions (in the frog). Since a living muscle obviously can perform many more contractions, the ATP that is broken down during activity must be rapidly restored, so that energy from other sources must be available for the recombination of ADP and phosphate into ATP. This is provided by the splitting of phosphocreatine, a reaction taking place while contraction is in progress. There is enough phosphocreatine available for nearly 100 contractions, but even the store of this substance must also be replenished and other sources of energy are required

for the resynthesis of phosphocreatine and further ATP. This is provided by the combustion of glycogen and other metabolites in the presence of oxygen, but only after the contraction has been completed. There is a large store of glycogen, which on oxidation may yield as much as 10,000 contractions. However, in case the supply of oxygen is insufficient, as may occur during exercise, energy may still be obtained from glycogen anaerobically; in this case glycogen is not oxidized but is transformed into lactic acid; the energy produced is now less, enough for only about 600 contractions.

The Components of Sarcoplasm

Although there are a few ribosomes and a small Golgi apparatus next to each one of the nuclei that are scattered along the periphery of striated muscle fibers, the most prominent organelles seen with the EM are (1) mitochondria, (2) transverse tubules that extend into the fiber from the sarcolemma, and (3) the smooth-surfaced endoplasmic reticulum which, in striated muscle fibers, is termed the *sarcoplasmic reticulum.*

Mitochondria and Glycogen. It was shown above that mitochondria are numerous, particularly in red fibers, and are disposed in rows between the myofibrils in the sarcoplasm (Fig. 18-5). Numerous particles of glycogen also are present in this region. The mitochondria play a role in the reactions involved in the production of the energy required for contraction.

Transverse Tubules. In the frog, in which they have been much studied, the transverse tubules, also known as T-tubules, may begin as a funnel-like invagination of the sarcolemma (Fig. 18-10, *lower left*). Another possibility is for a tubule to open into vesicles which themselves open at the surface. These vesicles, known as caveolae, are numerous below the plasma membrane (Fig. 18-10, *lower center* and *right*). The tubules enter the substance of the fiber more or less at right angles to the surface. They then branch so as to surround every myofibril, while remaining in the same plane as the Z lines, as is shown in the 3-dimensional drawing that comprises Figure 18-11. However, in mammals the tubules surround sarcomeres at the sites of the junctions between A and I bands (rather than at the level of the Z line as in frogs).

The opening of the transverse tubules at the surface of the fiber or in caveolae (Fig. 18-10) was further demonstrated by injection of ferritin, a finely granular but dense material that shows up as black dots in the EM. After injecting this material outside a fiber, it was shown to pass into the lumina of transverse tubules

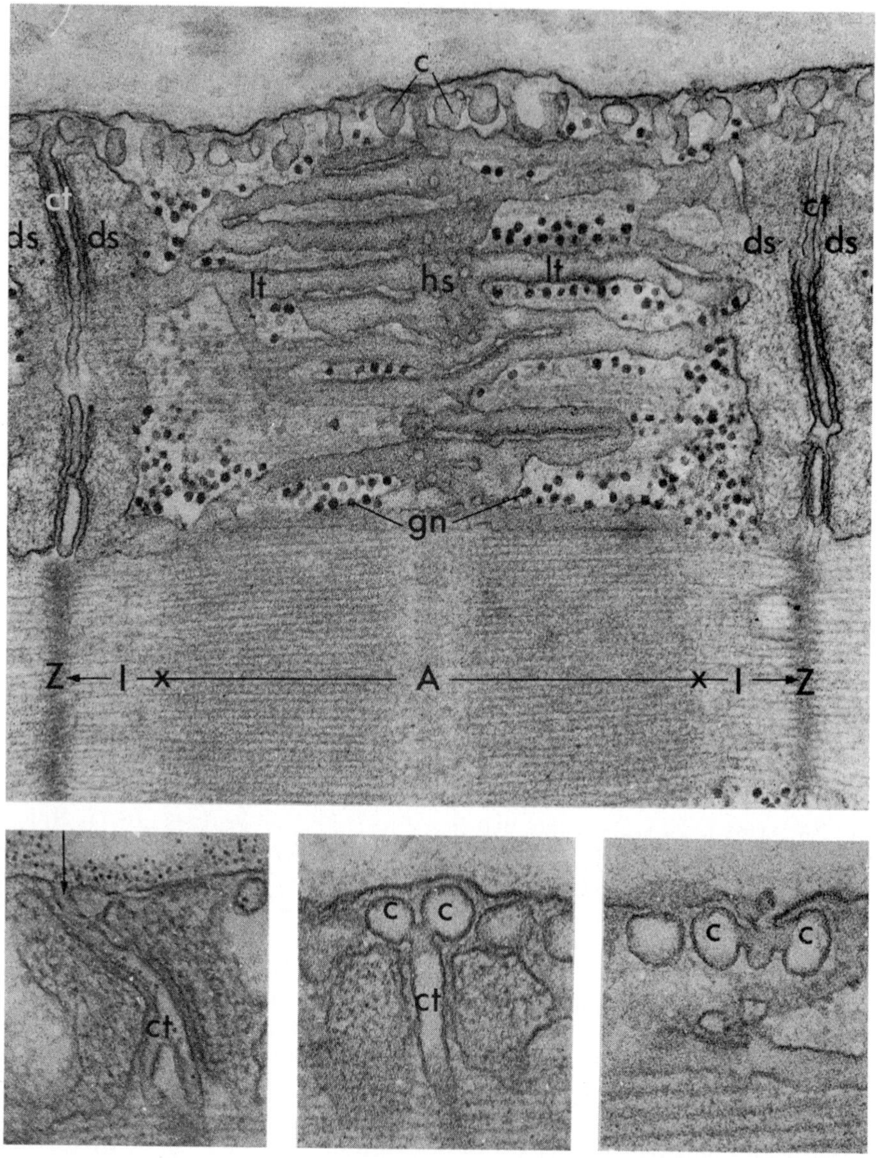

FIG. 18-10. In the top picture, two myofibrils are shown in frog skeletal muscle. The Z line as well as the A and I bands are labeled in the lower of the two myofibrils. The upper myofibril is cut tangentially and shows the sarcoplasmic reticulum. Corresponding to the Z lines are the transverse tubules (ct) at both ends of the sarcomere shown in the figure. These tubules lie closely apposed to the terminal cisternae (ds) of the sarcoplasmic reticulum. Longitudinal channels (lt) run from the terminal cisternae to the fenestrated portion or H-sacs (hs) of the sarcoplasmic reticulum at the center of the sarcomere. Densely stained glycogen (gn) particles are found in the sarcoplasm surrounding the tubules. Finally, the plasma membrane enclosing the muscle fiber is visible at top; immediately below, a number of caveolae (c) may be seen.

The three small pictures at the base of the figure show the plasma membrane. At left, it may be seen that ferritin particles injected into the extracellular space migrate into the transverse tubules (ct) via openings at the surface (arrow). Particles are not present in the terminal cisternae. Of the other two small pictures, the first one illustrates a transverse tubule (ct) opening into two caveolae (c), while the second shows two caveolae (c) opening into a duct connected with the outside. (Courtesy of Dr. R. I. Birks)

(Fig. 18-10, *lower left*), which are therefore continuous with the outside of the fibers. The system of transverse tubules represents, in effect, extremely complex invaginations of the sarcolemma.

The electrical charge on the outer surface of the sarcolemma is approximately the same as that on the outer surface of a nerve fiber, and for the same reasons. When a nerve impulse arrives at a motor nerve ending in a fiber (this will be described presently), the sarcolemma at this site becomes depolarized, and as a result a wave of depolarization progresses rapidly along the sarcolemma. As a result, the fiber contracts. Until relatively recently it was a mystery how the impulse for contraction could be conducted into the interior of the fiber quickly enough for all its parts to contract more or less simultaneously. It seemed impossible that ions could diffuse into the fiber from its surface quickly enough to accomplish this end. Now the system of transverse tubules has been shown to conduct the impulse for contraction into the fiber and into intimate contact with each and every sarcomere. Indeed, Andrew Huxley and his co-workers found that, provided that a tubule was present, a highly localized subthreshold depolarization of the muscle surface (produced by a 5-μm electrode) induced a contraction of individual sarcomeres. When the dose was increased, the contraction spread transversally across the fiber, that is, via the transverse tubules, but never longitudinally along myofibrils.

The manner in which a wave of depolarization conducted by transverse tubules causes the contraction of sarcomeres probably involves the next component of sarcoplasm to be described—the sarcoplasmic reticulum.

The Sarcoplasmic Reticulum. The smooth endoplasmic reticulum, referred to as sarcoplasmic reticulum in striated and cardiac muscle, consists of an array of connected membranous vesicles and channels that lie in the sarcoplasm around the myofibrils (Fig. 18-10, top figure). The membranous structures of the sarcoplasmic reticulum are of three different shapes and sizes. First, flattened cisternae known as terminal cisternae (400 to 1,000 Å wide) surround the I band regions of each sarcomere, so that there is one at each end of each sarcomere (ds in Figs. 18-10 and 18-11). These cisternae are in contact with the transverse tubule running along the Z lines limiting the sarcomere; their flat faces are in contact with one myofibril on one side and the adjacent myofibrils on the other side. Finally, the terminal cisternae connect with the second portion, which is composed of tubular channels (300 to 600 Å in diameter) running longitudinally over the A band (lt in Figs. 18-10 and 18-11).

These channels extend toward the middle of the sarcomere, where they connect with the third portion of the sarcoplasmic reticulum, an irregular branching system of channels that surrounds the myofibril at the level of the H zone; accordingly, these are called H-sacs (hs in Figs. 18-10 and 18-11); they are rather flat, being only 250 to 300 Å thick.

Relation Between the Transverse Tubules and the Sarcoplasmic Reticulum. Near the plasma membrane, the wall of a transverse tubule is smooth, but when it comes into contact with the terminal cisternae of the sarcoplasmic reticulum, the common wall has a beaded appearance (Fig. 18-10). This beaded appearance seems to be associated with the presence of minute units such as are encountered in gap junctions, which units, like those in gap junctions, allow the passage of ions and small molecules. A wave of depolarization coming from the fiber surface would be conducted from the transverse tubules through these minute units to the terminal cisternae of the sarcoplasmic reticulum.

With the EM it may be seen that there is granular material in the terminal cisternae. There is evidence that the granular material binds calcium ions, or at least that the cisternae somehow do so, because by differential centrifugation a calcium-binding fraction is obtained which the EM shows to be composed of large vesicles with the same diameter as the cisternae.

Contraction and Its Initiation. The arrival of a wave of depolarization conducted by a transverse tubule causes the sacs of sarcoplasmic reticulum to release calcium, which diffuses among the myofilaments and initiates contraction. This release of calcium couples the electrical and mechanical events of muscle contraction which, as mentioned above, consist of the following steps: (a) the calcium ions combine with the troponin complex; (b) this combination somehow elicits a release of the blocking by tropomyosin of the active sites of G-actin; (c) one of these active sites combines with a nearby myosin head, thus using up ATP energy as mentioned above. Contraction ensues.

After contraction is completed, the calcium ions leave troponin and diffuse back into the sarcoplasmic reticulum. As a result, tropomyosin again blocks the active sites of G-actin molecules. Relaxation results.

Development and Regeneration of Striated Muscle Fibers

The first sign of development of a striated muscle in embryonic life is the appearance of myoblasts; these are spindle-shaped cells, each with a single nucleus, and they undergo repeated mitosis at a rapid rate.

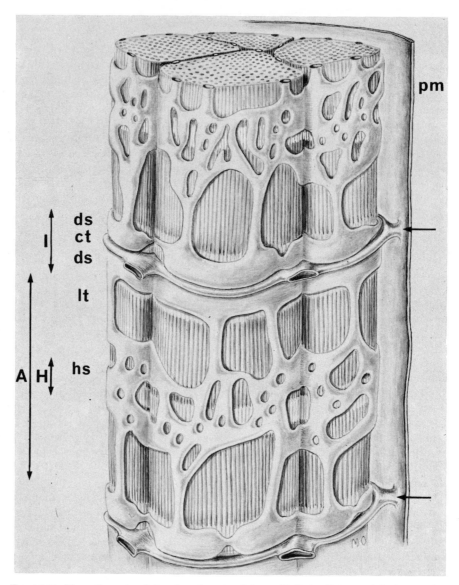

Fig. 18-11. Three-dimensional drawing of parts of 4 myofibrils to illustrate (1) the sarcolemma (labeled pm on the right), (2) the transverse tubules that extend into the substance of the fiber from the sarcolemma (from points indicated by arrows on the right) and (3) the sarcoplasmic reticulum which is interposed, and so lies, between myofibrils, over their I, A, and H portions (labels for the latter on left).

The transverse tubules are delicate tubules which are invaginations of the sarcolemma; hence their walls are composed of cell membrane, and their lumens open onto the outer surface of the sarcolemma. Transverse tubules (in the frog) enter the fiber at the level of Z line (indicated by arrows on right side), and each one branches as it extends across the fiber so as to surround myofibrils whose Z lines are in register with the site where it entered, as is shown by following the two tubules in this illustration, from right to left.

The sarcoplasmic reticulum consists of cisternae and channels of smooth-surfaced endoplasmic reticulum that lie between and so surround myofibrils. In the region of the I band, the extent of which is indicated at the left of the illustration, the cisternae, known as terminal cisternae, are large and flattened, but they may be more or less distended (ds); they lie to either side of the transverse tubule (ct). The cisternae, by means of channels which run longitudinally (lt) over the A band to the region of the H-zone, connect with a network of more or less flattened sacs called the H sacs (hs). The site of the H-zone in the A band is indicated at the left of the illustration. (Illustration courtesy of C. P. Leblond)

Eventually some of the myoblasts stop dividing and fuse into elongated structures known as myotubes. Addition of myoblasts to the myotubes continues; these eventually become long tubules containing large numbers of nuclei. In the myotubes, striated areas appear which become more and more numerous, and eventually each myotube becomes a muscle fiber.

It has been noted that the nuclei of the myotubes themselves do not divide nor do those of postembryonic muscle fibers. However, while the newly formed muscle fibers of the fetus contain relatively few nuclei, those of the adult contain many (Enesco, Moss). Moreover, MacConnachie, Enesco and Leblond observed mitoses within the basement membrane of muscle fibers of growing rats. They suggested that the mitoses were not of true muscle nuclei, but belonged to muscle satellite cells. These are small mononucleated cells located between the basement membrane and the plasma membrane of muscle fibers (Fig. 18-12). They were first observed in the electron microscope by Mauro and are not distinguishable from true muscle nuclei in the light microscope. Moss and Leblond injected ³H-thymidine in order to label the nuclei about to divide in young rats. One hour later many satellite cells, but no true muscle nuclei proved to be labeled. Hence, satellite cells divide, but true muscle nuclei do not. By 24 and 48 hours after the injection, however, both satellite and true muscle nuclei are labeled. Since a dose of ³H-thymidine is metabolized within 1 to 2 hours after injection, it follows that the true muscle nuclei showing label at 24 hours or later must have come from nuclei taking up label immediately after injection, i.e., from satellite cells that had subsequently been incorporated into the fibers. It is concluded that, although true muscle nuclei do not divide, their number increases as a result of division of satellite cells and the subsequent fusion of one or both of the daughter cells into the associated fibers. Satellite cells thus function as myoblasts.

Relation to Regeneration After Injury in Postnatal Life. During muscle regeneration, which may sometimes be seen after injuries to muscle, myoblasts appear which divide, whereas the nuclei in muscle fibers show no mitosis. These myoblasts are likely to be derived from satellite cells (although some believe that true muscle nuclei under these conditions may revert to a myoblast stage). It is more probable that the presence or absence of satellite cells explains why some muscles may and others may not regenerate!

Growth of Muscles in Postnatal Life. This matter is most easily described after we consider how muscles are attached to tendons.

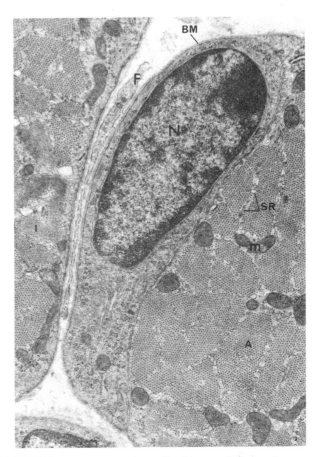

Fig. 18-12. A satellite cell with prominent nucleus (N) lies on the surface of a muscle fiber cut in cross section and is enclosed by the common basement membrane (BM). The myofibrils of this fiber are cut through the A band and show both thick and thin filaments (A). Mitochondria (M) and sarcoplasmic reticulum (SR) may also be distinguished. Some of the myofibrils of the fiber at left are similarly cut, but others are sectioned through the I band (I). A slip of fibroblast cytoplasm (F) lies in the extracellular space between the satellite cell and upper fiber. × 22,000. (Courtesy of Dr. E. Schultz)

How Striated Muscles Are Harnessed and Attached to Tendons

As noted previously, muscle *tissue* does not consist of muscle cells alone; it has a connective tissue component. This, as we shall see, serves several purposes.

Any given muscle may contain connective tissue, not only in its external wrapping but also in internal partitions, so that each one of the fibers of a muscle is embedded within a thin layer of connective tissue

(Fig. 18-1). This layer is associated with the basement membrane covering the sarcolemma.

The various connective tissue elements of a muscle are all continuous with the connective tissue structures to which the muscle is attached, and on which it exerts pull on contraction; this is illustrated very diagrammatically in Figure 18-13. Such a structure may be tendon, aponeurosis, periosteum, dermis of skin, a raphe, or almost any other kind of dense connective tissue structure found in the body. The connective tissue elements of muscle, by being continuous with the connective tissue structures on which muscle pulls, have a function something like a harness. But this is not the only way muscles are attached to the connective tissue structures on which they pull. The sarcolemma covering ends of muscle fibers themselves are also firmly attached to the connective tissue tendon on which they pull. The arrangement seen at the site where fibers are attached to tendons is of interest for another reason; it is here that muscle fibers grow in length, as will be described in the next section.

THE POSTNATAL GROWTH OF STRIATED MUSCLES

Muscles grow both in length and width during the postnatal period. Furthermore, the extent to which they grow in width depends to some extent on exercise. It is of interest to know something about how they grow in size.

It is generally agreed that the *number* of muscle fibers in any given muscle does not increase during the postnatal growing period or as a result even of continued exercise. Muscles become larger because their fibers become larger. The question, therefore, resolves itself into how muscle *fibers* increase in width and in length. We shall first consider growth in width.

Growth in Width of Muscle Fibers. Counts made from examining cross sections of muscle fibers in a given muscle at different times during the growing period have shown that the number of myofibrils in a fiber increases. In the very young there is relatively more sarcoplasm in a muscle fiber than there is later, and it is believed that new myofilaments are synthesized by ribosomes in the sarcoplasm, and that these new myofilaments are added to the exterior of existing myofibrils.

However, as myofibrils do not become larger and larger in diameter as a result of new myofilaments being added to their sides, but instead increase in number, it follows that after they reach a size beyond which they can no longer function efficiently, they split

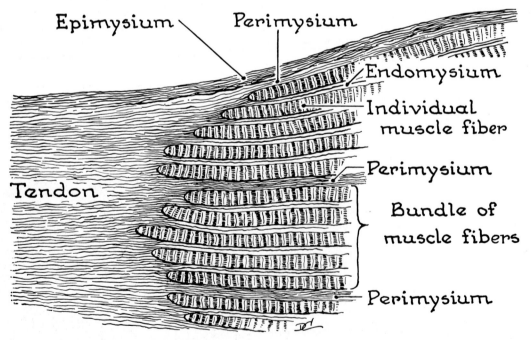

FIG. 18-13. Diagram of a longitudinal section of a muscle, showing how muscles terminate in tendons. The connective tissue embedding the muscle may be given different names: epimysium on the surface, perimysium for the broader partitions between muscle fibers, and endomysium for the thin layer of connective tissue at the surface of the fibers. Through these, the fibers are attached to the connective tissue of the tendon.

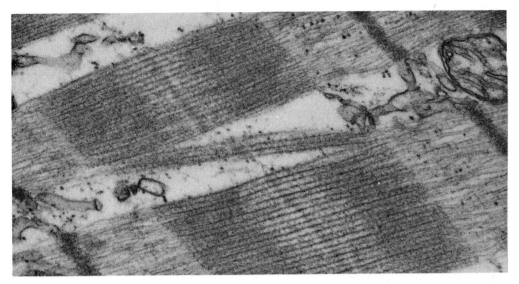

Fig. 18-14. Electron micrograph ($\times$ 43,000) of a portion of a striated muscle close to a tendon junction and from a growing animal. Myofilaments can be seen crossing from one myofibril to another. Such an arrangement of myofilaments might be expected in a region where myofibrils are increasing in number and where individual myofibrils were becoming thicker, and splitting. (Preparation courtesy of T. J. Harrop)

longitudinally, and thus increase in number. The illustration provided by Harrop (Fig. 18-14) shows that the myofilaments in growing muscles can sometimes be traced from one myofibril to another, a state that might well result from a myofibril having split into two myofibrils, but with the splitting process having begun from two different sites.

Growth in Length of Striated Muscles. Muscle fibers become longer during the period of postnatal growth. Goldspink showed that increase in sarcomere length was responsible for only about 25 percent of the lengthening of muscle fibers during that period. Hence the growth in length of a muscle is largely dependent on the production of new sarcomeres. The evidence available indicates that they are not formed anywhere along the course of myofibrils but instead at their ends near the site of insertion of fibers into tendons.

Electron micrographs of this latter site in young growing rats show first (Fig. 18-15) that the sarcolemma of the end of a muscle fiber that meets with a tendon becomes arranged so as to form a series of clefts

Fig. 18-15. An electron micrograph ($\times$ 25,900) showing the muscle-tendon junction in the rat. The muscle cell (at right) tapers quickly at its end where the sarcolemma is thrown into deep folds. In this region, myofibrils attach to the inner surface of the sarcolemma and, on the outer surface, darkly stained collagen fibrils penetrate deeply into the invaginations and attach to the basement membrane. (From Mackey, B., Harrop, T. J., and Muir, A. R.: Acta Anat., *73*:588, 1969)

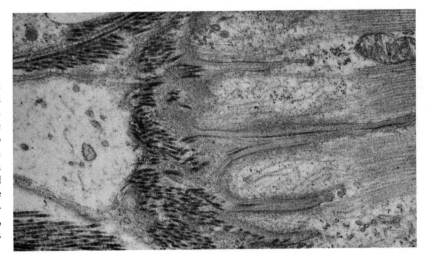

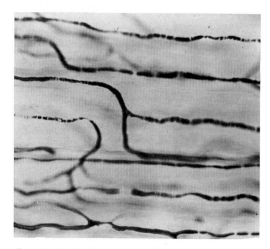

FIG. 18-16. Medium-power photomicrograph of a longitudinal section of striated muscle, the blood vessels of which were injected with India ink. The illustration shows how capillaries run between and parallel with the fibers. Some cross connections are also shown. (Preparation by W. S. Hartroft)

that project back into muscle fiber between adjacent myofibrils and sometimes even into a myofibril, thus splitting its end into two or more divisions. Figure 18-15 also shows that the ends of the myofibrils that reach the sarcolemma have only a scanty content of myofilaments. Furthermore, free ribosomes are to be seen in the sarcoplasm along with mitochondria in this site. It is likely that this is the site where the sarcoplasmic reticulum and myofibrils of new sarcomeres are synthesized.

Present evidence, therefore, suggests that new sarcomeres are added to myofibrils at the muscle-tendon junction, where the sarcolemma is adherent to the collagen of the tendon, and where the sarcolemma by forming long deep clefts in the muscle fiber provides some guidance for the diameter of sarcomeres that are to be synthesized and added to the ends of the pre-existing myofibrils in this site.

Blood Vessels and Lymphatics

Striated muscle has a rich blood supply. Arteries are carried from the surface connective tissue into the substance of the muscle. The arteries branch into arterioles and give off capillaries which run between and parallel with the muscle fibers (Fig. 18-16), but side branches from them often run at right angles to the fibers. The cross section appearance of muscle capillaries is illustrated in Figure 19-9 and their fine structure in Figure 8-7.

The lymphatics of striated muscle are confined almost entirely to its thicker connective tissue components. In this way it differs from cardiac muscle, which has lymphatics as well as capillaries between the fibers.

The Efferent Innervation of Striated Muscle

Motor Units. Nerves are conducted into muscles by the connective tissue components of muscle. The number of muscle fibers supplied by a single motor nerve fiber varies greatly. In one of the extrinsic muscles of the eye, in which the greatest delicacy of movement is required, there is a separate nerve fiber for every muscle fiber. The other extreme is represented by muscles that are not required to perform delicate movements, in which one nerve fiber may branch and supply over 100 muscle fibers. A nerve fiber, together with all the muscle fibers it supplies, is described as a *motor unit*.

If a single nerve fiber supplies many muscle fibers in a muscle, the latter do not, as might first be expected, constitute a localized group of fibers; instead the muscle fibers innervated by a single nerve fiber may have a considerable distribution throughout a muscle. However, they are either all red or all white. These findings are of importance because a single muscle fiber under the influence of a nervous stimulation always contracts to a maximum capacity; this is spoken of as the *all or none law*. Accordingly, the ability of a muscle *as a whole* to contract with different degrees of intensity is dependent, not on the ability of individual muscle fibers to contract with different degrees of intensity—for they cannot—but on the fact that different *numbers* of the fibers in the muscle can be stimulated to contract under different conditions. Hence, if a weak contraction is required, only a small proportion of the fibers in the muscle are stimulated to contract. Under these conditions it is desirable for those that do contract to be representative of the muscle as a whole so that the contraction is general rather than local. And since many fibers are supplied by a single nerve fiber, and since in minor contractions only a small proportion of the nerve fibers is stimulated, it is desirable that each fiber supply a group of muscle fibers that extend fairly well throughout the length of the muscle.

THE NEUROMUSCULAR JUNCTION

Most muscle fibers probably receive only a single nerve fiber; this ends on the muscle fiber in what was termed, from light microscopy, a *motor end-plate*.

There is some evidence to indicate that sometimes a muscle fiber may have more than one motor end-plate, but this is probably unusual.

With the LM, motor end-plates can be demonstrated by gold or silver impregnation technics. These technics show that a nerve fiber, as it ends on the surface of a muscle fiber, breaks up into several tiny terminal twigs which form a little cluster in a localized area on the fiber. Several pale muscle fibers disposed obliquely are shown in Figure 18-17 and almost each one shows a motor end-plate as well as the twigs connecting it to the nerve fiber.

Before the days of the EM, certain features of the neuromuscular junction were established: it was generally accepted that an axon, on approaching the muscle fiber, and before it branched into terminal twigs, loses its myelin sheath. The twigs, covered only with a sheath of Schwann, closely approach the surface of the muscle fiber.

With the EM, more detail was elicited, and this will be described here in relation to Figure 18-18, which shows a neuromuscular junction, below which a muscle fiber is easily identified by the myofibril (Mf). An axon (Ax) is seen approaching the muscle fiber from the right, and terminating in an expansion which covers the fiber over a distance of about two and a half sarcomeres in length. This is the motor end-plate.

The axon (Ax) that ends on the muscle fiber is covered on its free (upper) surface with a thin cytoplasmic coat provided by Schwann cells (SC). At the lower side of the end of the axon, the substance of the axon becomes expanded into terminations which closely approach the sarcolemma, as will soon be described. Each expanded ending contains many small vesicles similar to those seen in synapses (V). Several mitochondria can also be seen in these regions; their presence indicates metabolic activity.

The sheath of Schwann (SC), which covers the top of the nerve fiber that terminates in an end-plate, does not cover the bottom of the expanded endings of the nerve fiber; at this site, the axolemma of an expanded ending is naked, so far as a cellular covering is concerned.

The general area on a muscle fiber where an end-plate is located is commonly raised so as to form a little mound. Since the myofibrils pursue a straight course, the little mounds are filled only with sarcoplasm, and since this is disposed under the end-foot (the nerve ending), it is called *sole plasm*. The expanded terminal twigs of the nerve fiber are sunk into this sole plasm in little depressions termed gutters; these are shallow in Figure 18-18, there being one roughly under each V.

The sarcolemma that forms the floor of a gutter is

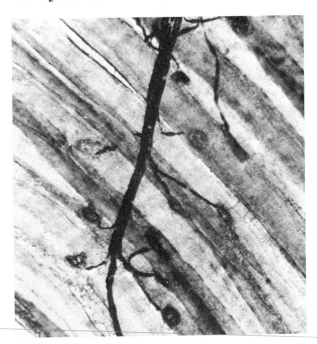

Fig. 18-17. Low-power ($\times$ 250) micrograph of a nerve fiber running diagonally across a bundle of muscle cells. Several fine twigs branch from the nerve and course to muscle fibers below, where they end in bulbous motor end-plates. (Courtesy of Dr. A. Hess)

thrown into numerous folds, called junctional folds (JF in Fig. 18-18), which extend toward the nerve ending; these increase the surface area of the sarcolemma that comes close to the nerve ending. The axolemma that covers each expanded nerve termination does not come into direct contact with the crests of the junctional folds; instead, the two cell membranes, that of the nerve fiber (called the presynaptic membrane) and that of the muscle cell (called the postsynaptic membrane), are always separated by a space that is about 200 Å wide and is termed the *synaptic cleft*.

The synaptic cleft is filled with an amorphous material of low electron density which seems to be composed of the basement membranes and cell coats found on the surface of both axon and muscle. The depression between adjacent junctional folds is filled with the same material; the axolemma does not follow the sarcolemma down into the depressions between junctional folds.

The neuromuscular junction is, in effect, a synapse between a nerve cell and a muscle cell. A nervous impulse arriving at an end-plate causes some of the vesicles (V), which are filled with acetylcholine, to open by exocytosis at the presynaptic membrane and

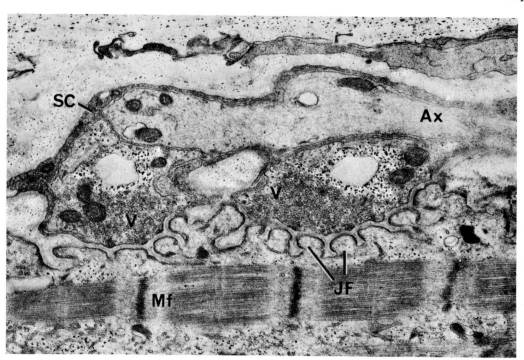

Fɪɢ. 18-18. Electron micrograph (× 20,000) of a neuromuscular junction from the newt *Triturus*. The motor axon (Ax) terminates in a slight depression or gutter on the muscle fiber surface. On its outer side the nerve is enveloped by a thin layer of Schwann cell (SC) cytoplasm. The nerve termination is filled with small synaptic vesicles (V) and contains mitochondria. Junctional folds (JF) extend outward from the muscle surface. The cleft between muscle and nerve is filled with amorphous material similar to a basement lamina. A myofibril (Mf) is found in the sarcoplasm. (Illustration provided by T. L. Lentz, Yale University)

thus release this chemical mediator. The acetylcholine thus appears in the synaptic cleft, where it affects the considerable amount of membrane of the muscle cell that is provided by this postsynaptic membrane being in the form of folds. The acetylcholine here seems to act by making the sarcolemma more permeable to sodium ions, and this in turn initiates a wave of depolarization that sweeps over the fibers via the sarcolemma and into the fiber via the system of transverse tubules. The acetylcholine liberated in response to a nervous impulse is promptly inactivated by cholinesterase.

Afferent nerve endings in muscle are described in Chapter 28.

Cardiac Muscle

For a long time it was believed that cardiac muscle differed fundamentally from both smooth and striated muscle in that its fibers were not individual cells but instead were all joined together in such a way that they formed a huge protoplasmic network called a syncytium (*syn,* joined together). The concept of cardiac muscle not being composed of individual cells arose because no ends of cells could be distinguished with the LM in the branching anastomosing fibers of cardiac muscle. The arrangement of the branching network of fibers is illustrated in Figure 18-19, where it can be seen that the fibers of the network are roughly parallel with one another, but that their branching and anastomosing account for the slits present between them. These slits contain loose connective tissue which is abundantly supplied with capillaries that are thereby brought into close contact with the muscle fibers of the network. Moreover, the space between cardiac muscle fibers is provided with lymphatic capillaries as well as blood capillaries, and it also carries nerve fibers.

The nuclei of cardiac muscle fibers tend to be disposed in the middle parts of the fibers (Fig. 18-20). They are usually ovoid and associated with a small amount of cytoplasm. In longitudinal sections, some cytoplasm free of myofibrils may often be distinguished at each pole of the nucleus. This feature helps in the identification of the tissue.

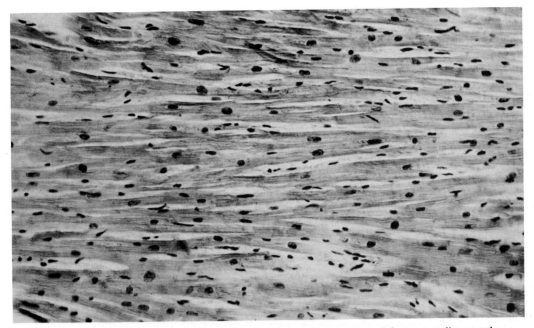

FIG. 18-19. Low-power photomicrograph of a longitudinal section of human cardiac muscle. Observe that the muscle fibers branch and anastomose, and that the interstices so created are filled with light-staining connective tissue. This carries the blood and lymph capillaries and the nerves.

The cytoplasm of cardiac muscle fibers contains myofibrils and sarcoplasm and shows cross striations similar to those described for striated muscle. The cross striations of cardiac muscle, although due to A and I bands and to Z lines similar to those of striated muscle, are not usually so distinct as those of striated muscle. In addition, cardiac muscle fibers are crossed every now and again by unique dark-stained bands called *intercalated disks* (*intercalated* means inserted) as may be seen in Figure 18-21. These disks, which are more or less inserted between some sarcomeres, are seen with the LM in suitably stained sections to be present at the sites of Z lines, but since they are thicker than Z lines, they encroach on each of their sides on the I band (Fig. 18-22, *inset*). Sometimes intercalated disks cross fibers in straight lines, but usually they cross in a stepwise fashion (Figs. 18-21 and 18-22, *inset*); this is due to the intercalated disks of different myofibrils of the fiber not being in register. There has been much speculation about their nature and function through the years. It was not until they were examined in thin sections with the EM that their true nature was definitely established, as will be described under Fine Structure.

Fine Structure. In many important respects, the fine structure of cardiac muscle is similar to that of striated skeletal muscle. The fibers of cardiac muscle

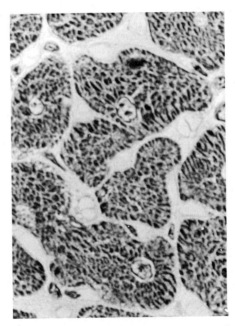

FIG. 18-20. Photomicrograph of cross section of cardiac muscle fibers. Note that the large nuclei tend to be in the more central parts of fibers. The myofibrils of the fibers show up clearly; the sarcoplasm between the myofibrils is not stained.

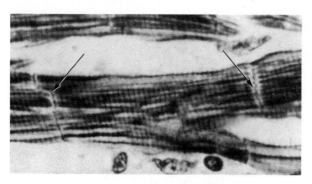

FIG. 18-21. A photomicrograph of a longitudinal section of a cardiac muscle cell stained with the TPA technic. By this method, cross striations stand out. Cross striations result from myofibrils being in register as in skeletal muscle. The end boundaries of the cell are demarcated by the presence of intercalated disks (arrows). These may cross the cell in a straight manner as does the right disk, or in a stepwise fashion illustrated on the left. Note the branching character of the cardiac muscle cell. (Courtesy of Dr. Y. Clermont)

are made up of myofibrils between which is sarcoplasm (Fig. 18-23). The I bands bisected by the Z line are in register with those of other myofibrils, and so are the A bands and their H zone. Mitochondria are abundant (Figs. 18-22 and 18-23), presumably owing to the energy requirements of cardiac muscle being at times great. In the atria, but not in the ventricles, the cytoplasm associated with the nucleus contains not only the usual organelles but also secretory granules arising in the Golgi apparatus (Cantin).

The Fine Structure of Intercalated Disks and Junctional Complexes in Cardiac Muscle. When intercalated disks were studied with the EM, it became apparent that they represented sites where the ends of individual cardiac muscle cells, each covered with its own cell membrane, were joined together by some type of junctional complex. However, since a cardiac muscle cell is covered on its sides as well as on its ends with a cell membrane, and since intercalated disks commonly cross fibers in a stepwise fashion, it follows that, in intercalated disks of the latter type, parts of one cardiac muscle cell overlap the next one, and that in these sites where two cells overlap, their sides are covered with cell membrane; and, further, these membranes are also joined together by some sort of junctional complex. So while the word *disk* was used originally to depict structures that crossed fibers at right angles, it has come to be used in connection with intercalated disks to include all sites of contact between the sides of two cardiac muscle

cells. The parts of the disks that cross fibers at right angles are termed *transverse parts* (Fig. 18-22, TR), whereas those that run parallel to myofibrils are termed *lateral parts* (Fig. 18-22, LAT).

Since the cell membrane follows the intercalated disks and these in turn are present at the sites of the Z lines, the transverse portions of the cell membrane are adjacent to dense material similar to Z line material (Fig. 18-24). Furthermore, the individual actin filaments terminate there. As a result, the zigzag appearance of the Z line depicted in striated muscle (Fig. 18-7) is often observed along the transverse portions of the cell membrane. Furthermore, three types of junction may be observed. Two are located in the transverse parts of the intercalated disks: tight junctions (5-layered), and desmosomes (as described in detail in Chapter 5); these are believed to provide close adhesion between successive cells, thus preventing them from being pulled apart when the cardiac muscle contracts. The third type is a nexus or gap junction (7-layered; Fig. 18-25) which serves to establish low resistance pathways between cells, and thus allows the conduction of the impulse from one cell to the next and, in this manner, propagates the impulse through large segments of the heart. The gap junctions are surrounded by a halo of clear cytoplasm and they are always placed along the lateral parts of the intercalated disks, that is, in a plane parallel to the axis of the myofibrils, which is probably their position of least stress; they may be considered to be "free floating," since, unlike tight junctions and desmosomes, they are not attached to fibrillar elements.

Sarcoplasmic Reticulum. Cardiac muscle fibers have a sarcoplasmic reticulum, which, although less well defined than in striated muscle, is associated with a system of *transverse tubules*. These are at the level of the Z line in cardiac muscle and are much wider than those found in skeletal muscle (1,000 Å vs 400 Å diameter). Also unlike the transverse tubules of skeletal muscle, they are lined with basement membrane material which is continuous with that of the sarcolemma. Finally, instead of being associated with large terminal cisternae of sarcoplasmic reticulum on both sides as in striated muscle, the transverse tubules are adjacent to small cisternae separated from one another. The remainder of the reticulum (Fig. 18-26) is a highly fenestrated complex of tubular cisternae which surround the myofibrils but show little regular arrangement.

The presence of a sarcoplasmic reticulum suggests that the impulse leading to cardiac contraction is not exclusively transferred by the cytoplasm of a cell

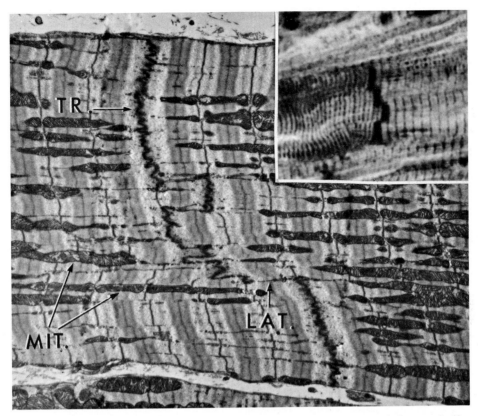

Fig. 18-22. Electron micrograph (× 5,100) of an intercalated disk in a ventricular muscle fiber of the canine heart. The disk passes across the fiber in a stepwise way. Each transverse portion of the disk replaces part of a Z-line. In this preparation the A and I bands of the myofibrils are evident. Fixed in sodium permanganate and stained with uranyl acetate and lead citrate. MIT., mitochondria; LAT., lateral parts; TR., transverse parts; see text.

(*Inset*) A light micrograph of a comparable intercalated disk in a ventricular fiber of the canine heart. Fixed in formol-sublimate and stained with toluidine blue and thizine red. (× 1,000). (Preparation courtesy of A. Spira)

Fig. 18-23. Electron micrograph (× 10,300) of a cardiac muscle cell from the atrium of a hamster. The nucleus (N) lies in the center of the cell and is bounded on its sides by myofibrils which show remarkable register of their sarcomeres and contain A bands (A), I bands (I) and Z lines (Z). At the nuclear pole shown at right is an area of sarcoplasm devoid of myofibrils and packed with mitochondria (M), a Golgi apparatus (G) and its associated darkly stained atrial granules (ag). These granules are also found scattered throughout the cell. (Courtesy of Dr. M. Cantin)

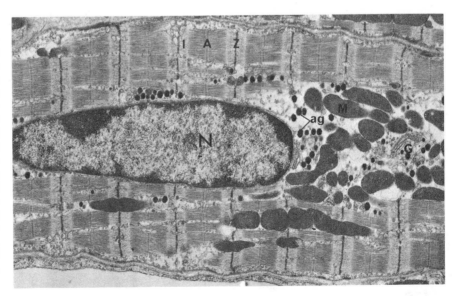

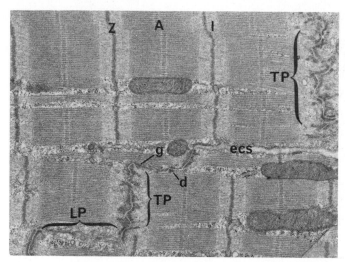

FIG. 18-24. Longitudinal section of cat ventricular muscle showing several sarcomeres of two myocardial cells. The end of the upper cell is demarcated, at the upper right of figure, by a transverse portion (TP) of an intercalated disk. This portion of the disk can be followed to a slip of extracellular space (ecs) that separates the upper and lower cells for a short distance. The space is obliterated, however, at the start of another intercalated disk which cuts stepwise to complete the boundaries shown between the upper and the lower cell. The lower disk shows transverse portions (TP) that are composed predominantly of junctions of the fasciae adherentes type (and are located at the level of the Z lines). The actin filaments of the I band insert into the filamentous mat of the fasciae adherentes. Lateral portions (LP) of the disks contain desmosomic junctions (d), as well as gap junctions (g). A gap junction from heart muscle at high magnification is seen in Figure 18-25. × 13,000. (Courtesy of Dr. N. S. McNutt)

through gap junctions to the cytoplasm of the next cell; there may in addition be a depolarization of the cell membrane transmitted to myofibrils through transverse tubule and cisternae as in striated muscle.

Finally, there are fibers specialized in conduction; these are characterized by various features, the most constant of which is the absence of sarcoplasmic reticulum. These will be described in Chapter 19 (The Circulatory System), which deals with the heart as an organ.

Pigment. Beginning at age 10, granules of golden-yellow pigments tend to accumulate in the sarcoplasm at each end of the nuclei of cardiac muscle fibers. It seems probable that these granules represent a type of "wear and tear" lipofuscin pigment described in Chapter 5. This pigment becomes very prominent in a condition termed "brown atrophy of the heart."

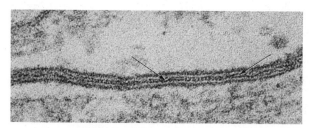

FIG. 18-25. Seven-layered junction (gap junction or nexus) from mouse heart at high magnification (× 200,000). This junction has a narrow electron-lucent zone (arrows) that appears to separate the apposed plasma membranes. More intense lead citrate staining often obliterates this central zone resulting in a 5-layered appearance. (Courtesy of Dr. N. S. McNutt)

Smooth Muscle

Smooth muscle is also called involuntary muscle; the reason is that it is not under the control of the conscious mind but under the control of the autonomic (involuntary) nervous system.

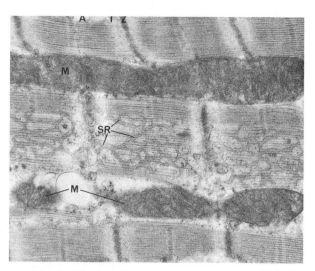

FIG. 18-26. Electron micrograph (× 22,000) of dog cardiac muscle. From top to base, this figure shows 3 myofibrils separated by rows of mitochondria (M). The A and I bands as well as the Z lines are labeled in the top myofibril. The middle one is cut tangentially in such a way that the sarcoplasmic reticulum (SR) is visible in relation to its 3 sarcomeres. The reticulum is relatively simple when compared to that of skeletal muscle and does not swell into large terminal cisternae as in skeletal muscle. Compare with Figure 18-10. (Courtesy of Dr. S. J. Phillips)

FIG. 18-27. A high-power photomicrograph ($\times$ 1,200) showing the circular layer (upper two thirds of figure) and the longitudinal layer of smooth muscle from mouse large intestine. Nuclei (n) are elongated but somewhat irregular in shape, possibly due to a partially contracted state of the muscle. The cytoplasm exhibits minute dark bodies visible in longitudinal sections as short rods or dots, and in cross section as small dots (db). The space separating the layers contains connective tissue, blood vessels and nerves. At the base of the picture a thin layer of mesothelium covers the longitudinal layer. S, the nucleus of a mesothelial cell. Iron hematoxylin. (Courtesy of Dr. J. E. Michaels)

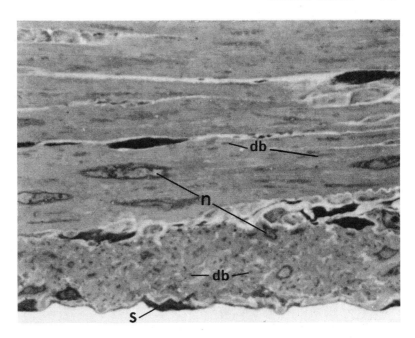

Size, Shape and Arrangement of Smooth Muscle Fibers

Smooth muscle fibers are mainly found in the walls of hollow viscera and blood vessels, where they play a major role in controlling the caliber of the lumens. Most hollow viscera are coated by two smooth muscle *layers,* an inner one composed of circularly arranged fibers and an outer one composed of longitudinally running smooth muscle fibers (Fig. 18-27). In stomach and in the lower portion of the ureter there is also a third layer of oblique or longitudinal fibers within the inner circular layer; in the upper portion of the ureter only this third layer and the circular one are present. In blood vessels, the layer of smooth muscle fibers is usually confined to the media, where the fibers are arranged in a spiral. The spiral causes the fibers to be at an angle with the axis of the vessel; in mice this angle was found to increase from the heart to vessels of the periphery—e.g., 30° in arteries, 72° in arterioles and a right angle in smaller arterioles. Hence, muscle fibers are slightly oblique in arteries but are arranged in a truly circular fashion in smaller arterioles (Rhodin).

The layers of muscle fibers are subdivided into *bundles* surrounded by sheaths of connective tissue (Fig. 18-28). In many cases—e.g., in the uterine wall—the bundles of a layer anastomose with one another.

Smooth muscle can exist in a state of sustained partial contraction that is called *tonus.* Hence the tonus of the smooth muscle in the wall of the tube is an important factor in regulating and maintaining the

size of the lumen in that tube. If the degree of tonus becomes increased, the lumen of the tube becomes narrower. However, too great a degree of tonus can have repercussions. For example, increased tonus in the smooth muscle that surrounds certain of the tubes that conduct air in and out of the lungs occurs in the condition called asthma, and the narrowing of the air passages so induced makes it difficult for the individual to expel air from his lungs. Increased tonus of the

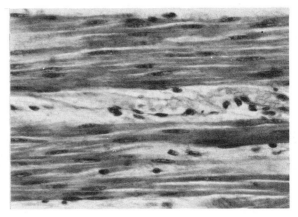

FIG. 18-28. A medium-power photomicrograph of portions of two bundles of smooth muscle cut longitudinally. In the space separating the bundles is a capillary filled with red blood cells. The remainder of the darkly stained fibers are separated by light areas filled with varying amounts of intercellular substance. (Illustration provided by E. Schultz and C. P. Leblond)

smooth muscle in the walls of arterioles restricts the outflow of blood from the arterial system, and this backs up the blood and raises the blood pressure. Finally, smooth muscle is an important component of the wall of the intestinal tract. Here it maintains tonus, but in addition waves of contraction of the circular layer of fibers can sweep down the intestines, squeezing the contents of the lumen ahead of them; these are called *peristaltic waves*. Smooth muscle is an important component of the wall of many other tubular structures that we shall study later. Its chief role is to maintain tonus and in some instances to undergo slow rhythmic contractions which involve a whole group of fibers.

The action of most smooth muscles, as compared to that of striated muscles, is sluggish. There are exceptions. Thus, the muscles that cause the pupil to contract (sphincter pupillae) function rather quickly.

Size Range of Fibers. Relaxed smooth muscle fibers have an elongated, tapered form (Fig. 18-28). Their size varies considerably according to their location. The smallest are those that encircle very small blood vessels; these may be only about 20 μm long. The largest are those that are encountered in the wall of the pregnant uterus; here they may be 0.5 mm. in length. However, the usual smooth muscle fiber is probably about 0.2 mm. long and at its widest part is somewhat wider than an erythrocyte.

Structure in LM

Seen with the LM the *cytoplasm* of smooth muscle cells (fibers) is characteristically pink or red in H and E sections. The *nucleus* lies in the widest part of the fiber (Fig. 18-28) and may be in the middle of the cell or may be located somewhat eccentrically. It may have pointed ends (Fig. 18-27) or rounded ends (Fig. 18-29) and may show indentations or even appear pleated along its longitudinal axis, particularly when the fiber is fixed in a state of contraction (Fig. 18-29).

Improved methods have revealed the existence in smooth muscle of tiny dark patches (Fig. 18-27). Studies of fibers in vitro have revealed that these patches play a role in contraction. These patches may be located along the surface or within the fiber. In contrast to the elongated shape of the relaxed fiber, the contracted one shortens into an ellipsoid. With contraction, the surface membrane, which is smooth at rest, becomes covered with bubblelike expansions, as shown in Figure 18-30. The bubbles are due to cytoplasm under pressure pushing the plasma membrane between the surface patches.

In most locations, particularly the uterus, the ends of smooth muscle fibers interdigitate with the other fibers of the bundle in which they are located. The interdigitation causes one end of the fiber to become displaced by two or three muscle diameters relative to the other end. This manner of packing results in numerous contacts from fiber to fiber so that a bundle of smooth muscle fibers forms a tightly bound group which in fact functions as a unit.

Between smooth muscle fibers there is a 500 to 800 Å space. This is filled by the basement membranes which cover the plasma membranes of each fiber and by collagenic and elastic fibers as well as intercellular substance. It is now known that smooth muscle cells can produce both collagen and elastin and it is believed that they give rise to the material in their interspace.

However, as already mentioned, there are tongues of frank connective tissue with its own fibroblasts that penetrate into the layers of smooth muscle fibers and subdivide them into bundles (Fig. 18-28). These tongues of frank connective tissue convey capillaries and nerve fibers to the bundles.

Some Points About the Recognition of Smooth Muscle. In routine sections, the appearance presented by elongated nuclei of fibrocytes that are lying between and hence are compressed by parallel collagenic fibers may sometimes simulate that of smooth muscle. Sometimes special staining is necessary to decide whether what is seen is the cytoplasm of smooth muscle fibers or collagen. Mallory's and Van Gieson's stains, the former of which color collagen blue and muscle red, are commonly used for this purpose.

Origin

Most smooth muscle develops from mesenchyme. In this process a mesenchymal cell becomes drawn out to form a long, tapering smooth muscle fiber. The nucleus as well as the cytoplasm becomes elongated. Since fibroblasts may arise from adjacent mesenchymal cells and make collagen, it is easy to understand why connective tissue and bundles of smooth muscle can become intimately associated and present difficulties with regard to distinguishing one from the other. In relation to some glands (e.g., salivary, sweat, lacrimal), cells are found around the secretory units embracing them, which have the appearance of smooth muscle cells and, like them, may contract, but are developed from ectoderm. Such cells are called myoepithelial cells.

Growth and Regeneration

The amount of smooth muscle in certain parts of the body may increase during postnatal life, and even in

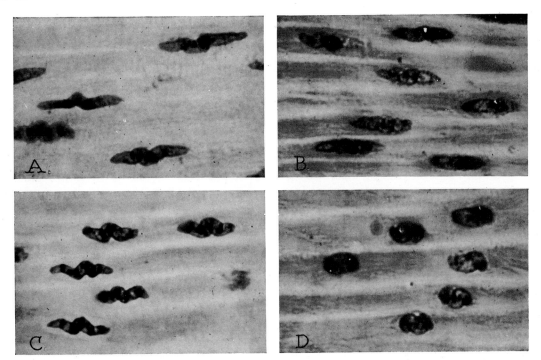

FIG. 18-29. High-powered photomicrographs of smooth muscle of the intestine, showing how the elongated nuclei of the fibers are thrown into folds (pleats) when the fibers, on contraction, become shorter and thicker. In D they are folded so tightly that they appear, on superficial examination, to be ovoid.

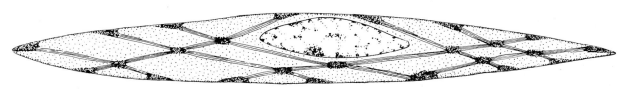

FIG. 18-30. A diagrammatic interpretation of the possible arrangement of the latticelike network of dark bodies and connecting filaments in the smooth muscle cell. Dark bodies are distributed throughout the cytoplasm and are interconnected with one another by 100-Å filaments. Thin actin filaments are also attached to the dense bodies (not shown), and interact during contraction with thick myosin filaments located in the sarcoplasm within the lattice. As the thin actin filaments are pulled toward the thick filaments, the dense bodies are also displaced due to the forces transmitted along the interconnecting cables. This eventually leads to a distortion of the cell surface as the pull of the lattice reaches a membrane-associated dense body. The sum total of the distortions around the cell periphery results in a shortening of the longitudinal axis. (Illustration courtesy of C. P. Leblond and E. Schultz)

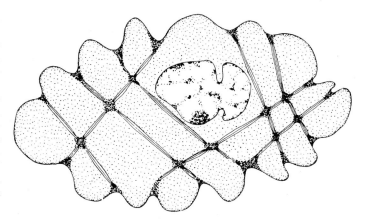

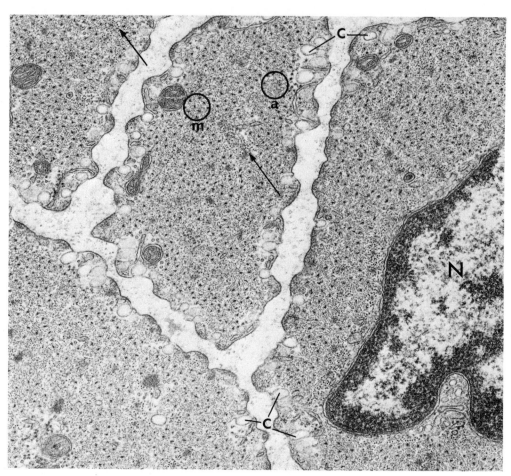

FIG. 18-31. Electron micrograph ($\times$ 34,000) of a transverse section of several smooth muscle fibers illustrating the fairly regular spacing of the thick filaments (m) and the relatively large number of thin filaments (a). Several groups of intermediate size (100 Å) filaments are shown by arrows. The large fiber at the right shows a centrally placed nucleus (N) and several caveolae (c) beneath the plasma membrane. (From Somlyo, A. P., Devine, C. E., Somlyo, A. V., and Rice, R. V.: Phil. Trans. Roy. Soc. London [B], *265:223*, 1973)

adult life. Some of these increases are physiologic—for example, that which occurs in the wall of the uterus during pregnancy. Others are pathologic, such as increase in the amount of smooth muscle that may occur in the arterioles of people suffering from long-continued high blood pressure. The amount of smooth muscle can increase not only by an increase in the size of individual fibers, but also by mitotic division. This is commonly seen in the walls of the pregnant uterus.

Fine Structure

In the EM smooth muscle fibers are seen to contain nucleus, mitochondria and glycogen as well as an endoplasmic reticulum. In addition, there are two main kinds of filaments, thick and thin, as well as anchoring filaments. In relaxed cells all are oriented more or less longitudinally.

The first kind, the *thin filaments* have a diameter that varies in different cells, from 30 to 80 Å. These filaments are readily seen in the EM (Fig. 18-31). They are believed to originate in the dark patches observed along the plasma membrane and within the cytoplasm but the other extremity would be free. The dark patches and bodies would correspond to the Z line of striated muscle and contain the protein actinin found by chemical methods in smooth muscle fibers (as well as in the Z line). The thin filaments themselves would be composed of actin, but an actin slightly different from that in striated muscle.

The second type, the *thick filaments,* have a diameter of 150 to 350 Å. They are fragile and difficult to fix. For reasons that are not clear, they are often not seen in the EM, except when the muscle is slightly stretched during fixation. They are then visible in cross section (Fig. 18-31) and longitudinal section (Fig. 18-32). However, they are now believed to be present in all fibers. They are not attached to the dark bodies. They are composed of a myosin which is of a slightly different type from that in striated muscles.

Because actin and myosin, as well as tropomyosin and troponin, are found in smooth muscle fibers it is widely believed that the process of contraction must be similar to that in striated muscle. The common view is that, even though the relations between actin and myosin filaments and their interaction with other smooth muscle proteins are obscure, the contraction of smooth muscle fibers is produced by the sliding filament mechanism.

Finally, the third type of filament has a diameter of about 100 Å and extends from one dark patch to another, being thus firmly anchored within the cell in both relaxed and contracted states (Fig. 18-30).

Endoplasmic Reticulum. There is a small amount of endoplasmic reticulum next to the nucleus. The rest of it runs longitudinally close to the cell surface between the dark bodies (Fig. 18-33). It is possible that the subsurface endoplasmic reticulum functions like the sarcoplasmic reticulum of striated muscle. The cisternae are often associated with structures known as caveolae, which are vesicles similar to the pinocytotic vesicles of capillaries (Fig. 18-33). Unlike pinocytotic vesicles, they all seem to open at the surface, since after deposition of ferritin in the intercellular space, they promptly become filled with this substance. The role of caveolae is thought by some to be one of decreasing the electric resistance of the cell surface and thus facilitating the response of the fibers to nerve impulses. Indeed, the caveolae may be involved in carrying the nerve impulse into the fiber. Since the cisternae of endoplasmic reticulum are closely related to the caveolae, and since they are known to be a site of calcium storage, it is widely believed that these cisternae play a role similar to that played by the sarcoplasmic reticulum in the initiation of striated muscle contraction.

Innervation and Conduction of Nervous Impulse. Since smooth muscle fibers are commonly packed together in sheets wrapping the walls of various kinds of tubes in the body (for example, in the walls of arteries

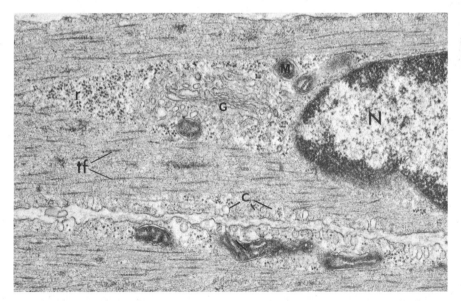

Fig. 18-32. Electron micrograph ($\times$ 38,000) of a longitudinal section of smooth muscle. Numerous thick filaments (tf) course through the cell. The apparent variability in lengths of these filaments is probably due to the obliquity of the section and to a somewhat different orientation of the filaments. Thin filaments are present in areas between the thick filaments. The sarcoplasm at the end of the centrally placed nucleus (N) contains ribosomes (r), mitochondria (M) and a Golgi apparatus (G). Note also the presence of caveolae (c) in the sarcoplasm beneath the plasma membrane. (From Somlyo, A. P., Devine, C. E., Somlyo, A. V., and Rice, R. V.: Phil. Trans. Roy. Soc. London [B] *265:223,* 1973)

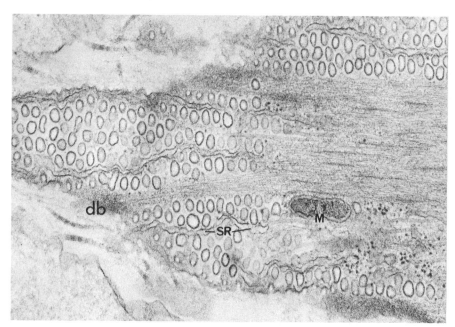

Fig. 18-33. An electron micrograph (× 53,000) showing a tangential section of a smooth muscle cell along its longitudinal axis. A large population of caveolae are located in the sarcoplasm immediately beneath the plasma membrane. Running in an intimate relationship among these caveolae are delicate tubules of sarcoplasmic reticulum (SR). These structures may represent the coupling site of the electrical and mechanical events of contraction. Note also the membrane-associated dark body (db) and the filaments extending from it into the interior of the cell. (From Devine, C. E., Somlyo, A. V., and Somlyo, A. P.: J. Cell Biol., *52*:690, 1972)

and the intestine), and since the smooth muscle fibers within a bundle contract more or less in unison to narrow the lumen of the tube in whose wall they are disposed, there must be some arrangement that permits adjacent fibers to contract simultaneously. There are two ways this could be accomplished: (1) by means of a separate nerve fiber passing to each muscle cell, with the impulses for contraction passing via these different nerve fibers simultaneously to all the smooth muscle fibers in a given area, or (2) by a nerve impulse that arrives at one muscle cell in a given area being conducted rapidly from this to other cells in the same area so that they again contract more or less simultaneously.

Recent studies indicate that both types of arrangement exist as well as intermediate conditions. In the first case, known as *multiunit type,* which is found, for instance, in the smooth muscle of vas deferens and sphincter pupillae, there is at least one nerve ending (comparable to a motor end-plate) for each smooth muscle fiber. Since these smooth muscles are geared for relatively fast and simultaneous contraction, the impulse must be passed on at the same time in all the nerve fibers of a given area. In the second case, known as *unitary* or *visceral type,* which is found, for instance, in the longitudinal layer of intestinal smooth muscle, only one or a few cells in a bundle are equipped to receive a nerve impulse; but these cells are coupled to all the other cells of the bundle and the impulse is transmitted rapidly enough for all of them to contract together. The coupling which allows conduction from

cell to cell is due to nexus or gap junctions (composed of 7 layers) between them at certain sites around their periphery. Contraction of the unitary type of smooth muscle fibers is rather slow and takes place spontaneously, sometimes continually. Finally, there are *intermediate types* in which many cells (20 to 50%) are adjacent to a nerve ending and are coupled with neighboring cells.

Neuromuscular Endings. Smooth muscle fibers are innervated by autonomic nerves. Their axons, instead of ending in a synapse or motor end-plate, terminate in a series of successive varicosities, one or several of which make contact with a smooth muscle fiber. An interspace of 100 to 200 Å is usually found between the varicosity and the fiber. However, particularly in the intermediate types, the interval may be much greater (up to 1,000 Å).

Smooth muscle fibers receive their impulses from the autonomic nervous system (sympathetic and parasympathetic nerves). Some of these nerves, known as cholinergic, contain acetylcholine bound in an inactive form in their terminal portions. This acetylcholine is contained in light vesicles measuring 250 to 600 Å, identical to the synaptic vesicles observed in motor end-plates. On stimulation of the nerve, the vesicles open into the interspace by a process of exocytosis; the acetylcholine is set free and reaches the membrane of the smooth muscle fiber which is thus activated.

Another form of innervation of smooth muscle fibers is by means of nerves which contain norepinephrine in their terminal portions and are known as noradrenergic. This substance is believed to be contained in vesicles which have the same size as those containing acetylcholine but differ by the presence of a dark core. Nerve stimulation cause these vesicles to release their norepinephrine content by exocytosis. This substance is set free and activates the smooth muscle fiber.

References

GENERAL REFERENCES ON MUSCLE

Bendall, J. R.: Muscles, Molecules and Movement. New York, American Elsevier, 1969.

Sandow, A.: Skeletal muscle. Ann. Rev. Physiol., *32:*87, 1970.

SOME REFERENCES ON STRIATED AND CARDIAC MUSCLE

Basmajian, J. V.: Control and training of individual motor units. Science, *141:*440, 1963.

————: Electromyography: Its structural and neural basis. Int. Rev. Cytol., *21:*129, 1967.

Betz, E. H., Firket, H., and Reznik. M.: Some aspects of muscle regeneration. Int. Rev. Cytol., *19:*203, 1966.

Bintliff, S., and Walker, B. E.: Radioautographic study of skeletal muscle regeneration. Am. J. Anat., *106:*233, 1960.

Cantin, M., Veilleux, R., and Huet, M.: Electron and fluorescence microscopy of hamster atrium after administration of 6-hydroxydopamine. Experientia, *29:*882, 1973.

Costantin, L. L., Frazini-Armstrong, C., and Podolsky, R. J.: Localization of calcium-accumulating structures in striated muscle fibers. Science, *147:*158, 1965.

Dreizen, P., and Gershman, L. D.: Molecular basis of muscular contraction—myosin. Trans. New York Acad. Sci., *32:*170, 1970.

Ebashi, S., Endo, M., and Ohtsuki, I.: Control of muscle contraction. Quart. Rev. Biophys., *2:*351, 1969.

Enesco, M., and Puddy, D.: Increase in the number of nuclei and weight in skeletal muscle of rats of various ages. Am. J. Anat., *114:*235, 1964.

Fawcett, D. W., and McNutt, N. S.: The ultrastructure of the cat myocardium. I. Ventricular papillary muscle. J. Cell Biol., *42:*1, 1969.

Forssmann, W. G., and Girardier, L.: A study of the T-system in rat heart. J. Cell Biol., *44:*1, 1970.

Frazini-Armstrong, C., and Porter, K. R.: Sarcolemmal invaginations constituting the T system in fish muscle fibers. J. Cell Biol., *22:*675, 1964.

Goldspink, G.: Sarcomere length during post-natal growth of mammalian muscle fibres. J. Cell Sci., *3:*539, 1968.

Hanson, J., and Huxley, H. E.: The structural basis of contraction in striated muscle. Sympos. Soc. Exp. Biol., *9:*228, 1955.

————: Structural basis of the cross-striations in muscle. Nature, *172:*530, 1953.

Huxley, A. F., and Taylor, R. E.: Local activation of striated muscle fibers. J. Physiol. (London) *144:*426, 1958.

Huxley, H. E.: The double array of filaments in cross-striated muscle. J. Biophys. Biochem. Cytol., *3:*361, 1957.

————: The contraction of muscle. Sci. Am., *199:*66, 1958.

————: The mechanism of muscular contraction. Science, *164:*1356, 1969.

————: The structural basis of muscular contraction. Proc. Roy. Soc. Lond., [B] *178:*131, 1971.

Knappeis, G. G., and Carlsen, F.: The ultrastructure of the Z disc in skeletal muscle. J. Cell Biol., *13:*323, 1962.

Lee, K. S., Ladinsky, H., Choi, S. J., and Kasuya, Y.: Studies on the in vitro interaction of electrical stimulation and Ca++ movement in the sarcoplasmic reticulum. J. Gen. Physiol., *49:*698, 1966.

Lowey, S., Slayter, H. S., Weeds, A. G., and Baker, H.: Enzymic degradation of myosin. J. Molec. Biol., *42:*1, 1969.

MacConnachie, H. F., Enesco, M., and Leblond, C. P.: The mode of increase in the number of skeletal muscle nuclei in the postnatal rat. Am. J. Anat., *114:*245, 1964.

MacKay, B., Harrop, T. J., and Muir, A. R.: An experimental study of the longitudinal growth of skeletal muscle in the rat. Acta anat., *73:*588, 1969.

Mauro, A.: Satellite cell of skeletal cell fibers. J. Biophys. Biochem. Cytol., *3:*193, 1961.

McNutt, N. S., and Fawcett, D. W.: The ultrastructure of the cat myocardium. II. Atrial Muscle. J. Cell Biol., *42:*46, 1969.

McNutt, N. S., and Weinstein, R. S.: The ultrastructure of the nexus. J. Cell Biol., *47:*666, 1970.

Moss, F. P.: Relationship between the dimensions of the fibers and the number of nuclei during normal growth of skeletal muscle in the domestic fowl. Am. J. Anat., *122:*555, 1968.

Moss, F. P., and Leblond, C. P.: Satellite cells as the source of nuclei in muscles of growing rats. Anat. Rec., *170:*471, 1971.

Sjostrand, F. S., Andersson-Cedergren, E., and Dewey, M. M.: The ultrastructure of the intercalated discs of frog, mouse and guinea pig cardiac muscle. J. Ultrastruct. Res., *1:*271, 1958.

Spira, D.: The ultrastructure of heart muscle. Trans. N.Y. Acad. Sci. [Ser. II], *24:*879, 1962.

Strickholm, A.: Local sarcomere contraction in fast muscle fibers. Nature, *212:*835, 1966.

Winegrad, S.: Autoradiographic studies of intercellular calcium in frog skeletal muscle. J. Gen. Physiol., *48:*455, 1965.

————: The location of muscle calcium with respect to the myofibrils. J. Gen. Physiol., *48:*997, 1965.

SOME REFERENCES ON MOTOR NERVE ENDINGS IN MUSCLE

Andersson-Cedergren, E.: Ultrastructure of motor end plate and sarcoplasmic components of mouse skeletal muscle fiber as revealed by three-dimensional reconstructions from serial sections. J. Ultrastruct. Res., Suppl. *1,* 1959.

Barrnett, R. J.: The fine structural localization of acetylcholinesterase at the myoneural junction. J. Cell Biol., *12:*247, 1962.

Coërs, C.: Structure and organization of the myoneural junction. Int. Rev. Cytol., *22:*239, 1967.

Couteaux, R.: Contribution a l'étude de la synapse myoneurale. Rev. Canad. Biol., *6:*563, 1947.

————: Localization of cholinesterases at neuromuscular junctions. Int. Rev. Cytol., *4:*335, 1955.

De Harven, E., and Coërs, C.: Electron microscopy of the human neuromuscular junction. J. Biophys. Biochem. Cytol., *6:*7, 1959.

Kelly, A. M., and Zacks, S. I.: The fine structure of motor endplate morphogenesis. J. Cell Biol., *42:*154, 1969.

Palade, G. E.: Electron microscope observations on interneuronal and neuromuscular synapses. Anat. Rec., *118:*335, 1954.

Reger, J. F.: Electron microscopy of the motor end-plate in rat intercostal muscle. Anat. Rec., *112:*1, 1965.

Richardson, K. C.: The fine structure of autonomic nerve endings in smooth muscle of the rat vas deferens. J. Anat., *96:*427, 1962.

Shanthaveerappa, T. R., and Bourne, G. H.: Nature and origin of perisynaptic cells of the motor end-plate. Int. Rev. Cytol., *21:*353, 1967.

Zacks, S. I.: The Motor End Plate. Philadelphia, W. B. Saunders, 1964.

SOME REFERENCES ON SMOOTH MUSCLE

Becker, C. G., and Nachman, R. L.: Contractile proteins of endothelial cells, platelets and smooth muscle. Am. J. Path., *71:*1, 1973.

Bulbring, E., Brading, A., Jones, A., and Tomita, T. (eds.) Smooth Muscle. London: Edward Arnold, 1970.

Cooke, P. H., and Fay, F. S.: Correlation between fiber length, ultrastructure and the length-tension relationships of mammalian smooth muscle. J. Cell Biol., *52:*105, 1972.

Devine, C. E., and Somlyo, A. P.: Thick filaments in vascular smooth muscle. J. Cell Biol., *49:*636, 1971.

Devine, C. E., Somlyo, A. V., and Somlyo, A. P.: Sarcoplasmic reticulum and mitochondria as cation accumulation sites in smooth muscle. Phil. Trans. Roy. Soc. Lond., [B] *265:*17, 1973.

Gabella, G.: Fine structure of smooth muscle. Proc. Trans. Roy. Soc. Lond., [B] *265:*7, 1973.

Kelly, R. E., and Rice, R. V.: Ultrastructural studies on the contractile mechanism of smooth muscle. J. Cell Biol., *42:* 683, 1969.

Lowy, J., and Hanson, J.: Ultrastructure of invertebrate smooth muscles. Physiol. Rev., *42* (Suppl. 5):34, 1962.

Oosaki, T., and Ishii, S.: The junctional structure of smooth muscle cells. J. Ultrastruct. Res., *10:*567, 1964.

Rice, R. V., Moses, J. A., McManus, G. M., Brady, A. C., and Blasik, L. M.: The organization of contractile filaments in a mammalian smooth muscle. J. Cell Biol., *47:*183, 1970.

Somlyo, A. P., Devine, C. E., Somlyo, A. V., and Rice, R. V.: Filament organization in vertebrate smooth muscle. Phil. Trans. Roy. Soc. Lond., [B] *265:223,* 1973. (Further references on smooth muscle are given in connection with arteries in Chap. 22.)

PART THREE

The Systems of the Body

The remaining chapters of this book will each deal with the histology of one of the systems. The term *system* is used in histology, physiology and other subjects to designate a group of organs and/or structures that collaborate to carry out some important function for the body. For example, the circulatory system consists of the heart and all the vessels that are concerned with circulating blood and lymph through all parts of the body. After we finish with the circulatory system, we shall take up the other important systems of the body one by one, a chapter at a time. It should be noted here, however, that in connection with our presentation of nervous tissue, in Chapter 17, we also dealt with the nervous system (brain, spinal cord and peripheral nervous system) to some extent; so there will be no separate chapter on the nervous system, which is a subject in itself and dealt with in other textbooks and courses.

19 The Circulatory System

General Function. In any population in which there is a division of labor, it is usual for raw materials to be produced in one place, manufactured goods in another place and so on. If all inhabitants are to receive some of a great variety of products that are produced in different areas, there must, of course, be an efficient transportation system. Whereas this is done by rail, truck, airplane, ship and pipeline in most countries to serve the people who work at various occupations in different localities, the transportation system which serves the specialized cells in different parts of the body, and permits them to exchange their particular products with cells in other parts, is all done by the equivalent of the pipeline. The tubes in this system are arranged in the form of a circuit by which blood is delivered to and brought back from all parts of the body. The circulation in the system is maintained by the pumping action of the heart. By this means oxygen taken into the blood in the lungs is delivered to the cells in all parts of the body. Food taken into the system from the lumen of the intestine is carried everywhere. The waste products formed by the cellular residents of the body are also emptied into circulating blood and eliminated from it in certain organs, most notably the kidney. The circulatory system therefore constitutes the transportation system for the variously located and specialized cells that make up the cellular population of the body. All cells have access to it, usually via tissue fluid. All take from it and pass products into it. If it fails in any part of the body, that part of the body soon dies.

The Parts of the Circulatory System and Their Particular Functions

THE HEART AND ITS FUNCTION

The heart is a muscular organ that consists of two halves, the right and the left. Each half is a pump in itself and has 2 parts, a reservoir with contractile walls into which blood from veins keeps collecting but which, by reason of its contractile walls rhythmically empties its contents into a strong pump which by reason of contractions of its thick muscular walls just as rhythmically pumps blood into an artery. The reservoir in each instance is called an atrium, and the strong pump in each case is called a ventricle. So the heart as an organ consists of a left half, the left atrium and the left ventricle, and the right half, the right atrium and the right ventricle.

The right atrium collects blood from the veins that drains all parts of the body except the lungs and empties this into the right ventricle. The latter pumps this blood via the pulmonary arteries through the capillary beds of the lungs, where carbon dioxide is released into the air of the lungs and oxygen is absorbed from it. The blood thus freshened passes via the pulmonary veins to the left atrium of the heart and from there to the left ventricle, which pumps it into the aorta. The aorta and its branches carry it to all parts of the body. Thus there are two circulatory systems, the pulmonary and the systemic. Blood is pumped through the pulmonary system by the right ventricle and through the systemic system by the left ventricle.

Each ventricle has certain features of a sac. However, a ventricle has thick walls; these are composed of cardiac muscle. Second, the end of each sac is sealed off except for two openings. One opening, which connects the ventricle with its respective atrium, in which blood collects, is guarded by an intake valve. The other opening leads to an artery—in the instance of the right ventricle, the pulmonary artery, and in the instance of the left ventricle, the aorta. The connection between the ventricle and the artery in each case is guarded by an exhaust valve. The valves are all more or less of the passive flap type, and whether they open or close is dependent on the relative pressures on their two sides as follows:

When a ventricle is full of blood, its muscular walls

contract, and this squeezes blood out through the exhaust valve into the artery that leads from that ventricle. When the ventricle finishes contracting and begins to relax, the exhaust valve closes because the pressure on its arterial side is now greater than that in the ventricle. The atrium of each side also has cardiac muscle in its wall, and the contraction of this, together with the fact that the ventricle is relaxing, causes the pressure in the atrium to be greater than that in the ventricle, so the intake valve opens, and the blood that has accumulated in the atrium is squeezed into the ventricle. The ventricle then contracts again; this closes the intake valve and opens the exhaust valve, and blood is once more forced into the arterial side of each circulation.

The Relation of the Structure of Blood Vessels to Their Particular Functions

The microscopic structure of all these will be described after the following general account.

Arteries

There are 3 main kinds of arteries. Although all conduct blood, the 3 kinds perform different and important functions, and their structure is particularly adapted to the performance of this function. They are: (1) elastic arteries, (2) muscular (distributing) arteries, and (3) arterioles. These types are not sharply divided, for type 1 merges with type 2, and type 2 with type 3. Examples of each type will now be described in turn.

Elastic Arteries. To simplify the following account, we shall deal only with the systemic circulation. The left ventricle functions much like a 1-cylinder pump; hence it delivers blood into the aorta in spurts, ordinarily slightly more than 70 spurts per minute. During the contraction of the ventricle, the pressure that is generated is relatively high. But between contractions the pressure in the arterial system would fall to zero if the walls of the arterial system were rigid, like the walls of metal pipes. The problem is essentially that of trying to maintain pressure in a system of pipes in which the taps are partly open, and in which pressure is generated by a 1-cylinder pump. However, the pressure in the arterial system during and between contractions of a ventricle is maintained more or less evenly because the walls of the arteries that lead directly from each ventricle are constructed chiefly of many layers of elastin called laminae. These are termed *elastic* arteries. Blood delivered into them by the contracting heart stretches the elastic tissue of their walls. Then, after the ventricle has finished contracting, its exhaust valve closes, and the walls of the elastic arteries, which were stretched when the ventricle contracted, passively contract to maintain pressure within the system for the short interval that elapses before the ventricle fills and contracts again.

Systolic and Diastolic Blood Pressure. The pressure within the arterial system generated during the contraction of the ventricle is called the *systolic* (*systole,* a contracting) blood pressure, and it is slightly more than half as much again as the pressure which is maintained by the stretched elastic tissue of the arterial walls between the contractions of the heart; the latter is called the *diastolic* (*diastole,* dilation) pressure.

It should be emphasized that the function of maintaining the pressure within the arterial system during diastole is performed chiefly by the largest arteries of the body because these are the only ones that have walls consisting chiefly of elastin. The branches that arise from the largest arteries to deliver blood to the different parts of the body have a function different from that of the elastic arteries, and it will be found that they have walls of a somewhat different character, as will now be described.

Muscular (Distributing) Arteries. Since different parts of the body under different conditions of activity require different amounts of blood, the arteries that supply them must be capable of having the size of their lumens regulated so that different amounts of blood can be delivered at different times. For example, the muscles in the right arm of a right-handed tennis player require more blood during a match than those of his left arm. Regulation of the size of the lumens of these *distributing* arteries is under the control of the autonomic nervous system, but for this to exert any effect it must do so through innervating smooth muscle. The walls of distributing arteries consist chiefly of circularly disposed smooth muscle fibers which, of course, are living cells and can respond to nervous stimuli and so regulate the size of the lumen of the artery that they surround. If their walls were made of elastin which is nonliving and can only contract passively, nervous control would not be possible. Distributing arteries are also called *muscular* arteries, and they variously regulate the flow of blood to different parts of the body according to the needs of these parts which are indicated by reflex phenomena.

Arterioles. Still other mechanical problems inherent

in a circulatory system must be considered. In order for man to stand erect, a substantial pressure must be maintained within the system; otherwise, blood would not be delivered in sufficient quantities to the various capillary beds of the body, particularly those of the brain, the supplying of which requires that the force of gravity be overcome. However, the maintenance of a relatively high pressure within the arterial system must be accomplished in such a way that blood is delivered into capillary beds under greatly reduced pressure because the walls of capillaries must necessarily be thin (and therefore weak) to permit ready diffusion through them. A high pressure within the arterial system, and the delivery of blood into capillary beds under relatively low pressure, could be accomplished in a mechanical model by inserting pressure reduction valves between the ends of arteries and the capillary beds. The same effect is achieved in the human body by *arterioles*. These, as their name implies, are very small arteries, but they are of a special construction, having relatively narrow lumens and relatively thick muscular walls. Since blood is of a certain viscosity, their narrow lumens offer considerable resistance to its flow, and this permits relatively high pressures to be built up behind them. The degree of pressure within the arterial system as a whole is regulated mainly by the degree of tonus of the smooth muscle cells in the walls of arterioles and this in turn is controlled by both the autonomic system and also by hormones as will be described in a later chapter. If the tonus of the smooth muscle cells becomes increased above the normal range, hypertension (high blood pressure) results.

Capillaries and Veins

Capillaries. The functions of capillaries, including the formation and the absorption of tissue fluid, were considered at length in Chapter 8.

Veins. Capillaries empty into small veins (venules) which join with others to form larger veins, and so on. The blood from all the veins in the systemic circulation eventually drains into either the superior or the inferior vena cava and so passes into the right atrium.

Blood enters venules from capillaries under such a low pressure that they do not require very thick walls. But since the blood in them is under very low pressure, it travels somewhat more slowly. For this reason, veins require lumens somewhat larger than those of arteries. Veins contain most of the blood that is in the circulatory system, probably about 70 percent. In a cross section seen with the LM, a vein always has a thinner

wall and a larger lumen than its arterial counterpart, as will be shown presently.

The pressure in veins draining dependent parts of the body overcomes the force of gravity only with difficulty. To assist, most of these veins are provided with simple flap-type valves to prevent backflow. Valves also have other functions, which will be discussed presently. Since there is no need for veins to cushion the contraction of the ventricle, there are no venous counterparts of elastic arteries. And since there is no need for a strong mechanism for narrowing their lumens against the force of arterial pressure, as is necessary in distributing arteries, there is no need for so much smooth muscle in their walls. However, there is evidence indicating that the tone of the smooth muscle in the walls of veins plays an important role in regulating the relative amount of blood held in the veins at any given time. Muscle tone is controlled by the sympathetic system. Collagen is used more extensively in the walls of veins than in arteries. We shall now discuss in some detail the histologic features of each of these various types of blood vessels.

The Histology of Arteries

The walls of arteries are described as consisting of 3 coats or tunics that are by no means always so clearcut as the following description may suggest. They are (1) the tunica intima (the innermost coat or layer), (2) the tunica media (the middle coat or layer), and (3) the tunica adventitia (the outermost coat or layer). The relative thickness of and the type of tissue in these different layers varies in relation to whether the vessel concerned is an elastic artery, a muscular artery or an arteriole.

BOUNDARIES AND CONTENTS OF THE THREE TUNICS AS SEEN IN SECTIONS

The three tunics are most easily distinguished in muscular arteries so we shall begin with them.

Muscular Arteries. The *intima* is bounded on its inner surface by endothelium (which is part of the intima) and at its outer surface by a substantial lamina of elastin; this lamina is regarded as part of the intima. This lamina of elastin is most easily seen in muscular arteries where it appears in an H and E section in an artery that has contracted after death (because there was no pressure within its lumen to keep its wall stretched) as a wavy bright pink line (Fig. 19-1, *left*). In many muscular arteries the endothelium

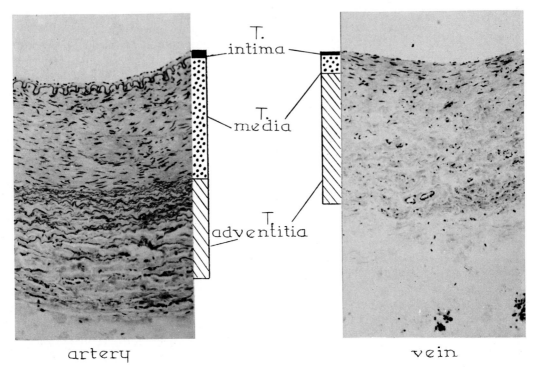

artery　　　　　　　　　　　　　　　　　　vein

FIG. 19-1. (*Left*) A medium-power photomicrograph of a cross section of the wall of a distributing artery. (*Right*) A photomicrograph, taken at the same magnification, of a cross section of the wall of one of its two companion veins. Note the great disparity between the thickness of the media of the artery and the vein.

lining the artery seems to lie directly on the internal elastin lamina. Sometimes the internal elastic in a muscular artery appears as two laminae; this is described as a split internal elastic lamina (Fig. 19-2).

The *media* of a muscular artery is composed essentially of more or less spirally disposed smooth muscle cells (Figs. 19-1, *left*, and 19-2). The intercellular substance between the smooth muscle cells holds them together. It is made by the smooth muscle cells and is chiefly elastin. There is relatively more elastin in the media of a large muscular artery than in a small one. The outer border of the media of a muscular artery is marked by a substantial lamina of elastin; this is called the *external elastic lamina* (Fig. 19-1, *left*, not labeled).

The adventitia of a muscular artery varies but usually it is from one half to two thirds the thickness of the media (Fig. 19-1, *left*). It consists chiefly of elastic fibers but it also contains collagenic ones. Elastin is condensed to form the noticeable external elastic lamina that is applied to and continuous with the outer border of the media. Vasa vasorum which are tiny blood vessels are present in the adventitia, particu-

larly in the larger arteries. Lymphatics are also present in the adventitia.

Coronary Arteries. Because thrombosis here is an important cause of disability and death, the coronary arteries, which supply the musculature of the heart, deserve special attention. They are of the muscular type. They differ somewhat, however, from the usual type of muscular artery. Usually the endothelium of a muscular artery lies directly on the internal elastic lamina as in Figure 19-2. This is true of the smaller ones and arterioles. However, it is not true for some parts of the coronary arteries of newborn children as will now be explained.

As described by Jaffé, Hartroft, Manning and Eleta there are intimal thickenings, termed musculo-elastic cushions, at the sites of branching of coronary arteries in the human newborn (Fig. 19-3). It is thought that the tissue in these sites has its origin from undifferentiated smooth muscle cells of the media, which migrate from the media through fenestrae in the internal elastic lamina (Fig. 19-3) to take up a subendothelial position. Here they produce elastin that is in the form of fibers or incomplete laminae. In addition, they probably produce most of the other types of intercellular substance (mostly a ground substance but sometimes a little collagen as well) in these cushions.

Cells other than the undifferentiated smooth muscle cells may also make their appearance in these thickenings very early in life. For example, monocytes are sometimes encountered. Since monocytes can develop into macrophages and since they gain entrance to this region of thickened intima, probably by penetrating the endothelium that lines the vessel, it seems likely that the macrophages that might be seen later in thickened intimas could have their origin from cells coming to the intima via the blood.

The musculo-elastic cushions, as may be seen at the lower left of Figure 19-3, tend to have two layers. The superficial layer contains more amorphous intercellular substance and fewer fibers than the deeper layer.

Next, as Jaffé, Hartroft, Manning and Eleta show, intimal thickening tends to become general along the coronary arteries in the early decades of life. The thickening is of the same nature as that seen in newborns at bifurcations, but it is not so pronounced. As a result of the thickening there are often elastic fibers rather than an internal elastic lamina directly beneath the endothelium, and there may also be little deposits of collagen in the intima in these sites. The cells in this subendothelial layer of the intima are mostly cells of the undifferentiated smooth muscle type already described. In the intima, however, they are disposed longitudinally, whereas in the media they are arranged at right angles to the direction of the lumen (Fig. 19-4).

In ordinary sections the internal elastic lamina of a muscular artery presents a wavy appearance (Fig. 19-1, *left*), but this appearance is due to the artery contracting after death, when arterial pressure within its lumen no longer exists.

Elastic Arteries. In these the intima is very much thicker than that of a muscular artery (Fig. 19-5). For example, the intima of the aorta of man makes up about one fifth or thereabouts of the total thickness of the wall of the aorta. In the H and E picture on the left of Figure 19-5, it appears paler than the media, and in the section stained for elastin on the right, it can be seen that the intima contains less elastin than the media.

The elastic component of that part of the intima between the endothelium and the internal elastic lamina is in the form of fibers and incomplete laminae which are embedded along with cells in an amorphous intercellular substance. It seems most probable that the main cell type in a normal intima is the same as

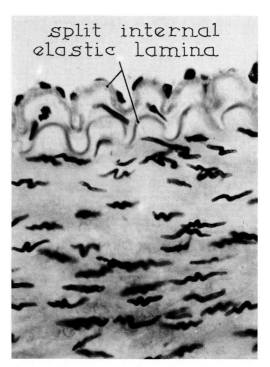

FIG. 19-2. High-power photomicrograph of a cross section of the wall of a distributing artery, showing a split internal elastic lamina.

that already described for coronary arteries, and that it is a relatively undifferentiated type of smooth muscle cell that can produce the various types of intercellular substance seen in the intima, including some of the small amount of collagen which is believed to be a normal component of the intima. However, other types of cells are commonly described as being present in the intima—for example, fibroblasts and macrophages; the latter may develop from monocytes that invade the intima through the endothelium.

The external border of the intima is marked by an internal elastic lamina; this is considered to be part of the intima, but it is similar to the other laminae that are such a prominent feature of the media and that will be described shortly. However, it is not always easy to distinguish the internal elastic lamina because there is so much elastin in the intima.

The media of an elastic artery constitutes the bulk of its wall and consists chiefly of concentrically arranged fenestrated laminae of elastin similar to the internal elastic lamina of the intima. They appear as dark lines in Figure 19-5, *right,* and as lighter ones in Figure 19-5, *left.* The number of these varies with age. There are about 40 in the newborn and up to 70 in

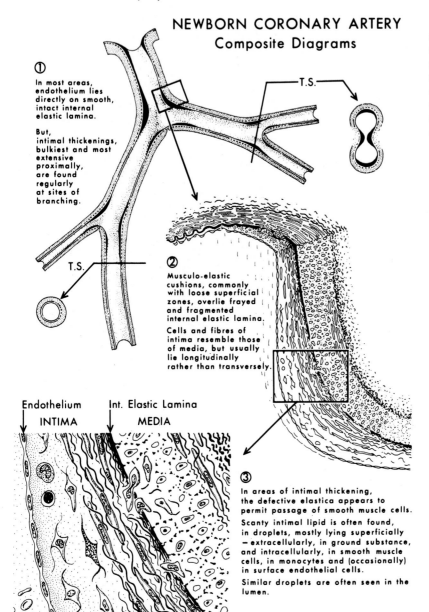

NEWBORN CORONARY ARTERY
Composite Diagrams

① In most areas, endothelium lies directly on smooth, intact internal elastic lamina.

But, intimal thickenings, bulkiest and most extensive proximally, are found regularly at sites of branching.

T.S.

T.S.

② Musculo-elastic cushions, commonly with loose superficial zones, overlie frayed and fragmented internal elastic lamina.

Cells and fibres of intima resemble those of media, but usually lie longitudinally rather than transversely.

Endothelium   Int. Elastic Lamina
INTIMA   MEDIA

③ In areas of intimal thickening, the defective elastica appears to permit passage of smooth muscle cells.

Scanty intimal lipid is often found, in droplets, mostly lying superficially — extracellularly, in ground substance, and intracellularly, in smooth muscle cells, in monocytes and (occasionally) in surface endothelial cells.

Similar droplets are often seen in the lumen.

FIG. 19-3. Diagram based on the study of the coronary arteries of 113 newborn children. The thickenings of the intima are often less or more than what is shown here. (Illustration based on study of Jaffé, D., Manning, M., and Hartroft, W. S.: Coronary arteries in the earlier decades of man. Fed. Proc., *27*:575, 1968)

the adult. The laminae become thicker in adulthood than they are in childhood.

The smooth muscle cells between adjacent laminae are of the type already described that produce, in addition to the elastin of the laminae and the fine elastic and collagenic fibers in the interstices between laminae, the considerable amount of amorphous intercellular substance that is also present between adjacent laminae in which the cells of the tunica media are immersed. The intercellular substance seen here commonly is more basophilic than the ground substance of ordinary connective tissue, and this fact suggests that it contains a greater percentage of sulfated mucopolysaccharide than ordinary connective tissue. Furthermore, there is additional evidence that the amorphous intercellular substance here is the product of a cell type that, in some species at least, has some of the attributes or at least the potentialities of a chondroblast. In experiments the author found that the administration of a very large dose of vitamin D to rabbits, a dose which caused calcification of the media, was followed afterward by the development of rings of cartilage in the aortic wall. Curiously enough, the rings were so regularly disposed as to mimic the distribution of rings of cartilage in the trachea. Hartroft has also found rings of cartilage forming in the aortic wall in animals in which arterial disease was produced by dietary means. As already noted, the undifferentiated smooth muscle cells of arteries seem to have a broad potentiality.

The outermost lamina of the media is termed the external elastic lamina of the artery. The coat to its outer side is termed the adventitia.

The adventitia of an elastic artery is thin (Fig. 19-5, *left*). It consists of irregularly arranged connective tissue which contains both collagenic and elastic fibers. Small blood vessels are present in it, and in suitable sections these may be followed into the outer parts of the tunica media. They are called the *vasa vasorum* (vessels of the vessels). These vessels supply capillary beds in the adventitia and in the outer parts of the media. Lymphatic capillaries are also present here. The reason capillaries and lymphatics are not present in the inner part of the wall of an artery will soon be described. The collagen in the adventitia of elastic arteries may serve as a sheath to restrain overexpansion of the artery.

Atherosclerosis. Since, of the patients that the medical student reader will have in due course, more will probably die of arterial disease than from any other cause, we shall here discuss some histological features of elastic and muscular arteries that may have a bearing on arterial disease. The kind of arterial disease that is so prevalent in our society involves a degeneration of portions of the intima and even deeper layers of important arteries and there is a good deal of evidence implicating a diet containing too much saturated fat as an important factor in bringing about this state of affairs. The lesions themselves suggest that lipid metabolism is involved in their formation; lipids—for example, cholesterol—often accumulate in them. Lesions of this type are commonly called atheromata because the contents, at least sometimes, have a gruel-like (*athero,* gruel) appearance.

Atherosclerosis would not be such a serious matter if it were not for the fact that platelets may begin to adhere to the rough inner surface of a vessel at the site of atherosclerotic lesions and there institute the formation of a thrombus (platelet plugs and thrombi were described in Chapter 11). So, from the standpoint of preventative medicine, there are really 2 interrelated problems: (1) that of preventing the development of

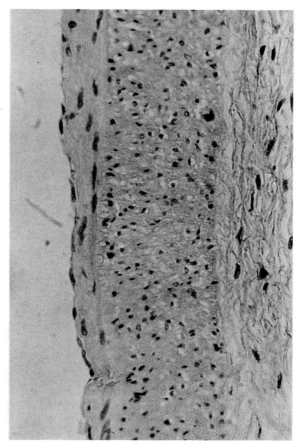

FIG. 19-4. Photomicrograph of longitudinal H and E section of coronary artery of a 5-year-old child. Endothelium is seen at the left. Beneath the endothelium is the intima with smooth muscle cells disposed longitudinally. The media runs up the middle of the picture; in it the muscle cells are cut in cross section because this is a longitudinal section. The adventitia is on the right. (Illustration courtesy of Dr. Doris Jaffé)

atherosclerosis, and (2) that of preventing the formation of thrombi on atherosclerotic lesions. It is the latter phenomenon—the formation of a thrombus—that causes the coronary thrombosis or cerebral stroke that may cause death, because the part of the heart or brain supplied by the affected artery dies.

So we might ask if there are any peculiarities about the histology of the walls of elastic and certain muscular arteries (for example, coronary arteries) that might give some clue to why they should so commonly be the sites of degenerative lesions and thrombus formations. In pursuing this thought, we shall consider briefly the mechanism by which artery walls must be nourished; this is different from most other body parts.

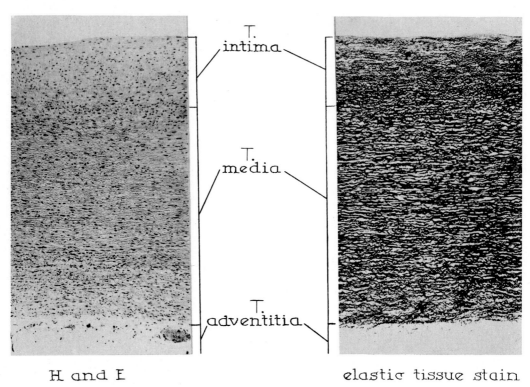

H and E   elastic tissue stain

FIG. 19-5. Low-power photomicrographs of 2 adjacent sections cut from the wall of the aorta; the elastic fibers and the laminae are stained specifically in the section on the right.

THE PROBLEM OF SUPPLYING OXYGEN AND NOURISHMENT TO, AND REMOVING WASTE PRODUCTS FROM, THE ARTERIAL WALL

The arterial wall, stretched by pressure from within the artery, presents unique problems for its nutrition.

The usual arrangement in the body for supplying any considerable mass of tissue abundantly with oxygen and nutrients is for it to be permeated with capillaries. Ordinarily, capillaries are supplied with blood under very low pressure. If low-pressure capillary beds were present in the inner parts of the walls of arteries, they would be collapsed because the relatively high pressure of the blood within the lumen of an artery is transmitted into at least the inner layers of the artery walls that contain the blood; this is a much greater pressure than exists in capillaries. In any event, low-pressure capillaries are not present in the walls of the arteries of man except as vasa vasorum in their outer layers; here they can remain open because the force of the pressure of the blood in the lumen of the artery is taken up by the inner and the middle layers of the artery walls. Lacking capillaries, cells in the inner and the greater part of the middle layers of the walls of arteries must be nourished by the diffusion of sub-

stances from the blood that is in their lumens; thus oxygen and nutrients, to reach the cells in artery walls, must diffuse from the lumen through the wet intercellular substances of the intima and most of the media. This is a long distance for a diffusion mechanism to operate effectively. The situation is reminiscent of that which exists in hyaline cartilage, where diffusion must occur over relatively long distances. It will be recalled that precipitation of mineral in the gelled intercellular substance of cartilage can interfere with diffusion and hence with the nutrition of its cells. It could be visualized that the slow deposition or accumulation of substances in artery walls likewise could interfere with the diffusion mechanism on which the cells in the wall are dependent.

The removal of waste products from the cells in the inner layers of arterial walls seems to be even more difficult. Waste products would surely have a difficult time diffusing through the substance of the wall back to the lumen of the vessel; to do so by means of a diffusion gradient, waste products would have to reach a high concentration within the substance of the wall. The problem is more complicated, moreover, because there can be no lymphatic capillaries in the wall to help remove waste products and, in particular, macromolecules, because the pressure within lymphatic capillaries is even less than that within blood capillaries; hence patent lymphatic capillaries, to carry off macromolecules that might get in, could not exist in those layers of the walls of arteries that bear the brunt of arterial pressure.

From the foregoing it might be expected that degeneration and necrosis would be more likely to occur in the tissues of arterial walls than in most sites in the body, and, further, that arterial walls might be more likely to become the sites of accumulation of materials of macromolecular dimension than the tissues of those parts of the body with lymphatic capillaries to drain macromolecules away. It seems to the author that in the study of atherosclerosis the mechanism of nutrition in artery walls deserves a great deal of attention.

The Endothelium of Arteries. Most of our knowledge of the fine structure of endothelium has come from the study of cross sections of endothelial cells of capillaries by means of ordinary transmission electron microscopy. Some of the findings have already been described in Chapter 8 in connection with the role of capillaries in the formation of tissue fluid and more will be described when we come to capillaries later in this chapter. More recently the scanning electron microscope has provided the means whereby a 3-dimensional view of the inner surface of the endothelium of an artery can be obtained. In a study by Smith, Ryan, Michie and Smith made on the lumen surface of the endothelial cells lining the pulmonary artery of the dog it was found that this surface was studded by little villuslike projections that were present over the whole lumen surface of the endothelial cells that made up the lining (Fig. 19-5A). They estimated the projections to be approximately 250 to 350 nm. in diameter and 300 to 3,000 nm. in length. The authors suggest that these would have an effect on fluid dynamics and could produce an eddying flow of plasma along the surface of the bodies of the endothelial cells. Such a state of affairs could assist in providing nutrition for the artery wall which, as was described above, is not provided with low pressure capillaries and hence is dependent on diffusion phenomena for its nutrition.

A basement membrane, visible with the EM, has been described as lying immediately beneath the endothelium in many arteries, but its existence in the aorta has been questioned.

The regenerative capacity of endothelial cells seems to be considerable, and, as a result, defects in the endothelial lining are repaired very quickly. Moreover, experiments have seemed to show that cells in the blood may settle out and form new endothelium where

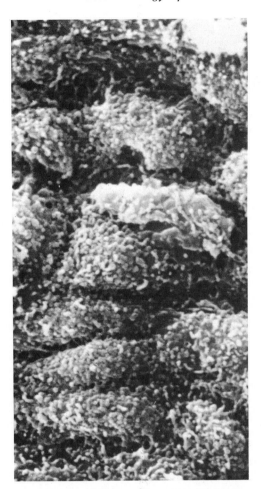

FIG. 19-5A. Low-power ($\times$ 3,000) scanning electron micrograph of endothelial surface of the pulmonary artery. About a dozen cells or parts of cells are shown with the borders between the individual cells being darker than the main bodies of the cells. The surface that the cell bodies present to the lumen of the artery is studded with almost innumerable tiny microvilli-like projections; these are light in the micrograph. (From Smith, V., Ryan, J. W., Michie, D. D., and Smith, D. S.: Science, *173:*925, 1971. Copyright 1971 by the American Association for the Advancement of Science)

there was none. It is conceivable that some endothelial cells become detached from some sites, circulate and become implanted at sites where endothelium is needed.

THE ELASTIN OF ARTERY WALLS

There is more elastin in the walls of the elastic arteries than in the walls of muscular arteries but there is a good deal in both. Because the elastin of elastic arteries can be stretched passively by the force generated by the pumping action of the heart, its subsequent passive contraction, as already noted, can maintain pressure in the arterial system during diastole. There is a second advantage in having elastin instead of collagen as the intercellular substance of choice in artery walls, and in particular in the intimas of arteries, where intercellular substance is guarded from platelets by only a thin film of endothelium. As noted in Chapter 11, and illustrated in Figure 11-12, collagen demonstrates a unique ability to induce the agglutination of platelets, which of course is the first step in the formation of a thrombus.

We might next inquire into the cellular mechanisms that account for the prevalence of elastin in arterial walls. This is to be explained by the fact that the intimas and medias of artery walls are built by a very special type of cell. There are both smooth muscle cells and intercellular substances in artery walls. But there are not (as might be thought) (1) smooth muscle cells to contract and (2) fibroblasts to secrete the intercellular substances. So far as the intimas and medias of arteries are concerned, one kind of cell both makes the elastin and serves as a smooth muscle cell. Moreover, this same cell probably accounts for the formation of such collagenic and reticular fibers as are found in normal intimas and medias and also for the special kind of amorphous intercellular (ground) substance in which all constituents of the intimas and medias are embedded.

When tissue—for example, the intima of an artery wall—is injured, repair processes are set into operation. When a special kind of tissue—for example, bone —is injured, the special cells that give rise to bone can generally repair the injury effectively (as in a simple fracture). When the effective repair of an injured tissue depends on the proliferating ability of the special cells of that tissue, there is always a danger that nearby fibroblasts will get into the act and produce collagen instead of the intercellular substances the special cells would have produced. Another possibility is that the environment might become so altered that osteogenic cells would differentiate into cells more like fibroblasts and produce only collagen instead of the special intercellular substance of bone. In fractures of bones this can lead to fibrous instead of bony union. In the repair of an intimal lesion, repair by fibroblasts or by smooth muscle cells influenced by a changed environment would result in the production of collagen instead of elastin, and the laying down of collagen that might therefore be exposed to platelets in the blood and could conceivably constitute the hazard of inciting platelet agglutination and thrombus formation. Hence injuries to the intima that institute a re-

pair process could lay a possible basis for platelet agglutination.

THE DEVELOPMENT OF ARTERIES AND THE FORMATION OF ELASTIN

In the formation of an artery, mesenchymal cells in the periphery of the developing endothelial tube become arranged so that they more or less loosely ring the tube. These mesenchymal cells differentiate into a type of cell that eventually will have the characteristics of a smooth muscle cell. It is now generally conceded that it is this type of cell that produces the elastin and probably the other intercellular substances in the intima and media of a developing artery. There is not universal agreement about endothelial cells also forming elastin; some think they can form the elastin that lies immediately beneath them.

EM studies show that elastin in a developing aorta is most easily recognized in sections as bands of a homogeneous material that are close to developing smooth muscle cells (Fig. 19-6). However, groups of fine electron-dense microfibrils, around 110 Å in diameter, can also be seen projecting from the developing smooth muscle cells and connecting with the less electron-dense islets of homogeneous elastin already mentioned; indeed, these can be shown to come first. The fine microfibrils which are arranged in swaths seem to originate, according to Fyfe, from the cytoplasm of the developing smooth muscle cells where dark areas can be seen. Ross and Bornstein visualize the microfibrils as appearing in troughs formed on the surface of the cell which elaborates them and tending to form cylindrical arrangements in which amorphous elastin is subsequently observed.

It was formerly assumed that the microfibrils were precursors of elastin but Ross and Bornstein showed that they are composed of a different type of material and they visualize their role as serving as guides or molds for the form that the elastin deposits will take.

It seems very probable that the processes of synthesis and secretion of a proelastin are very similar to those by which procollagen is synthesized and secreted, which processes were described in Chapter 9 and illustrated in Figure 9-6.

Ross and Bornstein have described features of the formation and structure of the elastin molecule that account for its unique stretchability and lack of solubility.

Growth of Elastin Laminae. Elastic laminae during the postnatal growth period have to become larger so as to encompass the lumen of arteries whose diameters continue to increase through that period. Some-

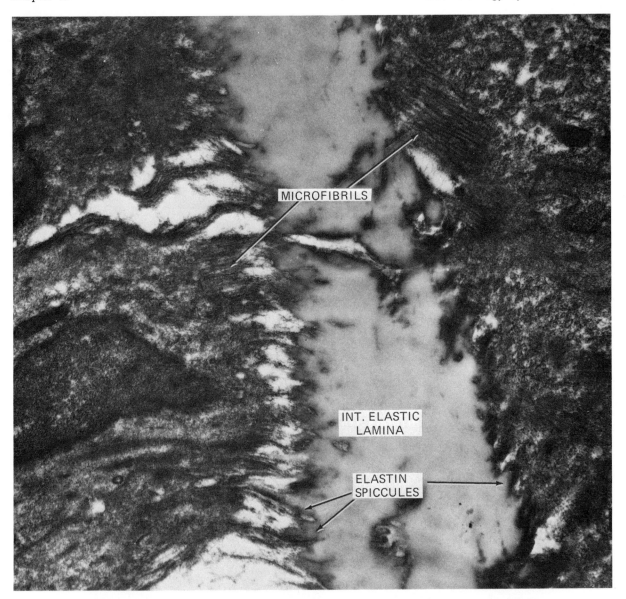

Fɪɢ. 19-6. Electron micrograph ($\times$ 33,000) of a longitudinal section of the aorta of a full-term mouse embryo. The pale material that extends from top to bottom in the middle of the micrograph is the elastin of the internal elastic lamina. The endothelium lies on the right and cells of the media type on the left; the nucleus of one is shown in the lower left. The microfibrils which are believed to influence the position where elastin is laid down appear as dark parallel lines and are labeled. The border of the forming elastic lamina is ragged because of the elastin extending outward in the form of spicules which consist of the most recently formed elastin. (Preparation by Dr. F. W. Fyfe)

how more elastic must make its appearance *within the substance* of a lamina if the first-formed elastin of that lamina is not to be unduly stretched as the artery becomes wider and longer. Yet elastin is formed by an appositional growth mechanism. In this connection it should be observed that elastic laminae are fenestrated.

It is usually and correctly assumed that the function of fenestrae is to serve as holes through which dissolved substances can diffuse to nourish cells deep to the lamina concerned. However, fenestrae may serve a second purpose, as follows:

During growth the aorta (for example) increases

both in length and in width. Hence the elastic laminae in its wall would have to stretch in two directions. If a lamina is stretched in both directions, its fenestrae would become increasingly larger holes. The inner surfaces of these holes would provide sites where elastin could continually be added to a surface to increase the amount in the lamina. So fenestrae may serve as sites where the appositional deposition of elastin can occur during growth.

Regeneration of Elastic Laminae. There has been some question as to whether new elastic laminae can form in arteriosclerotic arteries. The author's studies on arteriosclerosis produced in rats with a heavy overdose of vitamin D, by which method the greater part of the media of a coronary artery becomes almost immediately calcified, indicated that as time went on new elastin formed on each side of the calcified ring.

ARTERIOLES

Arteries with an over-all diameter of 100 μ or less are generally called *arterioles*, but some authors class considerably larger vessels as arterioles also. Cowdry has pointed out that the over-all diameter is not as important a criterion in determining whether any given vessel is an arteriole as is the thickness of its wall in relation to its lumen. Kernohan, Anderson and Keith measured this ratio in a large number of arterioles in muscle tissue obtained from both normal persons and from those suffering from hypertension (high blood pressure). They found that the ratio of the thickness of the wall of the vessel to the diameter of its lumen was 1:2 in normal persons, with variations from 1:1.7 to 1:2.7. They found that in hypertension the arterioles had thicker walls in relation to their lumens.

The walls of the larger arterioles have the usual 3 coats of arteries (Fig. 19-7, *left*). The intima consists of endothelium applied directly, or with a trace of intervening tissue, to an internal elastic lamina. The media consists of circularly arranged smooth muscle fibers. In the larger arterioles some intimation of an external elastic lamina is present (Fig. 19-7, *left*). The adventitia may be as thick as the media and it consists of a mixture of collagenic and elastic fibers.

As arterioles branch and become smaller, their walls become thinner and their lumens smaller. The internal elastic lamina becomes very thin in the smaller arterioles (Fig. 19-7, *right*), and in the smallest it is absent. The smooth muscle cells of the media are correspondingly small; if they were of the usual length, they

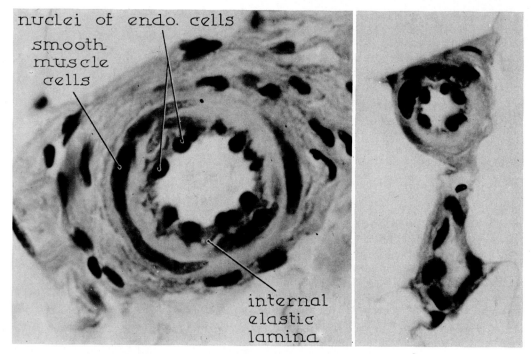

FIG. 19-7. (*Left*) A high-power photomicrograph of a cross section of an arteriole of moderate size. (*Upper right*) A photomicrograph of a cross section of a small arteriole. Its companion venule shows below.

would overlap each other in encircling the lumen (compare those on the left and the right sides of Fig. 19-7). In the smallest arterioles 1 or 2 smooth muscle cells constitute the media that is seen in a cross section (Fig. 19-7, *right*). The adventitia of small arterioles consists chiefly of collagenic fibers, and in the very small ones it is greatly reduced in amount.

A very small arteriole, with a lumen that in a section does not appear to be much larger than a red blood cell and a wall containing no internal elastic lamina and consisting of only a layer of smooth muscle surrounded by a little connective tissue, is sometimes termed a *precapillary* or *terminal arteriole*. Movat and Fernando in their EM study of the terminal vascular bed suggest that the terminal arterioles along their course soon turn into what are often termed *metarterioles*. Along metarterioles the smooth muscle cells of the terminal arterioles are replaced by cells that are probably even less differentiated; these are termed perivascular cells or pericytes. They neither form a continuous coat for the metarteriole nor are, according to Movat and Fernando, contractile. As will be described presently, they are also found along capillaries. They differ from the relatively undifferentiated smooth muscle cells of arteries and arterioles as follows:

Differences Between Smooth Muscle Cells and Pericytes. The relatively undifferentiated smooth muscle cells of arteries have the shape of fibers with elongated nuclei. The arrangements in which smooth muscle cells exist and their fine structure were described in the previous chapter.

The pericytes that are distributed along metarterioles, capillaries and venules (Fig. 19-8) have their organelles more diffusely distributed than those in smooth muscle cells. Their cytoplasm does not reveal myofibrils with the LM, filaments with the EM, or the dark bodies seen in smooth muscle cells. The pericytes, moreover, have long cytoplasmic processes that extend off from their cell bodies (Fig. 19-8, process of pericyte). The pericytes are each enclosed by a basement membrane.

The transition from arterioles into metarterioles is gradual. First, arterioles lose their internal elastic lamina to become terminal arterioles that have a continuous coat of smooth muscle cells. Then the coat becomes discontinuous, and the cells more or less gradually become changed in character, taking on the attributes of pericytes (which are described above) and losing the attributes of smooth muscle cells (described in the previous chapter).

The relation of the capillary bed to the arterioles and metarterioles (A-V bridges) will be described after capillaries.

Capillaries and Capillary Networks— the Terminal Vascular Bed

To visualize the function of, and circulation in, capillaries, it helps to examine under the microscope living preparations, such as the web of a frog's foot, or at least to see one of the motion pictures of capillary circulation. The study of thick cleared sections of material in which the capillaries have been injected with a colored material (Fig. 18-16) can also be helpful.

The Appearance of Capillaries in H and E Sections. Since capillaries are disposed in so many different planes in most tissues, and since most of them pursue irregular courses, it is seldom that they are seen cut longitudinally in thin sections. Striated muscle is an exception, for in this tissue they parallel the muscle fibers. For the same reason, the LM cross-section appearance of capillaries may be studied to great advantage in cross sections of striated muscle (Fig. 19-9). Such sections pass through most capillaries without passing through the nuclei of any of their endothelial cells; hence these capillaries appear as cytoplasmic tubes (Fig. 19-9, *lower right*). However, in many instances the nucleus of one of the endothelial cells making up a capillary wall will be cut, and, if so, it appears as a blue crescent partly encircling the lumen (Fig. 19-9, *slightly above center*). In cross sections some capillaries are seen to contain red blood cells (Fig. 19-9, *left of center*) and some, leukocytes (Fig. 19-9, *upper right*).

Control of the Capillary Circulation

The pink tinge to skin is due to blood in the capillaries and venules that lie below the epidermis. The fact that skin color changes under different emotional states (the white face of fear or the blush of embarrassment) proves that the flow of blood in the terminal vascular bed that lies beneath the epidermis must be under the control of the autonomic nervous system. Since the autonomic nervous system can regulate blood flow through vessels only by changing the tonus of the smooth muscle cells that surround blood vessels, there must be some place in the terminal bed where there are smooth muscle cells that surround vessels, and these are the ones that respond to nervous control (it is generally conceded that endothelial lining cells of capillaries or of other vessels are not under nervous control).

Decades ago it was shown that there were occasional contractile cells disposed along the sides of capillaries

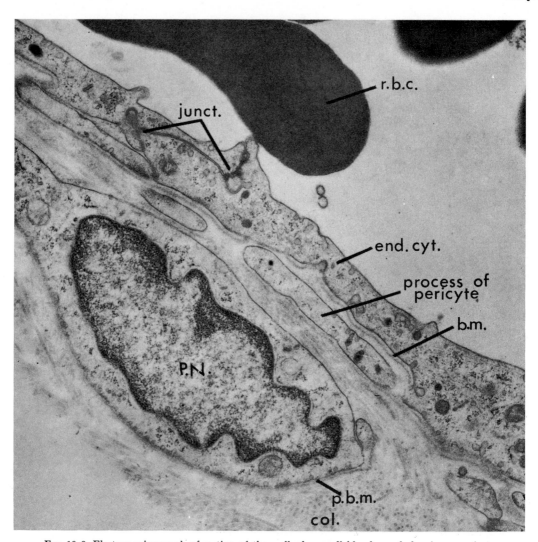

Fɪɢ. 19-8. Electron micrograph of section of the wall of a small blood vessel showing a pericyte. The lumen, shown at the upper right, contains a red blood cell (r.b.c.). The cytoplasm (end. cyt.) of parts of two endothelial lining cells lines the lumen. The site of contact between the two endothelial cells is labeled *junct*. There are junctional complexes at the sites of contact. The basement membrane of the endothelium is labeled b.m. Passing outward from the basement membrane, the process of a pericyte, labeled as such, is seen; farther outside is the nucleus of the pericyte. Basement membrane can be seen around the cell body of the pericyte (p.b.m.); outside this are some collagenic microfibrils (col.). (Preparation by N. S. Taichman and H. Z. Movat)

in the nictitating membrane of the eye of the frog. These were termed Rouget cells. So when occasional cells were demonstrated along the sides of capillaries in mammals, it was believed for a time that these were the counterparts of the Rouget cells, and that they, too, were contractile. However, it became established in due course that the cells distributed along the capillaries and venules were not Rouget cells but *perivascular cells* or *pericytes* (Fig. 19-8) and that they were not contractile.

Zweifach has made many studies on living preparations of circulation through the terminal vascular bed. He visualizes more direct and less direct routes through it. The more direct routes are composed of vessels of larger caliber. These larger vessels were first called A-V bridges and they are labeled as such in Figure

19-10. More recently, and more commonly, they are termed *preferred channels* or *thoroughfares*. The histologist would probably term them metarterioles. True capillaries branch off both from arterioles and from the preferred channels (Fig. 19-10) to join others and so form loops. From these loops some branch off to empty back into a preferred channel near its end, or into a venule (Fig. 19-10). We would assume that a continuous layer of contractile cells would be present only in the precapillary arteriole at the left and the largest venule shown on the right. However, it seems probable that occasional contractile (smooth muscle) cells could be present near the beginning or near the end of an A-V bridge (metarteriole). Under ordinary conditions blood would flow perhaps mostly through the direct route (labeled A-V bridge). But if the muscle cells around the precapillary arterioles and the metarteriole relax, the extra blood flowing through the bed would be partly diverted into the side roads (the true capillaries), which would open up to carry more of the traffic that was passing through the bed.

The role of the noncontractile pericytes disposed along the metarterioles, the true capillaries, and the smallest venules will be discussed presently.

THE FINE STRUCTURE OF CAPILLARIES AND VENULES

Types of Capillaries. The two types of capillaries, continuous and fenestrated, were described in Chapter 8 and illustrated in Figure 8-7.

Here we shall consider further the capillaries that have continuous endothelium.

The Fine Structure of Capillaries With Continuous Endothelium. The lumen of a typical functioning blood capillary is around 7 to 9 μ wide, slightly wider than the diameter of an erythrocyte. Erythrocytes may not be circulating through every capillary at any given time, and so many may not be fully open. The capillary shown in Figure 19-11 is partially collapsed. In some capillaries sites may be found where it seems one endothelial cell encircles the lumen. However, parts of 2 or more endothelial cells may often be seen in any given cross section of a capillary examined with the EM. The one shown in Figure 19-11 reveals parts of 2 endothelial cells. Since endothelial cells are fitted together in an irregular fashion, a very thin *cross section* would often cut through parts of 2 endothelial cells even if each of the 2 endothelial cells completely surrounded the capillary.

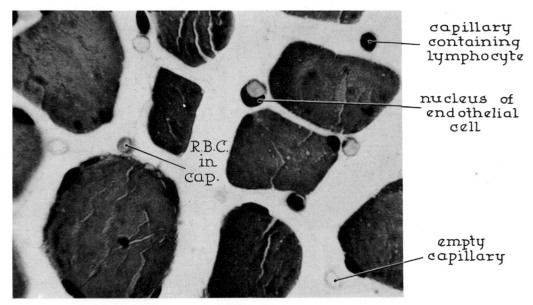

FIG. 19-9. Oil-immersion photomicrograph of a cross section of striated muscle, showing the various appearances presented by capillaries in cross section. In some instances the line of section passes through a capillary at a site where a nucleus of an endothelial cell is present; if so, the nucleus appears as a blue crescent, as may be seen above. If a capillary is cut at a site where no nucleus is present, it appears as a thin cytoplasmic ring. Either red blood cells or leukocytes may be present in capillaries at the sites where they are sectioned.

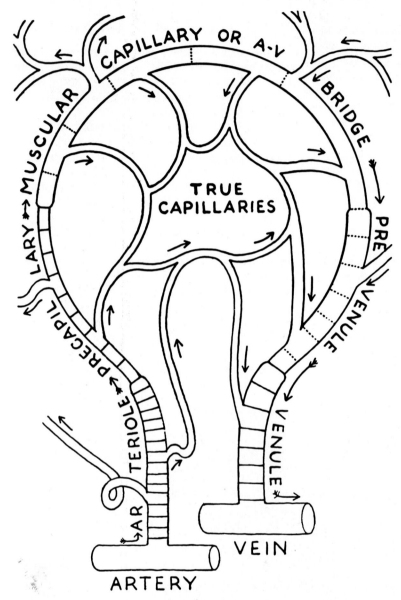

Fig. 19-10. Scheme showing the relationship between arterioles, metarterioles (also called A-V bridges or preferred channels), true capillaries and venules. (Zweifach, B. W.: Anat. Rec., *73*:478)

The nucleus of an endothelial cell creates a bulge in the endothelial wall. The nucleus is, of course, covered with cytoplasm on all its aspects (Fig. 19-11).

The cytoplasm of endothelial cells contains some representation of the usual organelles. Most notably, it is replete with pinocytotic vesicles, which are about 500 to 600 Å in diameter; these are indicated by arrows in Figure 19-11. These seem to arise as a result of invaginations of the cell membrane on either the inner or outer surface of the capillary. It is assumed that they could serve as a medium of transport, traversing the wall of the capillary in either direction.

Obviously, they would provide a good means of transporting macromolecules.

The edges of contiguous endothelial cells are often irregular and interdigitate or form overlap joints with one another. In most capillaries over most of their course the edges of contiguous endothelial cells appear as dark lines and are separated from each other by a space that is around 200 Å wide and is filled with a material of low electron density (Fig. 19-11).

As was described in Chapter 8, there are two main kinds of capillaries, the continuous and the fenestrated type. In most of both kinds the edges of contiguous

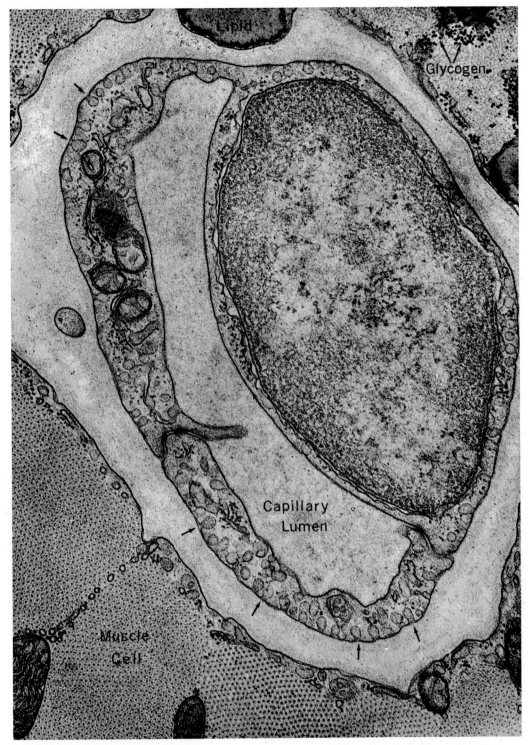

FIG. 19-11. Electron micrograph of a cross section of a partly collapsed capillary in cardiac muscle; the section passes through the nucleus of an endothelial cell. Parts of 2 endothelial cells can be seen; the junctions between them are both below the middle of the picture. A marginal fold projects into the lumen just above the one on the left. Note the very numerous pinocytotic vesicles; several sites where they are originating are indicated by arrows. (Fawcett, D. W.: J. Histochem. Cytochem., *13:*75, 1965)

endothelial cells are joined by tight junctions, but these are of the macula occludens type so there is not a continuous fusion of the outer laminae of the cell membranes of contiguous endothelial cells. Because of these spot-type junctions there is the 200-Å space between contiguous endothelial cells for the passage of tissue fluid from blood to the intercellular substance outside most capillaries. However, as already mentioned, the occludens junctions between the endothelial cells of capillaries of the brain are mostly of the zonula type and, furthermore, the capillaries are completely surrounded by a substantial basement membrane so there is an effective blood-brain barrier. At the point of contact between 2 contiguous endothelial cells, the

cytoplasm of one may form a fold or flap which projects from the inner surface of the endothelial cell into the lumen for a short distance. These little flap-like structures are termed marginal folds (Fig. 19-11, *near the center*) and their function has not been established.

The capillary as a whole is wrapped in a basement membrane which is only a fraction of the thickness of the endothelial cells. With the EM it appears as a seemingly structureless band that rings the capillary (Fig. 8-7, *upper left*). The basement membrane is separated from adjacent muscle fibers by a space that contains some amorphous material.

A few mitochondria are to be seen in the cytoplasm

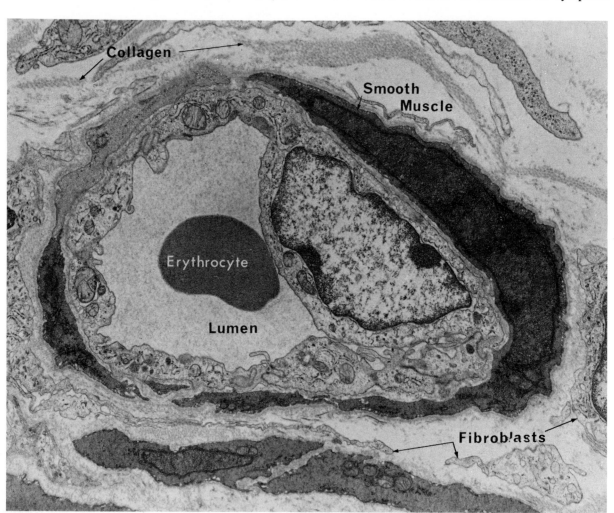

Fig. 19-12. Electron micrograph of venule or small vein in the lamina propria of the ascending colon of a mouse. Note that smooth muscle (dark) does not completely surround the lumen of the venule as it does in arterioles. To the right of the erythrocyte in the lumen the nucleus of an endothelial lining cell is present. Basement membrane can be seen between the endothelium and the smooth muscle. (Illustration courtesy of Melvin Weinstock)

of the endothelial cells (Fig. 19-11). Furthermore, the cytoplasm contains a small representation of almost all types of organelles, including microfilaments. Pinocytotic vesicles are a very prominent feature of the cytoplasm of most capillaries.

Pericytes (Fig. 19-8) may be seen along capillaries but are more characteristic of venules.

The Fine Structure of Beginning Venules. As has been emphasized by Movat and Fernando, venules may prove to be the most significant of all the vessels of the terminal vascular beds with regard to the study of inflammation. It is known that the migration of leukocytes can occur through the walls of venules, and they have also been shown to be sites where blood plasma passes out into the tissue in the inflammatory process.

Venules collect the blood from capillaries and preferred channels and are of a larger diameter than capillaries (Fig. 19-10). Their walls are best studied in the EM. As is shown in Figure 19-12, they are lined by endothelial cells. Except at sites where there are tight junctions, the cell membranes of the contiguous cells approach each other closely, so that there is a space of about 100 to 200 Å between them. As was shown in Figure 10-8, when endothelium is injured, leukocytes migrate through the walls of capillaries and venules, and to do so they effect a separation between the borders of contiguous cells and leave the vessels through the openings so formed; this in itself suggests that the tight junctions must be of the macula type and not in the form of zonulae.

Just outside the endothelium is a sheath of basement membrane (Fig. 19-8, b.m.). This is composed of an almost structureless fibrillar material. The basement membranes surrounding the endothelium of capillaries and venules are about 500 Å in thickness; they are thought to become thicker with age.

The large nucleus (Fig. 19-8, P.N.) at the lower left is the nucleus of a pericyte. The cytoplasm of the pericytes extends out from their main cell bodies in the form of processes. The processes in thin sections are often cut in oblique or cross section as they extend along or around the endothelial tube of the capillary or venule. The pericytes and their processes are also enclosed with basement membrane which is continuous with the basement membrane that surrounds the tube of endothelium. In this sense the basement membrane of the endothelial tube splits so as to envelop the pericyte and its processes as well as the endothelial tube. Basement membrane can be seen on the pericyte at the site marked p.b.m. in Figure 19-8. One process is labeled.

Some collagen can be seen surrounding the endothelial tube and the pericyte. This is in the form of fibrils that are mostly cut in cross section (Fig. 19-8, col.).

As venules become small veins, the character of the cells described as pericytes changes in that they become smooth muscle cells (Fig. 19-12).

As already noted, the function of the pericytes of capillaries and venules, unlike those of cells in a similar position in small veins and arterioles, is not generally believed to be contractile, as was once believed. The pericytes of capillaries and small veins are now generally regarded as relatively undifferentiated mesenchymal derivatives. In the growth of new veins from venules it is thought that they can develop into smooth muscle cells.

Veins

Venules have already been described.

Veins of Small and Medium Size. Their structure varies greatly. In general, their walls, like those of their corresponding arteries, consist of 3 tunics (Fig. 19-1, *right*). The intima consists of endothelium which either rests directly on a poorly defined internal elastic membrane or is separated from it by a slight amount of subendothelial collagenic connective tissue. The media is usually much thinner than that of a companion artery (Fig. 19-1). It consists chiefly of circularly disposed smooth muscle fibers. Smooth muscle cells, when present in the walls of venules, may not completely encircle the lumen as they do in arterioles (Fig. 19-12). More collagenic fibers and fewer elastic fibers are mixed with them than in arteries. In some veins the innermost smooth muscle fibers of the media have a longitudinal course. In general, the media is much less muscular and hence thinner in veins that are protected, for example, by muscles or by the pressure of the abdominal contents, than in veins that are more exposed. The cerebral and the meningeal veins have almost no muscle in their walls. The adventitia of veins of medium size is often their thickest coat (Fig. 19-1, *right*). It usually consists chiefly of collagenic connective tissue.

The muscular media is well developed in the veins of the limbs, particularly in those of the lower ones. This is particularly true of the saphenous veins. Being superficial, these are not supported by the pressure of surrounding structures to the same extent as deeper veins. Furthermore, when a person stands erect, their walls must withstand the hydrostatic pressure generated by a long column of blood. For these two reasons their walls must be thicker than those of most veins. This is accomplished chiefly by a very substantial media. The innermost part of this consists chiefly of

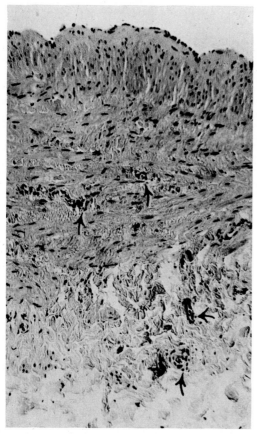

FIG. 19-13. Medium-power photomicrograph of the wall of the saphenous vein as it appears in a cross section. Note the inner layer of longitudinal muscle and note that the vasa vasorum, indicated by arrows, penetrate deeply into the media from the adventitia.

occasion than can be obtained by diffusion from the lumen of the vessel. Vasa vasorum carrying arterial blood into the substance of the walls of veins supply this need. Furthermore, since the blood in veins is under low pressure, vasa vasorum can approach the intima of the walls of veins without necessarily being collapsed by the pressure within the vein. Hence, the vasa vasorum of veins penetrate much closer to the intima than do those of arteries. They are seen to advantage in the thick walls of the saphenous vein (Fig. 19-13).

Lymphatics. Since the walls of veins do not have to withstand great pressures, as do the walls of arteries, lymphatics, as well as vasa vasorum, can be present in a patent state within the substance of their walls. Indeed, the walls of veins are supplied much more abundantly with lymphatic capillaries than are the walls of arteries. (This probably explains why tumors that spread by lymphatics invade the walls of veins but

longitudinally disposed smooth muscle fibers associated with elastic fibers (Fig. 19-13) and the outermost and thicker part of circularly disposed smooth muscle fibers (Fig. 19-13).

Large Veins. The structure of different veins varies considerably. In general, the tunica intima resembles that of veins of medium size, but the subendothelial layer of connective tissue is thicker. In most of the largest veins there is little smooth muscle in the media. The adventitia is the thickest of the 3 coats, and it contains both collagenic and elastic fibers. In many instances—for example, the inferior vena cava—its innermost part contains bundles of longitudinally disposed smooth muscle fibers (Fig. 19-14).

Vasa Vasorum of Veins. Veins are supplied much more abundantly with vasa vasorum than are arteries. Since veins contain poorly oxygenated blood, the cells of the walls of veins probably need more oxygen on

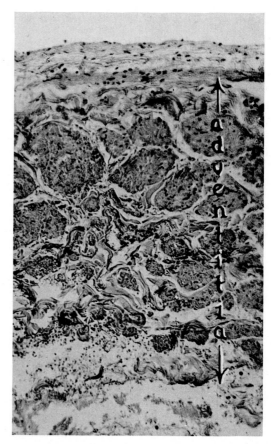

FIG. 19-14. Medium-power photomicrograph of the wall of the inferior vena cava, as seen in a cross section. Note the longitudinal muscle bundles in the adventitia.

never the walls of arteries.) Lymphatic capillaries may approach the inner surfaces of the veins so closely that the tissue fluid that enters them to become lymph is probably a filtrate or a dialysate of the blood in the lumen of the vein itself.

Valves of Veins. Many veins are provided with valves disposed so as to permit blood to flow toward the heart but not in the opposite direction. The valves of veins are of the flap (leaflet) type. Most valves have two leaflets, but some have only one. The leaflets are composed of folds of intima with some extra central reinforcements of connective tissue. Elastic fibers are disposed on the side of the valve that faces the lumen of the vessel.

Valves are especially abundant in the veins of the extremities, and they are generally absent from the veins of the thorax and the abdomen. Valves usually are placed immediately distal to sites where tributaries enter veins. Veins immediately proximal to the attachment of a valve are always dilated slightly to form a pouch or sinus. Hence, in distended superficial veins, localized swellings indicate the sites of valves.

The function of valves in veins is not completely understood. Obviously, valves must help to overcome the force of gravity by preventing backflow. But they may act in other ways. For example, valves in veins that are squeezed when surrounding muscles contract would enable the surrounding muscles to serve as pumps. Moreover, valves in such veins would prevent muscular contractions from creating back pressure on the capillary beds drained by the veins.

Varicose Veins. Superficial veins are relatively unsupported, and the force of gravity exerted through the blood within those below the heart is a more or less constant factor tending to cause their dilatation. Under conditions in which there is obstruction to the return of blood from a part, or in which the tissues of the walls of the veins are not as strong as usual, because of inheritance or disease, superficial veins gradually dilate. As dilatation proceeds, the valves become incompetent and, as a result, gravity exerts a still greater dilating force on their walls. Superficial veins that under these conditions become tortuous, irregular and wider than usual are called *varicose veins*.

The Transplantation of Blood Vessels

The transplantation of segments of blood vessels to bypass or replace segments of vessels that are malformed, diseased and weakened or occluded is now a relatively common surgical operation.

The use of autologous transplants of blood vessels is very limited because there is no source of autologous transplants for replacing any of the larger vessels of the body (except under certain circumstances when anastomoses are abundant). Some types of arterial defects can be repaired with autologous venous grafts, but the use of these is limited. Therefore, transplants of blood vessels are sometimes of the homologous variety, and, as has already been explained, there are serious problems associated with obtaining the survival of cells in this type of transplant. However, homologous transplants of blood vessels are effective, and for much the same reason that transplants of compact bone are effective: the intercellular substance in them survives for the time during which new tissue is growing into them. Elastin is probably the most important tissue component in the transplant, for it has been shown experimentally that it will remain intact for at least 6 to 9 months.

A homologous transplant is invaded by cells from the host site. These grow into the substance and form collagen. It is not believed that new elastin is formed in vessel transplants.

Since no cell survival is counted on in homologous transplants, they may be stored and treated in a variety of ways which might destroy any cells they contain. Homotransplants may be stored in the deep freeze, or may be frozen and dried, or treated in other ways.

Synthetic materials formed into the shapes of blood vessels are now widely used as substitutes for homotransplants. These are made of materials that do not stir up a tissue reaction. Furthermore, they are made so that they are porous; this permits cells from the host to grow into their substance and fill the interstices of it with cells and intercellular substance.

Arteriovenous Anastomoses

That arteriovenous anastomoses exist in many parts of the body, particularly in the distal parts of extremities, has been known for a very long time. Early evidence for their existence accumulated from experiments in which particulate matter, too large to pass through capillaries, was injected into an artery and recovered from the corresponding vein.

Grant first studied arteriovenous anastomoses in the living animal by subjecting carefully prepared rabbits' ears to direct microscopic observation by means of strong transmitted light. Grant and Bland later studied them in human skin and in the bird's foot. Clark and Clark, at almost the same time, studied them and their formation by means of transparent chambers inserted in rabbits' ears. Masson has described a special type

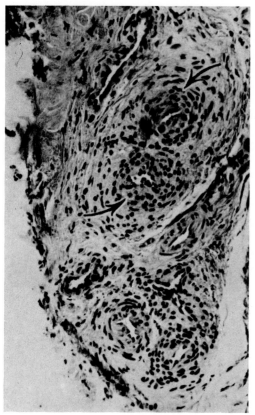

Fig. 19-15. Medium-power photomicrograph of a section of skin, showing a glomus. The thick-walled arterial vessel in the glomus (indicated by arrows) is coiled or convoluted; hence, cross sections of it appear in several sites.

of anastomosis seen in little organs in the skin called *glomi* (Fig. 19-15).

Arteriovenous anastomoses arise as side branches from arteries and arterioles and pursue either a tortuous or a fairly straight course to connect usually with the vein or the venule accompanying the arterial vessel from which they arise. Near the point where they empty into veins, their walls have the character of veins, and at their point of origin their walls have the character of arteries but are slightly thicker. But at the intermediate segment of transition, according to Grant, there is considerable muscular and adventitial thickening to be seen in the vessel. Moreover, this part of the anastomosis is particularly well supplied with nerve endings from the sympathetic division of the autonomic nervous system, and presumably it is more or less specialized to serve as a sphincter.

The dilatation of arteriovenous anastomoses in any part of the body permits a much greater amount of blood to pass through that part. It is obvious that arteriovenous anastomoses would serve a very important purpose in, for example, the tips of fingers or toes subjected to cold, because by their dilatation they could permit greatly increased amounts of warm blood to pass through the extremities and so help maintain their temperature. It is very likely that arteriovenous anastomoses do serve a very important function in this way. Furthermore, it is not unlikely that they serve important functions in certain structures in the body that indulge in intermittent activities. Moreover, the dilation of arteriovenous anastomoses in a normal body would have an effect in raising venous blood pressure and so aid the return of blood to the heart. Their closure under conditions of obstructed venous return similarly could help to diminish venous pressure. *Arteriovenous anastomoses are very different structures from A-V bridges, and to avoid confusion the latter are now commonly termed "preferred channels."*

Nervous Control of Arteries

Since the walls of distributing (muscular) arteries are composed primarily of smooth muscle, the size of their lumens can be regulated to allow for variations in the blood supply that may be required. Furthermore, if some given muscular artery or group of muscular arteries is to deliver more blood through some given part of the body—for example, the right arm of a right-handed baseball pitcher—the vessels beyond the distributing artery must also become more dilated to permit the increased flow of blood to be delivered to and pass through capillary beds. Both the distributing arteries and their branches, including the arterioles and even the terminal vascular bed, must cooperate if more blood is to flow through a part and adequately supply, say, muscle fibers with more oxygen and sugar.

Unmyelinated fibers from the autonomic nervous system (chiefly from the sympathetic division) supply the smooth muscle cells of blood vessels; they can be seen in the adventitia of arteries along which they course (Fig. 19-16). Nerve impulses reaching the smooth muscle cells influence them as described in the preceding two chapters.

Role of Arterioles in the Regulation of the Blood Pressure

The maintenance of a proper blood pressure depends on several factors including, for example, the strength of the pumping action of the heart, the amount of blood in the arterial system, the viscosity of the blood, and the degree to which the outlets of the arterial system, the arterioles, are contracted or dilated. All other things being equal, pressure within the system depends on the latter. Although temporary increases in blood pressure occur, and might normally be expected to occur under conditions which temporarily gear up a body for, say, fight or flight, there are some individuals in whom arteriolar constriction tends to be persistent, and so they have *hypertension.* The cause of a persistent hypertension due to constriction, but not to organic disease of arterioles, is not entirely clear. Some believe psychosomatic factors are involved; in particular, suppressed animosity has received mention in this respect. As we shall see when we consider the kidney, a humoral factor produced in that organ is also involved in controlling blood pressure. It should be mentioned that one of the most notable advances in treating disease has been in connection with treating hypertension; drugs are now available which have been widely and successfully used to ameliorate the condition. However, in some types of hypertension there are degenerative changes in the arteriolar walls, and this, of course, is a more serious condition and less amenable to treatment.

Heart

Pericardial Cavity. The heart is covered with a fibroelastic connective-tissue membrane, which, in turn, is covered with a single layer of mesothelium. This mesothelial-covered, fibroelastic membrane is termed the *epicardium* (*epi,* upon). The heart, so covered, is surrounded by another fibroelastic membrane, the *pericardium.* This is lined with mesothelium. Between the pericardium and the epicardium is a potential space, the pericardial cavity, which in health contains up to 50 ml. of fluid. This fluid is so distributed that it amounts to no more than a film in most places. The epicardium is continuous at the base of the heart with the pericardium. The lubricating film of fluid between the mesothelial lining of the pericardium and the mesothelial covering of the epicardium permits the heart to move freely during contraction and relaxation. In certain diseases the amount of fluid in the pericardial cavity becomes greatly increased; in others, the epicardium becomes united by fibrous connective tissue to the pericardium. Both deviations from the normal embarrass the action of the heart.

Epicardium. The character of the epicardium varies

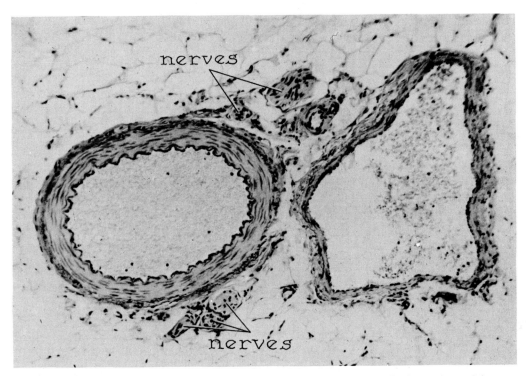

Fig. 19-16. Medium-power photomicrograph of a cross section of a distributing artery and its companion vein. Small nerves, cut in cross section, may be seen closely associated with the adventitia. Notice that the vein has a thinner wall and a larger lumen than the artery.

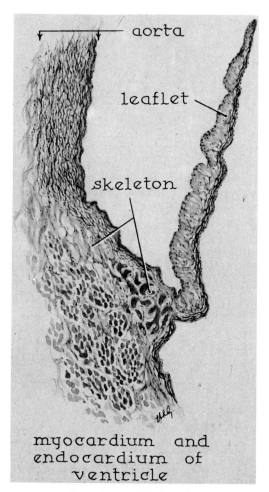

FIG. 19-17. Drawing of a longitudinal section of the heart (low-power) cut through the site where the wall of the ventricle continues an aortic valve leaflet. The tissue of the base of the leaflet merges into that of the skeleton of the heart.

somewhat over different parts of the heart. Its more superficial layer consists of mesothelium, beneath which is ordinary connective tissue; this contains some blood capillaries, lymphatic capillaries and some nerves. The deeper layer of the epicardium contains larger blood vessels and more fat and is continuous with the endomysium of the underlying cardiac muscle. Fat is particularly abundant along the course of the larger coronary vessels.

Myocardium. The muscular and thickest part of the wall of the heart lies deep to the epicardium. It is composed of cardiac muscle (as was described in Chap. 18). The arrangement of the various groups of fibers comprising the myocardium is considered in textbooks of gross anatomy.

Endocardium. This membrane forms a complete lining for the atrial and the ventricular cavities and covers all the structures that project into the heart (valves, chordae tendineae and papillary muscles). In general, the thickness of the endocardium varies inversely with the thickness of the myocardium it lines. The endocardium has 3 layers. The innermost consists of a delicate connective-tissue membrane lined with endothelium that is continuous with the lining of the blood vessels that leave the heart. The next (middle layer) is the thickest. It consists of dense connective tissue in which many elastic fibers are present, particularly in its inner part (Fig. 19-17). These commonly are disposed parallel with the surface, and in some sites where they are abundant, they alternate with layers of collagenic fibers. In the outer part of this layer some smooth muscle fibers may be present. The third and outermost (deepest) layer of the endocardium consists of more irregularly arranged connective tissue. Fat may be present here. This layer contains blood vessels and in certain sites it also contains cardiac muscle fibers of a special type (Purkinje fibers) to be described later. It is continuous with the endomysium of the myocardium.

Skeleton of the Heart. The aorta and the pulmonary artery arise from the left and the right ventricles, respectively. At its point of origin each is surrounded by a fibrous ring. The dense connective tissue (Fig. 19-17) of these rings is continuous, either directly or indirectly, through the medium of a triangular mass of dense connective tissue with some cartilaginous qualities, the trigonum fibrosum, with the connective tissue of fibrous rings that surround the atrioventricular orifices. The fibrous rings surrounding the outlets of the atria and the ventricles prevent the valve-containing outlets from becoming dilated when the muscular walls of the chambers contract and force their contents out through them. These fibrous structures, together with the fibrous (membranous) part of the interventricular septum, also provide a means for the insertion of the free ends of the fibers of the cardiac musculature. For this reason, these various fibrous structures sometimes are said to constitute the skeleton of the heart.

Valves of the Heart. Each ventricle requires an intake and an exhaust valve. The kind used is the leaflet (flap) type (Figs. 19-17 and 19-18). The leaflets consist essentially of folds of endocardium (Fig. 19-17). But, since 2 layers of endocardium would not be strong enough to withstand the pressures generated, each leaflet is reinforced with a flat sheet of dense connective tissue.

The intake valve of the right ventricle consists of 3

leaflets and is called the *tricuspid valve*. Although cusp means a point, it has become common to speak of the leaflets themselves as cusps. The intake valve of the left ventricle consists of only 2 leaflets; hence it is called the *bicuspid valve*. The leaflets of both of the atrioventricular valves have a similar histologic structure. They are covered on both sides with endocardium and have a middle supporting layer of dense collagenic connective tissue. On the ventricular side of the layer of collagenic tissue there are numerous elastic fibers. A few are also present beneath the endothelium on the atrial side of the leaflet.

At the bases of the leaflets, the middle collagenic supporting flat plate becomes continuous with the dense connective tissue of the rings surrounding the orifices. Smooth muscle fibers have been described at this site, and a sphincterlike action has been attributed to them. Capillaries may be present at the bases of the leaflets, where smooth muscle fibers are present, but capillaries do not extend into the valves proper in man. Such cells as are distributed throughout the dense connective tissue of the valves live in tissue fluid derived from the plasma of the blood that bathes the valves.

Tendinous cords of dense collagenic connective tissue (the chordae tendineae) covered with thin endocardium extend from the papillary muscles to connect with the ventricular surface of the middle collagenic supporting layer of each leaflet. It should be realized that the exhaust valves of the ventricles (the aortic and the pulmonary valves) open on ventricular contraction and that only the closed intake (atrioventricular) valves must withstand the full pressure of ventricular contraction. There is a danger, then, that unless they were specially protected, they might on strong ventricular contraction behave like umbrellas on windy days and be blown inside out. The chordae tendineae and the papillary muscles from which they arise limit the extent to which the portions of the valves near their free margins can be "blown" toward the atria. (See Fig. 19-19.)

The exhaust valve of the right ventricle is termed the *pulmonary semilunar valve* because of the shape of its leaflets. The exhaust valve of the left ventricle is termed the *aortic semilunar valve,* and it, too, has 3 leaflets (Fig. 19-18). The leaflets of these valves are thinner than those of the atrioventricular valves. However, they are of the same general construction, being composed essentially of folds of endocardium reinforced with a middle layer of dense connective tissue; the folds of endocardium at their bases become continuous with the skeleton of the heart (Fig. 19-17). They have no chordae tendineae. The leaflets contain

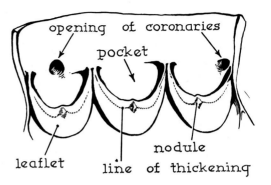
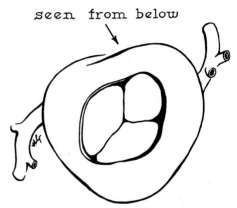

Fig. 19-18. (*Top*) The 3 leaflets of the aortic valve as they appear when the aorta is opened and spread out flat. (*Bottom*) The appearance of the closed valve as seen from below.

a considerable amount of elastic tissue on their ventricular sides (Fig. 19-17).

In a semilunar valve leaflet the dense middle layer becomes somewhat thickened along a line close to, and parallel with, its free margin, particularly near the middle of the leaflet. This is the line along which the leaflets touch one another when the valves close; hence the tissue here must be relatively strong. Between this line of thickened tissue and their actual free margins, the leaflets are filmlike. The very pliable free margins permit a more perfect seal than could be obtained by stiffer tissue unless it were perfectly "machined."

For the free edges of 3 "patch" pockets bulging inward from the lining of a vessel toward its center to make a perfect seal requires that each leaflet, when the valve is closed, must have the appearance, when seen from below (except for having a curved base), of a triangle with its apex reaching the center of the vessel (Fig. 19-18). Furthermore, the sum of the angles of the apices of the 3 triangular leaflets of a closed valve must be 360°. At the apex of each leaflet, the thickening along the line close to the free margin, described in the previous paragraph, is accentuated to form a nodule (Fig. 19-18). The free margin of a closed valve curves upward from both sides to a peak at this point; hence, this pointed portion of the free margin containing the nodule constitutes a true cusp (Fig. 19-18). However, as noted before, the whole leaflet is sometimes called a cusp.

Diseases affecting the valves of the heart may cause serious mechanical problems. In particular, in children suffering from rheumatic fever, the leaflets may become the seat of an inflammatory process. The healing of the leaflets often is associated with a considerable increase in their collagenic component; as a result, they may become stiffer and shorter or deformed in other ways. Leaflets sometimes become glued together with collagen. In any event, the end result is likely to be a valve that does not open or close properly. The student will see many examples of valves so affected in his clinical years.

Impulse-Conducting System of the Heart

In a cardiac cycle, the blood enters the right and the left atria from the venae cavae and the pulmonary veins, respectively. Part of this blood flows directly into the relaxed right and left ventricles, while the rest fills the atria. The two atria then contract simultaneously, squeezing their contents into the partially filled ventricles to complete the filling process. Contraction of the ventricles then follows, which closes the atrioventricular valves and opens the aortic and the pulmonary valves through which their contents are discharged into the aorta and the pulmonary arteries, respectively. In the meantime, the atria are filling again.

The efficiency of the heart depends to a great degree on these different events following each other in orderly sequence. Unfortunately, in certain all too common diseases the orderly sequence of events is disturbed. For example, instead of a wave of contraction sweeping over the atria and later over the ventricles, the atria may begin to contract more or less independently of, and at different rates from, the ventricles. Or the walls of the atria may only flutter instead of contracting properly. Indeed, there are far too many ways in which the normal order is disturbed to permit listing them here. But since the student will soon be seeing examples of these conditions in the clinic, at this time he should become as familiar as possible with the mechanism that permits different events to be synchronized properly in the normal heart.

Development of Knowledge. It was first realized that the orderly sequence of contractions to be observed in the hearts of cold-blooded animals depended on a wave of excitation sweeping first along the muscular tissue of the atria and then along that of the ventricles. But the theory of muscular conduction of the impulse for contraction could not be applied at that time to the hearts of mammals because these were thought to have a continuous connective-tissue partition between the atria and the ventricles. However, in 1893 W. His, Jr., demonstrated that the partition in the human heart was pierced by a bundle of muscle which passes from the atrial septum to the upper border of the interventricular septum (Fig. 19-19). (Earlier in the same year, Kent had shown that the partition in the monkey heart was pierced by bundles of muscle fibers which were somewhat different from those of ordinary cardiac muscle.) The *atrioventricular* (A-V) bundle of muscle or, as it is often called, the *bundle of His,* provides a means whereby each wave of contraction that sweeps over the atria can be conducted by muscular tissue to the ventricles to institute their contraction at precisely the time when they have been properly filled with blood by the contraction of the atria. The cardiac muscle fibers in the A-V bundle would, of course, be specialized to conduct (at a special suitable rate) rather than to contract, and, as we shall see presently, they have a different microscopic appearance from the fibers of ordinary cardiac muscle (Fig. 19-21).

It soon became apparent that there was further muscle tissue in the heart that was specialized for conducting instead of for contracting, and even some that was specialized for initiating the impulse for contraction. Indeed, it is now understood that the A-V bundle is only one important part of a whole system of fibers that are specialized for this purpose. These constitute what is termed the *impulse-conducting system of the heart,* and we shall now describe the various parts of this system and the microscopic structure of each representative division.

The Sinu-atrial (S-A) Node. This is a little mass of specialized cardiac muscle fibers that are contained in substantial amounts of dense fibroelastic connective tissue. It is abundantly supplied with nerve fibers from both divisions of the autonomic nervous system. It lies in the right wall of the superior vena cava at the upper end of the sulcus terminalis (Figs. 19-19 and 19-20) and was first described in 1907 by Keith and Flack, who considered that the impulse for the contraction of the heart arose in it. This concept soon received support because it was found in 1910 that the S-A node was the first region to become electronegative when a

Fig. 19-19. Drawing of the cut surface (striped) and the interior of the heart, as seen from the front. The cut was made so as to expose and extend along, so far as was possible, the main parts of the impulse-conducting system, which is shown in red.

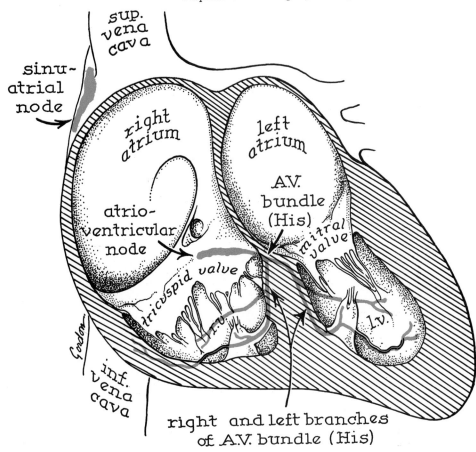

wave of contraction developed in the heart of the dog. It is now often described as the *pacemaker* of the heart, and it is generally believed that here nervous impulses make their influence felt by affecting the rate at which impulses for contraction develop in the node to sweep over the heart thereafter.

As Duckworth has described it, the connective tissue content of the node becomes considerably increased immediately after birth, and, at the same time, the muscular elements in the node develop into their adult form. The adult nodal fibers are small cross-striated fusiform fibers about half the size of the ordinary atrial fibers, and they lie parallel with the long axis of the nodal artery as it descends through the center of the node. These fibers are embedded in a relatively large amount of dense connective tissue which contains many capillaries (Fig. 19-20, *right*). Peripheral ganglia of the parasympathetic division of the autonomic system (of the vagus nerve) are present in close association with the node (Fig. 19-20, *left*), and, as has been noted already, the node is abundantly supplied with fibers from both divisions of the system. Parasym-

pathetic stimulation slows the rate of the heart, whereas sympathetic stimulation increases it.

No pathways of special fibers have as yet been satisfactorily demonstrated in the walls of the atria; hence it is assumed that the impulses that arise in the S-A node sweep through the ordinary muscle fibers of the atria to reach the next part of the impulse-conducting system, which is the atrioventricular node.

The Atrioventricular (A-V) Node. This was discovered in 1906 by Tawara, and it consists of a little mass of specialized tissue that is disposed in the lower part of the interatrial septum immediately above the attachment of the septal cusp of the tricuspid valve; anteriorly, it is continuous with the A-V bundle (Fig. 19-19). The cells of the node are cardiac muscle fibers but have fewer myofibrils than do ordinary cardiac muscle fibers. The fibers branch so extensively and in so many directions that the myofibrils of one cell are commonly seen to cross those of underlying or overlying cells at right angles.

The A-V Bundle. According to Duckworth, the fibers of the bundle during the first year of life become

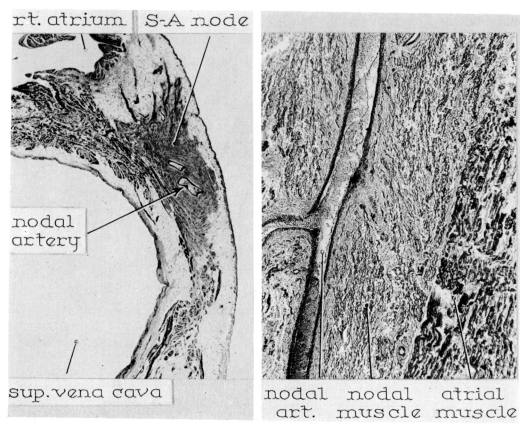

Fig. 19-20. (*Left*) Low-power cross section of the right wall of the superior vena cava at its junction with the right atrium, cutting through the sinu-atrial node. (*Right*) Low-power longitudinal section of the sinu-atrial node, showing the fine muscle fibers of the node, in contrast with the larger darker-staining atrial muscle. Note the nodal artery running through the center of the node. (Preparation by J. W. A. Duckworth)

fine in caliber (Fig. 19-21). They become arranged parallel with one another with little connective tissue but with many capillaries between them. Many of the fibers are no wider than the capillaries. However, like the fibers of the S-A node, they anastomose freely.

Purkinje Fibers. In the human heart the two branches of the A-V bundle run about halfway down the two sides of the interventricular septum before their fibers enlarge to become continuous with what are called Purkinje fibers. These were first seen by Purkinje in 1845 in the subendocardial region in the ventricles of the ungulate heart. Seen with the LM, they resemble ordinary cardiac muscle fibers in that they have centrally disposed nuclei and cross striations (Fig. 19-22). However, they differ from ordinary cardiac muscle fibers in that they are generally wider, and also in that the myofibrils in each fiber tend to be disposed around its periphery; this leaves the central core

of each fiber relatively empty of myofibrils, and their place is taken by considerable amounts of glycogen. In H and E sections the glycogen is not seen as such; hence the central part of each Purkinje fiber appears to be empty except where nuclei are present (Fig. 19-22).

As shown in red in Figure 19-19, Purkinje fibers supply the papillary muscles before they supply the lateral walls of the ventricles, up which they spread as a subendocardial network. Since these fibers conduct the impulse for contraction much more rapidly than the ordinary heart muscle, this arrangement ensures that the papillary muscles will take up the strain on the leaflets of the mitral and the tricuspid valves before the full force of the ventricular contraction is thrown against them.

The fine structure of Purkinje fibers is to a great extent what would be anticipated from their light microscopy in that they contain relatively few myofibrils (which demonstrate cross striations similar to those seen in cardiac muscle and are peripherally disposed), many mitochondria and much glycogen. Some lysosomes are present. The sarcoplasmic reticulum is not as well developed as in cardiac muscle and the fibers are relatively, if not completely, deficient with regard to transverse tubules.

The type of junctions that connect Purkinje fibers to one another and to cardiac muscle fibers would, it could be assumed, be similar to those of cardiac muscle fibers. It is incorrect to refer to the specialized muscle of the heart as the Purkinje system when only a part of that system is made up of true Purkinje fibers.

Electrocardiograms. The passage of a wave of excitation over either special or ordinary cardiac muscle fibers is associated with a changing electrical potential along the fiber. Essentially, the particular site over which the wave is passing at any given time is

always negatively charged in relation to the parts of the fiber over which it has passed, or which it has not yet reached. Hence, if a series of electrodes could be placed along the different parts of the conducting system and connected to different galvanometers, the passage of the impulse for contraction over the system could be followed by watching the galvanometers. Similarly, if electrodes are taken from the intact heart and connected to galvanometers, the passage of the impulse for contraction, plus the changing potentials due to waves of contraction occurring successively in different parts of the heart muscle on their reception of the impulse, could be followed by watching the galvanometers. However, in order to obtain a great deal of information about the passage of the impulse for contraction over the heart and the successive activation of the heart muscle of different parts of it, it is not necessary to connect electrodes to the heart. If leads are taken off different parts of the body that are projections, as it were, of 3 widely separated points on the

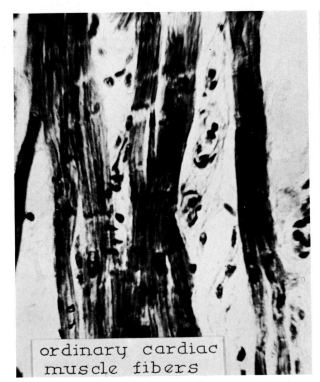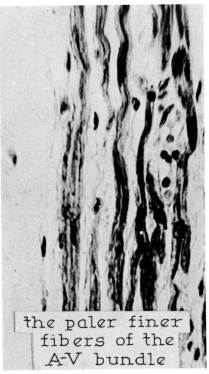

Fig. 19-21. Two high-power photomicrographs of the same magnification of adjacent areas in a section of the uppermost part of the interventricular septum of the heart of a human adult (Hollande's chlorcarmine stain). (*Left*) The muscle fibers are those of ordinary cardiac muscle. (*Right*) The muscle fibers of the A-V bundle; they may be seen to be both narrower and paler than those of ordinary cardiac muscle. The striations which they clearly exhibit in many instances cannot be seen in this illustration. (Preparation by J. W. A. Duckworth)

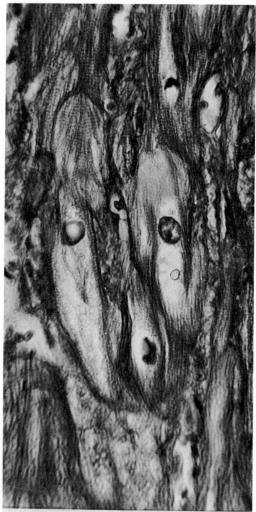

FIG. 19-22. High-power longitudinal section of human Purkinje fibers from the right ventricle. Note their large size and that the myofibrils occupy the periphery of the cell. (Preparation by J. W. A. Duckworth)

heart, they give somewhat similar information to leads taken directly from these 3 parts of the heart themselves. Originally, 3 standard leads were taken, but it has been found that a greater number give more detailed information. If any disease condition exists which interferes with the proper conduction of the impulse for contraction over the heart or the proper activation of its different parts, a deviation from the normal pattern of waves is apparent, and so electrocardiography is of great importance in helping to diagnose certain types of cardiac disease.

NERVOUS CONTROL OF THE HEART

In contrast to the control of the tonus of smooth muscle cells of arteries, which is a function chiefly of the sympathetic nervous system, the control of the heart rate is chiefly under the control of the parasympathetic division of the system. The heart has both sympathetic and parasympathetic innervation, but the parasympathetic fibers exert the greater regulatory influence. They are derived from the vagus nerve, and they act to depress heart action continuously. For example, if the vagus is paralyzed, the heart rate may be doubled. If afferent impulses from any part of the body were directed to the centers of the brain that control the tonus of arterioles and the heart beat, they could therefore by reflex mechanisms control arterial pressure within wide limits.

While it is probable that afferent impulses from many blood vessels, and from other sites, find their way to the centers in the brain that direct the flow of nervous impulses to the heart and arteries, there are a certain few sites in the vascular system where vessels are richly provided with afferent (receptor) nerve endings that are especially receptive to pressure changes. In other sites there are complex nerve endings sensitive to changes in the chemical composition of the blood. The *carotid sinus* and the *carotid body* serve as excellent examples of such structures, and we shall consider their structure.

The Carotid Sinus and the Carotid Body. The carotid sinus is the name given to a slight dilatation of one of the carotid arteries near the bifurcation of the common carotid artery. Usually, the site of the dilatation is the internal carotid artery immediately above its point of origin (Fig. 19-23). In the dilated part the tunica media of the vessel is relatively thin, and the tunica adventitia is relatively thick. Many nerve endings of afferent fibers from the carotid branch of the glossopharyngeal nerve are present in the adventitia. Since the media is thin at this site, the adventitia must bear more of the brunt of withstanding the pressure within the vessel than is usual in arteries; hence the nerve endings within it are readily stimulated by pressure changes. Nerve impulses set up by pressure changes within the sinus are conducted over nerve networks to the centers in the brain that control the heart and the arteries.

Green, and Boss and Green demonstrated that, in addition to the carotid sinus, there are other areas along the common carotid artery of the cat that have *baroceptor* (*baros*, weight) activity, Boss and Green have studied the histology of these baroceptor areas and have found that basically it is similar to that of

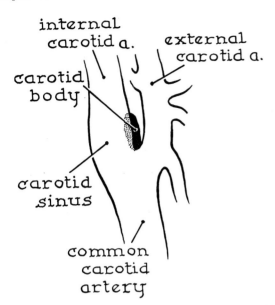

FIG. 19-23. Sketch of a carotid sinus and a carotid body.

the carotid sinus. In each area myelinated fibers ramify in the adventitia of the vessel in fibrillar arrangement. Furthermore, there are structural alterations in the arterial wall in each site in that there is generally less muscle and sometimes less elastin in the media, and the collagenic fibers of the adventitia are in the form of finer fibers than usual, and these are intricately interwoven.

The carotid body is a small condensation of tissue on the wall of the internal carotid artery (Fig. 19-23). It has a structure similar to that of an endocrine gland in that it consists of cords and clumps of epithelial-like cells and is abundantly provided with sinusoidal capillaries. The epithelial-like cells are richly supplied with nerve endings. These seem to be stimulated by changes in the concentration of carbon dioxide or oxygen tension in the blood. Nerve impulses arising from these endings, as a result of chemical changes in the blood, are also conducted to the centers in the brain that control the heart and the arteries.

Small structures similar to the carotid body are also present in the arch of the aorta, in the pulmonary artery and at the origin of the right subclavian artery. Delicate pressure receptors are also present in the walls of the great veins close to the heart.

The Lymphatic Division of the Circulatory System

Lymphatic Vessels. The vessels that conduct lymph are called *lymphatics*. The walls of the smallest

of these—the kind into which the lymphatic capillaries empty—consist of a thin layer of connective tissue and an endothelial lining. When lymphatics become somewhere between one fifth and one half a millimeter in diameter, their walls show indications of being composed of 3 layers: an *intima*, a *media* and an *adventitia*. The 3 layers are not well defined in the walls of the smaller lymphatics (Fig. 19-24); however, they may be distinguished fairly clearly in the larger ones. The intima commonly contains elastic fibers. The media of the larger vessels consists chiefly of circularly and obliquely disposed smooth muscle fibers. The muscle fibers are supported by some connective tissue which contains elastic fibers. The adventitia is relatively well developed, particularly in the smaller vessels, and it contains smooth muscle fibers; these run both longitudinally and obliquely. Small blood vessels are present in the outer coats of lymphatics of a medium and a large size.

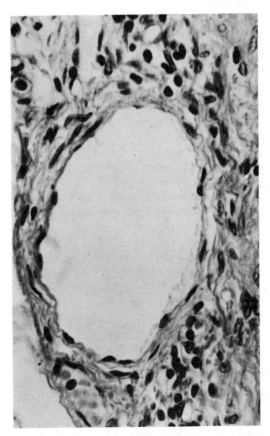

FIG. 19-24. High-power photomicrograph of a cross section of a small lymphatic vessel. The nuclei of a few smooth muscle fibers may be seen in its wall, but the layers of the wall are not clearly defined.

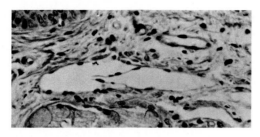

Fig. 19-25. Photomicrograph of an oblique section of a lymphatic showing a valve. (Illustration courtesy of Yves Clermont)

The lymphatics, which collect the lymph from the lymphatic capillaries and carry it to the larger lymphatic vessels that finally deliver it into the blood circulatory system, commonly pass through the tissue along with a vein and its companion artery. However, the lymphatic vessels do not show as much tendency to unite with one another to form a single large vessel as do small veins; hence, several lymphatics may be associated with a vein and its companion artery. The lymphatics, as they pass through the tissues, may unite with one another but they also branch again and so remain numerous.

Lymphatic vessels, except the smallest ones, commonly, but not always, possess valves. These are more numerous and hence closer together than the valves of veins. Indeed, the valves of lymphatics may be so close together that a distended lymphatic appears to be beaded, because dilated sections between the numerous valves are so close together. The valves commonly have 2 leaflets; these consist of folds of intima, so they have delicate connective tissue plates in their middles and endothelial coverings (Fig. 19-25). The endothelial cells are said, like those of the valves of veins, to be oriented differently on the 2 surfaces of a leaflet, their long diameters being parallel with the stream on the side of the leaflet that faces the stream and at right angles to the stream on its sheltered side.

It is easy to understand how each segment of a lymphatic that is situated between 2 valves could act as a pump if (1) the wall of the lymphatic in that segment contracted, or (2) that segment were squeezed because of compression developing outside the lymphatic. In frogs there are lymph hearts to propel lymph. It seems doubtful that lymph is propelled along the lymphatics of mammals by contractions of the smooth muscle in their walls. The compression of lymphatics occasioned by pulsating blood vessels in their vicinity, or by active or passive movements of the parts in which they are contained, may make lymphatic vessels serve as pumps to some extent and so aid in propelling lymph along them. This explains why massage may be employed to improve the lymphatic drainage of a part. It seems doubtful if there is very much lymph flow from normal tissues that are at rest. As we shall see when the intestine is studied, the lymphatics which drain it participate in the absorption of fat. After a fatty meal the lymph from the intestine is milky in color and is termed *chyle.*

The lymph that is collected in the body is finally returned to the bloodstream by means of 2 main terminal vessels; the *thoracic duct* and the *right lymphatic duct* (the latter may be represented by several vessels). At its beginning in the abdomen, the thoracic duct is somewhat dilated to form what is termed the *cisterna chyli,* and from here it extends for about 18 inches before it opens into the left innominate vein in the angle of its junction with the internal jugular and left subclavian veins. Sometimes it is represented by several smaller vessels which open separately into the great veins. The right lymphatic duct or, more commonly, several representatives of the right lymphatic duct enter the great veins on the right side at sites comparable with those at which the thoracic duct enters the great vessels on the left side. The tributaries that flow into the thoracic duct and the right lymphatic duct (or their representatives), respectively, are described in textbooks of gross anatomy; here it is enough to point out that the thoracic duct receives all the lymph that forms in the abdomen; hence, it is much the larger vessel of the two.

Fine Structure. Perhaps the most important point that should be made about the fine structure of lymphatics is that lymph capillaries lack the surrounding basement membrane that ensheathes blood capillaries; this fact probably accounts in part for their ability to absorb macromolecules more readily than blood capillaries from tissue fluid and inflammatory exudates. For details of their fine structure see Leak.

References and Other Reading

SOME REFERENCES ON ELASTOGENESIS IN ARTERIES

Bierring, F., and Kobayasi, T.: Electron microscopy of the normal rabbit aorta. Acta Path. Microbiol. Scand., *57:*154, 1963.

Fyfe, F. W., Gillman, T., and Oneson, I. B.: A combined quantitative chemical, light, and electron microscope study of aortic development in normal and nitrile-treated mice. Ann. N.Y. Acad. Sci., *149:*607, 1968.

Haust, M. D., More, R. H., Bencosme, S. A., and Balis, J. U.: Elastogenesis in human aorta: an electron microscope study. Exp. Molec. Path., *4:*508, 1965.

Paule, W. J.: Electron microscopy of the newborn rat aorta. J. Ultrastruct. Res., *8:*219, 1965.

Rhodin, J. A. G.: Fine structure of vascular walls in mammals with special reference to smooth muscle component. Physiol. Rev., *42*(5):447, 1962.

Ross, R., and Bornstein, P.: Elastic fibers in the body. Sci. Am., *224:*44, 1971.

SOME REFERENCES ON ARTERIES, VEINS AND LYMPHATICS

Abramson, D. I. (ed.): Blood Vessels and Lymphatics. New York, Academic Press, 1962.

Altschul, R.: Endothelium. New York, Macmillan, 1954.

Boss, J., and Green, J. H.: The histology of the common carotid baroceptor areas of the cat. Circ. Res., *4:*12, 1956.

Boyd, J. D.: Observations on the human carotid sinus and the nerve supply. Anat. Anz., *84:*386, 1937.

Buck, R. C.: The fine structure of endothelium of large arteries. J. Biophys. Biochem. Cytol., *4:*187, 1958.

Burton, A. C.: Relation of structure to function of the tissues of the wall of blood vessels. Physiol. Rev., *34:*619, 1954.

Clark, E. R.: Arterio-venous anastomoses. Physiol. Rev., *18:*229, 1938.

Franklin, K. J.: A Monograph on Veins. Springfield, Ill., Charles C Thomas, 1937.

Hollingshead, W. H.: Effect of anoxia upon carotid body morphology. Anat. Rec., *92:*255, 1945.

Jaffé, D., Hartroft, W. S., Manning, M., and Eleta, G.: Coronary arteries in newborn children. Acta Paediat. Scand., Suppl. *219:*1, 1971.

Kampmeier, O. F., and Birch, C. L. F.: The origin and development of venous valves. Am. J. Anat., *38:*451, 1927.

Keech, M. K.: Electron microscope study of the normal rat aorta. J. Biophys. Biochem. Cytol., *7:*533, 1960.

Lansing, A. I.: The Arterial Wall. Baltimore, Williams & Wilkins, 1959.

Leak, L. V.: Electron microscopic observations on lymphatic capillaries and the structural components of the connective tissue-lymph interface. Microvasc. Res., *2:*391, 1970.

Luft, J. H.: The fine structure of the vascular wall. *In* Jones, R. J. (ed.): Evolution of the Arteriosclerotic Plague. p. 3. Chicago, University of Chicago Press, 1963.

Nonindez, J. F.: The aortic (depressor) nerve and its associated epithelioid body, the glomus aorticum. Am. J. Anat., *57:*259, 1935.

————: Identification of the receptor area in the venae cavae and pulmonary veins which initiate reflex cardiac acceleration (Bainbridge's reflex). Am. J. Anat., *61:*203, 1937.

Parker, F.: An electron microscope study of coronary arteries. Am. J. Anat., *103:*247, 1958.

Pease, D. C., and Molinari, S.: Electron microscopy of muscular arteries: Pial vessels of the cat and monkey. J. Ultrastruct. Res., *3:*447, 1960.

Pease, D. C., and Paule, W. J.: Electron microscopy of elastic arteries: The thoracic aorta of the rat. J. Ultrastruct. Res., *3:*469, 1960.

Pritchard, M. M. L., and Daniel, P. M.: Arterio-venous anastomoses in the human external ear. J. Anat., *90:*309, 1956.

————: Arterio-venous anastomoses in the tongue of the sheep and the goat. Am. J. Anat., *95:*203, 1954.

Rhodin, J. A. G.: Fine structure of the vascular wall in mammals. Physiol. Rev., *42* (Suppl. 5):48, 1962.

Smith, V., Ryan, J. W., Michie, D. D., and Smith, D.: Endothelial projections, as revealed by scanning electron microscopy. Science, *173:*925, 1971.

Wollard, H. H.: The innervation of blood vessels. Heart, *13:* 319, 1926.

Wollard, H. H., and Weddell, G.: The composition and distribution of vascular nerves in the extremities. J. Anat., *69:*165, 1935.

SOME REFERENCES ON THE TERMINAL VASCULAR BED

Bruns, R. R., and Palade, G. E.: Studies on blood capillaries. I. General organization of blood capillaries in muscle. J. Cell Biol., *37:*244, 1968.

————: Studies on blood capillaries. II. Transport of ferritin molecules across the wall of muscle capillaries. J. Cell Biol., *37:*277, 1968.

Clark, E. R., and Clark, E. L.: Caliber changes in minute blood vessels observed in the living mammal. Am. J. Anat., *73:*215, 1943.

————: Microscopic observations on the extra endothelial cells of the living mammalian blood vessels. Am. J. Anat., *6:*1, 1940.

Farquhar, M.: Fine structure and function in capillaries of the anterior pituitary gland. Angiology, *12:*270, 1961.

Fawcett, D. W.: Comparative observations on the fine structure of blood capillaries. *In* The Peripheral Vessels, Internat. Acad. Pathol. Monograph No. 4. p. 17. Baltimore, Williams & Wilkins, 1963.

Fernando, N. V. P., and Movat, H. Z.: The smallest arterial vessels: Terminal arterioles and metarterioles. Exp. Molec. Path., *3:*1, 1964.

————: The capillaries. Exp. Molec. Path., *3:*87, 1964.

Florey, H.: Exchange of substances between the blood and tissues. Nature, *192:*908, 1961.

Karnovsky, M. J., and Cotran, R. S.: The intercellular passage of exogenous peroxidase across endothelium and mesothelium. Anat. Rec., *154:*365, 1966.

Kernohan, J. W., Anderson, E. W., and Keith, N. M.: Arterioles in cases of hypertension. Arch. Intern. Med., *44:*395, 1929.

Majno, G., Palade, G. E., and Schoefl, G. I.: Studies on inflammation. II. The site of action of histamine and serotonin along the vascular tree: a topographic study. J. Biophys. Biochem. Cytol., *11:*607, 1961.

Movat, H. Z., and Fernando, N. V. P.: Small arteries with an internal elastic lamina. Exp. Molec. Path., *2:*549, 1963.

————: The venules and their perivascular cells. Exp. Molec. Path., *3:*98, 1964.

Nelemans, F. A.: Innervation of the smallest blood vessels. Am. J. Anat., *83:*43, 1948.

Palade, G. E.: Blood capillaries of the heart and other organs. Circulation, *24:*368, 1961.

Zweifach, B. W.: Character and distribution of blood capillaries. Anat. Rec., *73:*475, 1939.

————: The structure and reactions of the small blood vessels in amphibia. Am. J. Anat., *60:*473, 1937.

————: The microcirculation of the blood. Sci. Amer., *200:*54, 1959.

Zweifach, B. W., Grant, L., and McCluskey, R. T. (eds.): The Inflammatory Process. New York, Academic Press, 1965.

SOME REFERENCES ON THE HEART AND THE IMPULSE-CONDUCTING SYSTEM

Bast, T. H., and Gardner, W. D.: Wilhelm His, Jr., and the bundles of His. J. Hist. Med., *4:*170, 1949.

Caesar, R., Edwards, G. A., and Ruska, H.: Electron microscopy of the impulse conducting system of the sheep heart. Z. Zellforsch., *48:*698, 1958.

Davies, F., and Francis, E. T. B.: The conducting system of the vertebrate heart. Biol. Rev., *20-21:*173, 1946.

Duckworth, J. W. A.: The Development of the Sinuatrial and Atrio-ventricular Nodes of the Human Heart, M.D. thesis, University of Edinburgh, 1952.

Gregg, O. E.: The coronary circulation. Physiol. Rev., *26:*28, 1946.

Harper, W. F.: The blood supply of human heart valves. Brit. Med. J., *2:*305, 1941.

Herman, L., Stuckley, J. W., and Hoffman, B. F.: Electron microscopy of Purkinje fibers and ventricular muscle of dog heart. Circulation, *24:*954, 1961.

His, W., Jr.: Die Thätikeit des embryonalen Herzens. Arb. Med. Klin., Leipzig, 1893. Cited by Mall, F. P.: Am. J. Anat., *13:*278, 1912.

Kaylor, C. T., and Robb, J. S.: Observations on the differentiation and connexions of the specialised conducting tissue in the human heart. Anat. Rec., *97:*31, 1947.

Keith, A., and Flack, M.: The auriculoventricular bundle of the human heart. Lancet, *2:*359, 1906.

Kent, S.: Researches on the structure of function of the mammalian heart. J. Physiol., *14:*233, 1893.

Kistin, A. D.: Observations on the anatomy of the atrioventricular bundle (bundle of His), and the question of other atrio-ventricular connexions in normal human hearts. Am. Heart J.. *37:*848, 1949.

Lewis, T., Oppenheimer, B. S., and Oppenheimer, A.: The site of origin of the mammalian heart beat; the pacemaker of the heart. Heart, *2:*147, 1910.

Mall, F. P.: On the development of the human heart. Am. J. Anat., *13:*249, 1912.

Muir, A. R.: Observations on the fine structure of the Purkinje fibers in the ventricles of the sheep's heart. J. Anat., *91:*251, 1957.

Purkinje, J. E.: Mikroskopisch-neurologische Beobachtungen. Arch. Anat. Physiol., *22:*281, 1845.

Rhodin, J. A. G., Delmissier, P., and Reid, L. C.: The structure of the specialized conducting system of the steer heart. Circulation, *24:*349, 1961.

Robb, J. S., Kaylor, C. T., and Turman, W. G.: A study of specialized heart tissue at various stages of development of the human heart. Am. J. Med., *5:*324, 1948.

Shaner, R. F.: The development of the atrio-ventricular node, bundle of His and sino-atrial node in the calf, with a description of a third embryonic node-like structure. Anat. Rec., *44:*85, 1929.

Stotler, W. A., and McMahon, R. A.: The innervation and structure of the conductive system of the human heart. J. Comp. Neurol., *87:*57, 1947.

Tawara, S.: Das Reizleitungssystem des Saugetierherzens. Jena, Fischer, 1906.

Walls, E. W.: The development of the specialized conducting system in the human heart. J. Anat., *81:*93, 1947.

(For fine structure of cardiac muscle, *see* References for Chap. 18.)

20 The Integumentary System (The Skin and Its Appendages)

Introduction

The skin consists of two layers of completely different kinds of tissue that are attached to one another over their whole extent. The outer layer consists of stratified squamous keratinizing epithelium (described in Chapter 7) and is derived from ectoderm. It contains no blood vessels so it must be nourished via tissue fluid from the second and deeper layer of the skin which consists of irregularly arranged connective tissue that is derived from mesoderm and which contains blood vessels.

Terminology. There are two ways this can be confusing. First the word *dermis* sometimes is used to refer to the skin as a whole—that is, as a membrane that consists of two layers. For example, this is the meaning of the word in the term dermatology, which is the branch of medical science that is concerned with diseases of the skin in which both layers of the skin may be involved. However, when a dermatologist, histologist or histopathologist studies skin with the microscope he will call the outer (epithelial) layer of the skin the *epidermis* (*epi,* upon) and the deeper connective tissue layer of the skin the dermis, thus using the latter term with a restricted meaning.

The second way the terminology may be confusing is due to a common error that is made even by learned individuals who sometimes say or write skin when they are really referring to epidermis. Indeed, the usual textbook classification of skin is based on this error because it is customary to classify skin into thick and thin types. In reality this classification refers to two kinds of skin that are distinguished from one another by whether or not they have a thick or a thin epidermis. These two types of skin will now be described.

The Structure and Distribution of So-Called Thick and Thin Skin

Thick skin is found on the palms of the hands and the soles of the feet; thin skin covers the remainder of the body. The skin of the palms of the hands and the soles of the feet has a thick epidermis with a particularly thick layer of keratin on its outer surface (Fig. 20-1, *left*). The skin covering the remainder of the body, although it has a thick dermis in some sites, as on the back, has a relatively thin epidermis, and the outer keratinized layer of this is relatively thin (Fig. 20-7, *top*). Note also the connective tissue dermis in Figure 20-1. The structure of thick and thin skin will be described in detail shortly.

Relation of Skin to Subcutaneous Tissue (Hypodermis). The two layers of the skin are firmly cemented together to form a cohesive membrane which varies in thickness from less than 0.5 mm. to 3 or even 4 mm. or more in different parts of the body. The skin rests on subcutaneous tissue, which varies, being of the loose, adipose, or dense varieties in different sites and in different people. The subcutaneous connective tissue (Fig. 20-1) is the superficial fascia of gross anatomy. It is sometimes called the *hypodermis,* but this terminology is confusing because, unlike the epidermis, it is not considered to be part of the skin. Irregularly spaced bundles of collagenic fibers extend from the dermis into the subcutaneous tissue to provide anchorage for the skin (Fig. 20-1, *left*). The subcutaneous tissue permits the skin over most parts of the body a considerable latitude of movement.

The Appendages of the Skin. During embryonic development, cells of the ectodermal derived developing epidermis grow down into the developing dermis to give rise to epithelial glands and glandlike structures which include sweat glands, hair follicles (that form hairs) and sebaceous glands. The way in which glands develop was described in Chapter 6 (review Fig. 6-1). Epidermal invasion of the connective tissue is also responsible for the grooves of epidermis that produce fingernails and toenails.

So a consideration of the skin includes the two more or less flat layers of tissue that constitute epidermis and dermis plus epidermal appendages. The

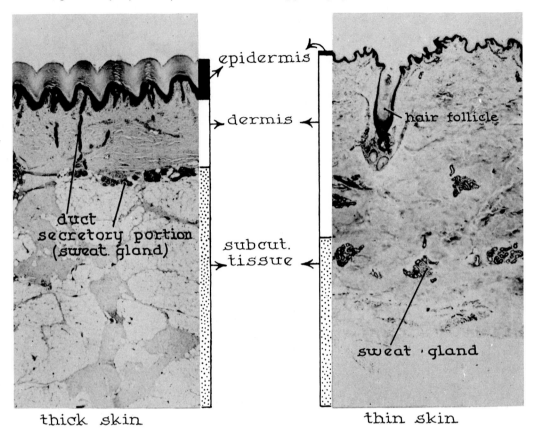

epidermis

dermis

hair follicle

duct
secretory portion
(sweat gland)

subcut.
tissue

sweat gland

thick skin

thin skin

Fig. 20-1. Low-power photomicrographs, taken at the same magnification, of sections of thick and thin skin. The skin at the left was taken from the sole of the foot, and that on the right from the abdomen. Note that thick skin has a relatively thick epidermis that consists chiefly of keratin, and that thin skin has a thin epidermis and a thick dermis.

latter are sweat glands, hair follicles, sebaceous glands, nail grooves and nails.

Some Functions of the Skin. The epidermis and particularly its layer of keratin is a barrier to disease organisms. Keratin is nearly waterproof; this permits a fluid body to exist in what is often very dry atmosphere. The keratin makes it possible to have a bath in fresh water without the body becoming swollen with water, or in salt water without the body becoming shrunken.

The epidermis, because it contains certain cells that can produce the dark pigment, melanin, can protect the body from the harmful effects of too much ultraviolet light.

The epidermis, however, is not impervious to everything; for example, certain chemicals can be absorbed through it into the capillaries and lymphatics of the underlying dermis. Accordingly, care has to be taken in many instances so that poisonous chemicals do not come into direct contact with epidermis.

The skin (epidermis and dermis) has many other useful functions. It is of the greatest importance in relation to the regulation of the temperature of the body; how it does this will be described later. By sweating the skin functions as an excretory organ. Vitamin D, the antirachitic vitamin, is made in skin exposed to ultraviolet light. Without vitamin D from other sources, children kept out of the sun develop rickets (Fig. 15-42). The skin contains nerve endings responsible for picking up stimuli that evoke many different types of sensation in consciousness (touch, pressure, heat, cold and pain). Hence the skin is of the greatest importance in permitting man to adjust to his environment.

Medical students will learn to appreciate the peculiar importance of the skin in a physical examination. No exploratory operations are necessary to see it; of all the important structures of the body, it alone is exposed so that it may be examined with the naked eye. Yet its appearance may reflect, just as truly as the appearance of deep-seated organs, the existence of a general disease. Its appearance often gives the physician a useful check on a patient's statement about his or her age. The way hair is distributed helps in estimating inherent degrees of masculine and feminine personality components. The presence and amount of hair in certain sites give some clue to the extent certain sex hormones are being secreted. The color of the skin may indicate a variety of conditions: it becomes yellow in jaundice, bronzed in certain glandular deficiencies, dry and hard in others, and warm and moist in still others. Cyanosis, already described, may give the skin a blue-gray appearance and so reflect impaired circulatory or respiratory functions. In vitamin A deficiencies the skin of extensor surfaces may lose its hair and become rough, like sandpaper. In certain other vitamin deficiencies the skin around the corners of the mouth may become cracked and scaly. Many infectious diseases that affect the whole body produce identifying rashes on the skin (for example, scarlet fever, measles, chickenpox, syphilis and others). The skin very commonly is affected when individuals are allergic (hypersensitive) to certain proteins and other substances; for example, some women develop rashes from certain kinds of face powder.

In addition to the involvement of the skin in conditions and diseases of a fairly general character, there are a whole host of skin diseases proper. The particular branch of medicine that deals with these and their treatment is called dermatology.

Since the skin is the most exposed part of the body, it is peculiarly susceptible to various kinds of injuries. The treatment of cuts, abrasions, burns and frostbites is part of the medical or paramedical life. Much skin often is destroyed by accidents and it is fortunate that it can be grafted readily from one part of the body to another; indeed, as will be described presently, one type of skin graft can be cut so that the skin at the site from which it is taken is renewed while that which is removed supplies skin for some site from which it has been lost. In this way areas of skin on a body can be, in a sense, multiplied.

Microscopic Structure of Thick Skin

The First Thief Identified by Fingerprints. In 1880 Henry Faulds, a Scottish medical missionary, published a note in *Nature* entitled "On the Skin Furrows of the Hand." He described these as "forever unchangeable" and pointed out that "finger marks" might be used for scientific detection of criminals. Indeed, he reported some experience in this matter and

described how greasy finger marks on a bottle had led to the identification of the individual who had been drinking the rectified spirits from their dispensary. From this beginning, fingerprinting developed into a most useful tool in crime detection.

Significance and Development of Surface Ridges and Grooves. If the palms of the hands (including the fingers) and the soles of the feet (including the toes) are examined with the naked eye or, better, with a magnifying glass, they are seen to be covered with ridges and grooves in a fashion reminiscent of a field plowed by the contour method. On the hands and the feet of the dark-skinned races the ridged area is clearly marked off by its lighter color.

Work by Cummins and others has shown that the ridges and the furrows develop during the 3rd and the 4th fetal months. The pattern that then forms never changes afterward except to enlarge. The patterns are determined chiefly by hereditary factors, as is shown by the close similarity of those of 1-egg twins and by the resemblances between those of the members of a family group. Racial differences are reflected in the patterns.

The patterns can be greatly modified by growth disturbances in the fetus during the 3rd and/or the 4th months. This is strikingly shown in children that are born with Down's syndrome (due to a chromosomal anomaly described in Chapter 2). Some 70 percent of such children show combinations of patterns not seen in normal babies; hence an analysis of the skin patterns of a newborn baby may give very important information on whether or not it has been born with this anomaly.

The epidermal ridges, which are the ones that can be seen with the naked eye, are caused by the epidermis following the contours of underlying dermal ridges. The latter may be studied in sections of skin cut at right angles to them. Sections so cut would be easier to interpret if they appeared as is illustrated in the upper drawing in Figure 20-2, which shows clear-cut *primary dermal ridges* underlying the epidermal ridges. However, actual sections of skin do not appear this way but as is shown in the lower picture in Figure 20-2. This—the real appearance—is due to the fact that epidermis grows down into the peak of each primary dermal ridge so that the primary dermal ridges are each split into two ridges. Each half of the split ridge, from the appearance it presented in a single section, was termed a papilla, and, as a consequence, the epidermal downgrowth that lies between each pair was termed an *interpapillary peg*. The structures termed papillae and interpapillary pegs are not actually cone-shaped papillae or pegs, because they

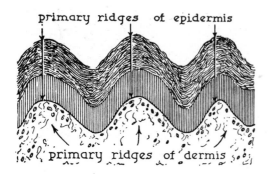

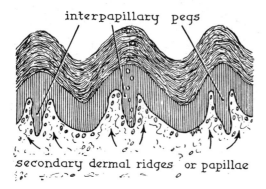

FIG. 20-2. Diagrams to show the relation between epidermal and dermal ridges. (*Top*) This diagram is not factual but is used to give the concept of a primary dermal ridge below each epidermal ridge. (*Bottom*) Actually, each primary dermal ridge is split into two secondary ridges as a result of the growth of the epidermis down into the primary ridge along its crest.

appear consistently in sections (see Fig. 20-1, *left*). If they were true papillae and pegs, they would be seen only on those occasions when the plane of the section happened to pass through one of them. That they appear consistently proves that they are actually ridges; however, they are deficient occasionally along their courses. As we shall see, the sweat glands of the skin open into the bottoms of the interpapillary pegs.

Epidermis. Since keratin is continuously worn away or shed from the surface, it must be continuously added to by means of the living cells beneath it turning into keratin. This requires that the living cells of the epidermis continuously proliferate to maintain their numbers. The living cells of plantar epidermis of rat have been shown to be completely renewed every 19 days.

Many processes, then, are in more or less continual operation in the epidermis: (1) cell division in the deep layers; (2) cells being pushed toward the surface as a result; (3) cells farthest from the dermis being transformed into keratin, and (4) keratin des-

quamating from the surface. If these 4 processes are not synchronized properly—and in many skin diseases they are not—the character of the epidermis changes greatly.

The various layers of the epidermis (stratified squamous keratinizing epithelium) were described in Chapter 7 and their features illustrated in detail in Figure 7-10.

For convenience the layers of epidermis are again shown as they appear in an H and E section of thick skin (Fig. 20-3). The description of these various layers was given in Chapter 7, and the description of

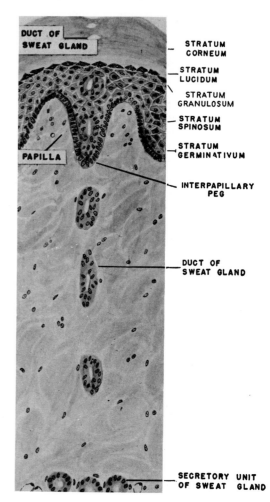

FIG. 20-3. Drawing of a section of thick skin (high-power) to illustrate the different layers of the epidermis, the way in which the duct of a sweat gland enters an interpapillary peg and how the wall of the duct thereafter is constituted by the cells of the different layers of the epidermis through which it passes. The thickness of the dermis is not in proportion; this was done to permit the secretory portion of the sweat gland to be shown.

desmosomes in Chapter 5 (Figs. 5-61, 5-62 and 5-63). Some further comment will be made here, particularly on the appearance of cells as seen with the LM.

Epidermis commonly is described as consisting of 4 or 5 layers, or strata, depending on whether or not the *stratum lucidum* is included (it can be seen only in certain examples of thick skin). The deepest stratum (germinativum) is separated from the dermis by a basement membrane which is seen to best advantage with the EM (Fig. 7-10). The surfaces of cells of the stratum germinativum that abut on the basement membrane are irregular (Fig. 7-10). On the inner aspect of the cell membranes of the cells that abut on the basement membrane there are hemidesmosomes (Fig. 5-61). The cells of the stratum germinativum are more or less columnar in shape (Fig. 7-10). The borders of these are not distinct in the usual H and E section, and the inexperienced student must avoid thinking that their nuclei, which are distinct, are the cells themselves. The deepest layer is called the *stratum germinativum* because it generates new cells.

The *stratum spinosum,* or *prickle cell layer,* is several cells thick (Figs. 20-3 and 7-10). The cells of this layer are of an irregular polyhedral shape. From appearances seen with the LM, such as the one illustrated in Figure 20-4, the individual cells of this layer often seem in sections to be slightly separated from one another, with the adjacent cells joined together only by fine lines (Fig. 20-4); the latter give the cells a prickly appearance, and this accounts for cells of this layer being called *prickle cells.* In the past it was believed that the fine lines were *tonofibrils* that actually crossed from the interior of one cell into the interior of the other. However, the EM has shown that the fine lines are actually very delicate strands of cytoplasm that extend out from each of two adjacent cells to meet and come into very close and firm contact at sites where the process from one cell is attached to the process of the contiguous cell by a desmosome (Fig. 5-63). Most of the substance of the fine lines that are seen with the LM is cytoplasm that has a considerable content of fibrillar material; these are the dense black fibrillar masses seen to either side of the desmosomes in Figure 5-63. These condensed bundles of tonofilaments are, in effect, the tonofibrils, but they do not pass from one cell into another, and they are always contained in cytoplasm. The intercellular spaces seen in Figure 20-4 are in part due to shrinkage artifact. If cells are separated slightly for any reason, the sites where cytoplasm is drawn out into fine lines are the sites where there are attachments between the cytoplasm of adjacent cells; in other words, at the sites of desmosomes, the cells do

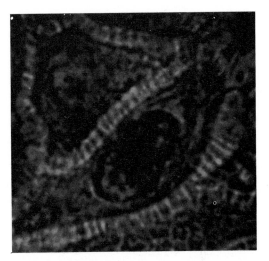

FIG. 20-4. Oil-immersion photomicrograph of section of thick human skin showing prickle cells. The fine lines that join adjacent cells, and which account for the prickly appearance of the cells, were once believed to be tonofibrils that passed from the cytoplasm of one cell into the cytoplasm of the next, and so anchored the cells together. It is now known that there is no cytoplasmic continuity between adjacent cells, but that they are held together by desmosomes, the fine structure of which is illustrated in Figure 5-63.

not pull apart, so the cytoplasm in these sites is drawn out into fine lines.

The details about the desmosomes seen in epidermis with the EM were described in Chapter 5 in relation to Figure 5-63 and in Chapter 7 in relation to Figure 7-10.

The *stratum granulosum* of thick skin is from 2 to 4 cells thick and lies immediately superficial to the stratum spinosum (Fig. 20-3). Its cells are roughly diamond-shaped (Figs. 20-3 and 7-11) and they are fitted together with the long axis of each paralleling the contour of the overlying ridge or groove. The cytoplasm of the cells of this layer contains granules that stain deeply with hematoxylin. These are called *keratohyalin* granules. The nature of these and their possible fates were described in Chapter 7 in relation to Figures 7-10 and 7-11.

The next layer is not always seen to advantage. When visible, it is thin and appears as a clear, bright, homogeneous line. For this reason it is called the *stratum lucidum* (Fig. 20-3). It is said to consist of eleidin, which is presumed to be a transformation product of the keratohyalin observed in the stratum granulosum.

The 5th and outermost layer of the epidermis is termed the *stratum corneum* (*corneus,* horny) (Fig. 20-3). Here the eleidin of the stratum lucidum (if this layer was present) has become transformed into keratin, and what were once living epithelial cells have become horny scales that adhere to one another tightly except at the surface, where they desquamate.

The formation of keratin was discussed in Chapter 7. Here it might be mentioned that epidermis transplanted into the subcutaneous tissue continues to form keratin. It is of interest that, specialized epithelium of certain other types in the body, that ordinarily are not keratinizing become so under conditions of prolonged vitamin A deficiency.

Dermis. This consists of two layers of connective tissue which merge into one another. The outer is by far the thinner and is composed of more or less the ordinary loose type of connective tissue. It is called the *papillary* layer because the connective tissue papillae that extend up into the epidermis are a prominent part of it (Figs. 20-1 and 20-2, *bottom*). This layer extends only slightly below the bases of the papillae, where it merges more or less insensibly with the thicker *reticular* layer, which consists of dense irregularly arranged connective tissue. It comprises the remainder of the dermis (the bulk of what is labeled dermis in Figure 20-1, *left*). It is called the reticular layer of the dermis because the bundles of collagenic fibers of which it is composed interlace with each other in a netlike manner.

Although both layers of the dermis consist of irregularly arranged fibrous tissue that of the papillary layer has a finer and looser texture, being more of the order of loose connective tissue than dense. It contains a representation of the cells of loose connective tissue described in Chapter 9 except that plasma cells are infrequent in normal dermis.

The Elastic Fibers in Dermis. Gillman describes the elastic fibers of skin as being in two locations—a network of very fine fibers in the papillary layer and coarser fibers randomly distributed in the reticular layer. It is believed this elastin is formed by fibroblasts. The elastin content of skin is, however, not very great, and it seems probable that past views about elastic fibers being chiefly responsible for the elasticity of the skin are incorrect. Gillman should be read for further information.

Capillary Content of the Two Layers. A very important difference between the papillary and reticular layers that should be mentioned here relates to their content of capillaries. As will be described in detail shortly, capillary blood supply of the papillary layer is extensive. One group extends in loops up into the so-called connective tissue papillae (ridges) which project into the epidermis; these provide nourishment for the epidermis and also act in heat regulation.

Another group, which is more in the nature of venules, forms a flat bed below the bases of the papillae. The papillary layer thus has a rich blood supply. Capillaries are scarce in the reticular layer, being numerous only in relation to epidermal appendages that project down into the reticular layer.

The cells of the dermis of thick skin are mostly fibroblasts, and these are scattered about sparingly. A few macrophages are also present. Fat cells may be present singly but are more commonly found in groups.

SWEAT GLANDS

Two Types. As was described in Chapter 7, there are several ways of classifying exocrine glands. One classification devised long ago divided glands into merocrine, apocrine and holocrine types. The distinction between merocrine and apocrine that was believed to exist was that in merocrine glands secretion is effected without any loss of cytoplasm from the secretory cell. In apocrine glands, however, it was believed that some fraction of the cytoplasm of the secretory cell was lost in the secretory process and became part of the secretion. This classification was of course made long before the EM became available, and, as was noted in Chapter 7, studies with this instrument have cast doubts on at least some of the secretions of apocrine glands requiring the detachment of cytoplasm for their cells to elaborate their secretions. However, this terminology is still used with regard to sweat glands, which are of two types that differ considerably in several interesting respects. The two types are classified as apocrine and eccrine. The latter term has the same meaning as merocrine, which we shall use, since we defined it in Chapter 7.

Apocrine Sweat Glands

This type probably evolved first and they are of considerably more practical use, and much more numerous, in lower animals than they are in man. Their chief function seems to be the production of relatively small amounts of secretions which, on reaching the skin surface, give rise to distinctive odors that enable animals to recognize the presence of others. In man, however, their distribution is very limited, for they are mostly confined to the axilla, the pubic region and the areola of the breasts. They develop from the downgrowths of epithelium that give rise to hair follicles and their ducts open, not onto the skin surface, as do the ducts of the ordinarily and infinitely more numerous merocrine sweat glands, but into hair follicles above the openings of the sebaceous glands soon to be described.

A sweat gland of the apocrine type has a secretory portion and a duct. Both are coiled; hence different coils of the same gland are often seen in the same section, where they appear as a group of secretory units. The secretory units have a wide lumen bounded by a layer of cuboidal to columnar secretory cells. Although it is believed they secrete more or less continuously, the secretion is not abundant and probably not under nervous control. The secretory units, however, are surrounded by myoepithelial cells which are innervated by the autonomic nervous system. Their contraction can express secretion from the secretory units under conditions of excitement or aroused emotions. The ducts are similar to those of ordinary merocrine sweat glands next to be described but (as already noted) they empty into the hair follicles.

Eccrine (Merocrine) Sweat Glands

These are the common type in man. They are simple tubular glands and are distributed all over the body except in a very few sites (lips and certain parts of external genitalia of both males and females). It has been estimated that there are around three million in the skin of man. They are particularly numerous in thick skin; it has been estimated that there are

3,000 per square inch in the palm of the hand. Each one consists of a secretory part and an excretory duct. The secretory part is usually situated immediately below the dermis in the subcutaneous tissue. The secretory part of the tubule is coiled on itself; hence in sections it appears as a little cluster of cross and oblique sections of tubes (Figs. 20-3 and 20-5). The secretory cells are of two types. Most are cuboidal or columnar in type, and have pale cytoplasm which contains some glycogen. These cells are wider at their bases than they are at the lumen surface. There are canaliculi between adjacent cells of this type which are believed to conduct sweat to the lumen. The other and less common type of cell is narrower at its base than at its lumen surface. Its cytoplasm can be shown to contain granules that stain well enough so that these cells are known as dark cells.

The lumen of the secretory part of a sweat gland is about as wide as its wall is thick. Spindle-shaped cells, which may have branches, and which resemble smooth muscle cells but are derived from ectoderm, are disposed obliquely and longitudinally around the secretory portions of the tubules to cover them, albeit incompletely, on the inner aspect of the basement membrane. These are commonly called *myoepithelial*

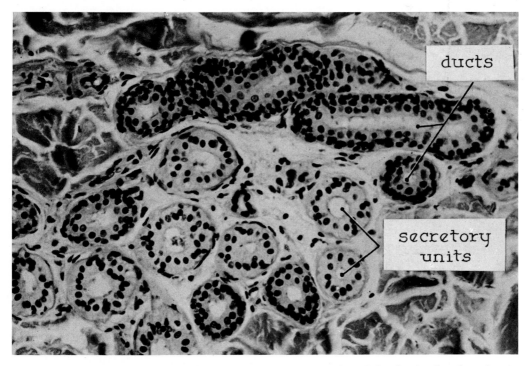

Fig. 20-5. High-power photomicrograph of an H and E section of dermis, showing the pale secretory units of sweat glands cut in cross section and the darker-staining ducts cut in both cross and oblique sections.

cells, and it is thought that their contractions may assist in expelling sweat. Immediately outside these flattened cells and the basement membrane of the tubule, connective tissue is condensed so as to form a sheath around the secretory portions of the glands.

After pursuing a tortuous course in a limited area, the secretory portion of the gland changes into a duct which passes toward the surface. The epithelial walls of ducts stain more deeply, on the whole, than those of the secretory cells because the lining cells of ducts form two layers and are smaller than those of secretory units and hence they contain relatively more nuclei to take up stain than do the walls of secretory units. Ducts, therefore, can be distinguished readily in sections (Fig. 20-5). Furthermore, the lumen of the duct is narrower than that of the secretory part of the gland; this is unusual, for in most glands the

lumens of ducts are much wider than the lumens of secretory units. The ducts, which follow a somewhat spiral course through the dermis, enter the tips of the interpapillary pegs of epidermis that project down between the double rows of papillae (Fig. 20-3). The epithelium of the ducts at this site merges with that of the interpapillary pegs, and, from this point on, the cells of the epidermis become the cells of the walls of the ducts. Ducts so constituted pursue a spiral course through the epidermis, and when the stratum corneum is reached, the spiral nature of their course becomes accentuated (Fig. 20-3). The ducts finally open on the surfaces of the ridges; their openings are obvious in a good fingerprint.

The nervous control of sweat glands and the way sweating acts to help control body temperature will be described after we consider the blood supply of the skin.

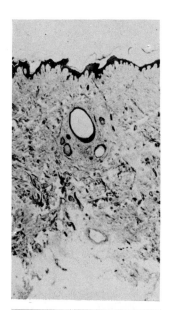
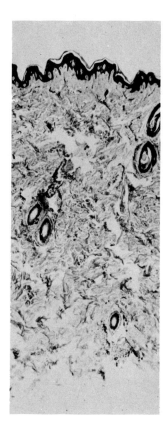
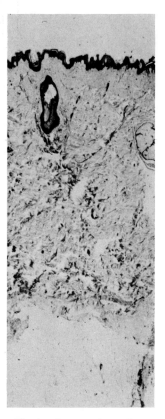
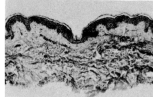

Fig. 20-6. The 3 large photomicrographs are all taken at the same magnification from sections of thin skin cut from different parts of the body. (*Left*) Skin from the inside of the leg. (*Center*) Skin from the abdomen which has been grafted to the wrist, where it has been in position for some time. (*Right*) Skin from the lateral side of the thigh. (*Lower left*) Photomicrograph of a section cut from a split-skin graft that was cut at $^{18}\!/_{1,000}$ of an inch in thickness. Notice that it contains a substantial content of dermis.

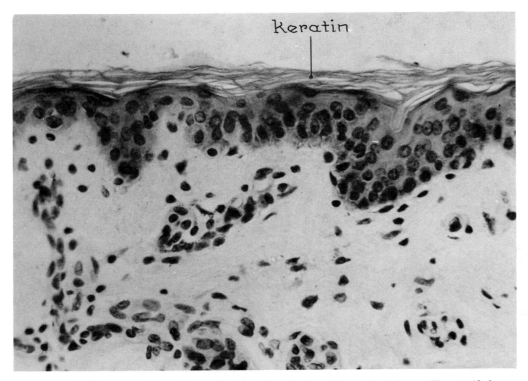

Keratin

FIG. 20-7. Low-power photomicrograph of a section of skin cut from the abdomen. The stratified squamous epithelium of thin skin, such as exists on the abdomen, is only a few cells thick. It runs across the upper part of the illustration, and at the surface the epithelial cells undergo a metamorphosis into keratin, which is labeled. The pale tissue on which the epithelium rests is the loose connective tissue of the papillary layer of the dermis.

Microscopic Structure of Thin Skin

Thin skin covers all of the body except the palms of the hands and the soles of the feet. As noted before, it should be understood that the adjectives "thick" and "thin" apply to the epidermis only, rather than to the skin as a whole. Actually, thin skin varies greatly in thickness in different parts of the body. These variations are due almost entirely to variations in the thickness of the dermis. The skin covering extensor surfaces is usually thicker than that covering flexor surfaces. The skin covering the eyelid is the thinnest in the body (0.5 mm. or less), and that covering the shoulders and the back is the thickest (up to 5 mm.) of the thin type. Figure 20-6 illustrates some specimens of thin skin obtained from different parts of the body.

Thin skin contains sweat glands (Fig. 20-1, *right*), but they are not so numerous as those in thick skin. Thin skin differs from thick in that it contains hair follicles. These are highly developed in the scalp and in certain other regions, but they are present in the thin skin over the whole body with a few minor exceptions (e.g., glans penis). Moreover, the surface of thin skin, unlike that of thick skin, is not thrown into ridges and grooves.

Epidermis. This has fewer layers than that of thick skin (Fig. 20-7). The stratum germinativum is similar to that of thick skin, but the stratum spinosum is thinner. The stratum granulosum may form a distinct continous layer; if not, numerous cells containing keratohyalin granules will be seen scattered along the line where this layer might be expected. No stratum lucidum is present, and the stratum corneum is relatively thin (Fig. 20-7).

Dermis. The surface presented by the dermis of thin skin to the epidermis is considerably different from that presented by the dermis of thick skin. Instead of being arranged in ridges, the dermis of thin skin projects here and there into the epidermis in the form of papillae. Their presence at any site is not reflected by any unevenness of the epidermal surface above them. The pattern seen on an epidermal surface is not due to underlying dermal papillae but is caused chiefly by lines that tend to connect the slightly depressed openings of the hair follicles.

Hair Follicles

Development. Early in the 3rd month of fetal life the epidermis begins to send downgrowths into the underlying dermis (Fig. 20-8). These develop first in the region of the eyebrows, the chin and the upper lip, and, soon after, they develop in all parts of the body that later will be covered with thin skin. These epidermal downgrowths become hair follicles, and give rise to hairs (Fig. 20-8, IV). By this means the fetus, at about the 5th or 6th month, has become covered with very delicate hairs. These constitute the *lanugo* (*lana,* wool) of the fetus. This coat of hair is shed before birth except in the region of the eyebrows, the eyelids and the scalp, where the hairs persist and become somewhat stronger. A few months after birth these hairs are shed and replaced by still coarser ones, while over the remainder of the body a new growth of hair occurs, and the body of the infant becomes covered with a downy coat called the *vellus* (fleece). At puberty, coarse hairs develop in the axilla and in the pubic regions and, in males, on the face and to a lesser extent on other parts of the body. The coarse hairs of the scalp and the eyebrows and those that develop at puberty are termed *terminal hairs* to dis-

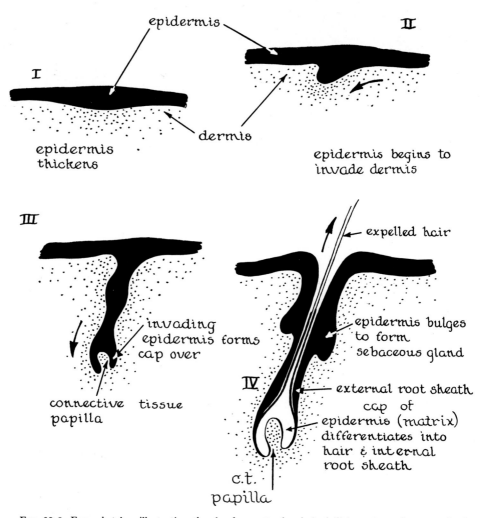

Fig. 20-8. Four sketches illustrating the development of a hair follicle and a sebaceous gland. (Redrawn and slightly modified from Addison: Piersol's Normal Histology. ed. 15. Philadelphia, J. B. Lippincott)

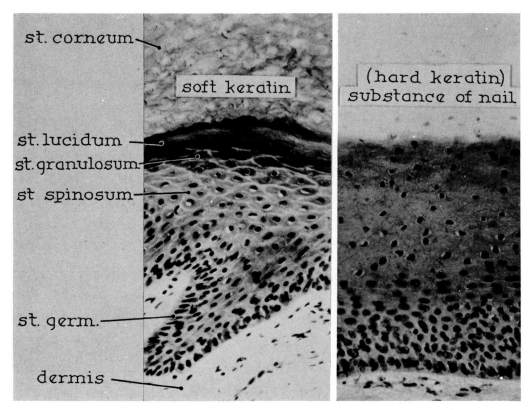

Fig. 20-9. (*Left*) The process by which the soft keratin of thick skin is formed. Note keratohyalin granules in the stratum granulosum and that a stratum lucidum is present. (*Right*) The process by which the hard keratin of the nail is formed. Note the gradual transition of cells into nail substances with no stratum granulosum or lucidum, and note that the hard keratin is more homogeneous than the soft.

tinguish them from those of the lanugo and the vellus.

The human species, of course, is not very hairy. Most of the body is not covered with anything more than the downlike vellus. Hair, then, is not a very important factor in keeping the body warm. It is, nevertheless, of the greatest importance that the skin of the human species should contain hair follicles. They, as we shall see, are instrumental in repairing epidermis injured by burns and abrasions, and they make split-skin grafting possible. We shall explain the reason for this presently.

The Two Kinds of Keratin in Hair Follicles and Hairs. There are two kinds of keratin. These, the *soft* and the *hard* types, can be distinguished by histological means, and they have different physical and chemical properties. Both types are encountered in hair follicles.

Soft keratin covers the skin as a whole; hard keratin is found only in certain of the skin appendages. The histologic changes that characterize the formation of

soft keratin are seen most easily in thick skin (Fig. 20-9, *left*). The formation of soft keratin here, as elsewhere, is characterized by the epidermal cells that are becoming keratinized accumulating keratohyalin granules (or their counterparts) in their cytoplasm. Hence, an area where soft keratin is being formed manifests a stratum granulosum or its counterpart. After this the cells become clear and glassy (stratum lucidum) before taking on the appearance which they characteristically present in the stratum corneum from which they continuously desquamate.

Hard keratin constitutes the fingernails and toenails and the cuticle and the cortex of the hairs of man, as well as the feathers, the claws or the hooves of certain animals. Its formation is manifested histologically by epidermal cells not passing through a phase in which they demonstrate numerous granules of keratohyalin in their cytoplasm or form a stratum lucidum; instead, in the formation of hard keratin there is a gradual transition from the living epidermal

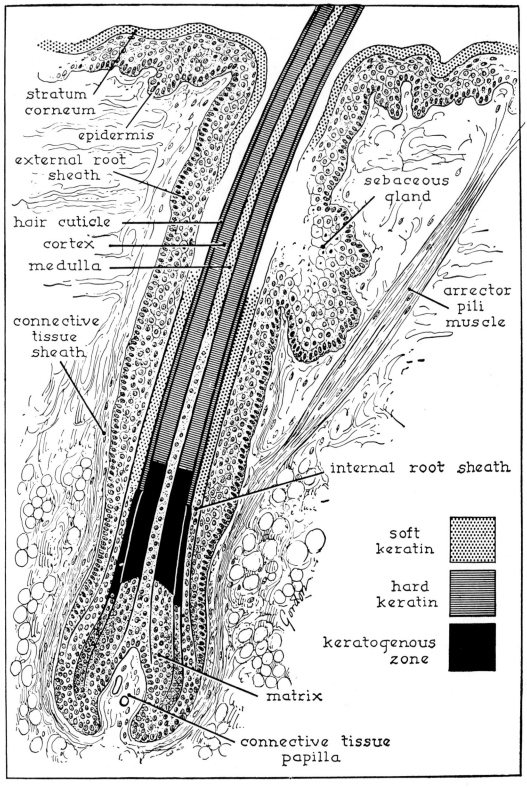

stratum corneum

epidermis

external root sheath

hair cuticle

cortex

medulla

connective tissue sheath

sebaceous gland

arrector pili muscle

internal root sheath

soft keratin

hard keratin

keratogenous zone

matrix

connective tissue papilla

Fig. 20-10. Diagram of a hair follicle, showing the distribution of soft and hard keratin and the keratogenous zone in which hard keratin is produced. (Based on Leblond, C. P.: Ann. New York Acad. Sci., *53*:464)

cells into keratin (Fig. 20-9, *right*). Physically, hard keratin appears to be solid, and it does not desquamate; hence, it is more permanent material than the soft keratin (nails and hair must be cut if they are not to grow too long). Chemically, hard keratin is relatively unreactive and contains more sulfur than the soft variety.

Structure of a Hair Follicle. A hair follicle involves the growth of cells of the epidermis into the dermis or even into the subcutaneous tissue.

The deepest part of the epithelial downgrowth becomes a knobby cluster of cells and is called the *germinal matrix* of the hair follicles (Figs. 20-8 and 20-10) because, as we shall see, it germinates the hair. This cluster of epithelial cells (the germinal matrix) becomes fitted over a *papilla* of connective tissue (Figs. 20-8 III and 20-10) which brings capillaries and, hence, a source of tissue fluid into its central part.

The External Root Sheath. The part of the epidermal downgrowth that connects the germinal matrix with the surface becomes canalized and thereafter is called the *external root sheath* of the hair follicle (Figs. 20-8 and 20-11). Near the surface of the skin, the external root sheath exhibits all the layers of epidermis of thin skin (Fig. 20-10, *top*). This, of course, is to be expected since the external sheath represents a downward continuation of the epidermis. Therefore the external sheath near the surface of the skin is lined with soft keratin that is continuous at the mouth of the follicle with the soft keratin of the epidermis of the skin (Fig. 20-10). But deep down in the follicle, the external root sheath becomes thinner and does not exhibit some of the more superficial layers of the epidermis. At the bottom of the follicle, where the external root sheath surrounds and becomes continuous with the germinal matrix, the external root sheath consists of only the stratum germinativum of the epidermis (Fig. 20-10).

Formation and Growth of a Hair. For hair to grow in a follicle, the cells of the germinal matrix must proliferate. This forces the uppermost cells of the germinal matrix up the lumen of the external root sheath. As the cells are pushed up, they get farther and farther away from the papilla, which is their source of nourishment, and they turn into keratin. Those cells that become the cuticle and the cortex of the hair, which is hard keratin, do so without developing any keratohyalin granules. The cellular area where the transition from cells into hard keratin occurs is called a keratogenous zone (Figs. 20-10 and 20-12). Hairs grow because of the continued proliferation of the epidermal cells of the germinal matrix and because

of the successive conversion of these cells into keratin as they are forced up the follicle (Fig. 20-12).

The Internal Root Sheath. The proliferating cells of the matrix form another structure in addition to a hair. This takes the form of a cellular tubular sheath which is pushed up around the hair to separate it from the external root sheath. This is called the *internal root sheath* (Figs. 20-10 and 20-11). It extends only partway up the follicle (Fig. 20-10). It is formed of soft keratin (Fig. 20-10); hence granules of keratohyalin can be seen in its cells as they become keratinized. In this region the granules are generally called trichohyalin (*thrix*, hair; *hyalin*, glass) granules, and instead of being basophilic they stain a bright red (Fig. 20-11).

The inner root sheath has 3 layers: an inner layer of cuticle, a middle Huxley's layer and an outer Henle's layer (Fig. 20-11). The student may have difficulty distinguishing these, but he should be able to recognize the internal root sheath by its contents of acidophilic trichohyalin granules (Fig. 20-11).

Development of Sebaceous Glands. As a hair follicle develops, cells from what will become the external root sheath of the upper third of the follicle grow out into the adjacent dermis and differentiate into sebaceous glands (Fig. 20-8, IV). When these are formed, their ducts open into the follicle at the site from which the outgrowth occurred; hence the sebaceous glands empty into the upper third of the follicle, below its mouth (Fig. 20-10). This part of the follicle is often called the *neck*.

Most hair follicles slant somewhat from the perpendicular. Therefore the angle between the hair follicle and the surface of the skin is acute on the one side and obtuse on the other. The sebaceous glands of a follicle usually are disposed on the side of the obtuse angle (Fig. 20-10).

The histology and other features of sebaceous glands will be described shortly.

The hair follicle is an epithelial structure. However, it is surrounded by a condensation of connective tissue which forms a *connective tissue sheath* about it (Figs. 20-10 and 20-11).

Arrector Pili Muscle. A little bundle of smooth muscle fibers, the *arrector pili* (erector of the hair), is attached to the connective tissue sheath of the hair follicle (about halfway down the follicle or deeper) and passes slantingly upward to reach the papillary layer of the dermis a short distance away from the mouth of the hair follicle (Figs. 20-10 and 20-13). This muscle, like the sebaceous glands, is on the side of the follicle that makes an obtuse angle with the surface. This bundle of muscle makes a third side to a

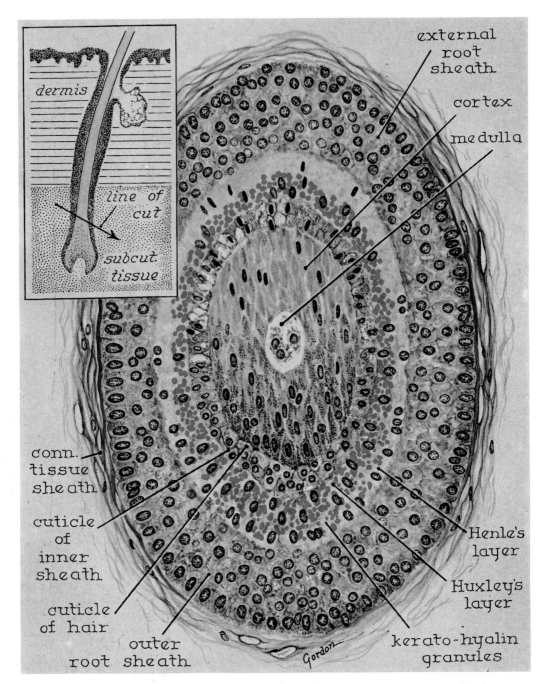

Fig. 20-11. High-power drawing of an oblique section cut through a hair follicle in the kera-togenous zone. The site and the plane of the section are shown in the inset at the upper left. (Hair follicles commonly extend into the subcutaneous tissue but usually not so far as the one shown in the inset.) Observe that the nuclei in both the internal root sheath and the hair are becoming pyknotic, and that red granules of trichohyalin (labeled kerato-hyalin) are present in the cells of the internal root sheath, thus indicating that it is forming soft keratin. No similar granules are to be seen in the cortex or the cuticle of the hair.

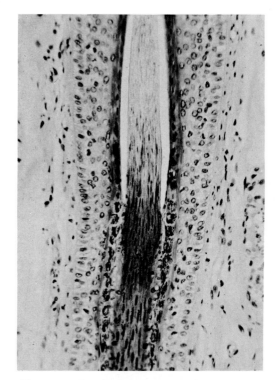

Fig. 20-12. Low-power photomicrograph of a longitudinal section of a hair follicle at the site where the cells from the matrix are losing their nuclei and becoming converted into keratin. The internal root sheath is thicker at the bottom of the figure than it is at the top.

triangle, the other two sides of which are the follicle and the surface of the skin. The sebaceous glands are situated inside this triangle (Fig. 20-10). When the arrector pili muscle contracts, it not only pulls the whole hair follicle outward but also, by pulling on its deeper part from one side, makes the follicle more perpendicular (the hair "stands up"). Moreover, contraction of the muscle tends to "dimple in" the skin over the site of its attachment to the papillary layer of the dermis. The net result is to produce on the skin a "gooseflesh" appearance or "goose pimples." Moreover, the contraction of the muscle squeezes the sebaceous glands contained in the triangle previously described (Fig. 20-10), and this causes their oily secretion to be expressed into the neck of the follicle and onto the skin.

The arrectores pilorum, being smooth muscle, are innervated by the sympathetic nervous system. Cold is an important stimulus for setting off the reflex that leads to their contraction. The purpose of this reflex may be to express more oil onto the surface of the body from the sebaceous glands so that less evaporation,

and hence less heat loss, can occur from the skin. Intense emotional states, as has been pointed out, tend to energize the body through the medium of the sympathetic nervous system, and these, too, cause the arrectores pilorum to contract. Fear can make one's hair "stand on end." This response is useful in the porcupine. Lower animals are also said to "bristle with rage."

SOME POINTS OF INTEREST ABOUT HAIR AND HAIR GROWTH

Cyclic Activity of Hair Follicles. The fact that hairs come out on a brush or comb does not indicate that baldness is inevitable. Reassurance is to be obtained from the knowledge that hair growth is cyclic. This is more obvious in animals that live in the far north than it is in man, for these northern animals commonly grow a new coat for each winter and lose it for each summer. The hair follicles of man also exhibit cyclic activity in that they alternate between growing and resting periods. During the growing phase of the cycle, the cells of the germinal matrix continue to proliferate and to differentiate, and as a result the hair is

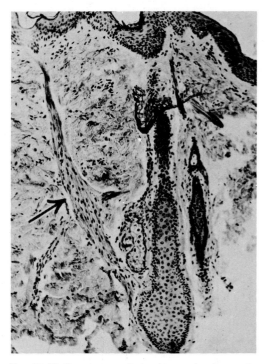

Fig. 20-13. Low-power photomicrograph of a section of thin skin at the site of an arrector pili muscle. The lumen and the upper part of the hair follicle do not show in this section. (Photomicrograph from Professor E. A. Linell)

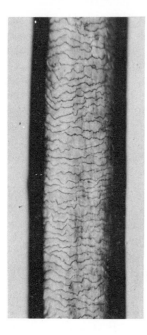

FIG. 20-14. Oil-immersion photomicrograph of the surface of a hair, showing its shinglelike cuticular scales.

continually elongated. However, the growing phase merges into a resting phase as the germinal matrix becomes inactive and atrophies. The root of the hair then becomes detached from its matrix and gradually moves up the follicle, gaining for a time a more or less secondary attachment to the external root sheath as the lower end of the hair approaches the neck of the follicle. Meanwhile, in the deeper part of the follicle, the epidermal external root sheath has retracted upward toward the surface. Finally, the hair comes out of the follicle. Either before or after this event, the deeper parts of the external root sheath grow downward again to cover either the old papilla, which becomes rejuvenated, or a new one. A new germinal matrix develops, and this leads to a new hair beginning to grow up the follicle again.

The cyclic activity of the hair follicles of man differs in 2 ways from that of animals that form and lose a coat of hair each year. First, the cycles are longer in man. The hairs of the scalp probably last from 2 to 6 years. Second, different, even adjacent, hair follicles in man tend to be in different phases of their cycles at any given time. For example, Trotter found that at a time when 45 percent of the hair follicles of the leg were in their growing phase, 55 percent were in their resting phase.

Common Baldness. That baldness is very uncommon in women suggested for long that male sex hormone might have something to do with its cause, and Hamilton first provided evidence to show that it has. His studies indicate that castration, and hence a lack of male sex hormone production in the male, tends to hold in check any hereditary tendency to develop baldness, and that the administration of male sex hormone to individuals deficient in the hormone permits a hereditary tendency toward baldness to become operative, with baldness resulting. In other words, the genetic factors which tend to cause baldness can be fully effective only if male sex hormone is present in the bloodstream of the individual concerned. Although baldness is an obvious sign of male sex hormone activity, the compensating conclusion should not be drawn by balding men that they are necessarily more virile than those with good heads of hair. Male sex hormone does not cause baldness unless the hereditary disposition to develop baldness is present.

The Effect of Cutting on the Growth of Hair. Another question about hair, probably of more interest to women than to men, is whether or not shaving or otherwise cutting hairs encourages their growth. This has been the subject of much careful enquiry that required long and painstaking experiments (see Trotter). The general conclusion from these experiments is that cutting or shaving hair has no effect on its growth.

Structure of Hair. The cross-section appearance and other features of hair vary in relation to race. In anthropology, 3 chief types of hair are recognized; straight, wavy and woolly. Straight hair is found in the members of the yellow or Mongol races, the Chinese, the Eskimos and the Indians of America. Straight hair is characteristically coarse and lank and is rounded in cross section. Wavy hair is found in a number of people, including Europeans, and woolly hair on nearly all the black races. A cross section of a wavy hair is oval and that of woolly hair, elliptical or kidney-shaped.

A hair consists of a central medulla of soft keratin (Figs. 20-10 and 20-11) and a cuticle and a cortex of hard keratin (Figs. 20-10 and 20-11). Many hairs contain no or, at most, a very poorly developed medulla; hence they show only a cuticle and a cortex of hard keratin.

The cuticle consists of very thin, flat, scalelike cells that are arranged on the surface of a hair like shingles on the side of a house, except that their free edges point upward instead of downward (Fig. 20-14). The free edges of these cells more or less interlock with the free edges of similar cells that line the internal root sheath and whose free edges point downward. The interlocking arrangement makes it difficult to pull out a hair without at least part of the internal root sheath coming with it.

The cortex consists of tapering cornified cells. It is the pigment in the cells of the cortex that gives color to hair.

The medulla consists of soft keratin. In it cornified cells are commonly separated from one another. Air or liquid may be present between the cells of the medulla.

Color of Hair. The color of hair depends on the quantity and the quality of the melanin pigment present in the cortex. White hairs mixed with pigmented hairs give what is commonly called gray hair (true gray hair is rare).

Sebaceous Glands

Usually, several form from each follicle. These open by very short but wide ducts (Fig. 20-15) into the neck of the follicle. These glands secrete a fatty material called *sebum;* this oils the hair and lubricates the surface of the skin. Sebum is said to possess some bactericidal and fungicidal properties but this has been disputed. Its chief function is probably that of acting as a natural "cold cream." It prevents undue evaporation from the stratum corneum in cold weather and so helps to conserve body heat. In keeping the stratum corneum oiled, it helps to keep it from becoming cracked and chapped, which can happen if it becomes too dry.

Sebaceous glands are holocrine glands; the mechanism of secretion in this type of gland was described in Chapter 7.

For a sebaceous gland (Fig. 20-15) to secrete sebum, many processes must be in progress more or less simultaneously. These are: (1) the proliferation of the cells of the basal layer of the gland; (2) the pushing of the extra cells formed as a result of the proliferation toward the center of the gland; (3) the synthesis and accumulation of fatty material in the cytoplasm of these cells as they move away from the basal layer, and (4) the necrosis of these cells as they

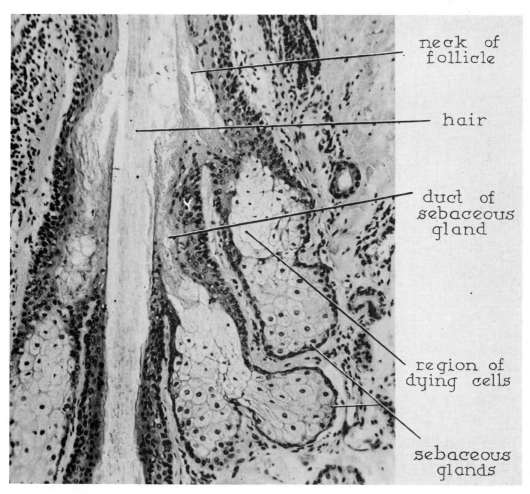

Fig. 20-15. Medium-power photomicrograph of a section of skin, showing a sebaceous gland opening into a hair follicle.

are pushed still farther toward the center of the gland (because they are so far removed from sources of nourishment) by the continuing proliferation and differentiation of cells behind them. As noted before, contraction of the arrector pili muscle can cause formed sebum to be expressed quickly from the gland into the hair follicle.

That sebaceous glands develop from hair follicles explains why no sebaceous glands are found in the skin that covers the soles of the feet or the palms of the hands. However, in a few sites in the body sebaceous glands develop without hair follicles (eyelids, papillae of breasts, labia minora and corners of lips near the red margins in some people). And in some sites, and in particular in the skin covering the nose, the sebaceous glands that develop from hair follicles become much more prominent than the hair follicles themselves; the hair follicle in these sites is, as it were, a means to an end.

The Hormone Control of Sebaceous Glands. As will be described in detail in subsequent chapters, sex hormones are secreted into the bloodstream in physiological amounts beginning at puberty (which they cause). Although the secretion of male hormones is predominant in males and female sex hormones in females, the chemistry of sex hormones is related and their metabolism complicated, and for one reason or another there is some female sex hormone activity in males and some male sex hormone activity in females. There is a substantial increase in the secretion of sebum at the time of puberty and experiments have shown that this is a result of male hormone. It has been shown moreover that this increased output of sebaceous glands is the result of a great increase in mitosis in sebaceous glands which brings about a more rapid turnover of the cell population of the glands. Unfortunately, the structural arrangements whereby this greatly increased production of sebum can be delivered to the skin surface freely do not seem to be adequate, with the result that sebum, instead of being freely expressed from the hair follicle, sometimes bulges into the skin so as to cause a condition called *acne* (pimples), and since this state of affairs is sufficiently abnormal to predispose to further problems such as local infections, it is a condition that requires medical attention. Although female sex hormone acts to depress the synthesis of sebum in sebaceous glands it apparently does not suppress mitosis and it seems that at the time of puberty girls as well as boys begin to secrete either enough male sex hormone or some female hormone that at this time acts similarly on sebaceous glands to stimulate mitosis in sebaceous glands, because they too are prone to acne at this time

of life. It should be mentioned that experimental work has shown that male sex hormone needs help from some pituitary hormones to achieve its effect; for male hormone in animals from which the pituitary gland has been removed is inactive so far as sebaceous glands are concerned.

The Healing of the Skin After a Surgical Incision or an Accidental Cut

This is a matter about which concepts of many decades ago have often continued to be taught.

The old, widely held view was that following a surgical incision closed with sutures some fibrin formed between the edges of the incision. The fibrin, it was thought, served as a weak bonding agent to help keep the cut edges of the skin together. It was assumed next that fibroblasts from the dermis on each side of the cut, together with some capillaries from the same source, grew into the fibrin between the two edges and joined the edges together with new collagen that was formed by the fibroblasts that grew in from each side. Meanwhile, the epidermis was believed to grow across the top of the incision, covering the new connective tissue that was forming below it and thus restoring the continuity of both the epidermis and the dermis. The subcutaneous tissue beneath the skin was assumed to heal by fibroblasts and by new capillaries growing across the region of the cut in this region.

Toward the end of the last decade Gillman reexamined the older concepts in the light of modern knowledge about the repair of tissue, and from experimental studies he found them wanting in several respects. More recently Lindsay and Birch were able to make a study of the subject on young children, and their results, like those of Gillman, indicate that there has been much misunderstanding in the past about what actually happens. The 4 illustrations used here (Fig. 20-16) are redrawn from those of Lindsay and Birch, and the sequence of events they illustrate is in general similar to that postulated by Gillman.

First, the role of fibrin in the repair of a simple skin wound has been overestimated, just as it has been in the repair of bone.

Second, the dermis of the skin is a poor source of fibroblasts, just as might be expected, because fibroblasts are scarce in the reticular layer of the dermis; it consists mostly of collagen. Third, the dermis is a poor source of new capillaries; this, too, should be expected because the reticular layer of the dermis is relatively nonvascular. Hence the old concept of the edges of dermis being glued together with fibrin, and then fibroblasts and capillaries invading the fibrin

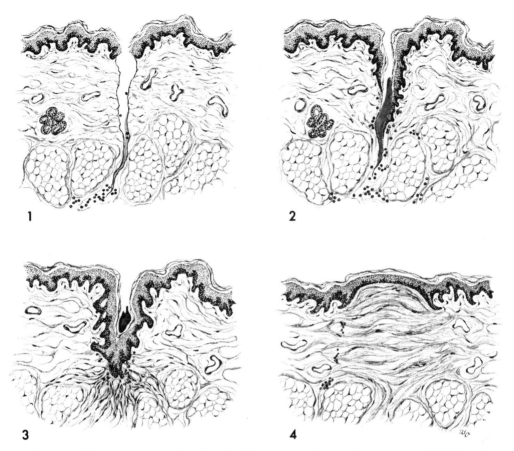

Fɪɢ. 20-16. Diagrammatic drawings showing the sequence of events that occur in the healing of an incision made in the skin of man under conditions in which the edges of the wound are approximated by catgut sutures. (1) State of affairs a few hours after the incision was made; (2) roughly a week afterward; (3) about 2 weeks afterward; and (4) 30 days afterward. The details shown in each illustration are described in the text. (Illustrations based on those of Lindsay, W. K., and Birch, J. R.: Canad. J. Surg., 7:297, 1964)

from each side to re-establish dermis continuity early in the repair process, is more of a myth than fact.

Next, the concept of the epidermis growing over the glued-together edges of the dermis is also not in accord with fact. What happens is that the edges of the dermis are not glued firmly together, and as a result there is a V-shaped slit that extends down from the surface right to the subcutaneous tissue (Fig. 20-16). A little fibrin soon forms near the bottom of this; this is the darker material seen in the slit near its bottom. Furthermore, the epidermis on each side of the slit begins to bend downward at each edge of the slit.

After several days the picture has changed somewhat. A prominent feature normally noticed about a week afterward is that the epidermis has extended down the sides of the slit in the dermis, adhering to sound tissue on either side (Fig. 20-16). If there is

fibrin present, the epidermis remains attached to healthy dermis (Fig. 20-16). It is obvious that the epidermis that both grows and slides down the sides of the wound would be in the way if fibroblasts from the dermis on either side of the cut tried to grow across the gap. By the end of about 2 weeks the epidermis that has grown down one side of the wound meets with that that has grown down the other side so that epidermal continuity is first restored deep down in the cleft (Fig. 20-16).

Meanwhile, fibroblasts and capillaries are engaged in repairing the connective tissue of the skin. However, the chief source of fibroblasts and capillaries is not the injured dermis but subcutaneous tissue. This is logical because the subcutaneous tissue has a much more abundant supply of capillaries and also many more pericytes than the relatively nonvascular and noncellular dermis. So at the junction between dermis and subcutaneous tissue there is an abundant growth of fibroblasts (Fig. 20-16) and capillaries; this forms a ridge of new tissue, which, as it grows, bulges up at the bottom of the epithelial lined cleft, pushing the bottom of the cleft toward the surface until the surface is level again (Fig. 20-16). This action requires, of course, that the area covered here by epidermis (that once lined the cleft) be enlarged, just as the surface of cloth is enlarged if it is pulled on each side to straighten out a depressed wrinkle. So in due course the area previously occupied by the epidermal-lined cleft becomes occupied by new connective tissue, which was derived chiefly from subcutaneous tissue, and which in the end is covered with thin epidermis (Fig. 20-16, 4)—thin because it is stretched as the connective tissue growth from below wells upward and expands the surface.

At least for a long time the epidermis over the widened area of new connective tissue that was derived from below is thin, and it also lacks the usual uneven undersurface occasioned by the connective tissue papillae that normally project into the epidermis of thin skin (Fig. 20-16, 4).

Lindsay and Birch give helpful advice on how skin may be sutured so as to diminish as much as possible the extent of the scar that can result from an unrestricted growth of connective tissue from the subcutaneous tissue, if the operative procedures do not take properly into account the way an incision heals.

Skin Grafting

Skin may be grafted from one part of the body to another by two general methods.

By the first method, much used, for example, in reconstructions of part of the face, skin is moved from one part of the body to another adjacent part (for example, skin of the arm is brought close to the face and kept there for some time) without the skin ever being severed completely from its blood supply. One edge of the graft is left connected with its original blood supply while the other edge of the graft is attached to a new bed. When the graft (after several days) has a sufficient blood supply from the site to which it has been attached, it can be severed from its original site and fixed in place in its new site. However, under most conditions where skin grafting is required—for example, the covering of a large area where the skin has been completely destroyed by a burn—*free* skin grafts, that is, grafts completely severed from their blood supply, are employed.

Free Skin Grafts

First, we must comment on autologous grafts and homografts. An autologous graft is skin taken from one part of the body and transplanted to some other site on the *same* body. The cells of autologous grafts, for the most part, continue to live in their new location, and the grafts become firmly attached to and part of the area where they are placed. They are said to "take." Homografts of skin are sometimes used more or less as a type of temporary dressing for a burned area. Under ordinary circumstances they do not take; instead, they are in due course rejected by the homograft reaction, as was described in Chapter 10 and illustrated in Figure 10-15.

Autologous grafts are of two general types: split grafts, and full-thickness grafts. Since in many kinds of accidents—in particular, thermal burns—large areas of skin may be destroyed, and since homografts do not take, it is fortunate that in the skin of man there is a provision for the surgeon to multiply its extent; this is done by means of split skin grafts. By the use of these it is possible for a patient eventually to have much more skin than he had before grafting.

How Skin Is Multiplied by Split Grafts

A split graft is a shaving cut from the skin. One is shown in the lower left corner of Figure 20-6. The left diagram in Figure 20-17 shows the state of affairs in skin if about half its thickness is taken as a shaving. The piece that is taken can be placed on an area that has been denuded of epidermis, and if it is kept in place in this area, its cells will be nourished via tissue fluid from the raw surface on which it has been placed, and in due course connective tissue cells from its bed will grow and form new intercellular substance to attach it firmly in place, and so it will provide a new epidermis for the skin. In due course it will become vascularized.

Next, let us consider the skin from which the superficial slice was taken, which, when the slice is taken, presents a raw surface, uncovered with epidermis (Fig. 20-17, *left, lower part*). The reason for this becoming re-covered with epidermis is that the hair follicles and sweat glands of the skin extend all the way through the skin. When the superficial part of the skin is removed to serve as a split graft, the external sheaths of the hair follicles and the ducts of sweat glands, as is shown in the right illustration in Figure 20-17, serve as sources of new epidermal cells which grow out from these structures to re-cover the surface with new epidermis. The author's studies in this connection were made on pigs, animals which have an

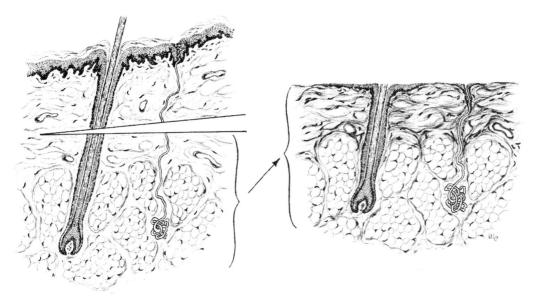

Fig. 20-17. Diagrammatic drawings of sections of skin. The left drawing depicts a split skin graft being cut at a level about halfway down the dermis. Such a graft (the part above the cut) can be transplanted to some site on the same individual and live. The site from which the graft is removed becomes covered in due course with new epidermis that grows up from hair follicles, and in man also from sweat glands, as is shown on the right. In due course the dermis becomes thickened.

excellent skin for skin-grafting experiments. In pigs the growth of new epidermis is chiefly, if not entirely, from the external sheaths of the hair follicles. It is said, however, that in man there is considerable growth of epidermis from the sweat glands (the counterparts in the pig of the sweat glands of man are different from those of man).

It should be appreciated that when the total thickness of the skin is destroyed, say, by a severe burn, there is no way for the epidermis to become regenerated except for it to grow from the edges of the denuded area from one side to the other. If the denuded area is large, the growth of epidermis from its edges is impracticable.

FULL-THICKNESS GRAFTS

In some instances, particularly for good cosmetic effects, full-thickness autologous free grafts are used. Here, however, there is no skin multiplying effect because the skin appendages as well as the epidermis and dermis are taken along as parts of the graft. So the edges of the site from which the full-thickness graft is cut must be sewn together, or the area must be covered with a split graft.

How Free Grafts Become Vascularized. It might be thought that a full-thickness graft would be too thick for its cells to be nourished by diffusion from tissue fluid from the bed on which the graft was placed. But full-thickness grafts do survive and soon develop a proper blood supply without their blood vessels having to be connected to those of the bed by the operator. Cloutier and the author showed by means of injection experiments in pigs that the capillaries of the graft and capillaries in its bed soon become joined, and that by 7 days blood would be flowing again in the larger vessels of the graft, which must have remained alive by diffusion phenomena through this period of time. It is of interest that the old vessels of the graft are used again. It seems probable that new vessels later on might grow into such a graft to supplement the functions of the original ones that became connected at the base of the graft by means of new capillaries. For those interested, photographs of specimens showing the revascularization of full-thickness grafts were published in an article in the *Journal of Bone and Joint Surgery*, vol. 34A, page 701.

Pigmentation of the Skin

The important pigment in the skin is melanin. Melanins are widely distributed in the animal kingdom and range from yellow, through brown, to black in color. In man, melanin occurs chiefly in the epidermis, and in the white race in the cells of the basal layers, where it tends to be disposed often, as a student once wrote on a histology examination, on the sunny side of the nuclei (Fig. 20-18, *right*). Melanin occurs in the form of fine brown to black granules, but these commonly clump together if the pigment is abundant. The content of melanin in the epidermis is responsible for the difference in the color of the skins of those different races (black, brown, yellow and white). All have some melanin in their skins. An inherent inability in any individual of any race to produce melanin results in an *albino* (*albus,* white).

Increased amounts of melanin appear in the epidermis of white skin when it is exposed to ultraviolet light. It is the ultraviolet light in sunlight that causes suntan to develop. Brunettes tan more readily than blonds. In some individuals melanin tends to form in little patches (freckles).

The Cells That Make Melanin Pigment. In the older literature the cells that manufacture melanin were generally termed melanoblasts; now they are termed *melanocytes.*

The term *melanoblast* is now used for cells that in embryonic life develop in the neural crest and then migrate to the epidermal-dermal junction. Until mel-

anoblasts take up a position at or in the basal layer of the epidermis, where they differentiate into melanocytes, they do not make melanin.

The cell bodies of melanocytes are disposed either just beneath or between the cells of the basal layer of the epidermis. Before they make melanin, they may appear in the basal layer as "clear cells" (Fig. 20-18, *left*). The cell bodies of melanocytes in either position send out long processes which extend between or under epidermal cells (Fig. 20-19), mostly those of the basal layer. The processes end on epidermal cells where the melanin granules, made by the melanocytes, are taken into the cytoplasm of the epithelial cells from the long processes of the melanocytes. By this means the ordinary epithelial cells of the basal layer come to contain melanin pigment. It follows, therefore, that melanocytes cannot be distinguished from true epidermal cells by, or because of, their containing pigment. Although it has been suggested that before they become functioning melanocytes, they may appear as "clear cells" (Fig. 20-18, *left*), functioning melanocytes can be distinguished from ordinary epidermal cells by a histochemical test which picks out cells that

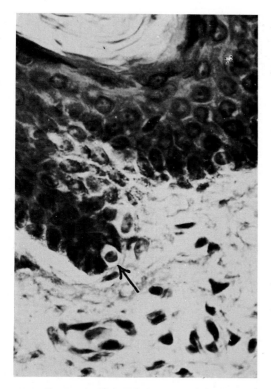 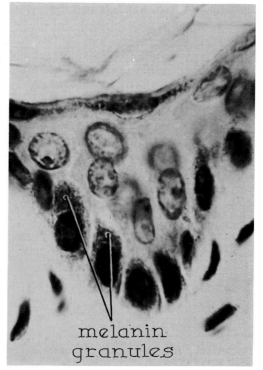

Fig. 20-18. (*Left*) High-power photomicrograph of a section of skin, showing a "clear cell" in the stratum germinativum. (*Right*) Oil-immersion photomicrograph of a section of pigmented skin, showing melanin granules in the cytoplasm of the cells of the stratum germinativum.

have the functioning metabolic equipment required to make pigment. This test, known as the "dopa reaction," will now be described.

Recognizing Melanocytes by the Dopa Reaction. The ability of melanocytes to produce melanin depends on their ability to synthesize the enzyme or the enzyme complex known as *tyrosinase.* If they possess this enzyme in active form, and are provided with the correct substrate, the tyrosinase will react with the substrate to form melanin. In man, however, the addition of tyrosine to preparations of epidermis does not lead, at least not immediately, to the melanocytes of the preparation forming melanin (the reactions involved are complicated). However, if dihydroxyphenylalanine, which is referred to as dopa, is added to a suitable preparation of epidermis, the tyrosinase within the melanocytes converts the dopa of the solution that penetrates into these cells into melanin, which then is seen in the cytoplasm of the melanocytes as a dark pigment. This test, which is termed the *dopa reaction,* can be used to distinguish cells that have the ability to make melanin from cells which merely take up melanin.

The dopa reaction has shown that melanocytes are very numerous in epidermis. According to Montagna, 1 out of every 4 to 1 out of 10 cells in the basal layer of the epidermis of man is a melanocyte. The dopa reaction has also been very helpful in demonstrating the complicated arrangements of processes that extend off from the cell bodies of melanocytes to intertwine with, and end on, epidermal cells and supply them with pigment. The processes are often termed dendrites, and in the past the cells that are probably now known as melanocytes were often termed dendritic cells.

Fine Structure. The biosynthesis of melanin by melanocytes has been studied by many methods including electron microscopy. Seiji *et al.* have suggested a sequence of events which occurs in cells that are producing melanin. It could be expected that the rough-surfaced vesicles of endoplasmic reticulum are concerned at least in the early steps of the synthesis of the enzyme, and that the protein products synthesized in rough-surfaced vesicles would be transferred to the Golgi region. Here the product that arrives from the rough-surfaced vesicles is probably condensed and packaged in the form of smooth-surfaced membranous vesicles, the content of which is now termed *protyrosinase.* The contents of these smooth-surfaced membranous vesicles are now changed further, and the vesicles with their contents are now known as premelanosomes. When this occurs, the contents become active; that is, active tyrosinase appears in the contents of the vesicles, and this results in melanin being synthesized in, or in association with, these vesicles. When this happens, the vesicles become known as melanosomes, which are oval, membrane-enclosed granules a little over half a micron in length. Before being obscured by melanin the granules reveal an internal arrangement of concentrically arranged lamellae. Soon, or later, each melanosome becomes converted into a melanin granule, and when this has happened, the structure no longer contains any demonstrable tyrosinase. The whole process appears to be similar to that which occurs in connection with the synthesis of secretory granules described in Chapter 5, except that the enzymes in membranous packages of secretion that appear in the Golgi region in melanocytes do their work while the packages (vesicles) are still within the cytoplasm.

Langerhans Cells. Cells in the epidermis with shapes and properties different from those already described were noted in the last century by Langerhans. These cells can be demonstrated to advantage by certain metallic impregnation methods which disclose that they have branching processes that extend (like those of melanocytes) from their cell bodies between adjacent epidermal cells. For a time the most widely accepted view about them was that they were old melanocytes, but modern studies with the EM have shown that they are healthy active cells (Fig. 20-19A).

Under conditions of vitamin A deficiency, various epithelial membranes not ordinarily of the stratified squamous type become stratified squamous; this can happen for example in the trachea, which is normally lined by pseudostratified columnar ciliated epithelium. Wong and Buck found that when this happens, Langerhans cells, which are not present in the normal type of epithelium in these locations, appeared in the stratified squamous epithelium that replaced the normal type and, furthermore, that Langerhans cells also made their appearance in the loose connective tissue underlying this stratified squamous epithelium.

Wong and Buck consider that the origin of Langerhans cells is more likely to be mesenchyme than epidermis. There is other evidence in addition to their findings that supports this view.

Langerhans cells are not connected by desmosomes to the epidermal cells with which they are in contact. They have a very irregular shape. Likewise their nuclei are greatly indented. With the EM the rER is not very prominent but the Golgi is well developed. The cytoplasm contains some microtubules. The cytoplasm contains characteristic granules not seen in melanocytes; these are elongated structures showing longitudinal striations. Occasionally some granules have a racquet shape.

Their function, and why they should have an association with stratified squamous epithelium, present problems. They are probably macrophages.

Melanin-Containing Cells of the Dermis. Such melanin-containing cells as are seen in the dermis, with one exception, are cells that have not made melanin but have phagocytosed it; hence, they are called *chromatophores* (*phoreo,* I carry). However, in infants of the Mongol race there may be true melanocytes deep in the dermis of the sacral region. Seen through the tissue that covers them, their pigment appears blue; this is the color of melanin that is seen through overlying tissue. The blue spot thus apparent is called a Mongol spot. Melanocytes are seldom seen in this site in children of the white race.

Function of Melanin. While in certain species melanin serves to camouflage an animal as was described in Chapter 5 in connection with microtubules, in man its primary function is to protect the deepest layers of the epidermis and the underlying dermis from excessive ultraviolet light. The fact that a person becomes tanned is evidence of the formation of an increased amount of melanin for this purpose. Ultraviolet light on the skin is, of course, helpful to a point, because it irradiates ergosterol, a derivative of cholesterol, and irradiated ergosterol is one form of vitamin D; this vitamin, which is absorbed from the skin, is

an essential factor in a proper mineral metabolism. A lack of vitamin D can cause rickets in children. It is of interest that it was noticed years ago that Negro children who are brought up in northern regions where there is not so much sunlight as there is in more southern regions, are more prone to develop rickets than children of the white race. Nowadays, of course, in order to prevent rickets, infants are given vitamin D preparations by mouth. The fact that some persons become tanned is probably an indication that, healthy as such people may appear, they have been getting enough ultraviolet irradiation of their skins for their melanocytes to begin to provide them with some protection.

The Pigmentation of Hair. The pigment of hair, like that of the epidermis, is primarily melanin. The melanin of hair is formed by melanocytes; these are distributed in the matrix of a hair follicle close to the papilla. The melanocytes in this region, like those of the epidermis, send out cytoplasmic processes that reach and provide melanin for the epithelial cells that will, by undergoing keratinization, become the cortex and the medulla of the hair. As the cells that formed by means of cell division in the matrix of the follicle move upward, they take up melanin in the upper part of the bulb, and then move up farther and become keratinized to become the cortex and the medulla of

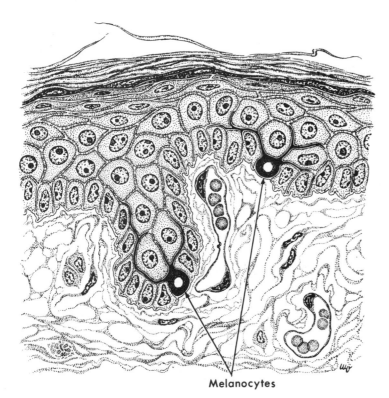

Melanocytes

Fig. 20-19. Diagram of epidermis and part of the papillary layer of the dermis showing the site where melanocytes (the cytoplasm of which is black in this illustration) are located, and also that their branching processes (also in black) extend between the epithelial cells to supply them with melanin.

FIG. 20-19A. Micrograph of stratified squamous epithelium. The large oval structure occupying the left side of the figure is the cytoplasm of a Langerhans cell featuring numerous lysosomes (L) and vermiform tubules (T) which are invaginations of the plasmalemma (note the line running along their axes). Possibly because of its tight confinement in the intercellular spaces of stratified epithelia, the Langerhans cell does not show the complex folds of plasmalemma typical of other macrophages. The adjacent stratified epithelial cells show tonofibrils cut in cross section (Tic) and longitudinal section (Tfl) as well as desmosomes (D) along the intercellular spaces. × 37,000 (Courtesy of C. P. Leblond)

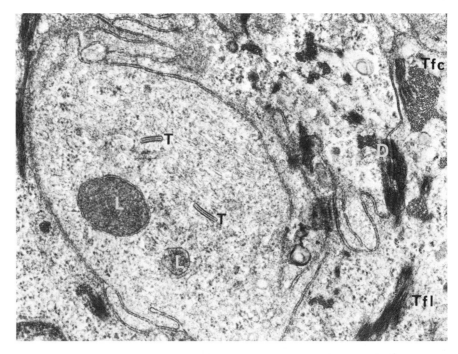

the hair. The melanin they contain becomes incorporated into the keratin of the hair to give it color.

There is evidence to indicate that the melanocytes of the bulb of the follicle divide by mitosis and so perpetuate themselves.

As people become older, their hair turns "gray." The lack of pigment in the hair of older people is ascribed to an increasing inability of the melanocytes of the bulbs of their hair follicles to make tyrosinase.

Although hair in the gross appears in different colors, hair pigments of only 3 colors can be seen with the microscope; these are black, brown and yellow. The yellow pigment is termed pheomelanin, and its formation seems to be under the control of genes other than those that control the formation of black and brown melanin. The metabolic pathways concerned in its formation are not thoroughly understood but are different from those concerned in the formation of black and brown melanin.

For a comprehensive consideration of the nature of hair pigment, those interested will find the chapter on this subject by Fitzpatrick, Brunet and Kukita in *The Biology of Hair Growth,* edited by Montagna and Ellis, most informative (see References).

Blood Supply of the Skin

Arteries. The largest arteries that supply skin are arranged in the form of a flat network in the sub-cutaneous tissue immediately below the dermis as is shown in Figure 20-19, B. This arterial network is called the *rete cutaneum*. From the rete cutaneum, branches pass both more deeply and toward the surface. Those that pass more deeply supply the adipose tissue of the more superficial parts of the subcutaneous tissue and the parts of such hair follicles as are disposed therein. Those that pass superficially supply the skin. As these arteries penetrate the reticular layer of the dermis, they generally pursue a curved course and give off side branches to the adjacent hair follicles, sweat and sebaceous glands. On reaching the junction of the reticular layer and the papillary layer, they form a second flat network, composed of smaller vessels, called the *rete subpapillare*.

Capillary Beds. An understanding of the site of the capillary beds of skin is of great importance in understanding how the temperature of the body is controlled and it is also of importance in knowing the sites of fluid loss from burns of different degrees.

First, as was already mentioned in connection with the healing of skin wounds, the dermis, since it consists chiefly of the relatively inert intercellular substance, collagen, does not require a very extensive capillary blood supply. Indeed, most of the dermis is very sparingly supplied with capillaries. As might be expected, the capillary beds of the skin are extensive only in that portion of the dermis that is in close association with epithelial cells that require abundant

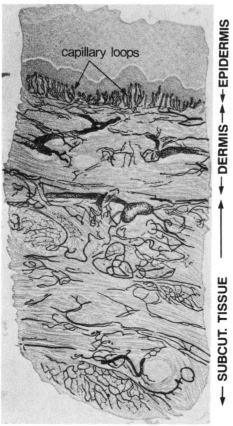

EPIDERMIS → DERMIS → SUBCUT. TISSUE →

FIG. 20-19B. Drawing of a section of thick skin and subcutaneous tissue the blood vessels of which had been injected with an opaque material. It shows the general disposition of the larger blood vessels in the dermis and subcutaneous tissue and also that there are very few capillaries in the intercellular substance of the dermis. The very numerous capillary loops that exist in the connective tissue papillae that project into the lower border of the epidermis are shown to advantage. (From Addison, W. H. F. (ed.): Piersol's Normal Histology. ed. 15. Philadelphia, J. B. Lippincott, 1932)

nourishment for their function and growth. The capillary beds of the skin, then, are confined to the connective tissue that (1) immediately underlies the epidermis, (2) surrounds the matrix of the hair follicles, and (3) surrounds the sweat and sebaceous glands.

The first capillary bed mentioned requires some further comment. Arterioles from the rete subpapillare pass toward the epidermis and give rise to capillaries that extend as loops up into the so-called connective tissue papillae (Figs. 20-19B and 20-20, *left*). These capillaries supply tissue fluid to the basal cells of the epidermis. However, the capillary loops in the papillae are not the cause of the pink color of the skin. This is

due to flat networks of small thin-walled vessels of the general nature of venules in the deeper part of the papillary and in the superficial part of the reticular layers of the dermis. These flat networks constitute the *subpapillary plexuses* of the skin. The small venules drain into larger ones, which, in turn, drain into small veins. In general, the veins leave the skin with the arteries.

Function of the Superficial Capillaries and Venules. In man, heat generated in the body is lost directly through the skin. If the temperature of the air is lower than that of the body, the rate of heat loss can be increased or decreased by the degree to which the capillaries and the venules of the papillary and the subpapillary regions of the skin are open to the circulation. If the temperature of the air is close to or higher than that of the body, the *effect* of a lower outside temperature can be achieved by the sweat glands pouring fluid onto the surface of the body, where it evaporates and so cools the outer part of the skin. Hence, blood circulating through the papillary and the subpapillary regions of skin from which sweat is evaporating loses heat. To keep down the temperature of an individual who performs violent muscular exercise on a very hot day and so generates a great deal of heat, both profuse sweating and dilation of the superficial blood vessels are needed. Some unfortunate individuals are born with very few or no sweat glands. When the temperature rises sufficiently, such individuals, while at work, can maintain their body temperature at correct levels only by frequently changing into fresh wet clothing.

The Nervous Control of Sweating. The secretory cells of the sweat glands are innervated by nerve fibers of the autonomic nervous system, chiefly cholinergic fibers of the sympathetic division. As already noted, the sympathetic fibers that innervate sweat glands produce acetylcholine at their endings, not norepinephrine as do most sympathetic fibers. The activity of the nerves and hence of the sweat glands is controlled by a heat-regulating center in the hypothalamus.

It should be pointed out that the skins of many animals cannot lose heat in this way in hot weather. The hairy coats of animals serve primarily as insulation. There is, then, no need for these animals to have sweat glands and extensive nets of capillaries and venules in the papillary and the subpapillary parts of the skin. (Dogs, for example, lose heat by panting.) And, indeed, the blood supply of the skin of most laboratory animals is very different from that of the skin of man. Therefore, deductions made from experiments performed on the skins of animals are not necessarily applicable to man. For example, a light burn on the shaved skin of a rat does not turn red as

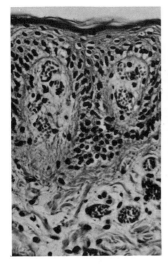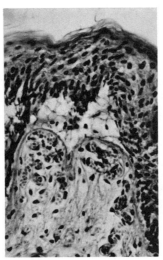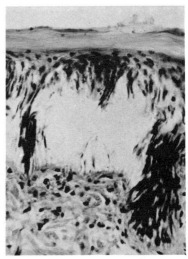

Fig. 20-20. Medium-power photomicrographs of sections of the skin of a pig, showing how a blister develops after a burn. (*Left*) Section taken from the skin 15 minutes after it suffered a light burn. Note that the capillaries in the dermal papillae, close to the epidermis, are dilated and congested with blood. (*Center*) Section taken 1 hour after the skin was burned lightly. The capillaries of the papillae are still dilated and congested, and, in addition, plasma has leaked from them and is accumulating between the dermis and the epidermis. (*Right*) Section taken 4 hours after the skin was burned slightly. It shows the epidermis lifted a considerable distance from the dermis by the plasma that has leaked from the injured capillaries of the dermis. (Ham, A. W.: Ann. Surg., *120*:692)

it does in man. The common pig is an exception. Its skin has an excellent supply of capillaries (Fig. 20-20). The blood supply of the skin of the pig is similar to that of the skin of man. It is one of the few animals that becomes sunburned.

Practical Application of Knowledge of Blood Supply. A light burn, such as is commonly obtained on the first visit of the year to the beach, produces enough injury to cause the capillaries and the venules in the papillary and subpapillary layers of the skin to become widely open to the circulation (Fig. 20-20, *left*). This makes the skin red.

The Nature of a Blister. In a slightly more severe burn, the capillaries and the venules of the papillary and the subpapillary regions, in addition to dilating, allow plasma to leak from them (Fig. 20-20, *center*). This causes an edema of the outer part of the skin and often results in blisters. In thin skin, blisters are the result of accumulations of plasma between the dermis and the epidermis (Fig. 20-20, *right*). In thick skin, blisters sometimes may be due to intra-epithelial accumulations of plasma.

The Regeneration of Epidermis After a Burn. If thin skin has been burned severely enough for blisters to have formed, it has been burned severely enough, we think, to have destroyed the epidermis. Under these

circumstances, a new epidermis must be regenerated from the living epithelium that persists in the hair follicles—just as it does when split skin grafts are cut from skin. Epidermis grows out from the external sheaths of hair follicles to cover the denuded dermis (Fig. 20-21). Even if a burn is severe enough to destroy the more superficial part of the dermis (as well as the epidermis), the epithelial cells from the deeper parts of the hair follicles will survive and grow out along the line between the living and the dead dermis (Fig. 20-21) to form a new epidermis at this level.

If a burn is severe enough to destroy the epithelium deep in the hair follicles, the burned area can become epithelized naturally only by epithelium growing in from the edges of the injured area. This is a slow process, and if the burned area is large, it would take months or years to heal, and it might never heal. In the meantime, the exposed dermis would become the seat of inflammatory process that, in all probability, would cause huge scars to form. Nowadays such burns are treated promptly by skin grafting, as has already been described.

Sites of Plasma Loss in Burns of Different Depths. In superficial burns, plasma leakage occurs chiefly from the dilated and injured capillaries and

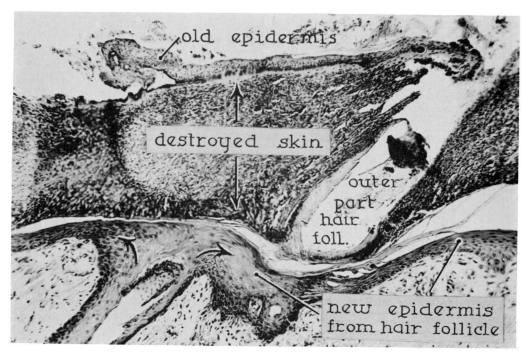

Fɪɢ. 20-21. Low-power photomicrograph of a section of the skin of a pig some days after it was burned sufficiently to destroy the epidermis and the outer part of the dermis. The original epidermis, now dead, may be seen in the upper part of the figure. Below it, a considerable layer of destroyed dermis, containing the destroyed outer part of a hair follicle, may be seen. Below the layer of dead dermis, a new thin line of epidermis growing out from the deeper part of the hair follicle may be seen. The newly formed epithelial cells push along the line between the living and the destroyed skin. The destroyed skin eventually is extruded as a scab when the new epidermis forms a continuous covering for the living skin below. Subsequently, the epidermis becomes thick, and the dermis beneath it also thickens, so that the thickness of the entire skin is restored.

venules of the papillary and subpapillary layers of the dermis. Such burns appear red because these superficial vessels become dilated by the injury (Fig. 20-20, *left*). In more severe burns these superficial vessels become coagulated by heat; hence, more severe burns may at first be *white in color*. In these, plasma leaks from deeper capillary beds associated with the hair follicles and sweat glands. In still more severe burns plasma leaks from the capillary beds that supply the fat cells in the subcutaneous tissue. If a large area of skin is burned, even if the burn is not deep, enough plasma may leak from injured capillaries and venules to cause the death of the patient (see Increased Permeability of Blood Capillaries, in Chapter 7). Consequently, in the modern treatment of burns, every effort is made to prevent hemoconcentration by administering blood plasma intravenously to the burned person. Extreme plasma leakage can be prevented to a considerable degree by applying pressure bandages

(plasma cannot very well leak out of the circulatory system into tissues unless it can expand the tissues).

Afferent Nerve Endings in Skin. See Chapter 28.

Nails

Toward the end of the 3rd month of embryonic life the epidermis covering the dorsal surface of the terminal phalanx of each finger and toe begins to invade the underlying dermis. The invasion occurs along a transverse curved line; hence, the invading epidermis has the form of a curved plate. Moreover, the invasion does not occur along a line at right angles to the surface but, instead, it slants proximally (Fig. 20-22). Later, the invading plate of epidermis splits so that it forms the nail groove (Fig. 20-22). The epidermal cells making up the deeper wall of this groove proliferate to become the matrix of the nail (Fig. 20-23). The cells in the matrix proliferate, and the upper ones differentiate into nail substance which is hard keratin (Fig. 20-9, *right*). With the continuing proliferation and differentiation of the cells in the lower part of the matrix, the forming nail is pushed out of the groove and slowly slides along the dorsal surface of the digit toward its distal part. Although it slides slowly over the epidermis of the dorsal part of the digit, it remains firmly attached to it all the while. The epidermis over which it slides is called the *nail bed* (Fig. 20-23). It consists of only the deeper layers of the epidermis; the nail, as it were, serves as its stratum corneum. The skin of the dorsal surface of the digits is formed into a groove along each side of the nail (Fig. 20-24). With sufficient growth, the *free margin* of the nail will project beyond the distal end of the digit (Fig. 20-24).

The *body* of the nail is the part that shows. The part that is hidden in the nail groove is called the *root*. Seen from above, a crescent-shaped white area appears on the part of the body nearest the root. This is called the *lunula* (Fig. 20-24); it is seen to best advantage on the thumb and the first finger. It is usually absent from the little finger. The nail, except for the lunula, is pink because the blood in the capillaries of the dermis under the nail bed shows through. The lunula is white because the capillaries under it do not show through. There are different theories to explain this. Some authorities think the lunula indicates the extent of the underlying matrix (Fig. 20-23).

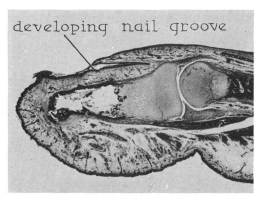

FIG. 20-22. Photomicrograph of a longitudinal section cut through a terminal phalanx of a fetus, showing how the epidermis invades the dermis proximally to form a nail groove.

Since the matrix is thicker than the epidermis of the nail bed, capillaries beneath it would not show through it as well as they would through the epidermis of the nail bed. However, the region of the lunula cannot always be correlated with the site of the matrix in sections. Hence some authors think that its whiteness is due to the nail substance, when it is first formed, being more opaque than the more mature nail substance found over the bed.

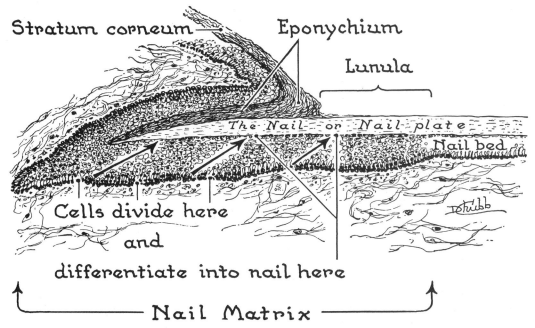

FIG. 20-23. Diagram of a longitudinal section (low-power) cut through the nail groove and the root of a growing nail.

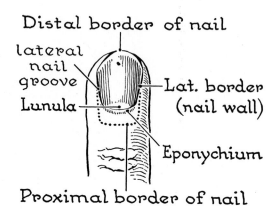

Distal border of nail

lateral
nail
groove

Lunula

Lat. border
(nail wall)

Eponychium

Proximal border of nail

Fig. 20-24. Diagram of the end of a finger and a fingernail.

At the proximal border of the nail, the stratum corneum of the epidermis of the skin of the dorsum of a finger or a toe projects over and is adherent to the nail. This, together with the stratum corneum of the epidermis that makes up the proximal and more superficial wall of the nail fold and is adherent to the proximal and outer surface of the nail root, constitutes the *eponychium* (*epi,* upon; *onyx,* nail) (Fig. 20-23), and it is soft keratin.

Infections in the region of the eponychium or along the lateral borders of the nail (Fig. 20-24) are not uncommon. Sometimes, in order to permit these infections to heal, it is necessary to remove the root of a nail. On being pulled out, the nail root will be seen to be shaped like the end of a curved chisel which does not extend into the nail groove as far as might be thought. Provided that the matrix is not destroyed, a new nail will grow out of the nail fold in due time. If the matrix is destroyed, a new nail will not form.

Sometimes, from wearing improper shoes, the curvature of toenails becomes accentuated, and they pierce the dermis along one of their lateral grooves (a normal groove is shown in Fig. 20-24). The condition is called an ingrown toenail. Sometimes it is necessary to cut away some matrix at one side of the nail groove to cure this condition. New nail will not grow from the region from which matrix is removed. Hence, the cutting away of matrix at one side of the nail groove results in the formation of a narrower nail, which therefore does not impinge on the skin at the bottom of the lateral groove, and so the pierced skin at this point can heal.

The dermis beneath the epidermis of the nail bed is arranged in longitudinal grooves and ridges. In cross sections the ridges appear as papillae. The dermis in this site is very vascular. The ridges and the grooves of dermis present under the bed do not continue proximally under the matrix, but there are some papillae in this region.

On the average, nails grow about 0.5 mm. a week. Fingernails grow more rapidly than toenails and both grow faster in summer than in winter. The rate of growth of nails is different at different ages. Nail growth may be disturbed when the body suffers from certain diseases. Even psychological upsets are said to be reflected sometimes by the pitting of nails. Certain hormone deficiencies and excesses affect the growth of nails; hence the condition of the nails sometimes may help to indicate an endocrine gland disturbance.

Chalones and the Control of Cell Multiplication in Epidermis. This matter was discussed in Chapter 6 where references to the literature were given.

Some References and Other Reading on Skin and Skin Appendages

Some Books

Champion, R. H., Gillman, T., Rook, A. J., and Sims, R. T. (eds.): An Introduction to the Biology of the Skin. Oxford and Edinburgh, Blackwell, 1970.
Della Porta, G., and Muhlbock, O. (eds.): Structure and Control of the Melanocyte. New York, Springer, 1966.
Elgjo, K.: Epidermal Cell Population Kinetics in Chemically Induced Hyperplasia. p. 116, Scandinavian University Books, Oslo, University Press, 1966.
Montagna, W., and Ellis, R. A. (eds.): The Biology of Hair Growth. New York, Academic Press, 1958.
———: Advances in the Biology of the Skin. vol. 6. New York, Pergamon Press, 1965.
Montagna, W., and Lobitz, W., Jr. (eds.): The Epidermis. New York, Academic Press, 1964.
Montagna, W. The Structure and Function of Skin. ed. 2. New York, Academic Press, 1962.
Riley, V., and Fortner, J. G. (eds.): Pigment cell. Ann. N.Y. Acad. Sci., *100:*1, 1963.
Rothman, S.: Physiology and Biochemistry of the Skin. Chicago, University of Chicago Press, 1956.
Zelickson, A. S. (ed.): Ultrastructure of Normal and Abnormal Skin. Philadelphia, Lea and Febiger, 1967.

Some Articles and Reviews

Bertalanffy, F. D.: Mitotic activity and renewal rate of sebaceous gland cells in the rat. Anat. Rec., *129:*231, 1957.
Billingham, R. E., and Silvers, W. K.: The melanocytes of mammals. Quart. Rev. Biol., *35:*1, 1960.
Breathnach, A. S.: The cell of Langerhans. Int. Rev. Cytol., *18:*1, 1965.
Brody, T.: The keratinization of epidermal cells of normal guinea pig skin as revealed by electron microscopy. J. Ultrastruct. Res., *2:*482, 1959.
Bullough, W. S., and Ebling, F. J.: Cell replacement in the epidermis and sebaceous glands of the mouse. J. Anat., *86:*29, 1952.

Butcher, E. O.: Development of the pilary system and the replacement of hair in mammals. Ann. N.Y. Acad. Sci., *53:*508, 1951.

Cauna, N.: Nature and functions of the papillary ridges of the digital skin. Anat. Rec., *119:*449, 1954.

Chacko, L. W., and Vaidya, M. C.: The dermal papillae and ridge patterns in human volar skin. Acta. anat., *70:*99, 1968.

Chase, H. B.: Growth of the hair. Physiol. Rev., *34:*113, 1954.

Chase, H. B., Montagna, W., and Malone, J. D.: Changes in the skin in relation to the hair growth cycle. Anat. Rec., *116:*75, 1953.

Clark, W. H., and Hibbs, R. G.: Electron microscope studies of the human epidermis. The clear cell of Mason (dendritic cell or melanocyte). J. Biophys. Biochem. Cytol., *4:*679, 1958.

Cummins, H., and Midlo, C.: Finger Prints, Palms and Soles. New York, Blakiston Division of McGraw-Hill, 1943.

Ellis, R. A.: Vascular patterns of the skin. *In* Montagna, W., and Ellis, R. A. (eds.): Advances in Biology of the Skin. vol. 2, p. 20. New York, Pergamon Press, 1961.

Edwards, E., and Duntley, S.: The pigments and color of living human skin. Am. J. Anat., *65:*1, 1939.

Fan, J., Schoenfeld, R. J., and Hunter, R.: A study of the epidermal clear cells with special reference to their relationship to the cells of Langerhans. J. Invest. Dermat., *32:*445, 1959.

Faulds, H.: On the skin-furrows of the hand. Nature, *22:*605, 1880.

Fingerman, M.: The physiology of chromatophores. Int. Rev. Cytol., *8,* 1959.

Fitzpatrick, T. B., and Szabo, G.: The melanocyte, cytology and cytochemistry. J. Invest. Dermat., *32:*197, 1959.

Gillman, T., *et al.:* A re-examination of certain aspects of the histogenesis of the healing of cutaneous wounds; a preliminary report. Brit. J. Surg., *43:*141, 1955.

Gillman, T., and Penn, J.: Studies on the repair of cutaneous wounds. Med. Proc. (South African), *2:*93, 1956.

Giroud, A., and Leblond, C. P.: The keratinization of epidermis and its derivatives, especially the hair, as shown by x-ray diffraction and histochemical studies. Ann. N.Y. Acad. Sci., *53:*613, 1951.

Ham, A. W.: Experimental study of histopathology of burns, with particular reference to sites of fluid loss in burns of different depths. Ann. Surg., *120:*689, 1944.

Hamilton, J. B.: Male hormone stimulation is prerequisite and incitant in common baldness. Am. J. Anat., *71:*541, 1942.

———: Patterned loss of hair in man: types and incidence. Ann. N.Y. Acad. Sci., *53:*395, 1968.

———: Quantitative measurement of a secondary sex character, axillary hair. Ann. N.Y. Acad. Sci., *53:*585, 1951.

Hibbs, R. G.: The fine structure of human exocrine sweat glands. Am. J. Anat., *103:*201, 1958.

Hibbs, R. G., Burch, G. E., and Phillips, J. H.: The fine structure of the small blood vessels of the normal human dermis and subcutis. Am. Heart J., *56:*662, 1958.

Hibbs, R. G., and Clark, W. H., Jr.: Electron microscope studies of the human epidermis. J. Biophys. Biochem. Cytol., *6:*71, 1959.

Leblond, C. P.: Histochemical structure of hair, with a brief comparison to other epidermal appendages and epidermis itself. Ann. N.Y. Acad. Sci., *53:*464, 1951.

Lindsay, W. K., and Birch, J. R.: Thin skin healing. Canad. J. Surg., *7:*297, 1964.

Lorber, M., and Milobsky, S. A.: Stretching of the skin in vivo, a method of influencing cell division and cell migration in the rat epidermis. J. Invest. Dermat., *51:*395, 1968.

McGuire, J., and Moellmann, G.: Cytochalasin B: Effects of microfilaments and movement of melanin granules within melanocytes. Science, *175:*642, 1972.

Odland, G. F.: The morphology of the attachment between the dermis and the epidermis. Anat. Rec., *108:*399, 1950.

Thodin, J. A. G., and Reith, E. J.: Ultrastructure of keratin in oral mucosa, skin, esophagus, claw and hair. *In* Fundamentals of Keratinization. p. 61. Washington, D.C., Am. Assoc. Adv. Sci., 1962.

Rodgers, G. E.: Electron microscope observations on the structure of sebaceous glands. Exp. Cell Res., *13:*517, 1957.

———: Some aspects of the structure of the inner root sheath of hair follicles revealed by light and electron microscopy. Exp. Cell Res., *14:*378, 1958.

Seiji, M., Shimao, K., Birbeck, M. S. C., and Fitzpatrick, T. B.: Subcellular localization of melanin biosynthesis. Ann. N.Y., Acad. Sci., *100:*497, 1963.

Southwood, W. F. W.: The thickness of the skin. Plast. Reconstr. Surg., *15:*423, 1955.

Storey, W. F., and Leblond, C. P.: Measurement of the rate of proliferation of epidermis and associated structures. Ann. N.Y. Acad. Sci., *53:*537, 1951.

Wolff, K., and Konrad, K.: Melanin pigmentation: an in vivo model for studies of melanosome kinetics within keratinocytes, Science, *174:*1034, 1971.

Wong, Yong-Chuan, and Buck, R. C.: Langerhans cells in epidermoid hyperplasia. J. Invest. Dermat., *56:*10, 1971.

Wyllie, J. C., More, R. H., and Haust, M. D.: Electron microscopy of epidermal lesions elicited during hypersensitivity. Lab. Invest., *13:*137, 1964.

For References about tonofilaments, tonofibrils and desmosomes see Chapter 5.

21 The Digestive System

Introduction

The digestive system (Fig. 21-1) consists of: (1) a long muscular tube that begins at the lips and ends at the anus, at which two sites its epithelial lining becomes continuous with the epidermis of the skin; and (2) certain large glands situated outside the tube proper (salivary glands, liver, gallbladder and pancreas) that empty their secretions into the tube because they develop from its epithelial lining.

Digestion Occurs Outside the Body Proper. It is important to realize that the fluid and semifluid material in the lumen of the tube is as much outside the body as the water in which an ameba lives is outside the ameba. Food must be absorbed through the epithelial lining of the tube before it can be said to have gained entrance into the body proper. But most food taken in at the mouth is not in a form that can be used by cells. The carbohydrate of bread and potatoes is in the form of starch which must be broken down to glucose before it can be absorbed and used by cells. The proteins of meat must be broken down to amino acids before absorption and use by cells. The process by which foods taken in at the mouth are converted into substances that may be safely absorbed and used by cells is known as *digestion*. Digestion occurs in the lumen of the digestive tube and is brought about by the food therein being acted upon by digestive juices that are secreted by the glands in the wall of the tube and by others situated outside the tube but emptying into it. The epithelial cells lining the tube are extremely selective in their absorptive functions; if they were not selective, and did absorb undigested substances, death could result.

Parts of the Tube. The digestive tube consists of the mouth, the pharynx, the esophagus, the stomach, the small intestine and the large intestine (Fig. 21-1). These different parts of the tube serve somewhat different purposes that will be described as we deal with each part in turn.

Definition and Description of a Mucous Membrane. The wet epithelial lining of the digestive tube and (as we shall see) of other internal passageways that open to the surface constitutes, like the epidermis of skin, a barrier between the community of cells that comprise the body and the outside world. The problem of providing protection along the vast wet epithelial surface of the digestive tube is considerably greater than that faced by the skin because a large part of the epithelial membrane of the intestinal tract must be thin enough to be absorptive. One of the chief agencies ensuring the integrity of the epithelium of a mucous membrane is its lubrication with mucus. From one end to the other, the digestive tube is richly provided with either individual cells or with glands that produce mucus. Wet epithelial membranes thus equipped are termed *mucous membranes*. But the term *mucous membrane* usually refers to something more than an epithelial membrane alone; it includes the underlying connective tissue that supports the epithelial membrane. This connective tissue layer is termed the *lamina propria* or *tunica propria* of the mucous membrane. In some instances mucous membranes are limited on the tissue side by some smooth muscle known as *muscularis mucosae* (muscle of the mucosa). The 3 layers of a mucous membrane are shown in Figure 21-21.

The Lips

The substance of the lips consists of striated muscle fibers and fibroelastic connective tissue. The muscle tissue consists chiefly of the fibers of the orbicularis oris muscle and is distributed in the more central part of the lip (Fig. 21-2). The direction of the fibers and their attachments are discussed in textbooks of gross anatomy.

The outer surface of each lip is covered with skin that contains hair follicles, sebaceous glands and sweat glands (Fig. 21-2, *right*). The red free margins of the lips are covered with a modified skin which represents a transition from skin to mucous membrane. The epithelium in this site is covered with a layer of dead cells, like that of the skin, but it is said that there is a high percentage of eleidin, which is relatively transparent, in it. The connective tissue

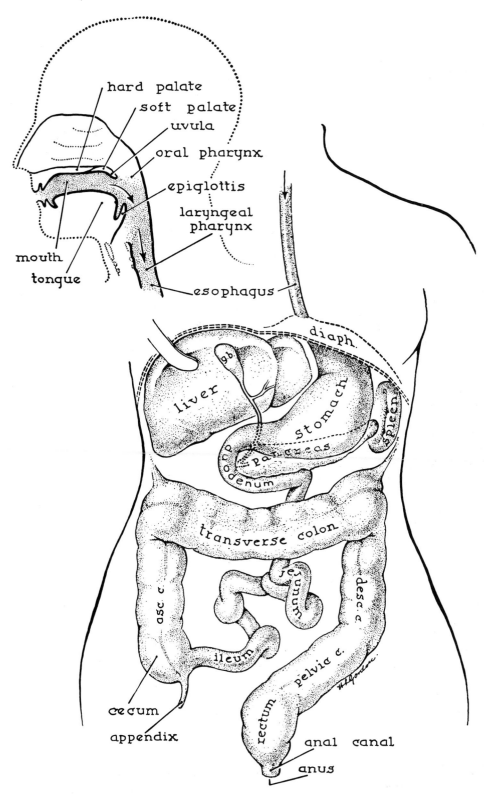

hard palate

soft palate

uvula

oral pharynx

epiglottis

laryngeal
pharynx

mouth

tongue

esophagus

diaph.

g.b.

liver

stomach

spleen

pancreas

duodenum

transverse colon

jejunum

asc. c.

desc. c.

ileum

pelvic c.

cecum

appendix

rectum

anal canal

anus

FIG. 21-1. Diagram of the parts of the digestive system. (Redrawn and modified from Grant, J. C. B.: A Method of Anatomy. ed. 4. Baltimore, Williams & Wilkins)

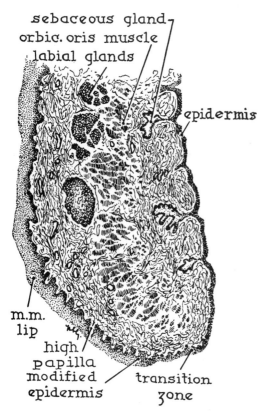

sebaceous gland
orbic. oris muscle
labial glands
epidermis
m.m.
lip
high
papilla
modified
epidermis
transition
zone

FIG. 21-2. Semidiagrammatic drawing of a sagittal section of a lip (low-power). (Redrawn from Huber: Piersol's Human Anatomy. ed. 9. Philadelphia, Lippincott)

papillae of the dermis beneath it are numerous, high and vascular (Fig. 21-2), and, as a result, the blood in their capillaries readily shows through the transparent epidermis to make the lips appear red. No sweat or sebaceous glands or hair follicles are present in the skin of the red free margins of the lips. Since the epithelium is not heavily keratinized and is not provided with sebum, it must be wetted frequently with the tongue if its integrity is to be preserved. "Chapped" and "cracked" lips are common under conditions which favor evaporation. The high papillae bring many nerve endings as well as capillaries close to the surface of the red margins of the lips; for this reason, they are very sensitive.

As the skin of the red free margin passes onto the inner surface of the lip, it becomes transformed into mucous membrane. The epithelium of this is thicker than the epidermis covering the outer surface of the lip (Fig. 21-2, *left*) and is of the stratified squamous nonkeratinizing type. However, some granules of keratohyalin may be found in the cells of the more superficial layers. High papillae of the connective tissue

lamina propria (which, in mucous membranes, replaces the dermis of skin) extend into it. Small clusters of mucous glands, the labial glands, are embedded in the lamina propria (Fig. 21-2) and connect with the surface by means of little ducts.

The Cheeks

The mucous membrane lining the cheeks has a fairly thick layer of epithelium of the stratified squamous nonkeratinizing type. This is the kind of epithelium that is characteristically found on wet epithelial surfaces where there is considerable wear and tear and from which no absorption occurs. The superficial cells of this epithelium are more or less constantly being rubbed off the surface and replaced from below. This, of course, requires that the cells in the deeper layers of the epithelium divide as rapidly as cells are worn away from the surface. If the ball of the finger is drawn across the inside of the cheek, many of the surface cells will be removed. If these are dabbed on a slide and stained with methylene blue, their flat bodies with their centrally disposed nuclei can be seen readily. As shown in Figure 4-2, chromosomal sex can be determined by examining stained smears of these cells.

The lamina propria here consists of fairly dense fibroelastic tissue and extends into the epithelium in the form of high papillae. The deeper part of it merges into what is termed the *submucosa* of the lining of the cheek. This layer contains flat elastic fibers and many blood vessels. Strands of fibroelastic tissue from the lamina propria penetrate through the fatty elastic submucosa to join with the fibroelastic tissue associated with the muscle that underlies the submucosa and forms the chief substance of the wall of the cheek. These strands fasten the mucous membrane to the underlying muscle at intervals, with the result that when the jaws are closed, the relaxed mucous membrane bulges inward in many small folds instead of in one large fold that would project inward so far that it would be an inconvenience and frequently would be bitten inadvertently.

There are small mucous glands, some of which have a few serous secretory demilunes, in the inner part of the cheek.

The Tongue

The tongue is composed chiefly of striated muscle, the fibers of which are grouped into bundles that interlace with one another and are disposed in 3 planes. Hence, if a longitudinal section is cut from the tongue, i.e., at right angles to the dorsal surface (a sagittal section), it will reveal both longitudinal and vertical muscle fibers cut longitudinally and horizontal fibers cut in cross section. Such an arrangement of striated muscle fibers is unique in the body, so that finding it in any given section permits that section to be identified as having been cut from the tongue.

The individual muscle fibers inside the bundles are each surrounded by endomysium which tends to be somewhat more substantial than that seen in most striated muscle. The endomysium brings capillaries close to the muscle fibers. The fibroelastic tissue between the muscle bundles can be thought of as constituting the perimysium. It contains the larger vessels and nerves and, in many sites, adipose tissue; in some parts of the tongue, glands are embedded in it.

Mucous Membranes. That covering the undersurface of the tongue is thin and smooth. The lamina propria connects directly with the fibroelastic tissue associated with the bundles of muscle. No true submucosa exists here.

The mucous membrane covering the dorsal surface of the tongue is of special interest (Fig. 21-3). The dorsal surface of the tongue may give the physician information because certain diseases—for example, scarlet fever and pernicious anemia—may cause certain specific alterations on the surface of the tongue.

The mucous membrane covering the dorsal surface of the tongue is divided into 2 parts: (1) that covering the anterior two thirds or oral part of the tongue (its body), and (2) that covering the posterior one third or pharyngeal part (its root). A V-shaped line, the sulcus terminalis, running across the tongue marks the border between these 2 parts (Fig. 21-3).

THE ORAL PART OF THE TONGUE

The mucous membrane covering the oral part of the tongue is covered by little projections of the mucous membrane called *papillae*. There are 3 kinds of these in man—filiform, fungiform and vallate.

(1) **Filiform papillae** (*filum,* thread) are relatively high, narrow, conical structures composed both of lamina propria and epithelium (Fig. 21-3, *upper left*). Each has a primary papilla of lamina propria from which much smaller secondary papillae of lamina propria may extend toward the surface. The primary papilla is covered by a cap of epithelium which breaks up to form separate caps over each of the secondary papillae. Sometimes the epithelial caps over the secondary papillae are threadlike which justifies the term *filiform*. The epithelium that caps the secondary papillae becomes very horny, but there is some question whether the surface cells become converted into true

keratin in man. In some animals the horny filiform papillae make the dorsal surface of the tongue distinctly rasplike, and it is said that a friendly lick from one may draw blood.

Filiform papillae are very numerous and are distributed in parallel rows across the tongue. Near the root these rows follow the V-shaped line that divides the body from the root of the tongue (Fig. 21-3).

(2) **Fungiform papillae** are so-called because they project from the dorsal surface of the oral part of the tongue like little fungi which are narrower at their bases and have expanded smooth rounded tops (Fig. 21-3, *upper right*). They are not nearly as numerous as the filiform papillae among which they are scattered; they are somewhat more numerous at the tip of the tongue than elsewhere. Each has a central core of lamina propria which is termed the *primary papilla,* and from this, secondary papillae of lamina propria project up into the covering epithelium. The epithelial surface does not follow the contours of the secondary papillae of lamina propria as it does in filiform papillae; hence the secondary papillae of lamina propria bring capillaries very close to the surface of the epithelium. Since the covering epithelium is not keratinized, it is relatively translucent; this permits the blood vessels in the high secondary papillae to show through, and as a result the fungiform papillae in life are red.

(3) **Vallate papillae.** From 7 to 12 are distributed along the V-shaped line that separates the mucous membrane of the body of the tongue from that of the root (Fig. 21-3). The name (*vallum,* a rampart) suggests that each, like an ancient city, is surrounded by a rampart. Actually, each is like a turreted castle because it is surrounded by a moat or trench (Fig. 21-3, *lower left*). The moat that surrounds each is kept flooded, and so cleansed of debris by glands which are disposed deep to the papilla, but which empty by means of ducts into the bottom of the moat.

Each vallate papilla has a central primary papilla of lamina propria (Fig. 21-3, *lower left*). Secondary papillae of lamina propria extend up from this into the stratified nonkeratinizing epithelium that covers the whole papilla. Vallate papillae are narrower at their points of attachment than at their free surfaces; hence their shapes are not unlike those of papillae of the fungiform type.

Functions of Papillae. Animals in which filiform papillae are highly developed are capable of licking layers off solid and semisolid material with a sandpaper-like efficiency. Even though filiform papillae are not very highly developed in man, they permit children to lick ice cream satisfactorily. Such papillae

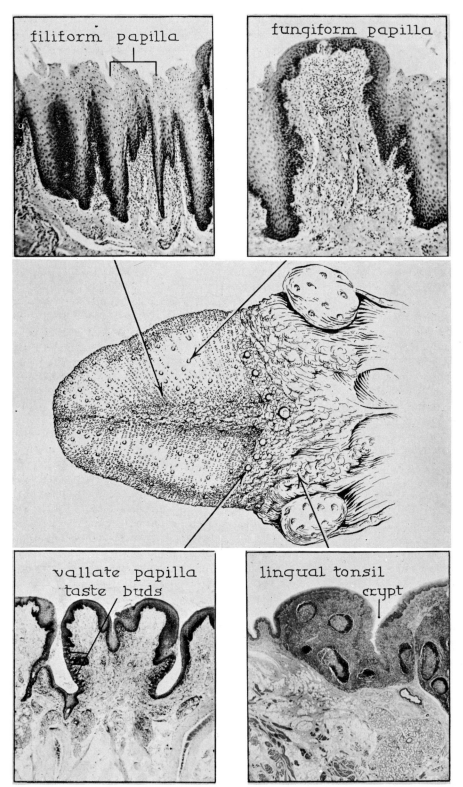

Fig. 21-3. Drawing of the dorsal surface of the tongue and photomicrographs of sections cut from its mucous membrane in 4 areas. See text for discussion. The sulcus terminalis is directly in front of the row of vallate papillae.

contain nerve endings specialized for touch (tactile sense). Most fungiform papillae and all the vallate papillae contain taste buds in which there are special nerve endings which, on being stimulated, give rise to the nervous impulses that result in sensations of taste. Taste buds will be described in Chapter 28.

ROOT OF THE TONGUE

Lingual Tonsil. No true papillae are present on the mucous membrane covering the root of the tongue. The small humps seen over this part of the tongue are due to aggregations of lymphatic nodules in the lamina propria beneath the epithelium (Fig. 21-3, *lower right*). Such an arrangement, i.e., aggregations of lymphatic nodules in close association with stratified squamous epithelium, is generally called *tonsillar tissue.* That over the root of the tongue constitutes the *lingual tonsil.* Many of the lymphatic nodules in the lingual tonsil have germinal centers. Diffuse lymphatic tissue fills the spaces between them. Along with the lymphocytes there are many plasma cells. The stratified squamous nonkeratinizing epithelium that overlies the lymphatic tissue extends down into it in many sites to form wells or pits (Fig. 21-3, *lower right*). These are called *crypts* (*kryptos,* concealed). Lymphocytes migrate through the epithelium covering these patches of lymphatic tissue, but more particularly through the stratified epithelial walls of the crypts, to gain entrance to their lumens. The superficial epithelial cells from the linings of the crypts desquamate into the lumens of the crypts, with the result that the lumens of crypts may show accumulations of debris formed from lymphocytes and desquamated epithelial cells. Ducts from underlying mucous glands open into the bottoms of many crypts; this arrangement, when present, serves to keep the lumens washed out and hence free from debris. For this reason, infected crypts are not so common in the lingual tonsil as in tonsillar tissue in certain other sites where there are no underlying glands that open into the crypts.

The Teeth

INTRODUCTORY DESCRIPTION OF THE PARTS OF AN ADULT TOOTH AND ITS ATTACHMENTS

The teeth are arranged in 2 parabolic curves, one in the upper jaw and one in the lower. Each of these 2 curved rows of teeth constitutes a *dental arch.* The upper arch is slightly larger than the lower; hence, normally, the upper teeth slightly overlap the lower teeth.

The bulk of each tooth is made of a special type of calcified connective tissue called *dentin.* Dentin normally is covered with a layer of one or the other of 2 calcified tissues. The dentin of that portion of the tooth that projects through the gums into the mouth is covered with a cap of very hard, calcified, epithelial-derived tissue called *enamel* (Fig. 21-4); this part of the tooth that is covered with enamel constitutes its *anatomic crown.* The remainder of the tooth, the *anatomic root* (Fig. 21-4), is covered with a sheath of a special calcified connective tissue called *cementum.*

The junction between the crown and the root of the tooth is termed the *neck* or *cervix,* and the visible line of junction between enamel and cementum is termed the *cervical line.*

Within each tooth is a space which conforms to the general shape of the tooth; this is called the *pulp cavity* (Fig. 21-4). Its more expanded portion in the coronal part of the tooth is called the *pulp chamber,* and the narrowed part of the cavity that extends through the root is called the *pulp* or *root canal.* The pulp consists of a mesenchymal-like connective tissue; this is what lay people call the "nerve" of the tooth because it is so sensitive. The pulp is well supplied with nerve fibers and small blood vessels. The dentin that surrounds the pulp cavity is lined with a layer of special cells called *odontoblasts* (Fig. 21-4) whose function, as their name implies, is related to the production of dentin. Odontoblasts bear much the same relation to dentin that osteoblasts do to bone and indeed are much like osteoblasts in several respects. The nerve and the blood supply of a tooth enters the pulp through a small hole (or holes) through the apex of the root called the *apical foramen* (Fig. 21-4, not labeled).

How the Roots of the Teeth Are Attached to Bone. The roots of the lower teeth are set into a bony ridge that projects upward from the body of the mandible, and the roots of the upper teeth are set into a bony ridge that projects downward from the body of the maxilla; these bony ridges are termed *alveolar processes.* In these processes are *sockets* (*alveoli*)—one for the root of each tooth. The teeth are suspended and held firmly in their alveoli by bundles of connective tissue fibers known collectively as periodontal membrane or preferably periodontal ligament (Fig. 21-4). This consists chiefly of dense bundles of collagenic fibers running in various directions from the bone of the socket wall to the cementum that covers the root. The collagenic fibers at one end are embedded in the calcified intercellular substance of the bone of the socket and at their other end into the cementum of the tooth. The embedded portions are

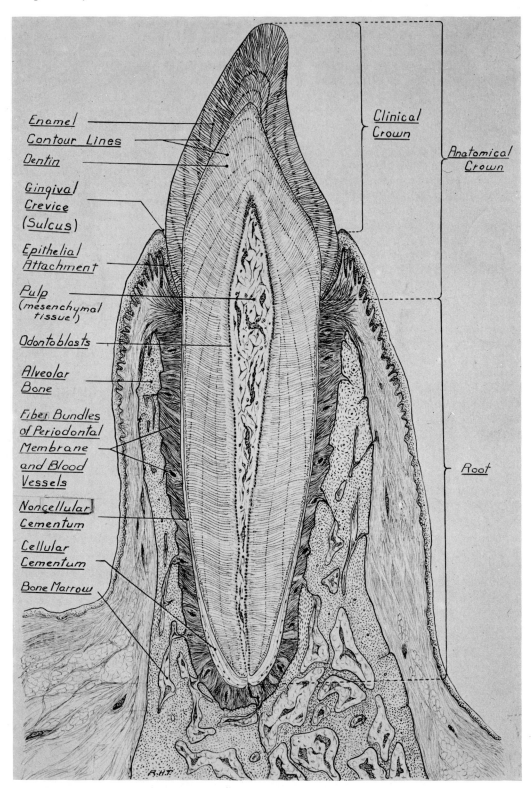

Enamel

Contour Lines

Dentin

Gingival
Crevice
(Sulcus)

Epithelial
Attachment

Pulp
(mesenchymal
tissue)

Odontoblasts

Alveolar
Bone

Fiber Bundles
of Periodontal
Membrane
and Blood
Vessels

Noncellular
Cementum

Cellular
Cementum

Bone Marrow

Clinical
Crown

Anatomical
Crown

Root

Fɪɢ. 21-4. Diagram of a sagittal section of a lower central incisor tooth and attachments.

called *Sharpey's fibers* (Fig. 21-15). The way in which Sharpey's fibers become embedded in bone and cementum will be explained later. The fibers not only hold the tooth in place, but they are arranged so that when pressure is exerted on the biting surface of the tooth, the tooth, being suspended by them, will not be pressed farther into the narrowing socket (which could squeeze the blood vessels in the periodontal ligament), and at the same time the tooth is permitted some slight movement within its alveolus.

The mucous membrane of the mouth forms an external covering for the bone of the alveolar process; these coverings constitute the *gums*. That part of the gum tissue extending coronally beyond the crest of the alveolar process is the *gingiva* (Fig. 21-4).

The part of the tooth that extends into the mouth beyond the gingiva is called the *clinical crown* (as distinguished from the anatomic crown described previously). The clinical crown may or may not be identical with the anatomic crown of a tooth. Soon after the tooth erupts into the mouth, the gingiva is attached to the enamel somewhere along the anatomic crown. As eruption proceeds, there is a time when the gingiva is attached to the tooth at the cervical line; at this stage the clinical and the anatomic crowns are identical. As the gingiva recedes still farther, as generally occurs in older people, the gingiva is attached to cementum, so the clinical crown is longer than the anatomic crown.

A General Description of Dentitions in Man

Two separate sets of teeth, or *dentitions*, develop during life. The first or *primary* dentition serves during the period of childhood. The teeth that develop in this dentition are called the *deciduous* (*decidere*, to fall down), *baby*, or *milk* teeth. These teeth are shed progressively and are replaced by the permanent teeth that are intended to last the individual for the remainder of his life.

There are 20 teeth in the primary dentition—10 in the upper and 10 in the lower jaw. The shape of these is not the same; each is modified for different functions related to mastication. The first 2 teeth on each side of the midline in the upper and the lower jaws are called *incisors* (*incidere*, to cut into). They appear in a baby at about the age of 6 months. The 2 incisors immediately next to the midline are the *central* incisors, and those next to them are the *lateral* incisors. The next teeth beyond the incisors are the *canine* or *cuspid* teeth; the free-biting surface of these has only a single *cusp* (conical projection). Next in line, in the

posterior part of a child's mouth, are 2 *molar* teeth on each side. Each molar tooth is modified for grinding food; hence its biting surfaces are wider and flatter than those of the other teeth and have 3 or more cusps projecting from them. They erupt at approximately 2 years. This set of teeth serves the child for the next 4 years or so, at which time the primary teeth begin to be shed and replaced by the permanent ones. This period of replacement of primary teeth extends over approximately 6 years, from about 6 through 12 years of age.

The permanent dentition consists of 32 teeth—16 upper and 16 lower. Their shape is similar to that of the primary teeth, but they are somewhat larger. The anterior or front teeth, as in the primary set, are the central and the lateral incisors and the cuspids. Immediately back of the cuspids are the 1st and the 2nd *bicuspids* or *premolars*, which are the teeth that occupy the spaces formerly occupied by the primary molars. Behind the bicuspids in each side of each jaw are 3 *molar* teeth. These are named the 1st, the 2nd and the 3rd molars; they have no predecessors in the primary dentition but erupt behind the last of the primary teeth in order. The 1st molar, or "6-year molar," erupts at about the age of 6 years. The 2nd molar erupts at about the age of 12 and is called the 12-year molar. The 3rd molar or "wisdom tooth" erupts considerably later, if it erupts at all. This tooth is subject to much variation in size and shape and all too frequently remains suppressed or impacted within the jaw.

The Development and Eruption of a Tooth

Two Germ Layers Participate in Forming a Tooth. The enamel of a tooth is derived from ectoderm. The dentin, cementum and pulp are all derived from mesenchyme. The covering of the gums is stratified squamous epithelium and is attached to the enamel around each tooth until later in life, when it becomes attached to cementum that covers the root.

The formation of a tooth—and to facilitate the description we shall here consider a lower tooth (so that we can speak of things growing up or down)—depends essentially on epithelium growing down into mesenchyme and assuming the form of the bowl of an inverted egg cup. Mesenchyme grows up into the bowl of the epithelial cup. Here inductive phenomena occur. The cells of the epithelium that line the cup become ameloblasts and produce the enamel. The mesenchymal cells in the bowl of the cup that are adjacent to the developing ameloblasts differentiate into odontoblasts and form successive layers of dentin to support the enamel that covers them. Thus the crown of a tooth develops from 2 different germ layers. We shall now consider development in more detail.

The following description will be limited to the development of the lower primary incisor. Other teeth develop in a similar manner in a regular chronologic sequence.

Early Development

During prenatal life, when an embryo is about 6½ weeks old, a section through the developing jaw cuts across a line of thickening of the oral ectoderm. Teeth will develop along and beneath this line. From this line of thickening an epithelial shelf called a dental lamina (Fig. 21-5, A) grows into the mesenchyme; and from the lamina little epithelial buds, called tooth buds, develop, and from each one a deciduous tooth will form (Fig. 21-5, A). Later, the dental lamina will give off similar epithelial buds which will give rise to the permanent tooth.

The dental lamina grows, and the tooth bud which is going to produce the deciduous tooth increases in size and penetrates deeper into mesenchyme, where it begins to assume the form of an inverted bowl (Fig. 21-5, B). It takes about 2 weeks for this structure to form, and it is then called the enamel organ, while beneath it the mesenchyme, which fills the bowl, is called dental papilla (Fig. 21-5, B).

During the next several weeks the enamel organ increases in size, and its shape changes somewhat. Meanwhile the bone of the jaw grows up to enclose it partly (Fig. 21-5, C). At this stage the line of contact between the enamel organ and the papilla assumes the shape and the size of the future line of contact between the enamel and the dentin of the adult tooth. By the 5th month of development (Fig. 21-5, D), the enamel organ loses any direct connection with the oral epithelium although remnants of the dental lamina may persist (sometimes giving rise to cysts in later life).

Just before this time, the cells of the dental lamina had also produced a second bud of epithelial cells on the lingual surface. This is the bud from which the permanent tooth will eventually develop (Fig. 21-5, C, D).

The dental papilla which will later become the pulp consists of a network of mesenchymal cells connected to one another by thin protoplasmic strands and separated from one another by an amorphous intercellular substance. This tissue becomes increasingly vascular as development proceeds.

Cellular Differentiation Within the Enamel Organ and the Beginning of the Hard Tissue Formation

At the end of the stage depicted in Figure 21-5, C, the cells of the enamel organ adjacent to the tip of the dental papilla become tall and columnar. These cells are called *ameloblasts* (*amel*, enamel, *blastos*, germ) (Fig. 21-6), and they become responsible for the production of tooth enamel. Next to these cells, a layer, 1 to 3 cells thick, is called the *stratum intermedium*. Next, the bulk of the dental cap is called the *stellate reticulum*, in which the cells assume a star shape and are connected to one another by long protoplasmic extensions (Fig. 21-6). The cells of the stratum intermedium are connected to ameloblasts and to each other by desmosomes. The cells of the stellate reticulum contain filaments similar to those making up tonofibrils. Finally, the outer edge of the dental cap is formed of a single layer of cells known as the *outer enamel epithelium*.

The ameloblasts first to appear are found next to the tip of the dental papilla. Further differentiation of ameloblasts proceeds down the sides toward the base of the crown. As this occurs, the mesenchyme cells of the dental papilla immediately adjacent to the ameloblasts also become tall columnar cells, which are known as odontoblasts (Fig. 21-6 and 21-8), for they will form dentin. Indeed, they start forming dentin before the ameloblasts form enamel. Dentin is first produced by odontoblasts at the tip of the papilla, as shown in white in Figure 21-5, C. After a thin layer of dentin is deposited, the ameloblasts start producing enamel matrix, shown in black in Figure 21-5, C. It should be pointed out here that the formation of dentin and enamel differs from bone formation in that no formative cells are trapped within the matrix that they produce. Instead, the cells, as they produce the hard tissue matrix, retreat away from it, the ameloblasts outward and the odontoblasts inward.

Formation of the Root and Its Role in Eruption

As dentin and enamel are deposited, the shape of the future crown appears (Fig. 21-5, D). New ameloblasts differentiate so that enamel begins to form all the way down to what will be the future line of junction of the anatomical crown and the root (Fig. 21-5, D), meanwhile inducing the cells of the dental papilla to differentiate into odontoblasts. It should be realized that the cells of the enamel organ that become ameloblasts and make up its inner layer are continuous at the site of junction between crown and root with those forming its outer layer (Fig. 21-5, D); that is, the

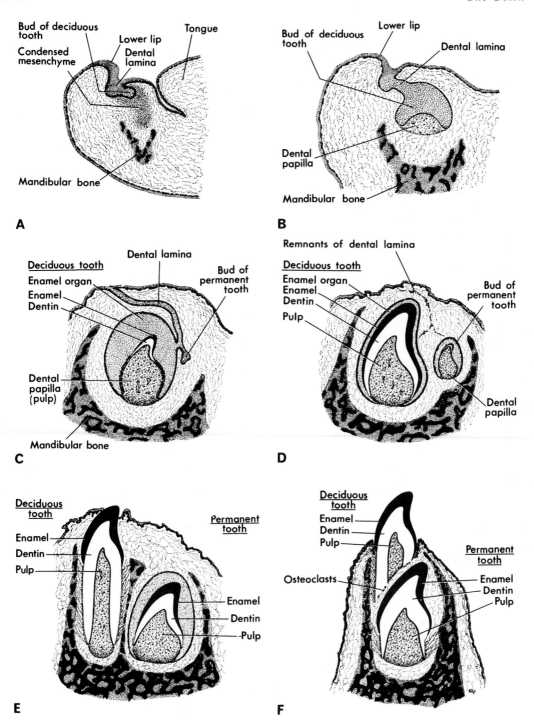

Fig. 21-5. Diagrammatic drawings illustrating the development and eruption of a lower incisor tooth of the deciduous dentition and also how a tooth of the permanent dentition develops and erupts to replace the deciduous tooth.

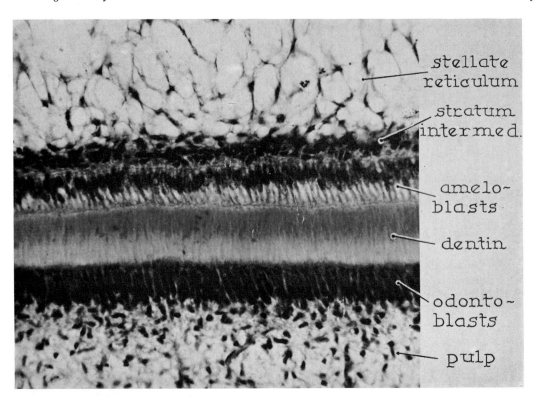

Fɪɢ. 21-6. High-power photomicrograph of a section cut through the dentino-enamel junction of a developing tooth shortly after dentin formation has begun. The light region between the odonto-blasts and the dentin is the predentin.

ameloblast layer is continuous with the outer enamel epithelium. The cells at the line of junction—that is, around the rim of the enamel organ—begin to proliferate and migrate down into the underlying mesenchyme. Since the rim of the enamel organ is ring-shaped (as seen from below), the proliferating cells arising from it form a tube that pushes down into the mesenchyme as it elongates. This tube is known as Hertwig's epithelial root sheath. As this sheath grows down, it sets the pattern outlining the shape of the root, and it organizes the nearest cells of the mesenchyme that it surrounds to differentiate into odontoblasts. However, there is little space here for the root to develop; hence, space is to be created by the crown being pushed out through the oral mucous membrane (Fig. 21-5, E). The formation of the root, therefore, is an important factor in causing the tooth to erupt. (Most permanent teeth have erupted and have been in function for about 2 years before the end of the root is completely formed.)

The root sheath grows downward by continuous proliferation of the cells at its leading ring-shaped edge. The older part of it, toward the crown, having served its purpose, becomes detached from the root of the tooth, and the epithelial cells of it remain within the confines of the periodontal ligament surrounding the tooth. They may be observed histologically within the ligament at any age after the roots have formed. They are called the *epithelial rests of Malassez,* and under proper stimulus they may give rise to dental cysts at any time in life.

The root sheath separates from the formed root of dentin; this allows cells from the mesenchymal connective tissues of the dental sac to deposit cementum on the outer surface of the dentin. As cementum is laid down, it traps the collagenic fibers of the periodontal ligament that the cells in this area are also forming. Thus the fibers of the periodontal ligament are firmly anchored in calcified cementum, which itself is firmly cemented to the dentin of the root.

The Permanent Tooth

By the time the deciduous tooth erupts into the dental arch, the tooth bud for the corresponding permanent tooth has been building up enamel and dentin in exactly the same manner as the deciduous tooth.

When the crown is complete and the root partly formed, the permanent tooth prepares to erupt. However, since one of Wolff's laws states that pressure causes the resorption of hard tissues, the growth of the permanent tooth and the pressure of its enamel against the root of the deciduous tooth causes the softer of the two tissues in contact—that is, the dentin of the deciduous tooth—to be resorbed by osteoclasts (Fig. 21-5, F). By the time the permanent tooth is ready to erupt into the dental arch, the root of the deciduous tooth above has been completely resorbed. The shed deciduous tooth is thus replaced by its permanent successor.

The Microscopic Structure and Functions of the Important Parts of the Tooth

(1) DENTIN

Odontoblasts begin to form dentin matrix (intercellular substance) very soon after they assume their typical form. Initially they are separated from the ameloblasts by only a basement membrane; but a layer of material rich in collagen is soon deposited by the odontoblasts next to the basement membrane, thereby removing these cells farther from the ameloblasts. This material comprises collagen fibrils, known as Korff's fibers, which are very long and thick and are seen between the odontoblasts. They are oriented perpendicularly to the basement membrane, but fan out before they reach it. Other collagen fibrils, which constitute the bulk of the fibrils of dentin, have a smaller diameter and arise from the apical end of the odontoblasts.

It will be recalled that a piece of bone becomes larger by the successive addition of new layers of bone tissue to one or more of its surfaces (Fig. 15-3). This

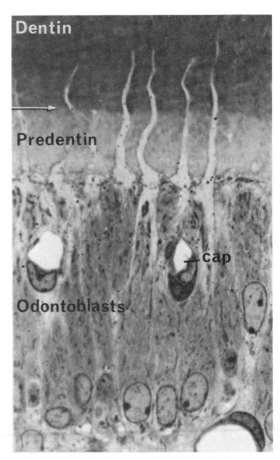

Fig. 21-8. Photomicrograph ($\times$ 1,000) showing odontoblasts, predentin and dentin from the growing end of the rat incisor. The cells are tall and well polarized and are arranged parallel to one another, each with a basally located nucleus. Extending into the predentin from the apical pole of each cell is a light-staining odontoblast process. Predentin extends from between the bases of the processes to a sharply defined predentin-dentin junction (arrow). The dentin is located beyond and stains darker than predentin. (Figure courtesy of M. Weinstock)

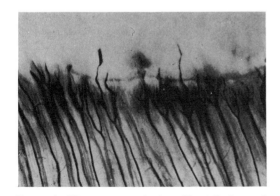

Fig. 21-7. The processes of odontoblasts lie in canals in the dentin. (Churchill, H. R.: Meyer's Histology and Histogenesis of the Human Teeth. Philadelphia, Lippincott)

is also true of dentin, except that growth is more limited because odontoblasts are present only along the inner (pulpal) side of dentin. Hence, any new layers of dentin that are formed can be added only on its pulpal surface. Therefore, the addition of new layers of dentin must encroach on the pulp.

It will be recalled also that osteoblasts possess cytoplasmic processes around which the organic intercellular substance is laid down. These are responsible for the canaliculi (Fig. 15-3). Each odontoblast is also provided with a cytoplasmic process (Figs. 21-7 and 21-8), which extends outward from the apex of the cell to the basement membrane that lines the concavity of the enamel organ. Thus, when material is deposited, these cytoplasmic processes are trapped in dentin and become enclosed in tiny canals called *dentinal tubules*. The processes are called *odontoblastic processes* (Fig. 21-7). With the addition of more and more dentin, the odontoblasts are displaced farther and farther away from the basement membrane that outlines the dentino-enamel junction. Concomitantly, the odontoblast processes maintain their connection with the basement membrane and, therefore, become increasingly elongated, as do the dentinal tubules containing them.

It has been pointed out above in this text that two steps occur as bone tissue is developing: the first is the manufacture of the organic substrate (bone matrix) and the second is its calcification. Similarly dentin matrix is formed first and calcifies somewhat later, usually about one day after it appears. The uncalcified layer of dentin matrix is called predentin and is located between the apex of the odontoblasts and the recently calcified dentin (Fig. 21-8). The oldest dentin is that in contact with the basement membrane which, at least in early stages, is recognizable at the dentino-enamel junction.

As most of us are well aware, teeth may be extremely sensitive to stimuli arising on a dentin surface. The ability of dentin to feel stimuli is attributed to the cytoplasmic processes of odontoblasts in the dentin, because nerve fibers have not been demonstrated in dentin except very close to the pulpal border. This sensitivity of dentin generally decreases with age, as a result of calcification within dentinal tubules.

Fine Structure of Odontoblasts

In contradistinction to the ameloblasts which are tightly apposed to one another, odontoblasts may be separated from each other by intercellular clefts which may contain Korff's collagenic fibers or even capillaries (Fig. 21-8). They are, however, held together by junctional complexes, visible in Figure 21-9 at each end of the terminal web. When viewed in the electron microscope (Fig. 21-9), odontoblasts consist of a long cell body (at the periphery of the pulp) and a longer odontoblastic process located within dentin. The cell body contains abundant profiles of rough endoplasmic reticulum which occupy most of the cytoplasm, except for a large Golgi region located toward the center of the cell. The odontoblastic process lies beyond the terminal web layer and contains no rough endoplasmic reticulum but mainly secretory granules, a few vesicles, microtubules and fine filaments.

The extracellular space above the apical junctions

and surrounding the base of the odontoblastic processes is occupied by predentin matrix. This at first consists of loosely arranged collagenic fibrils in an amorphous ground substance. Above and adjacent to this, the matrix is occupied by progressively denser arrangements of collagen. As stated above, the predentin matrix is not calcified, but the dentin matrix is, and the demarcation line between the two represents the calcification front. In the EM the predentin matrix shows a gradual increase in the concentration and size of collagenic fibrils, which are well packed at the predentin-dentin junction. When calcified, the crystals of apatite hide the underlying structures. After decalcification an accumulation of dense granular material appears on the surface of collagenic fibrils in dentin but not of those in predentin (Warshawsky).

After injection of tritium-labeled glycine or proline, a radioautographic reaction is seen within minutes over the cytoplasm of odontoblasts; a day later, the reaction is over predentin and later still over dentin (Carneiro and Leblond). Since both amino acids are far more abundant in collagen than in other proteins, the results indicate formation of collagenic fibrils. It is concluded that collagen precursor molecules are synthesized in the cytoplasm of odontoblasts and released to form the collagenic fibrils in predentin matrix, and that they are retained when the latter transforms into dentin matrix. Radioautography at the EM level revealed that a collagen precursor, that is, polypeptide chains known as pro-alpha chains, is synthesized in the rough endoplasmic reticulum. The pro-alpha chains differ from the alpha chains of extracellular collagen by the presence of a short tail piece containing —SH groups. Later, these pro-alpha chains join into a triple helix (starting with the —SH's of the three tail pieces forming —S—S— bridges), to make up a molecule known as procollagen. Although the exact place at which the coiling takes place is not known, the label has been seen to migrate from the rough endoplasmic reticulum to the spherical distentions of Golgi saccules, which later transform into cylindrical portions packed with parallel threads (Fig. 21-10). These threads are believed to consist of procollagen molecules. Later the cylindrical portions condense into secretory granules (Fig. 21-10) which pass into the odontoblast process. There they release their content into predentin by a process of exocytosis (M. Weinstock and Leblond).

After procollagen molecules are released to predentin, their tail piece is removed by an enzyme called "procollagen peptidase," thus giving rise to tropocollagen. The tropocollagen molecules polymerize into collagen fibrils.

Besides collagen, which makes up nearly 90 percent of the dentin matrix, about 10 percent is composed of phosphoprotein, with small amounts (probably less than 1 percent) of glycoprotein and mucopolysaccharide. The phosphoprotein is also synthesized by the cell and released to predentin but, unlike collagen, it does not stay there and diffuses to the dentin side of the predentin junction. Evidence was provided by M. Weinstock and Leblond that the phosphoprotein constitutes the granular material present at the surface of the collagenic fibrils on the dentin side of the predentin-dentin junction.

This is the site of mineralization of dentin. Immediately after injection of either ^{32}P-phosphate or ^{45}Ca salts, the radioautographic reaction is intense in this region, with no reaction on the predentin side of the junction and a weak one on the dentin side. It is, therefore, believed that the precipitation of the calcium phosphate of dentin does not occur within cells, but just beyond the predentin-dentin junction (Munhoz and Leblond).

(2) Enamel

After the odontoblasts have produced the first thin layer of dentin, the ameloblasts (Fig. 21-6) in turn begin to make enamel. Enamel then forms and covers the dentin over the anatomic crown of the tooth (Fig. 21-5, C). It forms first as a poorly calcified matrix, which later calcifies almost completely. The material of the mineralized matrix is in the form of rods. The enamel rods retain the shape of the cell; both are prismatic (Fig. 21-11). The elongated ends of the ameloblasts have been termed *Tomes' processes.*

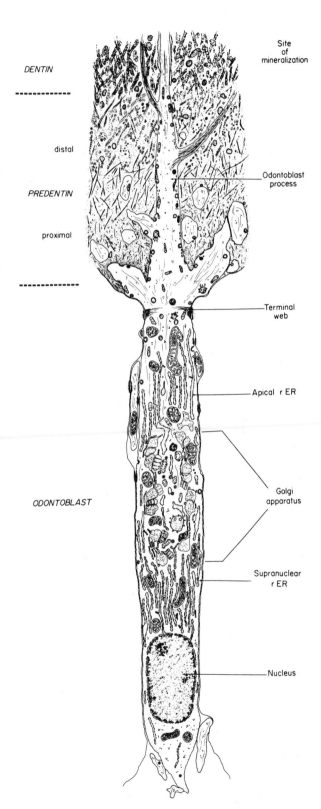

Fig. 21-9. Schematic drawing of an odontoblast, showing the usual arrangement of the organelles as well as the adjacent predentin and dentin matrix. The nucleus is basally located. An elaborate Golgi apparatus separates the supranuclear and the apical rER-rich regions. Both rER cisternae and Golgi saccules are absent from the odontoblast process which extends from the apical pole of the cell into the collagen-rich predentin and dentin. Peripheral branches of the process also project into the matrix. The small elongated profiles within the process and its branches are secretory granules originating in the Golgi apparatus. The secretory product is released from the granules into predentin by exocytosis.

Unlike the collagen fibrils of predentin, those of dentin possess a finely granular material on their surface. Dentin matrix also contains the calcium phosphate crystals of apatite. (Weinstock, M., and Leblond, C. P.: J. Cell Biol., *60*:92, 1974)

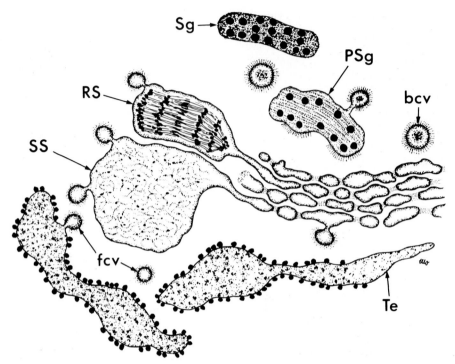

Fɪɢ. 21-10. Schematic drawing of a portion of the Golgi apparatus of an odontoblast showing the presumed sequence of events in the packaging of procollagen into secretory granules. Precursors of collagen are transported from the rER to the Golgi by way of transitional elements (Te) or fuzz-coated vesicles (fcv). They are sequestered into spherical portions of Golgi saccules (SS) where they appear as entangled threads, and then become organized into parallel threads, believed to be composed of procollagen molecules (RS). Cylindrical portions (RS) bud off from flattened saccules and form prosecretory granules (PSg). This formation includes condensation of the parallel threads with the release of bristle-coated vesicles (bcv). The secretory granules (Sg) formed carry the condensed parallel aggregates of procollagen to their site of secretion in the odontoblast process. (M. Weinstock and C. P. Leblond)

Individual ameloblasts are tall, columnar cells (Fig. 21-12). The mitochondria are close to the base of the cell (in some species mitochondria are found almost exclusively in this region). Above is an elongated nucleus associated with a few longitudinally oriented, narrow cisternae of rough endoplasmic reticulum (Figs. 21-12 and 21-13). The endoplasmic reticulum extends into the supranuclear region, where it follows the cell membrane, and terminates abruptly just below the apical web (Fig. 21-12).

An elongated Golgi apparatus is situated along the central axis of the cell in the supranuclear region (Fig. 21-12). When seen in cross section (Fig. 21-13, *top*), it appears roughly tubular in shape, and is surrounded by the peripheral network of rough endoplasmic reticulum. Membrane-bound granules originate within Golgi saccules (Fig. 21-14). These granules are seen scattered throughout the supranuclear region

of the cell and are clustered in the Tomes' process, soon to be described. Running through the middle of the Golgi and parallel to its long axis is a thick "axial fibril" composed of densely packed filaments. This fibril (Fig. 21-13, *top,* F) extends from the apical web region down to the nucleus, and then divides into several branches which continue downward along the sides of the nucleus (Fig. 21-14, *lower part*) to join the basal cell web (Kallenbach *et al.*).

Extending upward from the cell apex at the apical web is the cytoplasmic extension called Tomes' process (Fig. 21-12). This cell process is usually seen embedded in newly formed enamel during the stage of enamel matrix secretion. Numerous membrane-bound, dense granules similar to those seen in the Golgi region can be seen within Tomes' processes, and they are generally associated with elements of smooth endoplasmic reticulum, coated vesicles and microtubules.

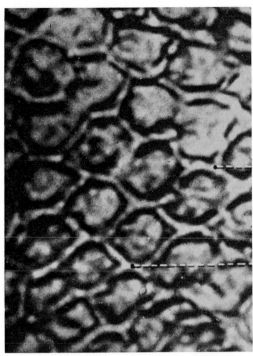

FIG. 21-11. This photomicrograph is from a cross section of formed enamel, showing the prismatic enamel rods and the interprismatic substance (indicated by a leader). Churchill, H. R.: Meyer's Histology and Histogenesis of the Human Teeth. Philadelphia, Lippincott)

The microtubules are long, and sometimes can be traced back almost the entire length of the cell.

Enamel is elaborated by the ameloblasts. It consists of an organic matrix composed of protein and carbohydrate, with calcium phosphate in the form of apatite: $Ca_{10}(PO_4)_6(OH)_2$. Each cell produces one enamel rod, the structural unit of enamel. In decalcified sec-

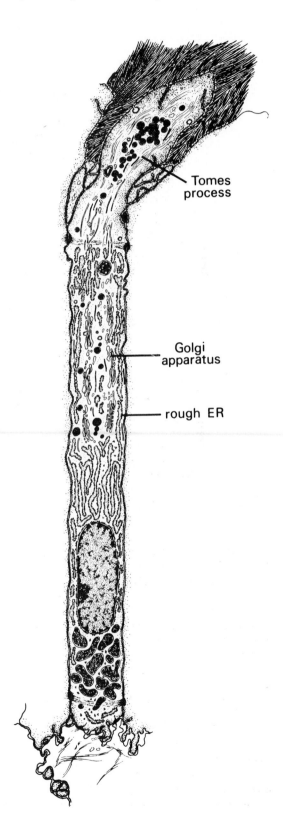

FIG. 21-12. Diagrammatic representation of the electron microscopic structure of a secretory ameloblast. The tall columnar ameloblast contains an oval nucleus situated close to the base of the cell. The mitochondria are located beneath the nucleus (infranuclear) whereas the bulk of rough ER is located above the nucleus (supranuclear). The supranuclear region also contains the Golgi apparatus which is made up of a series of flattened saccules arranged to form the peripheral walls of a tubule. Small numbers of membrane-bound secretory granules are located inside the tubular Golgi region. The apical projection of the ameloblast is called Tomes' process. It extends into the newly formed enamel matrix and contains large numbers of secretory granules in its core. The cell contains a basal web beneath the mitochondria as well as an apical terminal web beneath Tomes' process. (Illustration courtesy of H. Warshawsky)

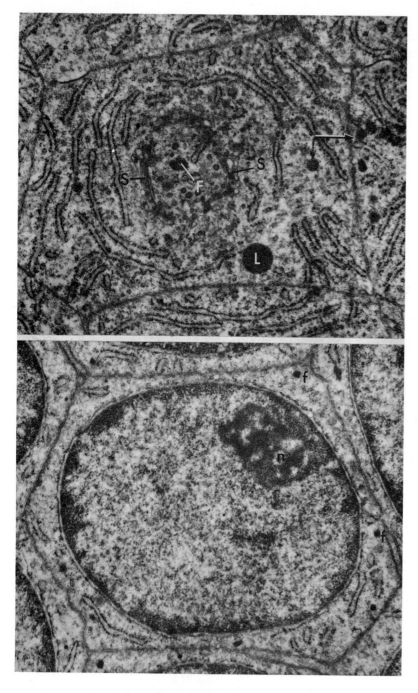

FIG. 21-13. The top electron micrograph represents a cross section of ameloblasts at the level of the Golgi region. The cell walls are distinct. Within the cell the rough endoplasmic reticulum is visible. The Golgi appears nearly circular because it is the cross section of a tubular arrangement of saccules (S). The cross section of an axial fiber is in the middle of the Golgi region (F). L is a dense body presumed to be a lysosome. Beyond the tips of the arrows secretory granules may be seen.

The lower electron micrograph represents a cross section of ameloblasts at the level of the nucleus showing the nucleolus with fibrillar and granular regions. Little may be seen in the cytoplasm except for a few cisternae of rough endoplasmic reticulum and longitudinal fibrils (f). (Illustration courtesy of H. Warshawsky)

tions examined in the EM, the matrix of the rod is seen to be composed of tiny tubular subunits with an oval diameter of about 250 Å. These are closely packed and run parallel to the axis of the rods. It is presumed that these tubules have a glycoprotein component. Warshawsky, after injecting rats with labeled amino acids, observed in radioautographs that a labeled protein arose in relation to ribosomes, which here as elsewhere are the site of protein synthesis. Within less than 5 minutes the radioactive protein appeared in the Golgi apparatus. There, radioautography showed that galactose and fucose are added to make the protein into a glycoprotein (A. Weinstock and C. P. Leblond), which is later packed into prosecretory granules at the mature face of Golgi stacks (Fig. 21-14). As mentioned above, these migrate rapidly while becoming mature secretory granules (G) and reach the Tomes' process (Fig. 21-12), where their content is released to the extracellular space to become the enamel matrix.

Calcification begins in relation to the tubules of the enamel matrix. It is discrete at first. As the rods lengthen and the whole layer of matrix thickens, calcification continues. As a result, the farther from Tomes' process the matrix is, the more intensely calcified it becomes. Hence, the mineral content increases as the dentino-enamel junction is approached. Along with the increase in mineral content, it is believed that there is a loss of water and a decrease in the organic portion. When the mineral content reaches about 95 percent of the total mass of enamel, no further calcification takes place; the enamel is said to be mature.

Besides secreting an enamel rod, each ameloblast provides enough material to build inter-rod substance, which also becomes calcified. The inter-rod substance appears to be identical to the material of the rods, but the tubular subunits run in different directions from the rods.

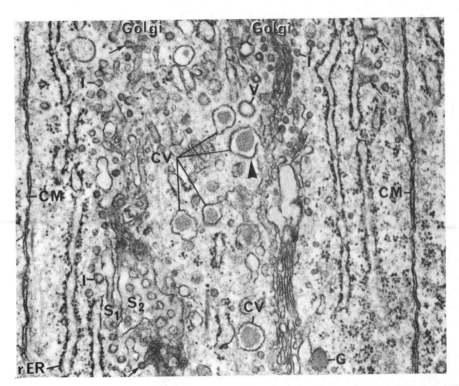

Fig. 21-14. Golgi region of an ameloblast cut along its length. The membranes of the cell (CM) may be seen along the left and right sides of the figure. Next and parallel to them run one or two rows of rER cisternae studded with ribosomes. At upper right, the cisternae show fuzz-coated buds (oblique arrows). The small, fuzz-coated circular profiles nearby are the vesicles known as transitional or intermediate vesicles (I).

More centrally, two incomplete rows of Golgi stacks run parallel to the cell membranes. They are longitudinal sections of the walls of the roughly tubular Golgi apparatus. The row at right is composed of longitudinal sections of saccules; at left, saccules may be cut longitudinally (S_1) or tangentially (S_2). The peripheral saccules, that is, those making up the forming face, often show fuzz-coated buds (ascending arrows, upper left and lower left). These are believed to represent fusion of intermediate vesicles with Golgi saccules.

In the center, a few prosecretory granules (also called condensing vacuoles) may be seen (CV); they arise from saccules at the mature face of Golgi stacks. Bristle-coated patches (arrowhead) give rise to bristle-coated vesicles (V); as a result the content of prosecretory granules condenses; they become secretory granules which migrate in the direction of the Tomes' process. One of these granules may be seen at lower right (G). (Illustration courtesy A. Weinstock and C. P. Leblond)

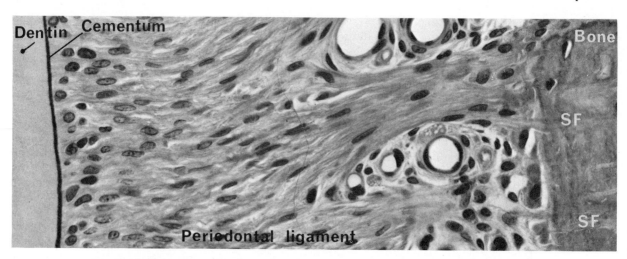

Fig. 21-15. High-power microphotographic montage of a portion of a decalcified tooth and associated alveolar bone from the rat, showing the collagenic fibers of the periodontal ligament. From left to right, it is possible to see the periphery of dentin, the cementum in the noncellular region, the periodontal ligament, and the edge of the alveolar bone. The fibers of the ligament abut on the cementum at left and extend between the blood vessels to reach the alveolar bone into which they are inserted (SF at *right center*). The fibers seen within bone (SF at *lower right*) are known as Sharpey's fibers. (Courtesy of H. Warshawsky)

The fully formed enamel is relatively inert; no cells are associated with it because the ameloblasts degenerate after they have formed all the enamel and the tooth erupts. Thus enamel is completely incapable of repair if it is injured by decay, fracture or other means. However, there is some exchange of mineral ions between enamel and saliva, and minute areas of recalcification can occur. This exchange predominates at the surface, but is negligible in the depth of the enamel.

(3) Cementum

Some cells of the mesenchyme of the dental sac along the side of the developing root differentiate to become cementoblasts. These are similar to osteoblasts, but are associated with the laying down of another special nonvascular calcified connective tissue called *cementum*. The role of cementum is to bury in its substance the ends of the fibers of the periodontal ligament and so attach them to the tooth (Fig. 21-15, *left*).

Cementum in the upper one third to one half the length of the root is noncellular (Figs. 21-15 and 21-4); the remainder has cells within its matrix. The latter are called *cementocytes*, and they, like osteocytes, reside in small spaces, called *lacunae*, within the calcified matrix and communicate with their source of nutrition through canaliculi.

Cementum, like bone, can increase in amount only by addition to its surface. The formation of cementum is required if the collagenic fibers of the periodontal ligament are to be attached to the root.

(4) Periodontal Ligament

As the root of the tooth forms and cementum is deposited on its surface, the periodontal ligament arises from the mesenchyme of the dental sac that surrounds the tooth during development and fills the space between it and the bone of the alveolar process. This tissue comes to consist of heavy bundles of collagenic fibers arranged in the form of a suspensory ligament between the root of the tooth and the bony wall of its socket (Fig. 21-4). The fiber bundles are embedded at one of their ends in the bone of the wall of the alveolus (Fig. 21-15, *right*) and at their other end in the cementum covering the root (Fig. 21-15, *left*). At both ends the parts of the fibers that actually are embedded in hard tissue are called *Sharpey's fibers* (Fig. 21-15).

There is a paradox in the fact that the collagen of the periodontal ligament seems to be the only one in the body that turns over rapidly, as shown by Carneiro. And yet the embedment of Sharpey's fibers suggests that both alveolar bone and cementum are laid down around pre-existing collagenic fibers, so that at least the embedded portions are unlikely to turn over.

Since the fibers are made up of polymerized tropocollagen molecules, it is possible that only a fraction of these molecules is subject to turnover.

The fibers of the periodontal ligament are generally a little longer than the shortest distance between the side of the tooth and the wall of the socket (Fig. 21-4). This arrangement allows for a certain limited movement of a tooth within its alveolus. The blood capillaries within the periodontal ligament form the only source of nutritive supply to cementocytes. The nerves of the ligament supply the teeth with their very important and remarkably sensitive tactile sense.

(5) The Epithelial Attachment and Periodontal Disease

The gingiva surrounds each tooth like a collar, and under normal conditions the inner surface of the collar is attached tightly to the tooth. If the tooth and its surrounding gingiva are sectioned longitudinally, the gingiva appears to extend up each side of the tooth as a narrow triangle, the apex of which is termed the *gingival crest* (Fig. 21-4). The side of the gingival triangle next to the tooth is covered with epithelium. This epithelium, as it extends down from the crest, is at first not adherent to the tooth; hence there is a crevice between it and the tooth surface. This is called the *gingival crevice* or *sulcus* (this rings the tooth) (Fig. 21-4). At the bottom of the sulcus the epithelium of the gingiva becomes adherent to the tooth. In erupting teeth, the epithelium, from here to the bottom of the anatomic crown, is attached to enamel. However, the epithelium extends a little below the enamel and is attached to the cementum of the root (Fig. 21-4). The attachment of the epithelium to the enamel is not nearly as strong as its attachment to the cementum because there is nothing on the surface of the enamel (except a little cuticle that is left over from the enamel organ) to which the epithelium can become firmly attached. However, the cementum in this region has been shown by Paynter to have some of the attributes of a basement membrane (it is PA-Schiff-positive), so it provides the same means for a firm attachment of epithelium as does the material of basement membranes elsewhere.

It is obvious that the gingival sulcus provides a site where debris might accumulate. Since there is calcium in saliva, it is not surprising that calcified material, called *tartar* or *calculus,* accumulates in the gingival sulcus, and expanding accumulations of this tend to separate the epithelial attachment from the tooth. Obviously, once the epithelial seal around the tooth is broken, bacteria could gain entrance to the connective tissue of the gingivae. Therefore the gingival crevice is a danger zone.

For the reasons given above, or for other reasons (perhaps systemic factors) which are not yet understood, the epithelium of the gingivae may become separated from the cementum, and what are called *pockets* may develop down the sides of a tooth. Pockets commonly separate the cementum-covered root from the fibers of the periodontal ligament, and this, of course, loosens the tooth. The gingival epithelium generally grows down the outer side of pockets, so that the pockets are bordered on their outer aspects by epithelium and on their inner aspects by cementum-covered dentin. The pockets become infected. Unfortunately, the type of periodontal disease produced by the above means is common in individuals in the middle and the older age groups; indeed, its prevalence in this age group is responsible for the loss of more teeth than any other condition. Another factor that has been considered as disposing to periodontal disease is malocclusion. Periodontal disease is commonly associated with a loss of alveolar bone. One factor in causing a loss of bone could be that the force of biting is not transmitted in such a way as to push the root squarely into its socket. In malocclusion the force of the bite may act to tip a tooth so that its crown is pressed toward one side and, because of a fulcrum effect, the deeper part of its root to the other. Force applied this way could cause resorption of alveolar bone at some sites and result in a poor attachment.

Nutritional factors—for example, a vitamin C deficiency—and metabolic factors can also be involved in causing periodontal disease.

(6) The Dental Pulp and Dental Caries

The life of the tooth depends on the health of the dental pulp. The health of the dental pulp is threatened all too commonly by the development of dental caries, so before discussing the pulp in detail, a few remarks will be made about this condition, which is probably the most common of all diseases.

Dental caries causes cavities to develop on exposed tooth surfaces. The disease begins on the outer surface of the enamel, commonly, in tiny pits or crevices, or between adjacent teeth, areas where food debris is not readily washed away by saliva or the toothbrush. The food in these tiny areas acts as a substrate for the metabolism of bacteria, which are abundant in the mouth. It is generally believed that the bacterial action leads to the formation of acid products that locally decalcify and destroy enamel. Cavities that thus develop tend to be progressive, for they retain food

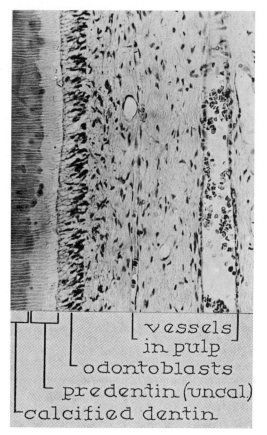

vessels
in pulp
odontoblasts
predentin (uncal)
calcified dentin

Fig. 21-16. High-power photomicrograph of a section of a child's tooth showing histology of pulp. Dentin is still forming. (Preparation by K. J. Paynter)

debris, which continues to be acted on by bacteria. Unless such cavities are treated, sooner or later they will reach the dentin and continue to extend through it to reach the pulp of the tooth. When they near the pulp, they are prone to cause inflammation of the pulp, and, as will be explained below, this can cause its death.

A developing cavity causes no pain when it is confined to the enamel. When it reaches the dentin, it may or may not give rise to increased sensitivity of the tooth; the increased sensitivity may be related to certain foods, for example, sweet materials. The presence of cavities is best determined by regular dental inspections. To treat them, all the surrounding enamel and dentin must be drilled away or otherwise removed. Then the cavity is shaped so that it will retain a filling. Fillings must be used because there are no cells on the outer aspects of the tooth to make new enamel and dentin.

Dental pulp is a connective tissue derived from the mesenchyme of the dental papilla (Fig. 21-5), and it occupies the pulp chambers and the root canals of teeth (Fig. 21-4). It is a soft tissue that retains its mesenchymal appearance throughout life (Fig. 21-16). The bulk of its cells appear stellate in sections, being connected to one another by long cytoplasmic processes. Pulp is very vascular; the main vessels enter and leave it through the apical foramina. However, the pulpal vessels, even the large ones, have very thin walls (Fig. 21-16). This, of course, renders this tissue very susceptible to changes in pressure because the walls of the pulp chamber cannot expand. A fairly mild inflammatory edema often can lead to compression of the blood vessels and hence to the necrosis and death of the pulp. Following pulp death, sometimes the pulp can be removed surgically and the space it occupied filled with an inert sealing material. Such a tooth constitutes what is commonly called a "dead" tooth.

The pulp is richly supplied with nerves, and nerve endings have been observed in close association with the odontoblast layer between the pulp and the dentin. Some authors have reported finding nerves actually entering the dentinal tubules, but, as mentioned above, there is no indication that they proceed more than a very short distance within the tubules.

It was explained before that any new dentin that is added to the walls of the tooth must be deposited on the surface of already existing dentin, and only on the surface abutting on the pulp, because this is the only place where odontoblasts exist. Dentin normally is produced throughout life, and under certain conditions it may form rapidly (for example, under a cavity), but under the latter conditions the dentin is of a more irregular character and is designated as *secondary dentin*. Dentin deposition leads to a gradual reduction in the size of the pulp chamber and the canals throughout life; hence, in older people the pulp is generally much reduced in size. The character of the pulp also changes in that it becomes more fibrous and less cellular.

The Salivary Glands

There are a great many glands that deliver their secretion into the oral cavity, so they are all salivary glands. However, most of these are small, and so the term *salivary glands* is commonly used to indicate the 3 largest: (1) the parotid, (2) the submandibular (also called the submaxillary) and (3) the sublingual.

Saliva and Its Functions. The mixed secretions of

all the salivary glands are called *saliva*. It usually contains some cellular and bacterial debris and leukocytes. In man the volume secreted in 24 hours varies from 1,000 to 1,500 ml. It may be thin and watery or viscous. Its composition varies with the type of stimulus that initiates its secretion. It contains salts, gases and organic material. Two enzymes (*ptyalin* or *salivary amylase,* and *maltase*) and mucus are present in it.

Saliva has several functions: (1) It provides for the lubrication and the moistening of the buccal mucosa and the lips, thus aiding articulation. This function must be carried on continuously because of the evaporation and the swallowing of saliva, and the providing of a more or less steady supply of saliva for this purpose is probably the chief function of the buccal glands. (2) It provides a means whereby the mouth may be washed clear of cellular and food debris which otherwise might provide an excellent culture medium for bacteria. (3) Another very important function of saliva is to moisten food and transform it to a semisolid or liquid mass so that it may be swallowed easily. It may be noted here that animals such as the cow, which live on a fairly dry diet, may secrete up to 60 liters of saliva daily. Moreover, moistening the food allows it to be tasted. Taste buds are stimulated chemically, and substances that stimulate them must be in solution. (4) The role of the salivary enzymes in the digestion of food is questionable. Amylase breaks down starch to maltose in an alkaline or slightly acid medium. The food is retained in the mouth for much too short a time for any significant digestion to occur there, and when food reaches the stomach, the acid reaction therein might be thought to inhibit any further amylase activity. But it has been shown that some of the starches that are consumed near the end of a meal may be broken down to maltose in the stomach because, being in the innermost part of the gastric contents, they are protected for a time from the gastric juice liberated from the stomach lining.

The Parotid Glands. These are the largest of the 3 pairs of salivary glands proper. Each lies packed in the space between the mastoid process and the ramus of the mandible. Each overflows onto the face below the zygomatic arch, and from this process of the gland, its duct (Stensen's), running parallel with and immediately below the arch, plunges through the buccinator muscle to open into the vestibule of the mouth opposite the 2nd upper molar tooth.

The gland is enclosed in a well-defined fibrous connective tissue capsule and is a compound tubulo-alveolar gland of the serous type. The microscopic de-

tails of the secretory units of such glands have been described in Chapter 7 and the mechanism of secretion in individual cells that secrete zymogen granules in Chapter 5. In addition to the usual features to be seen in a gland of this type, it is specially characterized by many and prominent intralobular ducts (Fig. 21-17). Accumulations of fat cells in the connective tissue septa are also characteristic of this gland.

The Submandibular (Submaxillary) Glands. These lie in contact with the inner surface of the body of the mandible, and their main ducts (Wharton's) open onto the floor of the oral cavity beside each other, anterior to the tongue and behind the lower incisor tooth. They are compound alveolar or tubulo-alveolar glands. Although of the mixed type, the majority of their secretory units are of the serous variety. Mucous units are usually capped by serous demilunes (see Chap. 7 for a description and illustrations of mixed glands). Like the parotid glands, the submandibular glands have well-defined capsules and fairly prominent duct systems.

The Sublingual Glands. Unlike the other salivary glands, the sublingual glands are not so definitely encapsulated. They lie well forward, near the midline, below the mucous membrane of the floor of the mouth, and their secretions empty by several ducts (Rivinus) that open along a line behind the openings of Wharton's ducts. They are compound tubulo-alveolar glands of the mixed type, but differ from the submandibular gland in that the majority of their alveoli are of the mucous type. Their microscopic appearance is different in different parts of the gland. In some areas only mucus-secreting units and mucous units with serous demilunes may be found. The connective tissue septa are usually more prominent than they are in the parotid or the submandibular glands.

Nervous Control of Salivary Secretions. Ordinarily, salivary secretion is controlled by nervous reflexes. Briefly, the efferent or secretory fibers to the salivary glands are derived from the cranial outflow of the parasympathetic system and the thoracic outflow of the sympathetic system. There are many afferent pathways that may be concerned in salivary reflexes. The stimulus that evokes secretion reflexly may be mechanical or chemical. For example, the presence of food (or even pebbles or dry powders in the mouth) stimulates the ordinary sensory nerve endings and causes salivary secretion. The taste buds are receptive to chemical stimulation. Stimulation of many sensory nerves other than those of the oral cavity may initiate a salivary reflex, provided that the reflex has been conditioned (Chap. 17). The amount and the

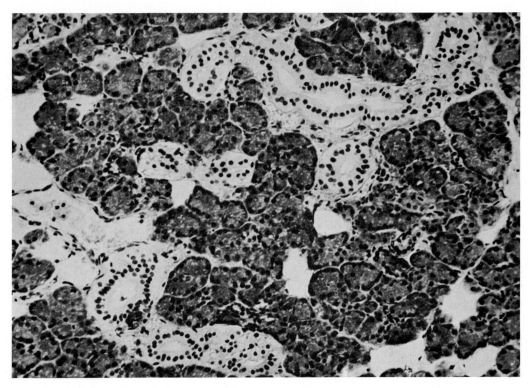

Fig. 21-17. Medium-power photomicrograph of a section of the parotid gland. The cytoplasm of the cells of the many ducts is light, and that of the cells of the secretory units, dark. The empty spaces represent fat, and a vein may be seen at the left.

composition of the saliva depends on the nature of the stimulus that initiates the reflex, and on whether sympathetic or parasympathetic fibers are predominantly involved in the efferent path. Stimulation of the sympathetic fibers is believed to cause vasoconstriction which would diminish the production of saliva. Parasympathetic stimulation gives rise to a copious secretion. The nerve endings which elaborate the chemical mediator in the parotid are shown in Figures 17-53 and 17-54.

It was mentioned in Chapter 7 that the acini of salivary glands include a cell flattened between acinar cells and basement membrane (Fig. 7-15), the cytoplasm of which contains myofibrils; this cell is accordingly called a *myoepithelial cell*. Myoepithelial cells are particularly well developed in serous acini. Both acinar cells and myoepithelial cells are under autonomic control.

RELATION OF SALIVARY GLANDS TO ENDOCRINE GLAND FUNCTIONS

Studies in rodents have shown that the histological structure of salivary glands is affected by sex hor-

mones. Lacassagne in 1940 first observed that certain tubular portions of the secretory units of the submandibular gland of the mouse were much more developed in a pregnant mouse than in a virgin mouse. Chaulin-Servinière in 1942 showed that the cells in these tubules were different in males and females, and that those of the male could be converted to the female type by castration, and that they could again become those of the male type if male sex hormone was administered. Grad and Leblond next showed in 1949 that both thyroid and male hormone were required to act together to restore the male type of tubule in animals from which both the thyroid and testes had been removed. In 1959 Baxter *et al.* showed that the removal of the pituitary gland led to an atrophy of the duct system of the submandibular gland and the loss of secretory granules in the parotid and submandibular glands, and that male sex hormone plus thyroxine would restore the normal picture. Still more recently, Travill in 1966 showed that the tubules of the submandibular glands of pregnant female mice increased in size and their appearance shifted toward the male type, and that by 6 weeks after the termination of pregnancy the glands had reverted to their normal size with the normal histological features of female glands.

The Hard Palate

It is desirable that the mouth (Fig. 21-1) should possess a strong roof so that the anterior part of the tongue, which is the part of the tongue that can move most freely, can bring force to bear against it in the process of mixing and swallowing food. It is also desirable that the mucous membrane lining the roof of the mouth in this site should be firmly fixed to the strong roof so that forceful movements of the tongue do not dislodge it, and that its epithelium should be capable of withstanding wear and tear. These desirable structural characteristics are realized by there being a bony roof over the mouth which is lined on its under-surface by a mucous membrane, the lamina propria of which is continuous with the periosteum of the bone above, and the epithelium of which is of the stratified squamous keratinizing variety.

Laterally, the mucous membrane is not so evenly adherent to the bony roof and is connected to it by strong bundles of connective tissue. Fat cells are disposed between these anteriorly, and glands, posteriorly.

In the median line is a ridge of bone to which the epithelium is attached by a very thin lamina propria. This ridge is called the *raphe*. Rugae with connective tissue cores radiate out from this laterally. They are more prominent in early life than thereafter.

The Soft Palate

The soft palate continues posteriorly from the hard palate (Fig. 21-1). Its functions are different from those of the hard palate. It does not have to bear the thrust of the tongue. It must be movable so that in the act of swallowing it can be drawn upward and thus close off the nasopharynx and so prevent food from being forced up into the nose. This requires that it contain muscle. It must be reasonably strong, and this requires that it contain connective tissue which is disposed in it as an aponeurosis.

The soft palate projects backward into the pharynx from the hard palate (Fig. 21-1). Hence, the mucous membrane on its upper surface forms part of the lining of the nasopharynx, and the mucous membrane on its lower surface forms part of the lining of the oral pharynx. From above downward it exhibits the following layers (Fig. 21-18): (1) stratified squamous or pseudostratified ciliated columnar epithelium; (2) a lamina propria which contains a few glands and, near the hard palate, has the form of a strong aponeurosis;

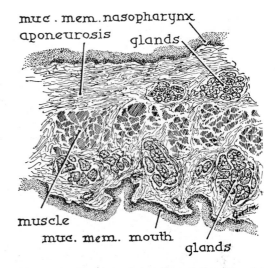

FIG. 21-18. Drawing of a section of the soft palate. (Redrawn and modified from Huber: Piersol's Human Anatomy. ed. 9. Philadelphia, Lippincott)

(3) a muscular layer (posteriorly); (4) a thick lamina propria containing many glands; and (5) stratified squamous nonkeratinizing epithelium.

The Pharynx

The pharynx is a somewhat conically-shaped chamber that serves as a passageway for both the respiratory and the digestive systems. Under conditions of nose breathing it conducts air between the nasal cavities and the larynx and to the eustachian tubes (Fig. 23-1). It also conducts food from the mouth to the esophagus, with which its apex is continuous (Fig. 21-1). But, since it is common to both systems, it permits an individual whose nasal passages are obstructed to breathe through his mouth or, when his mouth is immobilized for surgical reasons, to be fed with a tube through his nose.

The pharynx is divided into 3 parts. The *nasopharynx* lies above the level of the soft palate (Fig. 21-1). The posterior limit of the mouth is indicated by the glossopalatine arches, and the part of the pharynx behind these is the *oral pharynx* (Fig. 21-1). The *laryngeal pharynx* is the part that continues from the oral pharynx, from below the level of the hyoid bone, into the esophagus (Fig. 21-1).

The pharynx is lined with epithelium. This varies in the different parts in accordance with their various functions. Where there is wear and tear, such as that occasioned by food passing over a part or by parts rubbing together, the stratified squamous nonkeratinizing type of epithelium is found. Where the lining

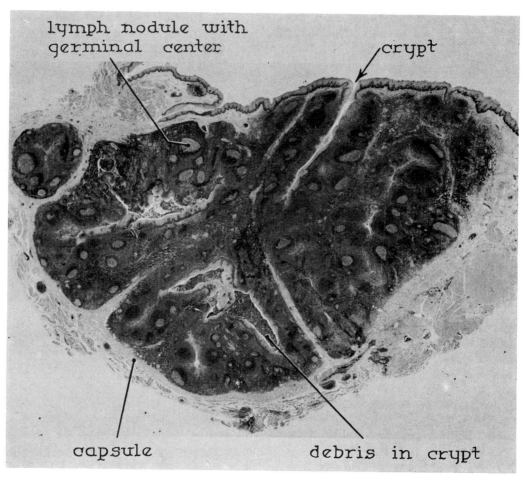

FIG. 21-19. Very low-power photomicrograph of a section of palatine tonsil.

epithelium comes into contact only with air, the pseudostratified columnar ciliated type is present. Stratified columnar epithelium is found in the transition zones between the other 2 types.

The lining of epithelium rests on a fairly dense connective tissue membrane which contains elastic as well as collagenic fibers. At the side of this farthest from the epithelium there is usually a stout layer of elastic fibers. Outside this again is striated muscle—the longitudinal and the constrictor muscles of the pharynx—and outside the muscles there is another fibrous layer that connects the pharynx to adjacent structures.

Glands are present deep to the epithelium of some parts of the pharynx, particularly near the openings of the eustachian tubes. In some instances the glands extend into the muscle coat. A slight rise along the midline of the nasopharynx indicates the location of the single *pharyngeal tonsil* (sometimes called ade-

noid, especially when hypertrophic). This is composed of a group of lymphatic nodules separated by loose lymphatic tissue under the pseudostratified columnar epithelium lining the nasopharynx.

The Palatine Tonsils

Far more prominent are the two palatine tonsils. These ovoid masses of lymphatic tissue are embedded in, and hence thicken, the lamina propria of the mucous membrane that extends between the glossopalatine and the pharyngopalatine arches. The epithelium here is of the stratified squamous nonkeratinizing type and dips into the underlying lymphatic tissue to form 10 to 20 little glandlike pits (*primary crypts*) in each palatine tonsil (Fig. 21-19). The stratified squamous epithelium lining the primary crypts may extend out into the adjacent lymphatic tissue to form secondary crypts. Either primary or secondary crypts may extend deeply enough to reach the outer limits of the tonsil.

The lymphatic tissue in the tonsil mostly lies directly below the epithelium and extends down along the sides of the crypts. It consists of primary nodules, with or without germinal centers, that may be so close together that they melt into one another, or they may be separated by loose lymphatic tissue. In addition to lymphocytes there are generally many plasma cells in this tissue.

The tonsillar tissue disposed near the beginnings of the digestive tube and the respiratory system seems to be designed to function as outpost on the watch for infective agents against which antibodies should be made as soon as possible. However, this is a hazardous occupation, and often the infective agents conquer the outpost and become so well established in the tonsils that the latter must be removed.

Many lymphocytes formed in the tonsil leave it by migrating through the crypt epithelium (Fig. 21-20). Lymphocytes may so infiltrate the epithelium that it becomes very difficult to establish its deep border. The lymphocytes that escape into the pharynx form degenerate bodies found in the saliva and called *salivary corpuscles.*

Glands are associated with the palatine tonsils, but their ducts open beside it and not into its crypts; hence, the crypts are not flushed out as they are in the lingual tonsil, and debris can accumulate in them and dispose them to infection.

General Plan of the Gastrointestinal Tract

The wall of the gastrointestinal tube consists of 4 main layers (see Fig. 21-21, *lower right*): the mucous membrane, the submucosa, the muscularis externa and the serosa. The relation of the structure to the function of these 4 layers will now be described.

Mucous Membrane

This consists of 3 layers: an *epithelial lining,* a supporting *lamina propria* and a thin, usually double, layer of smooth muscle, the *muscularis mucosae* (Fig. 21-21).

Epithelium. The type varies in relation to the function of the part of the tube it lines. In some sites it is primarily protective, in others it is absorptive, and in still others, secretory. In most of the gastrointestinal tract the surface-lining epithelial cells are unable to provide all the secretions that are needed. To supplement the secretions supplied by surface-lining cells, vast numbers of glands are present. The commonest ones are short and extend outward only

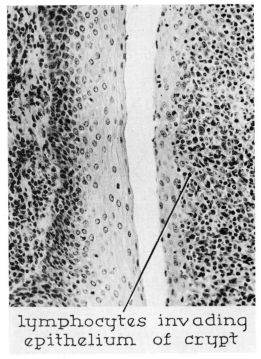

lymphocytes invading epithelium of crypt

Fig. 21-20. High-power photomicrograph of a section of palatine tonsil, showing lymphocytes migrating through the epithelial lining of a crypt.

to the muscularis mucosae; therefore they are wholly contained in the lamina propria of the mucous membrane (Fig. 21-21, labeled "gland in mucous membrane"). *The student, then, must expect to find the lamina propria of the mucous membrane of most parts of the gastrointestinal tract riddled with glands; indeed, in many parts the thin films of lamina propria between glands can scarcely be seen.* The second position occupied by glands that develop from the lining cells, to supplement their secretions, is the submucosa (Fig. 21-21, *middle left*). Glands in this position are found only in the esophagus and the duodenum. The third site occupied by glands that arise from the lining of the gastrointestinal tract is outside the tract altogether. The salivary glands, the liver and the pancreas are of this sort (Fig. 21-21, *upper left*). Since they all arise from the lining of the alimentary tract, they all drain into it by ducts which proclaim the sites of their origins.

Lamina Propria. This layer consists of connective tissue that is difficult to classify. It is what probably is best described as loose ordinary connective tissue with lymphatic tendencies.

The functions of the lamina propria are numerous. In order to support the epithelium and to connect it

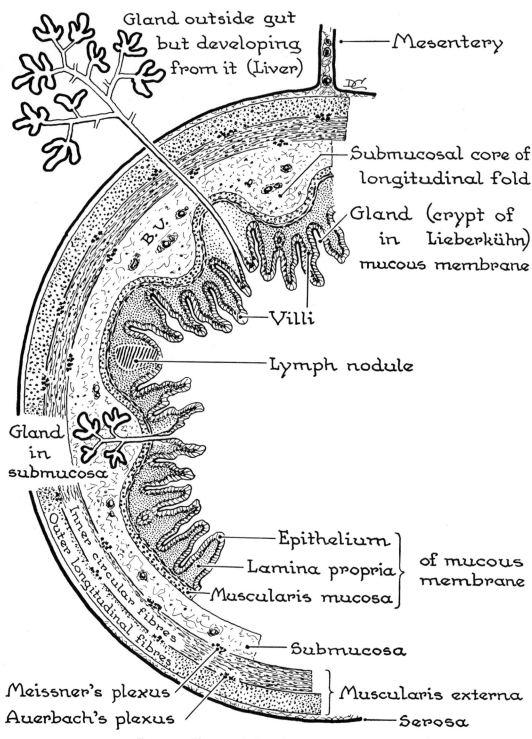

Gland outside gut but developing from it (Liver)

Mesentery

Submucosal core of longitudinal fold

Gland (crypt of in Lieberkühn) mucous membrane

B.V.

Villi

Lymph nodule

Gland in submucosa

Epithelium
Lamina propria
Muscularis mucosa
of mucous membrane

Inner circular fibres
Outer longitudinal fibres

Submucosa

Meissner's plexus
Auerbach's plexus

Muscularis externa
Serosa

FIG. 21-21. The general plan of the gastrointestinal tract.

with the muscularis mucosae, it contains collagenic, reticular and, in some sites, elastic fibers. The frank lymphatic tissue with which it is sprinkled is of the nonencapsulated type and hence typical of lymphatic tissue that is commonly disposed under wet epithelial surfaces and acts as a second line of defense against bacteria or other disease organisms that gain entrance to the tissues by invading the epithelial membrane, which, to be absorptive, must be relatively thin in much of the gastrointestinal tract.

The fact that lymphocytes are produced in numbers in the lamina propria of the digestive tube, and that many make their way through the lining epithelium to enter the lumen has often led to the suggestion that lymphocytes may play some nutritive function (often termed a trophic role) in connection with the maintenance of the lining epithelium.

The lamina propria carries both blood and lymphatic capillaries close to the epithelial surface, particularly in the little fingerlike villi that project into the lumen from the small intestine (Fig. 21-21). Consequently, the products resulting from the digestion of carbohydrates, proteins and fats do not have to diffuse any great distance through the tissue fluid of the lamina propria in order to gain entrance to either type of capillary.

Muscularis Mucosae. This, the third and outermost layer of the mucous membrane, consists generally of 2 thin layers of smooth muscle fibers together with varying amounts of elastic tissue. In the inner layer of muscle the fibers are circularly disposed, and in the outer, longitudinally (Fig. 21-21). The muscularis mucosae probably permits localized movements of the mucous membrane. Increased tonus of the circular fibers would tend to throw the mucous membrane into circular folds. The muscularis mucosae also could be visualized as acting on occasion to relieve the pressure on the veins in the submucosa caused by the tonus of the muscularis externa.

The muscularis mucosae sends off small bundles of smooth muscle fibers in the direction of the epithelium. The end of the fibers abuts on the basement membrane of the epithelium. In the small intestine where the mucosa forms fingerlike processes called villi (Fig. 21-21), one smooth muscle bundle from the muscularis mucosae goes to the tip of each villus where it ends on the basement membrane. These bundles contain the longest smooth muscle cells in the body. In the large intestine where the free surface is rather flat, the bundles end on the basement membrane of the epithelial cells on that surface.

Submucosa. This coat connects the mucous membrane to the muscularis externa. It consists of a loose pliable type of connective tissue. It houses the plexuses of larger blood vessels (Fig. 21-21). The elastic fibers of these impart an elastic quality to the coat as a whole. This is augmented, particularly in the upper part of the gastrointestinal tract, by a considerable number of elastic fibers distributed throughout its substance. The elastic quality of the submucosa permits it to form the cores of such folds of mucous membrane as are present in different parts of the tract (Fig. 21-21, *upper right*).

A plexus of nerve fibers with which some ganglion cells are associated is present in the submucosa. This is called *Meissner's plexus* or the *submucosa plexus* (Fig. 21-21). The fibers in it are mostly nonmyelinated and are derived chiefly from the superior mesenteric plexus (a prevertebral plexus); hence they are postganglionic fibers from the sympathetic division of the autonomic nervous system. The relatively few ganglion cells in the submucous plexus are of the nature of terminal ganglia of the parasympathetic division; the preganglionic fibers that synapse there are derived from the vagus nerve (cranial outflow).

Muscularis Externa. This coat consists characteristically of 2 fairly substantial layers of smooth muscle. The inner layer has circularly disposed fibers and is somewhat thicker than the outer layer, which has longitudinally disposed fibers (Fig. 21-21). However, it is probable that the fibers are not arranged precisely at right angles to, and parallel with, the tract, but that those of both layers tend to pursue a somewhat spiral course. By seeing whether the fibers in the inner and the outer coats are cut in cross or longitudinal section a student can tell whether he is examining a cross or a longitudinal section of any part of the tract (if in any section the fibers of the inner layer are cut in cross section, and the ones in the outer layer in longitudinal section, the section under view is a longitudinal section).

The muscularis externa is the primary instrument for propelling the contents of the tube downward from the pharynx to the anus. The orderly functioning of the muscularis externa is an important requisite for health and happiness. The various kinds of actions it performs and their control are complex, and only elementary comment will be made on them here.

1. The smooth muscle of the muscularis externa constitutes a surrounding sheath for the tract. Smooth muscle, it will be recalled, is adapted to maintaining different states of tonus (sustained contraction). The state of tonus of the muscularis externa is a very important factor in regulating the size of the lumen of the bowel.

2. Smooth muscle has the inherent property of undergoing spontaneous and rhythmic contractions. Moreover, when smooth muscle cells are arranged in laminae, as they are in the muscularis externa, contractions so initiated can spread from one cell to another. Even without the help of nerves, the smooth muscle of the muscularis externa can exhibit rhythmic contractions which spread over short distances. How impulses are conducted between smooth muscle cells was described in Chapter 18.

3. The muscularis externa engages in *peristaltic movements*. These are the primary cause of food being moved along the bowel. They consist of waves of constriction that sweep downward, pushing the contents of the bowel ahead of them. There are two kinds: slow gentle ones and vigorous rapid ones, called *peristaltic rushes*.

For waves of peristaltic contraction to sweep down the bowel, the help of a conduction system is required. This is provided chiefly by a plexus of nerve fibers, associated with numerous ganglia, that are situated chiefly between the circular and the longitudinal layers of the muscle. This plexus is called *Auerbach's plexus* or the *myenteric plexus* (Fig. 21-21). It contains preganglionic fibers of the parasympathetic division of the autonomic nervous system, which fibers (except in the distal part of the large intestine) are derived from the vagus nerve, and hence from the cranial outflow of the system. These fibers synapse with the cells of terminal ganglia in the plexus which are, therefore, parasympathetic cell stations. The postganglionic fibers given off by the ganglion cells terminate, for the most part, on muscle cells, which they stimulate. Postganglionic fibers of the sympathetic division of the autonomic nervous system, most of which arise from ganglion cells of the prevertebral ganglia, also contribute to Auerbach's plexus, though they have no cell stations there; they reach the muscle cells directly. Whether there are any afferent fibers in the myenteric plexus is a question that has been much discussed. Reflex actions seem to occur in the bowel, but there is little anatomic evidence to indicate a basis of afferent neurons to explain it. Perhaps something in the nature of an axon reflex that will be learned in physiology operates in this situation.

Impulses traveling down the vagus nerve (parasympathetic division) tend to augment both the tone and the peristaltic movements of the muscularis externa. Impulses traveling down the sympathetic fibers from the prevertebral ganglia tend to inhibit both tone and peristaltic movements. A vast amount of gastrointestinal malfunction seems to be due to emotional disturbances affecting the innervation of the bowel. Therefore many frustrated individuals must suffer not only the unhappiness for not having what they want but also gastrointestinal difficulties that develop as a result of their sustained emotional states.

Serosa or Adventitia. This, the fourth and outermost coat of the wall of the alimentary tube is of a serous character; that is, it consists of loose connective tissue, covered with a single layer of squamous mesothelial cells. In some portions of the tract that are affixed to adjacent tissues, the loose connective tissue is not covered by mesothelial cells, but merges into the connective tissue associated with the surrounding structures. It is then an *adventitia*.

Sheets of mesentery (Fig. 21-21, *top*) are covered on both sides by mesothelium and have a core of loose connective tissue containing varying numbers of fat cells, together with the blood and lymphatic vessels and the nerves that it conducts to the intestine.

The Esophagus

The *esophagus* (the *gullet*) is a fairly straight tube that extends from the pharynx to the stomach (Fig. 21-1). Its wall consists of the 4 layers described in connection with the general plan of the tract. Such variations from the general plan as are found in these layers are adapted to its special function.

The Epithelium and Its Renewal. First, food passes down the esophagus very rapidly. There is, then, no point in having absorptive columnar epithelium in the mucous membrane. Furthermore, since many individuals (from bad habit or lack of teeth) do not chew their food sufficiently, there is every reason to have a type of epithelium that is protective against the rough material often swallowed. Obviously, stratified squamous nonkeratinizing epithelium, or even the keratinized type, would be the logical choice for lining the esophagus. In man the epithelium is of the nonkeratinizing type (Figs. 21-22 and 21-23), but in many animals, which swallow rough material even more hastily, the keratinized type is employed. Even in the epithelium of man some keratohyalin granules sometimes may be seen.

The stratified squamous epithelium of the esophagus undergoes continual renewal. Mitosis occurs in the deeper layers while some of the superficial cells desquamate into the lumen. In the rat esophagus mitosis occurs only in the basal layer, whereas in other species 2 or even 3 of the deeper layers may show mitosis. In all cases the deep layers of cells where mitosis occurs are composed of small, deeply baso-

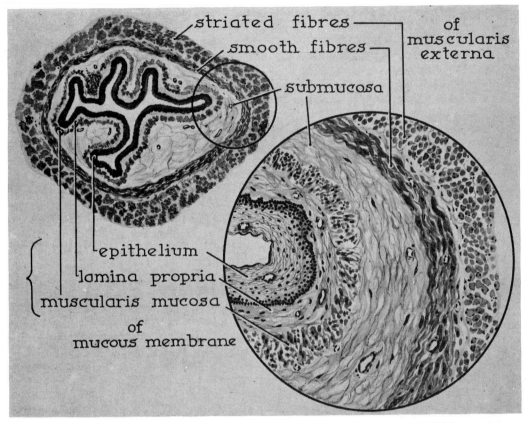

FIG. 21-22. A cross section of the esophagus (low-power) and a portion of its wall (high-power).

philic cells with rare tonofibrils. As cells are displaced toward the lumen, they lose their ability to divide; this is associated with loss of cytoplasmic basophilia and the appearance of tonofibrils in the cells and an over-all enlargement of the cells. The differentiation of the cells is eventually followed by their desquamation, as is described in Chapter 7.

The progeny of a mitotic division in a deep layer may take either of 2 courses: some remain in the deeper layers to divide again, whereas others differentiate in the manner just indicated, so as eventually to be shed at the surface. The mapping of cells labeled by thymidine-³H in the rat esophagus (Leblond, Greulich and Marques-Pereira) in 1964 made it possible to trace the 2 daughter cells from each mitosis. This showed that although a few mitoses led to 1 daughter cell differentiating and another remaining in the basal layer, many other mitoses resulted in the 2 daughter cells following the same course: that is, both differentiated, and in still other divisions both remained in the basal layer. Indeed, the frequency of

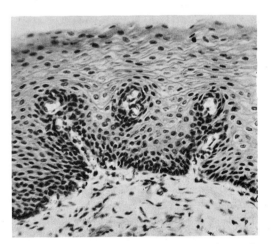

FIG. 21-23. High-power photomicrograph of a section of the lining of the esophagus. Notice a papilla of lamina propria extending up into the epithelium at the left. The light areas in the epithelium (*center* and *right*) are cross sections of papillae that ran into the epithelium at an angle.

the 3 occurrences was just as would have been expected if the decision of a cell for or against differentiation had been entirely a matter of chance.

Glands. Since the epithelium is thick, there is little need for lymphatic tissue to guard against the entry of pathogenic organisms. The relatively little lymphatic tissue is in areas where the ducts of glands pass through the lamina propria.

Since the food that enters the esophagus is lubricated with saliva and moves down it quickly, there is little need for esophageal glands to secrete either mucus or digestive enzymes. There are only a few mucous glands scattered here and there in the submucosa; these are called the *esophageal glands*. In addition, there are some glands in the lamina propria of the mucous membrane; these are most common near the stomach, and since they resemble the glands in the cardiac portion of the stomach, they are called *cardiac glands*. A few glands may also be present at a higher level; these also secrete mucus.

The muscle associated with the pharynx is striated, and this type continues into the upper part of the esophagus, where it forms the muscularis externa of the tube. In the middle third of the esophagus, smooth muscle makes its appearance in the muscularis externa to take the place of the striated, and in the lower third smooth muscle generally comprises all of the muscle present. Hence, cross sections from the upper third of the esophagus generally show all the muscularis externa to be composed of striated muscle; those from the middle third show a mixture, and those from the lower third show only smooth muscle. The section illustrated in Figure 21-22 was taken from the middle third and shows muscle of both types in the muscularis externa.

The striated muscle of the pharynx and of the upper part of the esophagus is an exception to the general rule that striated muscle is voluntary, that is, under the control of the will. That of the esophagus is innervated chiefly by parasympathetic fibers from the vagi and hence by the autonomic (involuntary) nervous system. Swallowing is, then, at least in part, an involuntary act of the nature of a reflex action set in motion by the stimulation of afferent nerve endings distributed chiefly in the posterior wall of the pharynx. An individual, because the striated muscles of the mouth are under the control of the will, can initiate swallowing, but its continuation from the pharynx onward is involuntary because of the autonomic operation of the reflex.

In man the muscularis externa of the esophagus is not thickened sufficiently at the point of entrance of the esophagus into the stomach (the cardia) to justify its being called the cardiac sphincter.

Since the esophagus is not covered with peritoneum, it has an adventitia rather than a serosa. This consists of loose connective tissue which connects the esophagus to its surrounding structures.

The Stomach

The stomach is the considerably expanded portion of the alimentary tract between the esophagus and the small intestine (Fig. 21-1). It has several functions. It acts as a reservoir. This function is facilitated by the elasticity of its walls, which can stretch sufficiently to give it a capacity of from 1 to $1\frac{1}{2}$ quarts; its contents are retained by the well-developed sphincter at its outlet. The stomach is also a digestive organ. Digestion is due to the action of the gastric juice that is secreted by the cells and the glands of the mucous membrane. Gastric juice contains 3 enzymes, hydrochloric acid and mucus. Of the 3 enzymes, *pepsin* is the most important. In an acid medium it begins the digestion of proteins. The other 2 enzymes are *rennin*, which curdles milk, and *lipase*, which splits fats. However, this last effect is probably not very extensive in the stomach.

The hydrochloric acid in the gastric secretion is present in sufficient concentration to kill living cells should they be ingested and it has long been a mystery as to why it does not destroy the cells that line the stomach and thus cause ulcers. Obviously there must be certain protecting mechanisms that operate in the normal individual to prevent this. It has long been assumed that the coating of mucus secreted by the pits and glands of the mucous membrane, soon to be described, is protective in this respect. But there must also be other protective mechanisms. Davenport has written an interesting article about this matter in *Scientific American* (see References) and points out certain factors that may be involved. First, the cells that line the stomach (which will be described in detail presently) are columnar mucus-secreting cells and they are joined near their free surface to one another by tight junctions. Second, the lipid content of the cell membranes of these cells that face the lumen would also seem to be a factor because it has been shown in experiments that the integrity of the lining membrane can be adversely affected by exposing it to the action of certain detergents. Davenport points out, moreover, that bile salts have a detergent action. Normally these are secreted into the intestine below the stomach so they would not enter it but it is possible that they could be regurgitated into the stomach and indeed there seems to be some indication that patients with stomach ulcers at least sometimes have been shown to have some bile salts in their stomachs. Finally, as will be described shortly, another protection is provided by the fact that the epithelial cells that line the stomach are completely replaced every three days.

The stomach acts as a mixer by virtue of its muscular movements, and it converts its contents, diluted with gastric juice, into a semifluid of an even consistency called *chyme*. The stomach is also concerned in the production of the factor necessary to permit the absorption of vitamin B-12. The stomach may also serve to some extent as an absorptive organ, but its function in this respect is limited to the absorption of water, salts, sugar, alcohol and certain other drugs.

Gross Characteristics. The shape of the stomach and the extent and position of its different parts are illustrated in Figure 21-24. The fundus is that part lying above a horizontal line drawn through the entrance of the esophagus. About two thirds of the remainder is called the *body of the stomach*. The third and last part of the organ is called the *pyloric antrum and canal;* these lead to the *exit,* or *pylorus* (= gate).

If an empty contracted stomach is opened, its mucous membrane is seen to be thrown into branching folds, most of which are disposed longitudinally. These are termed *rugae*. The cores of these consist of submucosa (Fig. 21-25, *top*). When the stomach is full, the rugae are almost completely "ironed out."

General Microscopic Features. The wall of the stomach is composed of the 4 usual layers already described. The mucous membrane is relatively thick and contains millions of little simple tubular glands. In some sites the muscularis mucosae has 3 layers instead of the 2 described in the general plan. The small bundles of smooth muscle fibers going from the muscularis mucosae to the surface travel between the glands and pits which will be described below. There are no glands in the submucosa except in the pyloric part adjacent to the duodenum. The muscularis externa consists of 3 instead of 2 layers. The fibers of the innermost layer are disposed obliquely; those of the middle coat, circularly, and those of the outermost coat, longitudinally. A serosa is present.

Pits and Glands of the Mucosa. If the gastric mucosa is examined with the LM, it is seen to be studded with tiny little openings through which the gastric juice wells up when the stomach is actively secreting. These little openings are the openings of what are termed *gastric pits* or *foveolae*. The pits descend into the mucous membrane to reach the upper ends of the glands, which extend more deeply still to

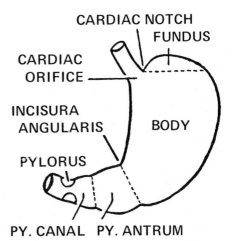

Fig. 21-24. Diagram of the parts of the stomach. (Grant, J. C. B.: A Method of Anatomy. ed. 4. Baltimore, Williams & Wilkins)

reach the muscularis mucosa. The glands deliver their secretion into the bottom of the pits, and the pits transport the secretion to the surface; see Figures 21-25 and 21-26. There is not universal agreement about the shape of the pits. Sometimes they are depicted as having a tubular form and sometimes as being crevices. Probably both kinds exist, with the percentage varying in relation to species, but it is also probable that many crevices are interpreted as tubules, because a section that cuts across a crevice makes it appear as a longitudinal section of a tubule. Unless tubules were arranged in perfect rows, it would be impossible to see so many in a single section as appear in Figure 21-25; the appearance shown here could result only from roughly parallel crevices being sectioned at right angles to their long diameters.

The lamina propria between the bottoms of the pits and the muscularis mucosae is literally packed with simple tubular glands that open into the bottoms of the pits. In their deepest parts these glands reach or almost reach the muscularis mucosae. There are so many glands in the zone between the bottoms of the crevices and pits and the muscularis mucosae that the student may have difficulty in thinking of this zone as lamina propria. And, indeed, the connective tissue of the lamina propria itself is so broken up by the glands that it can be seen only as thin films between glands (Fig. 21-25, *lower right*).

The Surface Epithelium (Which Also Extends Down the Sides of Pits To Line Them). The surface epithelium provides protection. Its cells are tall and all alike; the fact that they are all alike enables the student to distinguish at a glance a section of stomach

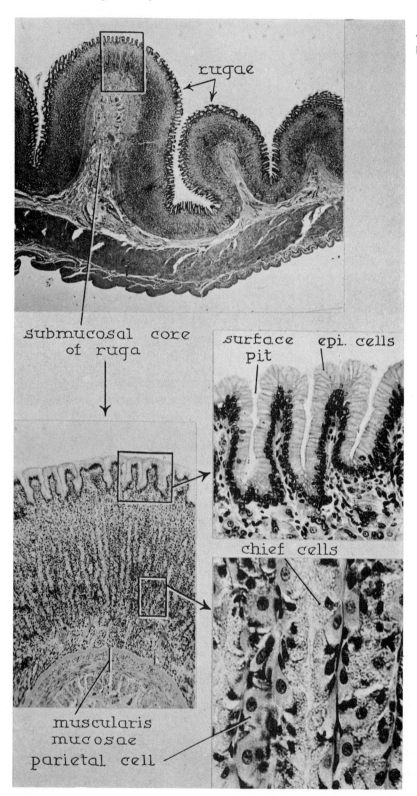

FIG. 21-25. Photomicrographs, taken at various magnifications, of a section of the body of the stomach of a cat.

from a section of small or large intestine. (In the small and the large intestine goblet cells alternate with nonmucus-producing columnar cells; this has a very different appearance from the lining cells of the stomach.) The surface epithelial cells form a membrane that, although it is only one cell thick, is fairly effective in protecting the rest of the wall. The apex of the cells is filled with mucus; and this mucus is secreted in such a way that it forms continuous sheets. When damage is produced to the mucous sheets and underlying cells by certain types of food and drink, particularly alcohol, some cells of the surface epithelium are shed in the stomach. The mortality of surface cells is compensated by the migration of new cells arising in the isthmus, as shown below. When more extensive wounds of the stomach are produced, for instance at surgical operations, they normally heal rapidly, presumably again because of the entry of new cells.

Glands of the Lamina Propria of the Cardia. The glands in the lamina propria in the area immediately surrounding the entrance of the esophagus into the stomach are somewhat different from those in the remainder of the organ. They are either simple or compound tubular glands composed of cells with pale cytoplasm. They secrete mucus and little enzyme and are, therefore, of little practical importance.

Glands of the Mucous Membrane of the Fundus and Body. These glands produce nearly all the enzymes and hydrochloric acid secreted in the stomach; they also produce some of the mucus. In the body of the stomach the pits extend into the mucous membrane for only a quarter to a third of its thickness (Fig. 21-25, *lower left*). Therefore the glands that extend from the bottoms of the pits to the muscularis mucosae are 2 to 3 times as long as the pits are deep. The glands here are straight except near the muscularis mucosae, where they may be bent (Fig. 21-26). Since they are straight over most of their length, they may be seen as reasonably complete longitudinal sections of tubules if sections are cut at right angles to the surface epithelium (Fig. 21-25, *lower left*).

According to Stevens and Leblond, each tubular gland here consists of 3 segments. The deepest part is the *base* (Fig. 21-26), the middle part is the *neck* and the upper part is the *isthmus* (Fig. 21-26). The isthmus is continuous with a pit. It should be understood that pits are not parts of glands; they are merely little wells and crevices sunk from the surface and lined by surface epithelial cells. Several glands may open into a pit.

The gastric juice is secreted by the glands. The glands contain 4 main kinds of secretory cells, but

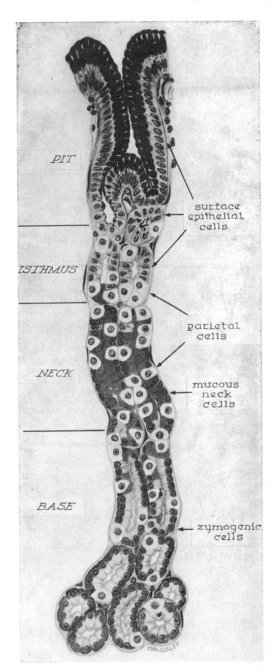

Fig. 21-26. Drawing of a section of the body of the stomach of a monkey, stained by the PA-Schiff method and by hematoxylin. (Preparation by C. P. Leblond)

these are not evenly distributed in the different segments. The 4 types can be demonstrated to advantage in sections stained by the PA-Schiff method and hematoxylin.

The isthmus contains 2 types of cells, surface epithelial cells and parietal cells. The surface epithelial cells along the sides of pits have a considerable apical content of mucus that is represented as black in Figure 21-26. In the deepest parts of the pits the amount of mucus in the apical parts of the cell is considerably less (Fig. 21-26), and in the isthmus the surface epithelial cells demonstrate only a few granules of mucus in their apical parts. Scattered between the surface epithelial cells of the isthmus are large *parietal cells* that have relatively clear cytoplasm when stained by the PA-Schiff method and hematoxylin. In good H and E preparations the cytoplasm of these cells is pink (Fig. 21-25). The parietal cells, as seen in a section, vary from being rounded to triangular in shape (Figs. 21-25 and 21-26). Their nuclei are dark and generally centrally placed. Their fine structure and function will be described presently.

The neck of a gland is made up chiefly of cells that were first described by R. Bensley as *mucous neck cells*. These are difficult to identify in H and E sections. With the PA-Schiff method the cytoplasm of the mucous neck cells is seen to be literally stuffed with pink mucus (dark in Fig. 21-26) and to have a foamy appearance. The nuclei of these cells are generally pressed against their bases, where they often have a more or less triangular shape (Fig. 21-26). Individual parietal cells are scattered between groups of mucous neck cells here (Fig. 21-26).

The base or body of a gland is made up mostly of *zymogenic (chief) cells*. These have accumulations of basophilic material in their cytoplasm near their bases. The cytoplasm between their nuclei and their free surfaces appears different with different fixatives and stains. In an ordinary H and E preparation it appears vacuolated and reticular (Fig. 21-25) because the secretion granules it contains are not well fixed or stained. The PA-Schiff and hematoxylin method demonstrates a similar appearance in it (Fig. 21-26). Parietal cells are sprinkled among the zymogenic cells. Not uncommonly a parietal cell will be seen that is roughly triangular and arranged so that one of its three sides is applied closely to the basement membrane of the gland, and its base extends between part of the base of a chief cell and the basement membrane on each side (Fig. 21-25). The apex of such a cell projects between the sides of the two chief cells that border it but not far enough to reach the lumen proper. The secretion from such a parietal cell then must pass between the two chief cells that almost cover it to reach the lumen. Since parietal cells have centrally disposed, rounded nuclei and decidedly acidophilic cytoplasm, in H and E sections they stand out as red cells among the paler chief cells. Under

special conditions, secretory canaliculi may be seen in their cytoplasm. These open on the side of the cell closest to the lumen of the gland.

The zymogenic (chief) cells produce the enzymes of the gastric secretion, and the parietal cells produce the hydrochloric acid. The other types of cells produce only mucus.

THE FINE STRUCTURE OF THE CELLS OF THE GLANDS

Parietal Cell. Under the EM the parietal cell is characterized by the presence of a branching canaliculus which extends into it from its apex, and by which it delivers its secretion into the lumen of the gastric gland (Fig. 21-27). In addition to intracellular canaliculi, there are intercellular canaliculi between adjacent parietal cells. A unique feature of the intracellular canaliculus is the tremendous number of microvilli which project into it (Fig. 21-27), and of fingerlike invaginations between them. Some believe these invaginations can be inverted to become microvilli and vice-versa, and that the phenomenon is related to acid secretion (about which more will be said below). The intracellular canaliculus takes up a considerable amount of space in a parietal cell and so encroaches on the cytoplasm, and the cytoplasm that remains is literally stuffed with mitochondria. There are a few ribosomes, little rough-surfaced endoplasmic reticulum and no secretory granules. A Golgi apparatus can be seen.

Mechanism of Secretion of HCl. Modern histological technics, in particular the use of the EM in revealing that parietal cells lack facilities for providing a protein type of secretion, and showing that the canaliculus provides a vast area for membrane phenomena, have considerably narrowed the number and kinds of hypotheses which have been held in the past about how parietal cells could secrete such a strong solution of a powerful acid.

The use of indicators on suitable sections shows that the cytoplasm of a parietal cell, as a whole, has a normal pH. However, the canaliculi have an extremely acid pH.

The enzyme carbonic anhydrase is abundant in parietal cells and is probably responsible for catalyzing the formation of carbonic acid. One theory is that hydrogen ions from this carbonic acid are transported, by an active transport mechanism, through the unit membrane that lines the fingerlike invaginations and covers the microvilli, where they combine with chloride ions. Although many details are vague or even unknown about the process, it seems clear that hydro-

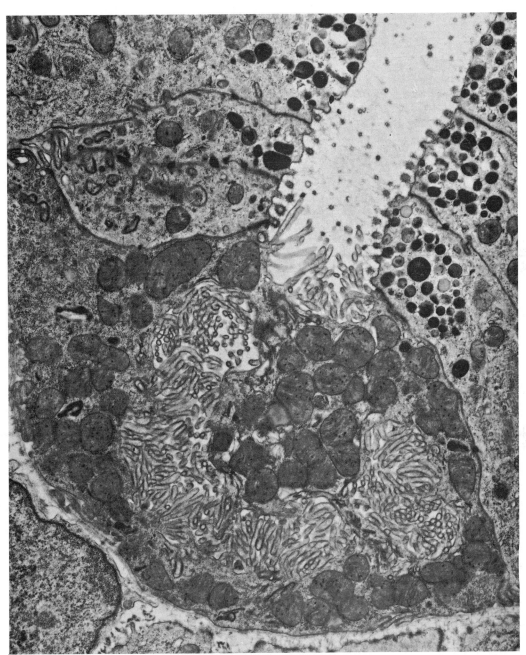

Fɪɢ. 21-27. Electron micrograph ($\times$ 9,500) of the bottom of a gastric gland of a bat. The clear area is the lumen of the gastric gland, lined on each side by mucous cells. Only the apical portions of these are shown. They contain many mucous granules and have short microvilli projecting into the lumen of the gland. The cell at the base of the gastric gland is a parietal cell. Its cytoplasm contains many round to ovoid mitochondria. Extending into this cell from the lumen of the gastric gland is a large C-shaped passageway which is an intracellular canaliculus. This does not appear empty, as might be expected, because it is filled with numerous microvilli projecting into it. These microvilli are cut in all planes, and more microvilli project from the surface of the parietal cell into the lumen of the gastric gland. (Preparation by Dr. S. Ito, Dr. R. J. Winchester and Dr. D. W. Fawcett)

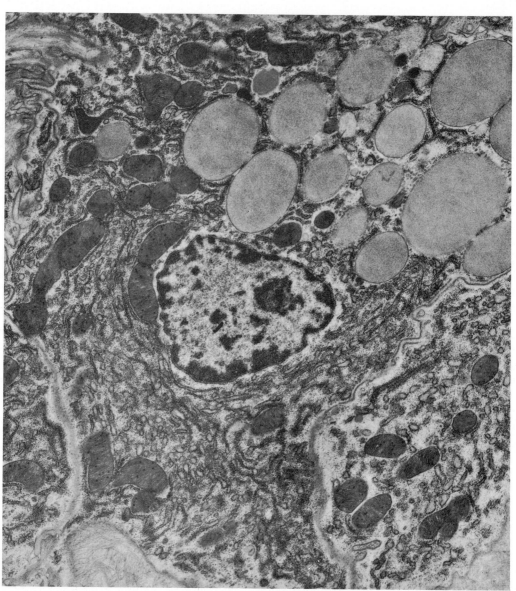

Fig. 21-28. Electron micrograph ($\times$ 14,000) of part of a zymogenic (chief) cell from the stomach of a bat showing nucleus, large secretory granules, granular endoplasmic reticulum and mitochondria. (Dr. S. Ito, Dr. R. J. Winchester and Dr. D. W. Fawcett)

chloric acid is secreted as free acid, and that its formation is dependent on the membrane between it and cytoplasm.

Zymogen Cells. These cells are characterized by an abundance of rough-surfaced vesicles and cisternae of endoplasmic reticulum (Fig. 21-28). The way these are concerned in the formation of the many secretion granules that are the precursors of the enzymes made by these cells (Fig. 21-28) was explained in Chapter 5.

Mucous Neck Cells and Surface Epithelial Cells. Both of these cell types show many mucigen droplets, particularly near the apex through which the secretion is delivered. Mucus-secreting cells have been dealt with in detail in Chapters 5 and 7.

Less Common Cell Types. It has long been known that the cytoplasm of some cells of gastric and intestinal epithelium contain granules capable of reducing silver nitrate. They were called argentaffin cells, also enterochromaffin cells because they are strongly stained also by bichromate salts. Slightly different cells can reduce silver nitrate only in the presence of a chemical reducer; these were called argyrophile cells. At a recent conference in Wiesbaden it was decided to group argentaffin and argyrophile cells under a single name, "endocrine cells" of the gastrointestinal tract. By analogy with the endocrine elements of the nervous system called "neuro-endocrine cells," it would be appropriate to call these *"entero-endocrine."* In the stomach several types are found: one, which is strongly argentaffin, produces serotonin (EC cell); another, which is argyrophile, secretes gastrin (G cell). All these cells are characterized by the presence of cytoplasmic granules accumulated in the base (Fig. 21-39), where these granules are believed to release their content into the extracellular space for passage into the circulation.

Toward the junction of isthmus and neck regions, a few cells are found which show the characteristic features of *immature cells* (abundance of free ribosomes, paucity of organelles, etc.). These cells give rise to the surface epithelial cells as will be mentioned presently; but there is evidence indicating that they may also produce the other cell types of the epithelium (mucous neck cells, parietal cells, and perhaps others). However, the situation is less clear than in the small intestine, where the problem of cell production will be examined in detail.

Renewal of Cells of the Gastric Mucosa. Stevens and Leblond, using the colchicine method, found that only the two mucus-containing types of cells showed active mitotic division. They found that the surface epithelial cells are maintained by divisions of the immature and partly mature cells occurring in the isthmus. The daughters of these divisions migrate into the pits, where they stop dividing, and, from there, to the free surface, where they are eventually lost to the lumen. They estimated that 5.87 percent of the surface epithelial cells enter mitosis every 4 hours. The mucous neck cells were found to divide less often; only 2.59 percent enter mitosis every 4 hours. The production of these cells is balanced by loss into the gland lumen. From the foregoing observations it appears that the surface epithelium in the stomach is renewed (in the rat) every 3 days, and that this is done by cells in the isthmus dividing, and the new cells formed here push up the sides of the crypts and then over the surface to replace those that are constantly being lost by desquamation.

Glands of the Pylorus. The pits and the crevices in the pyloric portion of the stomach are deeper than those in the body and the fundus. Furthermore, the glands that open into the pits and the crevices are much shorter than those in the body and the fundus. Hence, there is a considerable difference between the ratio of the depth of the crevices and the pits to the depth of the glands in the pyloric portion of the stomach and that in the body and fundus (compare Figs. 21-25 and 21-29). This point should enable the student to distinguish readily sections of pylorus from those of body and fundus. Another point of difference between the glands of the two regions is that the pyloric glands are coiled; hence, they never are seen in longitudinal section (the glands of the body and the fundus are, if sections are cut perpendicular to the surface). Still another point of difference is that the pyloric glands, except near the pyloric sphincter and the body, where a few parietal cells may be seen, consist of only one type of cell. In H and E sections, the cytoplasm of these cells is pale, but with special stains it may be shown to contain mucus. The nuclei are more or less flattened and pressed against the bases of the cells (Fig. 21-29). The lumens of the glands are wider than those of the glands in the body and the fundus. The occasional entero-endocrine cell may also be found.

Many observers have commented on the similarity between the cells of the pyloric glands and the mucous neck cells of the glands of the body and the fundus. They have the same function, for the pyloric glands do not produce enzymes but only mucus.

At the pylorus, the circularly disposed smooth muscle fibers of the middle coat of the muscularis externa of the stomach are increased so as to form a thick bundle which encircles the exit of the stomach. This is called the *pyloric sphincter.* The stout band of muscle of which it is composed bulges the submucosa and the mucous membrane inward so that these are thrown into a circular fold. The chief ingredient of the core of this fold, it should be noted, is the thickened middle coat of the muscularis externa. This fold differs from most folds in the alimentary tract, which have cores of only submucosa.

Peristaltic movements begin near the middle of the stomach and spread down to the pylorus. The pyloric sphincter automatically opens to permit such food as is sufficiently fluid and digested to enter the small intestine. At the same time it holds back solid undigested food. The precise way its operations are controlled is too complex a matter to discuss here.

Control of the Secretion of Gastric Juice. In dogs the surface of the resting stomach is coated with mucus; gastric juice wells up from the glands to flood the surface only when a meal is in prospect or is consumed. However, Carlson has shown that in man

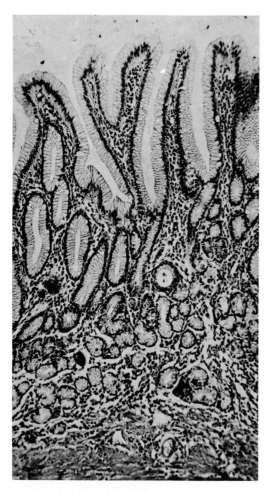

Fig. 21-29. Low-power photomicrograph of a section of the mucous membrane of the pyloric portion of the stomach of a man.

particularly when the breakdown products reach the small intestine, where they act on its mucosa possibly to make a substance that circulates by the bloodstream to reach the gastric glands. Accordingly, the gastric glands are said to secrete through 3 phases: (1) the cephalic (psychic factors), (2) the gastric, where consumed food either directly or indirectly stimulates the mucosa to induce secretion, and (3) the intestinal, where the breakdown products of digestion, and the gastric juice itself, reach and affect the intestinal mucosa to make it produce something that circulates by the bloodstream to stimulate further the gastric glands.

The Small Intestine

Relation of General Structure to Functions. The small intestine is about 20 feet long. Its first 10 to 12 inches constitute the *duodenum* (Fig. 21-1). This, except for its first inch or so, is relatively fixed in position, not being suspended by a mesentery. It pursues a horseshoe-shaped course around the head of the pancreas to become continuous with the *jejunum*, which constitutes the next two fifths of the small intestine (Fig. 21-1). The last three fifths is termed the *ileum* (Fig. 21-1). In general, the small intestine tends to become narrower throughout its course.

The small intestine has 2 chief functions: (1) completing the digestion of food delivered into it by the stomach, and (2) selectively absorbing the final products of digestion into its blood and lymph vessels. In addition, it also makes some hormones.

The structure of the small intestine is specialized in both its digestive and its absorptive functions. It will be more convenient to describe how its structure is specialized for absorption before describing how its structure is specialized for digestion.

To perform its absorptive function efficiently, the small intestine requires a vast surface of epithelial cells of the absorptive type. The great length of the small intestine helps considerably in providing such a surface, but this is not enough, and provision is made in 3 other ways for increasing the absorptive surface still further.

1. Beginning about an inch beyond the pylorus, the mucous membrane is thrown into circularly or spirally disposed folds called the *plicae circulares* or *valves of Kerckring* (Fig. 21-30). These folds are generally crescentic and extend from one half to two thirds of the way around the lumen. However, single folds may extend all the way around the intestine or even from a spiral of 2 or 3 turns; the highest ones project into the lumen for about a third of an inch.

there is a more or less continuous secretion of modest amounts of gastric juice, varying from 10 to 60 ml. per hour. This is augmented when food is about to be eaten or is eaten. Several factors are concerned in augmenting the secretion. Psychic factors, as shown by Pavlov, play an important part and so justify the imaginative cook. Psychic factors must operate through a nervous control of secretion by the vagus nerve. Certain foods, when they reach the stomach, have the ability to stimulate secretion further. These foods stimulate secretion even if the nerves to the stomach are cut. Hence, if they stimulate secretion by means of a reflex initiated in the mucosa of the stomach, the reflex concerned must have something of the nature of a local one. Then, in addition to certain foods stimulating secretion, the breakdown products of a wide variety of foods also have this property,

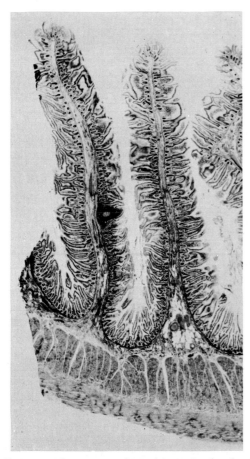

Fig. 21-30. Low-power photomicrograph of a longitudinal section of the wall of the jejunum of a dog, showing 2 plicae circulares cut in cross section. The plicae are studded with irregular villi.

These shapes are variable with the individual. More important are the length and surface of villi. In general, length and surface are maximal at the beginning of the small intestine, that is, immediately after the pylorus, and they decrease gradually to reach a minimum in the ileum just before the ileocecal junction (Fig. 21-32). At first, it would appear that the size of villi varies with the intensity of absorption phenomena. However, experimental work indicates that the large villus size in the duodenum is maintained by some factors present in the secretion arising locally as well as in that coming from stomach and pancreas. When the duodenum is connected to the terminal ileum in such a way that secretions are shared, ileal villi become taller and duodenal villi smaller than normally (Altmann and Leblond).

3. The absorptive surface is made still greater by the microvilli that are present on the free surfaces of the epithelial cells; these were described in Chapter 5. They are illustrated in Figures 5-8 and 21-35.

In order to perform its other chief function (completing the digestion of food received from the stomach), the small intestine requires large supplies of digestive enzymes and considerable quantities of mucus to protect its epithelial lining from injury. The digestive enzymes are provided by glands; mucus is provided both by proper glands and by innumerable goblet cells that are intermingled with absorptive cells

They all have cores of submucosa, are not ironed out if the intestine is full and, at first, are large and very close together (Fig. 21-30). In the upper part of the jejunum they become smaller and farther apart. In the middle or lower end of the ileum they disappear.

2. The surface of the mucous membrane over the folds and between the folds is studded with tiny leaf-, tongue- or fingerlike projections that range from ½ to 1 mm. or more in height. These are called the *intestinal villi* (Fig. 21-31). Since they are projections of mucous membrane, they have cores of lamina propria. The muscularis mucosae and the submucosa do not extend into them as they do into the plicae circulares.

The villi of the duodenum are broader than those elsewhere, and many examples of leaflike ones can be found in this region. In the upper part of the jejunum, the villi, in general, are said to be tongue shaped. Farther down, they become finger shaped. However,

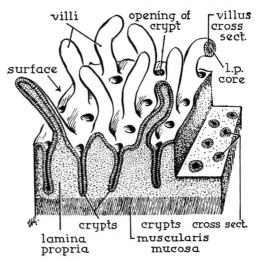

Fig. 21-31. Three-dimensional drawing of the lining of the small intestine. Observe that villi are fingerlike processes, with cores of lamina propria that extend into the lumen. Note also that crypts of Lieberkühn are glands that dip down into the lamina propria. Observe particularly the difference in the cross-section appearance of villi and crypts.

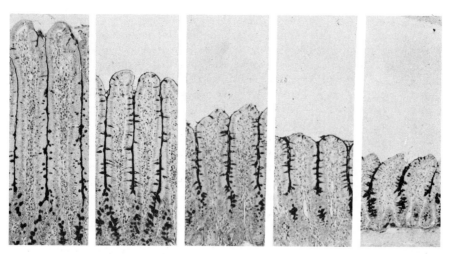

FIG. 21-32. Villi in different regions of rat small intestine. From left to right, the figures are taken from beginning of duodenum, jejunum, midportion of intestine (that is, junction of jejunum and ileum), midileum, and terminal ileum. It may be seen that villi are fairly close to one another, much more so than in the schematic drawing in Fig. 21-31. There is *a gradual decrease in villus size from pylorus to the ileocecal valve*. (G. Altmann and C. P. Leblond)

along the mucous membrane. The glands that provide the digestive juices and the mucus necessary for the function of the small intestine are distributed in 3 general sites: (1) outside the intestine, but connected with it by ducts, (2) in the submucosa and (3) in the lamina propria.

The microscopic structure of the pancreas and the liver, the two glands that are situated outside the small intestine and deliver their secretions into it, will be considered later. Here we are concerned only with the effect of their secretions on the digestive process. Their ducts, usually conjoined, open into the duodenum about 3 inches from the pylorus (Fig. 21-1). The secretion of the pancreas, delivered into the duodenum at this site, is alkaline (and so helps neutralize the acid stomach contents), and it contains enzymes concerned in the digestion of proteins, carbohydrates and fats; several enzymes that effect different steps in protein digestion probably are elaborated. The enzymes are not active until they reach the intestine, where some agency renders them potent. In their totality they can break down proteins to amino acids; it is in this form that proteins are absorbed. The pancreatic juice also contains enzymes that break down starches to sugars. Some sugars, for example, maltose, must be acted on further by enzymes secreted by glands in the lamina propria and must be converted to monosaccharides before they are absorbed. The pancreatic juice also contains lipolytic enzymes that both emulsify fat and break it down to fatty acids and 2-monoglycerides. The effect of these enzymes is facilitated by the presence of bile, the secretion of the liver.

The second group of glands to consider are those situated in the submucosa. Glands are found in this position only in the duodenum. These are compound tubular in type and are called the *glands of Brunner*

(Fig. 21-33). Their precise distribution varies considerably. They may extend into the pylorus for a short distance. Generally, they are most numerous in the first part of the duodenum and become less numerous and finally disappear in its more distal parts. Nevertheless, they have been observed on occasion in the first part of the jejunum.

The secretory portions of Brunner's glands are sufficiently expanded to have a somewhat alveolar appearance. The secretory portions are chiefly confined to the submucosa. The excretory ducts lead through the muscularis mucosae to empty into the crypts of Lieberkühn, to be described shortly. The muscularis mucosae does not always constitute a well-defined structure over them, for often it is so split up by glandular elements that it appears as a network of smooth muscle fibers whose interstices are filled with glandular elements.

The secretory cells are columnar and resemble those of the pyloric glands. Their nuclei are dark and flattened toward the bases of the cells. The cytoplasm is pale and finely granular in H and E sections (Fig. 21-33), but, with suitable stains, can be shown to contain mucus. The glands are obviously useful in producing extra mucus at the site where the pancreatic enzymes are emptied into the intestine.

The third set of glands to consider are those called *crypts of Lieberkühn;* these dip down from the surface between villi to reach almost to the muscularis mucosae (Fig. 21-21). Their openings on the surface of the intestine are shown in Figure 21-31, but their openings are in reality difficult to see in the living animal, because their mouths are tightly closed. It is known that some enzymes are secreted in the small intestine, particularly erepsin which acts in the later stages of protein digestion to produce amino acids. Enzymes that convert disaccharides into monosaccharides and others that transfer nucleic acids into nucleosides are also secreted. Of the cells in the crypts only some cells at their bottoms, the Paneth cells, to be described presently, show the features that are now associated with enzyme production. Yet there is also some evidence that the cells of the villi elaborate disaccharidase; this will be explained below.

Mucus is provided by the glands of Brunner and by innumerable goblet cells present both in the crypts of Lieberkühn and among the absorptive epithelial cells that cover the villi and otherwise line the interior of the intestine (Fig. 21-34).

Some Details Concerning the Structure of the Mucous Membrane

General Features of Epithelium of Villi. Whereas the surface epithelial cells of the stomach secrete mucus and are all of the same type (except for a rare entero-endocrine cell), the cells of the villi are of two main types. About 90 percent of them are tall cylindrical cells with a thick "striated border" described and illustrated, as it appears with the LM, in Chapter 7, Figure 7-6. The electron microscope shows the border to be composed of packed microvilli (Fig. 21-35); these cells are called "absorptive" or more commonly "columnar cells." The rest of the villus epithelium consists of mucus-secreting goblet cells (except for about 0.3% entero-endocrine cells).

Columnar cells have an abundant cytoplasm (cell to nucleus ratio, 3.5) and are enclosed on the sides by highly convoluted cell membranes; mitochondria are abundant (Fig. 21-35). Free ribosomes are scarce in all of them; there are cisternae of rough endoplasmic reticulum; these and the Golgi saccules are well developed in the epithelial cells at the base of the villi, but become less and less prominent as the villus tip is approached (Altmann). The difference may explain why cell coat production is intense in the cells at the base of the villi and decreases gradually to be insignificant in those near the tip.

In fact, the cell coat of villus columnar cells turns over. A method worked out to separate microvilli by centrifugation has revealed that their thick cell coat contains glycoproteins which are hydrolytic enzymes; one of them is alkaline phosphatase; others are disaccharidases. The turnover of these enzymes consists of production by the cell being balanced by shedding to the chyme. In the chyme, these enzymes exert their hydrolytic effect on the foodstuffs present.

Goblet cells (Fig. 5-36) are of two types. Those of the common type have been described previously. Their

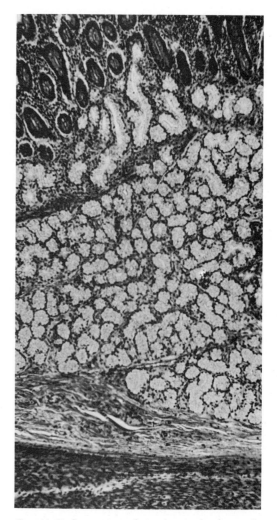

Fig. 21-33. Low-power photomicrograph of a section of the wall of the duodenum, showing Brunner's glands in the submucosa. The muscularis mucosae may be seen passing to the right and upward from above the middle of the left side. In the middle of the upper part of the figure, a gland of Brunner may be seen emptying into a crypt of Lieberkühn. The muscularis externa is seen at the bottom of the picture.

Golgi apparatus is prominent and the apical region of their cytoplasm is usually distended with mucous globules (Fig. 21-36, *top*). The cells of the other type show small dense granules within the mucous globules (Fig. 21-36, *bottom*); they are not numerous in villi.

Epithelium of Crypts. The epithelium lining the glands that dip down into the mucous membrane (the crypts of Lieberkühn) varies in relation to depth. The base of the crypts is composed of about equal numbers of Paneth cells with characteristic large secretion

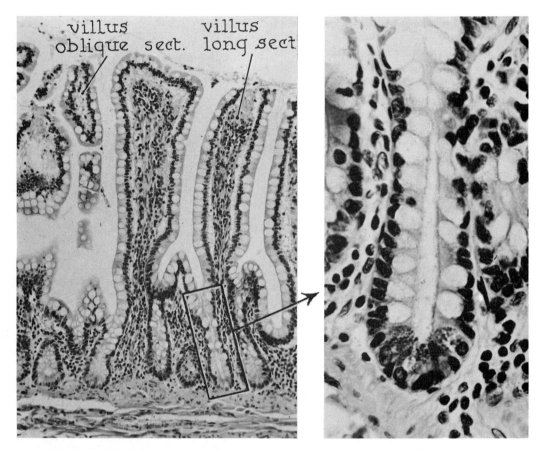

Fig. 21-34. (*Left*) Low-power photomicrograph of a section of the wall of the small intestine of a child, showing villi in longitudinal and cross section and crypts of Lieberkühn. Lymphocytes are numerous in the cores of villi. (*Right*) High-power photomicrograph of a crypt of Lieberkühn, showing goblet cells along its sides and some Paneth cells with cytoplasmic granules at its deepest part.

granules and of small columnar cells intercalated between them (Fig. 21-37). Examination of this region in the electron microscope (Fig. 21-38) demonstrates that the small columnar cells of the crypt base are poor in cytoplasm (cell nucleus ratio about 2) and are squeezed between Paneth cells. Unlike the villus columnar cells depicted in Figure 21-35, these small columnar cells have smooth lateral membranes. Their cytoplasm contains only few mitochondria and ER cisternae and a small Golgi apparatus, but is packed with free ribosomes. These features indicate that these cells exist in a relatively undifferentiated state and, as might be expected, they exhibit a high rate of division.

Paneth cells, in contrast, are highly differentiated as shown by an enormous development of rough endoplasmic reticulum and a prominent Golgi. Their zymogen granules, which are surrounded by a mucuslike

halo in the mouse (Fig. 21-38) but not in man, are released to the lumen by a process of exocytosis. Paneth cells contain zinc, but the significance of this fact is obscure. Nor is the nature of the enzyme they secrete known with certainty, although there is some evidence that they elaborate lysozyme (Erlandsen and Taylor).

The cells located above the crypt base are mostly columnar; they show a gradual transition between crypt base columnar cells and villus columnar cells— that is, the size increases progressively and the number of free ribosomes decreases, whereas the number of rER cisternae increases. Furthermore, the columnar cells present in the crypts divide, but those of the villi do not. Hence, these two types of columnar cells are somewhat different. However, the study of their embryologic development reveals that the epithelium of both crypts and villi have the same origin, and, furthermore, they transform into one another, as will be described below.

Next to the Paneth cell region, cells with just a few mucous globules may also be encountered. These cells, which are known as oligomucous cells, arise from the differentiation of some crypt base columnar cells (the type shown in Figure 21-37). Furthermore, they retain the ability to divide, but only temporarily; for as soon as the accumulation of globules is sufficient to produce some distention of the cell—the very distention which gave the cell its name, goblet cell—the ability to divide is lost. In the lower half of the crypts, most mucous cells contain only few mucous globules, while in the upper half they have the typical appearance of goblet cells (Fig. 21-36). Furthermore, in the crypts, one out of four goblet cells contains dense granules within mucous globules, as shown in the lower half of Figure 21-36.

In this region, entero-endocrine cells make up about 1 percent of the cells present. They are characterized by a narrow apex and a wide basal region packed with dense granules (Fig. 21-39), which, as in stomach, may be argentaffin or argyrophile. Some of these cells produce serotonin. Others are believed to produce the intestinal hormones: secretin, cholecystokinin, etc.

Even less common is another cell type, the caveolated cell, a strange cell (Fig. 21-40) characterized by invaginations of the surface membrane extending into the cytoplasm as irregular tubules, which are called caveolae (arrow at upper left corner, Fig. 21-40). Polyplike structures arise from the walls of the caveolae and become free in their lumen in the form of small spheres, which eventually come out between the microvilli to join the chyme. Other features of these cells are microvilli twice the length of those of nearby cells, long bundles of straight filaments extending from the core of microvilli deep into the cytoplasm, and also circular filaments following the surface of the cell in the apical region. The caveolated cells, although rare, are found in crypts and villi of small intestine as well as in stomach and large intestine (Nabeyama and Leblond).

Mention may also be made of migrating cells found within the epithelium. Not only lymphocytes and other blood-derived cells may be encountered, but also an interesting cell type known as "globule leukocyte." This cell is present in the epithelium of normal and, most commonly, parasite-infected individuals. The globule leukocyte (Fig. 21-41) is characterized by large inclusions with properties similar to those of mast cell granules. (Cells similar to globule leukocytes are occasionally seen in the lamina propria.)

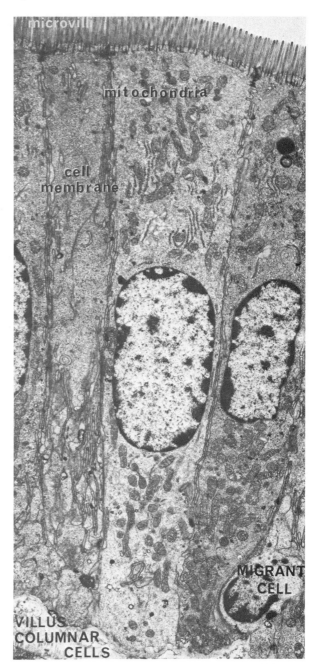

Fig. 21-35. Villus columnar cell of small intestine (mouse). This is a tall cylindrical cell with ample cytoplasm, numerous tall microvilli at the free surface, complex convolutions of the lateral membranes (well seen at left, particularly in the cell showing no nucleus), numerous mitochondria and very few free ribosomes. A few cisternae of rough endoplasmic reticulum are seen as thick threads between mitochondria in the supranuclear region of the central cell. (H. Cheng and C. P. Leblond)

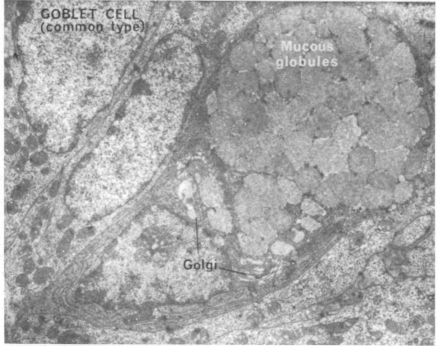

GOBLET CELL
(common type)

Mucous
globules

Golgi

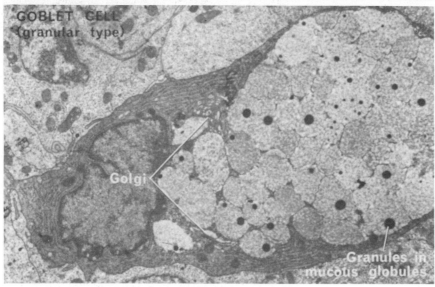

GOBLET CELL
(granular type)

Golgi

Granules in
mucous globules

Fig. 21-36. Goblet cells in the upper part of intestinal crypts (mouse small intestine).

These are mucous cells, whose apex is distended by mucous globules to the form of a goblet. In a prominent Golgi apparatus, the synthesis of the glycoprotein of mucus is completed and this is packaged into mucous globules. In about 1 in 4 of the mucous cells of the crypts, dense granules are present within the globules, as shown in the lower figure. However, the dense granules are infrequent in the mucous cells at the base of the villi and are completely lacking in those near the villus tip. This is taken to mean that, when granular mucous cells migrate out of the crypts and along the villus walls, they excrete the granule-containing globules and elaborate new mucous globules which are free of granules. (H. Cheng)

With radioautography, it was possible to show that columnar cells labeled by ^{3}H-thymidine before their division in the crypt appear on the villus surface within a day and by about 3 days have reached the villus tip (Fig. 21-42), where they are extruded. Hence the epithelium of the small intestine in experimental animals is renewed about every third day. Bertalanffy and Nagy reached similar conclusions for the intestine of man. The balance reached between cell production in the crypt and cell loss at the extrusion zone results in the familiar histological picture of the intestinal epithelium.

Goblet cells (Figs. 21-34 and 21-36), like columnar cells, arise from mitosis in the crypts of the small intestine. However, typical goblet cells do not divide; the mitoses occur only in the oligomucous cells mentioned above; and these, which retain the ability to divide, later transform into typical goblet cells. It is likely that the oligomucous cells come from the undifferentiated columnar cells at the base of the crypts (Cairnie; Merzel and Leblond; Cheng). Later, goblet cells migrate from crypt to villus in the same manner and at the same speed as the columnar cells to which they are bound by junctional complexes.

The least numerous of the cells of crypt and villi are the entero-endocrine cells. These cells may be of various types, as pointed out above. They all renew at about the same rate as the other cells (Ferreira and Leblond) to which they are also attached by junctional complexes. Incidentally, curious little tumors (carcinoids) not uncommon in the appendix, have been traced to entero-endocrine cells.

Summary. The types of epithelial cells found in the lining of the small intestine and their relationships and origin are shown in Figure 21-43.

Lamina Propria. The cores of villi are composed of lamina propria. In this particular site it consists of a loose connective tissue which has many of the attributes of lymphatic tissue. Its chief supporting element is a network of reticular fibers that extends throughout its substance and, at the sides and the tip, unites with the basement membrane under the surface epithelium. Branching cells with pale cytoplasm are irregularly scattered over the fibers in the reticular cells. In the network, lymphocytes are common (Fig. 21-34). Plasma cells are sometimes fairly abundant. Eosinophils that have migrated from the capillaries of the villus are also sometimes seen in the reticular net. Furthermore, smooth muscle fibers which extend from the muscularis mucosae have their long diameter parallel with that of the villus and are characteristically disposed along its central axis, usually around a single, large, lymphatic capillary that begins near the tip of the villus; this lymphatic capillary is usually termed the *lacteal* of the villus.

A single arterial twig from the submucosa usually penetrates the muscularis mucosae below each villus and ascends into it for some distance and then breaks up into a capillary network. The capillaries approach the epithelial cells very closely. Separate arterial twigs break up into capillary nets surrounding the crypts of Lieberkühn. Nerve fibers from Meissner's plexus in the submucosa likewise penetrate the muscularis mucosae to ascend into each villus. Here they break up into networks that are said to extend throughout all its substances. Frank nodules of lymphatic tissue are not uncommon in the lamina propria of any part of the digestive tract, but they are relatively more numerous in the small intestine, particularly in the ileum. They appear either singly, as "solitary" nodules, or in such close association with others that "confluent" masses

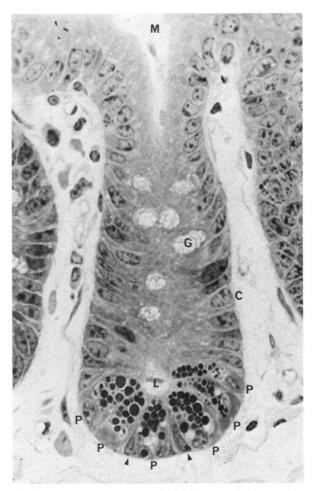

FIG. 21-37. Crypt of small intestine (mouse). From the base crowded with Paneth cells (P) to the mouth (M) of the crypts, cells are lined around a narrow lumen, part of which is shown in this section at the base (L). The Paneth cells of the crypt base are recognizable by their granules. Those Paneth cells that have small granules (as in the 2 cells at right) are younger than those with large granules. Between Paneth cells, small columnar cells are squeezed (arrowheads). Along the crypt walls, there are columnar cells (C) and mucous cells. The latter are recognized by light-staining groups of mucous globules (G). (H. Cheng, J. Merzel, and C. P. Leblond)

are formed. The possible function of lymphatic tissue in the lamina propria was discussed in the general plan.

Solitary lymphatic nodules may be present almost anywhere in the lamina propria in the small intestine. They range from $\frac{1}{2}$ to 3 mm. in width. The smaller ones are entirely confined to the lamina propria, but the larger ones may bulge through the muscularis mu-

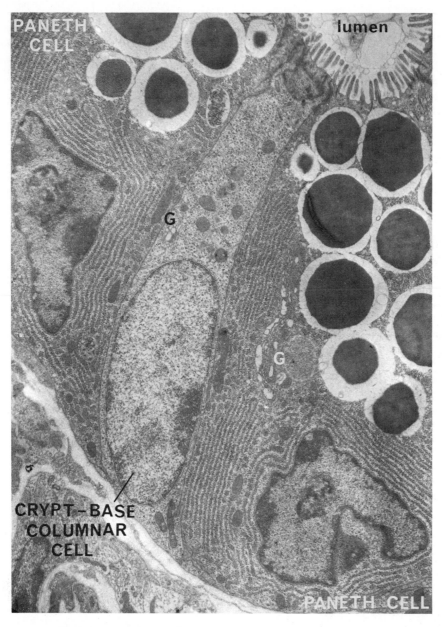

PANETH CELL

lumen

G

G

CRYPT-BASE COLUMNAR CELL

PANETH CELL

FIG. 21-38. Crypt base region, showing a small columnar cell intercalated between Paneth cells in mouse small intestine.

The crypt base columnar cell in the center of the figure has a regular nucleus and smooth lateral membranes. The cytoplasm is packed with free ribosomes, but otherwise contains a poorly developed Golgi (G) and few other organelles. This cell may be considered as being immature.

The cells on either side are Paneth cells characterized by their large granules, believed to be zymogenic. The one at right shows the irregular nucleus characterizing mature Paneth cells. The Golgi apparatus is extensive (G). To its right, a pale prosecretory granule separates it from the intensely dark secretory granules of the Paneth cell. (H. Cheng and C. P. Leblond)

cosae into the submucosa. The epithelium over them and the other tissues about them are usually infiltrated with lymphocytes derived from these nodules. When nodules are numerous, they tend to become confluent. The larger confluent masses have an elongated oval shape and are confined to the side of the intestine opposite the mesenteric attachment. They vary from 1 to 12 cm. in length and from 1 to 2½ cm. in width. They are called *Peyer's patches* after their discoverer. There are usually 20 to 30 of them, but more have been observed in young subjects. They are confined mostly to the lower part of the ileum, where they are largest, but they are also present in the upper part of the ileum and the lower part of the jejunum; they have even been observed in the lower part of the duodenum. Villi are usually absent over them. They were of particular interest when typhoid fever was a prevalent disease, for in this condition they exhibit a profound inflammatory reaction and are common sites of ulceration, hemorrhage and even of perforation. Like the lymphatic tissue as a whole, both the solitary and the confluent nodules become less prominent as an individual

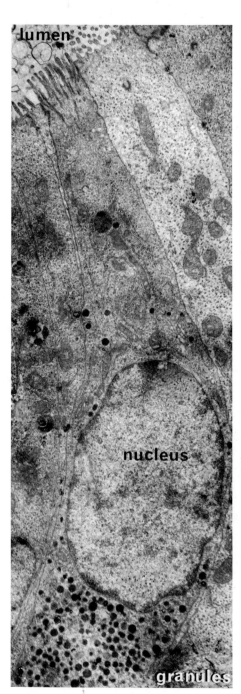

FIG. 21-39. Entero-endocrine cell of mouse small intestine, characterized by dense granules in the basal region and a narrow apex reaching the lumen.

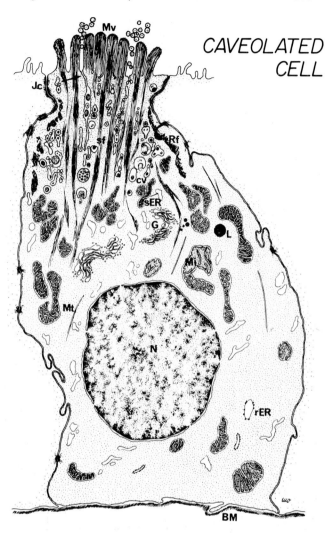

CAVEOLATED CELL

FIG. 21-40. Caveolated cell. This cell is found in stomach, and small and large intestine. It is the least common cell of the gastrointestinal tract and its function is unknown. It is characterized by: (a) caveolae, i.e., long irregular invaginations of the apical cell membrane opening between the bases of the microvilli (Mv) as shown at the arrow; most of the caveolae are seen in cross section as vesicular profiles of variable diameter; their lumens contain small spheres, which arise from polyplike expansions of the wall; the spheres are released from the caveolae between the microvilli and are seen next to their tips; (b) long and thick microvilli, the core of which consists of a bundle of straight filaments which extends deep into the supranuclear region; and (c) circular filaments around the apical region (Rf). (A. Nabeyama and C. P. Leblond)

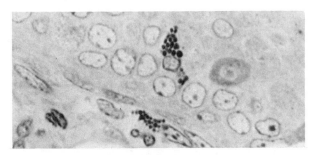

FIG. 21-41. Intestinal epithelium containing a globule leukocyte, recognized by large dense granules and a nucleus smaller than the nuclei of columnar cells nearby. Near the bottom of the illustration, the lamina propria contains a similar cell. This cell is often described as an atypical mast cell. (Illustration courtesy of Rosalie Alexander)

ages. In old age, Peyer's patches disappear almost completely.

The *muscularis mucosae* and the *submucosa* of the small intestine require no description other than that given in the general plan.

The *muscularis externa* of the small intestine exhibits no special features, but sections of the small intestine provide a good opportunity for the student to see and examine the ganglion cells and the nerve fibers of Auerbach's plexus, which is to be seen between the two muscle layers (Fig. 21-44).

Absorption From the Small Intestine. Under normal conditions, polysaccharides are broken down to disaccharides and monosaccharides in the lumen of the intestine. Monosaccharides are absorbed through the absorptive epithelial cells and into the blood capillaries

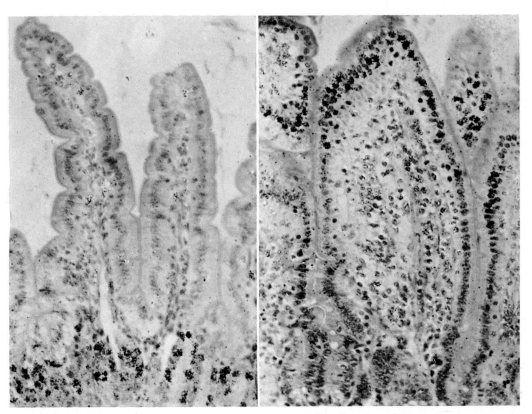

FIG. 21-42. H and E stained radioautographs of the jejunum of mice after ^{3}H-thymidine injection (1 month exposure, $\times$ about 150). At left, mouse sacrificed 8 hours, and, at right, 72 hours after injection.

At left, many clusters of silver grains are seen in the region of the crypts (exclusively over nuclei). At right, the clusters of silver grains are seen only in the epithelium of the upper third of the villi. From this region, a decreasing gradient of reaction extends along the epithelium down to the crypts. These radioautographs illustrate that many of the cells present in the crypts at the early time interval (*left*) eventually migrate to the tips of the villi (*right*). (Preparation from C. P. Leblond and B. Messier)

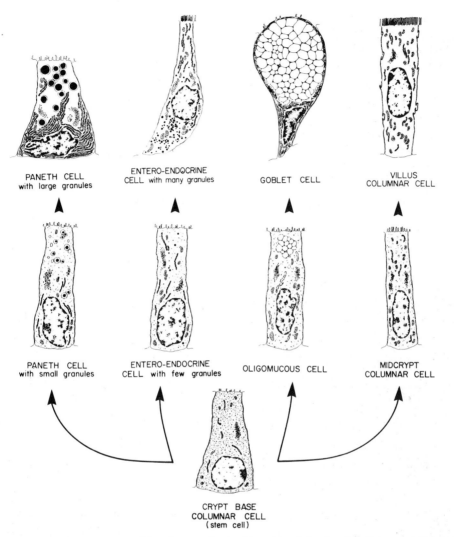

FIG. 21-43. Diagram summarizing the steps in the formation of the 4 main cell types of the small intestine. The top row shows mature cells; the second row, intermediate cell types; and the last row, a single cell, the crypt base columnar cell believed to be the "stem cell" of all cell types.

The crypt base columnar cell divides actively. As the diagram shows at left, a small proportion of the "cycling" cells acquire a few granules characteristic of either Paneth or entero-endocrine cells and later a full granule complement to become the corresponding mature cell. Some of the crypt base columnar cells acquire a few mucous globules (oligomucous cells in the third column); they retain the ability to divide and give rise to other mucous cells which accumulate more and more mucous globules. At about the time when the number of globules becomes large enough to distend the cell apex into a goblet, the ability to divide is lost. The majority of crypt base columnar cells give rise to the taller columnar cells found in the midcrypt region, as shown at right. These divide actively, giving rise to more and more columnar cells.

Paneth cells degenerate in about 3 weeks after they arise, but they do not leave the crypt base. The 3 other cell types are bound together by junctional complexes and desmosomes; they migrate together toward the villus tips where they are lost to the intestinal lumen. (Illustration courtesy of H. Cheng and C. P. Leblond)

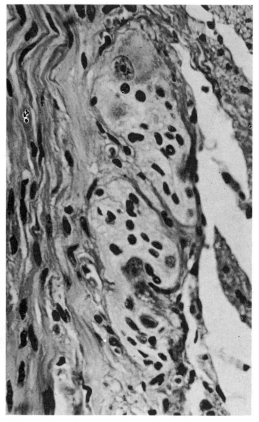

Fig. 21-44. High-power photomicrograph of a section of the small intestine of a child, showing a portion of Auerbach's plexus between the two layers of the muscularis externa. Note the large ganglion cell at the top. Its cytoplasm lies mostly above and to the right of its nucleus.

that are so close to them in the lamina propria. Probably some disaccharides are absorbed into the lining cells but are broken down in the cells to monosaccharides before they are delivered into capillaries. Proteins are absorbed as amino acids.

The digestion of fat in the intestine was described in Chapter 8 in connection with the account of adipose tissue. The role of the columnar absorptive cells of the small intestine in absorbing the products of the digestion of fat was also mentioned along with the formation of chylomicrons and their entrance into lymphatics. As was described there, it is well established that triglycerides as such are not taken up into columnar cells, but fatty acids, monoglycerides and possibly glycerol itself are. In the gut lumen, these substances are combined into 5-nm. particles (called micelles) which are produced under the influence of bile acids. There is discussion as to whether micelles are absorbed

as such by columnar cells or release their component fatty acids, monoglycerides and glycerol at the cell surface for absorption. It has been shown that, in their free or micellar state, these substances enter columnar cells readily by a diffusion process which does not require energy (taking place in vitro even at O°C. and in cells killed by heating); and, since this entry is not visible in the electron microscope, it is likely that the micelles are not taken up as such, but the free molecules themselves are involved in the absorption.

Once within the cells, fatty acids, monoglycerides and possibly glycerol find their way into the endoplasmic reticulum (both smooth and rough seem to be involved) where they are rebuilt into fats by a process that does require energy. The rebuilt fat is readily seen in the electron microscope within ER cisternae.

Some authors believe that the newly synthesized fat migrates from ER to Golgi and comes out of the Golgi in fat-containing vesicles which open by exocytosis at the *lateral* membranes and thus release their fat content to the intercellular spaces. Other authors deny the passage of fat through the Golgi apparatus, but all agree that the newly synthesized fat finds its way into the intercellular spaces.

The fat appearing outside the cell is readily seen in the electron microscope—for instance, one hour after a fatty meal. It is in the form of globules enclosed by a very delicate protein-containing membrane, the chylomicrons. The chylomicrons contain triglycerides, which make up 86 percent of their weight, and also 8.5 percent of phospholipids and 3 percent of cholesterol, as well as 2 percent of proteins (probably those associated with the membrane).

The chylomicrons then pass into the small lymphatic vessels of the lamina propria and, from there, mostly into the thoracic duct, which delivers them to the main circulation. Their fate was discussed in connection with mast cells in Chapter 9 and will be discussed further in connection with the liver in the next chapter.

The lymphatics that drain the intestine contain considerable amounts of emulsified fat after a fatty meal; this creamy lymph is termed *chyle*.

The Large Intestine

Parts. The large intestine consists of the cecum, the vermiform appendix, the ascending, transverse, descending and pelvic colons, and the rectum (including the anal canal). It terminates at the anus (Fig. 21-1).

Function. The unabsorbed contents of the small intestine are emptied into the cecum in a fluid state. By the time the contents reach the descending colon

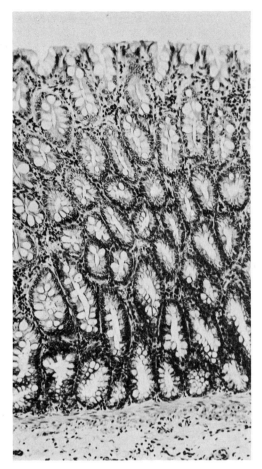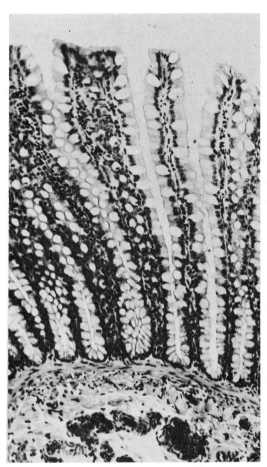

Fig. 21-45. Medium-power photomicrograph of sections of the wall of the large intestine, showing the mucous membrane. At the left, the crypts of Lieberkühn are cut in oblique section, and at the right, in longitudinal section. They are seen to extend down to the muscularis mucosae.

they have acquired the consistency of feces. Absorption of water by the mucous membrane is an important function of the large intestine.

Although a great deal of mucus is present in the alkaline secretion of the large intestine, no enzymes of importance are secreted with it. Nevertheless, some digestion occurs in the lumen. Part of this is due to enzymes derived from the small intestine remaining active in the material delivered into the large intestine, and part is to be explained by the putrefactive bacteria that thrive in its lumen, breaking down cellulose, which, if consumed in the diet, survives to reach the large intestine because no enzymes that attack it are liberated by the intestine of man.

Feces consist of bacteria, products of bacterial putrefaction, such undigested material as survives passage through the large intestine, cellular debris from the lining of the intestine, mucus and a few other substances.

Histologic Structure. The mucous membrane of the large intestine differs from that of the small intestine in many respects. It has no villi in postnatal life. It is thicker; hence the crypts of Lieberkühn are deeper (Fig. 21-45). The crypts, which are distributed all over the lining surface of the large intestine, contain no Paneth cells (except in the young), but they have more goblet cells than are present in the small intestine (Fig. 21-45). The ordinary surface epithelial cells have striated borders like those of the small intestine. Finally, entero-endocrine cells of the two main types are present.

Cell migration occurs in the large as well as in the small intestine, with the epithelial cells dividing in the lower half of the crypts and migrating from there to

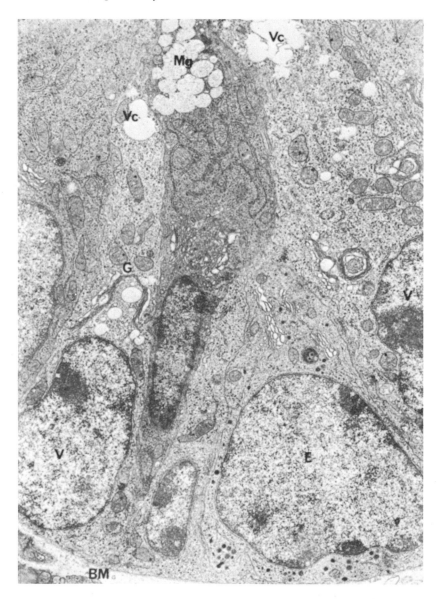

Fig. 21-46. Crypt base in descending colon. The columnar cells contain pale secretory vacuoles (Vc) and are often referred to as vacuolated cells (V). The Golgi apparatus (G) shows developing secretory vacuoles. The cytoplasm of these cells is lighter than that of the oligomucous cell seen in center and in which a small group of mucous globules (Mg) may be distinguished. At lower right, a young entero-endocrine cell (E) contains only a few dense granules.

As vacuolated cells migrate toward the crypt mouth, they become typical columnar cells with microvilli packed into a striated border. (A. K. Nabeyama)

the surface, where they are eventually extruded to the lumen.

At the base of the crypts in colon and rectum, there are immature-looking cells which are believed to function as stem cells for the epithelium. However, whereas the presumptive stem cells in the ascending colon appear to be small columnar cells, those of descending colon and rectum contain secretory vacuoles in their apex and, in fact, are often called vacuolated cells (Fig. 21-46). As these cells migrate toward the crypt mouth, they at first become filled with secretory vacuoles but, before approaching the surface, they lose all their vacuoles and become typical columnar cells with microvilli packed into a striated border (Chang and Leblond).

The crypts of Lieberkühn disappear in the anorectal canal at the junction of rectal and anal epithelium. The stratified squamous anal epithelium is not keratinized and extends over about 2 cm. At its outer border it becomes continuous with the keratinized epidermis of the skin and on its inner border with the columnar epithelium that lines the remainder of the rectum. At the junction between anal and columnar epithelium, circumanal glands are present. These glands have a stratified columnar epithelium and are of the branched tubular type but do not seem to be actively functioning. They probably constitute an atrophic organ, reminding one of the actively functioning glands of certain mammals.

In the anorectal canal, the mucous membrane is thrown into a series of longitudinal folds known as the *rectal columns* or *columns of Morgagni.* Below, adjacent columns are connected by folds. This arrangement produces a series of so-called anal valves. The concavities of the pockets so formed are called rectal sinuses.

The muscularis mucosae continues only to the region of the longitudinal folds, and in them it breaks up into bundles and finally disappears. Hence there is not the same demarcation between lamina propria and submucosa in this region as in other parts of the tract. The merging lamina propria and submucosa contain many convolutions of small veins. A very common condition, *internal hemorrhoids,* is the result of the dilatation of these veins so that they bulge the mucous membrane inward and encroach on the lumen of the anal canal. External hemorrhoids result from the dilatation of veins at, and close to, the anus.

Muscularis Externa. In the large intestine this layer differs somewhat from its arrangement in other parts of the tract. Beginning in the cecum, the longitudinally disposed fibers of the outer coat, though

present to a certain extent over the whole circumference of the bowel, are for the most part collected into three flat bands, the *teniae coli*. These are not as long as the intestine along which they are disposed; hence, they are responsible for gathering the wall of this part of the bowel into sacculations or haustra (Fig. 21-1). If the teniae are cut or stripped away, the bowel immediately elongates, and the sacculations disappear. The three teniae extend from the cecum to the rectum, where they spread out and fuse to some extent so as to form a muscle coat that is thicker on the anterior and the posterior aspects of the rectum than on its sides. The anterior and the posterior aggregates of longitudinally disposed smooth muscle are somewhat shorter than the rectum itself, and this results in a type of sacculation in this region; this causes the underlying wall of the rectum to bulge inward to form two transverse shelves, one from the right and a smaller one from the left, called the *plicae transversales* of the rectum. These help to support the weight of the rectal contents and so make the work of the anal sphincter less arduous.

The circularly disposed smooth muscle fibers of the inner coat of the muscularis externa form a thicker coat between sacculations than they do over the sacculations. In the anal canal they are increased to form

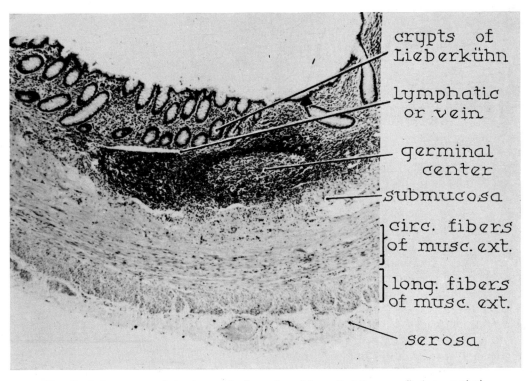

Fig. 21-47. Low-power photomicrograph of a portion of the wall of the appendix (cross section).

a sphincter muscle, the internal sphincter of the anus.

Serosa. Along the colon and the upper part of the rectum, the serous coat leaves the surface of the intestine at irregular intervals to form little peritoneal sacs that enclose fat. These peritoneal redundancies hang from the external surface of the bowel and are termed *appendices epiploicae.* In some sites they contain only areolar tissue.

Vermiform Appendix. This wormlike appendage of the cecum (Fig. 21-1) is the seat of so much disease that it merits a separate description. Developmentally, it is the lower, blind end of the cecum that has failed to enlarge as rapidly as the remainder, and as a result it appears as a diverticulum arising from the cecum an inch or less below the entrance of the ileum. In many lower animals it is larger than it is in man and so provides a good-sized pouch off the main track of the intestine where cellulose can be subjected to prolonged digestion. In man it is too short and has too narrow a lumen to serve a similar function. Indeed, its form is commonly so bent and twisted that there is grave danger of bacterial activity destroying not only the contents of the lumen but also the lining of the organ itself. As a result, organisms sometimes gain entrance to the tissues of its wall and lead to its infection. For this reason, surgical removal of the infected organ is one of the commonest abdominal operations.

The appendix usually is studied microscopically by means of cross sections (Fig. 21-47). In preparations of this sort, the lumen of the appendix of a young person often has a somewhat 3-horned instead of a circular appearance. In adults it is usually rounder, and in advancing years it may be obliterated by connective tissue's replacing the mucous membrane as well as filling the lumen.

The epithelium of the mucous membrane is similar to that of the large intestine (Fig. 21-47). However, the lamina propria contains much more lymphatic tissue; indeed, confluent lymphatic nodules may completely surround the lumen, though the amount diminishes with age. The muscularis mucosae is not well developed and may be missing in some areas. A few eosinophils are normal constituents of the lamina propria but, if present in the submucosa, are considered as being of some significance in indicating a chronic inflammatory condition of the organ. Neutrophils in any numbers in the lamina propria or any other layer indicate an acute inflammatory lesion (acute appendicitis). The muscularis externa shows no deviation from the general plan found in the intestine, and the longitudinal fibers form a complete coat. The appendix has a rudimentary mesentery.

References and Other Reading

THE ORAL CAVITY AND SALIVARY GLANDS

For Taste Buds *see* Chapter 28.
For Teeth *see* a following section.
Dewey, M. M.: A histochemical and biochemical study of the parotid gland in normal and hypophysectomized rats. Am. J. Anat., *102:*243, 1958.
Gairns, F. W.: The sensory nerve endings of the human palate. Quart. J. Exp. Physiol., *40:*40, 1955.
Jacoby, F., and Leeson, C. R.: The post-natal development of the rat submaxillary gland. J. Anat., *93:*201, 1959.
James, J.: Epithelium and lymphocyte in the development of the palatine tonsil. Acta anat., *27:*222, 1955.
Leeson, C. R., and Jacoby, F.: An electron microscope study of the rat submaxillary gland during its postnatal development and in the adult. J. Anat., *93:*287, 1959.
Parks, H. F.: Morphological study of the extrusion of secretory materials by the parotid glands of mouse and rat. J. Ultrastruct. Res., *6:*449, 1962.
Scott, B. L., and Pease, D. C.: Electron microscopy of the salivary and lacrimal glands of the rat. Am. J. Anat., *104:*115, 1959.
Travill, A.: The effect of pregnancy on the submandibular glands of mice. Anat. Rec., *155:*217, 1966.
Travill, A. A., and Hill, M. F.: Histochemical demonstration of myoepithelial cell activity. Quart. J. Exp. Physiol., *48:*423, 1963.

SOME GENERAL REFERENCES ON TEETH

Books and Symposia

Anderson, D. J., Estoe, J. E., Melcher, A. H., and Picton, D. C. A. (eds.): The Mechanism of Tooth Support—A Symposium. Bristol, England, John Wright and Sons, 1967.
Gaunt, W. A., Osborne, J. W., and Ten Cate, A. R.: Advances in Dental Histology. Bristol, England, John Wright and Sons, 1967.
Stack, M. V., and Fernhead, R. W. (ed.): Tooth Enamel. Its Composition, Properties and Fundamental Structure. Bristol, England, John Wright and Sons, 1965.
Symons, N. B. B. (ed.): Dentine and Pulp: Their Structure and Reactions. Edinburgh, E. & S. Livingstone, 1967.

See also textbooks of dental histology and oral histology.

SOME FURTHER REFERENCES ON TEETH

Bélanger, L. F.: Autoradiographic and histochemical observations on the mineralization of teeth in rats and hamsters of various ages. Anat. Rec., *114:*529, 1952.
Bélanger, L. F., and Leblond, C. P.: Mineralization of the growing tooth as shown by radiophosphorus autographs. Proc. Soc. Exp. Biol. Med., *73:*390, 1950.
Bevelander, G., and Johnson, P. L.: Alkaline phosphatase in amelogenesis. Anat. Rec., *104:*125, 1949.
Garant, P. R., and Nalbandian, J.: Observations on the ultrastructure of ameloblasts with special reference to the Golgi complex and related components. J. Ultrastruct. Res., *23:*427, 1968.
Garant, P., Szabo, G., and Nalbandian, J.: The fine structure of the mouse odontoblast. Arch. Oral Biol., *13:*857, 1968.

Kallenbach, E.: The cell web in the ameloblasts of the rat incisor. Anat. Rec., *153:*55, 1963.

Leblond, C. P., Bélanger, L. F., and Greulich, R. C.: Formation of bones and teeth as visualized by radioautography. Ann. N.Y. Acad. Sci., *60:*629, 1955.

Reith, E. J.: The ultrastructure of ameloblasts during early stages of maturation of enamel. J. Cell Biol., *18:*691, 1963.

———: Collagen formation in developing molar teeth of rats. J. Ultrastruct. Res., *21:*383, 1968.

Schour, I., and Massler, M.: Studies in tooth development; the growth pattern of human teeth. J. Am. Dent. Assoc., *27:*1778; *27:*1918, 1940.

Slaven, H. C., and Bavetta, L. A. (eds.): Developmental Aspects of Oral Biology. New York, Academic Press, 1972.

Warshawsky, H.: The fine structure of secretory ameloblasts in rat incisors. Anat. Rec., *161:*211, 1968.

———: A light and electron microscope study of the nearly mature enamel of rat incisors. Anat. Rec., *169:*559, 1971.

Weinstock, A.: Elaboration of enamel and dentin matrix glycoproteins. *In* Bourne, G. H. (ed.): The Biochemistry and Physiology of Bone. vol. 11. Physiology and Pathology. p. 121. New York and London, Academic Press, 1972.

Weinstock, M., and Leblond, C. P.: Radioautographic visualization of the deposition of a phosphoprotein at the mineralization front in the dentin of the rat incisor. J. Cell Biol., *56:*838, 1973.

———: Synthesis, migration and release of precursor collagen by odontoblasts as visualized by radioautography after ^{3}H-proline administration. J. Cell Biol., *60:*92, 1974.

SOME REFERENCES ON ESOPHAGUS AND STOMACH

Bensley, R. R.: The gastric glands. *In* Cowdry's Special Cytology. ed. 2, p. 197. New York, Hoeber, 1932.

Bertalanffy, F. D.: Cell renewal in the gastrointestinal tract of man. Gastroenterology, *43:*472, 1962.

Davenport, H. W.: Physiology of the Digestive Tract. ed. 2. Chicago, Year Book Medical Publishers, 1965.

———: Why the stomach does not digest itself. Sci. Am., *226:*86, 1972.

Ito, S.: The fine structure of the gastric mucosa. *In* Proc. Symp. Gastric Secretion; Mechanisms and Control. p. 3. Oxford, Pergamon Press, 1967.

———: Anatomic structure of the gastric mucosa. *In* American Physiological Society: Handbook of Physiology. Section 6 (Cole, C. F., ed.): Alimentary Canal. vol. 2, p. 705. Baltimore, Williams & Wilkins, 1967.

Ito, S., and Winchester, R. J.: The fine structure of the gastric mucosa in the bat. J. Cell Biol., *16:*541, 1963.

Marques-Pereira, J. P., and Leblond, C. P.: Mitosis and differentiation in the stratified squamous epithelium of the rat esophagus. Am. J. Anat., *117:*73, 1965.

Sedar, A. W.: The fine structure of the oxyntic cell in relation to functional activity of the stomach. Ann. N.Y. Acad. Sci., *99:*9, 1962.

———: Stomach and intestinal mucosa. *In* Electron Microscope Anatomy. p. 123. New York, Academic Press, 1964.

SOME REFERENCES ON THE SMALL AND LARGE INTESTINE

Altmann, G. G., and Enesco, M.: Cell number as a measure of distribution and renewal of epithelial cells in the small intestine of growing and adult rats. Am. J. Anat., *120:*319, 1967.

Bertalanffy, F. D., and Nagy, K. P.: Mitotic activity and renewal rate of the epithelial cells of human duodenum. Acta anat., *45:*362, 1961.

Cardell, R. R., Jr., Badenhausen, S., and Porter, K. R.: Intestinal triglyceride absorption in the rat. J. Cell Biol., *34:*123, 1967.

Chang, W. W. L., and Leblond, C. P.: Renewal of the epithelium in the descending colon of the mouse. I. Presence of three cell populations: vacuolated-columnar, mucous, and argentaffin. Am. J. Anat., *131:*73, 1971.

Creamer, B.: Variations in small-intestinal villous shape and mucosal dynamics. Brit. Med. J., *2:*1371, 1964.

Ferreira, M. N., and Leblond, C. P.: Argentaffin and other "endocrine" cells of the small intestine in the adult mouse. II. Renewal. Am. J. Anat., *131:*331, 1971.

Granger, B., and Baker, R. F.: Electron microscope investigation of the striated border of intestinal epithelium. Anat. Rec., *107:*423, 1950.

Grossman, M. I.: The glands of Brunner. Physiol. Rev., *38:*675, 1958.

Hally, A. D.: The fine structure of the Paneth Cell. J. Anat., *92:*268, 1958.

Irwin, D. A.: The anatomy of Auerbach's plexus. Am. J. Anat., *49:*141, 1931.

Kirkman, H.: The anal canal of the rhesus monkey with emphasis upon a description of bipolar, argyrophile cells in the zona columnaris. Am. J. Anat., *88:*177, 1951.

Landboe-Christensen, E.: The Duodenal Glands of Brunner in Man: Their Distribution and Quantity; An Anatomical Study. London, Oxford, 1944.

Leblond, C. P., and Messier, B.: Renewal of chief cells and goblet cells in the small intestine as shown by radioautography after injection of thymidine-H^3 into mice. Anat. Rec., *132:*247, 1958.

Leblond, C. P., and Stevens, C. E.: The constant renewal of the intestinal epithelium in the albino rat. Anat. Rec., *100:*357, 1948.

Leblond, C. P., and Walker, B. E.: Renewal of cell populations. Physiol. Rev., *36:*255, 1956.

Lesher, S., Fry, R. J. M., and Cohn, H. I.: Age and degeneration time of the mouse duodenal epithelial cell. Exp. Cell Res., *24:*334, 1961.

Lipkin, M., Sherlock, P., and Bell, B.: Cell proliferation kinetics in the gastrointestinal tract of man. II. Cell renewal in stomach, ileum, colon, and rectum. Gastroenterology, *45:*721, 1963.

McMinn, R. M. H., and Mitchell, J. E.: The formation of villi following artificial lesions of the mucosa in the small intestine of the cat. J. Anat., *88:*99, 1954.

Merzel, J., and Leblond, C. P.: Origin and renewal of goblet cells in the epithelium of the mouse small intestine. Am. J. Anat., *124:*281, 1969.

Moe, H.: The goblet cells, Paneth cells and basal granular cells of the epithelium of the intestine. Int. Rev. Gen. Exp. Zool., *3:*241, 1968.

Neutra, M., and Leblond, C. P.: Synthesis of the carbohydrate of mucus in the Golgi complex, as shown by electron microscope radioautography of goblet cells from rats injected with ^{3}H-glucose. J. Cell Biol., *30:*119, 1966.

Palay, S. L., and Karlin, L.: Absorption of fat by jejunal epithelium in the rat. Anat. Rec., *124:*343, 1956.

————: An electron microscopic study of the intestinal villus. I. The fasting animal. J. Biophys. Biochem. Cytol., *5*:363, 1959.

Palay, S. L., and Revel, J. P.: The morphology of fat absorption. *In* Meng, H. C.: Lipid transport. pp. 1-11. Springfield, Ill., C. C Thomas, 1964.

Quastler, H., and Sherman, F. G.: Cell population kinetics in the intestinal epithelium of the mouse. Exp. Cell Res., *17:* 420, 1959.

Richardson, K. C.: Electron microscopic observations on Auerbach's plexus in the rabbit, with special reference to the problem of smooth muscle innervation. Am. J. Anat., *103:* 99, 1958.

Spencer, R. P.: The Intestinal Tract; Structure, Function and Pathology in Terms of the Basic Sciences. Springfield, Ill., Charles C Thomas, 1960.

Strauss, E. W.: Morphological Aspects of Triglyceride Absorption. *In* Codel, C. F., and Heidel, W. (eds.): Handbook of Physiology. vol. 3, sec. 6, chap. 71. American Physiological Society, Washington, 1968.

Trier, J. S.: Studies on small intestinal crypt epithelium of the proximal small intestine of fasting humans. J. Cell Biol., *18:*599, 1963.

Weirnik, G., Shroter, R. G., and Creamer, B.: The arrest of intestinal epithelial "turnover" by the use of x-irradiation. Gut, *3:*26, 1962.

22 Pancreas, Liver and Gallbladder

The Pancreas

Introduction. The pancreas is a large and important gland. It lies in the abdomen with its head resting in the concavity of the duodenum and its body extending toward the spleen, which its tail touches (Fig. 21-1). A fresh pancreas is white with a pink tinge. With the naked eye its surface appears lobulated; it lacks a sufficiently substantial capsule to obscure the structure beneath it.

The pancreas is both an exocrine and an endocrine gland. The bulk of its cells are arranged in acini (Fig. 5-23) which produce its exocrine secretion. This is collected and delivered by a duct system into the second part of the duodenum. The functions of the pancreatic secretion in digestion have already been described. The endocrine secretion of the pancreas is made by little clumps of cells, richly supplied with capillaries, that are scattered throughout its substance (Fig. 22-1, islet) and are surrounded by exocrine glandular tissue. Hence these little endocrine units are appropriately termed *islets* and are named after Langerhans, who described them. The first hormone shown to be produced by the *islets of Langerhans* was called *insulin* (*insula,* an island). The insufficient production of this hormone leads to the development of diabetes mellitus, a disease that will be described when the islets of Langerhans are discussed in detail in Chapter 25 which deals with endocrine glands. The production of a second hormone, *glucagon* (also discussed in Chapter 25), has subsequently been attributed to the islets.

Development. The pancreas develops from 2 diverticula (outgrowths) that arise from the epithelial (endodermal) lining of the developing duodenum. The way that the respective parts of the pancreas develop from these 2 outgrowths is described in texts of embryology and gross anatomy, as is the way the duct system develops to drain different parts of the pancreas. In histology we are concerned with the fact that the developing duct system gives rise both to acini whose exocrine secretion drains into the duct system, and to little islands of cells that will be endocrine units and empty their secretion into the bloodstream.

The clumps of cells that arise from the developing duct system and are destined to become islets fail to develop a lumen. In many instances, though by no means always, these clumps of cells become completely detached from the duct system proper to become truly isolated islets of Langerhans. It should be mentioned, moreover, that the developing duct system gives rise to an ill-defined network of cords or tubules of cells that become disposed irregularly through the substance of the pancreas between acini. The cells of this network are relatively undifferentiated, and under certain circumstances they appear to give rise to new endocrine cells. This is the probable origin of those islet cells that sometimes seem to be scattered singly among the acini.

MICROSCOPIC STRUCTURE

Capsule. The connective tissue capsule that separates the pancreatic tissue from adjacent structures is remarkably thin; indeed it scarcely merits being called a capsule. The capsule is covered with peritoneum.

Septa. Partitions (septa) of connective tissue extend in from the capsule to divide the pancreas into lobules. These septa, like the capsule, are very thin (Fig. 22-1, interlob. septum). Furthermore, separation commonly occurs along them when pancreatic tissue is fixed. Consequently, in sections the lobules commonly are often clearly indicated because they are separated from one another by fissures of the nature of artifacts.

Although the septa are thin, there are considerable condensations of dense connective tissue often present around the main duct of the organ and its more immediate branches (Fig. 22-1, interlob. duct). These provide some internal support.

Acini. After the student has seen capsule, septa and ducts surrounded by connective tissue, he should next examine acini; these comprise most of the substance of lobules. The easiest way to find individual acini with the microscope was described in Chapter 5 in connection with Figure 5-23.

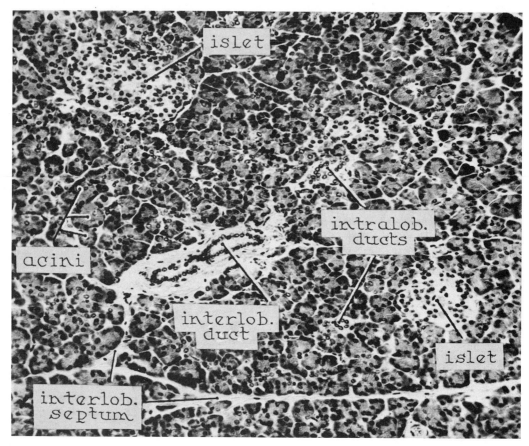

Fig. 22-1. Very low-power photomicrograph of a section of the pancreas, showing 2 islets, a large interlobular duct and smaller intralobular ducts, many acini and an interlobular septum.

Within the lobule acini are packed together in a most irregular way, with only a little reticular tissue which contains capillaries between them, so that a microtome knife in cutting a section of pancreas cuts across acini in almost every conceivable plane. Most, of course, are cut in oblique section. In many sections of pancreas the acini do not stand out at all clearly as individual structures. If you have difficulty in deciding just what constitutes an acinus, refer back to Figure 5-23. It may also be helpful to realize that under the high-power objective an acinus is approximately a tenth of the field in width. And since the nuclei of the secretory cells that make up the acinus lie toward their bases, the nuclei in a single acinus tend to be arranged so as to form a rough ring of nuclei in its outer part (Fig. 22-2).

The sides of the more or less pyramidal cells that are fitted together to form acini are so close together that cell boundaries between individual cells are not always distinct in the LM (Fig. 22-2). The apices of the cells of an acinus do not quite come together in the central part of each acinus; hence, a very small lumen is present in this site (Fig. 5-23). The cytoplasm between the nucleus and the apex of each secretory cell contains acidophilic zymogen granules (partly closing the condenser diaphragm may facilitate seeing these if they are not well stained). They are stained well in Figure 22-3. The nuclei are rounded and lie toward but not against the bases of the cells. They exhibit prominent nucleoli. The cytoplasm between the nuclei and the bases of the cells, as well as that on each side of the nuclei, is commonly basophilic because of its content of cytoplasmic RNA (Figs. 22-2 and 22-3), as might be expected in a cell that is synthesizing a great deal of protein (the zymogen granules which are secreted day by day are protein).

Centro-acinar Cells. Nuclei surrounded by pale-staining cytoplasm can often be seen in the central part of an acinus (Fig. 22-2). These are the nuclei of what are appropriately termed centro-acinar cells. If

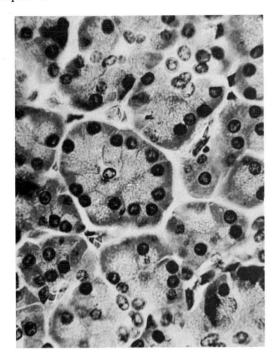

FIG. 22-2. High-power photomicrograph of a section of the pancreas, showing an acinus with the nucleus of a centro-acinar cell appearing in its center.

an acinus is cut in the proper plane (which happens once in a while), these cells can be seen to better advantage as being the cells of the little duct that drains the acinus (Fig. 22-3). The duct cells do not begin at an end of an acinus; the first ones, on what would seem to be one side of the little duct, are more or less invaginated into the lumen of the acinus on one side, as is shown in Figure 22-3. Since the duct cells thus begin in the center of an acinus, they are termed centro-acinar cells.

FINE STRUCTURE

The Fine Structure of Acinar Cells. This, together with the mechanism of secretion was dealt with in detail in Chapter 5 and illustrated in Figures 5-23 and 5-26, so this matter need not be considered further here. We shall, however, consider briefly some features of the acinus as a whole that have been revealed by the EM.

The Fine Structure of Certain Other Features of Acini. The junctional complexes between the borders of adjacent acinar cells close to the lumen of an acinus are illustrated in Figure 22-4. They are believed to be of the same type as those between the lining cells of the intestine, that is, there are zonulae occludentes

between the sides of their apices, and these are followed by zonulae adherentes and then desmosomes between the adjacent cell membranes deeper down toward the bases of the cells. Figure 22-4 also shows zymogen granules about to be secreted in the apices of acinar cells, and also that the centro-acinar cell in the illustration contains no zymogen granules; it is a duct type of cell. Both the centro-acinar cells and acinar cells reveal some short microvilli on their free borders (Fig. 22-4).

A delicate reticular connective tissue fills the space between individual acini and brings capillaries close to the bases of the secretory cells which are covered with a thin basement membrane (Fig. 22-3). Some of the capillaries have fenestrated endothelium. Nerve fibers of the autonomic system are also conducted in this reticular connective tissue.

Finding Islets of Langerhans. If in H and E sections enough lobules are inspected with the low-power objective, pale areas considerably larger than cross or oblique sections of acini will be seen (Fig. 22-1). These areas are *islets of Langerhans* and contain cords and irregular clumps of cells and capillaries. Red blood cells are present in the capillaries commonly enough for the capillaries to appear, even with the low-power objective, as pink or red streaks. However, it takes some practice to identify islets readily with the low-power objective; a beginner may confuse an islet with a duct or a little patch of connective tissue. With the high-power objective, the usual islet is a quarter to a half or more of the field in width, and its characteristic structure of cords and clumps of cells separated by capillaries can be seen clearly. Islets are *not* encapsulated and so are separated from acinar tissue by only

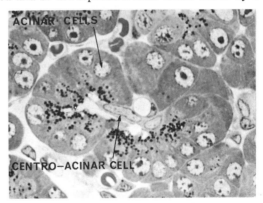

FIG. 22-3. Photomicrograph of a section of pancreas stained with toluidine blue. The section cut the acinus that is shown in such a way as to show a centro-acinar cell clearly and the beginning of the duct. Zymogen granules are stained and visible in the acinar cells. (Photomicrograph courtesy of Y. Clermont)

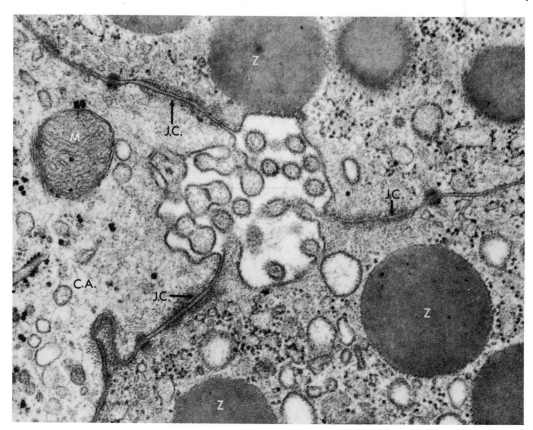

Fig. 22-4. Electron micrograph ($\times$ 50,000) of section cut through the lumen of a pancreatic acinus of a guinea pig. In the center, microvilli are seen projecting into the lumen. The cell at the left is a centro-acinar cell (C.A.); it is distinguished most readily by the fact that it contains no zymogen granules (Z) as do the other two cells whose apices abut on the lumen; it does, however, contain a mitochondrion. At the top a zymogen granule is about to be secreted. Junctional complexes (J.C.) are present at each site where the membranes of adjacent cells come into contact close to the lumen. (These are described in detail in Chap. 5.) (Farquhar, M. G., and Palade, G. E.: J. Cell Biol., *17*:375)

a film of reticular tissue. Internal support in islets is provided by reticular fibers that are associated with capillaries. But there is not much connective tissue in islets; otherwise, the secretion of the cells would have difficulty gaining entrance to the capillaries.

How the Amount of Islet Tissue in a Pancreas Is Determined. Any estimate of the relative amount of islet tissue made from a single section of any given pancreas has little more authority than a guess. The total number of islets and the total extent of islet tissue can be determined by cutting a whole pancreas into serial sections of known thickness and measuring the area of islets seen in each and every section. This, of course, is an enormous task. R. Bensley many years ago described a much simpler method. He perfused the blood vessels of the fresh organ with dilute solutions of either neutral red or Janus green. As reduction occurs on standing, the dye fades from the acinar tissue, so that the islets stand out as either red or blue areas, depending on the dye used (Fig. 22-5). Pancreas so prepared is cut into little pieces that can be mounted on slides, and a group of observers can soon count the number of islets in all the pieces and so determine the number of islets in the pancreas. Haist and Pugh devised a more elaborate technic based on the same staining principles; this permits them to estimate not only the number of islets in a pancreas but also the total volume of islet tissue.

The different types of cells in islets and their appearance in different physiologic states will be described in Chapter 25.

Ducts. Before describing the appearance of ducts

seen in a section of pancreas under low-power magnification, a few words about their general arrangement are in order. The main duct of the pancreas, the duct of Wirsung, is enveloped by connective tissue and serves more or less as a "backbone" for the organ through which it runs. From it, side branches emerge regularly at angles, so that the duct system, stripped clean of other tissues, resembles a herring bone. The side branches of the main duct run between lobules and hence are interlobular ducts. These branch to give rise to intralobular ducts which enter the substance of lobules. Intralobular ducts are not nearly so prominent in the pancreas as they are in salivary glands. A relative absence of clean-cut intralobular ducts is, then, an important criterion by which a student can quickly distinguish a section of pancreas from that of parotid gland. The presence of islets of Langerhans in the lobules is, of course, another, but in some preparations more than a glance is needed before islets can be identified with certainty.

The larger of the relatively few intralobular ducts can be seen under low power to be ensheathed by dense connective tissue derived from the septa from which they emerge (Fig. 22-1). The intralobular ducts give rise to very small ducts lined with flattened epithelium. These small ducts lead to the acini and are called *intercalated* (*intercalare,* to insert) *ducts* because they are inserted between the secretory units and the intralobular ducts proper. As noted before, the intercalated ducts often extend into the central part of acini to be known as centro-acinar cells (Figs. 22-2, 22-3 and 22-4).

The lumen of the main duct may be as much as $2\frac{1}{2}$ mm. wide. It is lined by columnar epithelium. Goblet cells may be interspersed between the ordinary columnar cells. Near the duodenum, small mucous glands may be associated with the main duct. The interlobular ducts are lined by low columnar epithelium. In the intralobular ducts, the epithelium is low columnar to cuboidal, and in the intercalated ducts, flattened cuboidal.

CONTROL OF EXOCRINE SECRETION

Since the pancreatic juice contains so many important enzymes needed to carry on the further digestion of food that has passed through the stomach, the need for some mechanism to regulate pancreatic secretion in accordance with deliveries of food into the duodenum from the stomach is obvious. Such a mechanism exists in the form of two hormones made by the mucosa of the duodenum when the acid contents of the stomach are delivered into it. The hormones circulate

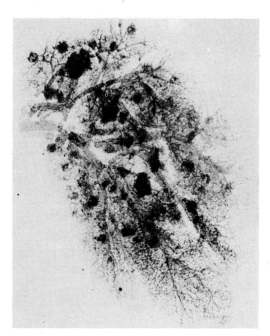

FIG. 22-5. Very low-power photomicrograph of a piece of a guinea pig's pancreas perfused with Janus green. The blood vessels subsequently were injected with carmine gelatin. The islets appear as dark patches, and the reticulated appearance of the background is due to the injected blood vessels. (Preparation of S. H. Bensley)

by the bloodstream to the capillaries of the pancreas and somehow stimulate secretion by duct cells and acinar cells.

Stimulation by *secretin* is chiefly manifested by its stimulating the secretion of the nonenzymatic ingredients of pancreatic juice so its action may be primarily on the cells of the small ducts. The second hormone, *pancreozymin,* has been shown to be much more effective than secretin in stimulating the secretion of enzyme-rich pancreatic juice, and so it is believed to act on acinar cells. Stimulation of the vagus nerve induces some secretion, but the control of secretion seems to be primarily hormonal.

MAINTENANCE OF THE ACINAR CELL POPULATION

It might be thought that acinar cells are such highly specialized secretory cells that they would have lost their ability to divide and that the formation of more of them would have to depend on the proliferation and subsequent differentiation of duct cells. However, in studies on diabetes induced with diabetogenic anterior pituitary extracts, Ham and Haist described and illustrated very numerous mitotic figures in the acinar

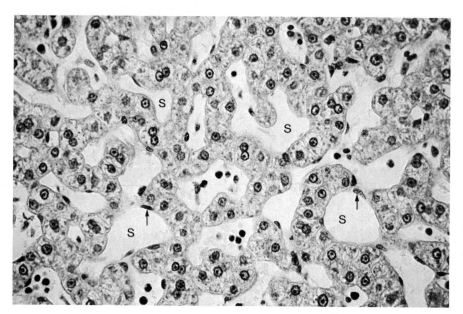

FIG. 22-6. Photomicrograph of an H and E section of human liver taken from an area where the sinusoids were somewhat distended and hence the liver cords were spread apart farther than is usual. Note that the cords are continuous with one another and hence that they always surround the sinusoids some of which are labeled with an S. The nuclei of endothelial cells lining sinusoids are indicated by arrows. Note that some liver cords appear to be one cell wide, some two cells wide, and some thicker still. (Illustration courtesy of H. Whittaker)

cells as well as in duct cells. This effect was probably due to the growth hormone in the extracts that were used. It therefore seems conceivable that under ordinary conditions mitosis occurs in acinar cells to replenish their numbers if others wear out.

The Liver

Some Gross Features. The liver is the largest gland in the body, weighing in the adult about 3 pounds. It performs both exocrine and endocrine functions. Its exocrine secretion is bile. Its endocrine function will be described later.

The liver is reddish brown. Most of it lies on the right side with its upper convex surface fitting the undersurface of the dome-shaped diaphragm (Fig. 21-1). It has 2 main lobes; the right is much larger than the left (Fig. 21-1). Its inferior surface is exposed in Figure 21-1 showing the impressions of the several organs which it normally contacts (parts of the alimentary tract and the right kidney, which are separated from it in Fig. 21-1), so its inferior surface is often called its visceral surface. This surface exhibits a short deep transverse fissure called the *porta* (door) of the liver (not shown in Fig. 21-1).

The Study of Liver With the LM

The liver, as we shall see, is both an exocrine and an endocrine gland and like other glands it is made up of a parenchyma and a stroma. The former is epithelial in nature and derived from entoderm. The

stroma is composed of connective tissue and is derived from mesoderm.

The Parenchyma. In the first chapter of this book the parenchymal cell of the liver was used as an example to describe and illustrate certain features of cells in general and also as an example of a kind of cell that can be found easily with the microscope by a beginner. In that chapter the parenchymal cells were termed liver cells. In our present study of the liver as an organ we shall refer to the parenchymal cells of the liver as *hepatocytes*.

As was pointed out in early chapters an examination of an H and E section of liver shows the hepatocytes to be arranged in what appear to be rows (also called cords) of cells that in a section often appear to be of only one cell in width. They commonly anastomose with one another as is shown in Figure 22-6 thus surrounding what were termed blood passageways in Figure 1-10. Here we shall refer to the blood passageways as liver sinusoids. Liver sinusoids are tubes that are wider than capillaries and their walls, as will be described in detail later on, are made up of two kinds of cells. One kind are similar to endothelial cells and the other kind are phagocytic and of the order of macrophages. It is by means of the sinusoids that blood circulates through the liver so that the hepatocytes of the cords have a means of obtaining nutrients and disposing of waste products as well as secreting certain of their products into the bloodstream in connection with their endocrine function.

In order to explain how the hepatocytes perform their exocrine function we have to do two things. First we have to discuss the stroma of the liver and second, we have to modify somewhat our conception of liver cords. We shall perform these tasks in that order.

The Stroma of the Liver. This consists of two main parts. First, the liver is covered with a thin connective tissue capsule (of Glisson) which contains regularly arranged collagenic fibers and scattered fibroblasts; this in turn is covered with a layer of mesothelial cells. Second, at the hilus of the liver the connective tissue of the capsule extends like the trunk of a tree into the parenchyma of the liver. In the parenchyma this tree of conective tissue branches very extensively, with branches extending in so many different directions that no parts of the liver parenchyma is ever farther than a millimeter away from one or more of these branches. Since these branches pursue somewhat irregular courses, thin slices cut for microscopic study commonly cut them in cross or oblique section and so they appear under the low or high power of the LM as little, more or less triangular patches of connective tissue which commonly contain what appear to be four holes. One is shown at the left side of the top illustration in Figure 22-7 and another in more detail in the lower left picture. These holes are the lumens of tubes that are housed in all branches of the connective tissue tree and this permits branches of these four kinds of tubes to reach all parts of the liver. The nature of these tubes will now be described.

The Tubes in Portal Tracts. The blood supply of the liver is derived from two sources. First, the greater part of it is derived from the portal vein which drains the food-laden blood from the intestine to the liver, since the portal vein is a large vein, the largest tube seen in every branch of the connective tissue tree is a branch of the portal vein. This is labeled PV in Figure 22-7, *left top* and *bottom left,* where it is shown at greater magnification. The second part of the blood supply of the liver is arterial blood, which is conveyed into the liver by branches of the hepatic artery. These, of course, have much smaller lumens than the branches of the portal vein as can be seen clearly in Figure 22-7, *bottom left,* where the branch of the hepatic artery is labeled A. It is thus by the branches of the connective tissue tree that blood from the portal vein and hepatic artery are conveyed to all parts of the liver, and, as we shall see presently, it is delivered from the end branches of the tree into the sinusoids to provide for the parenchymal cells.

The other two tubes seen in branches of the connective tissue tree permit certain fluids to leave the liver. The first of these tubes in each branch of the connective tissue tree is a duct made of epithelial cells (BD in Fig. 22-7, *bottom left*), and it drains the exocrine section of the parenchymal cells, which is bile, out of the liver. The little ducts in the various branches all join eventually in the trunk of the tree which they leave as main ducts to become the bile duct. The fourth type of tube seen in every branch of the tree has a very thin wall and is a lymphatic. The lymphatics in the various branches join up in the trunk and drain lymph from the liver. What is probably a lymphatic is labeled L in the lower left picture in Figure 22-7; the only other possibility would be that it is a tiny branch of the relatively large portal vein.

The Terms, Portal Tracts, Areas or Radicles. What is seen in a section at sites where a branch of the connective tissue tree containing the four tubes described above is cut is called a portal tract, portal area or portal radicle. One is seen at the left of the top picture of Figure 22-6 and in more detail in the bottom left picture in the same figure. It should be noted that the size of portal tracts seen in sections varies in relation to the size of the branch of the tree that happens to be cut. For example, a stout branch near the trunk would be large and contain large tubes while a section through a small branch near its termination would be small and have small tubes within it. Sometimes portal tracts are seen which represent cuts through sites where one or more of the tubes are branching and when this happens the portal tract reveals more than four tubes.

The Veins That Drain Blood From the Liver. As just described, blood is brought into the liver by the portal vein and the hepatic artery in portal tracts, and from these it is delivered as will be described presently into the sinusoids. It flows along these to reach what are called *central veins.* One is shown at the right side of the illustration at the top of Figure 22-6 where it is labeled CV and one is shown in greater detail at the bottom right of the same illustration. In the latter the sinusoids can clearly be seen emptying into it. Central veins drain into larger veins often called sublobular veins and these in turn drain into the hepatic veins which leave the back of the liver and empty their blood into the vena cava. The system of veins that drain the blood from the liver do not travel in any substantial tree of connective tissue as do the vein and artery that supply blood to the liver, and, furthermore, all through the liver the two systems of blood vessels remain apart from one another. The central veins of the liver, because they are not associated with any other vessels, constitute another type of landmark that is seen in sections which is used with regard to demarcating lobules of liver tissue, which we shall do presently.

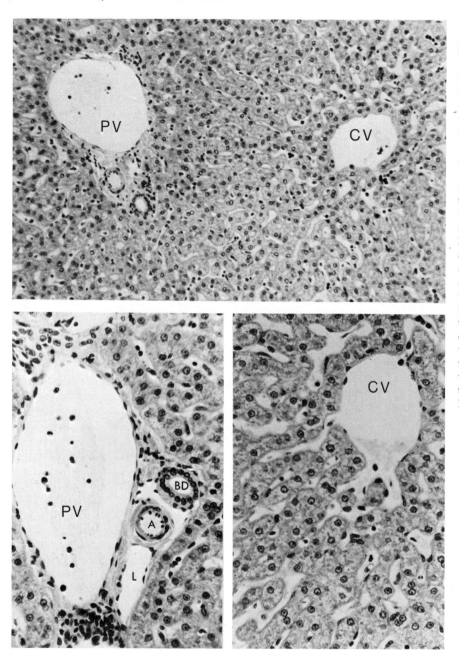

Fig. 22-7. (*Top*) Low-power photomicrograph of an H and E section of liver showing on the left a portal tract in which the branch of the portal vein is labeled PV and, on the right, a central vein labeled CV. Between the two there are cords of liver cells with sinusoids between them. (*Bottom, left*) A section through a portal tract taken at higher magnification. The branch of the portal vein is labeled PV, that of the hepatic artery, A, that of the bile duct, BD, and what is probably a lymphatic is labeled L. Note that the complex of vein, artery, bile duct and lymphatic are encased in a connective tissue stroma. (*Bottom, right*) A section through a central vein at magnification higher than that of the top illustration. Note sinusoids emptying into the central vein and that the endothelium that lines the latter is associated with very little if any connective tissue. (Illustrations by H. Whittaker)

How Bile Reaches the Bile Ducts in Portal Tracts. The next point to discuss relates to the exocrine function of the liver, which is the secretion of bile. This is done by the hepatocytes of the liver cords. As already mentioned, hepatocytes seen in any given section often seem to be arranged in rows of cells that are only one cell wide except at sites where they can be seen to anastomose with one another as seen for example in Figure 22-6. However the appearance of liver cords being composed of rows of cells only one cell wide or thick is misleading. The fact is that the hepatocytes are the secretory cells of an exocrine gland and so there must be a lumen into which every hepaocyte can secrete and, for there to be a lumen in a cord, every cord *must be at least two cells thick* in some plane. The misleading appearance is in part caused by the fact that the borders between adjacent liver cells in a row are not generally distinct (Fig. 1-11, *cell boundaries not apparent here*) so that what appears as the cytoplasm of a single cell in a row may actually be the cytoplasm belonging to two cells with one being above or below the one whose nucleus shows. Furthermore, since sections are thinner than liver cells, a slice cut through a row at least two cells deep could cut through only the top or the bottom cell in the row and so such a row would seem to be only one cell thick. In the simplest arrangement, a cord of liver cells of two cells in width or thickness can secrete bile into a duct system because there is a tiny cleft between the cell membranes of the two hepatocytes of the cord where their surfaces are otherwise in contact; two examples of clefts are shown as they are sometimes seen with the LM in Figure 22-8 where they are indicated by arrows. This little passageway that exists between hepatocytes where they are in contact with one another is called a *bile canaliculus*. It is not a duct but just a passageway. Sometimes the canaliculus is at the site where three hepatocytes meet as is shown in the electron micrographs, Figures 22-18 and 22-19. Since the hepatocytes that border a canaliculus secrete bile into it, the canaliculus can be considered to be the lumen of a secretory unit. The bile secreted into a canaliculus makes its way along liver cords to near a portal area where it enters a little ductule which in turn enters the portal tract to empty into a bile duct in the tract. The ductules will be illustrated when we later consider the fine structure of the liver.

Blood and Bile Flow in Opposite Directions. As is shown in Figure 22-9, blood from the portal vein and hepatic artery of a portal tract enters (but not as directly as is shown in this diagram) the sinusoids between the cords of hepatocytes and in these it is mixed and flows along them to reach and enter central veins. The bile that is secreted by the hepatocytes into the canaliculi of cords flows along between the hepatocytes of a cord to finally enter a bile duct in a portal tract. Hence between portal tracts and central veins blood and bile flow in opposite directions.

Liver Cords As Parts of Liver Plates. It has already been pointed out that liver cords seen in sections often appear to be rows of cells that are only one cell wide but that they must be at least two cells wide or thick if they are to be able to secrete bile into a canaliculus which they all do. The next point to make is that the appearance of a cord of cells as being one cell in width could be due to a slice having been cut from a plate of cells that was one cell thick but many cells deep as is shown in Figure 22-10. From studies made from reconstructing liver parenchyma from serial sections Elias suggested that the liver parenchyma should be considered as existing in the form of plates of hepatocytes, with the plates, however, being both perforated and curved and anastomosing with one

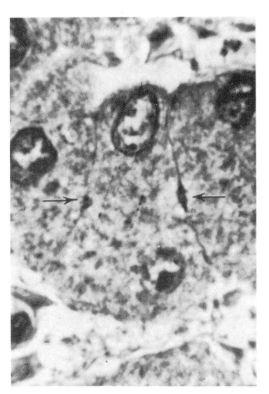

Fig. 22-8. Oil-immersion photomicrograph taken with the phase microscope of an H and E section of a liver plate, showing 2 bile canaliculi indicated by arrows.

another. This view thus goes a bit further than thinking of liver cords as being two or more cells in width or thickness and anastomosing with one another. Lest the student reader think this to be a completely different concept to be learned it should be pointed out that it is not as radically different a view as it might first seem because if it is accepted that liver cords must be two or more cells in width or thickness and that they anastomose with one another frequently, the structure visualized would not be very different from the one accounted for by anastomosing perforated curving plates. In any event the sinusoids are tubular structures surrounded by parenchyma (Fig. 22-6) and any parenchymal cells seen in a section must have other parenchymal cells beside them or beneath them or on top of them. We must next deal with the problem of the liver lobule which is important because various diseases of the liver affect some parts of lobules more than others.

THE LIVER LOBULE

Definitions of a Lobule. The term *lobule* means "little lobe." The term *lobe* seems to have been first

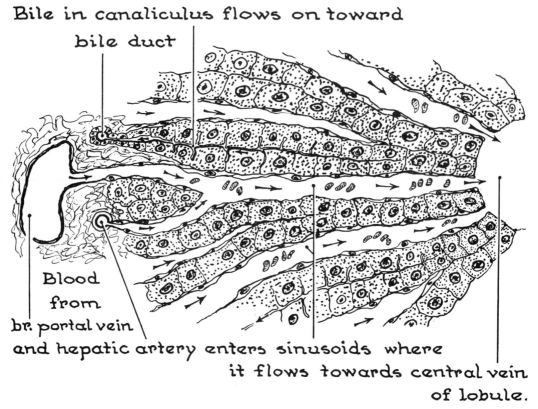

Bile in canaliculus flows on toward bile duct

Blood from br. portal vein and hepatic artery enters sinusoids where it flows towards central vein of lobule.

FIG. 22-9. Drawing (at high-power magnification) to show how blood from the portal vein and the hepatic artery (*left*) flows into sinusoids, lined by reticuloendothelium, that lie between liver cords, and empties into the central vein (*right*). The way that bile travels in the opposite direction in canaliculi to empty into bile ducts in portal areas is also shown.

used to describe any projecting rounded part of a structure—for example, the lobe of the ear (its rounded lowermost part). In connection with glandular organs it was employed to designate any part that projected from the main mass of an organ or was separated from other parts of the organ by fissures, connective tissue septa or indentations. The term *lobule* was first used to designate small parts of lobes that are separated from each other by a smaller order of fissures, septa or indentations. However, with the LM, lobules of *exocrine* glands were generally found to be not only parts that were separated from one another by partitions but also parts in which the secretory units all drained into a common intralobular duct or set of intralobular ducts. So, a second definition for lobules came into being—that lobules are small divisions of an organ that are constituted of groups of closely adjacent secretory units that drain into a common duct or set of ducts. This second definition proved useful; for example, it enables lobules to be identified

in the kidney even though they are not separated from one another by fissures, septa or indentations. However, the fact that there are two ways to define lobules causes complications with regard to the liver because the area defined one way is not the same as that which could be considered a lobule by the other way of defining one. Both kinds of lobules will now be described.

The Classic Lobule. Liver lobules were first described using the criterion that if small segments of liver parenchyma were separated from each other by thin partitions of connective tissue they represented lobules. The common pig probably played a prominent part in causing this concept of liver lobules to be adopted because the liver of this animal is broken up into little units of structure around 2 mm. in length and around 1 mm. in diameter and packed together with the sides of each being separated from adjoining lobules by partitions of connective tissue (Fig. 22-11). In cross sections these units of structure have a poly-

hydral outline; in the pig they are commonly hexagonal. At each angle of the hexagon there is a cross
section of a portal area (tract) so there are six around
each lobule. Furthermore in a cross section of a lobule
a central vein is seen; it, of course, runs longitudinally
along the axis of the lobule. Since hexagonal lobules
are packed together, it should be realized that the
portal vein, the hepatic artery and the bile duct in
each portal area, located at an angle of the hexagon,
serve not only the parenchyma inside the lobule we
have been describing but the parenchyma of the 2
other lobules that are in contact with that portal area.
The type of lobule we have described, which in the pig
is demarcated by partitions of connective tissue, is
called the classic lobule because it was the first type of
lobule described in the liver.

The Classic Lobule in Man. When however, we
turn from the liver of the pig to that of man, classic

lobules become more difficult to identify because they
are not separated from one another by partitions.
Hence to visualize a classic lobule the observer first
finds a central vein (Fig. 22-12). This is the center of
the lobule. The periphery of the lobule is established
by locating some portal areas in the parenchyma that
surrounds the central vein which are not too far away
from it. These portal areas are then connected together
with an imaginary line so that the central vein will lie
in the center of a polyhedral figure which with luck
could be a pentagon or a hexagon. If a continuous line
were drawn through the 5 portal areas indicated in
Figure 22-12, it would outline a pentagonal lobule
which would have a central vein in its center. It is
very difficult to find an example of a perfect hexagonal
lobule in man and a student should not be discouraged
if he doesn't encounter one. Often the best an observer
can achieve is to find a central vein that is cut in cross

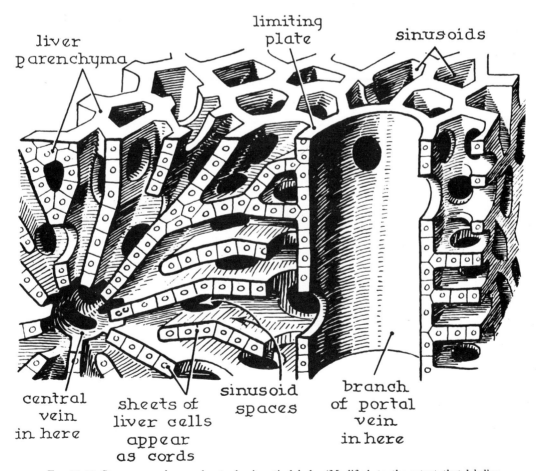

FIG. 22-10. Stereogram of a quadrant of a hepatic lobule. (Modified, to the extent that labeling
was added, from Elias, H.: Am. J. Anat., *85*:379)

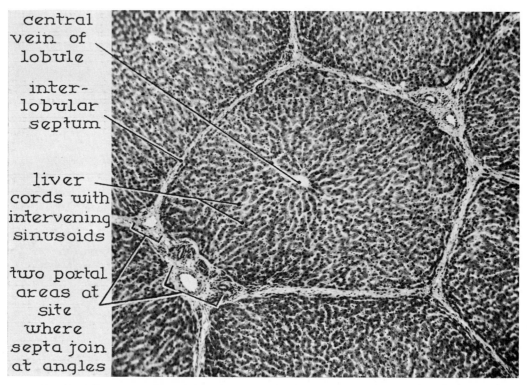

central vein of lobule

inter-lobular septum

liver cords with intervening sinusoids

two portal areas at site where septa join at angles

Fig. 22-11. Low-power photomicrograph of an H and E section of the liver of the pig, illustrating the classic hexagonal lobule.

section and mentally join up a few portal areas around it. One reason for this is that classic liver lobules are not rigid structures like cement blocks that can be stacked on top of each other in rows. Liver lobules are relatively soft, and if they are stacked side by side, they may not be stacked evenly (one may overlap the next); furthermore, they are not necessarily stacked side by side but instead, in such a way that one may point one way and the next one in a somewhat different direction. A second difficulty is that it is easy to think of their being 6 portal tracts that *belong* to each lobule. But even in an ideal arrangement a portal tract serves and so "belongs" to the 3 lobules it lies between. Portal tracts do not "belong" to any particular lobule; they merely run between lobules, and so if lobules are not stacked evenly, a portal tract that runs parallel with 1 lobule would not run parallel with the long axis of the other 2 lobules it lies between. There is a very small chance of the 6 portal tracts that run between such haphazardly stacked lobules ever running in the same direction, so that they would all be cut in cross section at once at 6 points around the lobule. More likely, portal tracts would be "missing" in any given section at several points around the periphery of a

lobule cut in cross section, because at these points— where they are "missing"—they are running in some other direction to parallel some other lobule and so would lie beneath or above the section that is being examined.

The reason that it is important to delve into this problem is that the liver can be affected by nutritional deficiencies, toxins, impaired circulation and other things, and it is very important in interpreting the cause of the damage observed in a liver to know which parts of the lobules that are seen in a section have the best and the poorest blood supply. We shall explain later why attempting to interpret lesions seen in liver lobules according to the concept of the classic lobule is not altogether satisfactory and why a different unit of structure proposed by Rappaport and called the *liver acinus* has proved to be helpful in this and other respects. But before describing the acinus we shall, in order to round out our account of lobules, comment on the second type of lobule, called the *portal lobule,* that has been described.

The Portal Lobule. As already noted, another way of defining a lobule of an exocrine gland is to consider that any group of secretory units that empty their

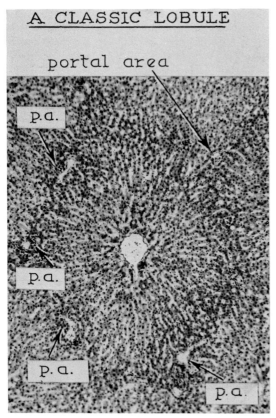

FIG. 22-12. Low-power photomicrograph of an H and E section of human liver, showing a classic lobule.

secretion into small ducts which in turn connect with one another so as to empty the secretion from a given area into a main duct constitutes a lobule. In many exocrine glands such areas are separated from one another by connective tissue partitions (septa) so the area defined by the term lobule is the same if either definition of a lobule is used. But the little portions of the liver whose secretory units (liver cords) empty into a common main duct (a bile duct in a portal area) are not the same portions of liver tissue that are surrounded by connective tissue partitions in the pig or are considered to constitute classic liver lobules in man. In the classic lobule the parenchyma of the lobule is that which surrounds a central vein (Fig. 22-13). But in the portal lobule the parenchyma of the lobule is that which surrounds a portal area because it contains the bile duct into which the surrounding liver cords empty their exocrine secretion (Fig. 22-13). As is shown in Figure 22-13, portal lobules are roughly triangular in cross section and there are twice as many of them as classic lobules (in species that have hexagonal classic lobules). As is shown at the left side of Figure

22-13, the liver cords (represented by lines) that lead from a central vein diverge and then converge again to empty their bile (via ductules to be described later) into the bile duct of the portal area.

It may seem—at least superficially—that, for anyone studying any aspect of the flow of bile through a lobule, the portal lobule would be the more suitable concept to employ. But if one were studying blood flow through the sinusoids of a lobule, the classic lobule would have certain advantages. However, in classic lobules it has often been more or less assumed that at any given site seen in a section blood derived from the hepatic artery and portal vein from the portal tract at the level seen in that section flows directly into the sinusoids that are seen around the portal area in that particular section. This simplified view proved to be a misconception and the elucidation of how blood from portal tracts is delivered into sinusoids led in due course to the concept of units of structure called acini instead of lobules and these will now be described.

The Liver Acinus

The subdivision of liver tissue known as an acinus is neither easy to explain nor easy to understand. It may help first to explain what it is *not*.

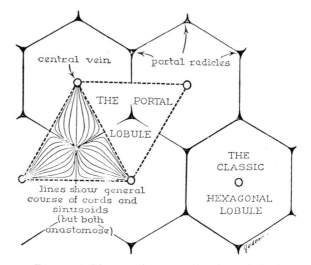

FIG. 22-13. Diagram of cross-section views of classic and portal lobules. Nodal points are not labeled but are present where the borders of portal and classic lobules bisect each other. Those interested will notice that this diagram differs from Mall's diagram of lobules (Fig. 1 of Mall's paper) but that it is in accord with his Figures 47 and 48, which were tracings of injected material, and his finding that there are twice as many portal radicles as central veins in the liver.

In studying the pancreas we learned that acini are small exocrine secretory units that are housed in lobules. There are hundreds or thousands of acini within a lobule of the pancreas and hence in the pancreas acini are much smaller subdivisions of structure than lobules. The liver acinus, on the contrary, is *not* an exocrine secretory unit. Furthermore, it is *not* a subdivision of a given classic lobule because, even though in a cross section of a classic lobule it is only one third of the size of the classic lobule, it is made up of parts of two adjacent classic lobules. So it is easiest to think of liver acini as subdivisions of liver structure in their own right and, instead of thinking of the liver as being made up of lobules, one can think of the liver as being made up of acini. But in order to describe how to locate liver acini, everyone assumes the reader knows about portal lobules. Furthermore, to locate acini we have to use the same guideposts that are used to locate, by the survey method, either of the kind of lobules that we have described. The guideposts are portal tracts and central veins. We shall describe how to locate acini after the following discussion.

Why It Is Advantageous To Think of the Liver As Being Composed of Acini Instead of Portal Lobules. It is obvious that the parts of the liver cords that are closest to central veins are exposed to blood of the poorest quality because to reach a central vein blood must have passed along a sinusoid that was at least as long as those that are seen extending from a portal area to the central vein. Along a sinusoid the blood would have continued to lose oxygen and accumulate carbon dioxide. We can conclude therefore that the parenchymal cells immediately adjacent to central veins are supplied by blood that would have the lowest oxygen content and also the lowest content of nutrients as compared to parenchymal cells situated closer to portal areas. Furthermore, it would have the greatest content of carbon dioxide and other waste products of metabolism.

Next, in days past before the concept of acini was developed, it was often assumed that the sinusoids of the parenchyma that immediately surrounds a portal area would receive the freshest blood; this concept was based on the idea that at any given site along a portal tract blood was emptied almost directly from the hepatic artery and the portal vein of that portal tract into the sinusoids that radiated from that portal tract. However, this view disregarded the fact that there must be smaller vessels that lead off from the vessels in the portal tracts to deliver blood into the sinusoids of the parenchyma. It would be an exception if, in any vascular tree, blood did not flow through smaller and smaller vessels until the peripheral circulation was reached where blood is emptied into either capillaries or sinusoids. The concept of acini takes into account the fact that in order for blood to be delivered from the hepatic artery and portal vein into sinusoids there must be branches of the hepatic artery and portal vein that periodically extend off more or less at right angles from the hepatic artery and portal vein in a portal tract, into the parenchyma, where they branch into small vessels that empty into sinusoids.

These side branches from the hepatic artery and portal veins of portal tracts constitute the backbone of the liver acinus and it is from these vessels that twigs empty blood into sinusoids and it is this blood that is the freshest of that in any part of the parenchyma. So to know where the best quality blood is to be found in liver we must ascertain where these vessels that are derived from those in well-defined portal areas are located.

How To Find an Acinus. As mentioned, finding six portal areas in any given section that can be connected by imaginary lines to form a hexagon, with a central vein in the center, is seldom possible in human liver, because classic lobules are not fitted together neatly in rows of even depth. Rappaport suggests that the observer is much more likely to find only 2, 3, or 4, instead of 6, well-defined triangular portal tracts around the periphery of any hexagon that is visualized around any central vein. In other words, if one thinks of hexagons around central veins, about half of the portal areas that should be at the angles of the hexagon are missing.

What could be considered to be a classic lobule showing only 3 portal areas in its periphery is illustrated in Figure 22-14, *right side;* this figure also indicates by an "M" where portal tracts are "missing." Rappaport believes that distributing terminal branches of the portal vein and hepatic artery in any portal tract extend out from them more or less at right angles to them (as is shown in the one just above the center of Fig. 22-14), toward angular points around the hexagon where well-defined portal areas are "missing" (labeled "M" in Fig. 22-14). Since these smaller terminal vessels grow out roughly at right angles from the main vessels, they are not cut transversely in cross sections of lobules. However, they are occasionally cut obliquely because they pursue irregular courses. On their arched and irregular course toward the points of the lobule where triangular portal tracts are "missing" (Fig. 22-14, "M"), they may be cut repeatedly or not at all in any given section. In their course toward "missing" portal tracts or corners of an imaginary hexagon, the terminal portal and arterial branches, in association with the terminal bile ductules, form the

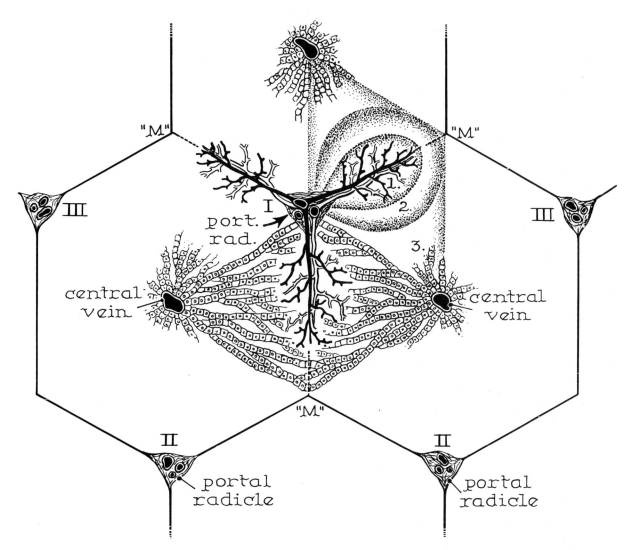

FIG. 22-14. Diagram illustrating the concept of liver substance being composed of units of structure called acini. So that the relation of acini to classic lobules can be visualized, lobules are outlined in the diagram. Only two acini are demarcated here; these are diamond-shaped in section. For details see text.

backbones of masses of hepatic parenchyma that are diamond-shaped in cross section and which constitute acini as is described below.

At the top of the middle of Figure 22-14 there is a central vein. A short distance below this there is a typical triangular-shaped portal tract. We shall concentrate first on the two small blood vessels that branch at right angles from the hepatic artery and the portal vein, respectively, of the tract to descend *vertically* toward an "M" (a site where a portal tract is "missing") to form the backbone of one acinus. The extent of this acinus (in 2 dimensions) is indicated in

the illustration because the area occupied by its parenchyma is shown complete with liver cords that extend out from its backbone toward both the left and the right, and on each side the liver cords of this acinus converge on central veins. The acinus is therefore roughly diamond-shaped in cross section and it includes liver parenchyma that is situated in parts of two different classic lobules, as is shown in Figure 22-14.

The parenchymal cells closest to the vascular backbone of the acinus would have the best blood supply of any of its parts. This part, which Rappaport terms

Zone 1 of an acinus, is more or less oval-shaped in cross section; it is shown by the shading and is labeled 1 in another diamond-shaped acinus that is present just above and to the right of the center of the Figure 22-14. The liver parenchyma that surrounds Zone 1 is roughly circular in cross section and is marked in the same acinus as 2. This zone has the second best blood supply in this acinus. The irregularly shaped outer part of an acinus that reaches to the central veins is termed Zone 3, and it has the poorest blood supply of any part of an acinus.

To Sum Up Some of the Foregoing. In cross section acini are more or less diamond-shaped, with each end of one converging on a central vein. A cross section view of one that is cut through its middle would probably show its backbone of blood vessels. But an acinus has thickness as well as width and length, and if it were too thick it would not be very efficient with regard to its backbone of vessels supplying blood to parenchyma that was relatively far away from them. Acini are therefore not as thick as classic lobules are long. So when we say there are three times as many acini as portal lobules we are only speaking of what is seen in a cross section. If they are not as thick as lobules are long there would, of course, be many more than three times as many acini along the length of a portal area that runs along the side of a classic lobule.

By thinking in terms of three dimensions it can be appreciated that since the vascular backbones of acini run more or less at right angles to the vessels in portal tracts, the parenchyma seen in the periphery of a lobule in a given section could be part of Zone 1, 2 or 3 of an acinus whose vascular backbone ran parallel to the plane of the section but might be considerably below or above the plane of the section. For this reason what appears as a peripheral part of a lobule in any given section, even a part adjacent to a portal tract, may not have the best blood supply because it may be relatively far off from the vascular backbone of an acinus.

The Acinus As a Metabolic Unit. There is now evidence indicating that the metabolic processes that occur in the 3 zones of an acinus are quantitatively different; this explains why different toxic agents or nutritional deficiencies affect different zones to different extents. For details Rappaport's various papers and his chapter in the general reference should be consulted.

The concept of the acinus helps in understanding why different areas of liver lobules are more damaged than others under different conditions, and why sites of damage within the periphery of lobules could seem to vary from section to section.

We shall now consider the lining of the sinusoids.

The Hepatic Sinusoids and the Space of Disse

With the LM sections of liver often suggested the existence of a space between the walls of sinusoids and the hepatocytes that bordered the sinusoids. Whether or not this space, called the *space of Disse,* as seen with the LM, was a shrinkage artifact was not established until the improved methods of fixation used for EM studies, and the EM itself, revealed that the space was real (Figs. 22-15 and 22-16). This space contains blood plasma but blood cells are normally not seen in it in postnatal life. It contains vast numbers of microvilli that project into it from the free surfaces of the hepatocytes that border it (Figs. 22-15 and 22-16).

The Cells of the Walls of Sinusoids

Development of Knowledge. Long ago it was observed with the LM that the lining of the liver sinusoids differed from the lining of ordinary capillaries because two morphological types of cells were involved in its structure. One type were relatively thin and flat, resembling those seen in the walls of ordinary capillaries but the other kind were much larger. In sections they often appeared to be stellate (shaped like a star) and they became known as the stellate cells of von Kupffer who, in the last century, was the first to describe them. They are now known as Kupffer cells.

In this century, with the advent of Aschoff's concept of a reticuloendothelial system the various parts of which could be identified by vital staining, it was observed that the Kupffer cells of the livers of animals injected with vital stains or particulates such as those of India ink where phagocytic (Fig. 22-17, *left*) and so the lining of the liver sinusoids was classified as part of the reticuloendothelial system along with the sinusoids of the spleen, bone marrow and lymph nodes, all of which had phagocytic cells associated with their sinusoids. The free macrophages of loose connective tissue were also included in the system, because they too phagocytosed vital stains. In due course the name macrophage system was also used for this system of cells.

It was noted that the formation of blood cells occurred in association with the sinusoids of many parts of what was visualized as the reticuloendothelial system. For example, blood cells are formed in the

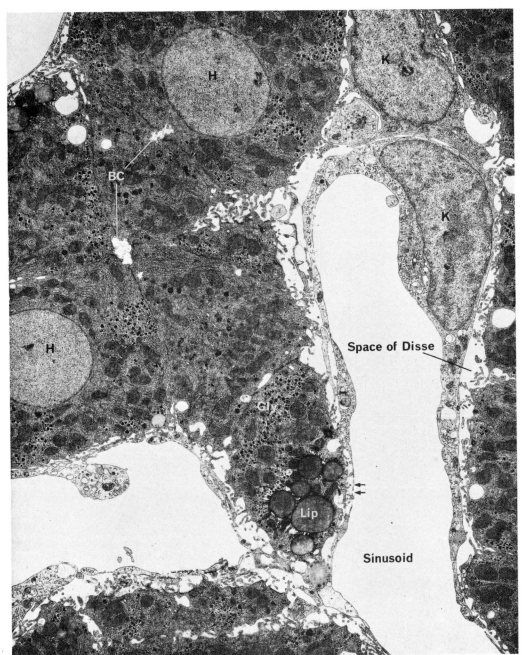

FIG. 22-15. Electron micrograph ($\times$ 5,100) of section of liver from young rat, fixed with para-formaldehyde, postfixed with osmic acid. The space of Disse between the lining cells of the sinusoids and the hepatocytes (H) is labeled. Between the hepatocytes, bile canaliculi (BC) may be seen. Within the hepatocytes glycogen areas (Gly) alternate with rough endoplasmic reticulum and mitochondria. A few lipid droplets (Lip) may be seen. (Courtesy of Miss Ethel Rau, McGill University)

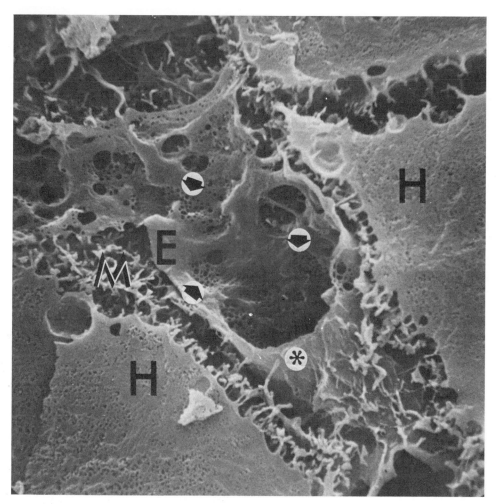

Fig. 22-16. Scanning EM micrograph. Rat liver was fixed by perfusion with glutaraldehyde, fractured after freeze drying and then coated lightly with carbon and gold under vacuum. The surface that is shown extends across a sinusoid and includes parts of two hepatocytes labeled H that are on the opposite sides of the sinusoid. The microvilli that extend from the surfaces of these into the space of Disse are seen to advantage; one site where they are very abundant is labeled M. The inner surface of the endothelial wall of the sinusoid (which was fractured obliquely) is labeled E. The outer surface of the sinusoid is seen a little lower down and it is indicated by an asterisk. Some reticular fibers are outlined here on the outer surface of the sinusoid. Fenestrated areas of the endothelium (sieve plates) are indicatd by arrows. (Brooks, S. E. H., and Haggis, G. H.: Scanning electron microscopy of rat's liver. Lab. Invest., *29*:60, 1973, © 1973, U.S.-Canadian Division of the International Academy of Pathology)

sinusoids of the liver in fetal life (Figs. 22-17, *right,* and 12-8). It was also noted that they are formed in the spleen and bone marrow close to sinusoids. There thus seemed to be some sort of an association between cells that had the great potentiality required to form blood cells and the phagocytic cells of the type described above, and this led to the suspicion that the blood cells and the phagocytic cells had a common

stem cell. It is of interest that it has now been shown that they have, but the common stem cell is not the one that it was conceived to be for many decades. In the instance of the liver, for example, it became fairly generally believed that the thin (endothelial type) lining cells that more or less alternate with Kupffer cells along the lining of the sinusoids were the relatively undifferentiated cells of great potentiality that could give rise not only to Kupffer cells but also, in fetal life, to blood cells. It was likewise assumed that as part of the stroma of bone marrow and spleen there were fixed primitive mesenchymal cells that could give rise to both the phagocytic cells of the sinusoids of these tissues and also to the types of blood cells formed in these tissues. Hence, until recently it was not uncommonly believed that the thin flattened (endothelial type) cells that form the chief lining of liver sinusoids possessed great mesenchymal potentiality and could give rise to Kupffer cells and also, under the proper stimulus, to blood cells.

The above-described concept is no longer considered to be valid for several reasons. First, as was described in Chapter 9, it has been shown that the cell that gives rise to blood cells is a free cell that arises in the yolk sac of the embryo, enters the circulation and seeds the various tissues that become hemopoietic.

Hence the blood cells that develop in the spaces between liver cords in the fetal liver (Fig. 12-8) do not arise from fixed cells of the thin flattened type of sinusoidal lining cell but from free cells from the yolk sac that seed these passageways. This finding, of course, detracts from the concept that the thin flattened endothelial-like cells of liver sinusoids have the potentiality to give rise to the Kupffer cells.

There is, moreover, further evidence against the older view. It has been established in recent years, by using cell markers, that macrophages in any part of the body originate from blood monocytes which on entering tissue develop into full-fledged macrophages. One way this has been shown is by means of labeling with tritiated thymidine the precursors of monocytes in the bone marrow. (Whereas blood monocytes and macrophages are not believed to divide, the precursors of monocytes duplicate their DNA and divide while in

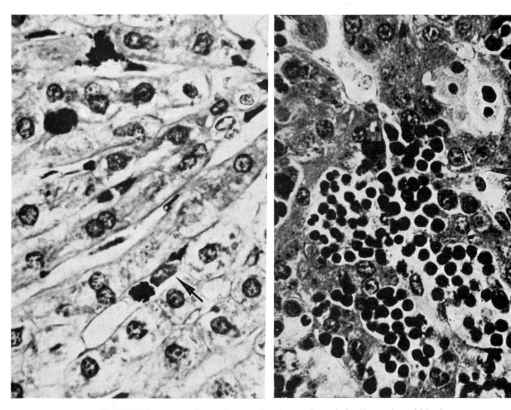

FIG. 22-17. (*Left*) High-power photomicrograph of a section of the liver of a rabbit that was previously injected intravenously with India ink. The arrow points to the nucleus of a reticuloendothelial cell that has phagocytosed India ink, which may be seen in its cytoplasm both to the left and the right of its nucleus. Two large masses of India ink in the cytoplasm of the reticuloendothelial cells may be seen in the upper part of the picture. (*Right*) High-power photomicrograph of a section of fetal pig liver, showing hemopoiesis in the sinusoids. The cells with the dark nuclei are mostly proerythroblasts and erythroblasts.

the bone marrow.) Labeled macrophages are subsequently found in various parts of the body, including the liver sinusoids where they appear as Kupffer cells.

It was noted in describing the sinusoids of both bone marrow in Chapter 12 and lymph nodes in Chapter 13 that current views are that the sinusoids in these tissues are lined with ordinary endothelial cells. It was formerly believed that at least some of their lining cells were phagocytic; these were called *littoral* cells. But EM studies, as was pointed out in Chapters 12 and 13 (Figs. 12-3 and 13-9), suggest that the phagocytic cells are only associated with these sinusoids. They may, however, give the appearance of being parts of their lining because although they lie against the outer surfaces of the sinusoidal walls they commonly, by means of pseudopodia, protrude between endothelial lining into the lumens of sinusoids. However, in the liver the Kupffer cells actually form part of the lining, being interposed between endothelial cells.

The Fine Structure of Kupffer Cells. Kupffer cells have an irregular outline; their cytoplasm projects from their cell bodies in the form of both pseudopodia and microvilli. Clefts extend into the cytoplasm between projections. Within the cytoplasm, membrane-enclosed spaces may be seen which could be pinocytotic or phagocytic vesicles. Phagocytosed material in the cytoplasm may be present—for example, iron in the form of hemosiderin, resulting from the phagocytosis and destruction of old erythrocytes. Mitochondria are not very numerous, and there is not very much in the way of rough-surfaced endoplasmic reticulum. The Golgi apparatus is not prominent. The latter points are to be expected, because the Kupffer cell is not specialized either to produce or to secrete protein substances. Wisse has found that the cytoplasm of Kupffer cells, unlike that of the endothelial cells, is peroxidase positive. This provides another means of distinguishing between Kupffer and endothelial cells and, of course, it also seems to suggest an origin from monocytes (which possess peroxidase-positive granules). The nucleus of a Kupffer cell, like the rest of the cell, resembles that of a macrophage; there is nothing unusual about it.

The Fine Structure of the Endothelial Cells of Hepatic Sinusoids

When tissue blocks fixed by immersion were studied with the EM it appeared that the cells that formed the walls of sinusoids formed a discontinuous lining in that small gaps were commonly seen between adjacent cells of the wall. Furthermore, it was noted that the cytoplasm of the endothelial cells of the wall was often attenuated and contained fenestrae. It was therefore considered that although there were no gaps in the sinusoid walls large enough to permit erythrocytes or other blood cells to enter the space of Disse, the gaps were of a size that could freely admit blood plasma into the space of Disse so that it would be in direct contact with the cell membranes of the hepatocytes which at this site extend into the space in the form of innumerable microvilli (Figs. 22-15 and 22-16).

Wisse, however, has studied the fine structure of the cells of sinusoid walls in tissue that was fixed by means of perfusing the vessels concerned and he came to somewhat different conclusions about its nature. First, in tissue fixed in this manner he did not find the gaps between cells that are seen in tissue fixed by immersion. He therefore conceived of the sinusoids having continuous walls. Next, he observed that the fenestrae were disposed in various very attenuated portions of cytoplasm that extend off from the perinuclear regions of endothelial cells. He described the site or portions of cytoplasm where fenestrae exist as *sieve plates* of around 500 Å in thickness (Fig. 22-16). The fenestrae in the sieve plates were therefore the only passageways that seemed to exist between the interior of the sinusoids and the space of Disse. Wisse found moreover that the fenestrae (which are not covered with diaphragms like those in the endothelial cells of some types of capillaries) were generally oval in shape with a diameter of around 1,000 Å and a length of around 1,150 Å. For more details see Wisse (1970).

If there are no other gaps in the sinusoidal walls except the fenestrae of *sieve plates*, the sinusoids could have a filtering function with a known pore size. There is no basement membrane surrounding the endothelial cells to interfere with the passage of particles of a size smaller than that of the pores. Chylomicrons are roughly about the same size as the pores and so they can gain entrance to the space of Disse.

In considering the problem of how the sinusoidal walls are supported, and what could prevent them from being flattened against the hepatocytes, thus obliterating the space of Disse, it should probably be mentioned that because of the pores in the endothelial cells which permit the free passage of plasma which always fills the space of Disse, the hydrostatic pressure in the space of Disse would be the same as that in the lumen of the sinusoid so that there would be no great force within the sinusoid to cause its expansion. However, the sinusoidal walls, according to Wisse, are often supported in their exteriors by what are called fat-storing cells (because they contain lipid droplets). These cells lie beneath the endothelium and could help provide it with support because they possess processes which could help support the endothelium. Wisse described both microtubules and filaments in the processes of the endothelial cells which could provide internal support for them. He also described the presence of bristle-coated pinocytotic vesicles in their cytoplasm.

The type of cell junctions between endothelial cells and between endothelial cells and Kupffer cells, where the latter are interposed between endothelial cells, does not seem to have been determined with precision. However, they do not seem to be of a continuous occludens type, because a narrow space between contiguous cell membranes has been observed, at least in many sites. Some reticular fibers (Fig. 22-16) have been demonstrated around sinusoids, which should help provide them with support.

The Histology of Hepatocytes

Hepatocytes illustrate so many features of general interest about cells that they were used in the early chapters of this book as models to describe various features of cells at the level of both the LM and the EM. It is therefore unnecessary to again describe and illustrate those features of hepatocytes that were dealt with earlier. However, for the convenience of the reader who may wish to review some of this material at this time the figures illustrating many of the features of hepatocytes previously dealt with will be mentioned again here.

The appearance of hepatocytes that are storing glycogen in sections stained and not stained for glycogen is shown in Figure 1-15 and the appearance of excessive amounts of fat in liver cells is shown in Figure 1-16. The differences between a hepatocyte that is in the prophase of mitosis and those in the interphase are shown in Figure 2-8. Hepatocytes frequently demonstrate polyploidy; one such is shown in Figure 2-27. One way that polyploidy can develop is shown in Figure 2-27. The effect of DNA-ase on hepatocytes is shown in Figure 2-5 and that of RNA-ase in Figure 4-7.

The fine structure of the nucleus of a hepatocyte is illustrated first in Figure 2-4. This shows the various ways in which chromatin is distributed in the interphase nucleus, as well as the general appearance of the nucleolus and the nuclear envelope. The nuclear envelope and the nuclear pores are shown in more detail in Figures 2-6 and 2-7.

The cytoplasm of hepatocytes abounds in organelles and inclusions. That mitochondria are very numerous in hepatocytes is shown in Figures 22-18 and 5-44; it has been estimated that each hepatocyte contains a thousand or more. The way they probably divide is illustrated in Figure 5-16 and their functions are dealt with in a separate section in Chapter 5. They are of particular importance in hepatocytes because of the great and varied types of metabolic activity that require their help. Free ribosomes and polyribosomes are well represented in hepatocytes. It is of interest that in malignant tumors of the liver of rats free ribosomes become relatively more prominent than the more complex types of organelles, as is shown in Figure 5-18: this seems to be due to energy in malignant tumor cells being directed into growth instead of into function. Rough endoplasmic reticulum is well represented in normal hepatocytes and sER is particularly prominent; their particular functions will be described when we soon discuss the endocrine functions of hepatocytes. Many Golgi stacks are scattered about in the cytoplasm; some are close to the nucleus and others close to bile canaliculi as in Figure 22-18. These are concerned with the endocrine function of the liver and probably with the exocrine function as well, as will be described in following sections. Lysosomes are present in hepatocytes, particularly close to bile canaliculi (Fig. 22-19) but, as described in Chapter 5, they may present a variety of appearances. When first seen in hepatocytes they were called pericanalicular dense bodies because most of them were dense and close to canaliculi. However, there are also many that contain lipofuscin, the wear-and-tear pigment. This is electron dense because of its fatty component combining with osmium in fixation. The lipofuscin in hepatocytes is taken up by lysosomes which are thereupon called lipofuscin bodies. Hepatocytes also contain a number of bodies that are smaller than mitochondria and are called microbodies (Fig. 22-19, *microbody*). In most species (but not in man) they have a dense body in their centers which may be crystalline. Microbodies have a surrounding membrane and have been shown to contain several enzymes. The crystalline structure seen in the centers of those of many species is due to uricase. This enzyme is concerned with metabolizing uric acid to a further state than occurs in man, thus making it easy for uric acid to be eliminated from the body. Man seems to lack this enzyme, so he has to secrete uric acid as such in his urine. The inability to metabolize or excrete effectively all the uric acid he produces and absorbs from his food leads to gout—which would seem to make man unique, although I have read that Dalmatian dogs are also prone to this disease.

Having given this general account of the organelles of hepatocytes we shall soon attempt to relate some of them more particularly to the functions of the hepato-

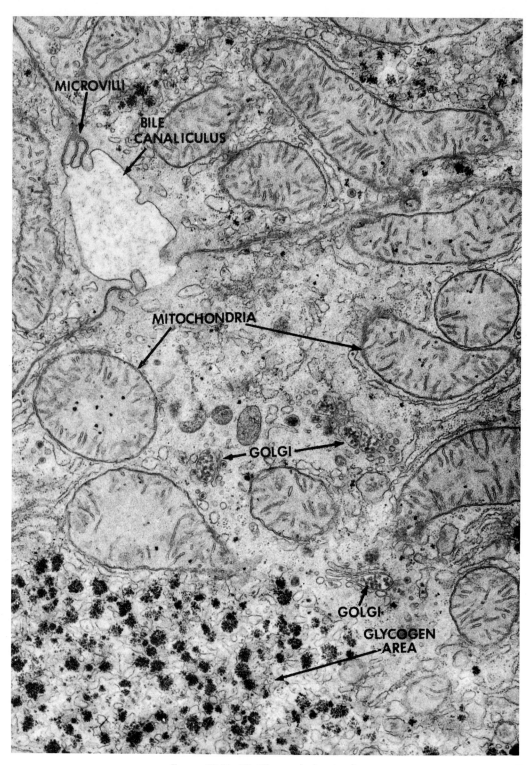

FIGURE 22-18. (*Caption on facing page*)

cytes. But first we must mention the surfaces of hepatocytes.

THE THREE SURFACES OF HEPATOCYTES

The cell membrane of a hepatocyte that faces the space of Disse has very numerous microvilli projecting from it into the space of Disse (Fig. 22-16), which, of course, provides each hepatocyte for a relatively enormous surface for absorption of substances from the bloodstream. Between the microvilli there is space for hepatocytes to secrete useful substances into plasma. The sides of hepatocytes in most species have many projections and indentations to fit complementary indentations and projections on the hepatocytes that are beside it, but these are not at all prominent along the sides of the hepatocytes of man. Presumably they help hold hepatocytes together in the liver plates. Third, at some site on the surface of a hepatocyte there is a bile canaliculus between it and one or two other hepatocytes (Figs. 22-18 and 22-19). Bile canaliculi will be described further in connection with the exocrine function of the liver.

The Functions of Hepatocytes

Without going into the subject of the functions of the liver in depth we shall now comment briefly on some of the kinds of functions it performs and relate these to the organelles concerned in the performance of these functions. We shall begin with the endocrine function of the liver.

SOME ENDOCRINE FUNCTIONS OF HEPATOCYTES AND THEIR RELATION TO ORGANELLES

As already noted, the liver is an exocrine gland because the hepatocytes secrete bile into canaliculi and this is carried away by a duct system to the intestine. But decades ago it was also described as an endocrine gland. At that time a gland was considered to be endocrine if it secreted any useful substance into the bloodstream. So when it was found that the liver secreted sugar into the blood it was listed as an endocrine gland as well as an exocrine gland. It is now known that it secretes several useful substances into the bloodstream as will next be described. It is noteworthy that its exocrine and endocrine functions are both performed by the same secretory cells—the hepatocytes. It should also be mentioned that although it is convenient here to discuss the liver as an endocrine gland, the latter term is now generally used in a more restricted way for those glands that secrete hormones and will be described in Chapters 25, 26 and 27.

The Synthesis of Glycogen and the Secretion of Glucose

After a substantial carbohydrate meal the blood glucose level would rise materially if it were not for the hepatocytes, in the presence of insulin, removing excess glucose from the blood and storing it as glycogen. When the blood sugar level begins to fall, they convert the glycogen back into glucose and release it into the blood. Several of the enzymes concerned in these reactions are probably synthesized in relation to the free ribosomes and polyribosomes which are relatively abundant in the cytoplasm of hepatocytes. Seen with the EM, the glycogen deposits formed from glucose are pale and seemingly amorphous in unstained material (Fig. 5-44) and are closely associated with tubules of sER. With special staining (lead citrate) the glycogen is shown to be present in black particles that are a little longer than free ribosomes and are arranged together to form rosettes (Fig. 5-46) which are closely associated with tubules of sER (Fig. 22-18).

The hormone *hydrocortisone,* of the adrenal cortex, also can cause glycogen to form in hepatocytes; but this is due to the glycogen being formed from proteins or protein precursors, and the glycogen in this instance results in the liberation of glucose into the blood and not in the subtraction of glucose from it. (This will be discussed more fully in Chapter 25.)

FIG. 22-18. (*On facing page*). Electron micrograph ($\times$ 30,000) of mouse liver cells. A bile canaliculus can be seen in the left upper corner. Its lumen contains a finely fibrillar material which is probably bile. Microvilli project into the lumen. Note that they vary considerably in size. This variability is often interpreted as being related to the functional state of the cells which constitute the lining. The cells show numerous mitochondria which are large and contain many cristae. Observe the rather prominent opaque granules in the matrix of the mitochondrion near the left center of the micrograph. Several Golgi zones are present, and their vesicles contain electron-opaque granules which are thought to be the excretion product of liver cells, possibly lipid in character. In the left lower corner is a group of glycogen granules which are arranged in rosettes of subunits. Between the glycogen particles are vesicles of the smooth-surfaced endoplasmic reticulum. (Preparation by Dr. A. M. Jézéquel)

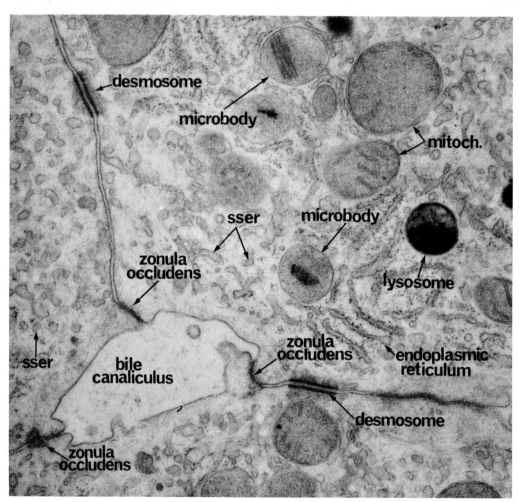

Fig. 22-19. Electron micrograph ($\times$ 17,550) of 3 liver cells of groundhog (*Marmota monax*) surrounding a bile canaliculus. The junctional complexes are seen as specializations of the cell membranes. The component of the junctional complex closest to the lumen is the zonula occludens, and
some distance away from this is a desmosome. In the cytoplasm of the cell just above is some
granular endoplasmic reticulum, a lysosome and 2 microbodies which show the crystalline structure
of their "nucleoid." On the left margin of the micrograph is an aggregate of agranular (smooth-
surfaced) endoplasmic reticulum (sser). Compare the agranular reticulum with the ribosome-studded
reticulum in the cell at the right margin of the micrograph. (Preparation by J. Steiner)

Why glycogen deposits are associated with sER is
not understood. It is, of course, suspected to have some
role in glycogen formation or the release of glucose
from glycogen.

Blood Proteins. Hepatocytes synthesize the albu-
mins, fibrinogen and most of the globulins, as well as
other proteins concerned in blood coagulation and
secrete these into the sinusoids. Hepatocytes do not,
of course, produce the immunoglobulins; these are produced by plasma cells.

The proteins secreted by hepatocytes into the blood
are synthesized in cisternae of the rER, stacks of

which are seen here and there in the cytoplasm. Some
are shown in Figure 5-46. After their synthesis it seems
probable that the blood proteins are delivered via the
Golgi to the cell surface and released in much the same
way as other secretory products contained in vesicles,
which process was described in Chapter 5.

The Lipoproteins. The hepatocytes are also concerned in controlling the level of lipids in the blood.
Although some lipid in the blood is in the form of a
loose complex of fatty acids and albumin, most lipid
is in the form of little particles in which lipid is combined in some fashion with protein. These particles

constitute the *lipoproteins* of the blood. Lipid particles by themselves would be hydrophobic and so would not remain in suspension in plasma. The protein with which they are associated acts so as to make the particles sufficiently hydrophilic to remain in suspension in plasma. There are four kinds of lipoprotein particles in blood. The chylomicrons, which were described in Chapter 9 in connection with adipose tissue, are the largest of these particles and, as already described, they are formed in the intestinal absorptive cells. The hepatocytes participate with other cells in the body in removing these from the blood after a fatty meal. Since they are suspended in blood plasma they readily enter the space of Disse and are probably absorbed as such by liver cells where they are broken down, with their constituents being utilized by the hepatocytes. The other lipoproteins are called pre-beta lipoprotein, beta lipoprotein, and alpha lipoprotein respectively. The particles of the pre-beta lipoprotein are somewhat smaller than chylomicrons and relatively richer in protein. They are believed to be made in the hepatocytes. The particles of beta lipoprotein are smaller still and denser and have less lipid. These, too, are synthesized by hepatocytes. These particles are the chief medium by which cholesterol is transported throughout the body. They are probably secreted along with, or as part of, the pre-beta lipoprotein. The alpha lipoprotein forms the smallest of all the types of lipoprotein particles and its lipid is chiefly in the form of phospholipid which is an essential component of cell membranes.

The lipoproteins that are made by hepatocytes seem to be assembled in a step-by-step manner. Their protein content is synthesized in the rER. Some rER in the liver is continuous with the sER. The sER is concerned with the synthesis of lipids. So it could be reasoned that the protein and lipid of the particles are synthesized in the same tubule, with the protein being formed where it is rough and the lipid where it is smooth. It seems probable, moreover, that the Golgi is also involved and that vesicles containing lipoprotein particles bud off from its saccules to move to the surface of the hepatocytes where the contained particle would be released into the blood. Within the cytoplasm the membrane-surrounded particles are believed to appear as dark granules.

SOME METABOLIC AND DETOXIFICATION
FUNCTIONS OF HEPATOCYTES AND ITS
RELATION TO ORGANELLES

Another function of hepatocytes besides their endocrine function just described and their exocrine secre-

tory function next to be described can only be touched on here; it involves transformations and/or conjugations which bring about the detoxification of certain undesirable products that, having been absorbed from the intestine or formed in the body, might otherwise exert a deleterious effect. For example, ammonia is formed in connection with the metabolism of amino acids, and ammonia is toxic in certain concentrations. The hepatocytes prevent such concentrations from being attained by using ammonia in the formation either of useful substances or of urea; the latter substance is nontoxic (unless concentrations are excessive) and is eliminated from the body by the kidney.

With regard to many chemical substances ranging from certain drugs often prescribed, or certain chemicals absorbed from various sources, in foods, from industrial contact, or from other sources, the hepatocytes are called upon to metabolize these and in such a way as to detoxify them. In some instances the metabolizing of some of these substances results in the formation of products that are more damaging than the one absorbed.

Steroid hormones are also metabolized in hepatocytes. In connection with their activity and in the detoxification of some of the categories of substances mentioned above there is a marked increase of sER in hepatocytes.

THE EXOCRINE SECRETION OF THE LIVER

The exocrine secretion of the liver is bile. About 500 to 1,000 ml. is formed and emptied into the intestine each day. Bile contains bile pigments (bilirubin), bile salts, protein, cholesterol and such crystalloids (dissolved in water) as are present in tissue fluid. Bilirubin pigment is primarily a waste product. It is formed not in hepatic cells but from the breakdown of the hemoglobin of erythrocytes in the macrophages that are closely associated with the sinusoids of the spleen and the bone marrow and to a less extent by the Kupffer cells of hepatic sinusoids. The non-iron-containing breakdown product of hemoglobin (bilirubin) passes into the blood and is absorbed from the blood by hepatocytes from the space of Disse. The hepatocytes change it slightly (by conjugation so as to make it water-soluble) and then secrete it as one component of bile. Bile salts, in contrast to bile pigments, are useful substances which in the intestine facilitate greatly the digestion of fats. Like cholesterol, a third component of bile, bile salts are produced in the hepatocytes.

There is another component of bile: The hormones produced by the adrenal cortex and the sex glands are constantly absorbed from the blood by hepatocytes

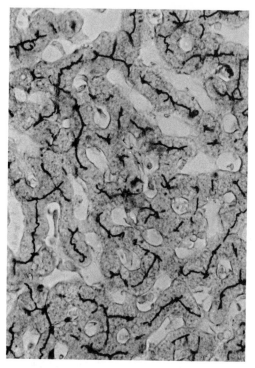

Fig. 22-20. Photomicrograph of section of liver. The anastomosing bile canaliculi within liver cords that must be two cells thick in some dimension are black. They are demonstrated here by the technic for alkaline phosphatase. The cells of the cords are gray (their nuclei do not show) and the sinusoidal spaces are pale. (Preparation by Drs. M. J. Phillips and J. W. Steiner)

trated in the gallbladder between meals, as will be described later in connection with the gallbladder.

Bile Canaliculi. The cell membranes of adjacent cells at either side of the lumen of a bile canaliculus are tightly bound together by a junctional complex (Fig. 22-19). There is a fusion of the outer (adjacent) lamellae of the two cell membranes that are in contact just before the two cell membranes diverge to form the canaliculus; thus the canaliculus begins on the lumen side with a zonula occludens. Farther away from the lumen of the bile canaliculus the junctional complex on each side only occasionally shows a zonula adherens. Farther out there are desmosomes (Fig. 22-19).

The cell membranes that form the wall of a bile canaliculus project irregularly into the lumen of the canaliculus as short microvilli (see Figs. 22-18 and 22-19). Histochemical studies indicate that there is a substantial amount of ATP-ase at the border of the cytoplasm that abuts on the bile canaliculus. There is also some condensation of cell web material in this location.

The Connections Between Canaliculi and Bile Ducts. Bile canaliculi can be demonstrated in the LM by different methods. Sometimes they can be seen in H and E sections, but their demonstration without special treatment probably depends on their being somewhat distended as in Figure 22-8. Gomori showed that histochemical methods for alkaline phosphatase revealed them; alkaline phosphatase is known to be present in bile (Fig. 22-20). Bile canaliculi can be injected with opaque materials through the bile ducts and studied in cleared thick and thin sections.

Although it was once believed that bile canaliculi were structures with cuticular walls of their own, the EM showed clearly that the bile canaliculi are merely spaces between the membranes of contiguous hepatic cells. There is, particularly in some species (but not much in man), a little condensation of cell web material around the cell membranes that border the canaliculi. This, together with the firm union that occurs between the cell membranes in the junctional complexes on each side of the canaliculi (Fig. 22-19), permits canaliculi to withstand considerable pressures without rupturing and also to remain more or less intact after the homogenization of liver cells or partial digestion of liver substance.

Bile canaliculi begin from blind endings in the hepatic plates in the region around the central veins of lobules. As they pass along liver plates toward the periphery of lobules, they anastomose freely (Fig. 22-20). The bile that flows along them drains finally into the bile ductules, which are the smallest branches of the bile ducts that are surrounded by connective

and metabolized to different extents. The products so formed, or even active unchanged steroid hormones, are partly secreted into the bile. From the bile in the intestine some hormone may be resorbed into the bloodstream. Hence, there is said to be an enterohepatic circulation of steroid hormones.

There is also an enterohepatic circulation of bile pigment, for when bilirubin reaches the intestine, it is changed into urobilinogen and stercobilinogen by the action of bacteria that live in the intestine. Part of the urobilinogen is subsequently reabsorbed into the capillaries of the intestine. These, of course, drain into the portal system, and as the blood containing the reabsorbed urobilinogen passes along the sinusoids of the liver, the urobilinogen is taken up by hepatocytes and changes into bilirubin again, after which it is again secreted into the bile.

Although bile is secreted by the liver at a fairly regular rate, it is delivered into the intestine irregularly, generally when it will do the most good; this requires that it be temporarily stored and concen-

tissue in portal tracts. The connections between the bile canaliculi of the plates and the bile ducts in the portal tracts has been studied vigorously over the years, and a certain amount of confusion about terminology has resulted. The use of the EM has clarified many of the points that were previously unsettled. The following description is based primarily on EM studies that have been made by Steiner and his associates.

First, the bile canaliculi in liver plates in man are bounded usually by 2 hepatocytes, and in some instances by 3 hepatocytes (Figs. 22-8 and 22-19). At sites where plates approach and abut on portal tracts, the canaliculi of the plates empty into what are called the *canals of Hering*. The canals of Hering along their short courses (Fig. 22-21) are bordered in part by hepatocytes and in part by a different kind of cell which is not a secretory hepatocyte but a *duct type* of cell. The important point here is that there are no types of cells in the walls of the canals of Hering that represent transitions between hepatocytes and duct cells. There is, however, a mixture of clear-cut hepatocytes and clear-cut duct cells along the course of the canals (Fig. 22-21). The canals of Hering are very short and connect with the bile ductules (the finest branches of the bile duct system); these are present in the connective tissue of portal radicles. However, the

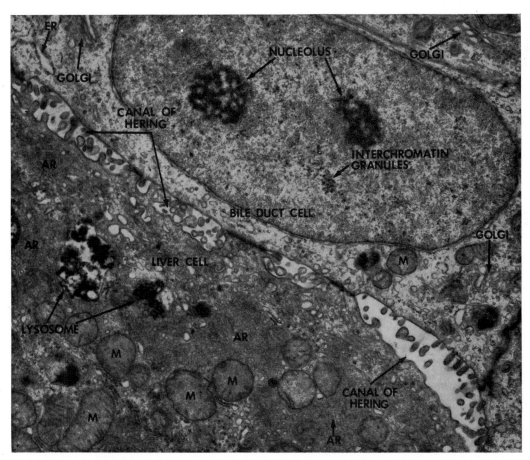

Fɪɢ. 22-21. Electron micrograph ($\times$ 13,300) of longitudinal cut of a canal of Hering in rat liver. These passages are difficult to find in normal liver. This picture is from an animal which received large doses of a chemical (alpha-naphthyl-isothiocyanate) which makes it easy to find them. In the left lower corner of the micrograph is a liver cell, and in the right upper corner is a bile duct cell. The channel between them, into which microvilli of both types of cells project, is the canal of Hering. Note that the mitochondria of the duct cell are somewhat smaller than those of the liver cell and that the structure of the duct cell is much simpler. The smooth-surfaced reticulum (AR) and the lysosomes of the liver cell are markedly increased in volume as a result of the effect of the chemical. (Preparation by Dr. J. W. Steiner)

canals of Hering are not the only channels by which bile from canaliculi reaches the bile ductules in the portal radicles, because leading off at angles from the canals of Hering there are little bypasses which are termed preductules, and these, too, drain into the bile ductules that are in the portal tracts. Preductules differ from canals of Hering because they have no hepatocytes along their course; their walls are made entirely of cells of the duct type (Fig. 22-22). The walls of the preductules are seen in cross sections to consist of no more than 2 or 3 cells of the duct type (Fig. 22-22). The bile ductules (small bile ducts) in the portal tracts, into which both the canals of Hering and the preductules drain, seen in cross section, always have more than 3 cells around their walls (Fig. 22-23). The bile ductules are merely the smallest branches of the branching tree of bile ducts that is contained in the connective tissue tree which sends its branches to the periphery of all liver lobules.

Cells of the duct type along the canals of Hering and in the walls of the preductules differ from hepatocytes in several ways. They are smaller and have much less cytoplasm in relation to their nuclei than hepatic cells (Figs. 22-21 and 22-22). Their cytoplasm contains only a few flattened rough-surfaced vesicles but

does contain a moderate number of ribosomes. The Golgi apparatus is not particularly well developed and is commonly disposed between the nuclei of the cells and their apices that abut on the lumen. They contain no glycogen, and their mitochondria are smaller than those of hepatocytes. Basement membrane is present at the bases of cells of the duct type but not in association with hepatocytes. Junctional complexes are present to hold the cell membranes of contiguous cells firmly together at the sites of canaliculi. Elsewhere the membranes of contiguous cells interdigitate to help hold the sides of contiguous cells together. Microvilli project into the lumens of bile ductules similarly to the way they project into canaliculi. All these points are shown by Figures 22-21 and 22-22.

BILE DUCTS

The bile ductules, the smallest branches of the bile duct system that is contained in the connective tissue tree, have walls of low cuboidal epithelium (Fig. 22-23). The slightly larger ducts seen in portal areas have walls of cuboidal epithelium (Fig. 22-7, *lower left*). Still larger bile ducts have columnar epithelium, so in general the height of the epithelium varies in relation

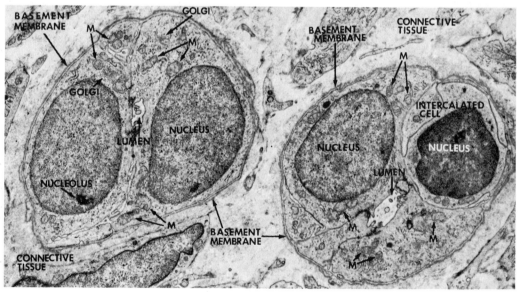

FIG. 22-22. Electron micrograph ($\times$ 8,320) of 2 bile preductules lying in the connective tissue of a portal tract. Each preductule is surrounded by a basement membrane. The lumen of the channel on the left side of the micrograph is lined by 2 biliary epithelial cells and the one on the right by 3. The channel on the right shows a cell which in this plane of section is not in contact with the lumen. Such cells are designated as intercalated cells. Note the rather simple structure of the cells with small, inconspicuous mitochondria, sparse Golgi vesicles and virtually no endoplasmic reticulum. This is thought to indicate that these cells are not metabolically very active. (Preparation by Dr. J. W. Steiner)

FIG. 22-23. Electron micrograph of section of portal tract in human liver showing a bile ductule. Notice the interlocking of folds along the cell membranes of the biliary epithelial cells; sites of these are indicated by arrows. Mitochondria are few. A bleb of cytoplasm (B), which is probably an expanded microvillus, lies in the lumen. (Preparation by Dr. H. Sasaki and Dr. F. Schuffner. *In* Steiner, J. W., Phillips, M. J., and Miyai, K.: The pathology of the liver. Int. Rev. Exp. Path., *3*:65)

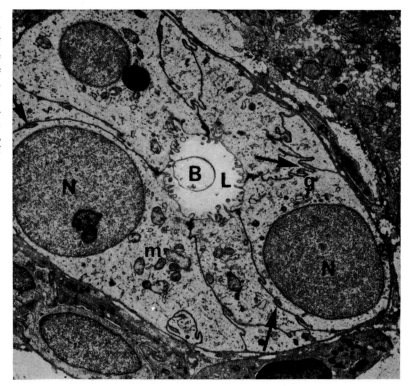

to the size of the duct. The two main hepatic ducts which leave the liver at the site of the porta (the transverse fissure) unite to form the *hepatic duct*. The extrahepatic ducts require more support than the intrahepatic ones that are embedded in the connective tissue of the portal tracts. This is provided by dense connective tissue and smooth muscle arranged so as to surround the epithelial-lined lumen of the tube.

When bile ducts are large enough to be lined by columnar epithelium, fat droplets within the cytoplasm of their lining cells are not uncommon. In the larger intrahepatic bile ducts, and in the extrahepatic ones, tubuloalveolar glands are present in a much-folded mucous membrane.

LYMPHATICS AND THE FORMATION OF LIVER LYMPH

There is nothing special about the appearance of the lymphatics in the portal tracts; their size and number vary with the size of the tract in which they are seen. There is, however, a problem—which is, to know the origin of the lymph they contain.

The liver produces a great deal of lymph, and it is relatively rich in protein. There has been controversy about where it is formed. Lymphatics as yet have not been demonstrated with certainty in or around liver

plates or sinusoids, but only in the connective tissue components of the liver, that is, in (1) the connective tissue of the capsule, (2) the tree of connective tissue that carries the branches of the portal vein, the hepatic artery and the bile duct to the sides of each lobule, and (3) the sparse connective tissue associated with the hepatic veins. The first question is whether liver lymph is formed in this connective tissue or elsewhere. Perhaps we should consider the "elsewhere" hypothesis first.

The "elsewhere" concept is that plasma could back up, as it were, in the spaces of Disse to sites where sinusoids begin—close to the connective tissue associated with portal tracts—and that the plasma would be under enough pressure in the spaces of Disse in this area to more or less filter through the delicate connective tissue at the edge of the tract to reach nearby lymphatic capillaries that begin in the connective tissue of the tract. The filter effect would hold back some but not all of the protein of the plasma.

Concerning the other hypothesis, that lymph is formed within the substance of the tract, it must be said that the number of blood capillaries in portal tracts seems to be far too small to account for the abundant liver lymph being formed in the way lymph is formed elsewhere (as shown and illustrated in Chapter 8). However, as noted in Chapter 19, lymph can be formed in the walls of veins as a filtrate of the blood in the lumens of the veins. Accordingly, the walls of the branches of the portal veins in the portal tracts also deserve some consideration as a possible source of liver lymph, particularly because blood in the portal vein is under much greater pressure than it is in most veins. Lymphatics within the capsule of the liver should also be considered. As yet the source or sources of liver lymph has not been established very clearly.

JAUNDICE

Jaundice means yellow. Under normal conditions the amount of yellow bile pigment in blood is not enough to give color to the skin. But under certain conditions blood can contain enough to cause the skin, the mucous membranes and the eyeballs to take on a yellow color. A person so afflicted is said to have jaundice.

Jaundice can occur in 3 different ways as will now be described.

(1) Normally, the hepatocytes remove bilirubin from the blood at the same rate at which it is produced by macrophages. But under conditions in which the rate of erythrocyte destruction becomes greatly increased, the uptake of bilirubin by hepatocytes may lag behind its rate of production by macrophages, with the result that the concentration of bilirubin increases in the blood sufficiently to cause jaundice. This type of jaundice is generally termed *hemolytic jaundice* because it is caused by the increased rate of hemolysis of red blood cells. (This is the mechanism responsible for the physiologic jaundice that occurs in the newborn, as all the nucleated red blood cells which still persist from prenatal life are quickly destroyed by macrophages.)

(2) The ability of the liver to absorb bilirubin, handle it metabolically and secrete it into canaliculi may become impaired in various ways. First, in a rare condition there is a block at the cell membrane of the hepatocytes, which become altered in such a way that bilirubin is prevented from entering them from the bloodstream as readily as it should. Next, hepatocytes may have hereditary enzyme defects which keep them from handling bilirubin properly, or hepatocytes may be injured from various causes so that there are not enough healthy cells to handle the bilirubin normally coming to them from blood. Finally, they may be injured in such a fashion that the bilirubin that they absorb is not properly secreted and leaks back into the sinusoids.

(3) Finally, both the production of bilirubin and its uptake and secretion by hepatocytes may be normal, but the bile secreted into the duct system is unable to flow to the intestine because of some obstruction to the duct system. The common obstruction is a stone in one of the main drainage ducts. Another cause of obstruction can be a malignant growth of cells in the head of pancreas which obstructs the duct entering the duodenum. Under these conditions bile is damned back through the hepatocytes into sinusoids.

THE REGENERATIVE CAPACITY OF THE LIVER AND THE PROBLEM OF CIRRHOSIS

Over 60 percent of the cells in the liver are hepatocytes. If a portion of the liver is excised from an experimental animal, the hepatocytes soon undergo mitosis and restore the liver to its normal size in a few days' time. The factors that operate to cause this rapid regeneration are not thoroughly understood. One concept is that the control of the cell population in the liver is performed by a chalone as was described in Chapter 6, and that when part of the liver is excised there is not enough chalone produced to restrain cell proliferation. If, however, hepatocytes are injured because of nutritional deficiencies, or toxic substances in the circulation or for other reasons, the problem of regeneration becomes much more complicated than it is when a portion of the liver is removed surgically; this is due primarily to the fact that all the structures essential for the regeneration of functional hepatic tissue may not be able to regenerate in a harmonious way so as to restore the normal complicated architecture of the organ; there are too many tubes and passageways within and without lobules to re-form and become connected together again properly.

In the healing of a fracture of a bone osteogenic cells may fail to grow from one fragment to the other to effect a cartilaginous and bony type of union. Under these circumstances fibroblasts from adjacent connective tissue may grow between the fragments at the fracture site and fill the gap with ordinary dense connective tissue, and this in turn impedes osteogenic cells from later growing across the gap to effect a bony union. Likewise, if the parenchyma of the liver is badly damaged, with much cell death, the reticular and connective tissue framework which supports lobules collapses. Regeneration of hepatocytes may begin in isolated areas where some healthy cells have remained. The nodules of new liver parenchyma that develop from these sources may be divorced from proper connections with the portal circulation, and hence they lack a proper organization of sinusoids.

Meanwhile, fibroblasts in the partially collapsed frame-work may variously proliferate and form much new connective tissue which interferes with new and normal connections being established between regenerating nodules of parenchyma and the system of bile ducts; the connective tissue also interferes with the develop-ment of proper connections being established between the sinusoids in regenerating parenchyma and the afferent venous and arterial vessels. Moreover, the in-creased amount of connective tissue prevents the liver from expanding as nodules of parenchyma become larger, and, furthermore, the connective tissue itself may shrink as it matures. This condition is termed cirrhosis. When the substance of the liver becomes compressed, blood flow through the affected liver is impeded.

As the student will learn if he studies pathology, degeneration of hepatocytes can occur from many different causes and can begin in different sites within lobules. As a consequence the cirrhotic process can be-gin in different parts of the liver lobule.

The Gallbladder

A side branch (the cystic duct) extends from the hepatic duct to a somewhat elongated pear-shaped sac, the gallbladder (Fig. 22-24). The gallbladder is lined by a mucous membrane which is thrown into so many folds when the bladder is contracted (Fig. 22-25) that a student, on seeing a section of the wall of the organ, might think its mucosa was riddled with glands (Fig. 22-25). Actually, there are no glands in the mucosa of the gallbladder except near its neck, and if the organ is distended, most (but not all) of its mucosal folds that give the mucosa a glandular appearance disappear.

The epithelium of the mucous membrane of the gall-bladder is high columnar (Fig. 22-26). Each cell in the membrane resembles the one beside it; in this respect it resembles the epithelium of the stomach. But the cells themselves are not like those lining the stomach. They resemble more closely the absorptive cells of the small intestine and, like them, are provided with microvilli. Secretory granules have been described in the more superficial parts of the cytoplasm of the cells, but the primary function of the lining cells is absorp-tive rather than secretory.

The epithelium rests on an areolar lamina propria (Fig. 22-25). There is no muscularis mucosae in the gallbladder; hence the mucous membrane rests on a skimpy layer of smooth muscle comparable in position, but not in thickness, with the muscularis externa of the intestine (Fig. 22-25). Some of the smooth muscle

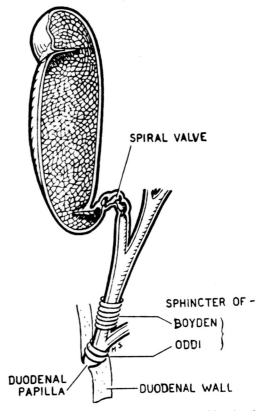

FIG. 22-24. Diagram of the gallbladder (showing its corrugated inner surface), the cystic duct, the bile duct and the sphincters of Boyden and Oddi. (Grant, J. C. Boileau, and Basmajian, J. V.: Grant's Method of Anatomy. ed. 7. Baltimore, Williams & Wilkins, 1965)

fibers of which the muscularis externa is composed run circularly and longitudinally, but most run obliquely. Many elastic fibers are present in the connective tissue which fills the interstices between the smooth muscle bundles of this coat.

Outside the muscle coat is a well-developed peri-muscular or subserosal coat (Fig. 22-25). This consists of areolar tissue, and it may contain groups of fat cells. It conveys arteries, veins, lymphatics and nerves to the organ. Along the side of the gallbladder that is attached to the liver, the connective tissue of its peri-muscular coat (which here cannot be termed properly its subserosal coat) is continuous with the connective tissue of the liver.

The neck of the gallbladder is twisted in such a fashion that its mucosa is thrown into a spiral fold (Fig. 22-24). Somewhat similar crescentic folds of mucosa are present in the lining of the cystic duct. More muscle appears in the wall of the gallbladder at

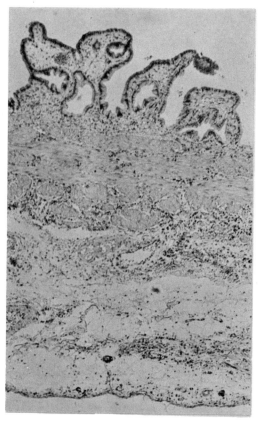

FIG. 22-25. Low-power photomicrograph of H and E section of human gallbladder. (Photomicrograph by H. Whittaker)

arrangement and the control of this muscle have been studied in detail by Boyden and his associates, whose papers (listed at the end of this chapter) should be consulted for full details. Briefly, these investigators have found that this muscle develops from mesenchyme independently and hence is not part of the muscle of the intestinal wall proper. That which develops around the preampullary part of the bile duct becomes strong and serves as a sphincter at the outlet of the bile duct; this may be called the *sphincter of Boyden* (Fig. 22-24). The muscle that develops around the ampulla itself and around the preampullary part of the pancreatic duct is not substantial enough to exert a very potent sphincteric action, except in a minority of individuals. The closure of the strong sphincter of Boyden, surrounding the preampullary part of the bile duct, prevents the secretion of the liver from entering the intestine, and, as a result, bile formed during its closure is bypassed, by way of the cystic duct, to the gallbladder, where it is stored and concentrated. There are

its neck, and in the wall of the cystic duct, than is present in the remainder of the gallbladder.

The Bile Duct and the Sphincter of Oddi. The duct that extends from the point of junction of the cystic and the hepatic ducts to the duodenum was, in the past, generally termed the *common bile duct*. In recent years there has been a tendency to omit the qualifying "common" from the term. This duct penetrates the outer coats of the duodenum close to the point of entry of the pancreatic duct. Part way through the duodenal wall the two ducts fuse, and the lumen of the fused duct is sufficiently expanded to be called an *ampulla* (*ampulla*, flask), the *ampulla of Vater*. The ampulla pursues an oblique course through the inner layers of the duodenal wall to open on the summit of a papilla that projects into the duodenal lumen, the *duodenal papilla*.

In the past, the muscle associated with the ampulla and the ends of the two ducts that enter the ampulla were said to constitute, collectively, the *sphincter of Oddi*. More recently, the development, the amount, the

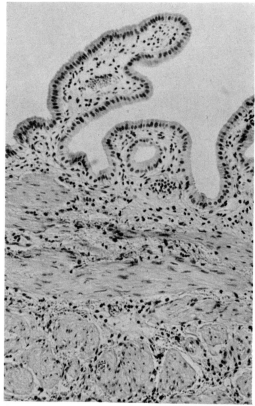

FIG. 22-26. Medium-power photomicrograph of an H and E section of the wall of the human gallbladder showing the epithelium, the lamina propria and most of the muscle coat. (Photomicrograph by H. Whittaker)

also smooth muscle fibers disposed parallel with the preampullary parts of the bile and the pancreatic ducts; their contraction shortens (and presumably broadens) the ducts so as to encourage flow through them.

Functions of the Gallbladder. The gallbladder stores and concentrates bile. Concentration is effected by the absorption of water and inorganic salts through the epithelium into the vessels of the lamina propria of its mucosa. This results in bile in the gallbladder coming to have an increased content of bile pigment, bile salts and cholesterol. Radiopaque substances of such a nature that they are excreted by the liver and so appear in the bile may be given to individuals. If the gallbladder is concentrating normally, these become sufficiently concentrated in the gallbladder to allow that organ to be outlined by x-rays. In this way, gallbladder function can be tested in the clinic. The reaction of bile becomes somewhat altered in the gallbladder; the absorption of the inorganic salts from it somehow results in its becoming less alkaline.

A hormonal mechanism is concerned in causing the gallbladder to contract. The feeding of fat is particu-larly effective in causing the gallbladder to contract. Boyden showed that if the blood of a recently fed animal is injected into the veins of another animal, such blood will cause the gallbladder of its recipient to empty. It is probable that a hormone is made by the intestinal mucosa under the influence of digesting food, and that this travels to the gallbladder by the blood-stream to cause its contraction. Ivy and Oldberg sug-gested *cholecystokinin* as a name for this hormone. Peristaltic waves in the intestine probably affect the opening and closing of the sphincter that lets bile enter the intestine, and so bile enters the intestine in squirts.

The muscle of the wall of the gallbladder is so thin that many investigators have doubted that its contrac-tion could be an important factor in emptying it. How-ever, considerable experimental work provides little ground for these doubts.

Development of Bile Ducts, Gallbladder and Liver

The liver originates from the entodermal epithelium of the developing duodenum; the epithelium here first

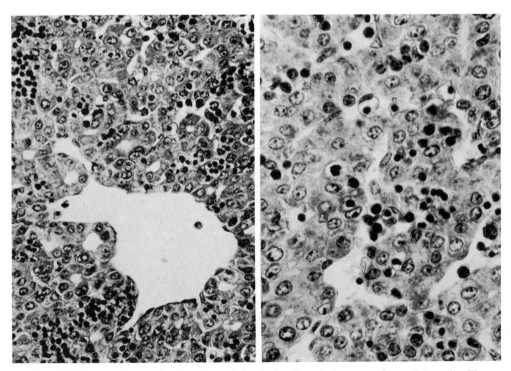

Fig. 22-27. Photomicrograph of sections of developing liver in human embryo of 8 weeks. The section at the left, which was taken closer to the source of the outgrowth, shows cells becoming arranged into tubules; these are future bile ducts. At the right, farther away from the source of the outgrowth, the cells are forming thick plates; these will later become split up to form liver plates only 1 cell thick. (Preparation from Dr. J. Steiner)

bulges outward to form what is termed the *hepatic diverticulum.* One branch of this forms the cystic duct and the gallbladder. The epithelial cells of another part grow in the form of projections into the splanchnic mesoderm and split it up. Branches from the veins which will become the portal vein grow into the area where the epithelium is splitting up the mesoderm, and the spaces between the developing epithelial projections become richly vascularized. The whole mass grows rapidly. The mesoderm provides a capsule for the organ and also the tree of connective tissue that forms in the interior of the organ.

In the development of exocrine glands the terminal outgrowths become secretory units, and the epithelial cells that connect these with the site from which the gland originates form the ducts. As is shown in the two pictures in Figure 22-27, there is a difference in the way the cells of the outgrowth differentiate in forming the liver. The cells closer to the site of origin of the outgrowth begin to differentiate to form tubules; the lumens of some of these are cut in cross section and can be seen in the left picture in Figure 22-27. Farther away from the origin of the outgrowth the cells become arranged into thick irregular clumps and plates (Fig. 22-27, *right*). At this time there is no difference in the appearance of the cells that form the tubules or the plates. Later their appearance changes, and the cells that in the left picture are forming tubules become the epithelial cells of bile ducts (ductular cells), whereas those shown in the right picture become the cells of the exocrine secretory units of the liver; these cells are called hepatic cells or *hepatocytes.* The thick plates in which the future hepatocytes are at first arranged become split up to form the parenchyma with blood vessels between them; the latter become the sinusoids of the liver.

References and Other Reading

PANCREAS

Caro, L. G., and Palade, G. E.: Protein synthesis, storage and discharge in the pancreatic exocrine cell. An autoradiographic study. J. Cell Biol., 20:473, 1964.
Ciba Foundation Symposium on the Exocrine Pancreas. Boston, Little, Brown & Co., 1962.
Ekholm, R., and Edlund, Y.: Ultrastructure of the human exocrine pancreas. J. Ultrastruct. Res., 2:453, 1959.
Farquhar, M. G., and Palade, G. F.: Junctional complexes in various epithelia. J. Cell Biol., 17:375, 1963.
Haist, R. E., and Pugh, E. J.: Volume measurement of the islets of Langerhans and the effects of age and fasting. Am. J. Physiol., 152:36, 1948.
Jamieson, J. D., and Palade, G. E.: Condensing vacuole conversion and zymogen granule discharge in pancreatic exocrine cells: metabolic studies. J. Cell Biol., 48:503, 1971.
Munger, B. L.: A phase and electron microscopic study of cellular differentiation in pancreatic acinar cells of the mouse. Am. J. Anat., 103:1, 1958.
Opie, E. L.: Cytology of the pancreas. *In* Cowdry's Special Cytology. ed. 2, p. 373. New York, Hoeber, 1932.

For further references on the fine structure of, and mechanism of secretion in, acinar cells, *see* Chapter 7.
For islets of Langerhans, *see* Chapter 27.

LIVER

A General Reference

Rouiller, C. (ed.): The Liver; Morphology, Biochemistry, Physiology. 2 vols. New York, Academic Press, 1963-64.

Special References

Biava, C. G.: Studies on cholestasis: A re-evaluation of the fine structure of normal human bile canaliculi. Lab. Invest., 13:840, 1964.
Bollman, J. L.: Studies of hepatic lymphatics. *In* Trans. of 9th Conf. on Liver Injury. p. 91. New York, Macy, 1950.
Brooks, S. E. H., and Haggis, G. H.: Scanning electron microscopy of rat's liver. Lab. Invest., 29:60, 1973.
Bruni, C., and Porter, K. R.: The fine structure of the parenchymal cell of the normal rat liver. 1. General Observations. Am. J. Path., 46:691, 1965.
Bucher, N. L. R.: Regeneration of mammalian liver. Int. Rev. Cytol., 15:245, 1963.
———: Experimental aspects of hepatic regeneration. New Eng. J. Med., 277:686, 1967.
Burkel, W. E.: The fine structure of the terminal branches of the hepatic arterial system of the rat. Anat. Rec., 167:329, 1970.
Carruthers, J. S., and Steiner, J. W.: Fine structure of terminal branches of the biliary tree. Arch. Path., 74:117, 1962.
Doljanski, F.: The growth of the liver with special reference to mammals. Int. Rev. Cytol., 10, 1960.
Elias, H.: Morphology of the stellate cells of Kupffer. Quart. J. Chicago Med. Sch., 13:13, 1952.
———: A re-examination of the structure of the mammalian liver: I. Parenchymal architecture. Am. J. Anat., 84:311, 1949.
———: A re-examination of the structure of the mammalian liver, II. Hepatic lobule and its relation to vascular and biliary systems. Am. J. Anat., 85:379, 1949.
Elias, H., and Petty, D.: Gross anatomy of the blood vessels and ducts within the human liver. Am. J. Anat., 90:59, 1952.
Elias, H., and Sokol, A.: Dependence of the lobular architecture of the liver on the portohepatic blood pressure gradient. Anat. Rec., 115:71, 1953.
Fawcett, D. W.: Observations on the cytology and electron microscopy of hepatic cells. J. Nat. Cancer Inst., 15:1475, 1955.
Frank, B. W., and Kern, F.: Intestinal and liver lymph and lymphatics. Gastroenterology, 55:408, 1967.
Hamilton, R. L., Regen, D. M., Gray, M. E., and LeQuire, V. S.: Lipid transport in liver. I. Electron microscopic iden-

tification of very low density lipoprotein in perfused rat liver. Lab. Invest., *16:*305, 1967.

Hard, W. L., and Hawkins, R. K.: The role of the bile capillaries in the secretion of phosphatase by the rabbit liver. Anat. Rec., *106:*395, 1950.

Harkness, R. D.: Regeneration of the liver. Brit. Med. Bull., *13:*87, 1957.

Hartroft, W. S.: Accumulation of fat in liver cells in lipodiastaemata preceding experimental dietary cirrhosis. Anat. Rec., *106:*61, 1950.

————: The escape of lipid from fatty cysts in experimental dietary cirrhosis. *In* Trans. of 9th Conf. on Liver Injury. p. 109. New York, Macy, 1950.

Howard, J. G.: The origin and immunological significance of Kluppfer cells. *In* van Furth, R. (ed.): Mononuclear Phagocytes. Oxford, Blackwell Scientific Publications, 1970.

Hruban, Z., and Swift, H.: Uricase, localization in hepatic microbodies. Science, *146:*1316, 1964.

Jéséquel, A., Arakawa, K., and Steiner, J. W.: The fine structure of the normal neonatal mouse liver. Lab. Invest., *14:*1894, 1965.

Jones, A. L., and Fawcett, D. W.: Hypertrophy of the agranular endoplasmic reticulum in hamster liver induced by phenobarbital. J. Histochem. Cytochem., *14:*215, 1966.

Knisely, M. H., Bloch, E. H., and Warner, L.: Selective phagocytosis: I. Microscopic observations concerning the regulation of the blood flow through the liver and other organs and the mechanism and rate of phagocytic removal of particles from the blood. Det. Kong. Dans. Videnskab. Selskab, Biol. Skr., *7:*1, 1948.

LeBouton, A. V.: Heterogeneity of protein metabolism between liver cells as studied by radioautography. Curr. Mod. Biol., *2:*111, 1968.

LeBouton, A. V., and Marchand, R.: Changes in the distribution of thymidine-³H labeled cells in the growing liver acinus of neonatal rats. Dev. Biol., *23:*524, 1970.

Lee, F. C.: On the lymph vessels of the liver. Contrib. Embryol., *74:*65, 1925.

Mall, F. P.: A study of the structural unit of the liver. Am. J. Anat., *5:*227, 1906.

Matter, A., Orci, L., and Rouiller, C.: A study on the permeability barriers between Disse's space and the bile canaliculus. J. Ultrastruct. Res., *11*(Suppl.), 1969.

Mosbaugh, M. M., and Ham, A. W.: Stimulation of bile secretion in chick embryos by cortisone. Nature, *168:*789, 1951.

Novikoff, A. B., and Essner, E.: The liver cell. Am. J. Med., *29:*102, 1960.

Paschkis, K. E., Cantarow, A., Walkling, A. A., Pearlman, W. H., Rakoff, A. E., and Boyle, D.: Secretion and excretion of carbohydrate-active adrenal compounds (oxysteroids). Fed. Proc., *7:*90, 1948.

Popper, H.: Correlation of hepatic function and structure based on liver biopsy studies. *In* Trans. of 9th Conf. on Liver Injury. p. 9. New York, Macy, 1950.

Porta, E. A., Hartroft, W. S., Gomez-Dumm, C. L. A., and Koch, O. R.: Dietary factors in the progression and regression of hepatic alterations associated with experimental chronic alcoholism. Fed. Proc., *26:*1449, 1967.

Rappaport, A. M.: The structural and functional acinar unit of the liver; some histopathological considerations (Monograph). Int. Symp. Hepatitis Frontiers. Boston, Little, Brown & Co., 1957.

————: The structural and functional unit in the human liver (liver acinus). Anat. Rec., *130:*673, 1958

————: Acinar units and the pathophysiology of the liver. *In* Rouiller, C. (ed.): The Liver. vol. 1. *See* General Reference, 1963.

————: The microcirculatory hepatic unit. Microvasc. Res., *6:*212, 1973.

Rappaport, A. M., Black, R. G., Lucas, C. C., Ridout, J. H., and Best, C. H.: Normal and pathologic microcirculation of the living mammalian liver. Rev. Int. Pathol., *16*(4):813, 1966.

Rappaport, A. M., Borowy, Z. J., Lougheed, W. M., and Lotto, W. N.: Subdivision of hexagonal liver lobules into a structural and functional unit; role in hepatic physiology and pathology. Anat. Rec., *119:*11, 1954.

Rappaport, A. M., and Hiraki, G. Y.: The anatomical pattern of lesions in the liver. Acta Anat., *32:*126, 1958.

————: Histopathologic changes in the structural and functional unit of the human liver. Acta Anat., *32:*240, 1958.

Rappaport, A. M., and Knoblauch, M.: The hepatic artery, its structural, circulatory and metabolic functions. 3rd Int. Symp. Int. Assoc. Study of Liver, Kyoto, 1966. T. Gastorent. p. 116, 1967.

Rhodin, J. A. G.: Ultrastructure and function of liver sinusoids. Proceedings IVth International Symposium of R.E.S., May 29-June 1, 1964, Kyoto, Japan.

Stein, O., and Stein, Y.: The role of the liver in the metabolism of chylomicrons, studied by electron microscope autoradiography. Lab. Invest., *17:*436, 1967.

Steiner, J. W., and Carruthers, J. S.: Studies on the fine structure of the terminal branches of the biliary tree. I. The morphology of normal bile canaliculi, bile pre-ductules (ducts of Hering) and bile ductules. Am. J. Path., *38:*639, 1961.

Steiner, J. W., Carruthers, J. S., and Kalifat, S. R.: The ductular cell reaction of rat liver in extrahepatic cholestasis. I. Proliferated biliary epithelial cells. Exp. Molec. Path., *1:*162, 1962.

Steiner, J. W., Jézéquel, A.-M., Phillips, M. J., Miyai, K., and Arakawa, K.: Some aspects of the ultrastructural pathology of the liver. Progr. Liver Dis., *2:*303, 1965.

Steiner, J. W., Phillips, M. J., and Miyai, K.: Ultrastructural and subcellular pathology of the liver. Int. Rev. Exp. Path., *3:*65, 1964.

Trump, B. F., Goldblatt, P. J., and Stowell, R. E.: An electron microscope study of early cytoplasmic alterations in hepatic parenchymal cells of mouse liver during necrosis in vitro (autolysis). Lab. Invest., *11:*986, 1962.

Wisse, E.: An electron microscope study of the fenestrated endothelial lining of rat liver sinusoids. J. Ultrastruct. Res., *31:*125, 1970.

————: An ultrastructural characterization of the endothelial cell in the rat liver sinusoid under normal and various experimental conditions, as a contribution to the distinction between endothelial and Kupffer cells. J. Ultrastr. Res., *38:*528, 1972.

Wisse, E., and Daems, W. Th.: Fine structural studies on the sinusoidal lining cells of rat liver. *In* van Furth, R. (ed.): Mononuclear Phagocytes. Oxford, Blackwell Scientific Publications, 1970.

GALLBLADDER

Boyden, E. A.: An analysis of the reaction of the human gallbladder to food. Anat. Rec., *40:*147, 1928.

————: The sphincter of Oddi in man and certain representative mammals. Surgery, *1:*25, 1937.

Chapman, G. B., Chiardo, A. J., Coffey, R. J., and Weineke, K.: The fine structure of the human gallbladder. Anat. Rec., *154:*579, 1966.

Hayward, A. F.: Aspects of the fine structure of gallbladder epithelium of the mouse. J. Anat., *96:*227, 1962.

————: The structure of gallbladder epithelium. Int. Rev. Gen. Exp. Zool., *3:*205, 1968.

Jit, I.: The development of the unstriped musculature of the gallbladder and the cystic duct. J. Anat. Soc. (India), *8:*15, 1959.

Kay, G. I., Wheeler, H. O., Whitlock, R. T., and Lane, N.: Fluid transport in rabbit gallbladder. A combined physiological and electron microscope study. J. Cell Biol., *30:*237, 1966.

Mueller, J. C., Jones, A. L., and Long, J. A.: Topographical and subcellular anatomy of the guinea pig gallbladder. Gastroenterology, *63:*856, 1972.

Ralph, P. H.: The surface structure of the gallbladder and intestinal epithelium of man and monkey. Anat. Rec., *108:* 217, 1950.

Yamada, E.: The fine structure of the gallbladder epithelium of the mouse. J. Biophys. Biochem. Cytol., *1:*445, 1955.

23 The Respiratory System

Introduction

General Function of the System. Blood leaves the capillaries of the systemic circulatory system with a diminished oxygen and an increased carbon dioxide content. This blood is emptied into the right heart, from which it is pumped via the pulmonary circuit through the lungs. The latter are two large organs, spongy because they contain innumerable little pockets of air and a vast number of capillaries which abut on the air pockets. Carbon dioxide diffuses from the capillaries into the air pockets, and oxygen from the air pockets diffuses into the blood that is circulating along the lung capillaries. The air in the pockets would, of course, quickly become highly charged with carbon dioxide and depleted of oxygen if there were no provision for constantly changing it. The latter action is accomplished by respiratory movements: inspiration, by which fresh air is drawn into the lungs; and expiration, by which vitiated air is expelled from the lungs.

The Lungs, Thoracic Cavity and Pleural Cavities. The lungs are contained in the thorax (Fig. 23-1). The thorax has a cagelike framework composed of the vertebral column, the ribs, the costal cartilages and the sternum. The bottom of the cage is a dome-shaped musculotendinous sheet, the diaphragm.

The two lungs fill two large compartments in the thoracic cavity. Each compartment is lined with a fibroelastic membrane, the *parietal pleura* (Fig. 23-1), which is provided with an internal layer of squamous mesothelial cells. Likewise, each lung is covered with a similar membrane, the *visceral pleura* (Fig. 23-1), the outermost layer of which consists of squamous mesothelial cells. A film of fluid is present between the parietal pleura that lines each cavity and the visceral pleura that covers each lung; this fluid has lubricating value and allows the visceral pleura covering the lungs —hence, the lungs themselves—to slide during respiratory movements along the parietal pleura that lines the cavities.

Except at its hilus, where a bronchus and blood vessels enter it (Fig. 23-1), each lung because of the slippery pleural surfaces, is freely movable within its

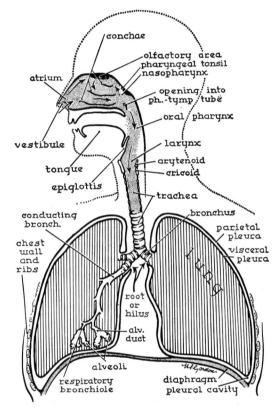

FIG. 23-1. Diagram of the parts of the respiratory system. (Redrawn and slightly modified from Grant, J. C. B.: A Method of Anatomy. ed. 4. Baltimore, Williams & Wilkins)

cavity. Around its point of attachment at the hilus, the visceral pleura covering each lung becomes continuous with the parietal pleura lining each cavity (Fig. 23-1). The space between the two layers of pleura contains, as was noted before, only a film of fluid; hence it is only a *potential space* or *cavity*. Under certain abnormal conditions the amount of fluid becomes increased; this converts the potential cavity into a real one. The potential or real space between the two layers of pleura is known as the *pleural cavity*. It should be understood that, although a lung occupies a cavity in the thorax, it does not lie in the pleural cavity but outside it, just as the intestines occupy the abdominal cavity but lie outside the peritoneal cavity.

Respiratory Movements

Inspiration. The ribs are disposed in such planes, and articulate with the vertebral column and the sternum at such angles, that the contraction of the muscles attached to them makes the thoracic cage both deeper in its anteroposterior diameter and wider. Moreover, contraction of the diaphragm (with the simultaneous relaxation of the muscles of the abdominal wall, which permits the diaphragm to descend) elongates the cage. Hence, by the contraction and the relaxation of muscles the thoracic cage can be made larger by becoming deeper, wider and longer. This is what occurs in inspiration.

In order for the thoracic cage to become larger on inspiration, something has to be drawn into it for the same reason that one cannot open a bellows if the inlet is closed. Inspiratory movements are not powerful enough to create a vacuum in the thoracic cage.

Normally, the thoracic cage can be enlarged by inspiratory movements only to the extent to which air can be drawn into its air spaces, which therefore expand, and blood can be drawn into its blood vessels to increase the amount they contain. Under normal conditions, air is drawn only into the lungs, but extra blood is drawn both into the vessels of the lungs and into those outside the lungs but inside the thorax. The reason for air not being drawn into any other part of the thoracic cavity except the lungs is that there is no opening to the surface from these other parts of the thorax through which it can be drawn. If an opening is provided—for example, a deep knife wound in the chest—air may be drawn by an inspiratory movement into parts of the thorax other than the lungs.

The lungs consist essentially of: (1) the spongy respiratory tissue in which gaseous exchange occurs between blood and air, and (2) a branching system of air tubes called *bronchioles* and *bronchi* which "pipe" air into and from the pockets and passageways of the spongy respiratory tissue. The main bronchus from each lung connects with the trachea (Fig. 23-1), and this, in turn, by means of the larynx, the nasopharynx and the nose (or the mouth if need be), connects with the outside air. Hence, on an inspiratory act, air is drawn through the nose, down the trachea, into the bronchial tree to its end branches and from there into the passageways and the pockets of the spongy, capillary-rich respiratory tissue, where, and only where,

gaseous exchange occurs (Fig. 23-1, alveolar duct and alveoli).

The Role of Elastin. Before briefly considering the mechanism of expiration, it is necessary to point out that the lungs would not fill the cavities in which they lie unless they were considerably stretched in all directions. A large amount of elastin is present in the visceral pleura that covers them, in the walls between the air pockets and in the bronchial tree. Since the lungs fill their respective cavities when they first develop in embryonic life, and since there is no easy way for fluid to be drawn into the pleural cavity during fetal life, the lungs are gradually stretched as the thoracic cavity increases in size. The same process continues in the growing period of postnatal life. As a result, the elastic tissue of the lungs, under normal conditions, is always stretched (even at the end of expiration), and the lung is always trying, as it were, to collapse and retract to the one point where it is attached (its root or hilus). Hence, if a hollow needle is inserted through the chest wall into the pleural cavity (between the parietal and the visceral layers of pleura), air immediately rushes through it into the pleural cavity, which thereupon, as the lung retracts toward the hilus, becomes a real (air-filled) cavity instead of being only a potential cavity. Letting air into the pleural cavity is a procedure sometimes used to put a lung at rest in the treatment of tuberculosis. The condition in which there is air in the pleural cavity is called a *pneumothorax*. In certain diseases the fluid in the pleural cavity, which is normally no more than a film, becomes greatly increased in amount. This, too, permits the lung to retract. This condition is known as a *hydrothorax*.

Expiration. Since the elastic tissue of the lungs is normally stretched even at the end of expiration, and becomes still more stretched on inspiration, it is scarcely necessary for an individual at rest to indulge in very much muscular movement to expel such air as is drawn into the lungs on inspiration. The elastic recoil of the lungs is almost enough to expel the air out through the bronchial tree and draw in the sides and the bottom of the thoracic cage. But during exercise expiration is facilitated—and probably also to some extent even in quiet breathing—by contractions of the abdominal muscles, which force the abdominal viscera against the undersurface of the diaphragm and so push it up into the thorax.

The Two Parts of the System: the Conducting and the Respiratory Parts. The system of cavities and tubes that conduct air from outside the body to all parts of the lungs constitutes the *conducting portion* of the respiratory system, and the pockets and the passageways of the respiratory tissue of the lung—the only sites where gaseous interchange occurs—are said to constitute the true *respiratory portion* of the system. The conducting part of the system consists of the nose, the nasopharynx, the larynx, the trachea, the bronchi and the bronchioles (Fig. 23-1). It is to be noted that some of these structures lie outside the lung, and others (some bronchi and all the bronchioles) within it. It should be realized that those parts of the conducting system that lie without the lung must be provided with reasonably rigid walls; otherwise, a strong inspiratory act might collapse them, as sucking a soft drink through a wet straw (dry straws have rigid walls) collapses the straw. Rigidity is provided by cartilage or bone. Moreover, it should be kept in mind that the conducting part of the respiratory system performs functions other than conducting air to and from the lungs. The mucous membrane lining the conducting passageways strains, washes, warms or cools, as the case may be, and humidifies the air that passes along it toward the respiratory portion of the system. In other words, the conducting portion of the respiratory system is an excellent air-conditioning unit. Its different parts and their microscopic structure will now be described.

The Nasal Cavities

The nose contains two nasal cavities, one on each side, separated from one another by the nasal septum. Each cavity opens in front by a *naris* or *nostril* and behind into the *nasopharynx* (Fig. 23-1).

Bone and, to a lesser extent, cartilage and, to a small degree, dense connective tissue provide rigidity to the walls, the floor and the roof of the nasal cavities and so prevent their collapse on inspiration.

Each nasal cavity is divided into two parts: (1) a *vestibule,* the widened part of the passageway encountered just behind the naris, and (2) the remainder of the cavity, called its *respiratory portion.*

The epidermis of the skin covering the nose extends into each naris to line the front part of each vestibule. It is provided with many large hair follicles together with some sebaceous and sweat glands. The hairs strain coarse particles from air that is drawn through the nostrils. Farther back in the vestibule, the stratified squamous epithelium is not keratinized, and, still farther back, the epithelium becomes pseudostratified ciliated columnar with goblet cells. This type of epithelium lines the remainder of each nasal cavity.

The mucous membrane lining the respiratory portion of the nasal cavities consists of pesudostratified columnar ciliated epithelium with goblet cells and a lamina propria that contains both mucous and serous glands, which is adherent to the periosteum of the bone, or the perichondrium of the cartilage, beneath it. The basement membrane separating the respiratory epithelium from the lamina propria is thicker than that for most epithelia.

The surface of the epithelium is normally covered with mucus provided by its goblet cells and by the glands of its lamina propria. Probably over a pint of fluid is produced by the nasal mucous membrane each day. The mucus, together with the particles of dust and dirt that are picked up by it, is moved backward through the nasopharynx to the oral pharynx by means of the cilia with which the epithelial lining cells, excepting the goblet cells, are provided. Each cell has between 15 and 20 cilia that are about 7 μ in height and are anchored in the cytoplasm by rootlets. The drainage of the nose depends to a great extent on orderly ciliary action, and a loss of cilia from trauma or disease can interfere with the proper drainage of the nose.

The lamina propria contains both collagenic and elastic fibers. In some sites, and evidently by no means regularly, the lamina propria forms a well-developed basement membrane with elastic properties. Lymphocytes, plasma cells, macrophages and even granular leukocytes may be seen in the lamina propria. In general, it is a very vascular membrane, and in cold weather it helps to warm the air that is to be drawn into the lungs. In some sites lymphatic nodules appear; these are most numerous near the entrance to the nasopharynx.

The mucous membrane of the respiratory portion of the nose has special characteristics in two places. That lining the upper parts of the sides and the roof of the posterior part of each cavity constitutes the organ of smell (the olfactory organ), and its special microscopic structure will be described in the chapter dealing with the system of sensory receptors (Chap. 28). The other site in which the mucous membrane is not typical will be dealt with now.

Three plates of bone, arranged one above the other like shelves, are disposed along the lateral wall of each nasal cavity. However, they are not flat like useful shelves; they are more like unsupported metal shelves which have had to bear too much weight, for they all curve downward. Since their curved form makes them look something like shells, they are called the *superior,* the *middle* and the *inferior conchae* (*concha* is Latin for shell), respectively (Figs. 23-1 and 23-2). They are also often referred to as the *superior,* the *middle* and the *inferior turbinate* (*turbinatus,* scroll-like) bones.

Although the mucous membrane of the nasal cavities is very vascular, containing many arteries, capillaries

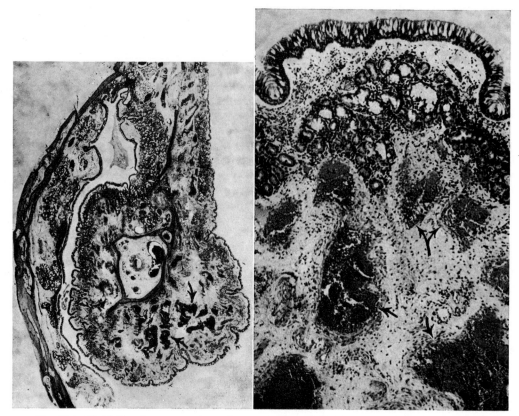

Fɪɢ. 23-2. (*Left*) Very low-power photomicrograph of a cross section of a concha. Thin bone may be seen in its central part. The blood in the venous spaces is dark. (*Right*) Medium-power photomicrograph of a section of the mucous membrane covering a concha. Glands may be seen in the upper region, and large venous spaces distended with blood (arrows) may be seen in the lower part of the figure.

and veins, that of the lamina propria of the mucosa covering the middle and the inferior conchae has, in addition, a large number of venous structures which, under normal conditions, are collapsed. However, under certain circumstances they can become distended with blood (Fig. 23-2), and this so increases the thickness of the mucosa that in some individuals it encroaches on the airway to such an extent that nose breathing is made difficult.

The term *erectile tissue* is usually used to designate any tissue that contains a large number of endothelial-lined cavities which, although they are on the circuit of the bloodstream, are usually collapsed and become distended with blood, to increase greatly the size of the tissue in which they lie, only as a result of special nervous stimulation. Most of the substance of the male copulatory organ, the penis, is erectile tissue; this accounts for the changes in the size and the consistency of this organ that can occur under conditions

of erotic stimulation. The lamina propria of the nasal mucosa of the conchae is not as typically erectile tissue as that present in the penis, and some observers consider that it is not true erectile tissue at all. Perhaps it is better described as possessing a great many thin-walled veins along which smooth muscle fibers are both circularly and longitudinally disposed (Fig. 23-2, *right*). Nevertheless, it reacts like erectile tissue in that it can rapidly become turgid with blood. Furthermore, in certain individuals the mucosa covering the conchae is affected by erotic stimuli. Mackenzie, many years ago, described individuals encountered in his own practice in whom erotic stimulation was associated with sneezing, with engorgement of the nasal mucosa covering the conchae and even with bleeding from this area; indeed, he even quotes one 16th century report of a youth who sneezed whenever he saw a pretty girl. It is difficult to understand the purpose served by having the erectile tissue of the nose linked nervously with that of the genital systems. The relationship probably hinges somehow on the fact that sex stimulation is so very dependent on the sense of smell in a large part of the animal kingdom.

Paranasal Air Sinuses of the Nose

The air *sinuses* (*sinus,* bay or hollow) are spaces in bones. There are 4 associated with each nasal cavity. They are named after the bones in which they are contained and hence are called the *frontal,* the *ethmoidal,* the *sphenoidal* and the *maxillary* sinuses, respectively. The maxillary sinus is the largest and is sometimes called the *antrum* (*antron,* a cavity) *of Highmore.*

The 4 sinuses on each side all communicate with the nasal cavity of that side. They are all lined by mucous membrane continuous with that lining the nasal cavity. The ciliated epithelium in the sinuses is not so thick as that in the nasal cavity itself, and it does not contain nearly so many goblet cells. The lamina propria is relatively thin and is continuous with the periosteum of the underlying bone. It consists chiefly of collagenic fibers and contains eosinophils, plasma cells and many lymphocytes in addition to fibroblasts. It has relatively few glands embedded in it.

The openings by which the sinuses communicate with the nasal cavities are not so large as to prevent their becoming closed if the mucosa at and around the opening becomes inflamed or sufficiently swollen for other reasons. Normally, the mucus formed in sinuses is moved to the nasal cavities by ciliary action. If the openings of the sinuses become obstructed, the sinuses may fill with mucus or, under conditions of infection, with pus. Drugs which act similarly to hormones of the adrenal medulla and cause contraction of the blood vessels of the part are often used locally to lessen the congestion about the openings of inflamed sinuses and so permit them to drain. Sometimes new openings must be made surgically to permit them to drain properly.

The Pharyngeal Tonsil

This consists of an unpaired median mass of lymphatic tissue in the lamina propria of the mucous membrane lining the dorsal wall of the nasopharynx (Fig. 23-1). A child who has an enlarged pharyngeal tonsil is said to have *adenoids* (*aden,* gland) because the enlarged lymphatic follicles of the tonsil give it a gland-like appearance. Adenoids may obstruct the respiratory passageway and lead to persistent mouth breathing. The muscular actions entailed in keeping the mouth always open, by changing the normal lines of

force to which the bones of the developing face are subjected, may prevent the bones of the face from developing as they otherwise would, and the effect produced is usually unfortunate. For this reason, and also for the reason that an enlarged pharyngeal tonsil is usually more or less persistently infected, the removal of adenoids is a relatively common operation.

The pharyngeal tonsil resembles the palatine tonsil in microscopic structure except that: (1) it is more diffuse, (2) its covering epithelium dips down into it as folds rather than crypts, and (3) its epithelium may be pseudostratified, at least in some areas, instead of stratified squamous nonkeratinizing.

The Larynx

The larynx is the segment of the respiratory tube that connects the pharynx with the trachea (Fig. 23-1). Its walls are kept from collapsing on inspiration by a number of cartilages that are contained in its wall and bound together with connective tissue membranes. Muscles that act on the cartilages are present both outside them (the extrinsic muscles of the larynx) and between them and the mucous membrane (the intrinsic muscles of the larynx). The larynx has many functions. It plays the most important part in phonation; however, this is phylogenetically a late development. A more fundamental function of the larynx is that of preventing anything but air from gaining entrance to the lower respiratory passages. It is said to be the watchdog for the lung, and if, in spite of its efforts, anything but air enters it, a cough reflex is set in motion immediately. It is of interest in this connection to note that some individuals who apparently have died from drowning are found at autopsy to have very little water in their lungs; they probably die from asphyxiation caused by laryngeal spasm induced by water gaining entrance to and irritating this organ.

The apex of a flaplike structure, the *epiglottis,* whose free portion projects upward and slightly backward, is attached anteriorly to constitute the uppermost part of the larynx (Fig. 23-1). In days past it was thought that the free part of this structure flapped down over the entrance of the larynx when food was swallowed and in this way kept food and fluid from gaining entrance to the larynx. Although this view has some modern supporters, it is now generally thought that the epiglottis plays a more subsidiary and passive role in keeping food and fluid out of the larynx during the act of swallowing, and that the main factor responsible for this latter effect is the larynx being brought upward and forward in the act of swallowing so that the upper end of its tubular part is pressed against

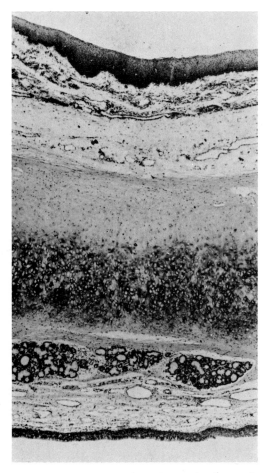

FIG. 23-3. Low-power photomicrograph of a section cut across the epiglottis. The anterior surface is above; the posterior below.

wear and tear. It, too, is of the stratified squamous non-keratinizing type. Taste buds are occasionally present in it. However, the epithelium covering the lower part of the posterior surface does not come into contact with food, and, since it constitutes the lining of part of the respiratory tube, it is lined with pseudostratified columnar ciliated epithelium with goblet cells (Fig. 23-3, *bottom*). The cilia beat toward the pharynx and wash mucus and particles picked up by the mucus in that direction. Mucous glands with some serous secretory units are present in the lamina propria under the posterior surface. They are said to be present also under the anterior surface. Glands are more numerous toward the attached margin of the epiglottis.

The lumen of the larynx is narrowed and made more or less slitlike (the slit being directed in an antero-posterior direction) in two sites by folds of mucous membrane that projects into the lumen from each side. The upper pair of folds constitute the false vocal cords (Fig. 23-4). The second pair of folds lie below the first pair, and their cordlike free margins constitute the true vocal cords (Fig. 23-4). The opening between the two vocal cords is termed the *rima glottidis*. It is slit-like when the vocal cords are close together but somewhat triangular in shape, with the apex of the triangle directed forward when the vocal cords are farther

the posterior aspect of the epiglottis, under the root of the tongue. Individuals who have had the epiglottis removed for one cause or another can still swallow without food entering the larynx.

A plate of elastic cartilage (Fig. 23-3) forms an internal support for the epiglottis. The perichondrium of this is continuous with the lamina propria of the mucous membrane which covers both its surfaces. The epithelium of the mucous membrane varies in relation to the function of the different parts of the epiglottis. On the anterior surface, where the epiglottis comes into contact with the root of the tongue in the act of swallowing, the epithelium is of the stratified squamous nonkeratinizing type (Fig. 23-3) that is so well adapted to cover wet surfaces subjected to wear and tear. The epithelium covering the upper part of the posterior surface comes into contact with things being swallowed and so is subjected to considerable

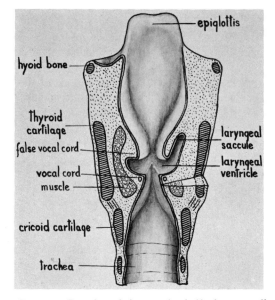

FIG. 23-4. Drawing of the anterior half of a coronally sectioned larynx as seen from behind. The cut is farther forward at the upper right side of the illustration so that the saccule is disclosed. (Redrawn and modified from Schaeffer, E. A.: Textbook of Microscopic Anatomy, published as Vol. 2, Part I, of Quain's Elements of Anatomy. ed. 11. New York, Longmans)

apart. The expansion of the lumen of the larynx between the two sets of folds is called the *sinus* or *ventricle* of the larynx (Fig. 23-4). Anteriorly, the sinus
of each side is prolonged upward. Each cul-de-sac, so
formed, is called the *laryngeal saccule* (Fig. 23-4).
The cores of the folds that comprise the false vocal
cords are composed chiefly of a somewhat loose lamina
propria which contains glands. The cores of the second and lower pair of folds consist of connective tissue
and muscle. The cores of the vocal cords themselves
(the parts of the folds nearest their free edges) consist of connective tissue that is composed chiefly of
elastic fibers. The aperture between the true vocal
cords, and the tension under which the cords exist, are
affected both by muscle fibers that act on the cords
directly and by muscle fibers that affect the cords indirectly by shifting the tissues to which they are
anchored.

The epithelium of the mucous membrane of the
larynx varies in relation to the functions performed
by its different parts. That covering the true vocal
cords, which are subjected to considerable wear and
tear, is of the stratified squamous nonkeratinizing
type. All the epithelium lining the larynx below the
true vocal cords is of the pseudostratified columnar
ciliated type with goblet cells. Most of that lining
the larynx above the true vocal cords is also of this
type, although patches of stratified squamous nonkeratinizing epithelium may be present in some sites. The
cilia beat toward the pharynx. Except over the true
vocal cords the lamina propria of the mucous membrane contains mucous glands. Lymph nodules occur
in the lamina propria of the mucous membrane. They
are more numerous along the lateral and dorsal wall
in the region of the ventricle and the false vocal cords.

The larynx is responsible for the phenomenon of
phonation, which is the ability to utter vocal sounds.
This ability hinges on vibration occurring in the vocal
cords. Vibrations are generated by air currents in a
somewhat complex manner and the pitch of the sound
depends on the extent to which the vocal cords are
stretched or relaxed and also on functional changes in
the arrangement of their edges. Vocalization is a
further complex matter. Lips, tongue, soft palate and
the various cavities with which these structures are
associated are all also involved. Special references
should be read for a satisfactory understanding of this
most interesting and important subject.

The Trachea

The trachea is a tube continuous with the larynx
above and ending below by dividing into two primary

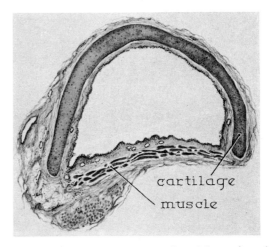

FIG. 23-5. Drawing of a cross section of the trachea of
an adult (very low-power).

bronchi which pass toward the right and the left lung,
respectively (Fig. 23-1).

The trachea is prevented from collapsing by about
20 U- or horseshoe-shaped cartilages that are set in
its wall one above the other so that each almost encircles the lumen. The open ends of these incomplete
cartilaginous rings are directed backward (Fig. 23-5),
and the gap between the two ends of each ring is
bridged by connective tissue and smooth muscle (Fig.
23-5).

If a *longitudinal section* is cut from the wall of the
trachea, the cartilaginous rings that encircle its wall
are cut in *cross section*. The cross-section appearance
of each ring is roughly ovoid (Fig. 23-6) with a greatest supero-inferior diameter of 3 or 4 mm. and a greatest mediolateral diameter of 1 mm. or thereabouts.
The inner surface of each ring is convex, and its outer
surface relatively flat (Fig. 23-6). The space between
adjacent rings is considerably less than the supero-
inferior diameters of the rings themselves and is filled
with dense connective tissue which is continuous with
that of the perichondrium of each ring (Fig. 23-6).
The bundles of collagenic fibers which make up this
connective tissue are woven in such a way that some
degree of elasticity is imparted to the tracheal wall.
Some elastic fibers, distributed among the bundles of
collagenic fibers, also may be of some importance in
this respect.

The trachea is lined by a mucous membrane. The
epithelium is of the pseudostratified ciliated columnar
type with goblet cells (Fig. 5-49). The lamina propria
on which the epithelium rests is condensed to form a

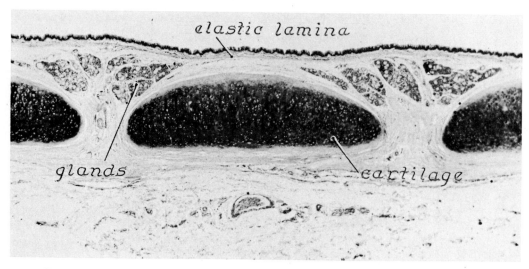

Fɪɢ. 23-6. Very low-power photomicrograph of a longitudinal section of the anterior wall of the trachea of an adult.

moderately distinct basement membrane. The remainder of the lamina propria contains a fairly high proportion of elastic fibers. A tendency toward a lymphatic character is indicated by the presence in the membrane of cells of the lymphocyte series and occasional true nodules. The deep border of the lamina propria is marked by a dense lamina or membrane of elastin (Fig. 23-6). The tissue just deep to this is termed *submucosa*. The secretory portions of many mucous glands, with some serous secretory units, are embedded in the submucosa. In longitudinal sections of the trachea the secretory portions of these glands are seen to be disposed chiefly in the submucosa that fills in the triangular spaces between adjacent cartilages (Fig. 23-6). The ducts from these glands pierce the elastic lamina of the lamina propria to empty on the inner surface of the trachea. Some secretory units may be present also in the lamina propria.

The posterior wall of the trachea is composed of interlacing bundles of smooth muscle fibers, arranged chiefly in the transverse plane and knitted together by connective tissue (Fig. 23-5). The inner surface of the posterior wall of the trachea is lined with a mucous membrane similar to that lining the remainder of its wall. The secretory units of glands are present in the mucous membrane, outside the mucous membrane in the interstices between the bundles of smooth muscle, and even outside the smooth muscle, in the connective tissue of the outer layers of the wall.

The fine structure of ciliated cells and cilia and of goblet cells was described in Chapter 5.

The Bronchial Tree

The trachea ends by dividing into 2 branches, the 2 primary bronchi, which pass to the roots of the lungs (Fig. 23-1). The microscopic structure of the walls of these is the same as that of the wall of the trachea.

Usually the right lung is made up of 3 lobes and the left lung of 2. Each primary bronchus, in a sense, continues into the lower lobe of the particular lung to which it passes. The right primary bronchus, before doing so, gives off 2 branches to supply the middle and the upper lobes, respectively, of that lung. Likewise, the left primary bronchus, before continuing into the lower lobe of the left lung, gives off a branch to supply the upper lobe of that lung. At the hilus of each lung the primary bronchus and its main branches become closely associated with the arteries which also enter the lung at this site and the veins and lymphatics which leave the lung, and all these tubular structures become invested in dense connective tissue. This complex of tubes invested in dense connective tissue is termed the *root* of the lung.

As stated above, a large bronchus enters each of the lobes of the two lungs. Within the lobes these branch to give rise to progressively smaller bronchi. The manner in which the first branchings occur to supply different parts of the different lobes of the lung is a matter of considerable interest, particularly in the surgical treatment of certain diseases of the lung. Although there is some variation, certain parts or areas of each lobe tend to be supplied by certain main branches of the bronchus that enters the lobe. These parts or areas represent units of lung structure that may be dealt with surgically and are of a smaller order of size than whole lobes. The pattern and the bronchial connections of these constitute a matter too specialized to discuss here.

Microscopic Structure of Intrapulmonary Bronchi. Although the bronchi that are within the lung have a microscopic structure similar to that of the trachea and the extrapulmonary portions of the 2 primary bronchi, they are somewhat different in a few respects, which will now be described.

(1) The U- or horseshoe-shaped cartilages of the trachea and the extrapulmonary parts of the primary bronchi are replaced in the intrapulmonary bronchi by cartilage plates of a most irregular shape. In a cross section of an intrapulmonary bronchus these may appear as crescents or ovals (Fig. 23-7), and the impression is given that several are required to encircle the tube. But, as Miller has pointed out, this appearance is deceptive, for he found from reconstructions that what seemed to be several cartilages in a single section are only the various prolongations of a single large cartilage of irregular shape. In many instances he found the irregular cartilages to encircle the lumen completely. Since cartilages are disposed around all parts of the walls of these bronchi, the latter are not flattened on one surface like the trachea and the extra-

pulmonary bronchi. At sites of branchings Miller found that special saddle-shaped cartilages were often present to support the 2 branches at the site where they make an acute angle with one another. The spaces between different cartilages and parts of the same cartilage which would otherwise be weak spots in the bronchial wall are filled with collagenic connective tissue which is continuous with the perichondrium of the cartilages concerned.

(2) The smooth muscle which is present only in the posterior part of the trachea and the extrapulmonary bronchi comes, in the intrapulmonary bronchi, to constitute a layer which completely encircles the lumen. This layer of muscle lies between the mucous membrane and the cartilages (Fig. 23-7). It does not appear as a complete layer in every section because it is composed of 2 sets of smooth muscle fibers that wind down the bronchial tree in a left and a right spiral, respectively. The arrangement of muscle can be roughly demonstrated by winding 2 shoelaces down a broomstick in fairly close spirals, one clockwise and the other counterclockwise.

(3) The contraction of this muscle after death, and perhaps to some extent during life, throws the mucous membrane into the longitudinal folds that are characteristic of intrapulmonary bronchi seen in cross sections (Fig. 23-7).

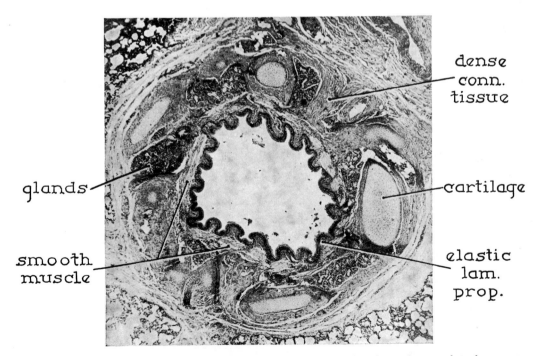

Fig. 23-7. Very low-power photomicrograph of a cross section of an intrapulmonary bronchus.

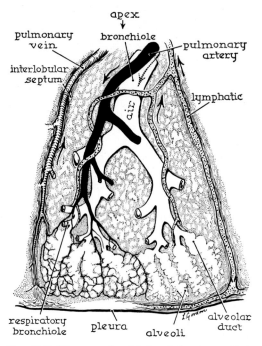

Fig. 23-8. Diagram of a lobule of the lung with its base abutting on the pleura. The size of the bronchioles and the air passages, as well as that of the blood vessels and the lymphatics, is out of proportion. To make it easier to follow the course of the blood vessels and the lymphatics, the former have been omitted from the right side, and the latter from the left side.

(4) The elastic lamina that marks the outer limit of the mucous membrane of the trachea is not present as such in the intrapulmonary bronchi, but instead elastic fibers are distributed in a way that will now be described. In the bronchi, the cartilages are bound together by coarse elastic fibers. Finer fibrils are present in the adventitia, between the muscle fibers and in the lamina propria. The most remarkable feature, however, is the presence of several strong stripes of elastic tissue situated in the lamina propria and running parallel to each other for the full length of the bronchial tree. They may easily be seen with the naked eye on inspection of the mucosa. They branch with the successive bronchial branches and are continuous with the elastic components of the terminal air passages.

The intrapulmonary bronchi are lined with ciliated pseudostratified columnar epithelium, and the secretion of the goblet cells disposed in this membrane is augmented by that of glands. The secretory portions of these are disposed, for the most part, outside the muscular layer (Fig. 23-7), particularly in sites where there are intervals between cartilages.

Both lymph nodes and individual nodules are scattered along the bronchi in the outermost fibrous parts of their walls.

Method of Branching. In general, the branching that occurs in the bronchial tree is of the *dichotomous* (*dichotomia,* a cutting in two) variety, with the total cross-sectional area of the lumens of each 2 branches that arise being greater than the cross-sectional area of the lumen of the parent tube. This fact has implications with regard to the relative speeds at which air travels in the smaller and the larger branches of the bronchial tree. Since the same amount of air (per unit of time) can pass through a parent tube as can pass through its 2 branches (which have a greater total cross-sectional area) only if it moves faster in the parent tube, it follows that air moves slowest in the smallest tubes of the bronchial tree and fastest in the largest. Keeping this in mind is of importance in interpreting the breath sounds heard with a stethoscope.

The Differences Between Bronchi and Bronchioles. The continued branching of the bronchial tree results in the formation of successively narrower bronchi. The smaller ones differ in structure from the larger ones, chiefly because their cartilages are not so large and do not extend around their walls so completely.

As will be explained later, the lung develops like a gland, and as a result its substance is made up of lobules. The bronchi of the lung are the equivalent of the extralobular ducts of glands because they are outside lobules. The branches of the bronchial tree that enter lobules, generally at their apices, are termed *bronchioles;* they are the counterparts of the intralobular ducts of glands. They differ in structure from bronchi in being smaller (generally bronchioles are less than 1 mm. in diameter), having ciliated columnar epithelium instead of pseudostratified columnar ciliated, and also by not having any cartilages in their walls. As will be explained later, bronchioles do not require cartilages in their walls to keep them from collapsing on inspiratory movements because they are inside the substance of the lung, which is opened up and hence expanded by inspiratory movements.

As is true in intralobular ducts, some connective tissue from interlobular septa extends along bronchioles to provide the larger ones particularly with support (Fig. 23-9).

Lung Lobules. Likening bronchioles to intralobular ducts is helpful because each of the bronchioles that arises from the branching of the smaller bronchi enters what is called a *lobule* of the lung to course thereafter, like an intralobular duct, through, and branch within, the substance of a lobule. Before discussing how the bronchioles connect with the air spaces where an interchange of gases between blood and air occurs, we shall discuss the structure of lobules in more detail.

Lung lobules, like pyramids, have apices and bases (Fig. 23-8). But here their resemblance to pyramids usually ends, for lobules are very irregular in shape. They vary greatly in size; their bases vary from somewhat less than 1 cm. to 2 or more cm. in diameter, and their height varies even more. Before considering how they are arranged within lobes, it may be helpful to compare each main bronchus with the trunk of a tree in that the bronchus "grows" from the root of the lung toward the central part of a lobe, and even beyond this point, branching as it grows. The smaller branches of the tree that are going to enter lobules and so become bronchioles mostly point outward toward the periphery of the lobe, but a considerable number of them point not outward, but inward, toward the central part of the lobe. The lobules fill the space that is available to them, and this affects their shape. The peripheral lobules tend to have the shape of elongated pyramids, as is illustrated in Figure 23-8, but the more central lobules in a lobe may be of irregular shapes and have angular contours. However, all the lobules are so arranged that their apices receive bronchioles (Fig. 23-8). This means that the bases of some lobules face the periphery of the lobe and those of others face its interior.

The bases of the peripheral lobules are visible as polygonal areas beneath the pleura. They are separated from one another by fibrous septa, which in man extend for only a short distance (as complete septa) into the lung. In some animals, however—for example, the pig—the lobules are completely separated from each other by interlobular septa of dense connective tissue. This is continuous with the connective tissue of the visceral pleura at the base of the lobule and with the dense connective tissue that ensheathes the bronchi at the apex of the lobule. However, in other animals—for example, the rabbit—the lobules are not separated from one another by septa. In man the septa are incomplete (Fig. 23-21).

Microscopic Structures of Bronchioles. A bronchiole on entering a lobule gives rise to many branches, and these extend in a treelike fashion to all parts of the lobule. Since bronchioles, like intralobular ducts, lie within the substance of lobules, they are attached on all sides to the elastic spongework of tissue that contains the air spaces where gaseous exchange occurs (Fig. 23-9). There is, then, no tendency for them to collapse on inspiratory movements; indeed, on an inspiratory movement they are "pulled on," all around their circumference, as the elastic fibers of the respiratory spongework are stretched. Hence, there is no need for the walls of the bronchioles to be protected against

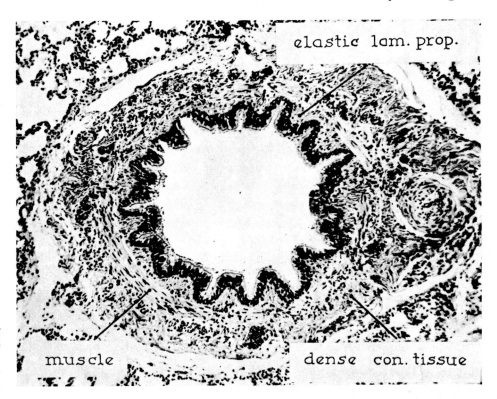

Fig. 23-9. Low-power photomicrograph of a cross section of a large bronchiole (Engel's bronchiolus) in the lung of a child.

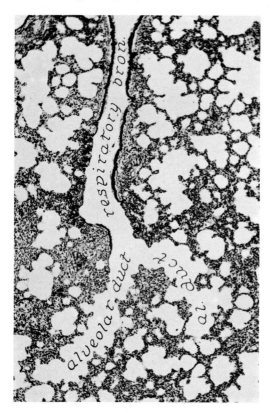

FIG. 23-10. Very low-power photomicrograph of a section of the lung of a very young child. A respiratory bronchiole is cut longitudinally and may be seen to be opening into 2 alveolar ducts.

collapsing on inspiratory movements by cartilaginous rings or plates, and they have none in their walls. They differ from bronchi also in not having any glands in their walls; perhaps they are so close to the respiratory spaces that secretions delivered into them from glands might be sucked into the respiratory spaces. Moreover, their epithelial lining is not as thick as that of bronchi. In the larger branches ciliated columnar cells are in the majority but nonciliated cells are scattered between them. These are tall and have been described as having a more or less serous secretory function. In the final branches, nonciliated cells that are of a high cuboidal type are present. To sum up, the walls of bronchioles consist of epithelium that rests on a thin elastic lamina propria, and this layer, in turn, is surrounded by the muscular coat previously described for bronchi (Fig. 23-9). The muscle is supported by connective tissue.

Orders of Bronchioles. Once inside a lobule, the bronchiole that enters it and which could be termed a preterminal bronchiole, gives off branches known as

terminal bronchioles, the number of which varies according to the size of the lobule. There are often 5 to 7 terminal bronchioles.

The next order of bronchioles arise, of course, from terminal bronchioles, and are called *respiratory* bronchioles (Figs. 23-8 and 23-10). The reason for their name is that as they branch and extend into lung substance they exhibit an increasing number of little delicate air-containing outpouchings from their walls. These little outpouchings are limited by capillary networks ensconced in delicate frameworks that will be described presently; the point to be made here is that gaseous exchange occurs between the blood in the capillaries in the walls of the outpouchings and the air they contain. Because respiration thus occurs in the outpouchings from these bronchioles they are called *respiratory* bronchioles. The free terminations of the respiratory bronchioles flare out to some extent and open into what are called alveolar ducts.

The Respiratory Portion of the Lobule; Alveolar Ducts, Alveolar Sacs (Saccules) and Alveoli. Before commenting on alveolar ducts, into which the respiratory bronchioles open, it may be helpful to emphasize that the bronchi and the bronchioles are tubes with walls of their own, and that they serve primarily to conduct air back and forth to the respiratory portions of the lobules. The terms that we shall now use to describe how air is conducted into all parts of the respiratory portion of the lobule (alveolar ducts, alveolar sacs [saccules] and alveoli), do not refer to structures that have walls of their own (as have bronchioles) but rather to spaces of various orders and shapes that exist in a huge elastic spongelike arrangement of capillary beds through which the right heart constantly pumps blood (Figs. 23-8 and 23-10). Alveolar ducts, alveolar sacs and alveoli all contain air that is more or less constantly being changed. The air in all these spaces is in close contact with the capillaries in the walls of the spongework that divide this portion of the lung into spaces, and since both the air and the blood are separated only by thin films of tissue through which diffusion occurs readily, a mechanism is provided for permitting blood to lose its carbon dioxide and take on oxygen as it passes through the capillary beds of the elastic spongelike respiratory portion of the lung.

Alveolar Ducts, Alveolar Sacs (Saccules) and Alveoli. The spaces into which the respiratory bronchioles directly open have the shape of long branching hallways along which there are many open doors of two general sizes. The long branching hallways are termed *alveolar ducts* (Fig. 23-10). The larger open doors communicate with rotundalike spaces which are termed *alveolar sacs* or *saccules*. Projecting inward from the periphery of the rotundalike saccules, spurlike partitions divide the peripheral zone of each saccule into a series of cubicles that open into the central part of the saccule. The cubicles are alveoli. It has been estimated that there are 300 million alveoli in an adult lung which present a surface area to air of 70 to 80 square meters.

Before describing the histologic structure of the walls that separate the air spaces from one another we shall comment briefly on units of respiratory structure smaller than lobules; these are of importance in understanding certain pathologic conditions of the lung.

Units of Structure Within the Lobule. It has been stated already that one bronchiole serves a unit of lung structure called the lobule. However, there never have been any generally agreed-upon terms for the units supplied by the succeeding divisions of the respiratory tree. The unit of lung served by a terminal bronchiole is now often termed an *acinus*. Millard suggests that this is the most practical unit of structure for dealing with pathologic conditions. There are no standard names for the more distal units, but Barrie has suggested that they should be designated according to the channel that supplies them. Thus the unit supplied by a respiratory bronchiole could be termed a respiratory bronchiolar unit, and the unit supplied by an alveolar duct a ductal unit.

The Microscopic Study of the Respiratory Portion of the Lung

The elastic fibers present in the spongework of the lung necessarily are stretched to enable a lung to fill the cavity in which it lies. Hence, when the pleural cavities are opened at autopsy the lungs collapse toward their roots. Sections cut from collapsed lungs do not give a representative picture of the structure of the respiratory spongework during life, for, when a lung collapses, the spaces in the spongework become smaller, and the partitions between the spaces become thicker. A better impression of the structure of the lung during life can be obtained from the study of sections cut from lungs that have been redistended to their original size immediately after death by injecting fixative through a cannula into a stem bronchus and subsequently tying off the bronchus so that the lung cannot collapse again.

Alveolar Walls or Septa vs. Interalveolar Walls or Septa. Most of the partitions seen in the spongework of the lung separate adjacent alveoli from one another. Some partitions, of course, separate the pas-

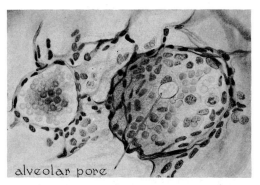

FIG. 23-11. Drawing of a thick section (high-power) of the lung of the rabbit. A venule shows at the left, and the floor of an alveolus is to be seen on the right. The blood cells in the floor are in capillaries. At one site, the floor of the alveolus exhibits a defect, an alveolar pore.

sageways of alveolar ducts from alveolar spaces that are just outside the duct but which communicate with some other duct. In general, all of these partitions are called *alveolar septa* or *alveolar walls*. However, it should be understood clearly that the word *alveolus* has two meanings: it can be used to depict either *a little space* or *a little vessel* (structure). In the instance of the postnatal lung, the word is used to depict a space. The structure that is termed an alveolar wall contains many components and is actually an *interalveolar* wall or septum; it lies *between* two alveoli.

The Structure of Interalveolar Walls or Septa

The Use of Thick Sections. In thin sections of distended lungs, interalveolar partitions are always cut in cross or oblique sections. The reason for this is that in distended lungs interalveolar partitions are as thin as the sections themselves, and since they are never perfectly flat (as sections are), it is impossible for a whole alveolar partition to be present in a thin section so that its full face may be examined. To see an interalveolar partition in full face it is necessary to cut sections of lung that are about as thick as the diameter of alveoli. In such sections, sites may be found where the top of one alveolus has been sliced off, together with the bottom of the alveolus immediately below it. One may then look down into an alveolus as one looks into a cup to inspect its bottom. In this instance the bottom of the cup is the interalveolar partition between the alveolus into which one is looking and the alveolus immediately below it (Fig. 23-11).

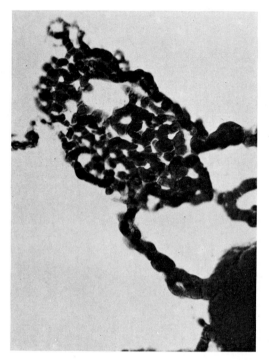

FIG. 23-12. High-power photomicrograph of a thick section of a lung, the blood vessels of which were injected with an opaque material. The figure shows the floor of an alveolus (an interalveolar partition in full face), and the injected capillaries may be seen to form an extensive and close mesh.

The Capillaries of the Walls. It is not easy to identify the various cells and structures in interalveolar walls seen this way. Many nuclei are seen; the various cells that contain these will be described presently. The extent of the capillary network in an interalveolar septum can scarcely be realized unless thick sections of lungs, the blood vessels of which have been injected with opaque material, are studied. Interalveolar walls seen in full face in such preparations show the networks in the interalveolar walls to be of a very close mesh (Fig. 23-12).

Alveolar Pores and Lambert's Sinuses. Some interalveolar partitions studied in full face in thick sections will be seen to be defective. The defects appear as little round or oval holes termed *alveolar pores* (Fig. 23-11). These were studied extensively by Macklin. Where present, they permit air to pass from one alveolus to another. Although some have argued that pores are always the result of a previous disease process, they are so abundant in the interalveolar partitions of so many different kinds of animals that the view that considers them all to be pathologic defects

no longer seems reasonable. Interalveolar pores may be regarded as allowing interchange of air in alveolar sacs whose own supply routes have been obstructed. Recently, further intercommunicating channels have been discovered in the lung by Lambert. These are short openings in the walls of bronchioles or respiratory bronchioles leading into alveolar sacs belonging to the same or to a neighboring unit. These channels, called Lambert's sinuses, provide an alternative route for entry or escape of air into the terminal units and probably play an important role when parts of the lungs become fibrotic.

How Interalveolar Walls Are Supported. The capillary networks of which interalveolar walls are chiefly composed have little tensile strength. If they were not supported in some fashion, individual alveoli might become so overexpanded with air that the capillaries would be torn. However, such support as is provided for interalveolar walls cannot be too rigid, lest it interfere with their normal expansion. The matter seems to have been solved by interalveolar walls having two kinds of support, *basic* and *intimate*. The

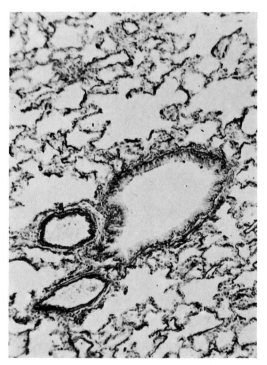

FIG. 23-13. Low-power photomicrograph of a section of rabbit lung stained with orcein to demonstrate elastic fibers. The elastic fibers appear as black lines and may be seen in the wall of the bronchiole, in the arteries, in the interalveolar partitions and along the alveolar ducts.

basic support consists of a skeleton of elastic fibers (Fig. 23-13). These are coarse and too infrequent to provide an intimate support for the many capillaries and cells in the walls; however, they do provide a backbone that would resist overexpansion. In addition to the occasional fibers that course along in walls, there are, according to Short, elastic fibers around the free margins of alveoli (where they open into alveolar sacs or ducts).

As noted above, the occasional elastic fibers that run in interalveolar walls provide a backbone for them but no intimate support for the capillaries and the cells

within the wall. Intimate support is provided for these by delicate fibrils of the reticular or the collagenic variety and by basement membranes, as will now be described. Some smooth muscle fibers may be seen along alveolar ducts, particularly around their doorways.

Concepts of the microscopic structure of interalveolar walls have changed considerably over the last decade because of research along two different lines. First, studies with the EM, beginning with the pioneer studies of Low, have shown clearly that alveoli are lined with a continuous layer of epithelium which, except

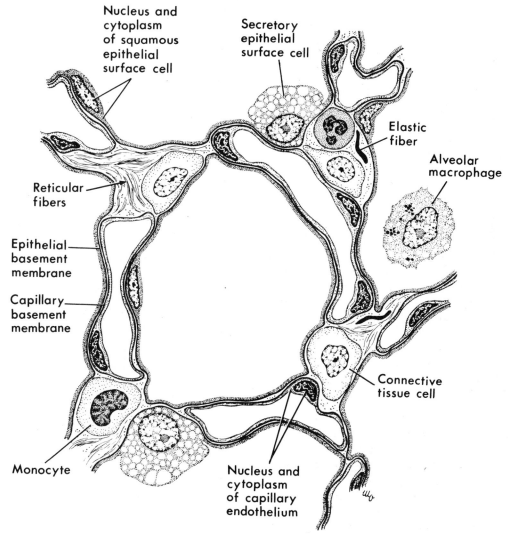

Fig. 23-14. Schematic drawing of a thin section of alveoli showing the modern concept of the structure and cell types of alveolar walls and the relation of cells to the basement membranes. (Modified, with additions, from illustrations by F. Bertalanffy and C. P. Leblond)

in sites where nuclei are present, is so thin that it would not be visible in ordinary sections examined with the LM. Second, the use of the PA-Schiff technic has made it possible, as has been shown so clearly by Leblond and Bertalanffy and their associates, to demonstrate the existence and the distribution of the basement membranes that underlie the epithelium and cover the capillaries in interalveolar walls (Fig. 23-14). Since experience with the basement membrane of the lens of the eye (which can be readily shelled out) indicates that it has some rigidity, it is likely that the basement membranes of the surface epithelium and the capillaries constitute important structural elements in the alveolar walls. It is now apparent that air in the alveoli is separated from blood in the capillaries, as can be seen in Figure 23-14 by: (1) the cytoplasm of the epithelial cells that line alveoli; (2) the basement membrane of the epithelium, which in some sites blends with the third component; (3) the basement membrane that covers the endothelium of the capillaries; and (4) the cytoplasm of the endothelial cells of capillaries. In some sites there are tissue spaces between the basement membranes of the epithelium and the capillaries, and some of these contain fine fibrils.

The Cells of Interalveolar Walls. The interalveolar walls, more commonly called alveolar walls, reveal nuclei which belong to two categories of cells: (1) those of the epithelial cells that line the alveoli, and (2) those of cells that are contained within the substance of the walls. With the LM it is, to say the least, difficult to distinguish between most of the nuclei of the two categories. Most of the nuclei seen appear as flattened or bent ovoids with fairly condensed chromatin, and most of these are the nuclei of the endothelial cells of the capillaries. Some of them, however, are the nuclei of the epithelial cells that line alveoli (Fig. 23-14).

The endothelial cells of capillaries were described in Chapter 19. We must here describe the epithelial cells that are found on the surface of alveoli.

THE TWO TYPES OF SURFACE EPITHELIAL CELLS

(1) **The Squamous Cells.** The alveolar walls are covered with a continuous epithelial membrane. Most of the cells of this membrane are of the simple squamous type (Fig. 23-15). Indeed, the cytoplasm of these cells is spread so thin that it cannot be resolved in ordinary sections with the LM. This fact led before the advent of the EM to a school of thought which subscribed to the view that alveolar walls did not possess a continuous epithelial covering. However, when

the EM became available, studies with the instrument, in particular those by Low, provided convincing evidence that a continuous epithelial indeed existed. Low estimated that the thickness of this sheet (except where there are nuclei) is approximately 0.2 μ in man and 0.1 μ in the rat. Underneath the epithelium there is a basement membrane which may be clearly seen at upper right in Figure 23-15, and which lower down fuses with the basement membrane of a nearby capillary to become a single membrane, a common ocurrence in the lung.

(2) **The Secretory Cells.** These are often referred to as great alveolar cells. The LM had shown that there are occasional, fairly large, rounded cells that project from the surface of alveoli into their lumens (Fig. 23-14). The EM has shown (Fig. 23-16) that these are epithelial cells, and that they are part of the membrane because they are connected on either side to adjacent squamous cells by junctional complexes which show both tight junctions and structures of the adhaerens type. The EM has shown, moreover, that these larger cells are secretory. Their cytoplasm is characterized by their containing what are termed *lamellar bodies* (Fig. 23-16), which are globules of dark laminated material believed to be phospholipidic. Some authors (i.e., Collet) have seen examples of lamellar bodies opening on the surface of the cell and releasing their contents onto the surface of the epithelial lining of the alveolus. Hence it has been suggested that the content of the lamellar bodies is of the nature of a secretory product that spreads over the surface of the squamous epithelium of each alveolus in a thin film and acts as a surfactant. It is thought that if the surface tension on the fluid-coated alveolar walls was not reduced by a surfactant, it would be of sufficient force to bring about the collapse of small alveoli at the end of expiration. The surfactant is of particular importance in the newborn infant in connection with air having access to alveoli that in fetal life contained fluid.

THE CELLULAR CONTENT OF ALVEOLAR WALLS

An alveolar wall is covered on both its sides with continuous epithelium, and the two types of cells in this epithelial membrane have been described. Within the substance of the alveolar walls are capillaries which, in the usual section, are cut in a variety of planes. The endothelial cells of the capillaries have been described previously. Between the basement membrane that underlies the epithelium and the basement membrane that covers the capillaries there is a space (Fig. 23-15, *upper right*) which is not continu-

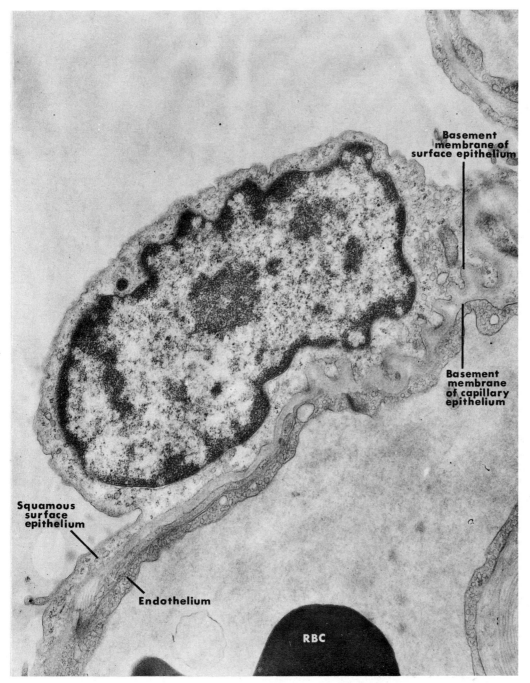

FIG. 23-15. Electron micrograph ($\times$ 11,900) of section of alveolar wall of lung of a cat showing the nucleus and cytoplasm of a squamous epithelial cell (*above*) and a capillary (*below*). Note the basement membranes of the squamous epithelium and the endothelial cells of the capillary, and that in some sites they separate to enclose a space and in other sites they fuse. (Collet, A.: Infrastructure du poumon normal et pathologique. Arch. Ital. Anat. Istol. Pat., *39*:119, 1965)

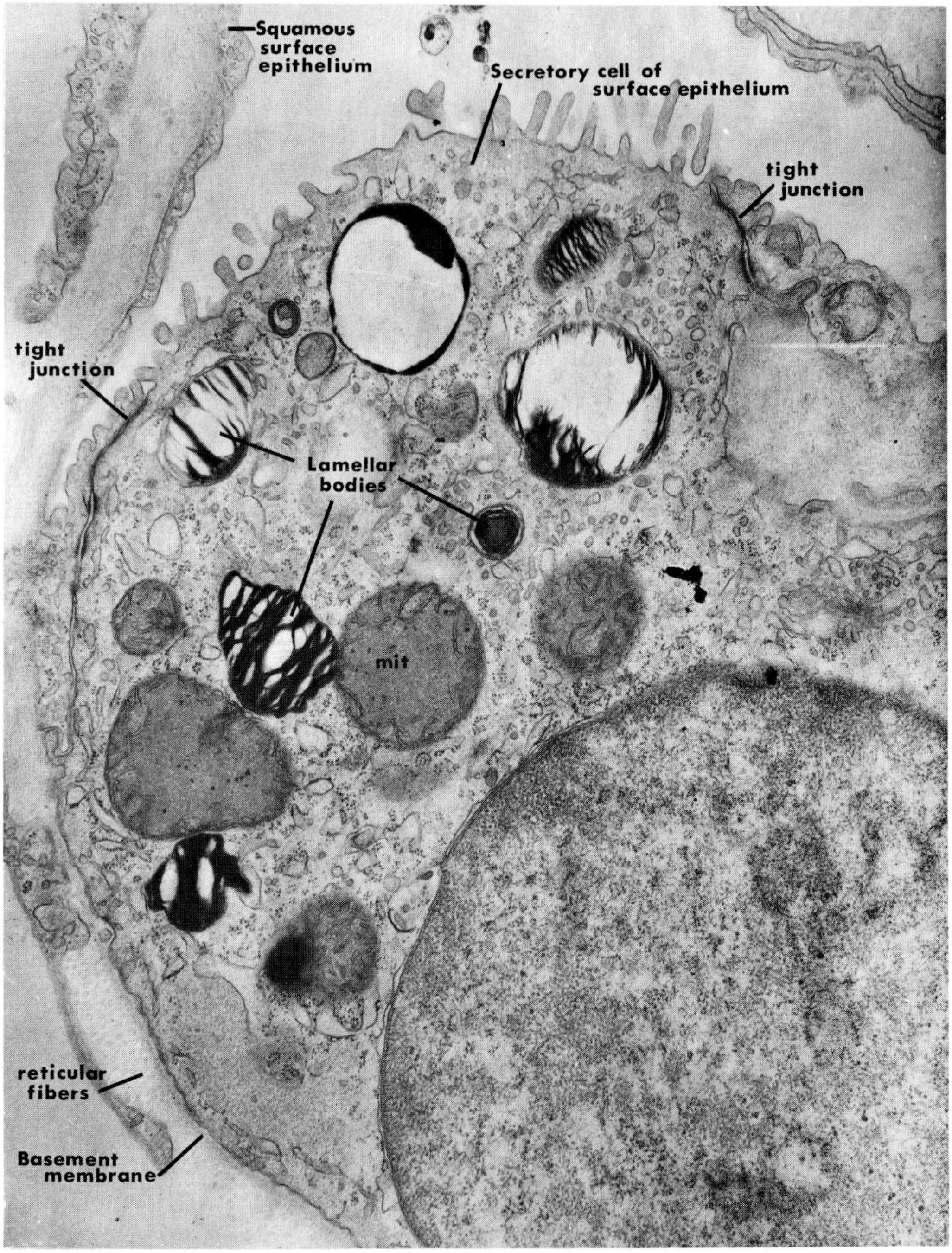

Fig. 23-16. Electron micrograph ($\times$ 13,300) of an alveolar wall of the lung of a cat showing a secretory cell. Note in particular the lamellar bodies; these constitute its secretory product. Note also that the secretory cell is joined to squamous cells by junctional complexes on each of its sides, and that it has microvilli on its free surface. The reticular fibers (*lower left*) are in the space described in the text. (Collet, A.: Infrastructure du poumon normal et pathologique. Arch. Ital. Anat. Istol. Pat., *39*:119, 1965)

ous because in some sites the basement membrane of
the epithelium is fused with the basement membrane
of the capillaries (Fig. 23-15, *middle*). In some sites
where this space is apparent there may be an elastic
fiber, or a few reticular fibers (Fig. 23-16, *lower left*)
and, in addition, in all probability some amorphous
intercellular substance. Moreover, there are cells sometimes to be seen in this space. In the development of
the lung, as will be described shortly, this site where
the space exists was previously occupied by a soft mesenchyme, and it seems most probable that occasional
descendants of the original mesenchyme persist as
fibroblasts here and there in the space, and that these
are responsible for making the elastic and reticular
fibers and the amorphous intercellular substance sometimes to be observed in these spaces.

In addition to the fibroblasts which may be found
here and there in the space, there are also some leukocytes that migrate from the capillaries into the space.
There is also one further kind of cell here that we
must consider.

Alveolar Phagocytes. Next, it is common to see
fairly large, rounded cells bulging from alveolar walls
into the alveolar space, and it is common to see the
same kinds of large cells free in the alveolar space.
These cells often contain carbon pigment which they
have phagocytosed from smoke-containing air that has
been drawn into the alveoli on inspiratory acts (Fig.
23-17). Because of their pronounced phagocytic properties these cells have long been termed alveolar phagocytes. The origin of these cells has been a matter of
dispute for many decades. In particular, it has been
difficult to determine whether they originate from (1)
either of the types of epithelial cell that line alveoli,
(2) mesenchymal-derived cells that persist in the alveolar wall from the developing lung, or (3) monocytes
that migrate through the walls of the capillaries of the
alveoli.

Studies with the EM have clarified the problem to
some extent. It has been shown that the squamous
cells give no evidence of having phagocytic ability.
Next, the EM has shown that the other kind of epithelial cells are first of all secretory cells rather than
phagocytic cells, and second, that they are part of the
continuous epithelium, being connected to squamous
cells by junctional complexes. Before the days of the
EM these cells were suspected of being the forerunners of the phagocytes. The current view is that the
alveolar phagocytes develop from monocytes that come
to the alveolar wall by way of the bloodstream, pass
out into the alveolar space from a capillary, and then
move out through the epithelial covering of the wall
to enter the lumen of an alveolus. Two lines of evi-

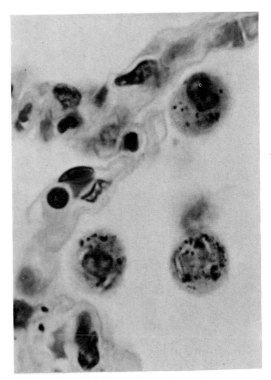

Fig. 23-17. Photomicrograph of section of lung showing three alveolar phagocytes free in an alveolar space.
Each contains some phagocytosed carbon in its cytoplasm. (Photomicrograph courtesy of Y. Clermont)

dence support this view. First, when mice are given
total-body irradiation and then kept alive by giving
them an infusion of bone marrow cells from an isologous mouse whose bone marrow cells bear a marker,
washings from the lungs of the transfused animal subsequently reveal cells (presumably alveolar phagocytes) which bear the marker. This experiment seems
to indicate that cells from the bone marrow could become alveolar phagocytes. The other evidence was
derived from an experiment of Osmond, in which he
labeled, with tritiated thymidine, cells developing in
the bone marrow of the hind legs of guinea pigs. Later,
labeled cells appeared both within the alveolar wall
and in alveolar lumens. It would therefore seem that
monocytes arising from bone marrow migrate to the
alveolar wall and, from there, break through to the
alveolar space to become the alveolar phagocytes,
which are therefore macrophages.

The function of the alveolar macrophages is to serve
as phagocytes so that any dust particles or other types
of debris that gain entrance to alveolar spaces can be
removed (Fig. 23-17). They are mobile. First, they
have to break through the epithelial basement mem-

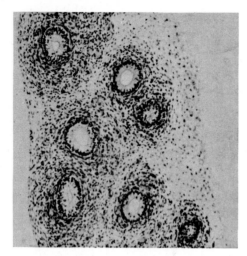

FIG. 23-18. Low-power photomicrograph of a section of the lung of a pig embryo in an early stage of development. Epithelial tubules (future bronchi) are growing and branching into the mesenchyme. (Ham, A. W., and Baldwin, K. W.: Anat. Rec., *81:*377)

brane. Eventually, they move up along the air passages to reach bronchioles and eventually bronchi, where their future progress is aided by the cilia. They may be lost to the outside as sputum or pass into the esophagus and stomach.

When lungs are congested with blood because of an incompetent heart, blood often escapes into alveolar spaces, where the alveolar phagocytes engulf the erythrocytes and form iron pigment from the hemoglobin they contain. The pigment-containing cells are commonly coughed up in large numbers under these conditions, and they give positive histochemical tests for iron. Such cells are called heart-failure cells.

The Development of the Lungs

The lungs develop like exocrine glands. The outgrowth responsible for them arises from the epithelium of the anterior wall of the foregut. The epithelial outgrowth first assumes the form of a longitudinal bulge but this, before long, becomes pinched off from the foregut except at its cephalic end. The tube formed as a result of the pinching-off process is the forerunner of the larynx and the trachea. Its caudal end is closed, but cell proliferation at this site soon results in two hollow epithelial bulges forking out from it, one being directed toward the left, and the other to the right. These bulges are commonly termed the lung buds, but they are better termed the *primary bronchial buds* because they are the forerunners of the 2 primary bronchi.

The 2 primary bronchial buds, because of the continued proliferation of cells in their ends and walls, advance toward the sites at which lungs will develop. Bulges appear on these advancing tubes; these subsequently grow and elongate to give rise to the secondary bronchi. These, in turn, usually by pairs of bulges which appear at their blind ends, continue to branch and grow to give rise to the smaller bronchi (Fig. 23-18). The branching then becomes more irregular but continues to give rise to the forerunners of bronchioles.

Although it simplifies matters to say that the growing, branching, hollow epithelial tree that develops originally from the epithelium of the foregut gives rise to the bronchi and the bronchioles of the lungs, and that these are comparable with the interlobular and intralobular ducts of exocrine glands, this is not the whole truth, for the epithelial outgrowth gives rise to only the epithelial lining and the glands of the bronchi and the bronchioles. The connective tissue and the smooth muscle of the walls of the bronchi and the bronchioles, and the cartilages of the bronchi, develop from the mesenchyme that is invaded by the growing, branching, hollow epithelial tree. The mesenchyme, as it is invaded, becomes condensed around the epithelial tubes (Fig. 23-18) and there differentiates into the connective tissue constituents of their walls.

It is believed that all the orders of bronchioles that will form in a human lung are present by the end of the 16th week in man. The number of generations of bronchi and bronchioles differs, of course, in different species and it is greater in the lower lobes than in the upper lobes of the lungs of man. From the time all the bronchioles have formed until around the 24th week of development the epithelium of the bronchioles grows into the mesenchyme to form what would be the counterparts of secretory units if one thinks of the lung at this time of development as a gland. In the pig embryo, these are rounded structures whose walls are composed of cuboidal cells that have very pale cytoplasm. In Figure 23-19 they are labeled as alveoli and it is presumed that the larger tubular structures that are cut in cross section are future bronchioles as they are labeled in this figure.

That the lung attains a stage of development, sometime during the 5th month, when it is clearly glandlike, possessing a branching duct system (the bronchial tree), the terminal branches of which connect with epithelial structures that are the equivalent of secretory units (alveolar ducts and alveoli), is generally accepted (Fig. 23-19). However, there was a difference of opinion as to whether the lung remains glandlike throughout the remainder of prenatal development. It was sometimes said that the lung retains its glandlike character until the time of birth; that is, until the time of birth the alveoli of the fetal lung are *rounded* hollow epithelial structures, being made of cuboidal to columnar epithelial cells. According to this view, the gland-like nature of the lung disappeared only when respiratory movements began after birth.

However, many investigations of lung development made with the LM, including our own, yielded results at variance with the concept described above. If *gland-like* refers to the alveoli remaining rounded, like secretory units, until the time of birth, the lung does not remain glandlike, for in the later stages of development the alveoli become angular, taking on the appearance that they have in postnatal life (Fig. 23-20, *top*). This fact has implications both with regard to how alveoli increase in number and as to whether a newborn infant that dies has breathed air or not.

The thoracic cage can become larger in prenatal or postnatal life only if something can enter it to let it enlarge. For all practical purposes only two things can enter the thoracic cage in postnatal life to permit it to enlarge with inspiratory movements—air and blood. In prenatal life the only two things that can be drawn into the lungs to let the cage expand are amniotic fluid and blood. Therefore, it is obvious that, if there were inspiratory movements in fetal life, amniotic fluid would be drawn into alveolar ducts and alveoli to let them expand, and blood would be drawn into the capillaries of interalveolar walls to let them expand. It seems not improbable that slight inspiratory movements in late fetal life assist in opening up alveoli so that they become angular rather than round, and that the movements also play a part in filling and expanding the capillary bed of the lungs, which may stimulate its growth, for it develops very rapidly in the interalveolar walls as the lung changes its character.

According to the more modern concept of the development of the lung, birth is not such an important milestone as it is according to the older view. According to the newer view, the developing lung ceases to be glandlike, not at birth, but approximately two thirds of the way through fetal life (Fig. 23-20, *top*). At this time it goes through most of the preparations for birth so that a baby born prematurely has a chance of living. If sections of a fetal lung show it to be glandlike throughout, it can be assumed with much justification that the fetus concerned never breathed air. But if a lung is not glandlike, but instead opened-up, as in Figure 23-20, *top*, it cannot be assumed that the fetus concerned has breathed air. If a newborn baby has breathed air and subsequently dies, its lungs, when removed at autopsy, will not sink if they are placed in a pan of water, because the air they contain makes

them lighter than water. If a baby has not breathed air, its lungs will sink. This test is probably much more reliable than that afforded by microscopic examination. The medicolegal significance of interpretations of sections of lungs of the newborn with reference to whether the infants concerned breathed air or not has been thoroughly investigated and discussed by Shapiro in the light of the newer knowledge of lung development.

A fetus of 7 months is generally said to be *viable;* that is, it is capable of living by means of breathing air if it should be born. The great development of the capillary beds of the interalveolar walls that begins about two thirds of the way through fetal life is an important factor in permitting the fetus to attain this state.

Changes at Birth. The future air spaces of the fetal lung are filled with what is termed alveolar fluid at the time of birth. These spaces are expanded further when air is taken into the lungs after birth. Their greater

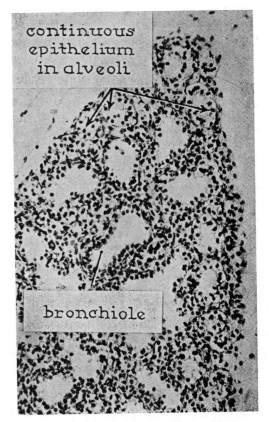

Fig. 23-19. Medium-power photomicrograph of a section of the lung of a pig embryo about halfway through prenatal development. Notice that the developing bronchioles have given rise to epithelial alveoli, which are structures comparable to the secretory alveoli or glands.

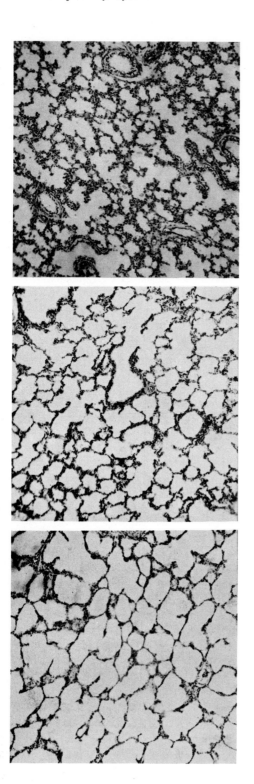

expansion after birth (Fig. 23-20, *center*, and *bottom*) is brought about by the respiratory movements that occur when a baby is born. It is of interest that these inspiratory movements not only draw air into the lungs but also more blood. This may explain why a newborn baby will increase its weight by several ounces if the umbilical cord is not cut too soon after a baby is born. Every effort is made by the doctor who delivers a baby to remove all the fluid that he can from the upper respiratory tract and so assist its displacement by air. However, only about 30 percent of the fluid in the air spaces of the lung is drained away through the upper respiratory tract after birth (Avery et al.); so most of it is absorbed into lymphatics and into the bloodstream.

The Importance of Surfactant at Birth. It is very important that the secretory cells have developed in the lung before a baby is born because the surfactant they produce is of the greatest importance in reducing the surface tension which might otherwise hold interalveolar walls together at the end of expiration and prevent them separating so that air spaces could open up in the following inspiratory act. Avery, Wang and Taevsch have written a most interesting article about this matter and how serious problems that may arise in prematurely born infants that could be due to the cells that produce the surfactant not yet having developed sufficiently. Some encouraging results with regard to the possible use of certain steroid hormones to cause the more rapid development of surfactant-secreting cells are also mentioned.

POSTNATAL GROWTH OF THE LUNG

The Problem of How Alveoli Increase in Number. As already noted, new bronchioles do not form after the 16th week of fetal life. However, alveoli continue to develop, both until the time of birth and thereafter. It has been estimated that at birth there are about 20 million alveoli in the human lung but by the age of 8 there are 300 million. After this they do not increase in numbers but they become larger.

Just how 280 million new alveoli develop between birth and the age of 8 has not, in the opinion of the

FIG. 23-20. (*Top*) Low-power photomicrograph of a section of the lung of a pig about two thirds of the way through prenatal development. It is not glandlike, and the alveoli are angular. (*Center*) Photomicrograph of a section of the lung of a pig killed 3 hours after birth. The alveoli are larger. (*Bottom*) Photomicrograph of another area of a section of the lung of a pig killed 3 hours after birth. The alveoli here are greatly expanded. (Ham, A. W., and Baldwin, K. W.: Anat. Rec., *81*:377)

author, been explained very satisfactorily, for two reasons: First, it has been assumed that alveoli must develop as they do in glands, that is, that they are rounded epithelial structures that bud off from pre-existing epithelium, instead of accepting that alveoli are primarily angular spaces separated from each other by common interalveolar walls. Second, in most explanations given, no account is taken of how easy it is for air to permeate a soft tissue as is shown in the process by which the condition known as interstitial emphysema develops. That the latter process should be taken into account was suggested by the author and Baldwin in 1941. Much has been learned about the lung since then and it is time that the hypothesis should be restated in the light of this new information. First, we shall describe the phenomenon of what is called interstitial emphysema.

Interstitial emphysema is a condition that can occur in infants who have some obstruction to their airway and try to overcome it by strong expiratory movements. These can result in the positive pressure that is generated causing air to break into the connective tissue of the pleura or septa, or that which wraps the bronchi and blood vessels. Moreover, the condition can occur at any age by some sort of injury that allows air from the respiratory portion of the lung to gain entrance to the connective tissues of the lung mentioned above, or, in some instances, it is due to injuries that permit air from the lungs to gain entrance to the connective tissue of the thoracic wall.

If air gains entrance to soft tissues under positive pressure, it readily infiltrates by opening up spaces in it. By this means it can extend through soft tissues for long distances. For example, it has been recorded that an ancient form of torture was carried out by making a small incision into the soft tissue of the victim, inserting a straw into the little incision, and then blowing through the straw until the body of the victim became swollen with air. Moreover, in the scientific literature there are accounts of males who after an accident involving the chest wall and lungs developed interstitial emphysema which spread so much that the tissues of the scrotum became so swollen with air that incisions has to be made in it to allow some of the air to escape.

Now it might be asked what this has to do with the formation of 280 million new alveoli between the time of birth and the age of 8. As already mentioned, if alveoli are thought of as structures, as for example, the alveoli of glands, it is very difficult to conceive of how this great number could be formed. But if we think of alveoli as spaces in a 3-dimensional sponge

that is stretched in all directions, with every inspiratory act, it becomes easier to visualize how new alveoli could form. The substance of the sponge is continually increasing in size because of the proliferation of the endothelial cells of its capillaries and its fibroblasts which make its elastic and reticular fibers and amorphous intercellular substance. The epithelium that covers interalveolar septa and hence lines alveolar spaces is a most tenuous membrane with almost no tensile strength. At each inspiratory act the 3-dimensional spongy substance of the lung, consisting of capillaries, elastic fibers, some fibroblasts and amorphous intercellular substance, is stretched in three directions. All that would be required to start a new alveolar space on its way would be for a microscopic crevice to appear in some place where the substance of the sponge was becoming relatively thick because air would immediately be sucked into the crevice to expand it until further expansion put surrounding elastic and reticular fibers on sufficient stretch to limit still further expansion. The epithelium through which the crevice appeared would then grow along the sides of the new space and line it with epithelium. The question then regarding the formation of this enormous number of new alveoli in a growing lung is whether they develop as *spaces* in a soft tissue which thereupon become lined with epithelium or whether they are formed by epithelial buds that arise from somewhere that invade the soft tissue of the 3-dimensional sponge of capillaries, elastic and reticular fibers and amorphous intercellular substance. It seems to the author that the most logical view is that the 280 million alveoli that develop between birth and the age of 8 can best be accounted for by new slitlike spaces being opened up in a 3-dimensional sponge as it is stretched in three directions with every inspiratory act and with the slit-like spaces appearing in sites where recent cellular proliferation has made the substance of the sponge thick enough for it to be opened up further. The new angular spaces would then quickly become lined with pulmonary epithelium which would grow into them to line them. The same general process would also account for some former alveoli becoming alveolar ducts as the substance of the sponge continued to open up in the manner described above.

The process described above is the same as that which accounts for air opening up soft connective tissue in the spread of interstitial emphysema. But the process does not lead to the lung being the site of interstitial emphysema because each new crevice or defect in the spongework of the lung that is opened up by air becomes lined by pulmonary epithelium so the air in any

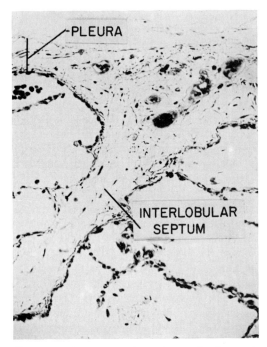

FIG. 23-21. Low-power photomicrograph of a section of the human adult lung showing the pleura at the top and the interlobular septum extending down from the pleura into the substance of the lung.

new space that opens up is thereafter not in the substance of the sponge but in spaces separated from the sponge substance by epithelium.

If the substance of the spongework of the respiratory tissue of the lung is opened up so as to contain more alveolar spaces by the same kind of process that enables air to spread in soft tissue, the question arises as to why the process does not extend into the pleura, septa, the connective tissue wrappings of the bronchioles and bronchi and even into lymphatics so that from the respiratory tissue of the lungs air would spread all over the body. The reason is that the respiratory tissue of the lung is encased by a layer of relatively dense connective tissue; this is found in the pleura beneath the mesothelium and it extends into septa. It is continuous with the relatively dense connective tissue that forms the wrapping for the vessels and bronchi and bronchioles. It is significant that lymphatics are not found in the pure respiratory tissue of the lung; if they were they would be a hazard with regard to the spread of air to the lymphatic system. They are confined to denser connective tissue which ordinarily prevents the spread of air from the respiratory tissue.

BLOOD SUPPLY OF THE LUNG

Blood from the right ventricle is delivered by the pulmonary artery and its branches to the capillary beds of the respiratory tissue of the lung to be oxygenated there. Oxygenated blood is collected from the capillary beds of the lung by the branches of the pulmonary vein and delivered to the left atrium of the heart. It is to be kept in mind that, in the instance of the pulmonary circulation, the arteries carry what is ordinarily called venous blood, and the veins, arterial.

The pulmonary artery to each lung enters it at its root, and within the lung it branches along with the bronchial tree so that each branch of the bronchial tree is accompanied by a branch of the pulmonary artery. The small branches that reach the respiratory bronchioles break up into terminal branches which deliver blood into the capillary beds of the alveolar ducts, the alveolar sacs and the alveoli (Fig. 23-8, *left*).

Blood from the capillary beds of the respiratory tissue of the lungs is collected by the smallest branches of the pulmonary vein. These begin within the substance of lobules and in this region are supported by thin connective tissue sheaths. Supported in this fashion, they travel to and enter interlobular septa, where they empty into interlobular veins (Fig. 23-8, *left*). These in turn are conducted by the septa to the site where the apices of the lobules concerned meet. Here the veins come into close association with branches of the bronchial tree. From this point to the root of the lung, the veins follow the bronchi. In other words, except within lobules, the branches of the pulmonary artery and the pulmonary vein follow the branches of the bronchial tree, but within lobules only the arteries follow the bronchioles.

Oxygenated blood is supplied to parts of the lung by the bronchial arteries. These also travel in close association with the bronchial tree and supply the capillary beds of its walls. They also supply the lymph nodes that are scattered along the bronchial tree. Moreover, branches of the bronchial arteries travel out along the interlobular septa and supply oxygenated blood to the capillaries of the visceral pleura.

LYMPHATICS OF THE LUNG

General principles are easier to remember than details. It could be said that there is a rough general principle about the distribution of lymphatics in the lung: they are confined to the relatively dense connective tissue structures that confine air to the respiratory tissue of the lung. Hence they are present in the visceral pleura (Fig. 23-21), in the interlobular septa

(Fig. 23-21), and in the dense connective tissue wrappings of the bronchioles, the bronchi, the arteries and the veins (Fig. 23-8, *right*). They are not present in the interalveolar partitions. However, Miller has described lymphatics in the tissue bordering the alveolar ducts. Lymphatic capillaries in alveolar walls might very well constitute a hazard because, if air were sucked into a lymphatic on inspiration, expiratory movements would pump it along the lymphatic so that it would go for long distances. If it got into the bloodstream, it could cause air embolism.

It is customary to describe the lung as having a superficial and a deep set of lymphatics. The superficial ones are contained in the visceral pleura (Fig. 23-8, *bottom*). In city dwellers these are usually blackened by carbon particles which have become incorporated into their walls. The larger ones follow the lines where interlobular septa join the pleura; hence the bases of those lobules which are projected onto the pleura may be outlined by dark lines. Smaller lymphatics in the pleura form a pattern of closer mesh than those which surround the bases of lobules. The pleural lymphatics join up with one another to form vessels that are conducted by the pleura to reach and empty into the lymph nodes at the hilus of the lung.

The deep set consists of 3 groups: (1) those in the outer layers of the walls of bronchioles and bronchi (Fig. 23-8); (2) those that accompany the branches of the pulmonary artery (Fig. 23-8)—these anastomose with those in the branches of the bronchial tree; and (3) those that run in the interlobular septa, particularly in association with the interlobular veins (Fig. 23-8, *right*). All 3 groups drain toward lymph nodes at the hilus of the lungs.

The lymphatics of the interlobular septa (which belong to the deep set) communicate with those of the pleura (which belong to the superficial set) at sites where interlobular septa join the visceral pleura (Fig. 23-8, *lower right corner*). It has been taught for years, largely because of Miller's influence, that the lymphatics of the interlobular septa have valves that are disposed close to the pleura (Fig. 23-8, *lower right corner*), and that these valves prevent lymph from the pleural lymphatics from draining into the lymphatics of the septa. In other words, it has been generally conceded that although lymph could pass from the lymphatics of the interlobular septa outward into the pleural lymphatics, because of the direction of the valves it could not pass the other way, and hence that lymph in the pleural lymphatics, to reach the hilus of the lung, would have to pass by way of the pleural lymphatics over the whole surface of a lobe to reach the hilus. However, Simer has shown that this older view is fallacious, and that the valves that were generally believed to prevent flow from the pleural lymphatics into the lymphatics of the interlobular septa (Fig. 23-8, *lower right corner*) (1) are not always present; (2) if present, they are often poorly developed and (3) do not always point toward the pleura. Simer showed that India ink injected into the pleural lymphatics does not usually pursue a course around the periphery of the lobe in order to reach the hilus, but instead passes into the lymphatics of the interlobular septa and from there into the lymphatic vessels associated with the bronchial tree and its vessels, and so it takes a direct rather than a roundabout course to the hilus of the lung.

EFFECTS OF RESPIRATORY MOVEMENTS ON LUNG STRUCTURE

The descent and the expansion of the lungs on inspiration require that the bronchial tree be elastic. Macklin showed that bronchi become longer and wider on inspiration. The root of the lung also descends on inspiration. Recoil from these movements is accomplished chiefly by the already described elastic tissue of the tracheobronchial tree. Macklin's papers should be consulted for details of this and the recoil mechanism.

It is probable that the expansion of the respiratory tissue itself, that occurs on inspiration, is due more to the elongation and the dilatation of alveolar ducts than it is to expansion of alveoli.

Innervation of the Smooth Muscle of the Bronchi and the Bronchioles

Fibers from both divisions of the autonomic nervous system pass to the bronchial tree. The parasympathetic supply is brought by branches of the vagus nerve. Stimulation of the efferent fibers causes the bronchiolar musculature to contract. Stimulation of the fibers of sympathetic nerves causes the bronchiolar musculature to relax. In the condition known as asthma, the smooth muscle of the smaller bronchioles contracts, and the mucous membrane of the affected tubes swells. This narrows the passages by which air can enter or leave alveolar ducts and makes breathing exceedingly difficult. Adrenalin, or a similarly acting substance, is often given to relax the bronchiolar musculature and so widen the lumens of the bronchioles of an individual suffering an attack. It is of interest that it is more difficult for an individual with asthma to expel air from his lungs than it is to draw it in; the reason is that inspiratory movements tend to expand such tubes as lie within lobules and so enlarge their lumens, while powerful expiratory movements, such as occur in asthma, tend, if air cannot be forced out freely through the bronchial tree, to compress such tubes as lie within lobules and so make their lumens still narrower.

References and Other Reading

Some General References on the Lung

Avery, M. E., Wang, Nai-San, and Taeusch, H. W., Jr.: The lung of the newborn infant. Sci. Am., *228:*75, 1973.

Bertalanffy, F. D.: Respiratory tissue: structure, histophysiology, cytodynamics. I. Review and basic cytomorphology. Int. Rev. Cytol., *16:*233, 1964; II. New approaches and interpretations. Int. Rev. Cytol., *17:*213, 1964.

Engel, S.: The Child's Lung. London, Arnold, 1947.

Krahl, V. E.: Microscopic anatomy of the lungs. Am. Rev. Resp. Dis., *80:*24, 1959.

————: Anatomy of the mammalian lung. *In* American Physiological Society: Handbook of Physiology. Section 3 (Fenn, W. O., and Rahn, H., eds.), Respiration. vol. 1, p. 213. Baltimore, Williams & Wilkins, 1964.

Miller, W. S.: The Lung, ed. 2. Springfield, Ill., Charles C Thomas, 1947.

von Hayek, Heinrich: The Human Lung, trans. by Vernon E. Krahl. New York, Hafner, 1960.

Some Further References on the Lung and Some References on Other Parts of the Respiratory System

Barrie, H. J.: The acinus: The architecture of caseous nodules in the lung and the place of the word "acinar" in describing tuberculous lesions. Canad. Med. Assoc. J., *92:*1149, 1965.

Bertalanffy, F. D.: Dynamics of cellular populations in the lung. *In* The Lung. Int. Acad. Path. Monograph No. 8. pp. 19-30. Baltimore, Williams & Wilkins, 1967.

Boyden, E. A.: Development of the human lung. *In* Kelley, V. C. (ed.): Brennemann's Practice of Pediatrics. vol. 4, Chap. 64. New York, Harper and Row, 1971.

————: Notes on the development of the lung in infancy and early childhood. Am. J. Anat., *121:*749, 1967.

Burnham, H. H.: An anatomical investigation of blood vessels of the lateral nasal wall and their relation to turbinates and sinuses. J. Laryng. Otol., *50:*569, 1935.

Collet, A., Basset, F., and Normand-Reuet, C.: Etude au microscope électronique du poumon humain normal et pathologique. Poumon Coeur, *23:*747, 1967.

Collet, A., and Reuet-Normand, C.: Aspects infrastructuraux de la traversée de la paroi alvéolaire du poumon par des cellules migratrices. Sem. Hôp., Paris, *29:*1928, 1967.

Duguid, J. B., and Lambert, M. W.: The pathogenesis of coal miner's pneumoconiosis. J. Path. Bact., *88:*389, 1964.

Dunnill, M. S.: Postnatal growth of the lung. Thorax, *17:*329, 1962.

Flint, J. M.: The development of the lungs. Am. J. Anat., *6:*1, 1906.

Godleski, J. J., and Brain, J. D.: The origin of alveolar macrophages in mouse radiation chimeras. J. Exp. Med., *136:*630, 1972.

Greene, M.: The Voice and its Disorders. ed. 2. Philadelphia, J. B. Lippincott, 1965.

Ham, A. W., and Baldwin, K. W.: A histological study of the development of the lung with particular reference to the nature of alveoli. Anat. Rec., *81:*363, 1941.

Hartroft, W. S., and Macklin, C. C.: The size of the human lung alveoli expressed as diameters of selected alveolar outlines as seen in specially prepared 25 micron microsections. Trans. Roy. Soc. Canada, Sec. V (Biol. Sci.), *38:*63, 1944.

Karrer, H. E.: The ultrastructure of mouse lung. J. Biophys. Biochem. Cytol., *2:*241, 1956.

————: The ultrastructure of mouse lung. J. Biophys. Biochem. Cytol., *2* (Suppl.):287, 1956.

————: The ultrastructure of mouse lung: the alveolar macrophage. J. Biophys. Biochem. Cytol., *4:*693, 1958.

Karrer, H.E.: The fine structure of connective tissue in the tunica propria of bronchioles. J. Ultrastruct. Res., *2:*96, 1958.

————: The experimental production of pulmonary emphysema. Am. Rev. Resp. Dis., *80:*158, 1959.

Krahl, V. E.: Current concept of the finer structure of the lung. A.M.A. Arch. Int. Med., *96:*342, 1955.

————: The respiratory portions of the lung. Bull. Sch. Med. Univ. Maryland, *40:*101, 1955.

Lambert, M. W.: Accessory bronchiolo-alveolar communications. J. Path. Bact., *70:*311, 1955.

————: Accessory bronchiolo-alveolar channels. Anat. Rec., *127:*472, 1957.

Loosli, C. G., and Potter, E. L.: Pre- and postnatal development of the respiratory portion of the human lung. Am. Rev. Resp. Dis., *80:*5, 1959.

Low, F. N.: Electron microscopy of the rat lung. Anat. Rec., *113:*437, 1952.

————: The electron microscopy of sectioned lung tissue after varied duration of fixation in buffered osmium tetroxide. Anat. Rec., *120:*827, 1954.

————: The pulmonary alveolar epithelium of laboratory mammals and man. Anat. Rec., *117:*241, 1953.

Low, F. N., and Sampaio, M. M.: The pulmonary alveolar epithelium as an entodermal derivative. Anat. Rec., *127:*51, 1957.

Lucas, A. M.: The nasal cavity and direction of fluid by ciliary movement in Macacus rhesus (Desm.). Am. J. Anat., *50:*141, 1932.

Luchsinger, R., and Arnold, G.: Voice-Speech-Language: Clinical Communicology—Its Physiology and Pathology. Wadsworth Publishing Co., 1965.

Mackenzie, J. N.: The physiological and pathological relations between the nose and the sexual apparatus of man. Johns Hopkins Hosp. Bull., *9:*10, 1898.

Macklin, C. C.: Alveolar pores and their significance in the human lung. Arch. Path., *21:*202, 1936.

————: The dynamic bronchial tree. Am. Rev. Tuberc., *25:*363, 1932.

————: The mechanics and dynamics of the human lungs and bronchi. Med. Rec., *143:*89, 1936.

————: The musculature of the bronchi and lungs. Physiol. Rev., *9:*1, 1929.

Millard, Max: Chapter on Lung, Pleura and Mediastinum. *In* Anderson, W. A. D. (ed.): Pathology. ed. 6, vol. 2, p. 875. St. Louis, C. V. Mosby, 1971.

Reynolds, S. R. M.: The fetal and neonatal pulmonary vasculature in the guinea pig in relation to hemodynamic changes at birth. Am. J. Anat., *98:*97, 1956.

Rhodin, J., and Dulhamn, T.: Electron microscopy of the tracheal ciliated mucosa in rat. Z. Zellforsch., *44:*345, 1956.

Scarpelli, E. M.: The Surfactant System of the Lung. Philadelphia, Lea and Febiger, 1968.

Schaeffer, J. P.: The mucous membrane of the nasal cavity and the paranasal sinuses. *In* Cowdry's Special Cytology. ed. 2, p. 105. New York, Hoeber, 1932.

Shapiro, H. A.: The limited value of microscopy of lung tissue in the diagnosis of live and stillbirth. Clin. Proc., *6:*149, 1947.

Short, R. H. D.: Alveolar epithelium in relation to growth of the lung. Phil. Trans. Roy. Soc. London, *235:*35, 1950.

Sorokin, S.: The Cells of the Lungs. *In:* Nettesheim, P. Hanna, M. G. Jr., and Deatherage, J. W. Jr. (eds.): Morphology of Experimental Carcinogenesis, page 3. CONF 700501, Atomic Energy Commission, Oak Ridge, Tenn. 1970.

Sun, C. N.: Lattice structures and osmiophilic bodies in the developing respiratory tissue of rats. J. Ultrastruct. Res., *15:*380, 1966.

van Furth, R., and Cohn, Z. A.: The origin and kinetics of mononuclear phagocytes. J. Exp. Med., *128:*415, 1968.

Woodside, G. L., and Dalton, A. J.: The ultrastructure of lung tissue from newborn and embryo mice. J. Ultrastruct. Res., *2:*28, 1958.

24 The Urinary System

Some General Considerations

The metabolism of food by body cells produces both energy and waste products. The latter seep from cells through tissue fluid into the bloodstream. From there, as was described in the previous chapter, one important waste product, carbon dioxide, is eliminated from the lungs. For the elimination of certain other waste products, particularly those that result from the metabolism of proteins, the body is equipped with two specially constructed organs of substantial size—the kidneys—through which more than one fifth of the total blood of the body circulates every minute.

Parts of the Urinary System. In the kidneys, waste products from the blood become concentrated in a fluid called *urine,* which is carried away from each kidney by a tube called a *ureter.* The ureter from each kidney leads to the *urinary bladder;* here urine can accumulate so that it can be evacuated from the body periodically and at will through another single tube, the *urethra.* The two kidneys, the two ureters, the urinary bladder and the urethra comprise *the urinary system.*

The Kidney Has Many Functions. It should be emphasized that the kidneys perform other functions of very great importance in addition to that of ridding the body of the waste products of metabolism. For example, they can vary the amount of water that is lost from the body in urine. Hence, the kidneys play a very important part in regulating the *fluid balance* of the body. Likewise, the kidneys can vary the amounts and the kinds of electrolytes that are eliminated from the body in urine; thus they assist in maintaining a proper *salt balance* in blood and tissue fluid. The kidneys also act in many other ways to maintain in the body a fluid environment which is suitable for the life of body cells. To perform these functions they conserve some things and eliminate others.

The Basic Mechanisms Involved in the Excretion of Waste Products by the Kidney

In simpler organisms, in which blood circulatory systems are not highly developed, tissue fluid is the dominant fluid. The waste products from the metabolism of cells seep into and tend to accumulate in tissue fluid, and from it they must be excreted. A relatively simple mechanism for this is seen in the earthworm. Its segments are provided with tubules, both ends of which are open. One end of each tubule is open to tissue fluid in the interior of the worm, and the other end opens onto the exterior of the worm. Tissue fluid enters the open internal end of each tubule and passes slowly along the tubule to be eliminated at the exterior of the worm as a sort of urine.

Since the tubules are long and coiled, it takes some time for tissue fluid to pass along them. This provides an opportunity for the tissue fluid *to be altered as it passes along the tubule,* because the epithelial cells lining the tubule either (1) *absorb* certain valuable constituents of the fluid back into the organism or (2) *excrete* further things into the fluid in the tubule. It might be anticipated, then, that the fluid that finally emerges from the external end of the tubule onto the surface of the organism (and this, for all practical purposes, is urine) contains fewer valuable constituents than the tissue fluid that enters the internal end of the tubule, and also that the fluid that leaves contains waste products in greater concentration. We shall see that in man, as in the earthworm, *urine is tissue fluid that has been modified* in the above described fashion by passing along a tubule.

Evolution of the Glomerulus. As organisms became more complex, the blood circulatory system became of increasing importance in distributing oxygen and food to cells in different parts of the body and in carrying away their waste products. This required some mechanism by which waste products could be removed from the blood more or less continuously. In the arrangement that evolved in mammals excretory tubules were retained, but they are all segregated and housed in the kidneys. Furthermore, instead of each tubule being open at both ends, the innermost end of each tubule was closed. The arrangement that evolved to permit each of these tubules to have access to the blood was that of having a little cluster of capillaries form in association with the blind end of each one of these tubules in the kidney, and push, as it were, into its blind end, so that the thin epithelium of the blind end of the tubule covers each of the capillaries that push into it. The little cluster of capillaries that projects into the blind end of each tubule is called a *glomerulus* (*glomus,* a skein) (Fig. 24-1), and the tissue fluid that is formed by the capillaries of the glomerulus passes into the lumen of the tubule and is called *glomerular filtrate*. Glomeruli, for reasons to be given shortly, cause vast amounts of tissue fluid to be delivered into excretory tubules. As this filtrate passes along the remainder of the long tubule, valuable substances are resorbed, and so the fluid that emerges from its external end as urine, and drains via the ureter into the urinary bladder, has waste products concentrated in it.

The Nephron. An excretory tubule with a glomerulus pushed into its blind end is the unit of structure of the kidney and is called a *nephron* (Fig. 24-1). There are over a million of these in each kidney in man.

Why Glomerular Capillaries Produce More Tissue Fluid Than Ordinary Capillaries. Tissue fluid is formed at the arterial ends of most capillaries in the body and resorbed at their venous ends (Fig. 8-6). The reasons for this are explained in Chapter 8. They are essentially that the hydrostatic pressure in the arterial ends of ordinary capillaries is a stronger force that is directed toward pushing fluid out of the capillary than the osmotic pressure imparted to blood by its colloids (protein) that is directed toward drawing fluid into the capillary. At the venous end of ordinary capillaries the hydrostatic pressure falls, and so the osmotic pressure of blood becomes the dominant force and draws fluid back in. But if the drainage of capillaries is impeded, as occurs, for example, in venous obstruction, tissue fluid is formed along the whole length of the capillary (Fig. 8-8, *upper left*) because the hydrostatic pressure along the whole length of the capillary is greater than the osmotic pressure imparted by colloids to the blood. In glomerular capillaries hydrostatic pressure is high (60-70 mm. Hg) and, moreover, remains high along their whole lengths. The reason the pressure is high in glomerular capillaries, and high along their entire lengths, is that they drain, not into a wide unobstructed venule, but into an arteriole that offers resistance to the outflow of blood. Since glomerular capillaries are supplied by an arteriole and also drained by an arteriole, they represent, as it were, a tuft of capillaries interposed along the course of an arteriole (Fig. 24-1). The arteriole that supplies the glomerular capillaries is termed the *afferent arteriole* of the glomerulus, and the arteriole into

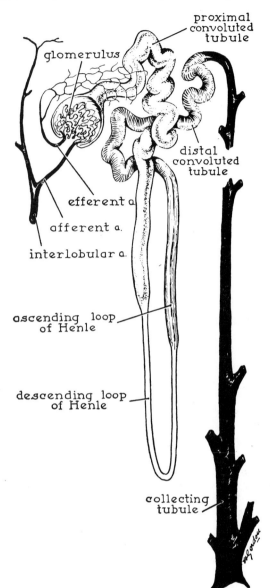

FIG. 24-1. Diagram of a nephron—a tubule with a glomerulus at its blind end, connecting with a collecting tubule. To make this diagram less complex, the ascending limb of the loop of Henle is not shown in its normal relation to the vascular pole of the glomerulus; actually it should return to the glomerulus and fit into its vascular pole to form a macula densa before continuing on as the distal convoluted tubule.

which the glomerular capillaries empty is termed the *efferent arteriole* of the glomerulus (Figs. 24-1 and 24-6). Since the lumen of the efferent arteriole is not much larger, or even any larger than that of the afferent one, a situation exists in glomerular capillaries that

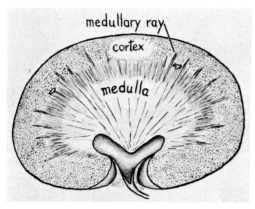

FIG. 24-2. Drawing of the cut surface of a split kidney of a rabbit. Notice that medullary rays appear to be extensions of the striated medulla into the granular cortex.

would be comparable to venous obstruction in ordinary capillaries; the resistance to the exit of blood from them is enough to maintain a sufficiently high hydrostatic pressure throughout their whole lengths to permit them to exude tissue fluid along their whole lengths. The tonus of the muscle in the walls of the efferent arteriole can change so as to vary the amount of resistance it offers.

As a result of this arrangement, glomerular capillaries produce vast amounts of tissue fluid which instead of causing edema, as it would in ordinary capillaries, passes through the epithelium that covers the capillary to enter the blind end of the nephron (Fig. 24-7). As soon as the tissue fluid passes through the epithelium covering the capillary, it is called glomerular filtrate.

Resorption as the Filtrate Flows Along the Tubular Part of the Nephron. According to Allen, from the 1,700 liters of blood that passes along the glomerular capillaries of the two kidneys every 24 hours, 170 liters of tissue fluid (glomerular filtrate) are formed. It follows, then, that every 24 hours 170 liters of glomerular filtrate are delivered into the tubular portions of nephrons. As this passes along the nephrons, over 168 liters of it are resorbed back into the bloodstream so that only about $1\frac{1}{2}$ liters of it emerge into the two ureters each 24 hours to constitute the daily output of urine. Obviously, there must be as efficient a mechanism for the *tubular resorption* of fluid as there is in glomeruli for its production. Resorption involves the activities of the epithelial cells that line the nephron and also the absorptive function of the extensive low-pressure capillary bed in which the tubules lie, as will be described later.

The various specialized resorptive and excretory functions performed by the tubular portion of the nephron are not performed with equal facility along its whole length. The tubular portion of each nephron (Fig. 24-1) exhibits 3 consecutive segments which reveal somewhat different structural features and perform somewhat different functions. These are termed the *proximal convoluted segment, the loop of Henle* and the *distal convoluted segment,* respectively (Fig. 24-1). Their particular structure and functions will be described in some detail somewhat later when the nephron of the human kidney is considered.

The Unilobar Kidney

It is customary in many schools to begin the laboratory study of the histology of the kidney, not with that of man, but with the kidney of a rat or rabbit. There are good reasons for this practice. The gross unit of structure of the kidney is the lobe. The kidney of man contains many lobes whereas the kidney of the rat or rabbit consists of only one lobe. Next, the kidney of a rat, or even a rabbit, is small enough for a single section to be cut along its long axis and through its greatest diameter and mounted on a slide, as is shown diagrammatically at the top of Figure 24-3. In such a section all parts of a lobe and all its connections with the ureter can be seen in the one slide. Since the kidney of man is large and multilobed, any single section shows only one small part of it, and generally the section includes incomplete parts of more than one lobe, which makes the section difficult to interpret unless the observer has seen a section of a complete lobe, as can be done so easily in a section of a unilobar kidney. The author's students have always found it helpful to approach the study of the multilobar kidney after a preliminary study of the unilobar kidney. To prevent undue repetition, the description of the unilobar kidney that follows will be kept at the level of the low power of the LM.

Naked Eye Inspection. The unilobar kidney is shaped like a lima bean; hence, if one is laid flat on a table and viewed from above, it is seen to have an extensive convex, and a smaller concave, border. Considerable fat is generally present in its concavity, which is called its *hilus.* The drainage tube of the kidney, the *ureter,* together with the renal artery and vein and a surrounding plexus of fine nerves, reach the kidney through the fat at the hilus.

If such a kidney is laid flat on a table and then cut in half by keeping the blade of a knife parallel with the surface of the table, the cut surface, when viewed with the naked eye, as is shown in Figure 24-2, shows the kidney substance to consist of two chief parts. The first is called the *cortex* (Fig. 24-2); it consists of a broad red-brown granular layer of tissue that lies immediately beneath the convex border and follows its contours (Fig. 24-2). The remainder of the kidney is shaped like a broad pyramid that is upside down. The base of the pyramid is convex rather than flat and is fitted up against the concave inner border of the cortex (Fig. 24-2). The apex of the pyramid points downward in Figure 24-2 and juts into the concavity or hilus of the kidney (Fig. 24-3, *top*). In contrast with the darker and granular cortex, the cut surface of the medulla is lighter and has a striated appearance, with the striations fanning out from the apex of the pyramid to all parts of its broad base (Figs. 24-2 and 24-3).

A pyramid of medullary substance, together with the cap of cortical substance that covers its base, constitutes a *lobe* of kidney tissue, and one lobe, of course, constitutes the whole kidney of the rat or the rabbit. We shall now consider how nephrons are disposed in a lobe of a kidney; this will explain an important point, namely, why the cut surface of the cortex has a granular appearance, and the surface of the medulla of a kidney cut as described has a striated appearance. It will also reveal the way in which a kidney lobe is divided up into lobules.

Disposition of Different Parts of the Nephrons in the Kidney Substance. Nephrons are so long that they can fit into a kidney only by pursuing a devious course in its substance. Figure 24-3, *bottom*, shows two complete nephrons in solid black; the remainder of the illustration shows the cortex and medulla as seen in an ordinary section under low power.

The glomeruli of the two nephrons depicted in solid black are shown as black balls (Fig. 24-3). The glomeruli, represented in the drawing as they appear in an H and E section, are tufted structures lying in circular cavities (Fig. 24-3). All glomeruli are always in the cortex.

As can be seen by following either of the two nephrons outlined in black in Figure 24-3, a tubule (the proximal convoluted tubule) leads off from the glomerulus and pursues a looped and very tortuous course in the cortical tissue close to the glomerulus from which it originated. It then turns down to pursue a fairly straight course toward and into the medulla. This segment of the nephron that passes straight down into the medulla is termed the descending limb (or arm) of the loop of Henle. The reason for the term *loop* is that the tubule, after descending for various distances into the medulla, loops back and ascends into the cortex again: the part that ascends is called the ascending limb of the loop of Henle. In the lower part of the descending limb, the epithelial wall, which up to this time has been relatively thick, becomes very thin and then, part way up the ascending limb, it becomes thick again (Fig. 24-3).

The ascending limb of the loop of Henle, on approaching the glomerulus of the nephron, curves in to touch the root of the glomerulus between the site of entry of the afferent arteriole and the site of exit of the efferent arteriole. The portion of the wall of the tubule that comes into contact with the glomerular root becomes heavily nucleated and constitutes a thick spot known as the *macula densa* (Figs. 24-3 and 24-6).

The segment of the nephron that continues on from the macula densa is known as the *distal convoluted tubule*. It pursues a mildly tortuous course in the neighboring cortical tissue (Fig. 24-3). It then joins a little side branch of one of the members of a branching system of long straight *collecting tubules* that extend from the cortex down through the medulla (Fig. 24-3) to open through the apex of the pyramidal medulla; this apical part of the pyramidal medulla is called its papilla (Fig. 24-3).

Collecting Tubules. The collecting tubules are not parts of nephrons. They convey fluid from the nephrons into the pelvis and the ureter, thus bearing a relation to nephrons similar to that which ducts bear to secretory units of glands. Indeed, they have a different developmental origin from that of nephrons. A nephron develops from mesodermal cells which become organized into a tubule; this later becomes associated with blood capillaries that are forming a renal corpuscle in the kidney cortex. On each side of the body a tube grows up from the developing bladder into the developing kidney, where it branches. This tube becomes the ureter and the pelvis of the kidney, and each of its many branches becomes a collecting tubule which later connects with nephrons in such a way that the lumens of the two become continuous.

Why the Cortex Is Granular and the Medulla Striated. The cortex contains all the glomeruli and all the convoluted parts of the proximal and distal tubules; hence, except for some of the straight parts of the loops of Henle, the cortex consists of a mixture of glomeruli and convoluted tubules; these constitute most of the bulk of the cortex (Fig. 24-3). If a slice is cut through a kidney, the proximal and distal convoluted tubules, being tortuous, are cut in cross and oblique section. Tubules cut this way, with glomeruli scattered among them, give a granular appearance to the cortex when its cut surface is examined with the naked eye.

The parts of the nephrons in the medulla are the

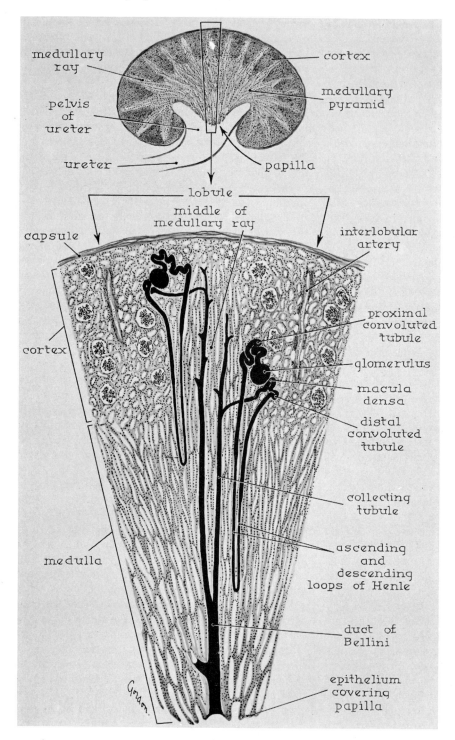

medullary
ray

cortex

medullary
pyramid

pelvis
of
ureter

ureter

papilla

lobule

middle of
medullary ray

capsule

interlobular
artery

cortex

proximal
convoluted
tubule

glomerulus

macula
densa

distal
convoluted
tubule

collecting
tubule

ascending
and
descending
loops of Henle

medulla

duct of
Bellini

epithelium
covering
papilla

Fig. 24-3. Semidiagrammatic drawings of sections of a unilobar kidney. Two complete nephrons (in black) have been inserted into the drawings so that their course in the kidney may be followed. Of course, complete nephrons cannot be seen in any single section.

loops of Henle. Since these and the collecting tubules that are mixed with them all run fairly straight courses, the medulla, when sliced roughly parallel with them, has a striated appearance, with the striations fanning out from the apex of the medullary pyramid toward the base of the pyramid, which, as has been noted before, fits into the concave border of the cortex.

The Connection Between the Ureter and the Kidney. In a fresh unilobar kidney the ureter is seen to extend out from the kidney through the fat at its hilus (Fig. 24-2). If this tube is traced back up into the fat of the pelvis of the kidney, it will be seen to become expanded to form a cap which fits over the papilla of the pyramid (Fig. 24-3). This expanded end of the ureter is called its *pelvis* (basin). Urine formed by nephrons passes into collecting tubules which carry it out through the papilla of the pyramid, and here it is collected by the caplike basin portion of the ureter. Urine here can only enter the lumen of the expanded end of the ureter because the epithelium that lines the pelvis is continuous with the epithelium covering the papilla of the pyramid, and this, in turn, is continuous with that lining the collecting tubules (Fig. 24-3). The papilla is so riddled with the collecting tubules that pass through it that it is called the *area cribrosa* (*cribrum*, a sieve). Smooth muscle has been described in the wall of the pelvis of the ureter, and it has been suggested that its contraction may exert a milking influence on the papilla and so squeeze urine out of the collecting tubules into the pelvis.

Lobules and Medullary Rays

It is important not to confuse lobules with lobes.

A *lobe* of kidney tissue is a medullary pyramid with its cap of cortical tissue (Fig. 24-3). Accordingly, a unipyramidal kidney is a unilobar kidney. (Each kidney of man consists of a dozen or more lobes; each of these lobes in itself greatly resembles a whole unipyramidal kidney.)

The Two Definitions of a Lobule. As was explained in connection with the discussion of liver lobules, a lobule can be defined as a small part of some organ that is separated from other parts by a connective tissue partition or by an indentation or by some other means. However, in glandular tissue the small parts that are separated from one another by partitions are generally constituted of secretory units that drain into a single common duct that leaves the lobule. Hence the parts of glands that drain into a single common duct came to be called lobules in the kidney even though these parts are not separated from one another by partitions or indentations. This is the definition of

a lobule that is used in the kidney; in this organ lobules are considered to be parts of the organ in which the nephrons all drain into the same collecting tubule. Since areas of tissue (lobules) are not separated from one another by partitions or indentations, it is not easy to find them; it is much easier to locate their central cores, which are known as *medullary rays,* and these will now be described.

Medullary Rays As the Cores of Kidney Lobules. The cortex of a freshly cut kidney has been said to be granular. But it is not *evenly* granular because *raylike* extensions of the light-colored striated medullary substance project up into it at intervals from the base of the medullary pyramid (Figs. 24-2 and 24-3). These raylike extensions of medullary substance that are *projected* into the cortex are termed *medullary rays,* and the student must take care to remember that these are not, as their name might be thought to imply, in the medulla but in the cortex.

In order to explain medullary rays, it is necessary to amplify somewhat the description already given of the disposition of nephrons in the kidney. A proximal convoluted tubule leads off from a glomerulus and then after pursuing a tortuous course in the vicinity of the glomerulus it dips down toward the medulla as the descending limb of a loop of Henle. It then returns to the cortex as an ascending limb of the loop of Henle and after touching the glomerulus again at the macula densa becomes the distal convoluted tubule which pursues a tortuous course and empties, together with many other nephrons, into a *common collecting tubule,* which, in turn, descends into and through the medulla to open through the papilla of the pyramid into the pelvis of the ureter. *Many nephrons drain into each collecting tubule* (Fig. 24-3).

The core of a lobule is a medullary ray, and the core of a medullary ray is the branched collecting tubule into which the distal convoluted segments of the many nephrons that surround it empty. The branched collecting tubule in the kidney cortex is the counterpart of a branched *intralobular* duct of an exocrine gland. In addition to a branched collecting tubule, a medullary ray contains the descending and the ascending limbs of the loops of Henle of the nephrons that, in the cortex, empty into the branched collecting tubule that the ray contains. The medullary ray, *plus* the surrounding glomeruli and proximal and distal convoluted tubules of the nephrons that empty into its branched collecting tubule, constitutes a *lobule* of kidney tissue (Fig. 24-3). As noted, kidney lobules are not clearly delineated. However, when we study the blood supply of the cortex, we shall find that interlobular arteries ascend into the cortex roughly between lobules, and these are seen occasionally in sections where they serve as landmarks to indicate the margins of lobules (Fig. 24-5).

The narrowest part of a medullary ray is the part that most closely approaches the capsule of the kidney. The reason is that medullary rays in the outer part of the cortex contain, in addition to collecting tubules, which narrow as they approach the cortex, only the descending and the ascending limbs of loops of Henle of the nephrons whose glomeruli are in the outermost zone of the cortex. But as medullary rays descend in the cortex toward the medulla, they are added to by the descending and the ascending limbs of loops of Henle of the nephrons whose glomeruli are in the deeper parts of the cortex, and this, of course, makes the rays broader (Fig. 24-3).

A medullary ray, on entering the medulla, is no longer called a ray, because it does not stand out like a ray against a background of a different character; the substance of the medullary continuation of the ray is the same as that of medullary substance in general (Fig. 24-3). This leads to students visualizing kidney lobules as purely cortical structures. However, it should be remembered that the bundle of tubules that enters the medulla from each medullary ray, even though its limits can no longer be identified, is as much a part of the lobule as the bundle that projects into the cortex as the medullary ray. In other words, kidney lobules have medullary as well as cortical components.

The Multipyramidal or Multilobar Kidney of Man

Some General Features. The kidney of man contains from 6 to 18 lobes—individual pyramids of medullary tissue capped by cortical tissue. These are arranged within the kidney so that the tip of each pyramid points toward the pelvis (Fig. 24-4) of the ureter. In fetal life, and for at least part of the first year of postnatal life, the lobes are sufficiently distinct for their limits to be seen on the surface of the kidney. This condition occasionally persists into adult life and accounts for what is termed *fetal lobulation*. This term is not apt because *lobes,* not *lobules,* are demarcated. Normally, however, as growth continues, the surface distinctions between lobes is lost in early childhood, *and the cortical tissue that covers each pyramid comes to merge smoothly into that which covers adjacent ones.*

Columns of Bertin. A lobed appearance is retained in the medulla, for although some pyramids fuse during development and come to have a common papilla, many remain separated and provide the basis for a multilobar structure. Individual medullary pyramids, curiously enough, are separated from one another *by partitions of cortical substance* that extend down between them for some distance from the cortex proper. When a kidney is sliced, these partitions of typical cortical substance between pyramids appear as columns and are called the *columns of Bertin* (columni Bertini) (Fig. 24-4).

The Cortical Labyrinth. Medullary rays extend from the base of each pyramid of medullary tissue into cortical substance as they do in unipyramidal kidneys to form the cores of lobules (Fig. 24-5). In sections of cortex a ray is seen to be surrounded by cortical substance composed of the convoluted tubules and glomeruli of the nephrons that empty into its branched collecting tubule (Fig. 24-5). Since convoluted tubules pursue such tortuous courses, the cortical substance of lobules that surrounds the medullary rays is termed the *labyrinth* (*labyrinthos,* a maze) of the cortex (Fig. 24-5), to distinguish it from the substance of the ray.

The Calyces of the Pelvis of the Multilobar Kidney. Since the multilobar kidney has many medullary pyramids, each of which elaborates urine through its papilla, the pelvis of the ureter of the multilobar kidney is more complex than that of the unipyramidal organ. The ureter, on approaching the hilus of a multilobar kidney, becomes expanded into a pelvis as it does in the instance of a unipyramidal kidney. But, since there are many papillae from which urine must be collected, the pelvis of the ureter of the multilobar kidney divides into several large primary branches. Each of these, in turn, branches into a set of smaller tubular branches so that a separate tube (with an open end) is provided to fit over the papilla of each pyramid. Since these tubular branches from the pelvis fit over the individual papillae like cups, they are termed *calyces* (*kalyx,* the cup of a flower). Each one that fits over a papilla is termed a *minor calyx* (Fig. 24-4), and the main (primary) branches of the pelvis, from which the minor calyces arise, are termed *major calyces* (Fig. 24-4). Each papilla is, as it were, pushed for a short distance into the open end of its calyx. Of course, it cannot be pushed into the open end of the tubular calyx for any great distance because of its pyramidal shape (the tip of a sharpened pencil can be pushed into the open end of a glass tube for only a short distance). The walls of the open end of a calyx come into contact with the sides of the papilla a short distance up from its tip, and here the tissues of the wall of the calyx become continuous with those of the papilla. In particular, the epithelium that lines the calyx loops back to become the covering of the papilla.

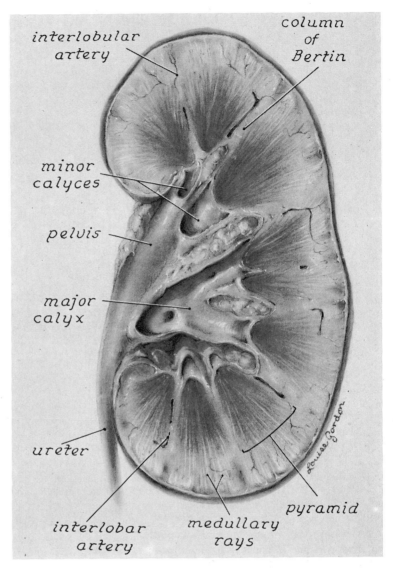

FIG. 24-4. Drawing of the cut surface of a human kidney. The granular cortex is streaked with medullary rays.

interlobular artery

column of Bertin

minor calyces

pelvis

major calyx

ureter

interlobar artery

medullary rays

pyramid

The Nephron of the Kidney of Man: Its Parts and Their Functions

Methods of Study. Knowledge about the parts and the courses of nephrons was worked out, not by making reconstructions of nephrons from serial sections of kidneys, which would be an almost impossible task, but by the method of maceration and dissection. This was employed close to the turn of the century by both Huber and Peter, and our knowledge of the morphology and the course of the normal nephron stems from this work. More recently, Jean Oliver, by employing maceration and dissection, combined with staining technics, has investigated nephrons in many types of diseased kidneys and kidneys altered by ex-perimental procedures and so has made an enormous contribution to an understanding of the pathology of this organ.

Some General Features. Nephrons of the kidney of man are said to be of an average length of 50 to 55 mm. Their general microscopic structure and disposition within lobes and lobules is similar to those of unipyramidal kidneys. Those nephrons that begin from glomeruli situated in the zone of cortex that is close to the medulla (the juxtamedullary glomeruli) have longer loops of Henle than those nephrons that begin from glomeruli nearer the exterior of the kidney (see nephrons in black in Figure 24-3). There are probably about 1,300,000 nephrons in each kidney; some estimates run as high as 4,000,000. Allen gives the total

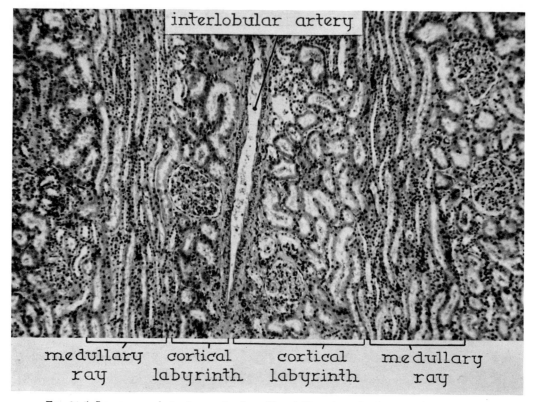

FIG. 24-5. Low-power photomicrograph of an H and E section of a human kidney showing 2 lobules separated by an interlobular artery. The 2 medullary rays that form the central cores for the 2 lobules are each surrounded by the glomeruli and convoluted tubules of the nephrons that empty into the collecting ducts of the ray; these comprise what is termed the cortical labyrinth.

length of all the tubules of both kidneys as approximately 75 miles. The nephron of the kidney of man (Fig. 24-1) consists of 4 chief parts: (1) the malpighian or renal corpuscle, which contains the glomerulus, (2) the proximal convoluted tubule, (3) the loop of Henle and (4) the distal convoluted tubule (Fig. 24-1). The microscopic structure of each of these parts of the nephron will now be described and related, so far as is practicable, to its particular function.

THE MICROSCOPIC STRUCTURE OF THE MALPIGHIAN OR RENAL CORPUSCLE

Definition and Development. A glomerulus, as has been noted, is a tuft of capillaries supplied by an afferent arteriole and drained by an efferent arteriole —an arrangement admirably suited for the production of tissue fluid. When, during development, a glomerulus forms in the blind end of an epithelial tubule, the structure that comes into existence is known as a *malpighian* or *renal corpuscle* (Fig. 24-6). This structure is composed of capillaries, probably with some associated mesangial cells (to be described later), plus the epithelium that comes to cover them, plus the expanded blind end of the epithelial tubule into which the epithelial-covered capillaries project. The epithelium that comes to cover each capillary is known as the *visceral layer of Bowman's capsule,* or more commonly, as the *glomerular epithelium* (Fig. 24-6). It is important to appreciate that the epithelium insinuates itself over the individual capillaries of the glomerulus (Fig. 24-6) so that, except in certain sites to be described later, each capillary will be completely covered with basement membrane, as will be explained in detail later. The epithelium that lines the bulged end of the nephron, into which the epithelial-covered glomerulus is invaginated, is known as the *parietal layer of Bowman's capsule* or, more commonly, as the *capsular epithelium* (Fig. 24-6). It is continuous with the glomerular epithelium. The lumen of the tubule, which in effect consists of all the spaces between the epithelial-covered capillaries and the parietal layer of Bowman's capsule, constitutes *Bowman's* or the *capsular space* (shown but not labeled in Fig. 24-6).

Renal corpuscles range from about 150 to 250 μ in diameter. They are oval rather than spherical. The juxtamedullary corpuscles are generally larger than those nearer the capsule, probably because the juxtamedullary ones are the first to form during development and hence are the oldest.

Course and Character of the Larger Glomerular Blood Vessels. The over-all diameter of the afferent arteriole of a glomerulus is generally about twice that of the efferent arteriole. However, the lumen of the afferent arteriole of most glomeruli is probably about the same as that of the efferent one during life, because R. D. Bensley found that in preparations fixed by injection while under pressure, they were of about

the same size. More recently, Trueta and his associates have shown that the lumens of the efferent arterioles of the juxtamedullary glomeruli may even be wider than those of the afferent arterioles. Since the over-all diameter of the afferent arterioles is so much greater than that of the efferent arterioles, it is obvious that afferent arterioles must have thicker walls than those of efferent arterioles. Since the adventitia and the intima of afferent arterioles is poorly developed, it is obvious that the great difference in the thickness of the walls of the two vessels is due to the afferent arteriole having a more substantial muscular media. Although the muscular media of the efferent vessel is not well developed, Bensley provided definite evidence of contractile cells in the wall of this vessel.

Glomerular Root, Vascular Pole and Macula

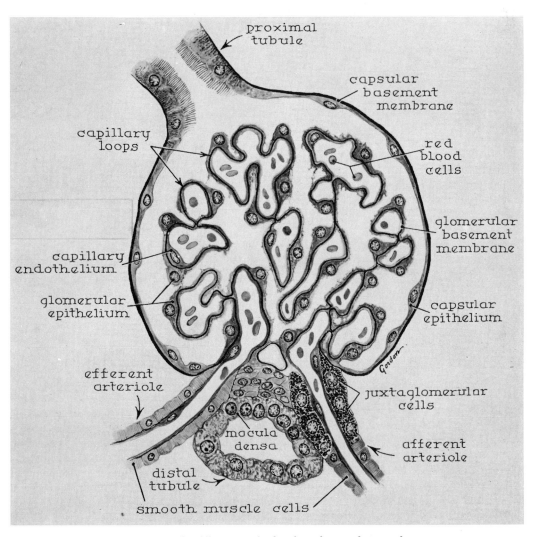

Fig. 24-6. Semidiagrammatic drawing of a renal corpuscle.

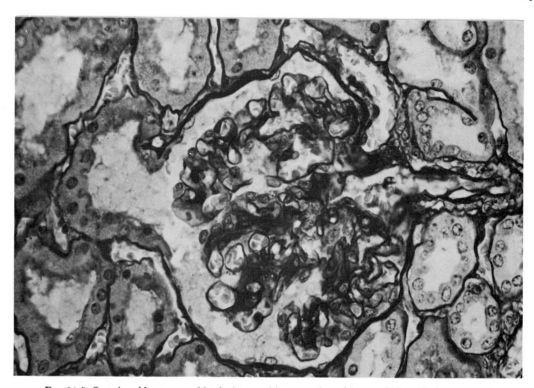

FIG. 24-7. Once in a blue moon a histologist searching a section of human kidney finds an example of a renal corpuscle having been cut in such a plane that it shows both the afferent and efferent arteriole, respectively, entering and leaving the glomerulus, the macula densa, and the beginning of the proximal convoluted tubule with its lumen connecting with the glomerular space. All of these features, together with well-stained basement membranes, are to be seen in the above illustration, which is a photomicrograph ($\times$ 750) of a section of human kidney stained with the PA-Schiff technic and hematoxylin. (From A. L. Burton of the University of Texas)

Densa. The afferent and the efferent arteriole generally pursue curved diverging courses as they respectively enter and leave glomeruli close to one another (Figs. 24-6 and 24-7). This site is termed the *vascular pole* of the glomerulus. The ascending limb of the loop of Henle of each nephron returns to the glomerulus of that nephron, and before it continues on as the distal convoluted tubule it bends in between the afferent and the efferent arterioles at the vascular pole so that its wall, on one side, comes into close contact with the root of the glomerulus and also with the wall of the afferent arteriole (Figs. 24-6 and 24-7). The epithelial cells of the wall of the nephron, where it touches the root of the glomerulus and the afferent vessel, as has been mentioned before, exhibit a concentration of nuclei (Figs. 24-6 and 24-7). This relatively heavily nucleated portion of the wall of the nephron constitutes a structure which, although not sharply defined in ordinary sections, can be seen very clearly and measured in Oliver's preparations. It appears as a group of

epithelial cells that are higher than those in other parts of distal convoluted tubules. It is termed the *macula densa* (thick spot). Between it and the glomerulus proper, in the concavity between the afferent and the efferent arterioles, is a curious little aggregation of small cells with pale nuclei (Fig. 24-6). This little area or group of cells is termed the *polkissen*. There is as yet no certainty about the nature or function of these cells.

The Juxtaglomerular Complex. The cells of the media of the afferent arterioles of glomeruli, in the region of the glomerular root, are distinctly different from ordinary smooth muscle cells. Their nuclei, instead of being elongated, are rounded, and their cytoplasm, instead of containing myofibrils, or as many as usual, contains granules (Fig. 24-6). The cells are known as JG (juxtaglomerular) cells. They have been found in all species that have been examined, including reptiles, birds and mesonephric fish. The cytoplasmic granules of JG cells are not visible with many of the usual histologic technics. The granules can be demonstrated with the PA-Schiff technic. However, the best method for their demonstration in the LM is the one evolved by Wilson working with the Hartrofts and is a modification of Bowie's neutral stain that has been commonly used for the demonstration of beta granules in the islets of Langerhans. The granules are clearly seen in the EM.

There are several peculiarities about the position of the JG cells. (1) They are to be found only in the walls of afferent arterioles and not in the walls of the efferent ones. (2) The internal elastic lamina of the afferent arteriole disappears at the site where they are present; therefore, they are in very close contact with the endothelium lining the afferent arteriole and hence with the blood in its lumen. (3) They are in very close contact with the macula densa (Figs. 24-6 and 24-7), which, as has been described, nestles into the depression between the afferent and the efferent arterioles of the glomerulus. (4) McManus has shown that the basement membrane which otherwise surrounds the nephron throughout its whole length, which will be described presently, is absent at the macula densa; hence, the JG cells come into intimate contact with the cells of the distal convoluted tubule at this site. Finally, McManus has also shown that the Golgi network, which in the cell of a nephron generally is situated between its nucleus and the lumen, is situated in the cells of the macula densa between the nucleus and the outer border of most of its cells—in fact, on the side of the cell that faces the JG cells. In due course it became established that the JG cells are concerned in the control of blood pressure, as will now be described.

The student doubtless understands that a condition termed *high blood pressure* or *hypertension* is by no means uncommon in individuals who have passed the prime of life, and that it may also occur, but less commonly, in younger people. Hypertension is due to the arterioles of the body becoming constricted; this raises the pressure within the arterial system. This, of course, puts more work upon the heart, which therefore tends to become hypertrophied. The arteriolar constriction may be due, at least for a time, to increased tonus or hypertrophy of the muscle cells of the arteriolar walls, with the cells of the wall remaining healthy. But in all too many instances the cells of the arteriolar walls become diseased, and deposits of abnormal materials accumulate in and beside them; these encroach on the lumens of the vessels and narrow them further. This type of hypertension is almost always associated with kidney disease; indeed, the relation between kidney disease and hypertension has been so noticeable

through the years that each has been suggested as the cause of the other.

In 1939 Goldblatt made a brilliant discovery in this field; he showed that if the arterial blood supply of the kidneys was not entirely cut off, but only diminished, the blood pressure of an animal would rise. Moreover, he showed that this was due to the kidneys liberating into the blood, under these ischemic conditions, a substance called *renin* (*renis,* kidney). In the bloodstream renin acts on another substance, *angiotensinogen,* to convert it to *angiotensin I,* which is inactive but when affected by an enzyme (converting enzyme) is changed to angiotensin II (previously called angiotonin), which causes arteriolar constriction and so raises blood pressure. It has, however, only a transient effect, so if it is to cause a sustained hypertension, it must be formed continuously. Renin can be extracted from kidneys; indeed, it was demonstrated in 1898, many years before Goldblatt's discovery.

Relation of JG Cells to Renin. Only natural was the conjecture that the JG cells make renin, and that the granules in them (Fig. 24-6) are either renin or its precursor. Goormaghtigh, in Belgium, was the first to suggest that the JG cells make a hypertensive substance. Dunihue, in America, also found indications of hypertrophy of the JG apparatus in animals made hypertensive. There now are three types of evidence that JG cells elaborate renin. Pitcock and Hartroft have shown that there is a correlation between the amount of renin in the kidneys of man and the degree of granulation of their JG cells. Second, Bing and Kazimierczak, using microdissection technics, have demonstrated that the concentration of renin is highest in the region of the JG cells. The third type of evidence for secretion of renin by JG cells has been obtained by Edelman and Hartroft, using the immunofluorescence technic. Antiserum to renin prepared in the dog was coupled with a fluorescent dye and then used to locate renin in kidney sections. This showed that the fluorescent antibody attached itself chiefly to the JG cells.

The Functions of the JG Cells. It now seems that the JG cells are involved in two ways in a homeostatic mechanism that is concerned in the control of blood pressure. If the blood pressure falls, the afferent arterioles of the glomeruli are not stretched from within as much as they would be normally. It has been suggested that the JG cells, in the walls of these arterioles, are baroreceptors—sensitive to the degree to which they are stretched by the pressure within the afferent arteriole. If they are not stretched by a normal pressure, they respond by secreting more renin; this results in there being more angiotensin II in the blood, and this has two effects, both of which would seem to be directed toward raising the blood pressure.

First, angiotensin II has a direct effect on arterioles, stimulating their muscular walls to contract, which decreases the size of the arteriolar lumens, and this raises the blood pressure in the circulatory system as a whole.

Second, the angiotensin II stimulates the adrenal cortex to secrete increased amounts of a hormone known as aldosterone (which will be described in the next chapter). Aldosterone acts on the tubular parts of nephrons, causing them to conserve more sodium and water. This increases the fluid content of the circulatory system (and the tissue fluid content of the body as well). Increasing the amount of fluid in the circulatory system serves to increase the pressure within the system.

The fundamental role of JG cells would therefore seem to be that of responding to a fall in blood pressure by secreting renin, which by producing angiotensin II acts to bring blood pressure up to normal. The effect would not be permanent because the extra sodium in the blood or in the filtrate passing the macula densa, and the increased pressure within the arteriole would act to cause the JG cells to slow down their secretory activity and in due course contain fewer granules. These negative feedback mechanisms would prevent the blood pressure from being maintained at an excessive level.

The JG mechanism can, however, cause a sustained hypertension in some animals at least, if the arterial circulation through one or both kidneys is diminished, not temporarily by some transient event, but permanently. Disease in one or both kidneys of man may permanently obstruct the arterial flow. Experimentally, a permanently diminished arterial flow and pressure can be achieved by applying clips to the renal arteries and by other means. Under these circumstances, the JG cells of the affected kidney or kidneys try to raise the pressure by secreting renin, but if the higher pressure thus generated in the circulatory system as a whole cannot be transmitted to the arterioles of both of the two kidneys because of the arterial circulation in even one kidney being impeded, the JG cells of that kidney will continue to secrete renin, and, as a result, the blood pressure in the body as a whole will remain high.

Seen with the EM, the granules of the JG cells of mammals are round to oval in shape, large, covered with membrane but not particularly homogeneous. However, in 1966 P. Hartroft noticed that the JG cells of the American bullfrog revealed two types of granules, which, of course, could conceivably be related to two different types of secretion. This observation may

be of interest with respect to the possibility of JG cells being the source of erythropoietin as well as renin. It has been thought for some time that the kidney is the source of erythropoietin, and now there is some experimental evidence suggesting that the cellular source of this substance is the JG cell. (See reference to Hartroft, Bischoff and Boucci, 1969.)

(Lest by discussing one histological feature of the kidney, namely, JG cells, that affects blood pressure, the impression may inadvertently be given that excessive and sustained secretion of renin is the basis for the usual instance of hypertension in man, it should perhaps be said that, as will be learned in other courses, the basis for the usual instance of hypertension in man is complex, and that the development or continuance of the condition may be dependent on various factors. Salt and water metabolism, aldosterone secretion, kidney disease and even emotion all seem to be factors that can variously be involved.)

Glomerular Capillaries and Glomerular Lobules. The most widely held early view was Vimtrup's. He postulated that the afferent arteriole on entering the glomerulus branches into a few primary branches, and that from these about 50 single capillary loops arose which drained into primary branches of the efferent arteriole. According to this view, there were no anastomoses between individual capillary loops. Subsequent studies led to a modification of this view. First, it was shown that there were, indeed, primary branches from the afferent arterioles, and that these gave rise to capillaries that drained to primary branches of an efferent arteriole. This finding suggested that there were what might be termed lobules in a glomerulus, a lobule consisting of the capillaries that hung from one primary branch of an afferent arteriole and drained into one primary branch of an efferent arteriole. It became accepted that there were anastomoses between the capillaries within any given lobule, but not between the capillaries of different lobules. Figure 24-8 shows the appearance sometimes seen in sections, which suggest that the capillaries are arranged into lobules. However, further work has shown that there may be anastomoses between the capillaries of adjacent so-called lobules. The conclusion is, therefore, that whereas there is a suggestion of the glomerular capillaries being arranged to some extent into so-called lobules, there are enough anastomoses between lobules for the glomerular capillaries to constitute an anastomosing network.

The Mesangium and Mesenchymal Cells. The glomerulus hangs from the vascular pole. The sites where the afferent arteriole branch to deliver blood into the capillary loops of lobules, and where the capillary loops of lobules drain into the branches of the efferent arteriole, can be considered as the stalks from which the lobules hang. In this region capillaries arise from the afferent vessel, and capillaries converge on the efferent vessel; and so in this region capillaries are often in intimate contact with one another. Whereas glomerular epithelium covers all the exposed surfaces of glomerular capillaries that are close together, it does not always, in this region, penetrate far enough between the capillaries that are adjacent to one another in a stalk to provide a complete covering for each capillary of that stalk. Instead, the glomerular epithelium surrounds little groups of contiguous capillaries as a whole; this is shown in Figure 24-9.

In such sites, the basement membrane that is derived from the epithelial cells therefore does not completely surround each capillary (gray in Fig. 24-9). Hence, the parts of the walls of the grouped capillaries that are not covered with glomerular epithelium, and epithelial-derived basement membrane, are relatively weak. Some support is provided in these sites, however, because of mesangial cells being disposed between the contiguous capillaries (Fig. 24-9). The mesangial cells make an intercellular substance (Fig. 24-9) that is similar to basement membrane, and this covers the endothelial cells of the capillaries where they are not covered by epithelial-cell-derived basement membrane. The endothelial cells of capillaries are, of course, covered with a thin basement membrane on their outer aspects (dark line in Fig. 24-9), and this fuses with the epithelial-derived basement membrane where there is epithelium. Where there is not epithelial basement membrane, it more or less fuses with the matrix of mesangial cells.

Mesangial cells tend to have more or less of a stellate shape. Sometimes a cytoplasmic process can be seen to reach between endothelial cells to abut directly on the lumen of a capillary.

The general nature of the mesangial cell seems to be similar to that of a pericyte or an undifferentiated smooth muscle cell. There is also some suggestion that mesangial cells represent a continuation into the glomerulus of a type of cell similar to the JG cells of the afferent arteriole. Granules have been seen in them, and they behave in certain ways like JG cells. However, they possess, or can develop, phagocytic properties and cope with macromolecular materials that enter the intercapillary spaces where they are present. Their supportive role, as noted above, seems to be that of providing support where the usual relatively strong basement membrane component that is provided by the glomerular epithelial cells is not present.

Whether or not mesangial cells are associated with

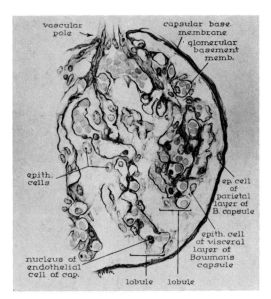

Fig. 24-8. Drawing of a portion of a renal corpuscle as seen under oil-immersion in a section of human kidney stained by the PA-Schiff method and by hematoxylin. Three lobules are to be seen hanging from the vascular pole.

free capillaries in a glomerulus is perhaps open to question. If they are ever present in such sites, they would in effect be pericytes and be located on the outer surface of the basement membrane produced by endothelial cells, and hence between this basement membrane and that made by the epithelial cells. Mesangial cells are easier to demonstrate in some species —for example, rats and mice—than in man.

The Respective Roles of Endothelium and Epithelium in the Formation of Basement Membranes. As described in Chapter 8, there is evidence indicating that the epithelium plays a major role in the formation of basement membranes that lie between epithelium and connective tissue. At the same time it is true that endothelial cells of capillaries can produce a very thin basement membrane on their outer surface even though the capillary is in contact only with connective tissue. The capillary basement membrane, however, is so thin it can be seen only with the EM.

In examining a PA-Schiff-stained section of kidney with the LM, well-defined basement membranes can be seen only where epithelial cells abut on connective tissue cells (including endothelium). Thus, a well-developed basement membrane can be seen in renal corpuscles in two sites. First, there is a substantial basement membrane between the continuous squamous epithelium that constitutes the parietal layer of Bow-

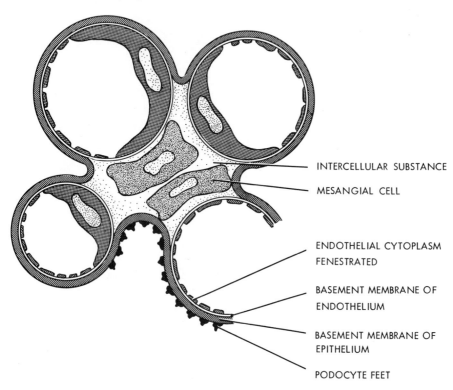

INTERCELLULAR SUBSTANCE

MESANGIAL CELL

ENDOTHELIAL CYTOPLASM
FENESTRATED

BASEMENT MEMBRANE OF
ENDOTHELIUM

BASEMENT MEMBRANE OF
EPITHELIUM

PODOCYTE FEET

Fig. 24-9. Diagram to illustrate the position of mesangial cells in relation to the surrounding capillaries in a tuft. Note that, whereas the basement membrane of the endothelial cells of the fenestrated capillaries completely surrounds each individual capillary, the basement membrane beneath the podocyte feet of the epithelium does not surround each capillary completely but is present only where the capillaries are covered with podocyte feet. The mesangial cells are essentially macrophages and are immersed in an amorphous type of intercellular substance which more or less forms the core of a capillary tuft.

man's capsule and the connective tissue that supports this epithelium (Figs. 24-6, 24-7, and 24-8). Second, there is a continuous basement membrane interposed between the walls of glomerular capillaries (endothelium with some pericytes) and the epithelium (the so-called visceral layer of Bowman's capsule or the glomerular epithelium) that covers the capillaries. An important fact to take into account in attempting to visualize the arrangements of glomerular capillaries in 3 dimensions is that, except where a mesangial cell lies between two or three contiguous capillaries, *every capillary appearing in a cross or oblique section is seen in a good PA-Schiff preparation to be completely surrounded with a basement membrane* (Figs. 24-6 and 24-8).

In other parts of the cortex, a basement membrane, visible with the LM, is *not* seen around capillaries that are associated with the tubular parts of the nephron. The tubules themselves, however, are each surrounded with a substantial basement membrane that can be demonstrated with the PA-Schiff technic and the LM, as is seen in Figure 24-12.

Accordingly, it seems that epithelium interacting somehow with a connective tissue is a requisite for the formation of substantial basement membranes in the kidney.

The Surface Area of Glomerular Capillaries. The total surface area of the capillaries of a glomerulus has been both estimated and measured. The latter procedure involves making exact large models of each section cut successively through an injected glomerulus and measuring the surfaces of the capillaries of the models. The procedure is so laborious and fraught with difficulties that few have attempted it. Book, two of whose preparations are shown in Figure 24-10, injected the blood vessels of a kidney of a child of 6 and made wax replicas of each section cut through one glomerulus. On these replicas he measured the capillary surfaces. Allowing for certain corrections, he calculated the capillaries of the glomerulus to have a surface area of 0.3813 sq. mm. More recently, Kirkman and Stowell have measured painstakingly the capillary surface area of several rat glomeruli and find that it averages 0.19 sq. mm. They suggest that Book's illustrations indicate that the injection distorted the capillary loops to some extent, and that injected material is not suitable for this type of study. However, they state that his figure is the most reliable one available for the human glomerulus. Rat glomeruli are smaller than human glomeruli; hence, there is surprisingly good agreement between Book's findings and those of Kirkman and Stowell. Since it has been estimated that there are well over a million glomeruli in each human kidney, it seems probable that the total filtration surface of all the glomeruli of both kidneys is well over a square meter.

It has been estimated that the glomerular capillaries of all the renal corpuscles of the two kidneys produce from 170 to 200 liters of tissue fluid each 24 hours. As this fluid moves along through proximal convoluted tubules, loops of Henle and distal convoluted tubules, almost 99 percent of it is resorbed through the walls of the tubules back into the bloodstream. After considering the fine structure of the glomerulus we shall consider the structures of these parts of the nephron where resorption occurs and how their structure is related to their functions.

RELATION OF THE FINE STRUCTURE OF THE GLOMERULUS TO ITS FUNCTION

The problem of what constitutes the filtration barrier of the glomerulus is complicated by the fact that there are 3 layers to consider: (1) the endothelium, (2) the basement membrane between the endothelium of the capillaries and the epithelium on the outer aspects of the capillaries, and (3) the epithelium that covers the capillaries (the visceral layer of Bowman's capsule). Before considering their respective roles in filtration we shall describe each layer.

The Endothelium of Glomerular Capillaries. First, the cytoplasm of the endothelial cells (except in sites that contain nuclei and in cytoplasmic sites adjacent to the nuclei, where most of the organelles of the endothelial cells are contained) is attenuated and riddled with pores (Fig. 24-11, *left side*). The pores have a diameter of around 1,000 Å.

The Basement Membrane. The basement membrane with the EM appears as a complex of amorphous material and extremely fine filaments. Since the endothelium is weak and the glomerular epithelium frankly discontinuous (as will be described shortly), it seems evident that the basement membranes of glomerular capillaries must possess a good deal of tensile strength. Blood is pumped into the capillaries under a pressure of about 60 to 70 mm. Hg, which would stretch the capillaries both in width and length if their walls were not reasonably strong and maintained in a good condition. The role of preventing their stretching seems to be allotted to the basement membrane.

The Turnover of the Substance of Basement Membrane. Experiments performed by giving animals silver salts which deposit in glomerular basement membranes have shown that new basement membrane forms in due course to cover, on the epithelial side of the membrane, the site where the deposit occurred. It therefore seems probable that the epithelial cells are active in the formation of new membrane.

If new layers are added to the exterior of the basement membrane by the epithelial cells, it seems reasonable to assume that some of the material of the basement membrane would be just as continuously lost from its inner surface if it was not to become unduly thick. Mesangial cells and pericytes may act on the inner part of the basement membrane to phagocytose and remove accumulation of debris or old altered membrane. So there may be processes operating here that are reminiscent of those that operate in the appositional growth of bone, with the formation of new layers on one surface and the removal of old layers from the other. Indeed, Walker has very recently shown that new basement membrane is formed continuously on the epithelial side of the membrane and

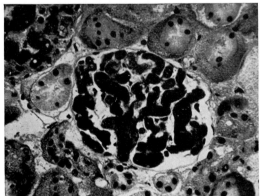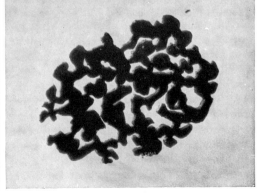

FIG. 24-10. (*Left*) A medium-power photomicrograph of a section cut through a glomerulus in a kidney whose blood vessels were injected with a material that shows black in the photomicrograph. (*Right*) A photograph of a wax plate made from an enlargement of a section of an injected glomerulus (but not the same one). (Preparation by M. H. Book)

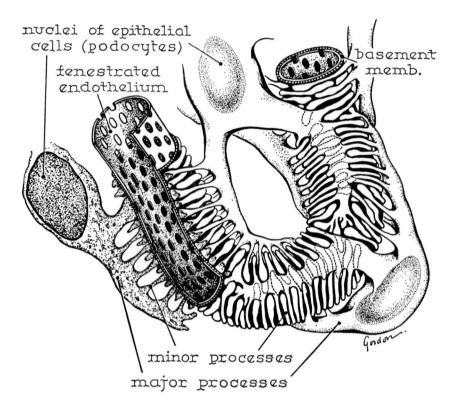

nuclei of epithelial
cells (podocytes)

fenestrated
endothelium

basement
memb.

minor processes

major processes

FIG. 24-11. Schematic diagram devised to give a 3-dimensional concept of part of a capillary loop in a glomerulus with its covering of podocytes and its fenestrated endothelium. At the upper left, part of a podocyte and part of a capillary have been cut away. (Based on electron micrographs from D. C. Pease and a diagram in Pease, D. C.: J. Histochem., *3:*295)

that in the rat the basement membrane is thus replaced every year. Old material is disposed of by mesangial cells. There is also some, and a more rapid, turnover of basement membrane material associated with the endothelial cells.

The Epithelial Cells of the Visceral Layer of Bowman's Capsule (the Glomerular Epithelium): the Podocytes. Although some histologists who studied the kidney through the years with the LM suggested that the epithelial cells that comprise the visceral layer of Bowman's capsule were of an unusual form, having many processes that were attached to the basement membranes that overlie the capillaries, not much attention was paid to their views, and there was a general belief that these cells were squamous in type, and that they formed a continuous covering for the capillaries. With the EM it has become evident that this view was incorrect on both counts, for the cells are not squamous in type, and they do not provide a continuous covering for the capillaries. They have a most unusual form and, because they have feet, are now generally termed *podocytes* (*podos,* foot). See left side of Figure 24-11.

The main cell body of a podocyte (which contains its nucleus) is separated from the capillary over which it lies by what was originally termed the *subpodocytic*

space; it is, of course, filled with glomerular filtrate (Fig. 24-12, *bottom,* subpodocytic space). Numerous arms of cytoplasm, which we shall call *major processes,* extend from the cell body (Figs. 24-11 and 24-12); these tend to run roughly parallel with the long axis or the circumference of the capillary, and they, too, tend to be separated from the capillary by spaces (Figs. 24-11 and 24-12); these spaces also are filled with glomerular filtrate and, of course, are continuous with the glomerular space proper (Figs. 24-11, 24-12 and 24-13). From the major processes, delicate minor processes extend in orderly array to the capillary; these are labeled in Figure 24-11 and unlabeled in Figures 24-12 and 24-13. The minor processes terminate in *feet* (pod. feet are labeled in Fig. 24-12 and seen to advantage in Figs. 24-11 and 24-13); the soles of these are firmly planted on the basement membranes of the capillary and follow its curvature (Figs. 24-11, 24-12 and 24-13). The minor processes and feet from different major processes interdigitate with one another as they approach and come into contact with the capillary (Figs. 24-11 and 24-13). The minor processes and feet that interdigitate with one another may be derived from two or more major processes of the same podocyte or from the major processes of two or more podocytes (Fig. 24-11). Such evidence as is

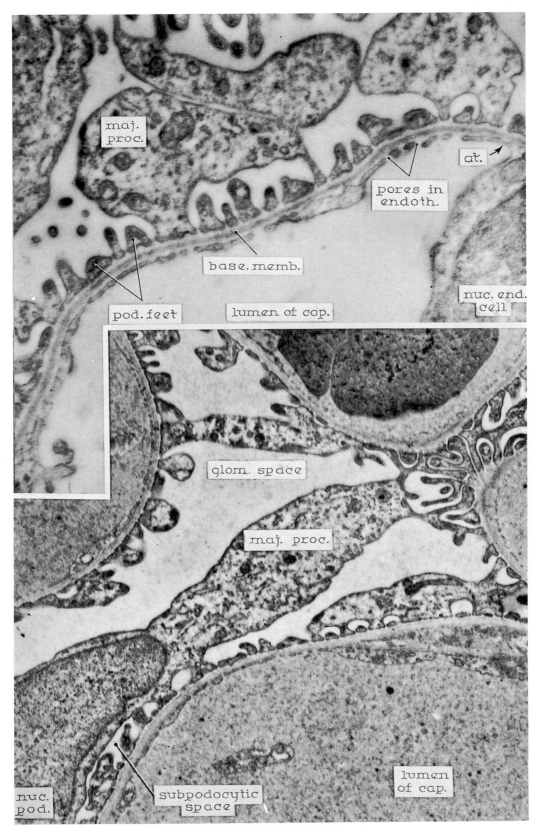

FIG. 24-12. Electron micrographs (*top*, $\times$ 30,000; *bottom*, $\times$ 22,000) of sections of glomerular capillaries and podocytes. (Pease, D. C.: J. Histochem., *3:295*, with labeling added)

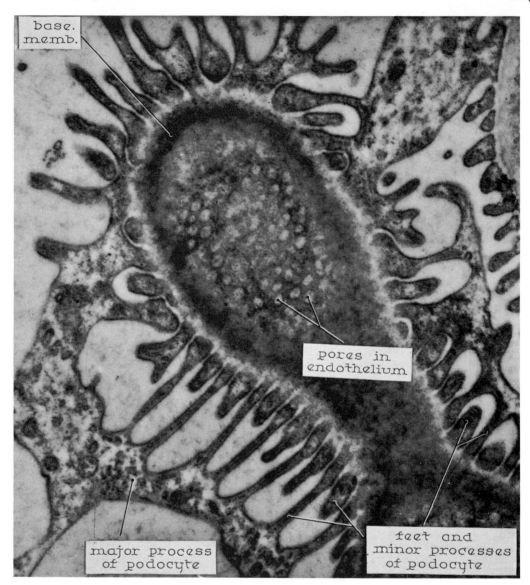

base. memb.

pores in endothelium

major process of podocyte

feet and minor processes of podocyte

FIG. 24-13. Electron micrograph ($\times$ 40,000) of a tangential section through a glomerular capillary, showing pores in the endothelium as well as the interdigitating processes and the feet of podocytes. (Pease, D. C.: J. Histochem., *3:295*, with labeling added)

available suggests that one podocyte can send processes to two capillaries, although generally their processes probably all go to one.

As may be seen in Figures 24-11, 24-12 and particularly in 24-13, the interdigitating feet do not come into contact with one another; there are tiny slits between them; these are believed to be from 200 to 500 Å wide.

Respective Roles of the Three Layers of the Membrane in Filtration. The fluid that passes through the glomerulus has in general the composition of tissue fluid that forms from capillaries elsewhere, which means that water and substances in simple solution pass through it readily but the protein content of the blood plasma is mostly held back by the filter so that it does not appear to any great extent in the glomerular filtrate. Since the endothelium of the membrane is fenestrated with pores that measure around 1,000 Å in diameter (Figs. 24-11 and 24-13) and since these pores are not covered by membranes as are the pores in many of the fenestrated endothelial membranes of capillaries elsewhere in the body, it could not be expected that the glomerular endothelium would hold back anything more than the cells of the blood. It follows therefore that either the basement membrane or the slits between the feet of the podocytes that rest on the basement membrane, must account for holding back proteins.

The size of protein molecules is indicated by their molecular weights. So proteins of various molecular weights can be injected into the bloodstream of experimental animals and it can then be determined with the EM whether or not they are held back by the glomerular filter. However, to do this the proteins must be of a sort that can be recognized with the EM. Ferritin is one that can be used for this purpose because it is a protein that is combined with iron. It has a molecular weight of around 460,000. Studies with it showed that it was arrested by the basement membrane which suggested this was the important layer so far as filtration of the glomerular membrane is concerned. But the molecular weights of the proteins in the blood are for the most part considerably smaller than that of ferritin. So to study this problem further Graham and Karnovsky used two types of peroxidase, one with a molecular weight of around 40,000 and another with a molecular weight of from 160,000 to 180,-000. They used a technic which they had developed by which the sites to which these two peroxidases penetrated could be identified by their reacting with a substance which rendered the sites of their presence visible with the EM. Their results seemed to show that the one with the smaller molecular weight (40,000) passed fairly freely through all three layers of the membrane. However, the one with the molecular weight of from 160,000 to 180,000, while it passed through the endothelium and the basement membrane, was impeded in its further passage through the membrane by the slits between the feet of the podocytes that rest on the basement membrane. Their results therefore seemed to show first that there is no substantial barrier to proteins having a molecular weight of less than 40,000 and, secondly, that somewhere between molecular weights of 40,000 and 160,000 the slits between the podocyte feet on the basement membrane become the important barrier. Taking the earlier studies performed with ferritin into account it would therefore seem also that for proteins having a molecular weight of somewhere between 460,000 and 160,000 the basement membrane ceases to be the effective barrier. To investigate the matter more closely Venkatachalam, Karnovsky, Fahimi and Cotram modified somewhat the technic used by Graham and Karnovsky and employed beef liver catalase (which has peroxidase activity) and has a molecular weight of 240,000.

They also repeated the work previously performed with the horseradish peroxidase having a molecular weight of 40,000 but in their experiments used smaller doses. With the catalase they found a progressive reaction through the substance of the basement membrane. This reaction extended to the slits between the podocyte feet but not through them. The peroxidase with the molecular weight of 40,000 in this experiment was found to permeate the whole thickness of the basement membrane but gradients of staining of the membrane were noticed. It therefore seems that the general conclusion to draw is that the basement membrane restrains the passage of large molecules over a considerable range, with its filtering effect increasing in relation to the size of the molecules, and that the slits account for the filtration of molecules in a size range that pass the basement membrane. However, the precise limits of the size of molecules that can pass both barriers readily is difficult to establish. Certainly at least a little protein from blood plasma passes the filter under normal conditions.

The various proteins in plasma differ in their molecular weights. For example albumin has a molecular weight of 69,000 while the immunoglobulins have molecular weights around 160,000, with the macroglobulins having a molecular weight of 930,000.

In view of the findings described above, certain questions may arise in the mind of the reader. First, why would plasma proteins, most of which have molecular weights of less than 160,000, not pass through fenestrated capillaries in other parts of the body where there would be no podocyte feet to arrest their passage? It might be thought that at these sites there would be a free passage of plasma out into the tissues. One factor that may prevent this could be that the fenestrae in these capillaries outside the kidney are closed with diaphragms even though these may not always be detected with the EM. Another reason could be that the blood in capillaries in sites other than the glomerulus are not under the considerable hydrostatic pressure that exists in glomerular capillaries. This, however, is a question for which the answers as yet are not as satisfactory as might be wished.

Another question that might come to mind is why the glomerular filters would not become plugged or otherwise affected by straining out molecules and other particulates too large to pass clearly through them. In connection with this latter question it should be mentioned that antigen-antibody complexes that form in other parts of the bloodstream or gain entrance to it, may be filtered out by the glomerular filter where they form irregular deposits underneath the podocyte feet where the latter rest on the base-

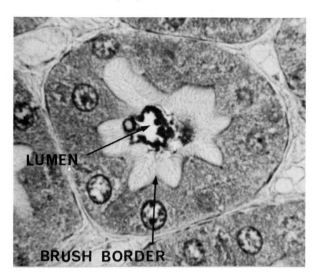

FIG. 24-15. Photomicrograph of a section of rat kidney stained by the TPA technic and showing a cross section of a collapsed proximal convoluted tubule. In this state the cells assume a truncated appearance; that is, they appear as pyramids with their apices cut off. The brush border is visible and so extensive there is little space left in the lumen; in the latter precipitated TPA protein, which is black, is easily seen. The cell borders between contiguous cells cannot be seen; the reason is that the borders of contiguous cells interdigitate so extensively with one another. (Photomicrograph courtesy of Y. Clermont)

ment membrane. It is important to realize that the antibody component of these complexes is not directed against any component of the basement membrane itself but that complexes formed elsewhere are merely trapped here as they attempted, as it were, to pass through the filter. However, such antigen-antibody complexes may activate the complement system which could then at this site attract polymorphs. The degranulation of these could in turn damage the glomerulus. (It should be mentioned also that there is another type of damage to glomeruli, less frequent than the above described type, which is due to antibodies directed against the basement membrane itself; this would be of the nature of an auto-immune reaction. The complement system can be activated by this type of reaction also, with resulting inflammatory disease.)

THE PROXIMAL TUBULE

The proximal convoluted tubule is about 14 mm. in length and has an over-all diameter of about 60 μ. The first part of it, which leads off from the glomerulus, is sufficiently narrow and straight in some species to con-

stitute a neck for the tubule. But in man this portion of the tubule differs little from the remainder of the tubule (Fig. 24-7). Proximal convoluted tubules get the convoluted parts of their names from their looped and tortuous courses in the immediate vicinity of the renal corpuscles from which they originate (Fig. 24-1). They then enter medullary rays (Fig. 24-3) and descend in these as the upper thick parts of descending limbs of loops of Henle. The descending limbs enter the medulla and extend into it for different distances before looping back as ascending limbs (Fig. 24-3). The character of the proximal convoluted tubule does not change materially as it becomes the first part of the descending loop of Henle. Only when it becomes thin do its character and functions change. Hence, the thick segment of the descending loop of Henle, though straight, has the same character and presumably performs the same function as the convoluted part of the tubule proper and so should be considered to be part of the proximal tubule.

Some Aids To Recognizing and Studying Proximal Tubules in Sections With the LM. (1) For the most part proximal tubules are seen in sections of cortex as oblique cuts through curved tubes (Fig. 24-14). (2) Oblique and cross sections of proximal convoluted tubules are the most common sight in a section of kidney cortex (Fig. 24-14), and indeed they are the only kind seen between the outermost glomeruli and the capsule of the kidney in the normal. (3) The cells of proximal convoluted tubules become altered very rapidly as a result of postmortem degeneration; however, even if fixation has not been prompt, their cytoplasm is generally more acidophilic and more granular than that of other tubules; accordingly, proximal convoluted tubules are not only the most numerous tubules seen in an H and E section of kidney cortex, but they are also the pinkest (Fig. 24-14). (4) Finally on their free surfaces, the cells of the proximal tubules have a striated border (Figs. 24-14 and 24-15).

Some Details About the Cells. The cells of the walls of proximal convoluted tubules are broader at their bases, which lie against a basement membrane, than at their free margins, which abut on the lumen. In good preparations a striated (brush) border can be seen on the free surface of each cell (Figs. 24-14 and 24-15). The boundaries between adjacent cells cannot be seen to advantage because the edges of any two cells that touch each other are serrated, with the projections from the edge of one fitting into the notches of the other. In tissue fixed immediately after death and suitably stained, the appearance of proximal convoluted tubules varies between two extremes. At one extreme the epithelium is low, and the lumen wide and

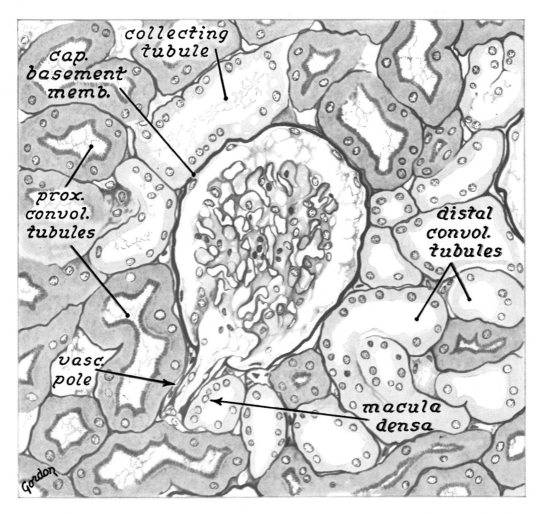

Fig. 24-14. Drawing of a section of human kidney fixed in formalin and stained by the PA-Schiff technic followed by hematoxylin. Note the PAS-positive brush borders of the proximal convoluted tubules and that the cytoplasm of the cells of these tubules stains more deeply than that of the cells of the distal convoluted or collecting tubules. Note the PAS-positive basement membranes that surround the tubules. Basement membrane is also present under both the visceral and the parietal layers of Bowman's capsule. The numerous capillaries that lie between adjacent tubules are collapsed and hence not seen in this preparation. The vascular pole of the glomerulus has been cut obliquely and is not as prominent as it otherwise would be.

round; at the other, the epithelium is high, and the lumen small and triangular (Fig. 24-15). These two extreme appearances, as well as intermediate ones, are to be explained by two factors: (1) the state of functional activity of the epithelial cells of the tubule, and (2) the degree to which the lumen of the tubule is distended by glomerular filtrate; the latter is affected by whether or not the glomerulus of the nephron is producing much or little filtrate. It is believed that the low epithelium and the wide round lumen is associated with the production of much filtrate.

The nuclei of the cells of proximal convoluted tubules are disposed toward the bases of the cells. They are large and spherical and possess nucleoli (Fig. 24-15).

Proximal convoluted tubules are ensheathed in a substantial basement membrane which is beautifully demonstrated by the PA-Schiff technic (Fig. 24-14).

Fine Structure and Its Relation to Function. The cell surfaces that face the lumen are covered with thin microvilli about 1 μ long, which in many respects are similar to those of the lining cells of the small intestine (Fig. 24-16, *lower right*); these, of course, account for the appearance of the striated or brush border seen with the LM in Figures 24-14 and 24-15. There is a sort of matrix that fills in the spaces between them. Accordingly, in electron micrographs of cross sections of microvilli, the matrix between individual microvilli may appear as prominent as the microvilli themselves, and this appearance suggested a view held in the past, that the microvilli, instead of being fingerlike structures that project into the lumen from the cell surface, were actually pits, lined with cell membrane, that project inward into the cytoplasm from the free surface of the cell. However, it is now accepted that the brush border consists of countless microvilli with some sort of jellylike matrix between them. The number of microvilli is enormous, and obviously they increase the surface area greatly. In man, the total surface of the brush border of the proximal tubules of both kidneys is about 50 to 60 square meters.

Mechanisms of Absorption. The proximal convoluted tubules absorb about $\frac{7}{8}$ of the water and sodium that pass along them. The explanation for this enormous resorption of sodium and water by the cells of the proximal convoluted tubules is to be found at their bases, for it is in this location that the sodium pump (described in Chap. 5) operates to pump sodium out through the cell membrane into the tissue fluid at the bases of the cells, where there are many capillaries. The sodium that is pumped out, together with chloride ions, attracts water and draws this from the cytoplasm

out through the base of the cell. There is therefore both a concentration and an electrical gradient set up between the fluid in the lumen of the tubule and the cytoplasm of the cell, a gradient which results in water and sodium moving into the cytoplasm from the lumen of the tubule. It seems, then, that it is the sodium pump operating at the bases of these cells to pump sodium out of the cell that accounts for the remarkable absorption of water and sodium that occurs here.

The operation of the sodium pump requires both a cell membrane and the expenditure of energy. It is therefore not surprising to find that the mitochondria are both long and abundant in the cytoplasm at the bases of these cells (Fig. 24-17). To provide abundant cell membrane, there are also what seem at first glance to be very numerous infoldings of the cell membrane at the bases of these cells, which would, of course, increase greatly the surface area of cell membrane through which a sodium pump could operate (Fig. 24-17). However, as has been shown by Bulger, these infoldings are not as simple as they might seem to be in a single section. To understand them it may help to reiterate that the cell membranes of the *lateral* sides of contiguous cells in both proximal and distal tubules interdigitate with one another in a very complex fashion so that the sides of these cells are thrown into many complex ridges and grooves. Moreover, near the bases of the cells, the infoldings of the lateral and basal membranes split the basal aspect of these cells up further into what are termed basal processes. These are so extensive that the basal processes of contiguous cells may, to some extent, interdigitate. Hence, a basal process that in a single section might seem to belong to the cell whose cytoplasm seems to surround it in that particular section may actually belong to a contiguous cell.

The Absorption of Glucose, Amino Acids, etc. Active transport mechanisms, descriptions of which are more suited to a biochemistry than a histology text, operate in the cells to absorb many useful substances back into the body. However, the absorption of protein involves histological considerations and will now be described.

The Absorption of Protein. A not inconsiderable amount of protein (derived from blood) normally leaks through the glomeruli of the kidneys every 24 hours, and this in the normal is all absorbed by the proximal convoluted tubule. Protein is absorbed at the free surface by pinocytosis, that is, by means of little membranous vesicles or tubules, containing protein, being formed at and pinched off from the cell membrane between microvilli. The protein-filled vesicles pass into the cytoplasm, where they fuse with

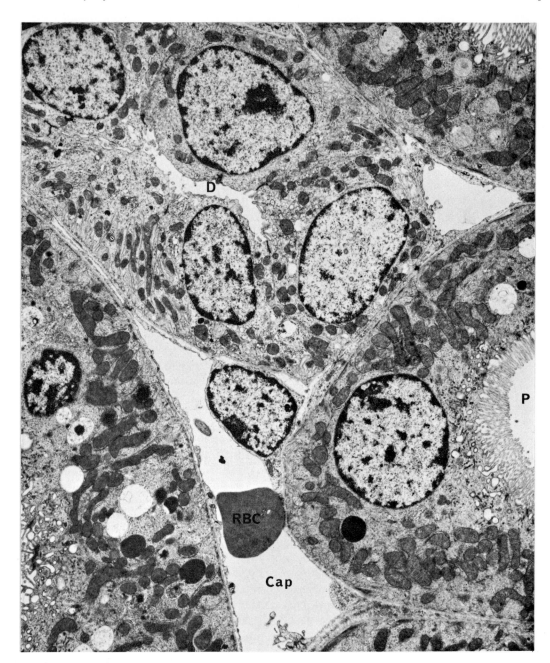

Fɪɢ. 24-16. Electron micrograph ($\times$ 7,100) of section of kidney from young rat fixed with glutaraldehyde and postfixed with osmic acid. At the top left is a distal tubule (D) with a narrow lumen. There are also portions of several proximal tubules (P) with capillaries in the spaces between tubules (Cap). Note the microvilli lining the proximal tubule, lower right, and the concentration of mitochondria in the more basal parts of the cells. (Courtesy of Miss Ethel Rau, McGill University)

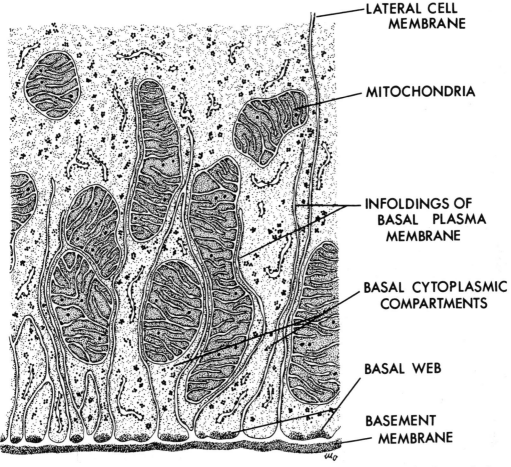

Fɪɢ. 24-17. Drawing illustrating the appearance of the basal portion of the cells of a proximal convoluted tubule as seen in the EM. (Illustration provided by Miss Ethel Rau)

lysosomes. The enzymes of the lysosomes digest the protein, so that soluble products of digestion (probably amino acids) are formed, and they are presumably freed in the cytoplasm to be absorbed into capillaries (or perhaps used to some extent by this cell).

Excretory Functions. The cells of the proximal convoluted tubules can also perform excretory functions. Evidence has accumulated to establish the excretory capacity of tubular cells from several sources and procedures: (1) species whose kidneys have tubules but no glomeruli; (2) species in which the glomeruli and the tubules of the kidney have a different blood supply and so permit the glomeruli to be put out of action by experimental procedures; (3) by lowering the blood pressure of animals in whose kidneys the glomeruli and the tubules have a common blood supply below the point at which glomeruli continue to produce tissue fluid, and (4) from the study of tubules in tissue culture. But while proximal convoluted tubules can excrete as well as resorb, their excretory function is limited to a few substances. Their resorptive function is their chief one.

THE LOOP OF HENLE

Although glucose and amino acids, and calcium, phosphate and some other ions are resorbed in the proximal tubule, the fact that so much water and sodium are resorbed (and in approximately the same proportions) results in the fluid that remains in its distal portion, soon to enter the thin descending limb of the loop of Henle, having approximately the same osmotic pressure as the glomerular filtrate that entered the proximal tubule. Although the total amount of fluid that enters the descending limbs of the loop of Henle is only about $\frac{1}{8}$ of the glomerular filtrate, it would still constitute an enormous amount of urine unless it were reduced further. The further reduction in its amount requires that it be concentrated.

Mechanisms Involved in Concentrating Urine. Many years ago Crane observed that only animals that have loops of Henle in their nephrons excrete urine that is hypertonic to blood. It was therefore natural to assume for many years that water must be selectively reabsorbed along the course of the loops of Henle, with the result that electrolytes in solution in tubular fluid, for example, sodium and chloride, became more concentrated as the fluid passed along the loops. This led to the further assumption that the fluid delivered into distal convoluted tubules was hypertonic. But when methods were evolved to provide information about the osmotic pressure of fluid along various parts of the nephron, and the osmotic pressure of the tissue fluid present between the tubules in various parts of medullary pyramids, some surprising results were obtained, one result being that the fluid that entered the distal convoluted tubule was even less concentrated and even of a lower osmotic pressure than that which left the proximal tubule.

Before describing what happens in the loop of Henle, we shall deal briefly with what happens in the distal convoluted tubule and the collecting tubules. As fluid passes along the distal convoluted tubule, more water than salt is reabsorbed from its contents, and so in this tubule the fluid once more becomes isotonic. The reabsorption of fluid in the distal convoluted tubule is regulated by the antidiuretic hormone of the posterior lobe of the pituitary (ADH). If the pituitary gland is removed, this reabsorption does not occur, and hence an animal passes great quantities of dilute urine (as will be explained in connection with diabetes insipidus, which will be discussed in connection with the posterior pituitary in Chap. 25).

Since the fluid becomes isotonic again in the distal convoluted tubule, the concentration of urine which accounts for its finally becoming hypertonic must occur as the fluid passes along the collecting tubules. In order to account for this, we now have to consider what happens in the loops of Henle, for what happens in the loops of Henle is indirectly responsible for what happens in the collecting tubules.

The function of the loops of Henle would seem to be that of creating a hypertonic environment in the tissue fluid that surrounds them, so that the collecting tubules that pass through this same environment (consult Fig. 24-3) will have water drawn out of them into the tissue fluid that surrounds them. This extra water in due course passes into the capillaries and is thus taken back into the circulation. It is easiest to describe what happens in the loops of Henle if we begin with what happens as fluid passes up the ascending limb of the loop.

It seems that the lining cells of the ascending loops have the ability to pump sodium from the fluid in the lumens of these tubules out into the tissue fluid in which they and the descending loops are both bathed. It seems, moreover, that the walls of the ascending loops hold back water in their lumens. As a consequence, the fluid contained in the ascending loops would, since it is losing sodium (and, as a result, chloride), become increasingly hypotonic as it ascends ·toward the distal convoluted tubule; and, indeed, this is what happens, and why the fluid delivered into the distal convoluted tubule is hypotonic. However, what happens in the ascending tubule has another effect, which we shall describe next.

As a result of the ascending limb of the loop of Henle pumping sodium out into the tissue fluid, but at the same time holding back water, the tissue fluid in the surrounding area becomes hypertonic. The walls of the thin descending limbs of the loops of Henle, unlike those of the ascending limbs, can let water pass from their lumens out into this tissue fluid. Accordingly, the extra sodium chloride in this tissue fluid withdraws water from the fluid in the descending limb of the loop of Henle and as a result the fluid in the descending limb of the loop becomes increasingly hypertonic as it nears and reaches the bottom of the loop. But, as already noted, as the fluid begins to ascend, the cells of the tubule pump out sodium, and so the fluid first becomes isotonic, and then, as it reaches the proximal convoluted tubule, it becomes hypotonic.

The whole purpose of these activities that occur in the thin loops of Henle and in particular in the loops of the nephrons that begin at the juxtamedullary glomeruli, which have loops that descend deep toward the apex of a medullary pyramid, would seem to be that of making the tissue fluid which surrounds them in the part of the medullary pyramid situated toward its apex more salty and hence hypertonic. Since the collecting tubules pass through this same territory (see Fig. 24-3), the hypertonic tissue fluid acts to draw water from the previously isotonic fluid in the lumens of the collecting tubules, with the result that by the time the fluid in the collecting tubules has passed down through this hypertonic area, it, too, has become hypertonic. Hence the urine delivered into the pelvis of the kidney by the collecting tubules is hypertonic. The antidiuretic hormone, as well as acting on the distal convoluted tubule, controls the permeability of the cells of the collecting tubules in the extent to which they permit the hypertonic tissue fluid to draw water through their walls into the tissue fluid.

All the capillary loops present in this area contain blood that has passed through glomeruli (Fig. 24-20). As blood passes along capillaries (Fig. 24-20) toward the tip of the pyramid it gains sodium but as it passes up again toward the cortex it loses sodium, thus more or less duplicating what happens in the descending and ascending arms of the loop of Henle.

A more precise and detailed account of the mechanisms involved will be found in reference books on the kidney and in textbooks of physiology; what is given here is only intended to provide a rough idea of what is involved.

Microscopic Appearance. Loops of Henle are either short or long. The majority of those nephrons, the glomeruli of which are in the outer part of the cortex, have short loops that do not extend for any great distance into the medulla; perhaps the reason is that they were the last nephrons to develop, and their loops had to accommodate themselves to such space as was available. The nephrons that arise from glomeruli near the medulla, the juxtamedullary glomeruli, have long loops that extend well down toward the apex of the medulla (Fig. 24-3).

The first part of the descending loop is the straight continuation of the proximal convoluted tubules (Fig. 24-1). As it passes down into the medulla—a short distance in the instance of tubules that arise from glomeruli in the outer part of the cortex, and a greater distance in the instance of tubules that arise from glomeruli near the medulla—its lumen rather abruptly becomes narrower, and the cells of its walls squamous (Fig. 24-3). After this change has occurred, the tubule is known as the *thin segment* of the descending limb of the loop of Henle. The thin segments of nephrons that arise from juxtamedullary glomeruli are much longer than those that arise from glomeruli in the outer part of the cortex (Fig. 24-3).

The appearance of a thin loop of Henle is so similar to that of a large capillary that the student may not be able to distinguish easily these tubules in the medulla from the capillaries that run between them (Fig. 24-18). It may be of help to understand that the tubules are wider than capillaries, but they may be partly collapsed. In general, the nuclei of the epithelial cells of the tubules bulge into the lumen of the tubule somewhat more than the nuclei of the endothelial cells of the capillaries. The nuclei of the squamous cells of the tubules are somewhat closer together than the nuclei of the endothelial cells of capillaries. Red blood cells in the capillaries may also be helpful toward identifying them, but artifact may lead to red blood cells being present in the tubules.

In the instance of long loops, the first portion of the ascending limb may be similar to the thin portion of the descending limb. But this soon gives way, in the ascending limb, to a wider tubule with thicker walls; this is known as the *thick segment* of the ascending limb (Fig. 24-18, *bottom*). The character of the thick segment is very similar to that of the distal convoluted tubule, next to be described. In the instance of nephrons with short loops of Henle, the epithelium may change from the thin to that of the thick type even before the nephron has looped back to begin its ascending arm.

Munkacsi and Palkovits have provided evidence to indicate that the ability of animals to live in a desert environment is related to the degree to which their juxtamedullary nephrons, with long thin loops of Henle, are developed. The better they are developed (and they are well developed in desert rats), the more able they are to conserve water.

THE DISTAL CONVOLUTED TUBULE

As has been described already, the thick segment of the ascending loop of Henle returns to the glomerular root of the glomerulus from which the nephron has its origin, and there the part of its wall which comes into contact with the glomerular root becomes heavily nucleated and forms a thick spot, the *macula densa* (Figs. 24-6 and 24-7).

Some authorities define the distal convoluted tubule as only that part of the nephron which extends from the macula densa to a collecting tubule. However, more authorities classify the thick ascending arm of the loop of Henle as part of it. Distal convoluted tubules differ from proximal convoluted tubules in several respects, which are listed below:

1. They are not so long; hence, cross and oblique sections of them are not seen nearly so often in a section of kidney cortex (Fig. 24-14).

2. Their cross-section diameters are generally not quite as great, but since the cells of their walls are generally lower, their lumens tend to be larger (Fig. 24-14).

3. The cells of their walls are smaller in all directions; hence a cross section through a distal tubule reveals many more nuclei than similar sections of proximal convoluted tubules (Fig. 24-14).

4. The cells of their walls have no brush or striated borders on their free surfaces, and their cytoplasm is not nearly so acidophilic (Fig. 24-14).

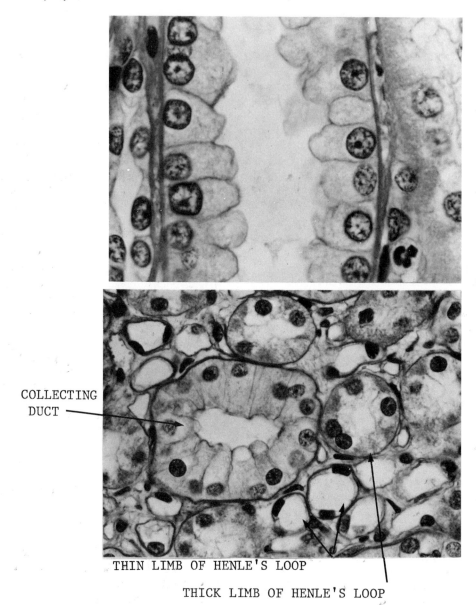

COLLECTING
DUCT —

THIN LIMB OF HENLE'S LOOP

THICK LIMB OF HENLE'S LOOP

FIG. 24-18. (*Top*) Photomicrograph of a section of the medulla of a monkey kidney showing a portion of a collecting tubule cut in longitudinal section in the middle of the picture. To the left of the collecting tubule is a thin portion of a loop of Henle. (*Bottom*) A cross section of the medulla of the kidney of a dog, stained with H and E, and showing a cross section view of a collecting tubule and thin and thick portions of loops of Henle, all of which are labeled.

5. Since the borders between contiguous cells do not interdigitate as extensively as those of cells of the proximal tubules, cell borders can be distinguished more clearly than in proximal tubules.

Like proximal convoluted tubules, the distal ones have a pronounced basement membrane encircling them (Fig. 24-14).

Fine Structure and Relation to Function. The cell surfaces that face the lumen show only a few minor villous projections (Fig. 24-16). The basal parts of the cells show very highly developed infoldings of the cell membrane, which are even more highly developed than those seen at the bases of proximal convoluted cells and illustrated in Figure 24-17; these more or less divide this portion of the cytoplasm into basal processes which contain large long mitochondria. Here also sodium is pumped out of the tubular cells into the tissue fluid, but its place is taken by other cations. As already noted, the withdrawal of water from the tubule is regulated by the antidiuretic hormone of the posterior pituitary.

OTHER FEATURES OF THE KIDNEY

Collecting tubules are not to be thought of as parts of nephrons, even though they absorb water, a process controlled by the antidiuretic hormone, as has been described. They comprise a series of drainage ducts into which urine is delivered by distal convoluted tubules and conducted to medullary papillae, where it is emptied into the calyces of the ureter (Figs. 24-3 and 24-1).

The collecting tubules form a branched system. The largest ones are known as the *ducts of Bellini*. These are easily seen in the apical part of a medullary pyramid where they empty through its papilla. They are large ducts with wide lumens and thick walls composed of pale-staining, high columnar cells with a thin cuticle on their free border. In contrast with the different parts of the renal tubules, the borders between the cells that make up the walls of the ducts of Bellini and the smaller collecting tubules that empty into them are distinct in the ordinary section (Fig. 24-18). The pale cytoplasm of these cells is illustrated in Figure 24-18. With the EM, the cells of the collecting tubules have been found to have only moderately deep infoldings of the cell membrane at their bases.

In the medulla the ducts of Bellini branch at very acute angles (Fig. 24-3). Several generations of branches arise to provide a sufficient number of collecting ducts to supply each medullary ray in the kidney. In the rays the ducts give off side branches. There each pursues a short arched course before becoming continuous with the termination of a distal convoluted tubule (Fig. 24-1).

Although each nephron is provided with an individual arched collecting tubule, several arched tubules empty into a single straight collecting tubule. Hence there are not nearly so many straight collecting tubules as nephrons in the kidney.

Casts. In connection with the kidney, the term cast is used to describe coagulated material, usually protein, that is seen sometimes in the lumens of the more distal parts of nephrons and in collecting tubules. Casts are not seen in the strictly normal kidney. But material obtained at autopsy and used for teaching kidney histology may not always be strictly normal; hence, some casts may be seen in the lumens of the tubules in it.

The Connective Tissue of the Kidney. The kidney is covered with a thin translucent *capsule* that consists of fibrous connective tissue; the intercellular substance in it is chiefly collagen, but a few elastic fibers may be present. In health the capsule is smooth and glistening and can be stripped easily from the cortex. In some kinds of kidney disease fibrous connective tissue forms in the parenchyma of the cortex and extends out to the capsule to bind it firmly to the organ. Under these conditions the capsule cannot be stripped readily from the organ, and this fact is noted at autopsy as an indication that the kidney has become diseased.

The basement membranes that surround the tubules are supported on their outer surfaces by delicate reticular fibers. More substantial fibrous types of intercellular substance may be found in association with the larger vessels of the kidney. But, all in all, the fibrous connective tissue of the kidney parenchyma, except between the ducts of Bellini in the papilla, where there is some loose connective tissue, is extraordinarily scanty, a fact which suggests that there is a great amount of osmotic activity requiring that only substances through which diffusion can occur (amorphous types of intercellular substances) be present between the tubules and the capillaries. Increased fibrous tissue in the kidney is a manifestation of past disease, and in itself it can further interfere with function.

The Circulation of Blood Through the Kidney

Each kidney is supplied by a renal artery. These are relatively large vessels that arise from the aorta, so each kidney receives large amounts of blood delivered under high pressure.

According to Sykes, a renal artery divides close to or within the hilus into 2 large branches. From these 5 end arteries originate; these are called segmental arteries and each of these supplies a particular part of the kidney. All of these are end arteries. From these 5 segmental arteries further branches arise; these tend to ascend toward the cortex as interlobar arteries (Fig. 24-19).

Arcuate Arteries. Some of the interlobar arteries break up into main branches as they ascend in the columns of Bertin, but most of them do so only when they have almost reached the corticomedullary border. Here their branches are given off at wide angles and in all directions but more or less in the same plane. These main branches, into which the interlobar arteries break up, arch over the bases of the medullary pyramids and are called *arcuate (arcuatus,* arched) arteries (Fig. 24-19). Just as there is no continuity

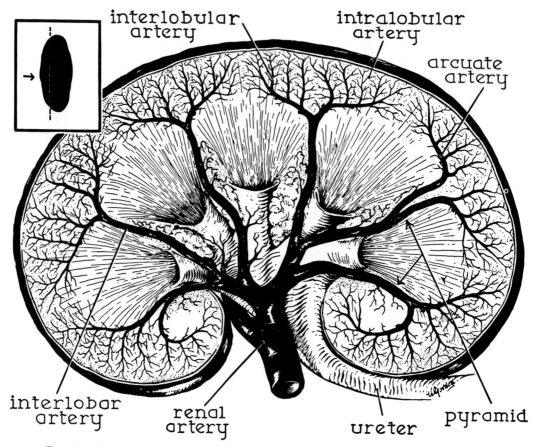

FIG. 24-19. In order to show certain principles essential to understanding the histological aspects of the blood supply of the kidney, this diagram was greatly simplified. For exact knowledge of the precise distribution of the larger arterial vessels, works on gross anatomy and original studies should be consulted.

between the branches of adjacent trees, there is no continuity between the arcuate arteries that arise from adjacent interlobar arteries. Hence, there are no anastomoses between interlobar arteries through arcuate arteries (Fig. 24-19). Accordingly, if an interlobar artery becomes plugged with a thrombus, a pyramidal-shaped segment of kidney tissue dies (the area supplied by the arcuate arteries from that particular interlobar artery); this area of dead tissue is called an infarct.

Interlobular Arteries. The arcuate arteries give off branches that ascend into the cortex (Fig. 24-19). These vessels run between lobules and are termed interlobular arteries (Figs. 24-19 and 24-20). They mark the boundaries between lobules and so alternate with the medullary rays that form the central cores of lobules (Fig. 24-5).

The interlobular arteries give off branches at wide angles on every side. Since these immediately enter the substance of surrounding lobules (the cortical labyrinth), they are called *intralobular arteries* (Fig. 24-20). These give rise to the afferent vessels of glomeruli. However, the terminal branches of the interlobular arteries continue on to the capsule to supply its capillary bed.

How the Capillary Beds of Cortex and Medulla Are Supplied. The efferent arterioles of glomeruli in different parts of the cortex deliver blood into different capillary beds. As may be seen in Figure 24-20, which is based on the study of Morison, the efferent arterioles from glomeruli in the outer part of the cortex (Fig. 24-20) empty their blood into the capillary beds that surround the proximal and the distal convoluted tubules in the cortex. Those from glomeruli somewhat deeper in the cortex (Fig. 24-20) contribute to the capillary bed of the cortex but also to long straight

Fig. 24-20. Diagram to show how the capillary beds of the cortex and the medulla are supplied with blood. (Based on Morison, D. M.: Am. J. Anat., *37*:93)

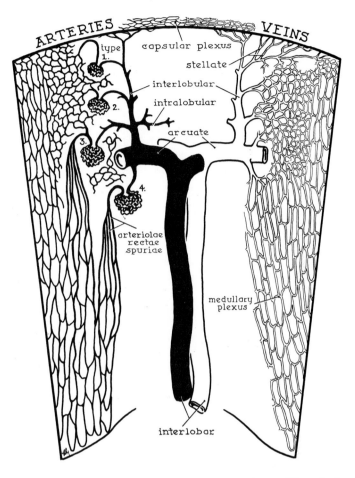

capillarylike vessels that descend into the medulla and are called *arteriolae rectae spuriae* (false straight arterioles) for reasons that will become obvious later. The efferent vessels from the deepest glomeruli in the cortex, some of which are below the level of the arcuate arteries, deliver most or all of their blood into the arteriolae rectae spuriae (Fig. 24-20).

The return of the blood from the capillary beds of the cortex and the medulla is illustrated on the right side of Figure 24-20. In general, the veins correspond to the arteries already described. It is to be noted that at the surface of the kidney little veins arise from the capillary beds of the capsule and the superficial part of the cortex to pass in a converging fashion to interlobular veins. Since these end branches radiate out in a starlike fashion from the ends of the interlobular veins, they are called *stellate veins* (Fig. 24-20).

Since the arteriolae rectae spuriae, which supply the capillary beds of the medulla, are all supplied by the efferent vessels of glomeruli in the deeper part of the cortex (Fig. 24-20), it follows that all the blood that is delivered into the capillary beds of the medulla,

like that which is delivered into the capillary beds of the cortex, has passed immediately beforehand through glomeruli. However, this concept has been contested from time to time. It has been claimed by some who have investigated the circulation of blood through the medulla that arterioles arise directly from the arcuate and the interlobular arteries to pass directly to the capillary beds of the medulla. To distinguish these from the arteriolae rectae spuriae (the false straight arterioles), they are called the *arteriolae rectae verae* (true straight arterioles). If these exist, it would mean that medulla was supplied with some blood that had not passed through glomeruli. Most modern students of this matter do not believe that enough of these exist to be of any functional significance. Hartroft's study shows how some vessels, apparently of this nature, could arise through the fusion of the afferent and the efferent arterioles of the juxtamedullary glomeruli that undergo a physiologic atrophy during the growth of the kidney. Moreover, MacCallum's study shows how estimates of the number of arteriolae rectae verae present in normal kidneys might be overestimated because of their being investigated in kidneys that have been injured throughout life by disease. He has shown that the capillaries of glomeruli that are affected by certain disease processes tend to atrophy and disappear, and at the same time a more or less direct connection becomes established between their afferent and efferent vessels. Unless an observer looked very carefully, he might fail to see these atrophied glomeruli —and there are some, according to MacCallum, even in apparently normal kidneys (Hartroft's physiologic atrophy?)—and so the observer might conclude that what is really an afferent arteriole joined to an efferent arteriole at the site of a defunct glomerulus is an arteriole that has extended from an interlobular artery directly to the capillary bed of the medulla without there being a glomerulus inserted along its course. Therefore, general opinion is that for all practical purposes the blood in the capillary beds of the medulla has passed through glomeruli.

It is possible that a small amount of blood that has not passed through glomeruli may be delivered to the capillary beds of the cortex by means of branches of afferent arterioles that have long been described as emptying into these beds. Such a branch of an afferent arteriole is known as a *Ludwig's arteriole.*

The Two Circulatory Pathways Through the Kidney. During World War II, attention was focused on the study of those unfortunate individuals who were partly buried by rubble when buildings collapsed from bombing. It was found that an individual whose legs had been crushed by a great weight but not necessarily irreparably injured would, in some instances and some days after the event, fail to excrete urine. Many injured in this fashion died after a short period of apparent recovery, not from their primary injuries but from kidney failure. This condition, termed *crush syndrome,* inspired Trueta, a surgeon, and his associates to make investigations which have thrown light upon how the route taken by blood through the kidney may be altered in what is generally termed *shock.*

To understand this matter the student should refer back to Figure 24-20. This shows that the efferent vessels of the glomeruli in the outer part of the cortex (labeled 1 and 2) empty into the capillary bed of the cortical labyrinth, whereas those of the glomeruli near the border of the medulla, which Trueta terms the *juxtamedullary glomeruli* (labeled 3 and 4), empty almost entirely into the arteriolae rectae spuriae which supply the capillary beds of the medulla (the capillary beds of both the cortex and the medulla are, of course, continuous) (Fig. 24-20). Furthermore, it is to be observed that the juxtamedullary glomeruli are larger than those nearer the surface of the kidney, and, as

has been noted, the lumens of their efferent vessels may be larger than the lumens of their afferent vessels.

Trueta and his associates found that injuries, such as those occasioned when limbs are crushed, can reflexly cause spasm of certain blood vessels in the kidney. In general, the chief effect is on the peripheral two thirds of the interlobular arteries, which become constricted. Another factor that can have much the same effect as spasm of these vessels is a loss of plasma from the circulatory system, for the amount of fluid in the circulatory system is an important factor in keeping blood vessels open. Accordingly, it is easy to visualize that spasm in the smaller arterial vessels in the kidney and a lack of fluid in the circulatory system (as can occur in untreated shock) could result in the smaller arterioles becoming pinched off, and this could lead to impaired function in or even the death of kidney tissue. Since the greatest effect would be exerted on the smaller arterial vessels, the impairment of circulation would be greatest toward the periphery of the kidney. Conditions can arise, therefore, when it is possible for blood to continue to circulate through the juxtamedullary glomeruli while ceasing to circulate through the glomeruli in the outer part of the kidney. Under these conditions the whole outer part of the cortex becomes relatively pale and bloodless. Thus, all the blood that circulates through the kidney passes through the more deeply disposed glomeruli (the juxtamedullary ones), and since the efferent vessels of these empty almost entirely into the arteriolae rectae spuriae, the blood from them is conducted to the capillary beds of the medulla rather than to those of the cortex; thus the proximal and distal convoluted tubules would have no or little blood supply.

Lymphatics of the Kidney

The distribution of the lymphatics of the kidney has been investigated in recent years by Peirce and by Rawson. Peirce, using stab injections and other methods, could not satisfy himself that there were any lymphatics in the kidney other than those that accompany the blood vessels. He found that the periarterial plexuses were richer in lymphatics than the perivenous plexuses, and that the lymphatics of the plexuses could be traced from the renal artery and vein along the interlobar, arcuate and interlobular vessels to the capsule of the kidney, where they communicated with capsular lymphatics. However, they were not found to extend into the actual parenchyma of the cortex or the medulla from these vessels. He found valves in the larger lymphatics in the hilus of the kidney. Rawson, somewhat later, studied the lymphatics of a kidney which had been invaded by cancer cells, and he used their presence for mapping out the lymphatics. In general, Rawson found lymphatics in the same sites as those described by Peirce, but he also found evidence of some lymphatic capillaries which began beneath the epithelium of the tip of the medullary pyramid and extended toward the base of the medullary pyramid, where they emptied into the lymphatics associated with the arcuate vessels. However, none was found in the actual parenchyma of the cortex.

Postnatal Development and Growth of Nephrons

The growth of the kidney in early postnatal life has been investigated more extensively in the rat than in any other species; hence, most of the information given here relates to the studies made on this animal.

It has been shown by both Kittelson and Arataki that only about one third of the number of glomeruli that are to be found in the adult are present at birth. Glomeruli continue to be formed for about 100 days after birth, but the majority are formed in the first 3 to 4 weeks.

The first-formed glomeruli are in the region close to the medulla, and many of these undergo a physiologic atrophy (Hartroft) and disappear. However, in some instances their afferent and efferent vessels may remain and fuse to constitute a few arteriolae rectae verae. The oldest glomeruli, which are also the largest, are to be found near the arcuate vessels. At birth, the outer part of the cortex of the kidney is undifferentiated, and it is here that new nephrons are formed. After birth, renal corpuscles develop in the outer cortex of the kidney (the nephrogenic zone). The tubule of each new nephron then becomes connected to the duct system. The youngest nephrons are those situated in the outer cortex immediately beneath the capsule, and these are not fully differentiated for about 3 months after birth. The glomeruli of these nephrons are the smallest in the kidney. The renal corpuscle develops more or less as a unit and not by capillaries invaginating the blind end of a previously formed tubule. In the renal cortex a clump of cells is associated with the end of a developing tubule. Some of these cells become the parietal and visceral epithelial cells of Bowman's capsule, and others become endothelial cells. The capillaries so formed later connect with the vascular system.

The size of the kidneys in postnatal life is affected both by the diet and by hormones. High protein diets make the kidneys become larger. Injections of male sex hormone also make the kidneys of experimental animals become larger. The increase in size that occurs with high protein diets or male hormone treatment is brought about by nephrons increasing in size and not in number.

If one kidney is removed from adult animals, the remaining kidney becomes larger. The increase in size is due to the nephrons becoming larger and not more numerous. However, in individual nephrons there is an increase in the number of cells of which they are composed, and mitotic figures can be seen in the nephrons of the remaining kidney for a period following the removal of the other. The kidneys also become larger during pregnancy; this is termed a physiologic hypertrophy, and mitotic figures have been found in the nephrons as they enlarge in this condition.

The Ureter

The wall of the ureter has 3 coats: (1) a mucous membrane, (2) a muscular coat and (3) a fibroelastic adventitia.

Mucous Membrane. This consists of only 2 layers, an epithelial lining and a lamina propria. The epithelium is of the transitional type (Fig. 7-8) and is from 4 to 5 cells in thickness, except in the pelvis, where it is somewhat thinner. Transitional epithelium is described in detail in Chapter 7, and information is given there on the polyploidy that occurs in it. The lamina propria consists of fairly dense connective tissue, except in its deepest part, next to the muscular coat, where it is of a somewhat looser texture. Some elastic fibers are mixed with the abundant collagenic ones. Occasional lymphatic nodules are encountered in it.

The mucous membrane of the ureter, except in the pelvis, is thrown into longitudinal folds which give its lumen a stellate appearance in cross sections (Fig. 24-21). The combination of transitional epithelium (which can stretch without rupturing) and longitudinal folds makes it possible for the lumen of the ureter to become considerably expanded without the mucous membrane rupturing. This is an asset should concretions (kidney stones) form in the pelvis, as they do under various abnormal conditions. These are sometimes "passed" by way of the ureter, the bladder and the urethra.

Muscular Coat. In approximately the upper two thirds of the ureter the muscular coat consists of 2 layers: an inner one of longitudinally disposed smooth muscle fibers and an outer one of circularly disposed fibers (Fig. 24-21). It may be helpful to remember that this is the reverse of the arrangement seen in the intestine. Moreover, the layers of smooth muscle in the ureter are infiltrated by connective tissue from the lamina propria and adventitia; hence they are not

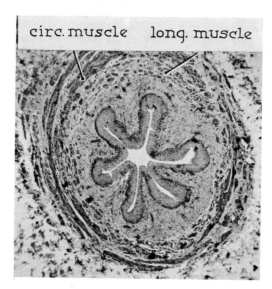

FIG. 24-21. Very low-power photomicrograph of a cross section of the ureter.

nearly so compact and distinct as those in the intestine. The amount of smooth muscle in the wall of the pelvis is less than that in the remainder of the ureter, except where the calyces are attached to the pyramids. At this site the circularly disposed fibers are prominent, and it could be assumed that if this muscle contracted, the papilla it surrounds would be squeezed. A sustained, pronounced contraction of this muscle conceivably could shut off the flow of urine from the papilla concerned. However, occasional and not so severe contractions conceivably could have a "milking" effect on a papilla and squeeze urine out of the ducts of Bellini into the calyx concerned. It is likely that some action of the latter type is of physiologic importance.

In approximately its lower third, a third coat of muscle fibers is present in the ureter. This forms the outermost layer of the muscular coat, and its fibers are longitudinally disposed.

The ureters pierce the bladder wall obliquely. This, together with little valvelike folds of bladder mucosa that guard their entrance into the bladder, prevents contractions of the bladder wall from forcing urine back up the ureters (the contraction of muscle fibers arranged in a thick sheet tends to close the lumen of a tube that passes through the sheet obliquely). As each ureter enters the bladder wall, it loses its circularly disposed fibers. However, its longitudinal fibers continue through the wall to the mucous membrane of the bladder, where they are attached. Urine does not drain from the kidney to the bladder because of

gravity as at first might be thought; this is convenient for astronauts traveling through weightless space. Peristaltic-like waves of contraction sweep down the muscle of the ureter and force urine into the bladder. The contraction of the longitudinal smooth muscle fibers in the part of the ureter that passes through the wall of the bladder helps open the lumen of that segment of the tube so as to permit urine to be delivered into the bladder.

Adventitia. This, the outermost coat of the ureter, consists of fibroelastic connective tissue. At its periphery it merges into adjacent areolar tissue, which, in turn, is connected to other structures.

The Urinary Bladder

The wall of the urinary bladder must accommodate itself to great changes occurring in the size of the cavity that it encloses because this cavity is very much larger when the bladder is distended with urine than when it has been emptied. It is relatively easy to understand how the muscularis could accommodate itself to these changes, and also how the more or less elastic lamina propria together with its lining of transitional epithelium could be thrown into some folds in a contracted bladder which would be ironed out as the bladder became distended with urine. But it is not so easy to understand how the transitional epithelium that lines the bladder becomes stretched as the bladder becomes distended and at the same time remains intact so that urine cannot leak through it. Furthermore, since transitional epithelium is not keratinized, it is difficult to understand why the surface epithelial cells exposed to the urine do not absorb urine as such or fluid from it. Various studies with the EM have contributed to increasing information on this subject.

Staehelin, Chlapowski and Bonneville have recently reviewed past work in this field and described an EM study which they made using a variety of technics to investigate primarily the surface epithelial cells. It should be mentioned in this connection the large surface cells of the epithelium in a contracted bladder are rounded and large (Fig. 7-8) but they become squamous when the bladder is distended. For a round cell to assume the form of a squamous cell requires that its cell membrane must stretch just as the rubber wall of a blown-up balloon must stretch if anyone happens to sit on it to make it squamous in shape. However, the surface cells of the bladder do not burst when they are stretched because their surrounding membranes can accommodate themselves to this change and still remain intact. In this connection it was found that the lamella of the cell membrane that faces the urine—and this lamella of the cell membrane will hereafter be termed the lumenal lamella—is made up of polygonal plaques which are much thicker than the inner cytoplasmic lamella of the cell membrane that lies beneath the plaques; indeed, the lumenal lamella in the region of a plaque is 80 Å thick, and the cytoplasmic lamella of the cell membrane underlying the site of a plaque is only around 10 Å in thickness. The plaques are composed of hexagonal particles oriented at right angles to the surface, and around 73 percent of the lumenal surface of the cell membranes of the surface cells is made up of plaques. Between adjacent plaques the cell membrane is smooth and not unusual in appearance. Next, they have shown the existence of cytoplasmic filaments as shown in Figure 24-22, F, which run in various directions with some of them having anchorage in the cytoplasmic membrane at the sites of plaques and possibly having anchorage in the plaques themselves.

It is believed that as the bladder becomes distended the lamellar layer of the cell membrane of a surface cell would become relatively flat (Fig. 24-22, a) and that undue stretching would be restrained by the cytoplasmic filaments (black lines in Fig. 24-22) which have anchorage in the membrane. Then when the bladder is contracted, the surface cells could accommodate themselves to assuming a more globular form because their lumenal cell membranes would become folded, with the bends occurring not in the plaques but at the sites of the normal cell membrane between the plaques; these latter sites would act more or less as hinges as is shown in Figure 24-22 (b). In other words, the lumenal cell membrane of the surface cells, on contraction of the bladder, would fold in an accordion-like fashion, as is shown in Figure 24-22.

The transitional epithelium rests on a lamina propria which is collagenic in character and has only a few elastic fibers in it. Its deepest layer is somewhat looser in texture and has more elastic fibers in it than are found in its more superficial part; this is sometimes termed the *submucosa layer* of the bladder. This extends up into such folds as form in the lining of the contracted organ. The muscular coat consists of 3 layers, but in sections these cannot be distinguished from one another to advantage. Their respective thicknesses vary in different parts of the bladder. In general, the middle coat is the most prominent one, and its fibers are mostly circularly disposed. Around the opening of the urethra, muscle fibers are usually aggregated to form an internal sphincter. The adventitia is fibroelastic in nature. Over part of the bladder it is

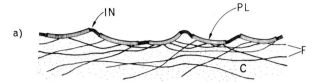

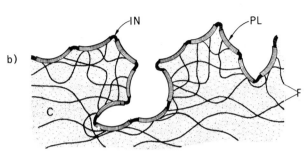

Fig. 24-22. A simplified diagram of the lumenal region of a surface cell of the urinary bladder epithelium, as it would be in a distended bladder (a) and a collapsed bladder (b). C, cytoplasm; F, cytoplasmic filaments; PL, the plaques; IN, interplaque regions. (From Staehelin, L. A., Chlapowski, F. J., and Bonneville, M. A.: J. Cell Biol., *53*:73, 1972)

covered with peritoneum. Over the remainder it blends into adjacent areolar tissue.

The Urethra

The urethra is a tube which extends from the bladder to an external orifice and so permits urine contained in the bladder to be evacuated from the body. In the male, the urethra courses through the male genital copulatory organ, the penis; hence the male urethra will be dealt with in Chapter 27 which deals with the male reproductive system. However, the urethra of the female serves no genital function but only a urinary one; hence its structure will be described here.

The female urethra is said to vary in length from 2 to 6 cm. There is some difference of opinion about its average length, different estimates ranging from about 3 cm. to about 4½ cm. It is a fairly straight muscular tube lined by mucous membrane. The musculature of its wall consists of 2 coats of smooth muscle fibers; those of the inner one are disposed longitudinally, and those of the outer coat, circularly. At its external orifice striated muscle fibers reinforce the smooth ones to form an external sphincter.

In cross section the lumen of the urethra is seen to be roughly crescentic. The mucous membrane is thrown into longitudinal folds. The epithelium of most of the urethra is stratified or pseudostratified columnar in type. However, transitional epithelium is present near the bladder and stratified squamous near the external orifice. The relatively thick connective tissue lamina propria, particularly in its deeper part, which is sometimes called the *submucosa,* is rich in elastic fibers and plexuses of veins; the latter are sufficiently extensive to give the deeper portions of the lamina propria a resemblance to erectile tissue.

In many sites the epithelium extends into the lamina propria to form little outpocketings. These little gland-like structures commonly contain mucous cells. In the aged, concretions may form in them. True glands, opening by fine ducts into the lumen of the urethra, have also been described as being present, particularly in its upper part.

Innervation of the Urinary System

Nerve fibers reach the kidney by way of the renal plexus. This is a network of nerve fibers that extends along the renal artery from the aorta to the kidney. The bodies of ganglion cells also may be present in the renal plexus; if so, they are to be regarded as out-lying cells of diffuse celiac and aortic ganglia. Most of the fibers in the renal plexus are those of the sympathetic division of the autonomic system and are derived from the cells of the celiac and the aortic ganglia. Parasympathetic fibers occur in the renal plexus in smaller numbers. These are derived from the vagus nerve, whose fibers, to reach the renal plexus, course through the celiac plexus without interruption.

The nerve fibers from the renal plexus follow the arteries into the substance of the kidney. Harman and Davies have described their distribution within the organ. They penetrate glomeruli to form extensive perivascular networks in these structures. They also supply the epithelium of the convoluted tubules, the transitional epithelium of the pelvis and the walls of the arteries and the veins.

Since transplanted kidneys, which are necessarily removed from a nerve supply, and kidneys left in situ but with the nerves that supply them cut, both function in a fairly normal fashion, it is obvious that the functions of the kidney are not fundamentally dependent on nervous mechanisms. However, nervous mechanisms control kidney function to some extent. It seems likely that most of the control is mediated by way of the sympathetic fibers that terminate in the blood vessels. The way in which this nervous regulation can operate to cause the blood to circulate chiefly through the juxtamedullary glomeruli, as in crush syndrome, has already been described. The part played by the parasympathetic, vagus-derived fibers in the kidney is obscure.

Afferent impulses travel over nerves in the renal plexus, for cutting the fibers of the plexus abolishes pain of renal origin.

Both sympathetic and parasympathetic fibers course along the ureter. But they do not seem to be particularly concerned with the normal peristaltic movements that sweep down the musculature of this tube, for the movements continue if these nerves are cut. Some of the nerves here carry afferent impulses.

The bladder is supplied by fibers from both the sympathetic and the parasympathetic divisions of the autonomic system. The parasympathetic fibers are derived from the sacral outflow. The terminal ganglia to which they lead are present in the bladder wall; hence, in sections of bladder the student may occasionally observe ganglion cells.

References and Other Reading

SOME GENERAL REFERENCES ON THE KIDNEY

Dalton, A. J., and Haguenau, F. (eds.): Ultrastructure of the Kidney. New York, Academic Press, 1967.

Oliver, J.: New directions in renal morphology: a method, its results and its future. Harvey Lect., *40:*102, 1944-45.

Rouiller, C., and Muller, A. F. (eds.): The Kidney: Morphology, Biochemistry, Physiology. vols. 1 and 2. New York, Academic Press, 1969.

Smith, H. W.: The Kidney—Structure and Function in Health and Disease. ed. 2. New York, Oxford Univ. Press, 1956.

———: Principles of Renal Physiology. New York, Oxford University Press, 1956.

Symposium: Histochemistry and the elucidation of kidney structure and function. J. Histochem., *3:*243, 1955.

SPECIAL REFERENCES ON THE GLOMERULUS

Books, M. H.: The secreting area of the glomerulus. J. Anat., *71:*91, 1936.

Boyer, C. C.: The vascular pattern of the renal glomerulus as revealed by plastic reconstruction from serial sections. Anat. Rec., *125:*433, 1956.

Elias, H.: The structure of the renal glomerulus. Anat. Rec., *127:*288, 1957.

Farquhar, M. G., and Palade, G. E.: Glomerular permeability. II. Ferritin transfer across the glomerular capillary wall in nephrotic rats. J. Exp. Med., *114:*699, 1961.

———: Functional evidence for the existence of a third cell type in the renal glomerulus. Phagocytosis of filtration residues by a distinctive "third" cell. J. Cell Biol., *13:*55, 1962.

Farquhar, M. G., Wissig, S. L., and Palade, G. E.: Glomerular permeability. I. Ferritin transfer across the normal glomerular capillary wall. J. Exp. Med., *113:*47, 1961.

Graham, R. C., and Karnovsky, M. J.: Glomerular permeability: ultrastructural cytochemical studies using peroxidases as protein tracers. J. Exp. Med., *124:*1123, 1966.

Hall, B. V.: Studies of normal glomerular structure by electron microscopy, Proc. Fifth Ann. Conf. Nephrotic Syndrome. p. 1. New York, National Nephrosis Foundation, 1953.

————: Further studies of the normal structure of the renal glomerulus, Proc. Sixth Ann. Conf. Nephrotic Syndrome. p. 1. New York, National Nephrosis Foundation, 1964.

Kirkman, H., and Stowell, R. E.: Renal filtration surface in the albino rat. Anat. Rec., *83:*373, 1942.

Lewis, O. J.: The vascular arrangement of the mammalian renal glomerulus as revealed by a study of its development. J. Anat., *92:*433, 1958.

Menefee, M. G., and Mueller, C. B.: Some morphological considerations of transport in the glomerulus. *In* Ultrastructure of the Kidney, 1967 (see General References). p. 73.

Michielsen, P., and Creemers, J.: The structure and function of the glomerular mesangium. *In* Ultrastructure of the Kidney, 1967 (see General References). p. 57.

Richards, A. N.: Urine formation in the amphibian kidney. Harvey Lect., *30:*93, 1934-35.

Suzuki, Y., Churg, J., Grishman, E., Mautner, W., and Dachs, S.: The mesangium of the renal glomerulus. Electron microscope studies of pathologic alterations. Am. J. Path., *43:*555, 1963.

Trump, B. F., and Benditt, E. P.: Electron microscopic studies of human renal disease. Observations on normal visceral glomerular epithelium and its modifications in disease. Lab. Invest., *11:*753, 1962.

Venkatachalam, M. A., Karnovsky, M. J., Fahimi, H. D., and Cotran, R. S.: An ultrastructural study of glomerular permeability using catalase and peroxidase as tracer proteins. J. Exp. Med., *132:*1153, 1970.

Vimtrup, B.: On the number, shape, structure and surface area of the glomeruli in the kidneys of man and mammals. Am. J. Anat., *41:*123, 1928.

Walker, F.: The origin, turnover and removal of glomerular basement membrane. J. Path., *110:*233, 1973.

Some References on the Vascular Pole and JG Cells

Bing, J., and Kazimierczak, J.: Renin content of different parts of the periglomerular circumferences. Acta Path. Microbiol. Scand., *50:*1, 1960.

Dunihue, F. W.: The effect of adrenal insufficiency and desoxycorticosterone acetate on the juxtaglomerular apparatus (abstr.). Anat. Rec., *103:*442, 1949.

Dunihue, F. W., and Robertson, Van B.: The effect of desoxycorticosterone acetate and of sodium on the juxtaglomerular apparatus. Endocrinology, *61:*293, 1957.

Garber, B. G., McCoy, F. W., Marks, B. H., and Hayes, E. R.: Factors that affect the granulation of the juxtaglomerular apparatus. Anat. Rec., *130:*303, 1958.

Goldblatt, H.: Experimental hypertension induced by renal ischemia. Harvey Lect., *33:*237, 1937-38.

Goormaghtigh, N.: Existence of an endocrine gland in the media of the renal arterioles. Proc. Soc. Exp. Biol. Med., *42:*688, 1939.

————: La fonction endocrine des arterioles renales. Louvain, Fonteyn, 1944.

————: Histological changes in the ischemic kidney with special reference to the juxtaglomerular apparatus. Am. J. Path., *16:*409, 1940.

————: Facts in favour of an endocrine function of the renal arterioles. J. Path. Bact., *57:*392, 1945.

Hartroft, P. M.: Juxtaglomerular cells of the American bullfrog as seen by light and electron microscopy. Fed. Proc., *25:*238, 1966.

————: The juxtaglomerular complex as an endocrine gland. *In* Bloodworth, J. B. (ed.): Endocrine Pathology. p. 641. Baltimore, Williams & Wilkins, 1968.

Hartroft, P. M., Bischoff, M. B., and Boucci, T. J.: Effects of chronic exposure to high altitudes on the JG complex and the adrenal cortex in dogs, rabbits and rats. Fed. Proc., *28:*1234, 1969.

Hartroft, P. M., and Edelman, R.: Renal juxtaglomerular cells in sodium deficiency. *In* Moyer, J. H., and Fuchs, M. (eds.): Edema. pp. 63-68. Philadelphia, W. B. Saunders, 1960.

Hartroft, P. M., and Hartroft, W. S.: The effects of dietary factors and administration of desoxycorticosterone acetate (DCA) on juxtaglomerular cells of the rat (abstr.). Anat. Rec., *112:*39, 1952.

————: Studies on renal juxtaglomerular cells. J. Exp. Med., *102:*205, 1955.

Hartroft, P. M., Newmark, L. N., and Pitcock, J. A.: Relationship of renal juxtaglomerular cells to sodium intake, adrenal cortex and hypertension. *In* Moyer, J. (ed.): Hypertension. pp. 24-31. Philadelphia, W. B. Saunders, 1959.

Hatt, Pierre-Yues: The juxtaglomerular apparatus. *In* Ultrastructure of the Kidney, 1967 (see General References). p. 101.

Marks, B. H., and Garber, B. G.: The juxtaglomerular apparatus as an extra adrenal site of ACTH action. Anat. Rec., *133:*306, 1959.

McManus, J. F. A.: Further observations on the glomerular root of the vertebrate kidney. Quart. J. Micr. Scn., *88:*39, 1947.

Pitcock, J. A., and Hartroft, P. M.: The juxtaglomerular cells in man and their relationship to the level of plasma sodium and to the zona glomerulosa of the adrenal cortex. Am. J. Path., *34:*863, 1958.

Pitcock, J. A., Hartroft, P. M., and Newmark, L. N.: Increased renal pressor activity (renin) in sodium deficient rats and correlation with juxtaglomerular cell granulation. Proc. Soc. Exp. Biol. Med., *100:*868, 1959.

Tobian, L., Janecek, J., and Tomboulian, A.: Correlation between granulation of juxtaglomerular cells and extractable renin in rats with experimental hypertension. Proc. Soc. Exp. Biol. Med., *100:*94, 1959.

Wilson, W.: A new staining method for demonstrating the granules of the juxtaglomerular complex. Anat. Rec., *112:*497, 1952.

Some References on the Tubular Parts of the Nephron, Including Fine Structure

Gottschalk, C., and Mylle, M.: Micropuncture study of the mammalian urinary concentrating mechanism: evidence for the countercurrent hypothesis. Am. J. Physiol., *196:*927, 1959.

Gottschalk, C. W.: Micropuncture studies of tubular function in the mammalian kidney. Physiologist, *4:*35, 1961.

Latta, H., Maunsbach, A. B., and Osvaldo, L.: The fine structure of renal tubules in cortex and medulla. *In* Ultrastructure of the Kidney, 1967 (see General References). p. 2.

Marshall, E. K., Jr.: A comparison of the function of the glomerular and aglomerular kidney. Am. J. Physiol., *94:*1, 1930.

Munkácsi, I., and Palkovits, M.: Study of the renal pyramid, loops of Henle, and percentage distribution of their thin segments in animals living in desert, semidesert and water-rich environments. Acta Biol. Hung., *17:*89, 1966.

Pease, D. C.: Electron microscopy of the tubular cells of the kidney cortex. Anat. Rec., *121:*723, 1955.

————: Fine structures of the kidney seen by electron microscopy. J. Histochem., *3:*295, 1955.

Pitts, R. F.: The Physiology of Body Fluids. New York, Year Book Medical Publishers, 1963.

Rhodin, J.: Correlation of ultrastructural organization and function in normal and experimentally changed proximal convoluted tubule cells of the mouse kidney. Karolinska Institutet, Stockholm, Aktiebolaget Godvil, 1954.

————: Anatomy of the kidney tubules. Int. Rev. Cytol., *7:*485, 1958.

————: An Atlas of Ultrastructure. Philadelphia, W. B. Saunders, 1963.

Richards, A. N., and Walker, A. M.: Methods of collecting fluid from known regions of the renal tubules of amphibia and perfusing the lumen of a single tubule. Am. J. Physiol., *118:*111, 1937.

Ruska, H., Moore, D. H., and Weinstock, J.: The base of the proximal convoluted tubule cells of rat kidney. J. Biophys. Biochem. Cytol., *3:*249, 1957.

Sjöstrand, F. S., and Rhodin, J.: The ultrastructure of the proximal convoluted tubules of the mouse kidney as revealed by high resolution electron microscopy. Exp. Cell Res., *4:*426, 1953.

Smith, H. W.: The fate of sodium and water in the renal tubules. Bull. N.Y. Acad. Med., *35:*293, 1959.

Wirz, H.: Introduction—Tubular transport mechanism with special reference to the hairpin countercurrent. *In* Duyff, J. W., *et al.* (eds.): XXII International Congress of Physiological Sciences, Symposium VII. vol. 1, p. 359. New York, Excerpta Medica Foundation, 1962.

Some References on the Renal Circulation

Barclay, A. E., Daniel, P., Franklin, J. K., Prichard, M. M. L., and Trueta, J.: Records and findings obtained during studies of the renal circulation in the rabbit, with special reference to vascular short-circuiting and functional cortical ischaemia. J. Physiol., *105:*27, 1946.

Baringer, J. R.: The dynamic anatomy of the microcirculation in the amphibian and mammalian kidney. Anat. Rec., *130:*266, 1958.

Bensley, R. D.: The Efferent vessels of the renal glomeruli of mammals as a mechanism for the control of glomerular activity and pressure. Am. J. Anat., *44:*141, 1929.

Bialestock, D.: The extra-glomerular arterial circulation of the renal tubules. Anat. Rec., *129:*53, 1957.

Daniel, P. M., Peabody, C. N., and Prichard, M. M. L.: Cortical ischaemia of the kidney with maintained blood flow through the medulla. Quart. J. Exp. Physiol., *37:*11, 1952.

————: Observations on the circulation through the cortex and the medulla of the kidney. Quart. J. Exp. Physiol., *36:*199, 1951.

Daniel, P. M., Prichard, M. M. L., and Ward-McQuaid, J. N.: The renal circulation in experimental hypertension. Brit. J. Surg., *42:*81, 1954.

Graves, F. T.: The anatomy of the intrarenal arteries and its application to segmental resection of the kidney. Brit. J. Surg., *42:*132, 1954.

————: The anatomy of the intrarenal arteries in health and disease. Brit. J. Surg., *43:*605, 1956.

Grollman, A., Muirhead, E. E., and Vanatta, J.: Role of kidney in pathogenesis of hypertension as determined by study of effects of bilateral nephrectomy and other experimental procedures on blood pressure of dog. Am. J. Physiol., *157:*21, 1949.

MacCallum, D. B.: The arterial blood supply of the mammalian kidney. Am. J. Anat., *38:*153, 1926.

————: The bearing of degenerating glomeruli on the problem of the vascular supply of the mammalian kidney. Am. J. Anat., *65:*69, 1939.

Machado, Simoes de Carvalho, A. A.: Contribuicao para o estudo da circulacao renal. Coimbra, Imprensa de Coimbra, 1954.

More, R. H., and Duff, G. L.: The renal arterial vasculature in man. Am. J. Path., *27:*95, 1950.

Morison, D. M.: A study of the renal circulation, with special reference to its finer distribution. Am. J. Anat., *37:*53, 1926.

Pease, D. C.: Electron microscopy of the vascular bed of the kidney cortex. Anat. Rec., *121:*701, 1955.

Sykes, D.: Some aspects of the blood supply of the human kidney. Symp. Zool. Soc. London, *11:*49, 1964.

————: The correlation between renal vascularization and lobulation of the kidney. Brit. J. Urol., *36:*549, 1964.

Trueta, J., Barclay, A. E., Daniel, P., Franklin, K. J., and Prichard, M. M. L.: Renal pathology in the light of recent neurovascular studies. Lancet, *2:*237, 1946.

————: Studies of the Renal Circulation. Oxford, Blackwell Scientific Publications, 1947.

Some References on the Connective Tissue, the Lymphatics and the Nerves of the Kidney and Other Parts of the Urinary System

Gruber, C. M.: The autonomic innervation of the genitourinary system. Physiol. Rev., *13:*497, 1933.

Harman, P. J., and Davies, H.: Intrinsic nerves in the kidney of the cat and the rat. Anat. Rec., *100:*671, 1948.

Kirkman, H.: The number and distribution of macrophages and fibroblasts in kidneys of albino rats with emphasis on twenty-five day males. Am. J. Anat., *73:*451, 1943.

Leeson, T. S.: An electron microscopic study of the postnatal development of the hamster kidney, with particular reference to intertubular tissue. Lab. Invest., *10:*466, 1961.

Peirce, E. C.: Renal lymphatics. Anat. Rec., *90:*315, 1944.

Rawson, A. J.: Distribution of the lymphatics of the human kidney as shown in a case of carcinomatous permeation. Arch. Path., *47:*283, 1949.

Some References on the Development and the Growth of the Kidney

Arataki, M.: On the postnatal growth of the kidney, with special reference to the number and size of the glomeruli. Am. J. Anat., *36:*399, 1926.

Clark, S. L., Jr.: Cellular differentiation in the kidneys of newborn mice studied with the electron microscope. J. Biophys. Biochem. Cytol., *3:*349, 1957.

Hartroft, W. S.: The vascular development of the kidney of the pig. Trans. Roy. Soc. Canada, Sec. V (Biol. Sci.), *35:*67, 1949.

Kittelson, J. A.: The postnatal growth of the kidney of the albino rat, with observations on an adult human kidney. Anat. Rec., *17:*385, 1917.

Kurtz, S. M.: The electron microscopy of the developing human renal glomerulus. Exp. Cell Res., *14:*355, 1958.

Leeson, T. S.: Electron microscopy of the developing kidney: an investigation into the fine structure of the mesonephros and metanephros of the rabbit. J. Anat., *94:*100, 1960.

Leeson, T. S., and Baxter, J. S.: The correlation of structure and function in the mesonephros and metanephros of the rabbit. J. Anat., *91:*383, 1957.

MacDonald, M. S., and Emery, J. L.: The late intrauterine and postnatal development of human renal glomeruli. J. Anat., *93:*331, 1959.

Sulkin, N. N.: Cytologic study of the remaining kidney following unilateral nephrectomy in the rat. Anat. Rec., *105:*95, 1949.

Urinary Bladder

Staehelin, A., Chlapowski, F. J., and Bonneville, M. A.: Lumenal plasma membrane of the urinary bladder. I. Three-dimensional reconstruction from freeze-etch images. J. Cell Biol., *53:*73, 1972.

25 The Endocrine System

Introduction

Development and General Structure. As explained in Chapter 6, some glands lose their connection with the epithelial surface from which they develop and become islands of epithelium surrounded by connective tissue (Fig. 6-1). Since such glands possess no ducts, they are termed *ductless glands;* and since they secrete into the substance of the body rather than through a duct onto a surface, they are called *endocrine glands* or glands of *internal secretion.* To secrete internally, the cells of endocrine glands must abut directly on blood capillaries. This leads to endocrine glands, in general, having a very simple microscopic structure; they consist of either cords or small solid or hollow clumps of cells interspersed between capillaries and supported by delicate connective tissue (Fig. 6-1).

Although a gland that secretes any useful product into the blood, as, for example, the liver does by secreting glucose into the blood, can be termed an endocrine gland, the term is commonly associated with those glands that secrete general hormones.

The Nature of Hormones. Hormones are chemical substances so named because *hormao* means "I arouse to activity." Different hormones affect different kinds of cells and their effects are also different but, in general, they are all of the "arousing to activity" sort. The cellular activity and, to a large extent, the normal microscopic structure of many parts of the body are dependent on these parts of the body being supplied more or less continuously by way of the bloodstream with small amounts of certain hormones. Only minute quantities are necessary in the bloodstream for hormones to exert their normal effects.

How Hormones Exert Their Effects. This subject is under intensive investigation at the level of molecular biology. It should be said here, however, that hormones include a variety of types of chemical compounds. Some (for example) are peptides, some proteins, some glycoproteins, some steroids (steroids will be described when we come to steroid hormones), some are catecholamines (to be described later) and still others represent less familiar types of chemical substances. Next, many are specific in that they act only on certain types of cells. One way this is conceived of as occurring is through the cells that are sensitive to a particular hormone having special receptors on their cell membrane by which they "recognize" the presence of the hormone and through which a series of reactions are instituted within the cell in response to the hormone. As was described in Chapter 6, cyclic AMP is involved in many of the reactions that are instituted by hormones meeting their special receptors. In at least some instances it is believed that the reactions instituted by a hormone on a specific cell are such that as a result certain genes may be turned on or off so as to bring about the response the hormone is known to cause in the cell that it affects. Some further comment will be made on the effects of certain of the hormones as we take them up in turn.

A Very Brief Survey of the Role Played by Hormones in the Body. The hormones produced by some endocrine glands are essential to life. Others are responsible for growth and for the development of such physical differences as exist between the male and the female and for most other male and female characteristics. Hormones play a very important role in the intermediate metabolism of carbohydrates, proteins and fats and in maintaining the mineral and water balance of the body. One hormone controls the metabolic rate of cells in general. In addition to affecting the growth and the form of the individual, hormones affect the temperament, the feelings and the emotions. Experimentally, they may be used to convert a male animal into a motherly creature solicitous for the young. Indeed, the former male, given the proper hormones, will feed the young at its breasts, for the development of the breasts and their capacity to produce milk are also due to hormones. It seems possible that a good many of the physical and emotional differences between people have their bases in people inheriting different types of endocrine constitutions. The particular effects of the different hormones will be described as each endocrine gland is described.

Diseases Caused by Hypofunction and Hyperfunction. Since there are many hormones, there is a large group of diseases that are caused by different endocrine glands secreting either too little or too much of the hormone or one of the hormones they produce. The study and the treatment of these constitute much of the subject matter of the branch of medicine termed *endocrinology.*

Development of Knowledge About Endocrine Glands and Hormones. Details will often be given as we discuss individual glands. But, in general, progress depended on certain observations being made and procedures performed, roughly, but not always exactly, in the order that follows.

(1) Observing at autopsy that some clinical syndrome (some particular group of signs and symptoms) observed during life was associated with a diseased state of one of the organs we now know to be endocrine glands.

(2) Development of surgical technics which made it possible to remove a gland from an experimental animal and see what happened.

(3) Noticing that the removal of a gland from an animal simulated the state of affairs seen in people who when they died revealed some lesion that had impaired, or destroyed, the function of that gland.

(4) Development of the concept of there being such a thing as an internal secretion on which the body is dependent in some particular way.

(5) The preparation of an extract of a gland and showing that it would on being injected into an animal restore the health of the animal from which that gland had been removed.

(6) Showing that administering excessive amounts of the extract would simulate a condition sometimes seen in people who when they died showed enlargement of a gland or a tumor of that gland.

(7) With improvements in biochemical methods, isolating the active principle or principles in pure form from extracts of a gland.

(8) Determining the chemical structure of the hormone.

(9) Synthesizing the hormone.

(10) Trying to determine how it exerts its effects at the level of the cell it affects.

The latter steps have not been achieved as yet for every hormone. New hormones are still being found. Perhaps the most important relatively recent development in endocrinology has been the increasing elucidation of how the activities of the hormone-secreting cells of the anterior lobe of the pituitary gland are controlled by neurohormones which reach the anterior lobe by way of the bloodstream from the hypothalamus.

This subject will be outlined briefly after we consider the development of the pituitary gland—for, as we shall see, the two subjects are related—and then it will be dealt with in more detail later.

The endocrine glands listed below will be considered in this chapter. These plus the ovary of the female and the testis of the male (to be considered in the next two chapters) constitute what might be termed the classic endocrine glands. The pineal body or gland will also be considered in the present chapter although its endocrine status in man is perhaps open to question. (Hormones, however, are also made in the body by cells other than those of the classic endocrine glands. The placenta of pregnancy is, in the human female, a veritable hormone factory. Hormones are made by cells in the digestive tract, as was described in the chapters dealing with the digestive system. Perhaps the JG cells, described in the previous chapter, should be thought of as making a hormone or hormones. Then there are local as well as general hormones.) In this chapter we shall consider the following endocrine glands:

(1) The pituitary gland and hypothalamus
(2) The thyroid gland
(3) The parathyroid glands
(4) The adrenal glands
(5) The islets of Langerhans of the pancreas.

The Pituitary Gland or Body (Hypophysis Cerebri)

If there is such a thing as a master endocrine gland, it is the pituitary gland. It is of enormous importance.

Some Gross Features. The pituitary gland is ovoid. It measures about 1.5 cm. in the transverse plane and about 1 cm. in the sagittal plane and is from 0.5 to 0.75 cm. or more thick. It becomes larger during pregnancy. It lies immediately below the base of the brain, to which it is attached by the pituitary stalk (Fig. 25-1). It rests in a depression in a bony prominence on the upper surface of the sphenoid bone. This bony prominence is shaped something like a Turkish saddle with a high back and a high front, and for this reason it is termed the *sella turcica.* The pituitary gland sits, as it were, in the saddle and so has bony protection in front, below and behind. The dura mater dips down to line the seat of the saddle and so envelop the pituitary gland. Furthermore, a shelf of dura mater, the diaphragma sellae, extends over most of the top of the gland to complete its enclosure (Fig. 25-1, DS). The degree of protection that it is afforded is in relation to its importance.

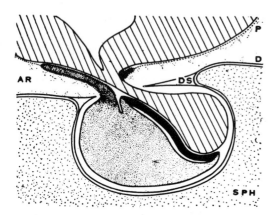

FIG. 25-1. Diagram of a sagittal section of the hypophysis cerebri, showing relation of the pars tuberalis to the meninges. *Lines,* brain floor and pars nervosa; *fine stipple,* pars anterior; *coarse stipple,* pars tuberalis; *solid black,* pars intermedia; SPH, sphenoid bone; P, pia mater; D, dura mater; DS, diaphragma sellae; AR, arachnoid spaces. (Atwell, W. J.: Am. J. Anat., *37*:174)

The Four Anatomical Parts of the Gland. In a sagittal section the pituitary gland of many animals can be seen to be separated into an anterior and a posterior lobe by a cleft that runs downward and posteriorly from near the attachment of the stalk (Fig. 25-1). Such a cleft may be seen in the pituitary gland of a young child, but in the human adult it is replaced by a row of follicles. There are four parts of the gland, as follows: (1) The main body of the gland anterior to the cleft or row of follicles is termed its *pars anterior* (Fig. 25-1, *fine stipple*). (2) A projection from this, the *pars tuberalis* (Fig. 25-1, *coarse stipple*) extends up along the anterior and lateral aspects of the pituitary stalk. (3) A rather narrow band of glandular tissue disposed along the posterior border of the cleft or row of vesicles comprises the *pars intermedia* (Fig. 25-1, *solid black*). (4) The remainder of the gland (all that is posterior to the narrow cellular band that makes up the pars intermedia) is called its *pars posterior* or *pars nervosa* (Fig. 25-1, *lined*). The pars nervosa is not so wide as the pars anterior and more or less fits into a concavity on the posterior aspect of the pars anterior but is separated from it, of course, by the pars intermedia.

Development. The pars anterior, the pars tuberalis and the pars intermedia all have a microscopic structure fairly typical of endocrine glands. However, the pars nervosa does not; it resembles nervous rather than glandular tissue (Fig. 25-13, *right*). Its origin provides the reason. It develops as a downgrowth from the base of the brain. The other parts of the gland

develop from an epithelial membrane, as do endocrine glands in general. We shall elaborate:

The anterior part of the mouth results from the inward bulging of ectoderm to form the oral fossa. Very early in development, before the bones of the skull have formed, the ectodermal lining of the roof of the oral fossa is in very close contact with the floor of the developing brain (which at this stage has a tubular form), and indeed the ectoderm of the roof of the oral fossa soon becomes adherent to the lower surface of the developing brain. This connection does not break as mesenchyme proliferates and gradually separates the developing brain from the developing mouth. As a consequence, the gradual separation of the brain and the mouth causes both the lining of the oral cavity and the floor of the brain to be drawn out into funnel-shaped structures with their tips in contact. The funnel-shaped extension of the roof of the oral fossa that points toward the brain is called *Rathke's pouch*. By the end of the second month of development this pouch breaks away from the oral ectoderm and thereupon becomes a hollow island of epithelium surrounded by mesenchyme except at its uppermost part, where a

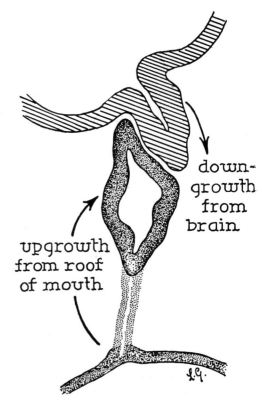

FIG. 25-2. Diagram illustrating the development of the pituitary gland from its two main sources.

peninsula is attached to the downward extension of the floor of the brain (Fig. 25-2). The main body of the hollow island of epithelium becomes more or less flattened around the anterior surface of the downgrowth of the brain. The cells of the anterior wall of the hollow epithelial island proliferate so that its anterior walls become greatly thickened. This becomes the pars anterior of the pituitary gland, and an upward extension of it becomes the pars tuberalis. The posterior wall of the island becomes the pars intermedia. The central cavity of the epithelial island between the pars anterior and the pars intermedia becomes flattened to form the cleft previously described, and the downward extension from the floor of the brain becomes the pars nervosa of the gland.

A residuum of cells of a character similar to those of the pars anterior may be present in the pharynx at the site from which the anterior lobe develops (Fig. 25-2). If so, they are said to constitute the *pharyngeal hypophysis.*

The part of the pituitary gland that develops from the epithelium of the pharynx (pars anterior, intermedia and tuberalis) is often referred to as the *adenohypophysis,* and the part that develops from the brain as the *neurohypophysis.*

THE HYPOTHALAMUS AND ITS RELATION TO PITUITARY GLAND FUNCTION

The possibility of there being some significance in the facts that the anterior lobe of the pituitary gland develops from an epithelial membrane as do other endocrine glands but the posterior pituitary develops as part of the nervous system, and that the two parts remain in juxtaposition throughout life intrigued many scientists throughout the years. The reason for this anatomical arrangement has only become apparent in the relatively recent past. It had previously become known, as the anterior lobe was studied, that it produced several important hormones—for example, the hormone that is required for the growth of the body and also the one required for lactation in females. It was also found to produce, as will presently be described in detail, what are called trophic hormones that control the functions of the thyroid gland, the cortex of the adrenal gland and the sex glands. Indeed its central role in endocrinology often inspired musically inclined lecturers to refer to the anterior pituitary gland as the conductor of the endocrine orchestra.

In recent years, however, this expression has fallen into disuse because it has become apparent that all this time the real conductor of the endocrine orchestra was, as it were, hiding in the wings—in the hypothalamus.

Many observations had to be made before this was established, and, for purposes of perspective, some of these will here be mentioned because they show why it is important that the pituitary gland should have a dual origin, from epithelium and nervous tissue respectively, and why the anterior lobe should occupy the position that it does.

It was known for a long time that two hormones termed oxytocin and vasopressin (to be described later) could be extracted from the posterior lobe of the pituitary gland and it was at first assumed that this is where they were made. However, in due course it was shown that these two hormones were produced in the cell bodies of neurons that were located in the hypothalamus as shown in Figure 25-16 and that the reason for their presence in the posterior lobe of the pituitary was that axons from the bodies of these nerve cells passed down the pituitary stalk to reach the posterior lobe where they ended in association with capillaries into which they elaborated the hormones that were made in their cell bodies. Since the hormones sometimes accumulated near the endings of the axons, the hormones could, of course, be extracted from the posterior lobe. As a result of these findings it became obvious that nerve cells could produce what were called *neurosecretions* and that these could be delivered into the bloodstream and act as hormones in various sites to which they were carried.

In the meantime some findings were made about the anterior pituitary that were puzzling. It was found, for example, that if it was transplanted to some other site it did not function properly. It was found, however, that if it was removed and then placed back in its normal environment it would function. It seemed as if it had to be close to the nervous part of the pituitary if it was to operate properly. One thought that was explored was that its cells must be innervated by nerve fibers for it to work properly. But no nerve fibers could be found to extend into it from the nervous tissue that could explain how its hormone-producing cells were controlled. During this time it was pointed out, as will be noted in more detail later, that the blood that coursed through the wide capillaries of the anterior lobe had already passed through capillary tufts in nervous tissue (Fig. 25-14). It was then found that there were nerve cell bodies in the hypothalamus (not the same ones that make the posterior lobe hormones but others not far away) that had short axons and that they made neurosecretions also and that these flowed down their short axons that ended on the capillaries that drained into the capillaries of the anterior lobe. These neurosecretions that reached the anterior lobe by way of the bloodstream were found to be the hor-

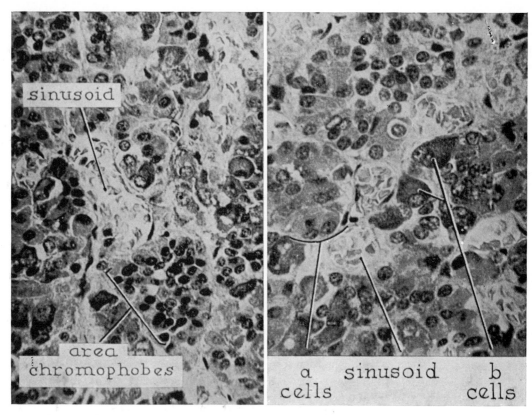

Fig. 25-3. Two high-power photomicrographs of an H and E section of the anterior lobe of the hypophysis. (*Left*) An area of chromophobes, with their nuclei close together. A sinusoid and some chromophils may be seen also. (*Right*) Acidophils, basophils and sinusoids (a, acidophils, b, basophils).

mones that controlled the secretory activities of the various cells of the anterior lobe. These neurohormones were thus called *hormone-releasing factors* because they controlled the release of hormones from the cells of the anterior lobe. With this introductory information about the role of the hypothalamus we shall now comment on the hormones produced by the anterior lobe and the cells that produce them, after which we shall discuss the hormone-releasing factors further.

The Anterior Lobe of the Pituitary (Pars Distalis)

Microscopic Structure. In an H and E section viewed with the LM the anterior lobe is seen to be composed of thick branching cords of cells (Fig. 25-3). Between these there are capillaries that are wide enough to have often been called sinusoids; they are so-labeled in Figure 25-3. With the EM it can be shown that the endothelial walls of the capillaries are surrounded by a basement membrane (Fig. 25-6) and that

between the borders of the epithelial cells of the cords and the basement membranes of capillaries there is at least a potential pericapillary space which presumably contains a little tissue fluid. The secretion of the epithelial cells passes through this space, the basement membrane and the endothelial walls of capillaries to enter the bloodstream.

Classifications of Cells of the Anterior Lobe

There are at least six and possibly seven different hormones produced by the cells of the anterior lobe. The first question that had to be solved as to their respective origins was whether or not all the cells of the anterior lobe were hormone producers or whether some served some other purpose. Hence, the first step made in classifying the cells was to divide them into two types. The cytoplasm of one kind of cell was seen to be relatively abundant and to have an affinity for some, but not necessarily the same, kind of stain so cells of this kind were called *chromophils* because their cytoplasm "liked" color, and the cells whose cytoplasm did not stain were called *chromophobes* because they "disliked" color. The impression was gained that the chromophils were the cells that secreted hormones and the chromophobes did not. It was proposed, however, that chromophobes had the ability to become chromophils and it was also suggested that chromophils could revert back to being chromophobes. In other words the view arose that chromophobes and chromophils were the same kind of cells but in different states of functional activity. This view received support from EM studies.

The cells classed as chromophobes with the LM are considerably smaller than chromophils. Indeed the easiest way for a student to identify in an H and E section the cells classed in the past as chromophobes is to look for a group of cells within a cord in which the nuclei are close together—which means, of course, that the cytoplasm of such cells is relatively small in amount (Fig. 25-3, *area chromophobes*).

Acidophils and Basophils. The first way that the chromophils were classified depended on whether the granules they contained had an affinity for basic stains or for acid stains. Hence the chromophils were divided into two types, basophils and acidophils; this terminology is still used to some extent. The next problem that was suggested was to see if acidophils and basophils made different kinds of hormones. The eventual problem was to try to find out if each hormone made by the anterior lobe was made by a separate kind of cell which could be identified histologically. Tracing different hormones to different cell types was first attempted by utilizing a great many different staining methods. While much success was obtained, this method led to a confusing nomenclature which was partly due to the finding that the same staining methods did not produce the same results in different species. Two further methods have subsequently been employed with considerable success in distinguishing the different kinds of chromophils; these are, first, electron microscopy and secondly, immunofluorescence technics. The latter type of technic was described in Chapter 13; in this instance antibodies are prepared from the plasma of animals injected with a particular pituitary hormone and the antibody is then conjugated with a fluorescent dye; when sections of the anterior pituitary are flooded with the fluorescent antibody, it attaches to the type of cell that contains the hormone that was used as the antigen to induce the antibody, and hence the type of cell that makes this hormone can be identified. As a result of studies with stains, with the EM and with fluorescent antibodies it is now generally conceded that each hormone, with perhaps

one exception to be mentioned later, is made by a special and separate type of cell.

Development of Knowledge About the Hormones Produced in the Anterior Lobe

Learning about the hormones produced by the anterior lobe of the pituitary was much more difficult than learning about the hormone or hormones produced by other endocrine glands, for several reasons. First, because of its location, it was much more difficult to surgically remove the pituitary gland than it was to remove any of the other endocrine glands from an experimental animal to learn what effects were suffered by the animal from a loss of the hormone it produced. It took time to develop technics which made it possible to perform hypophysectomies fairly readily on animals such as rats so that the effects of a loss of anterior lobe hormones could be precisely determined. Furthermore, the fact that the anterior lobe produced so many hormones resulted at first in the extracts made from anterior lobes of the pituitaries of animals being of a shotgun variety—they contained so many different hormones it took a great deal of time before pure extracts could be obtained of each of these hormones so that the specific effects of each could be ascertained.

When it became obvious that the anterior lobe produced and secreted several different hormones another problem became obvious; this related to the particular cells in the anterior lobe that produced them. At present it is conceded that there are seven different hormones made by cells of the pars distalis. It seems also that these are produced by at least six different cell types. However, some of the cell types are not absolutely specific, for it seems there are some examples of one fairly specific cell type being able to make not only its specific hormone but also at least a little of some closely related hormone. The hormones produced by the pars distalis are:

Growth Hormone (GH) also called Somatotrophin (STH)

The Lactogenic Hormone (also called Prolactin or Mammotrophin)

Thyrotrophin (TSH)

The Follicle-Stimulating Hormone (FSH)

The Luteinizing Hormone (LH)

Adrenocorticotrophin (ACTH) also called Corticotrophin

The Melanocyte-Stimulating Hormone (MSH)

These will be discussed briefly in turn before we attempt to attribute their origin to specific cell types.

Growth Hormone (GH). (Somatotrophin—STH). A young animal stops growing after its pituitary gland is removed and thereafter remains a dwarf unless ex-

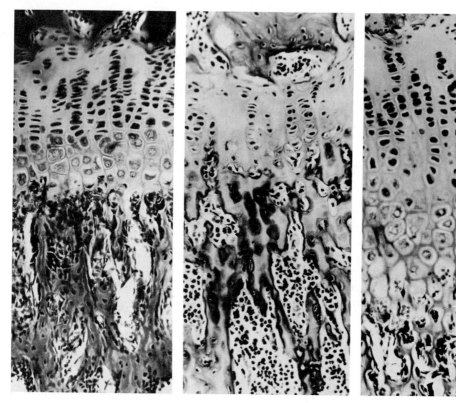

FIG. 25-4. (*Left*) Low-power photomicrograph of a longitudinal section of a metaphysis of the tibia of a rat nearing full growth. (*Center*) A similar photomicrograph of a metaphysis of a rat of the same age that received large injections of female sex hormone; the sex hormone suppressed the secretion of the growth hormone in the animal concerned. Observe that the epiphyseal disk is thinner, and that it lacks a zone of maturing cells. (*Right*) A similar photomicrograph of a metaphysis of the tibia of a rat of the same age as the other two but which received injections of anterior pituitary extract containing growth hormone. Observe that the epiphyseal disk is thicker than at the left. High-power inspection shows many mitotic figures in the disk. (From experiments in collaboration with Dr. W. Harris)

tracts of the pars anterior are given to it. The most striking cessation of growth is observed in the cartilage cells of the epiphyseal disks of the long bones. When the young cells in the zone of proliferation stop dividing, no new cells are produced to mature and so add to the thickness of the disk. Since calcification does not cease, the zone of calcification continues to advance into the zone of maturation, and as a result the zone of maturing cells becomes greatly thinned. (Compare *left,* which is normal, with *center* in Figure 25-4.) Since this zone is an important factor in the thickness of the disk, a reduction in the thickness of this zone makes the disk, as a whole, thinner.

In a normal person, either the secretion of growth hormone decreases somewhat and/or that which is secreted becomes less effective in the face of other developments at a certain time of life, and at that time the individual stops growing. The cells of certain rare tumors that may develop in the anterior lobe keep on secreting beyond the time when the cells of a normal pars anterior would stop secreting enough hormone to cause more growth. A person so afflicted keeps on growing; the condition is termed giantism.

If growth-hormone-producing tumors develop after the epiphyseal disks of the long bones have become replaced by bone—that is, after normal growth is over —or if growth hormone is given to a normal animal after its growth is over, no further growth in stature occurs. However, although cartilage would seem to be the primary target for the growth-stimulating effect of growth hormone, some growth of bone can still be stimulated because the bones, particularly those of the hands and feet, tend to become thicker, and there is a great overgrowth of the mandible and a lesser growth of certain other bones in the face. Other tissues (e.g., the skin) are affected as well; the condition as a whole is termed *acromegaly* (*akron*, extremity, *megas*, large) because the growth of the bones in the head, the hands and the feet makes these extremities large.

The epiphyseal disks of some laboratory animals are unusual in that they do not ordinarily become replaced by bone when their normal growth is over. For example, the epiphyseal disks persist for a long time in the female rat; hence, if female rats which have stopped growing (these are called plateaued rats because their growth curve has reached a plateau) are given growth hormone preparations, they will begin to grow again (Fig. 25-4, compare *left* and *right*). Therefore plateaued rats can be used for determining whether any given preparation contains growth hormone, but they are not as good for assaying growth hormone as hypophysectomized rats. They are, however, much easier to obtain. It has also been shown that growth hormone causes a rapid uptake of radioactive sulfur in cartilage.

Growth hormone prepared from the pituitary glands of cattle and pigs produces growth and other metabolic effects in laboratory animals, but it is virtually ineffective in man and monkeys. It has now been shown that growth hormone prepared from pituitary glands of monkeys and from human pituitary glands obtained at autopsy is effective metabolically in man and monkeys.

For information on the metabolic effects of growth hormone, textbooks on endocrinology should be consulted. It should be mentioned, however, that growth in fetal life, and for a brief period after birth, is not dependent to any great extent on the hormone.

Lactogenic Hormone (Prolactin). During pregnancy several hormones are required to cause the mammary glands of the female to grow and develop greatly as will be described in the next chapter. Hence, when a baby is born, the mammary glands are large enough to supply it with an adequate amount of milk. However, a particular stimulus is required for the glands to begin secreting milk and to continue performing this function. This stimulus is provided by a hormone called the *lactogenic hormone,* or *prolactin,* which is made by the pars anterior of the pituitary gland by cells that are believed to secrete large amounts of it at the termination of pregnancy. Thereafter they continue to secrete this hormone in quantities as long as the offspring is fed at the breast. Lesser amounts are secreted during pregnancy; this probably assists in causing the breasts to develop, and part of this is derived from the placenta.

The lactogenic hormone has been prepared in crystalline form by White and his associates. In addition to stimulating milk secretion, it arouses a maternal attitude in the individual exposed to its action; it will even do this if it is injected into males. It induces broodiness in hens.

In fowl, where the young are fed in part with the epithelial debris that desquamates from the lining of the crop gland of the mother, administration of the lactogenic hormone has been found to increase greatly the rate of epithelial proliferation of the thick lining epithelium of the gland. Indeed, the effect of the lactogenic hormone on the crop gland of the pigeon constitutes one biologic method by which this hormone, which causes milk secretion in mammals, may be assayed.

The lactogenic hormone will be discussed further in the next chapter in connection with the mammary gland.

Trophic Hormones. In addition to growth hormone and lactogenic hormone, the pars anterior secretes other hormones, each of which stimulates the growth and function of some one particular endocrine gland; for this reason they are termed *trophic* (*trophe,* to nourish) hormones. (Some authors substitute *tropic* for *trophic,* and the student who encounters these different spellings of the word may wonder which is correct. This matter was the subject of an article and several subsequent letters in *Science* in 1963. In the opinion of the author, *trophic* clearly vanquished *tropic*.)

Four trophic hormones have been identified by their effects, and are named according to the particular gland that they affect: (1) thyrotrophin (TSH for thyroid-stimulating hormone), which affects the thyroid gland; (2) adrenocorticotrophin (ACTH), also called corticotrophin, which affects the cortex of the suprarenal (adrenal) glands; and (3) and (4) two gonadotrophins, the follicle-stimulating hormone (FSH) and the luteinizing hormone (LH). Both of the gonadotrophins are produced in females and also in males, and discussion of their actions on the respective gonads of the two sexes will be postponed to the next two chapters. The endocrine gland that is affected by any particular trophic hormone is referred to as its target gland. Thus the thyroid gland is the target gland for TSH (the thyrotrophic hormone).

In order to describe how trophic hormones control the growth and secretory activities of the cells of their respective target glands, and how the concentration of the hormones of the target glands control the secretory activities of the respective cells of the pars distalis that secrete trophic hormones, we must explain what is termed feedback inhibition.

A very simple type of feedback inhibitory mechanism that operates to control the secretion of an endocrine gland was described in Chapter 7 where it was pointed out that the level of calcium ions in the blood controls the secretory activity of the cells of the parathyroid gland. If there is too little calcium in the blood the cells of the parathyroid gland secrete more hormone and this acts to raise the blood calcium level. If there is too much calcium in the blood the activity of the parathyroid gland tends to be suppressed (feedback inhibition).

With regard to at least some of the trophic hormones, the secretory activity of the cells that secrete them is suppressed if the amount of the hormone of the target gland with which they are concerned rises above its normal level in the blood. Likewise, if there is not enough of the target hormone in the blood the cells that produce the trophic hormone that stimulates that target gland secrete more trophic hormone. For example, the secretion of female sex hormone by the ovaries of women decreases very substantially after women reach the menopause. The cells of the anterior pituitary that secrete the trophic hormone that stimulates female sex hormone secretion in the ovary immediately notice this and secrete more trophic hormone. They do this so actively that there is so much of this trophic hormone in the blood that it escapes into the urine. Hence, if one injects some urine from an older woman into an immature female mouse it will cause the mouse to prematurely produce female sex hormone.

It was at first thought that the interaction between target hormone and the cells that make the trophic hormone concerned was direct. But with the new knowledge of the existence and function of hormone-releasing factors from the hypothalamus it appears that the negative feedback mechanisms may act via the hypothalamus or at least in cooperation with it. In other words, it may be that too much of a hormone of a target gland decreases the release of the hormone-releasing factor that controls the secretion of the trophic hormone concerned. However, the situation is complicated, because feedback mechanisms are not always negative and also some releasing factors are inhibitory instead of stimulatory. Furthermore, the secretion of releasing factors is in part controlled by nerve pathways that affect the hypothalamus. For these and other reasons the subject dealing with the control of the secretory activity of the cells of the anterior lobe that produce trophic hormones is not one that can be dealt with here in more than a very general way.

The Melanocyte-Stimulating Hormone (MSH). Whether this should be classed as an anterior lobe hormone is doubtful. In certain species (fish and amphibia) it is produced in the pars intermedia. But in man the pars intermedia is not very well developed and it has been suggested that in man the cells of the pars intermedia that produce MSH have migrated into the pars anterior.

The action of MSH in causing the dispersion of melanin pigment in fish was described in Chapter 5 in connection with microtubules. In man MSH has been shown to stimulate pigment formation and its dispersion in melanocytes. Molecules of MSH and ACTH contain some similar amino acid sequences and it seems probable that both hormones are made by the same cell type in man. It has been established that both ACTH and MSH can cause increased pigmentation in man, but as yet the respective roles of these two hormones in patients with increased pigmentation is not clearly established.

Having named and described some effects of the anterior lobe hormones, we shall now turn our attention to the cells that produce them.

How Different Hormones Were Traced to Different Cells by Light Microscopy

As already noted, with ordinary stains two types of chromophils can be distinguished, acidophils (sometimes termed alpha cells as in Fig. 25-3, *right*) and basophils (sometimes termed beta cells as in Fig. 25-3, *right*). An early development in tracing a particular hormone to a particular cell depended on the fact that tumors of acidophils occasionally develop in the pituitary and people who are found to have had such tumors at autopsy have undergone certain physical changes which indicated the action of excessive amounts of a particular hormone as follows:

After it became known that giantism or acromegaly was due to the anterior pituitary gland secreting extra growth hormone, and that this was often due to a tumor having begun to grow in that gland, the anterior pituitary glands of those who had been afflicted in this way were studied histologically and found to usually reveal some overgrowth of acidophils. This finding, of course, strongly indicated that acidophils secrete growth hormone.

Next, acromegaly in women is occasionally associated with persistent lactation; this is termed galactorrhea (*galactos,* milk, *rhoia,* flow), which may or may not be related to a previous pregnancy; this suggested that the cells producing growth hormone may also produce lactogenic hormone. Furthermore, the pituitary glands of women during the later stages of pregnancy and in the several weeks following childbirth contain increased numbers of lightly granulated acidophils. These were originally termed pregnancy cells by Erdheim.

Types of Acidophils. The question then arose whether the same acidophils secrete both growth and lactogenic hormones, or whether there are normally separate types of acidophils to secrete the two different hormones, and the reason for two hormones being secreted by acidophil tumors was that differentiation into both types may occur in tumors. The matter has been investigated by different staining methods. It was found in due course that a combination of erythrosin and orange G would distinguish between the two cell types clearly. With this combination of stains, the granules of the cells that produce prolactin stain with the erythrosin and the granules of the cells that produce growth hormone stain lightly with orange G. The EM has permitted a distinction to be made between the two types of acidophils by the size and variation of size of the granules they contain as will be described shortly. Hence the type of acidophil that secretes growth hormone can be distinguished and is termed a *somatotroph* while that which secretes lactogenic hormone is termed a *mammotroph*.

Different Types of Basophils. The problem of distinguishing different kinds of basophils and correlating different types with different functions has been even more difficult than it is with acidophils.

First, it became established from chemical studies that whereas the growth and the lactogenic hormones are proteins, the trophic hormones—TSH, FSH and LH—are *glycoproteins*. Accordingly, since the PA-Schiff method specifically stains certain reactive carbohydrate groups present in glycoproteins, it could be expected to stain specifically the granules of the basophils that produce these three types of glycoprotein hormones, and indeed it was found it did (Fig. 25-5). The Gomori method also distinguishes clearly between acidophils and basophils (see Fig. 25-17, *bottom left*).

Once this was established, attempts were made to see if further staining methods could be combined with the PA-Schiff method to distinguish subtypes among them. However, the problem of interpreting what is seen as a result of various stains used in various species is beyond the scope of a student's book.

Even if staining methods can distinguish different types of basophils a problem arose in connection with tracing specific hormones to specifically stained cells. However, by studying the pituitaries of people who died with various clinical conditions due to special hormone deficiencies, and by removing various target glands of the different trophic hormones from animals

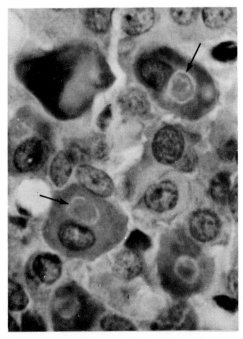

Fig. 25-5. Photomicrograph of section of anterior pituitary gland of rat stained by the PA-Schiff technic and hematoxylin. Notice that the cytoplasm of the cells that secrete glycoprotein hormones is deeply stained by the PA-Schiff method. Negative Golgis, indicated by arrows, can be seen to advantage in them. (Preparation courtesy of Y. Clermont)

(which leads to the cells in the pituitaries that produce the particular trophic hormones working harder), and by suppressing the secretion of different trophic hormones by giving the hormone made by the target gland to animals (this leads to a storage of the trophic hormone in the cells that made it), much information was obtained to indicate the particular cells that make these three trophic hormones.

It is now considered that the cell that makes TSH, and which is therefore termed a *thyrotroph*, is a large cell of irregular shape which, after PA-Schiff staining combined with aldehyde thionin, reveals blue-purple granules. The cells that make FSH and LH are rounded rather than angular, and their granules with the combined PA-Schiff and aldehyde thionin technic are roughly halfway between red and blue while the cell that makes ACTH and MSH retains the red color and does not take up any blue. As already noted, there are similarities in the amino acid sequences in the structure of the melanocyte-stimulating hormone and ACTH, and this makes it less certain that there are two cell types for the respective production of these

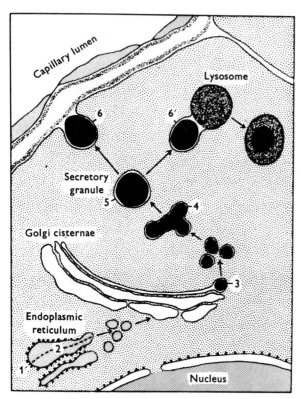

FIG. 25-6. Diagrammatic representation of proposed events in the secretory process of mammotrophs in the anterior pituitary of the rat. MTH is synthesized on ribosomes (1), segregated and transported by the rough ER (2) and concentrated into granules by the Golgi complex. Small granules arising within the inner Golgi cisterna (3) aggregate (4) to comprise the mature secretory granule (5). During active secretion, the latter fuse with the cell membrane (6) and are discharged into the perivascular spaces by exocytosis. When secretory activity is suppressed and the cell must dispose of excess stored hormone, some granules fuse with lysosomes (6) and are degraded as depicted in Figure 25-8. (From Farquhar, M. G.: Processing of secretory products by cells of the anterior pituitary gland. *In* Heller, H., and Lederis, K. (eds.): Subcellular Organization and Function in Endocrine Tissues. Mem. Soc. Endocrinol., *19:*79, 1971. London, Cambridge University Press)

two hormones. Indeed, there is some uncertainty about whether or not FSH and LH cannot be made by the same cell. It is difficult to distinguish two types of gonadotrophs.

After having described in the foregoing what special staining and light microscopy has achieved in tracing different anterior lobe hormones to different cell types, we shall now describe how studies with the EM have provided further information.

The Fine Structure of, and the Mechanism of Secretion in, Chromophils

These two subjects have been investigated in depth by Farquhar on whose findings most of the following account is based; her papers should be read for further information.

Distinguishing Different Types of Chromophils. The EM permits the size and shape of various cells of the anterior lobe to be ascertained more accurately than does the LM. Furthermore, the size and shape of the granules they contain are revealed so clearly that different types of chromophils can be recognized by the kind of granules they contain. The granules of the mammotrophs, the chromophils believed to secrete prolactin (lactogenic hormone) have a maximum diameter of around 400 to 700 nm. and are somewhat irregular in shape (Fig. 25-8); those of the somatotrophs (which secrete growth hormone), 300 to 400 nm. (Fig. 25-10); those of gonadotrophs, 200 to 250 nm. (Fig. 25-11); those of thyrotrophs, 140 to 200 nm. (Fig. 25-12) and those of corticotrophs (the cells that secrete ACTH), 100 to 200 nm. Comment on the size and shape of the cells that synthesize and secrete these different types of granules will be given later, for, as noted, this also helps in distinguishing them from one another.

The Mechanism of Secretion and the Effects of the Stimulation and Suppression of Secretion. Farquhar points out that the mammotroph is the most favorable cell type for investigating these matters because its secretory activity can be easily manipulated under physiological conditions and the formation and secretion of its granules can be most easily followed because of their distinctive features. As is shown in Figure 25-8 they are large and dense and often of an irregular shape, which is in contrast to the shape of the granules of certain other chromophils—for example, those of somatotrophs, which are somewhat smaller and more evenly spherical (Fig. 25-10).

As is shown in Figure 25-6, the process of the synthesis and mechanism of secretion of the granules of mammotrophs is similar to the synthesis and secretion of zymogen granules described in detail in Chapter 5 and illustrated in Figure 5-25. Prolactin is a protein hormone. Its synthesis begins as shown in Figure 25-6 (1) by amino acids being linked by the polyribosomes of the rER so that the assembled product comes to be contained in the lumens of cisternae of rER as indicated by (2) in Figure 25-6. By means of transfer vesicles the assembled product is carried to the saccule on the convex aspect of a Golgi stack and, when this saccule has become the one on the concave aspect of the stack, a vesicle containing mature protein hormone buds off from the saccule (Figs. 25-6 (3) and 25-7). Small secretory vesicles of this type containing the hormone fuse with one another to make larger vesicles (Figs. 25-6, (4) and (5), and 25-7). The larger secretory vesicle approaches the cell membrane where the lamellae of its surrounding membrane fuse with the lamellae of the cell membrane as was described in Chapter 5 and illustrated in Figure 5-37. In this fusion (Fig. 25-8) its membrane adds to the cell membrane with the outer lamellae of the membrane of the vesicle joining with the inner lamella of the cell membrane. Immediately afterward the inner

lamella of the membrane surrounding the vesicle joins with the outer lamella of the cell membrane. The membrane can then open out to the surface at the site where the two fused so that the naked granule is discharged. The process by which the granules are discharged is often termed *exocytosis* (Fig. 25-8).

As is shown in the diagram (Fig. 25-6) and in the micrograph (Fig. 25-8) the granule enters an ill-defined pericapillary space that exists between the cell border and the basement membrane of the capillary. The granule, or its substance, penetrates the basement membrane and capillary wall so that the hormone gains entrance to the circulation.

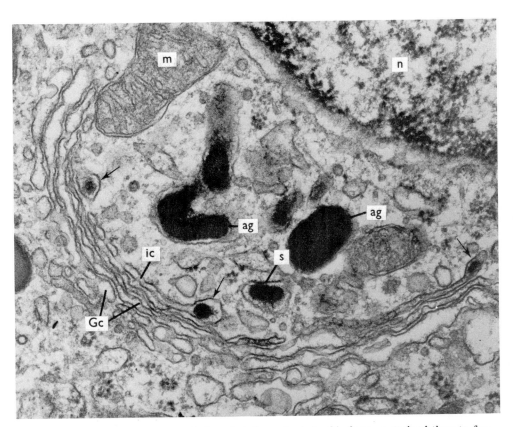

FIG. 25-7. Portion of mammotroph from lactating animal. In this figure, a stack of three to five slightly curved Golgi cisternae (Gc) occupies the center of the field. The central core of cytoplasm circumscribed by the cisternae contains several immature secretion granules (ag). The outer cisternae along the convex surface of the Golgi stack are dilated or vacuolar whereas the inner ones (ic) along the other surface of the Golgi stack are more flattened. Three small, rounded (100-200 nm) masses (arrows) of condensing secretory material are present within the innermost Golgi cisterna and another small granule (s) is seen along the concave Golgi surface. The polymorphous granules in the Golgi "core" appear to be formed by fusion and aggregation of several of the smaller units which bud from the inner cisterna. (From Farquhar, M. G.: Processing of secretory products by cells of the anterior pituitary gland. *In* Heller, H., and Lederis, K. (eds.): Subcellular Organization and Function in Endocrine Tissues. Mem. Soc. Endocrinol., *19*:88, 1971. London, Cambridge University Press)

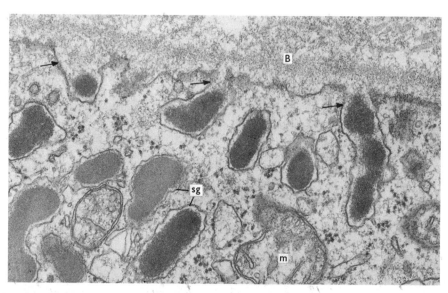

FIG. 25-8. Peripheral cytoplasm of a mammotroph from a lactating rat, depicting several secretory granules (sg) lined up facing the perivascular spaces and undergoing discharge by exocytosis. The membranes of several granules are in continuity with the cell membrane at the points indicated by arrows. B, basement membrane. × 42,000. (From Farquhar, M. G.: Processing of secretory products by cells of the anterior pituitary gland. *In* Heller, H., and Lederis, K. (eds.): Subcellular Organization and Function in Endocrine Tissues. Mem. Soc. Endocrinol., *19*:89, 1971. London, Cambridge University Press)

Suppression of Secretion. The foregoing account deals with what occurs in a mammotroph that is producing hormone under physiological stimulation (suckling). The next matter to be discussed is what happens when the young are removed from the mammary gland so that the stimulus for function would no longer exist.

Farquhar found that during the first 12 to 18 hours secretory granules continued to accumulate. However, their numbers soon decreased. But what is of the greatest interest is that, 24 hours afterward, lysosomes were found in the cytoplasm of mammotrophs with granules inside them. The mechanism involved was seen to be that of the membrane that surrounds a mammotroph granule fusing with the membrane that surrounds a lysosome so that the membrane of the two previously separate vesicular structures becomes continuous so that a single continuous membrane now surrounds the contents of both of the two pre-existing vesicles. The process is illustrated in the diagram, Figure 25-6, (6) and in the micrograph, Figure 25-9, which shows two lysosomes, the upper a multivesicular body, and the lower a dense body, which contain remnants of secretory granules.

Somatotrophs. The fine structure of a somatotroph is illustrated in Figure 25-10, which shows it to contain parallel cisternae of rER, a Golgi, some mitochondria and an abundance of specific granules which are somewhat smaller and much more regularly rounded than those of mammotrophs. The mechanism of synthesis and secretion of granules is the same as in mammotrophs. Furthermore, the granules leave the cell similarly by entering a pericapillary space by exocytosis.

The effects of suppression are not so easy to study as in mammotrophs but removal of the thyroid gland or the adrenal glands suppresses secretion in somatotrophs and after either procedure, according to Farquhar, lysosomes dispose of the excess granules in a fashion similar to that described for mammotrophs. Farquhar notes that in the instance of somatotrophs, the removal of excess granules by lysosomes results in the latter showing a great many lamellar residues of the type often termed myelin figures which were illustrated in Figure 5-42. It is not known in this instance what components of somatotroph granules could lead to their formation.

Gonadotrophs. As previously noted, the functions of gonadotrophs will be considered in the next two chapters. In contrast to mammotrophs and somatotrophs which synthesize and secrete protein hormones, the granules synthesized and secreted by gonadotrophs consist of glycoprotein. The normal functioning gonadotroph of the female rat is a rounded cell with some rER and a centrally disposed Golgi (Fig. 25-11). The granules are all rounded and vary somewhat in size with the largest, however, being smaller than those of mammotrophs or somatotrophs. Moreover, gonadotrophs tend to contain some larger dense droplets of a glycoprotein material (dr in Fig. 25-11) in addition to granules.

There are probably two types of gonadotrophs, one that secretes a trophic hormone termed the follicle-stimulating hormone (FSH) and another which secretes what is termed a luteinizing hormone, termed LH. The mechanism of secretion in gonadotrophs is similar to that of other pituitary basophils but, in the nonpregnant female, as will be described in detail in the next chapter, the secretory activity of both types of gonadotrophs follows a cyclical rhythm during the years between puberty and the menopause.

Effects of Castration. The function of the gonadotrophic hormones (FSH and LH) is to stimulate the sex glands so as to bring about the development and maturation of germ cells and the secretion of sex hormones. Under ordinary circumstances there is a negative feedback sort of arrangement whereby the increased concentration of sex hormones in the bloodstream prevents the gonadotrophs from oversecreting. However, if the sex glands are removed from an individual so that they can no longer produce sex hormone, this inhibitory effect on gonadotrophs is lost and, as a consequence, they work harder and oversecrete. This phenomenon is usually studied by castrating female animals and it is found that when this is done the gonadotrophs become considerably larger. Studies with the EM have shown that this is due largely to a great development of the rER, the cisternae of which become dilated. The Golgi also becomes more prominent and the number of granules in the cytoplasm increased.

Thyrotrophs. The secretion of thyrotrophs is a glycoprotein hormone (TSH) which controls the activity of the follicular cells of the thyroid gland which, in turn, secrete the thyroid hormones which will be described shortly.

With the EM thyrotrophs present angular contours (Fig. 25-12) and the granules they contain are in a smaller size range than any of the other chromophils which we have already considered, having a maximum diameter of from 150 to 200 nm. The mechanism of secretion of these granules seems to be the same as that described for the other chromophils.

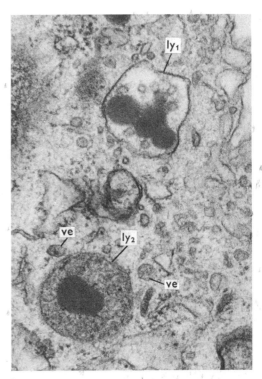

FIG. 25-9. Cytoplasm of a mammotroph from a lactating rat killed 24 hours after separation from its suckling young, showing lysosomes. A multivesicular body (ly₁) is shown as well as a dense body (ly₂). The small vesicles labeled ve that have a finely granular content are probably primary lysosomes. (From Farquhar, M. G.: Processing of secretory products by cells of the anterior pituitary gland. *In* Heller, H., and Lederis, K. (eds.): Subcellular Organization and Function in Endocrine Tissues. Mem. Soc. Endocrinol., *19*:91, 1971. London, Cambridge University Press)

The secretion of TSH is normally controlled by the amount of thyroid hormone in the blood, the control being effected by a negative feedback mechanism already described. Hence it is relatively easy to study either the stimulation or the suppression of secretion in thyrotrophs, the former by removing the thyroid and the latter by administering thyroid hormone to the animal involved.

When the thyroid gland is removed, the thyrotrophs become greatly enlarged and Farquhar describes this as being due chiefly to a ballooning of the cisternae of rER with a material of moderate density. However, the number of granules in the cytoplasm becomes decreased. It seems probable that under these conditions the Golgi is more or less bypassed and that the contents of the dilated cisternae of the rER somehow

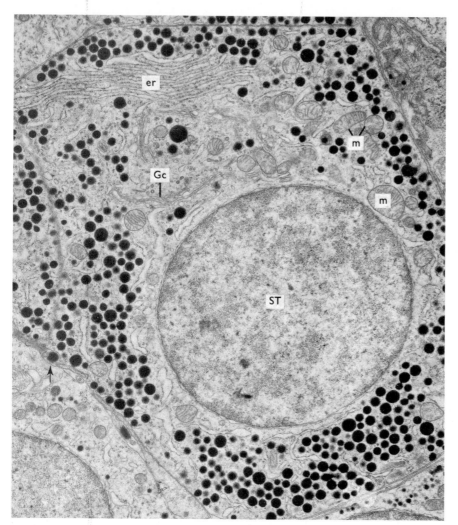

Fig. 25-10. Somatotroph (ST) or growth hormone-producing cell from a young growing rat. The cytoplasm contains abundant secretory granules which are smaller (maximal diameter = 350-400 nm) and more regularly round than those of mammotrophs. The cell shows a number of mitochondria (m), a Golgi complex (Gc), and stacks of rough ER cisternae (er). On either side of the cell are seen images of granules in the process of undergoing discharge by exocytosis (arrows). × 6,900. (From Farquhar, M. G.: Processing of secretory products by cells of the anterior pituitary gland. *In* Heller, H., and Lederis, K. (eds.): Subcellular Organization and Function in Endocrine Tissues. Mem. Soc. Endocrinol., *19:*97, 1971. London, Cambridge University Press)

make their way into the capillaries as an incomplete type of secretory product, but further work is indicated before this particular situation is clarified.

As noted, secretion by thyrotrophs is easily suppressed by giving an animal extraneous thyroid hormone. The suppression is due to the negative feedback mechanism which operates partly at least by shutting off the TSH-releasing factor from the hypothalamus as will be commented on further later. In any event, if thyroid hormone is given an animal from which the thyroid gland has been removed, the factor which stimulates the thyrotrophs is removed and the thyrotrophs begin to assume their normal appearance, with the product of the rER being increasingly processed by the Golgi with the formation of normal granules. The disposal of excess granules and the material that has accumulated in the enlarged cisternae of

rER involves the activity of lysosomes but the manner in which this disposal of the latter is effected is not entirely clear.

THE PARS TUBERALIS

Although this is an upward extension of the pars anterior, it has a different microscopic structure. The cells it contains are roughly cuboidal and contain no cytoplasmic granules. Their cytoplasm is diffusely and mildly basophilic. The pars tuberalis is fairly vascular. Its function, if any, is unknown.

THE PARS INTERMEDIA

This is not nearly so well developed in man as in many animals. In man, what is often interpreted as the pars intermedia consists chiefly of (1) an irregular row of follicles which contain pale-staining colloidal materials and are made of pale cells (Fig. 25-13) and (2) a few rows of moderate-sized cells with strongly basophilic granular cytoplasm (Fig. 25-13, *center*). (The granules disappear very quickly unless fixation is prompt.) These cells may extend into the pars nervosa (Fig. 25-13, *upper right*).

In certain species (for example, fish and amphibia) the cells of the pars intermedia produce the melanocyte-stimulating hormone (MSH) or intermedin. As already noted, it is not clear in man as to whether or not MSH is made by the same cell as that which makes ACTH. Furthermore, it appears that the cell or cells that make these hormones in man are basophils that are present in the pars distalis. The suggestion that these cells may have migrated in man from the pars intermedia into the pars distalis seems logical.

INFLUENCE OF HYPOTHALAMUS ON SECRETION OF ANTERIOR LOBE HORMONES

In order to discuss this matter further we must first describe the blood supply of the pituitary.

The Blood Supply of the Pituitary Gland

Two main groups of vessels, the *superior* and the *inferior hypophyseal arteries,* supply the gland.

The *superior hypophyseal arteries,* of which there are several, take origin from the circle of Willis. They approach the gland as an anterior group and a posterior group of vessels (Fig. 25-14).

The arteries of the *anterior* group penetrate the upper part of the pars tuberalis (Fig. 25-14) and, in general, turn downward. As they pass downward toward the pars anterior, they give off numerous

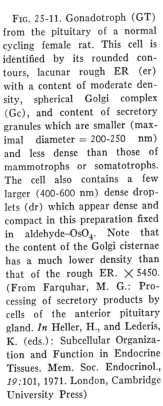

FIG. 25-11. Gonadotroph (GT) from the pituitary of a normal cycling female rat. This cell is identified by its rounded contours, lacunar rough ER (er) with a content of moderate density, spherical Golgi complex (Gc), and content of secretory granules which are smaller (maximal diameter = 200-250 nm) and less dense than those of mammotrophs or somatotrophs. The cell also contains a few larger (400-600 nm) dense droplets (dr) which appear dense and compact in this preparation fixed in aldehyde–OsO₄. Note that the content of the Golgi cisternae has a much lower density than that of the rough ER. × 5450. (From Farquhar, M. G.: Processing of secretory products by cells of the anterior pituitary gland. *In* Heller, H., and Lederis, K. (eds.): Subcellular Organization and Function in Endocrine Tissues. Mem. Soc. Endocrinol., *19*:101, 1971. London, Cambridge University Press)

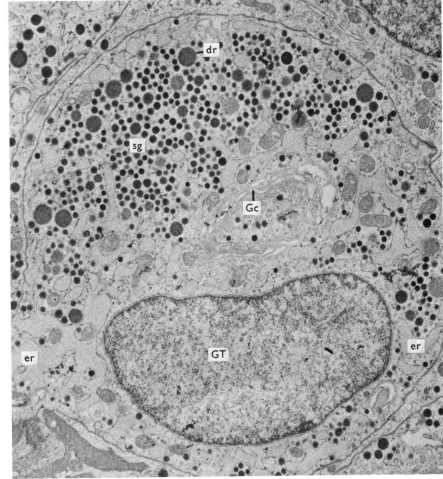

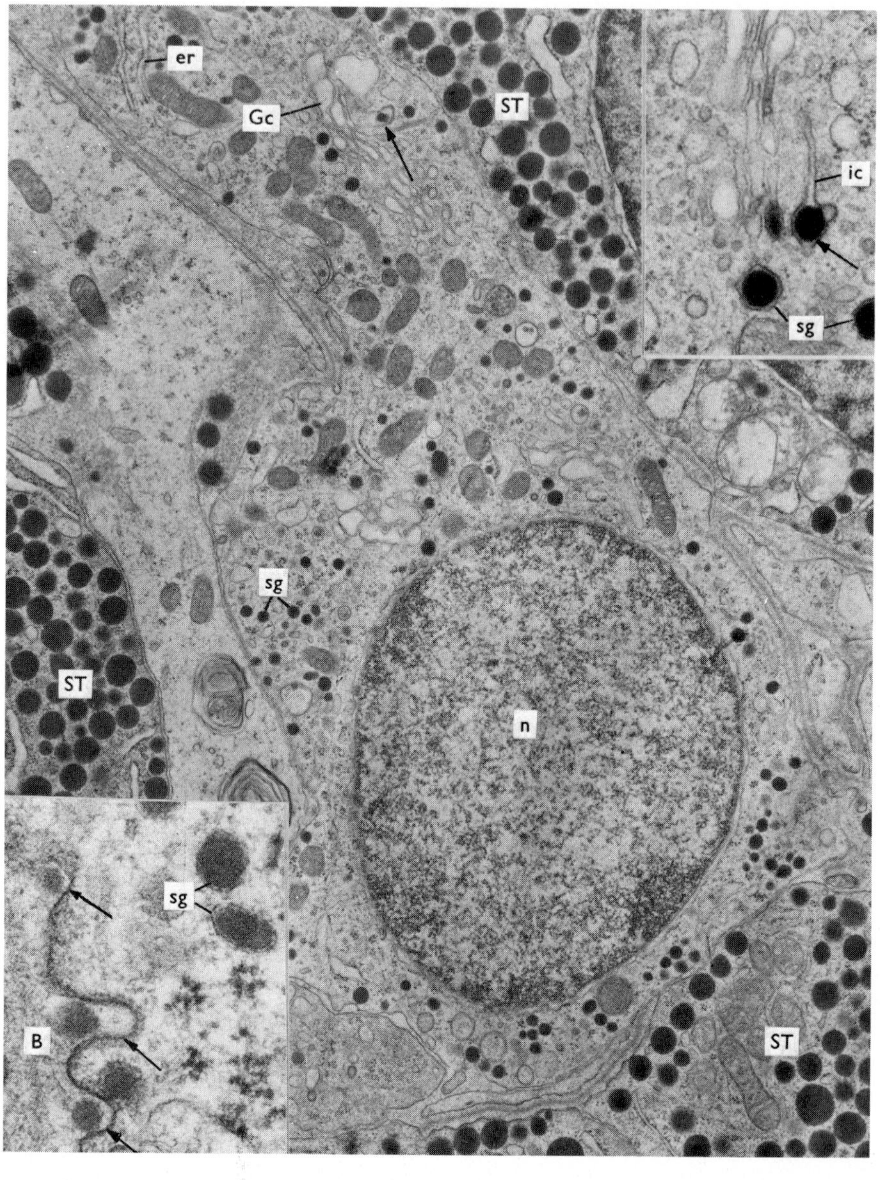

FIG. 25-12. Thyrotrophs from the pituitary of a normal rat. The cell in this figure can be identified by its angular contours and content of secretory granules, which are smaller (maximal diameter = 150-200 nm) than those of the surrounding somatotrophs (ST). It contains a small Golgi complex (Gc) and relatively few elements of the rough ER (er). In the normal gland thyrotroph secretory granules, like those of mammotrophs, somatotrophs and gonadotrophs, arise in the inner Golgi cisterna (arrows upper right inset), and are released by exocytosis (inset, lower left). The latter inset shows several thryotroph secretory granules in the process of undergoing discharge by fusion of the granule membrane with that of the cell (arrows). B, basement membrane. Central figure: × 6,400; upper inset: × 36,000; lower inset: × 60,000. (From Farquhar, M. G.: Processing of secretory products by cells of the anterior pituitary gland. *In* Heller, H., and Lederis, K. (eds.): Subcellular Organization and Function in Endocrine Tissues. Mem. Soc. Endocrinol., *19*:105, 1971. London, Cambridge University Press)

branches. The uppermost of these pass into the region of the median eminence (Fig. 25-14), and the ones at lower levels pass into the neural stalk (Fig. 25-14). All of these vessels end in clusters of tortuous wide capillaries; these have been a subject of much study, in particular by Wislocki and by Green, who should be read for details. Green describes the arterial vessels and the capillary clusters in which they terminate as being enclosed in a curious connective sheath; this has also been described as a glial sheath. The capillary clusters empty into venules which run back in the same sheaths toward the pars tuberalis (Fig. 25-14, dotted lines), where they join with one another to form larger venules (Fig. 25-14, dotted lines), which pass down to empty into the sinusoids of the pars anterior of the gland. Since the system of venules that drains the capillary clusters of the median eminence and the stalk contain venous blood which they empty into a second capillary bed, they constitute a *portal* system, a term which should be familiar from study of the portal circulation in the liver.

The *posterior* group of superior hypophyseal arteries penetrate the posterior aspect of the stalk (Fig. 25-14). The upper branches from these supply the median eminence, and the lower branches supply lower levels of the stalk. Here again the branches end in clusters of tortuous wide capillaries which, with the vessels that supply and drain them, lie in a connective tissue sheath. The venules from these capillary clusters pass forward to the pars tuberalis (Fig. 25-14, dotted lines) to drain down into the pars anterior: hence these venules also constitute a part of the hypophysioportal system.

There appear to be no connections other than capillary anastomoses between the median eminence and the remainder of the hypothalamus. Therefore, the hypophysioportal circulation is concerned not with delivering blood from the bulk of the hypothalamus to the pars anterior but with delivering blood from the median eminence and the neural stalk into the pars anterior. According to Green, the portal circulation is not concerned with draining blood from the pars nervosa into the pars anterior. Consequently it is thought that hormone-releasing factors are produced by nerve cell bodies in different parts of the hypothalamus and that the axons from these cell bodies end in the median eminence or possibly neural stalk, where the releasing factors enter the capillaries that drain into the anterior lobe.

It is to be noted that not all of the blood that reaches the pars anterior from the superior hypophyseal arteries has passed through capillary clusters in the median eminence and/or stalk because some arterial branches pass directly down the pars tuberalis to the pars anterior (Fig. 25-14).

The second blood supply of the pituitary gland is obtained from the inferior hypophyseal arteries. There are two of these, one on each side. Each arises from the internal carotid artery (of the same side) as it lies in the posterior part of the cavernous sinus. Each inferior hypophyseal artery passes medially into the floor of the pituitary fossa and reaches the lower part of the gland at its inferolateral aspect. Here each gives off one or two small branches which enter the inferior aspects of the anterior and the posterior lobes. The main vessel on each side passes upward in the groove between the anterior and the posterior lobes, giving off numerous branches to the posterior lobe as it does so. At the upper part of each groove each main vessel passes forward between the corresponding lateral lobe and the stalk and then dips down into the lateral connective tissue cores of the anterior lobe. Therefore the inferior hypophyseal vessels provide the chief blood supply for the pars nervosa of the gland and also the arterial blood for the pars anterior. There does not seem to be any evidence that the blood from this source enters the hypophysioportal system; in other words, the blood supplied to the pars nervosa by these

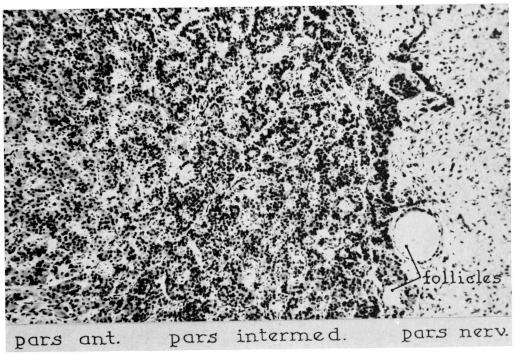

FIG. 25-13. Low-power photomicrograph of a section extending from the pars anterior (*left*) through the pars intermedia (*center*) into the pars nervosa (*right*) of the hypophysis cerebri.

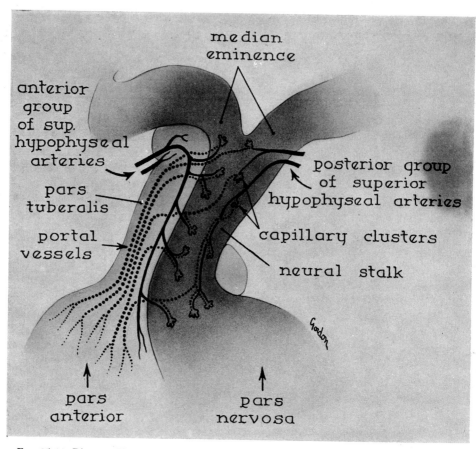

FIG. 25-14. Diagram illustrating Green's concept of the blood supply of the hypophyseal stalk. The course of arterial blood is indicated by straight lines and that of venous blood by dotted lines. (Redrawn and slightly modified from Green, J. D.: Anat. Rec., *100:273*)

vessels is collected into veins that do not empty into the pars anterior.

The Source of the Hormone-Releasing Factors and Their Entry Into the Portal Circulation

The relation of the hypothalamus to the pituitary stalk is shown in Figure 25-16. As already mentioned, the posterior pituitary hormones, to be described in the next section of this chapter, are produced in the bodies of nerve cells that are located in what are termed the supraoptic and paraventricular nuclei of the hypothalamus (the term *nucleus* is used here to denote a group of more or less contiguous nerve cell bodies). However, the position of the bodies of the nerve cells whose *terminal axons* liberate the hormone-releasing factors in close association with capillaries in the median eminence and pituitary stalk is not very clearly defined; they are somewhere in roughly the same regions as those of the supraoptic and paraventricular

nuclei. They are, in any event, in a position to be the recipients of nervous stimulation. This causes the expanded ends of their short axons to release granules or globules of neurosecretion, possibly as shown in Figure 25-15, at a site where in man the termination abuts on one of the specialized capillary arrangements from which blood flows into the portal circulation to reach the secretory cells of the anterior pituitary. The neurosecretions that the terminations of the axons liberate here are the hormone-releasing factors.

The hormone-releasing factors are mostly stimulatory in their effects; these include the specific releasing factors that respectively stimulate secretion by corticotrophs, thyrotrophs, somatotrophs and gonadotrophs. In the instance of prolactin and MSH the releasing factor from the hypothalamus that affects their secretion does so by inhibiting the secretion of anterior lobe cell types concerned. The fact that there are so-called releasing factors that are able to suppress as well as stimulate secretion of pituitary cells may be one reason for the present tendency to term what were first called releasing factors, hormones in their own right.

It may be of interest to comment here on how afferent nervous impulses arising in some part of the body can bring about the secretion of a releasing factor. One of the earliest examples of this phenomenon was observed in the virgin rabbit.

As will be described in the next chapter, the trophic hormone LH, when secreted in sufficient amounts, causes a ripe ovarian follicle (or follicles) on the surface of the ovary to burst and so liberate an ovum (or ova) so that it or they would be available for fertilization should the female mate with a male at that time. It was found that a female virgin rabbit during summer is generally in a state in which there are several ripe follicles available for rupture on the surface of its ovaries. However, they require LH to make them rupture. It was next noticed that if such a female mated with a male, even with a sterile male, the follicles ruptured. It was therefore evident that afferent nervous impulses set up from the act of coitus must somehow have stimulated the secretion of LH by cells of the anterior pituitary gland and in due course it was shown that this was to be accounted for by the afferent nerve impulses being relayed to the hypothalamus and causing the secretion by an axon of a releasing factor. What is even more interesting, moreover, is that some virgin rabbits will ovulate in response to the presence of a male in their immediate vicinity.

Another example is provided by stress. This can be of physical or mental origin. Physical injury or disease causes stress. Psychological situations in which people sometimes find themselves may cause mental stress. It has already been mentioned that in certain situations an individual may experience the emotion of rage or fear and that under these conditions the body becomes geared for fight or flight; this is accomplished by the sympathetic division of the autonomic nervous system being stimulated. Sympathetic stimulation brings about many functional changes in the body which may be of temporary help for fighting or running away but, if long continued, can cause undesirable symptoms. However, in addition to activating the sympathetic division of the autonomic nervous system, stress can also cause the hypothalamus to liberate more of the releasing factor that causes the cells that make the trophic hormone ACTH to liberate more of it and this, in turn, causes the cortex of the adrenal gland to liberate more hydrocortisone. This has many metabolic effects. This is an example of how stress can cause changes in the function of certain endocrine glands. With continued

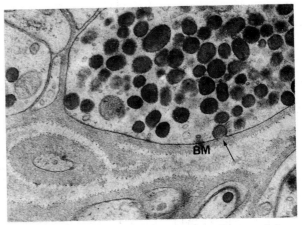

Fig. 25-15. Axon terminal of a neurosecretory cell in the blow-fly showing neurosecretory granules, one of which has fused with the membrane to release its content to the outside. A thick basement membrane (BM) is visible. (From Normann, T. C., Z. Zellforsch, *67*:461, 1965)

stress the histological picture in many endocrine glands becomes altered; this is one reason why many of the endocrine glands obtained from autopsies in hospitals of persons who have died after long illnesses are not suitable for students in histology courses to study in order to learn about their normal structure.

THE PARS NERVOSA
THE NEUROHYPOPHYSIS

The pars nervosa of the hypophysis is involved in the endocrine system in an unusual way, for it does not contain the cell bodies of the nerve cells whose hormones enter the bloodstream from it. The bodies of the nerve cells are located in supraoptic and paraventricular nuclei (groups of nerve cell bodies) in the hypothalamus (Fig. 25-16). The hormones are synthesized in them (Fig. 25-17, *top left*). There are two posterior lobe hormones produced in the cell bodies of these nerve cells, *vasopressin* and *oxytocin*. From the cell bodies, the hormones pass down their axons which are in the hypothalamo-hypophyseal tract into the pars nervosa of the hypophysis (Fig. 25-16), where the axons terminate in association with capillaries at the ends of axons (Fig. 25-17, *right, top* and *bottom*).

Development of Knowledge About Its Endocrine Functions. It was known for a long time that a disease, *diabetes insipidus,* could result from lesions of the pars nervosa. (This is a very different disease from "sugar" diabetes, which will be described later in this chapter.) Diabetes insipidus is characterized

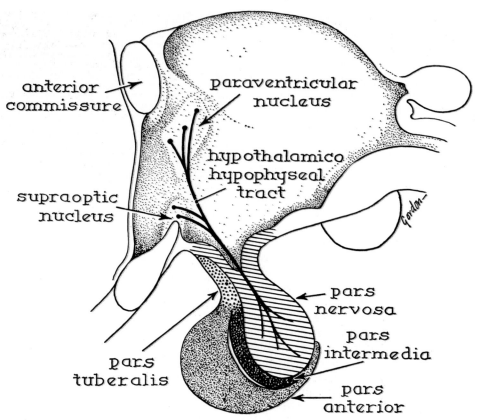

F𝚒ɢ. 25-16. Drawing showing the hypothalamo-hypophyseal tract and the course of neurosecretion from hypothalamic nuclei into the pars nervosa.

by a great production of urine of low specific gravity. For many years it was believed that this disease was due to the failure of the pars nervosa to make a hormone called the *antidiuretic hormone*. If the antidiuretic hormone is not present in the bloodstream in sufficient quantities, the distal convoluted and collecting tubules of the kidney do not absorb their proper share of the glomerular filtrate; hence the volume of urine is many times greater than normal.

However, there were many puzzling things about the relation of this disease to the pars nervosa. It was known, for example, that the disease could be caused by injuries to the hypothalamus and also by interrupting the nerve tract that leads from the hypothalamic nuclei to the pars nervosa (Fig. 25-16). Nevertheless, the disease could be alleviated by means of extracts prepared from the pars nervosa. Hence it was incorrectly assumed that the antidiuretic hormone was made by the pars nervosa, but that the pars nervosa required proper innervation from the hypothalamic region if it was to make its hormone.

In addition to containing an antidiuretic hormone

which came to be termed vasopressin, extracts of the pars nervosa, on being injected into animals, were found to cause smooth muscle to contract or develop increased tonus. The hormone causing these effects was termed oxytocin (*oxys*, swift, *tosos*, labor) or *pitocin*, and, as its name implies, it acts chiefly on the smooth muscle of the wall of the uterus where its action may help in expelling a fetus. Oxytocin is also believed to be released under the stimulus of nursing (or milking), and it acts by causing myo-epithelial cells that embrace milk-secreting alveoli of the mammary glands to contract; this causes them to express the milk they contain into the duct system of the mammary gland. Both hormones have been shown to be peptides.

A puzzle was presented by the fact that although hormones could be extracted from the pars nervosa, its microscopic structure was not that of an endocrine gland. However, in due course it became established that the hormones that can be extracted from the pars nervosa are not made in the pars nervosa but in the bodies of nerve cells in the paraventricular and supra-

Figure 25-17

Fɪɢ. 25-17. (*Top, left*) Drawing of a nerve cell in the human hypothalamus, showing neuro-secretory granules and Nissl bodies in the cytoplasm of the nerve cell. The section was stained with Klüver and Barrera's luxol fast blue-cresyl violet. (Prepared from a section provided by Louis Poirier) (*Center, left*) Drawing of a part of a section of the anterior pituitary of man, stained by the method employed by Ezrin and Wilson (see text). The acidophils are a yellow-orange color. Two types of basophils are to be seen: red and purple. The distinction between chromophobes and chromophils is not so distinct as with most stains. (Preparation supplied by W. Wilson) (*Bottom, left*) A section of the anterior pituitary of man, stained by the Gomori method. The acidophils are red, and the basophils are a light blue-purple. (*Top, right*) Section of the posterior lobe of the pituitary gland of man, stained by the Gomori method. The illustration shows the terminal branchings of a nerve fiber and neurosecretory material around them. A Herring body is also present. (*Bottom, right*) A section of the posterior pituitary of man, stained by the Gomori method. The termination of a nerve fiber, with an accumulation of neurosecretory material around it, is seen beside a capillary into which the neurosecretory material probably passes.

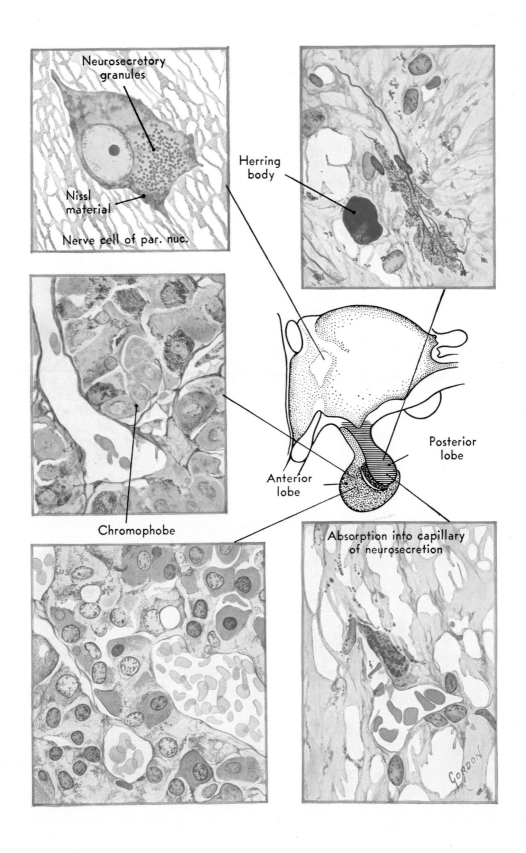

Neurosecretory granules

Nissl material

Nerve cell of par. nuc.

Herring body

Chromophobe

Posterior lobe

Anterior lobe

Absorption into capillary of neurosecretion

GORDON

optic nuclei of the hypothalamus and only reach the pars nervosa of the hypophysis by passing down axons in the hypothalamo-hypophyseal tract. If the hypothalamo-hypophyseal tract is interrupted, the neurosecretion cannot reach the pars nervosa to be absorbed, and diabetes insipidus results (unless new absorptive sites are built up).

By means of the chrome alum hematoxylin technic, neurosecretory granules have been observed in hypothalamic nuclei in every species studied, including man, where they were first seen by Scharrer and Gaupp. In mammals they are very small granules (Fig. 25-17, *top, left*). The nerve cells that produce them possess all the ordinary features of nerve cells, including Nissl bodies in their cytoplasm (Fig. 25-17, *top, left*).

Microscopic Structure of the Pars Nervosa. In most species it does not exhibit a very well organized structure. However, in the opossum it is much more clear-cut, and this has been studied by Bodian in the light of knowledge about neurosecretion.

Bodian has shown that the pars nervosa of the opossum is divided into lobules by septa; the latter contain many small blood vessels, and it is into these that most of the neurosecretion is delivered (Fig. 25-18). The more central part of each lobule constitutes a hilus, and this is made up chiefly of bundles of fibers of the hypothalamo-hypophyseal tract. By means of Gomori's staining method, fine granules of neurosecretion can be seen in these nerve fibers. From the region of the hilus the fibers diverge to approach the septum that surrounds the lobule at right angles to it. Near their terminations each one is coated with a wrapping of neurosecretory substance; hence, near their terminations the fibers exist as the central cores of cylinders of neurosecretory material which comes into contact with the septa more or less at right angles to them. The neurosecretory material is absorbed from the ends of these cylinders into the blood vessels of the septa. Bodian terms the zone that consists of cylinders that abut on the septa the *palisade zone* of the lobule (Fig. 25-18).

In the hilus of each lobule the nuclei of *pituicytes* can be seen (Fig. 25-18). Pituicytes are a type of neuroglia cell and probably serve a supporting function. Their cytoplasmic processes (fibers) may extend out between the cylinders of neurosecretory material in the palisade zone (Fig. 25-18).

Bodies of material that stain with the Gomori technic, which have been known as Herring bodies, are to be seen in the pars nervosa (Figs. 25-17, *top, right*, and 25-18). These are probably terminal bulb formations of fibers of the hypothalamo-hypophyseal tract that end within the substance of the gland, and in which there are accumulations of neurosecretory material.

It seems probable that the microscopic structure of the pars nervosa of other species is basically similar to that of the opossum but not organized so clearly into lobules by orderly septa; hence there is probably more absorption of neurosecretory material from the end

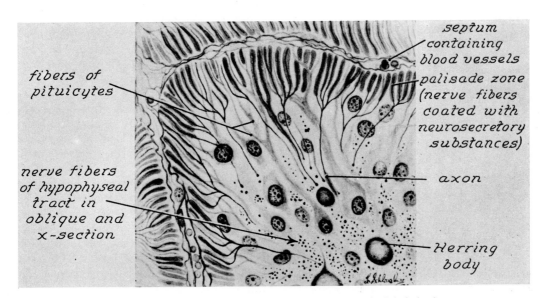

FIG. 25-18. Schematic representation of the histologic organization of a lobule in the pars nervosa of the opossum. (Bodian, D.: Bull. Johns Hopkins Hosp., *89*:354)

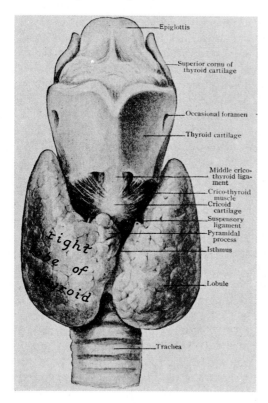

FIG. 25-19. The thyroid gland in situ. (Huber: Piersol's Human Anatomy. ed. 9. Philadelphia, Lippincott)

regions of the fibers into blood vessels that are more irregularly disposed (Fig. 25-17, *bottom, right*).

The Thyroid Gland

Gross Anatomy. This gland was called *thyroid* (*thyreos,* an oblong shield; *eidos,* form) because it is shaped like a shield (Fig. 25-19). It has two lobes of dark red glandular tissue joined together by an *isthmus* (Fig. 25-19). The isthmus lies over the 2nd and the 3rd cartilaginous rings of the trachea; and the two lobes, for the most part, fit over the front and around the sides of the trachea just below the larynx, but their upper parts extend for a short distance up its sides (Fig. 25-19).

MICROSCOPIC STRUCTURE OF THE THYROID GLAND AS SEEN WITH THE LOW-POWER OBJECTIVE OF THE LM

The gland is covered with two capsules. The outer one is continuous with and is part of the pretracheal fascia, which in turn is part of the deep cervical fascia. The inner capsule is to be regarded as the true capsule of the gland. It consists of fibroelastic connective tissue, and it sends septa into the gland, providing internal support and carrying blood vessels, lymphatics and nerves into its substance. The septa divide the gland into lobules, the limits of which may be dimly apparent on the surface of the gland (Fig. 25-19). However, the lobules are not discrete because the septa do not join with one another in the substance of the gland in such a way as to enclose completely limited areas of tissue; hence the thyroid gland is not truly lobulated but pseudolobulated.

The Follicles of the Gland. Figure 7-19 illustrates how a clump of cells in an endocrine gland can become a follicle, permitting its secretion to pour into a central lumen. Follicles are the units of structure of the thyroid gland, and the secretion product within them is called colloid. Each follicle is therefore not only a structural unit but also a functional unit. In the thyroid there are no cords of secretory cells, as there are in so many endocrine glands.

In normal gland the follicles vary from being irregularly rounded to tubular in shape (Fig. 25-20). According to Marine, they measure from 0.05 to 0.5 mm. in diameter. In a section they appear to vary even more in size. This is due to the fact that in cutting a single section, the knife passes through the centers of some follicles, through the edges of others, and through others at various levels between their centers and their edges. Those follicles whose edges are merely shaved by the knife appear in sections as solid clumps of cells (Fig. 25-20, *left*) for the same reason that a thin shaving cut from an orange shows only skin and no pulp.

Marine, who did such impressive pioneer work on the thyroid, estimated that there were about 3 million follicles in the human thyroid. This was probably an underestimate; it is likely that there are 10 times this number. Follicles are packed fairly close together in a delicate reticular network that contains *an extensive capillary bed.* However, this does not appear to advantage in an ordinary section; for some reason, probably shrinkage, the blood is squeezed out of most of the capillaries, and so they are collapsed and not obvious.

Each follicle is surrounded by a basement membrane which is PA-Schiff-positive. However, if careful reconstruction studies of the thyroid gland are made, it is possible, as Isler showed, to find apertures in the basement membranes of adjacent follicles where two neighboring follicles may be continuous. This feature makes it difficult to outline follicles and count them accurately.

Colloid contained within the follicles, after fixation, appears in sections as a solid, structureless, acidophilic

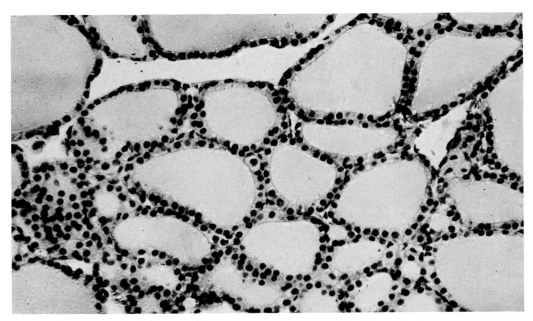

Fig. 25-20. Low-power photomicrograph of a section of the thyroid gland of a normal dog. Two light cells are visible in the lower central part.

material (Fig. 25-20). However, in sections of fixed tissue, the colloid is often seen to have shrunken away from the follicular epithelium in such a way as to present a serrated rather than a smooth outline. This is particularly true when the gland is very active. (Fig. 25-24). Colloid before fixation is a viscous homogeneous fluid. The protein in colloid consists chiefly, if not exclusively, of a glycoprotein which becomes combined into a complex with iodine and is called *thyroglobulin*. Because of the carbohydrate content of the thyroglobulin, colloid stains very well with PA-Schiff.

Thyroglobulin is synthesized by the ordinary cells of follicles and secreted into the lumens of follicles. Its further fate will be described presently.

The Cell Types in Follicles. Two fundamentally different kinds of cells can be seen in the epithelial walls of follicles, even with the low-power objective.

(1) The great majority—about 98 percent in the rat, for example—are all of the same type: normally, low cuboidal epithelium. These cells are the kind that are concerned in the production and resorption of the colloidal material (thyroglobulin) contained in the follicle. They are called follicular cells.

(2) The second kind of cells present in the thyroid are known as light, parafollicular or C cells. They are larger and have paler cytoplasm than the ordinary low cuboidal epithelial cells.

Two light cells are easily seen in the central part of the low-power illustration, Figure 25-20. As may be seen in a higher-power illustration (Fig. 25-26), these cells are placed in the outer aspect of the wall of a follicle so that they do not abut on its lumen. Hence they are always separated from colloid by ordinary follicular cells. These cells have nothing to do with producing or absorbing constituents of colloid. As will be described later, these cells secrete a hormone completely different from the hormones secreted by ordinary follicular cells. As we shall see, too, they also develop from a source different from that of the ordinary follicular cells.

DEVELOPMENT OF KNOWLEDGE ABOUT THE HORMONES MADE BY THE FOLLICULAR CELLS

The first clue about the function of the thyroid gland was due to the observation that a small but fixed number of people became afflicted in a special way. The condition they developed was called myxedema because their connective tissues—for example, that of their skin—become thickened with a firm type of edema (*myxo* refers to the edema fluid being mucoid). They would become somewhat obese, tend to lose their hair, become slow of speech and mentally and physically sluggish. When they died, it was found at autopsy that their thyroid glands had either atrophied or were absent or destroyed for some reason. Subsequently, it was found that children who were born with no or an incompetent thyroid gland became dwarfs and did not develop mentally. This latter condition is termed *cretinism*.

In due course it became recognized that the thyroid gland produces an internal secretion that affects the general metabolism of the body, and it became possible to treat both myxedema and cretinism with extracts made from thyroid glands. In 1914 Kendall at the Mayo Clinic extracted an iodine compound from the thyroid in crystalline form which he termed thyroxine, and it proved to be the active principle of the gland. In 1927 Harington and Barger determined its formula and accomplished its synthesis.

Throughout recorded history a considerable number of people in many parts of the world have developed greatly enlarged thyroids, which are called goiters. In this era, the fact that thyroxine, the hormone of the gland, was known to contain iodine, pointed to the possibility of a basic cause of goiter being a deficiency of iodine in the food and water in many parts of the world. Surveys in different regions of the iodine content of water and the distribution of goiter supported this view. For example, some of the areas close to the Great Lakes in North America proved to be iodine-deficient. The author, shortly after graduating in medicine, worked as assistant to the surgical pathologist in a large hospital close to the Great Lakes, and one of his duties each day was to collect all the specimens removed at operation from the various operating rooms of the hospital and cut pieces from each specimen for sectioning. He well remembers what a large proportion of the specimens at that time were goiters. Marine in particular did a great deal during this era to indicate the need for more iodine in the diet in many parts of the world. Eventually it became customary to add iodine to common salt, and this over the years has changed the picture very substantially. That people do not now develop goiters as before is just another of the vast number of accomplishments in medical research that everyone now takes for granted.

For many years it was believed that thyroxine was the only hormone made by the ordinary cells of the thyroid. But in the early 1950's the work of Gross, in Leblond's laboratory, led to the discovery of a second hormone secreted by the ordinary cells of the thyroid, which in general has the same kind of action as thyroxine but is more potent. It is termed triiodothyronine.

Although the exact mode of action of these two hormones is not known, speaking generally, they control the rate of metabolism in body cells. The basal metabolic rate of any individual can be determined by a breathing test which is based on determining the rate at which the individual, while at rest, uses up oxygen. This test in the past was much used to determine the state of the thyroid function in people who were suspected of having altered thyroid function. However, determining the basal metabolic rate of a person gives only indirect information about the functioning of his thyroid gland; now, as will be explained presently, there are more direct methods for establishing how well the thyroid gland of any individual is functioning.

Hypothyroidism and Hyperthyroidism. Disorders of thyroid function may vary from the norm in either direction; the thyroid glands of some individuals secrete too little of these hormones, whereas those of others secrete too much. The two conditions so produced are termed *hypothyroidism* and *hyperthyroidism,* respectively. Both can vary in severity. These terms apply only to the metabolism-affecting hormones, thyroxine and triiodothyronine.

SOME IMPORTANT STEPS IN THE SYNTHESIS
AND RELEASE OF THYROID HORMONES
EXPLORED BY THE EM AND RADIOAUTOGRAPHY

Two important components that enter into the chemical structure of thyroid hormones are (1) the amino acid tyrosine, and (2) iodine. However, the formation of the hormone is not brought about by a simple process whereby tyrosine is linked directly to iodine. Tyrosine first must be incorporated into glycoprotein molecules as tyrosyl radicals. Iodide brought to cells also has to be changed. First we shall follow the process whereby thyroglobulin is formed in follicular cells and secreted into the lumens of follicles. This has been described by Nadler and his associates, who used labeled leucine, an amino acid, which, like tyrosine, is incorporated into glycoprotein molecules.

1. **The Fine Structure of Follicular Cells and the Synthesis of Thyroglobulin.** Figure 25-21 shows a follicular cell as it appears in the EM. Just below the base of the cell, which is at the bottom of the picture, a capillary (cap) containing a red blood cell (RBC) is present. Running along the base of the cell is a delicate basement membrane (bm). The nucleus (N) is near the base of the cell. The most prominent feature of the cytoplasm seen over a little more than the bottom half of the cell is the presence of many dilated cisternae of rER; one in this illustration is labeled c. Toward the upper right side of the cell some smooth-surfaced vesicles of the Golgi apparatus (g) can be seen. Near the lumen there are many small vesicles that are filled with a material of slight-to-moderate electron density; these are termed apical vesicles (av). Microvilli (mvl) are seen on the surface that abuts on the colloid, which is above and labeled C.

Fig. 25-21. Electron micrograph (× 9,000) of section of rat thyroid, showing a follicular cell. The basement membrane (bm) that is immediately below the base of the cell can be seen at the bottom of the picture along with a capillary (cap) that contains a red blood cell (RBC). The nucleus (N) lies close to the base of the cell. The most prominent feature of the cytoplasm that is near the nucleus is the presence of numerous more or less distended rough-surfaced vesicles of endoplasmic reticulum; one is labeled c. Some mitochondria are evident (m). Toward the right, parts of the Golgi apparatus can be seen (g). Close to the apex of the cell, numerous small vesicles filled with some moderately dense material are evident; these are apical vesicles (av). Numerous microvilli (mvl) extend from the inner border (the apex) of the cell into the colloid (C). (Nadler, N. J., Young, B. A., Leblond, C. P., and Mitmaker, B.: Endocrinology, *74*:333)

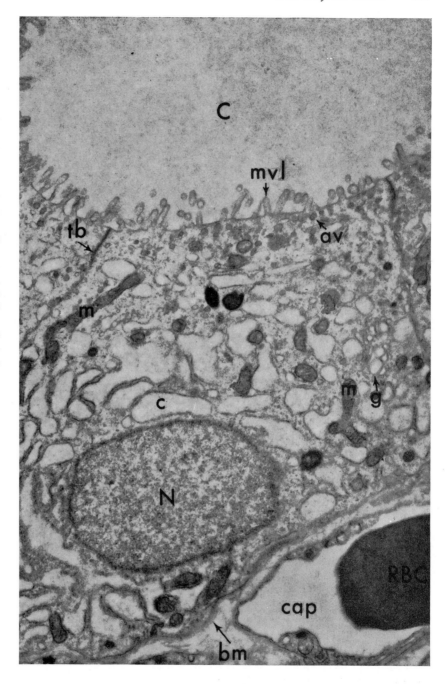

It is thus seen that follicular cells have a series of morphologic features which can be expected to be observed consistently as they are viewed from the basement membrane at the base of a cell to its apex that abuts on the colloid.

The process here, as described by Nadler and his associates from their radioautography and EM studies of how thyroglobulin is synthesized, seems to be much like that concerned in the synthesis and the secretion of other proteins or glycoproteins in that the labeled amino acid is incorporated into a protein that is synthesized in association with rough-surfaced cisternae of endoplasmic reticulum. The polypeptide portion of thyroglobulin is synthesized as subunits and later aggregated to give rise to the whole protein. Meanwhile, the carbohydrate side-chains are added in step-

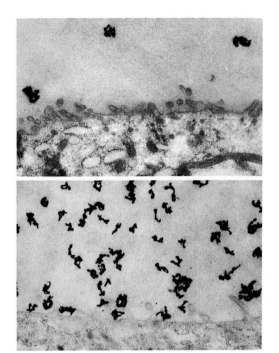

Fig. 25-22. Electron micrographs of radioautographs prepared from sections of thyroid gland of animal injected with radioactive iodine (^{125}I). (*Top*) Section taken 2 minutes after the injection of radioiodine. A few grains indicate that incorporation of iodine into thyroglobulin is beginning in the colloid close to the apical borders of the follicular cells. (*Bottom*) Section taken 12 hours after radioiodine was given. Grains are now numerous and widely distributed in the colloid. (Preparation from Dr. H. E. van Heyningen)

the blood of capillaries. As already noted, the thyroid gland has an extremely good blood supply, and hence much blood regularly courses by follicular cells, which manifest a remarkable ability to extract iodine from it. If radioactive iodine is injected into an individual, it is picked up and concentrated in the thyroid gland very quickly.

By some mechanism not as yet clearly understood, but perhaps through the action of a peroxidase enzyme, the iodide taken up by follicular cells from the bloodstream is converted to iodine which becomes bound to the tyrosyl radicals of the glycoprotein molecules. The site of iodination of the tyrosyl radicals in thyroglobulin molecules can be explored by giving animals radioactive iodine and then examining radioautographs made at different time periods after the radioactive iodine was given. Before this technic was more or less perfected, it was thought, chiefly from the earlier radioautographs examined in the LM, that iodination began within the cytoplasm of the follicular cells; that is, *before* the thyroglobulin was secreted into the lumen of the follicle. But increasingly, precise studies with the LM and newer studies made with the EM (Fig. 25-22, *bottom*) show that silver grains, which indicate incorporation of the labeled iodine into a product, are first seen, not in cells but in the colloid, close to the lumen borders of the follicular cells, and that, soon after, the label is seen throughout the colloid (Fig. 25-22, *top*). So this step in the formation of thyroid hormone occurs in the colloid.

3. **The Breakdown of Thyroglobulin and the Release of the Thyroid Hormones.** The next and final step in the formation of the thyroid hormones involves the proteolysis of the thyroglobulin molecules with the release of its component amino acids. For those who wish the details, the latter step involves the liberation of free mono- and diiodotyrosine and tri- and tetraiodothyronine. Triiodothyronine and tetraiodothyronine leave the thyroid gland to constitute the thyroid hormones; the first one is called triiodothyronine or T_3, and the second, thyroxine or T_4. On the other hand, free mono- and diiodotyrosine do not leave the gland, for there is a dehalogenase enzyme or desiodase enzyme which acts specifically on these two substances. As a result, the iodine is detached from them and presumably goes back into the general iodide pool of the thyroid gland.

The mechanism by which the breakdown of thyroglobulin occurs is as follows:

The surface of the cells in contact with the colloid each sends off narrow streamers which enclose small amounts of colloid; the colloid droplets thus formed are then brought into the cytoplasm (Fig. 25-23, *top*)

wise fashion. The mannose component of the sidechains is added on the subunits soon after their synthesis, probably in the cisternae. Galactose is added on in the Golgi apparatus at about the time when the subunits aggregate to form thyroglobulin. Finally, the glycoprotein thus formed is packaged into small secretory vesicles and transported in these, which in follicular cells are termed *apical vesicles* (av in Fig. 25-21), to the inner surface of the cell, where the contents of the vesicles are discharged into and so become part of the colloid. As a result of all this activity, tyrosine, like leucine, enters the base of the cell and becomes incorporated into huge molecules of thyroglobulin which are secreted into the lumens of the follicles, where they help to constitute the colloid.

2. **The Uptake of Iodine by Follicular Cells and the Iodination of Tyrosyl Radicals in Thyroglobulin Molecules.** The cells of the thyroid follicles have a unique ability to trap iodide that passes by them in

as would occur in ordinary phagocytosis or pinocytosis. Within the cytoplasm the membrane-surrounded droplets combine with lysosomes; and under the influence of their enzymes the droplets break down and release thyroid hormones. This sequence of events is readily seen shortly after a single injection of TSH, which enhances thyroglobulin breakdown and hormone release.

It is to be emphasized that all processes involved in the synthesis and the secretion of thyroid hormones take place continuously and simultaneously; that is, while there is a synthesis of glycoprotein in the follicular cells, there is also its secretion into the colloid, its iodination there and finally the breakdown of the iodinated thyroglobulin. The net result is a continuous release of thyroid hormone. By chance, some newly formed thyroglobulin molecules in the lumen may break down as soon as they are formed, while others may survive longer. In general, a measure of their mean survival is their turnover time. The faster the gland is working, the less is the turnover time of the average molecule in the thyroid follicle.

FACTORS AFFECTING THE HISTOLOGY OF THE THYROID GLAND

In the embryo, follicles are small because they have little colloid in their lumens. During growth, the thyroid gland increases in size because all the components of the thyroid follicles increase in size and also because of the occasional formation of new follicles. In the young, when the follicles are small, the gland has a uniform appearance. However, with age, considerable variation appears in the size of follicles. In old age, previously spheroidal follicles often take on an irregular appearance.

TSH. The histological structures of the thyroid gland are profoundly affected by TSH. After hypophysectomy, the follicular cells become less active and change in appearance. Without the stimulus of TSH the cells gradually change from cuboidal to squamous, and the nuclei flatten.

These various changes that occur in the thyroid gland after hypophysectomy can be repaired by giving the animals TSH. TSH augments the iodide-accumulating ability of the follicular cells, increases the rate of synthesis and secretion of glycoprotein by the cells into the colloid, increases the rate of iodination of glycoprotein in the colloid, and, finally, increases the rate of breakdown of thyroglobulin and the liberation of hormones. Morphologically, the effect of TSH is to increase the size of the follicular cells, to decrease the volume of the colloid and to increase the number of intracellular colloid droplets.

Experimental work by Nadler and collaborators demonstrated that colloid droplets make their appearance in the follicular cells as a result of pinocytosis (Fig. 25-23). It has been pointed out above that, shortly after a TSH injection, the follicular cells send out streamers of cytoplasm that take up colloid droplets (Fig. 25-23, *top*), which then pass into the cytoplasm (Fig. 25-23, *bottom*). Thirty minutes after a large dose of TSH, nearly one half of the whole content of the colloid in the lumen of a follicle may be resorbed into the follicular cells in this fashion. Within the cytoplasm the colloid droplets release hormone as already described.

HOW A DIFFERENT IODINE INTAKE CAN AFFECT THE HISTOLOGY OF THE THYROID —PARENCHYMATOUS AND COLLOID GOITER

If a person is on a low iodine diet, there is too little iodine available to the thyroid gland for it to make adequate amounts of hormone. As a result of the decreased amount of thyroid hormone in the blood, the anterior pituitary gland begins to secrete increased amounts of TSH. This stimulates the cells of the thyroid follicles both to secrete and grow in all the ways just described. As a result of increased secretory activity, the colloid content of the follicle becomes reduced, and the colloid itself becomes thin and pale-staining (Fig. 25-24). As a result of the stimulation of growth, the epithelial cells of the follicles become taller and increase in number by mitotic division. The follicles thus come to have thicker walls and to be composed of far more cells than before (Fig. 25-24); this is reflected in an increase in the size of the gland as a whole, although as the follicles grow, they lose most of their colloid, there being little within them to keep them distended. As a consequence, their walls become collapsed and infolded to a considerable extent. Since the enlargement of the gland is due chiefly to an increase in the number and the size of the epithelial cells of the follicles (the parenchyma of the gland) and not to an increased amount of colloid, the enlarged gland that results from thyrotrophic stimulation is termed a *parenchymatous* goiter. Before the days of iodized salt such goiters were common in many regions. Probably because the body's demands for thyroid hormones are greater at certain times, such as at puberty and during pregnancy, parenchymatous goiters are more likely to develop at those times than others.

From a Parenchymatous to a Colloid Goiter. On the assumption that a parenchymatous change has developed to some degree in an individual at a time

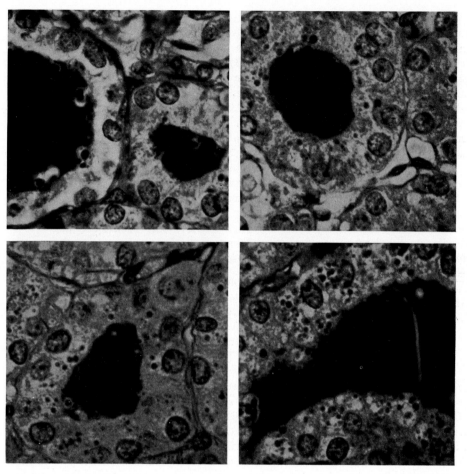

Fig. 25-23. Photomicrographs ($\times$ 1,000) of sections of central follicles of thyroid glands taken at various times after giving the animal TSH. Sections stained by the PA-Schiff method. (*Top, left*) Eight minutes after TSH. Note colloid droplets in lumen being taken up by streamers of cytoplasm from follicular cells. (*Top, right*) Twelve minutes after TSH. Colloid droplets have by now been taken into the apical halves of the cells. (*Bottom*) Thirty minutes and 4 hours, respectively, after TSH. Droplets of colloid have reached the basal parts of the cells and are disintegrating. (Nadler, N. J., Sarkar, S. K., and Leblond, C. P.: Endocrinology, 71:120)

when the supplies of iodine were not adequate for the amount of hormone needed—for example, at puberty —and then that subsequently either the needs for thyroid hormone became less, or a little more iodine was taken in the diet, the microscopic structure of the thyroid would change once more. With a lessened demand for hormone, or with more iodine with which to make hormone, the gland would be able gradually to raise the concentration of hormone in the bloodstream. As the concentration of hormone in the bloodstream rises, the secretion of thyrotrophic hormone by the pars anterior is gradually suppressed. With lessened thyrotrophic stimulation, the cells of the follicles of the thyroid gland would then revert to their former state; instead of being high cuboidal or columnar, they would become low cuboidal again (Fig. 25-25). It has been generally assumed that since the follicles would no longer be stimulated to secrete so much hormone into the bloodstream, they would be able to store more thyroglobulin within their follicles, and as a result that the follicles would increase in size (Fig. 25-

25). It has been generally assumed, further, that since the follicles, as a result of the preceding proliferation of the cells of their walls, would have more cells in their walls than before, they would be much larger than before when they became distended with colloid. As a result, the gland as a whole would become larger than it was when it was primarily a parenchymatous goiter. Further, since its increase in size would now be due primarily to its large content of colloid (instead of parenchyma as previously), it would now be termed a *colloid* rather than a parenchymatous goiter (compare Figs. 25-24 and 25-25). The concept elaborated by Marine, and given above, of how a colloidal goiter develops at first did not seem to lend itself to experimental verification in rats. However, Fallis produced colloidal goiters in hamsters by this means, which substantiates Marine's concept of how colloid goiters develop.

The type of parenchymatous goiter described above can be thought of as a physiologic response to a lack of iodine intake. It is not a spontaneous disease state of the thyroid and not in itself a cause of hyper-thyroidism.

Hyperthyroidism. Excessive secretion of thyroid hormones occurs mostly in a disease called exophthalmic goiter (Graves' disease) or as a result of little, generally benign, tumors called toxic adenomas, developing in the thyroid gland. Hyperthyroidism is associated with clinical signs and symptoms as will be learned about in later courses. The point should be made here, however, that hyperthyroidism is not, or is very rarely caused, by excessive TSH stimulation of the gland. In exophthalmic goiter, so called because the eyes protrude, the thyroid gland has a histological picture similar to that of a parenchymatous goiter but there is no excessive TSH secretion. For some years it has been more or less accepted that in this condition there was a factor in the blood which has an effect similar to TSH except that it acts more slowly and is more long lasting. It is termed LATS for long-acting thyroid stimulator. It, however, has been identified as an antibody and doubt has been cast on its being the actual cause of the great activity in the thyroid.

The follicular cells of adenomas, since the latter are tumors, are not under the control of regulatory mechanisms to the same extent as normal cells, so the cells of these can secrete more independently and at an abnormal rate, and so cause hyperthyroidism.

Drugs That Interfere With the Formation of Thyroid Hormones. It is now possible to treat certain kinds of hyperthyroidism with certain drugs, most notably thiouracil, which prevents the thyroid gland from properly synthesizing thyroid hormone even if the diet contains adequate amounts of iodine. Therefore the administration of thiouracil can cut down the production of hormone by the gland and so allay hyperthyroidism. It is of interest that thiouracil administered to a normal animal with an adequate iodine intake will soon cause its previously normal thyroid gland to assume the microscopic appearance of a parenchymatous goiter. The explanation for this is self-evident.

The Testing of Thyroid Function. This was done first by determining the *basal metabolic rate* of an individual under conditions of complete rest by measuring his oxygen utilization over a given period of time. This test, however, is neither as accurate nor as specific as might be wished. Information about the thyroid can also be gained in other ways: Thyroid hormones, upon leaving the gland, for the most part become linked to proteins of the globulin type in the blood. The iodine that is in this way attached to protein (serum protein-bound iodine, abbreviated to PBI) can be measured, and its level gives an indication of the function of the thyroid gland. However, there are conditions under which this test can be misleading. New and more direct tests of the

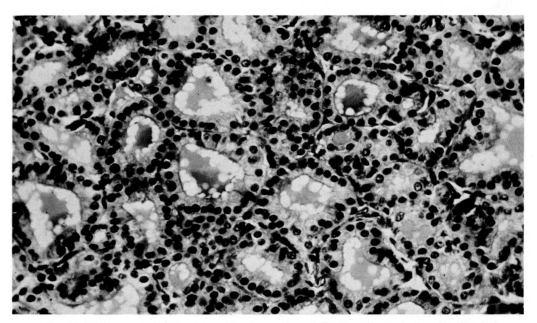

Fig. 25-24. Low-power photomicrograph of a section of the thyroid gland of a dog that had received 7 daily injections of anterior pituitary extract containing thyrotrophin. This is the type of histologic picture seen in parenchymatous goiter.

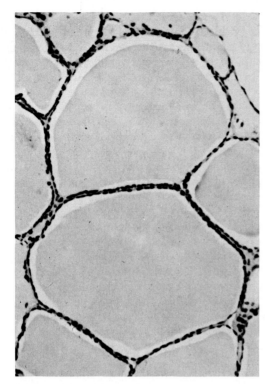

Fig. 25-25. Medium-power photomicrograph of a small area of a section of a simple colloid goiter.

amounts of the two thyroid hormones in blood are becoming available.

The Case of the Secluded Antigen— Autoimmune Disease

As was explained in previous chapters, immunologic tolerance develops to macromolecules to which a fetus (or, in many species, a newborn animal) is suitably exposed, and as a consequence of this the animal in postnatal life will lack the capacity for reacting immunologically against any of these macromolecules. This is true of heterologous antigens which are suitably injected into the fetus or the newborn animal, and it is reasonable to assume that it is also true of those macromolecules which develop normally in the fetus, and which would be antigens if they were injected into other hosts. Therefore, as a general rule, it seems that an animal does not react against any of its *own* macromolecules in postnatal life because it has been suitably exposed to them in fetal life and has thus become immunologically tolerant of them.

However, if a fetus is to become tolerant to macromolecules that develop within it during fetal life, these macromolecules must gain entrance to the tissue fluid or the lymph or the blood of the fetus, so that somehow they can give information to the precursors of B and T lymphocytes so that neither will form mature cells that would be programmed to react to these macromolecules. As has already been explained, the period during which immunologic tolerance can be induced terminates close to the time of birth. Accordingly, if any antigen forms in the fetus but is kept hidden from the tissue fluid, the lymph or the blood of the body, so that it does not come in contact with the precursor cells of B and T lymphocytes there will be some of these that are programmed to react against this antigen. Hence, if previously *secluded antigens* gain entrance to one of the fluids of the body and so make their presence known to cells and precursor cells of the lymphocyte series for the first time in postnatal life, it could be expected that the lymphocytes would react against them as it would against any foreign antigen.

The thyroid gland provides an example of a secluded antigen. Thyroglobulin or its precursor is a glycoprotein that is secreted by follicular cells into the lumens of follicles, and under normal conditions this glycoprotein does not as such enter any of the fluids of the body. Accordingly, an animal body may not be immunologically tolerant to the glycoprotein in the follicles of its thyroid gland. Experimental evidence provided by Witebsky and his associates and by others indicates very strongly that an animal injected with a suitable extract prepared from its own thyroid gland will react immunologically against it.

There is now some reason to believe that the development of autoimmunity against thyroglobulin or its precursor is a contributing factor to the development of a disease of the thyroid gland occasionally seen, which is called Hashimoto's disease. In this disease the thyroid gland becomes enlarged; this is due primarily to the stroma of the gland becoming increased in amount and heavily infiltrated with lymphocytes and plasma cells and even giving birth to lymphatic nodules. The thyroid follicles become atrophic and contain little colloid, and thyroid function is generally impaired. Antibodies to some thyroid proteins have been demonstrated in the blood of patients with this disease. Experimentally, it has been shown that if part of the thyroid gland of an animal is excised, disease can be produced in the remaining part by immunizing the animal with extracts prepared from the excised portion. Therefore Hashimoto's disease seems to have its origin in thyroglobulin or its precursor somehow gaining access to the stroma of the thyroid gland. It is not clear as to whether autoimmune disease of the thyroid is due primarily to antibodies or whether it is a cell-mediated type of reaction, or both.

Other Secluded Antigens

Another example of the secluded antigen is provided by the lens of the eye. Several factors are probably involved in keeping its proteins secluded: (1) its proteins are relatively insoluble; (2) the lens is enclosed by a capsule; and (3) the encapsulated lens lives in a bath of a special fluid, aqueous humor, which provides a more secluded environment than does ordinary tissue fluid. In any event, there is evidence that if lens protein escapes—for example, during an eye operation—it can serve as an antigen in the body in which it was formed.

Spermatozoa (male germ cells, to be described in Chapter 27) provide another example of a secluded antigen, for they are formed inside tubules and hence are not in contact with tissue fluid, lymph or blood. It has been shown experimentally that a male can develop antibodies against his own spermatozoa. However, there is additional reason for a body's not being tolerant to its own spermatozoa: it is that spermatozoa do not develop in the body until postnatal life and then not until the time of puberty. Hence there is no opportunity for the body to become immunologically tolerant to spermatozoa in fetal life.

Secluded antigens are not the only cause for host immunological reactions being directed against body components, but further discussion of this matter would be out of place here.

CALCITONIN AND THE C CELLS OF THE THYROID

As noted at the beginning of this section, thyroid follicles reveal two types of cells. The ordinary follicular cells and their activities have been described, so we can now discuss what have been termed, light, parafollicular, or C cells.

The light cells are larger than the ordinary follicular cells (Figs. 25-20 and 25-26). They do not abut against the lumens of the follicles, being always separated from the lumen by ordinary follicular cells; this is the reason that they were termed parafollicular cells. However, like the ordinary follicular cells, they are situated on the inner aspect of the PA-Schiff-positive basement membrane that surrounds the follicle (Figs. 25-26 and 25-27). With the LM the clear cells in ordinary sections have pale cytoplasm. With the EM (Fig. 25-27) the cytoplasm contains prominent Golgi and mitochondria, but the characteristic feature is the presence of a large number of vesicles containing particularly fragile material. After fixation in osmic acid alone, the vesicles lose their content, so that the cells look light in the EM as in the LM. However, after a brief formalin fixation followed by postfixation in osmic

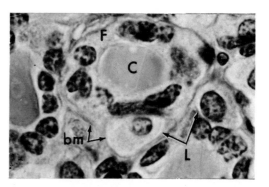

FIG. 25-26. Photomicrograph of section of rat thyroid showing a follicle which has two light cells (labeled L), one beneath it and the other toward its right. Note that the basement membrane of the follicle extends over the light cells, which indicates they are part of the follicle, but they are always separated from colloid by the follicular cells. Masson trichome stain. (Young, B. A., and Leblond, C. P.: Endocrinology, *73:*669, 1963)

acid, the content of the vesicles is retained and stains intensely, as may be seen in Figure 25-28. It is postulated that the content is calcitonin, a hormone which will now be described.

Development of Knowledge About Calcitonin, the Hormone of the Parafollicular, Light, or C Cells, Which Acts To Control Hypercalcemia

As previously noted, it has been believed for a long time that the delicate control of the blood calcium level is achieved by means of feedback mechanisms that operate between the calcium of the blood and the cells of the parathyroid gland that secrete parathyroid hormone. If the level of the calcium of the blood begins to fall, the parathyroid gland secretes more parathyroid hormone, which probably acts chiefly on the cells that cover and line bone surfaces and in such a way that their differentiation is directed into the formation of osteoclasts as well as stimulating the activities of osteoclasts already present (Fig. 15-18). This would result in bone resorption and the addition of calcium to the blood. Another effect of increased parathyroid hormone secretion has been suggested—that is, that it affects osteocytes in lacunae so that they cause some resorption of, and liberation of calcium from, the intercellular substance around them.

The second tenet of the negative feedback theory held some years ago was that the cells of the parathyroid gland were just as sensitive to the level of the calcium of the blood becoming increased over normal as they were to its dropping below normal, so that if the calcium level of the blood rose above normal, the

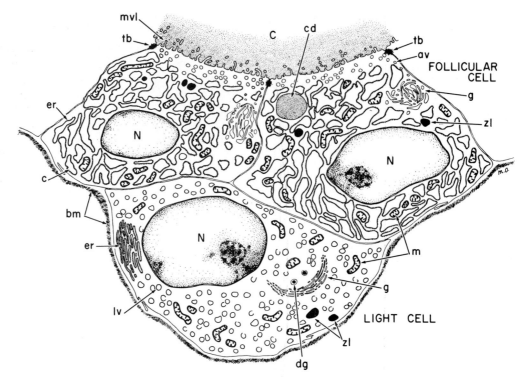

Fig. 25-27. Drawing illustrating the relation between a light cell (*below*) and two follicular cells (*above*) in a thyroid follicle. Note that the follicular cells have microvilli (mvl) that project into the colloid and other cytoplasmic structures already illustrated in Figure 25-21. Note that both the follicular cells and the clear cell are contained by the basement membrane (bm) of the follicle, but that the clear cell is not in contact with the colloid. The clear cell is characterized particularly by numerous vesicles, most of which lose their content after osmic acid alone, as is represented here; those labeled *dg* are exceptions. Their contents are preserved in Figure 25-28. (Young, B. A., and Leblond, C. P.: Endocrinology, *73:*669, 1963)

cells of the parathyroid gland would stop secreting their hormone, and so the blood calcium level would then fall as calcium was either used in the body or excreted. Although it is still possible that this second tenet of the feedback theory may be true, to some extent at least, it is now obvious that there is another mechanism for lowering the blood calcium level when it exceeds normal, namely the secretion by clear cells of the hormone calcitonin. It took a long time for this hormone to be discovered for several reasons, which are of interest to describe.

First, one factor that held back progress in research in this area is the fact that in most animals the thyroid and parathyroid glands are very closely associated, and they are supplied by the same arteries. So if, for removal of the parathyroid glands, it is usual in many example, experiments are performed requiring the species (for example, in rats, in which the parathyroids are buried in the thyroid) to remove the whole complex of thyroid and parathyroid glands together, and if the

experiment is prolonged, to give the animal thyroxine. Likewise, if perfusion experiments are performed (through arteries), both glands are necessarily perfused simultaneously.

Next, the story begins with Copp and his associates performing some experiments which need not all be described here, but which gave rise to the surprising finding that if measures were taken to raise the blood calcium level of animals, the blood calcium level subsequently fell much more quickly in animals in which the thyroid-parathyroid complex was still present than in animals from which it was removed after the hypercalcemia had been obtained. Thus the thought arose that there might be some humoral factor secreted by the complex of parathyroid and thyroid that has a positive action in bringing down the level of the blood calcium when it exceeds normal limits.

Copp and his associates next did experiments in which they perfused the thyroid-parathyroid complex, which, as noted, has a common arterial supply. Although the experiments were of a nature too complicated to give the details here, they showed essentially that perfusing the glands with a fluid with a high calcium content would cause the level of calcium in the blood of the animal to fall, and that this fall in the calcium level did not occur if the glands were immediately removed. It became obvious that if the blood or perfusing fluid flowing through the glands had a high calcium content, some humoral substance was secreted by the glands which acted to lower the blood calcium. This is now known to be the hormone *calcitonin*.

At this time, of course, it was assumed that the thyroid gland was concerned only with producing iodine-containing hormones that affect the metabolic rate, and that the parathyroid glands were concerned with secreting a hormone that controlled calcium metabolism. It was therefore very natural for it to be assumed by its discoverers and nearly everyone else that calcitonin, since it affected calcium metabolism, was a second secretion of the cells of the parathyroid gland. But in 1963 and 1964, two groups of investiga-

tors provided evidence indicating that the hormone was produced by cells of the thyroid gland, and one of these groups, Hirsch and his associates, devised a biological assay method for it. Further evidence for a thyroid origin was soon forthcoming, and as a result many began to refer to the hormone as *thyrocalcitonin* instead of *calcitonin*. At this time, however, there was still some confusion on whether or not there were two hormones, calcitonin from the parathyroids and thyrocalcitonin from the thyroid. In the next few years this matter was clarified, as follows:

When it was discovered that a calcium-lowering factor was produced by the thyroid gland, the first assumption, as might be expected, was that the ordinary cells of thyroid follicles produced the hormone along with thyroxine and triiodothyronine. But in 1964 Foster, MacIntyre and Pearse suggested from their cytological studies on light cells that the clear cells were the cells of the thyroid that produced the hormone. Then in 1967 Bussolati and Pearse made antibodies to calcitonin in one animal and then, using the immunofluorescence technic, showed that fluorescent

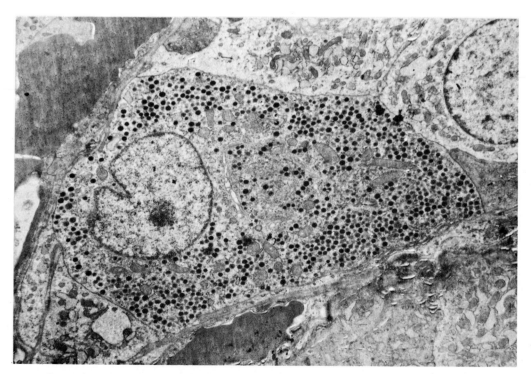

FIG. 25-28. Electron micrograph (approx. × 6,000, as reproduced here) of a section of dog thyroid fixed in purified buffered formalin. This fixes the electron-dense material in the vesicles in the clear cells, as can be seen in the clear cell that occupies most of the field. A capillary is present at the upper left and another at the bottom of the picture; they are separated from the clear cell by a basement membrane. (Illustration courtesy of Dr. B. A. Young, University of Cambridge)

antibody made to calcitonin attached itself to the light cells and not to the ordinary thyroid cells, a finding which showed definitely that the clear cells made the hormone. Pearse suggested that these cells, previously termed clear or parafollicular cells, should hereafter be termed C cells to indicate that they produce calcitonin.

The next step in the story placed emphasis on the origin of the clear cells.

The thyroid gland develops as a result of a downgrowth of endodermal cells from the floor of the pharynx into the neck. The cells that mark the course of the downgrowth constitute the thyroglossal duct. In man this normally atrophies and so becomes obliterated, but sometimes some of its cells remain, and these may later in life give rise to cysts.

The downgrowth of cells destined to form the bulk of the thyroid comes into contact with cells that develop from certain of the 5 pairs of pharyngeal pouches that develop from grooves along each side of the developing pharynx. In man the cells of the 3rd pharyngeal pouches give rise to the epithelial component of the thymus and also to the inferior parathyroid glands. The 4th pouches in man give rise to the posterior parathyroid glands. In man both parathyroid glands are associated closely with the thyroid. In some species—for example, rats—the parathyroid glands commonly become buried within the substance of the thyroid gland.

The cells of the 5th pharyngeal pouch (which pouch is often considered to be a further part of the 4th pouch) give rise to what is termed the *ultimobranchial body*. In fish, amphibia, reptiles and birds, the ultimobranchial bodies are structures that constitute separate glands. But in mammals the cells that grow out from the 5th pharyngeal pouch become intimately associated with the developing thyroid gland. It was suggested many years ago that these cells were probably the cells that accounted for the light cells of the thyroid gland. That this indeed is the origin of C cells has been confirmed recently by Pearse and Cavalheira. So attention has very recently been paid to obtaining ultimobranchial glands from birds and fish (large ones) in which they are separate from the thyroid, and extracting calcitonin from them. Work in this area by Copp and his associates indicates that substantial amounts of calcitonin can be obtained this way. It is hoped, of course, that calcitonin will be of use in clinical medicine—for example, in conditions in which bone resorption has taken precedence over bone formation.

The Ways Calcitonin Could Reduce High Blood Calcium Levels. This matter was discussed in the chapter on Bone (Chap. 15) but will be reviewed briefly here.

It must always be remembered that for a hormone to achieve any action whatsoever, it must act on living cells of some type and affect their behavior in some way.

The cells for calcitonin to act on are, obviously, the osteoclasts which by eroding bone liberate calcium into the bloodstream which tends to raise and/or help maintain the blood calcium level. Moreover, there is evidence that calcitonin has a direct effect on osteoclasts, for it has been shown by electron microscopy that it brings about the virtual disappeaarnce of their ruffled borders which are normally instrumental in dissolving bone surfaces.

There are also indications that calcitonin cán stimulate bone formation. (For some references see the chapter on calcitonin by Copp in "The Biochemistry and Physiology of Bone," which is listed in the references.) In order to do so it would have to act on such osteoblasts as were already present on bone and hence encourage them to deposit new bone intercellular substance which would, in its subsequent calcification, absorb calcium from the blood and hence lower the blood calcium level. However, if calcitonin acts so as to encourage bone formation as well as inhibiting resorption by osteoclasts, if seems very probable that it would also stimulate osteogenic cells to form more osteoblasts so as to increase their numbers. Osteoblasts, it will be recalled, cannot divide. So if calcitonin does encourage new bone formation, its general effect would seem to consist in swinging cell differentiation and function in the bone cell lineage toward bone formation instead of resorption. The next hormone that we shall consider—the hormone of the parathyroid glands —tends, as we shall see, to have an opposite kind of effect.

The Parathyroid Glands

Introduction. There are usually 4 parathyroid glands in each person, but there may be more. They are so-named because they are *beside* the thyroid gland. More precisely, they are usually arranged 2 on each side, on the backs of the lobes of the thyroid gland, immediately outside the true capsule of the thyroid gland but to the inside of its outer capsule of fascia. The upper parathyroids lie about midway between the upper and the lower poles of the lobes, while the lower ones are near the lower poles of the lobes. The upper ones are of a flattened ovoid shape, and the lower ones roughly that of a somewhat flattened sphere. Their length or greatest diameter is slightly more than

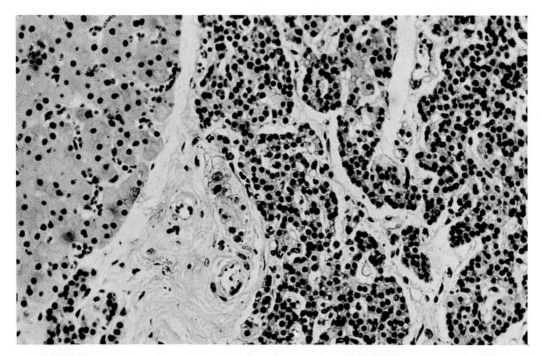

Fɪɢ. 25-29. Medium-power photomicrograph of a small area of a section of the parathyroid gland. An area of oxyphil cells may be seen at the left. The right side shows chief cells.

half a centimeter. They are yellow-brown when seen in the fresh state. Both the upper and the lower parathyroids are supplied by twigs from the inferior thyroid artery, and it is said that these small glands can sometimes be found conveniently by tracing the arterial twigs that arise from the inferior thyroid artery to their terminations.

The numbers and the sites of parathyroid glands vary in different kinds of experimental animals. In the rat there are only 2 glands, and these lie buried in the substance of the thyroid gland, one in each lobe. In the dog parathyroid glands may sometimes be found as far down as the bifurcation of the trachea. Even in man, aberrant parathyroid glands are not uncommon, and if a tumor develops in one of these, it may be difficult to find.

Microscopic Structure. Each parathyroid gland is covered by a delicate connective tissue capsule. Septa from it penetrate the gland to carry blood vessels and a few vasomotor nerve fibers into its substance. The septa do not divide the gland into distinct lobules. Until a few years before puberty, only one type of secretory cell is found in the gland. This is termed the chief or principal cell. It is smaller than the secretory cells of most endocrine glands; hence *in the parathyroid gland the nuclei of the parenchymal cells are generally very close together* (Fig. 25-29). No granules can be

seen in the cytoplasm of chief cells in H and E preparations, but some visible with the LM can be demonstrated by special staining. Although their cytoplasm is never very dense or dark-staining, that of some chief cells is darker than that of others. Those with the darker cytoplasm are called *dark chief* cells; and those with very pale cytoplasm, *light chief* cells. Some light chief cells have so little stainable substance in their cytoplasm that they are called *clear* cells. Part of the clear appearance of the light cells in H and E sections is due to their content of glycogen, which, of course, is not stained by H or E and is translucent.

Although chief cells are smaller than the cells of most endocrine glands, they are arranged in clumps and irregular cords that are wider than those of most endocrine glands. The cells within the cords and the clumps are supported by reticular fibers. Large capillaries are present between the cords and the clumps.

A few years before puberty, clumps of cells with much larger amounts of cytoplasm than chief cells make their appearance in the gland. In contrast to that of chief cells, the cytoplasm of these is acidophilic; hence the cells are termed *oxyphil* (*oxys,* acid) cells. The easiest way for the student to detect clumps of these is to look for sites in the gland where nuclei are more widely separated from each other than they are in areas of chief cells (Fig. 25-29). Such areas are

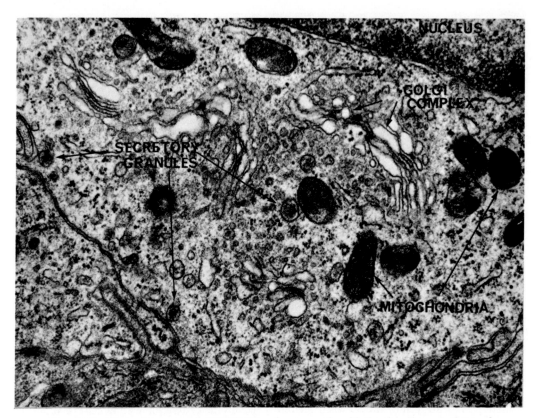

Fɪɢ. 25-30. Electron micrograph ($\times$ 35,000) of rat parathyroid showing the cytoplasm of a chief cell. The Golgi complex (labeled) is well-developed, and a few secretory granules which have dense material in their more central parts, and which are surrounded by membrane, are also labeled. (Illustration courtesy of Dr. Nakagami)

more common in the periphery of the gland. Oxyphil cells are not nearly so numerous as chief cells. Oxyphil cells are not present in the parathyroid glands of most animals. In man transitions between chief and oxyphil cells are commonly seen; since chief cells appear in the gland first, this suggests that oxyphil cells probably arise from chief cells. The function of oxyphil cells, if any, is unknown. One interesting feature of them that has been shown is that they have an extremely abundant content of mitochondria.

In the parathyroid glands of older people, occasional clumps of chief cells may form follicles. In addition, the glands of older people often contain considerable amounts of fat.

The Fine Structure of Chief Cells. The chief cells produce the hormone of the gland. Their cytoplasm, as is shown in Figure 25-30, contains a normal-appearing content of mitochondria and rough-surfaced vesicles of endoplasmic reticulum. The Golgi apparatus is well developed (Fig. 25-30). The secretory granules have a dense material in their more central parts and

a pale rim between this and their surrounding membranes (Fig. 25-30). They are few in number. The chief cells do not seem to store granules of secretion to any extent, which was probably one reason for the hormone not having been extracted from glands by earlier experiments.

Development of Knowledge About the Parathyroid Glands and the Hormone They Produce

Only a few decades ago there was a good deal of controversy about the function of the parathyroid glands. It was known that if they were removed from an animal, the animal would develop a condition called tetany (not to be confused with *tetanus,* which is an infection). Tetany is characterized by the development of prolonged or convulsive spasms of certain muscles. When it is very severe, spasms of muscles of the larynx or those responsible for respiratory movements may cause death. It became known that the immediate cause of tetany is a lack of a sufficient concentration of calcium ions in the blood. Since the level of calcium in the blood falls when the parathyroid glands are removed, it seemed obvious that the parathyroid glands must in some way help to maintain a proper level of calcium in the blood. That the glands did this by producing a hormone, however, was not established until 1925, when Collip succeeded in making an extract of parathyroid glands that would raise the level of the blood calcium in dogs from which the parathyroid glands had been removed, and so prevented tetany from developing in them. It is now known that the hormone is a polypeptide.

Although it was obvious that one effect of parathyroid hormone was to raise the level of the blood calcium, it was difficult to establish that this was its primary effect, and it is still questioned if this is its only effect. The difficulty arose from the fact that there is an inverse reciprocal relation between the level of the blood calcium and the level of the blood phosphorus that confuses the answer to many types of experiment. Under many conditions, when the level of calcium in the blood becomes increased, the level of phosphorus in the blood falls, and vice versa.

For example, it was noticed that the parathyroid glands often became enlarged in children with rickets. This finding was, of course, interpreted to indicate that the glands were working harder in rickets. It was shown that a similar enlargement of the parathyroid glands could be produced experimentally in animals either by putting animals on a low calcium diet or by giving them injections of phosphate. The difficulty of interpreting these findings was that the reciprocal relation between calcium and phosphorus confused the issue: animals on a low calcium diet develop an increased level of blood phosphate, and the giving of phosphate injections to animals lowers the blood calcium level. So a case could be made out for the parathyroid glands becoming enlarged in response to a low blood calcium level or to a high blood phosphorus level. Both views were entertained. In 1940 Ham, Littner, Drake, Robertson and Tisdall showed (1) that parathyroid enlargement did not occur in low phosphorus rickets but only in low calcium rickets, and (2) that it was possible to devise a diet to produce a relatively high blood phosphorus level while at the same time keeping the blood calcium at a normal level, and under these conditions parathyroid hyperplasia did not occur. The fact that the parathyroid glands proved to be responsive only to calcium and not to phosphorus suggested that the parathyroid hormone acts primarily on calcium and not on phosphorus metabolism.

Next, it was argued that parathyroid hormone became ineffective in raising blood calcium levels if the kidneys of an animal were removed, and hence that this showed that its primary action was on the kidneys, where it is assumed to cause increased phosphate excretion. However, it was shown eventually by Grollman that if animals from whom the kidneys had been removed were kept alive by peritoneal lavage, parathyroid hormone would raise their blood calcium levels.

It is still the usual opinion that parathyroid hormone acts on the kidney to diminish the reabsorption of phosphorus by the tubules so that the effect is to increase the excretion of phosphorus. But it is now conceded that the effect of parathyroid hormone on the blood calcium level or on bone is not to be explained by the inverse reciprocal relation brought about by excreting more phosphorus.

Effects on Bone. It was observed that individuals with tumors of parathyroid tissue often suffered from a disease termed generalized osteitis fibrosa, in which there was widespread resorption of bone, together with the formation of new poor quality bone intercellular substance or fibrous tissue as a substitute for normal, well-calcified bone in the skeleton. The presence of this disease and the presence of a parathyroid tumor in a patient have sometimes been suggested to physicians because the patient had experienced fractures of bone which could not readily be explained by the small degree of trauma sustained. It was observed on histological examinations of bone obtained from individuals with generalized osteitis fibrosa that there were, as might be expected, many osteoclasts.

The injection of parathyroid hormone, particularly into young animals, quickly changes the picture in sites of bone formation to that of bone resorption, as is illustrated in Figure 15-18. As was described in detail in Chapter 15, there is much reason to believe that the primary action of parathyroid hormone is on the cells that normally cover and line all bone surfaces. There is some reason to think that in sites where bone is forming and being calcified, some of the most recently deposited mineral can be removed without any or very much disruptive effect on the surface cells, but it is very easy to show that the way in which parathyroad hormone removes any substantial amount of mineral from bone is by its acting on covering and lining cells to cause them to fuse together and become osteoclasts, and that the presence of osteoclasts is associated with the removal from the bone they overlie of both its organic intercellular substance and its mineral.

Why It Is Important To Have an Adequate Dietary Source of Calcium. Since a lowered level of calcium in the blood stimulates parathyroid secretion, and since increased parathyroid secretion can cause the withdrawal of calcium from the bones, it is obvious that a diet that does not contain enough calcium could lead to increased parathyroid activity and increased bone resorption. An important concept here is that this state of affairs might exist without the level of the blood calcium being reduced. In other words, the parathyroid gland by some extra activity could maintain the level of the blood calcium but at the expense of continued loss of calcified intercellular substance from the skeleton. So the fact that a person has a normal blood calcium level does not necessarily prove that his dietary calcium intake is adequate, and that he will not in due course suffer from having his bones weakened because of his having been subjected to the prolonged resorptive activities required to maintain normal calcium levels in his blood.

Some Factors Affecting Calcium Absorption. It is generally believed that parathyroid hormone, as one of its effects, activates the absorption of calcium from the intestine; this would be a bone-sparing effect. But if there is not enough calcium in the diet, this effect does not, of course, spare the bones.

It should be mentioned that vitamin D also facilitates calcium absorption from the intestine. Indeed, vitamin D and parathyroid hormone exert many of the same effects. If great overdoses of vitamin D are given an animal, the effects seen are in many respects the same as those seen in hyperparathyroidism. In both conditions the blood calcium level is raised to the point at which the blood seems unable to retain all its calcium in solution, and, as a consequence, calcium salts precipitate into the walls of arteries and the heart and into the kidneys.

The antagonistic effects of calcitonin and parathyroid hormone are discussed in the preceding section on calcitonin and also in Chapter 15.

The Adrenal (Suprarenal) Glands

SOME GROSS CHARACTERISTICS

The adrenal glands are paired, flattened yellow masses of tissue that lie, as their name implies, in contact with the upper poles of the kidneys (Fig. 25-31). The right gland—sometimes described as having the shape of a cocked hat—is wedged in the interval between the upper pole of the right kidney and the adjacent inferior vena cava; the left gland—roughly crescentic—occupies the medial border of the left kidney from pole to hilum. Each gland is about 5 cm. long, 3 to 4 cm. wide and somewhat less than 1 cm. in thickness. In many animals the glands, although situated close to the kidneys, do not lie above them; hence the term *adrenal* (*ad,* to) has a more general application than suprarenal.

Each gland consists of a cortex and a medulla. These two parts have different origins, characters and functions. Therefore each suprarenal gland is to be thought of as two glands in one. Indeed, in some animals cortical tissue and medullary tissue form separate bodies no more related to one another anatomically than they are functionally. Many investigators have suspected that there is some reason for the close anatomic association of the two parts of the gland in so many animals.

DEVELOPMENT

The first intimation of the development of the cortices of the glands is a thickening that occurs in the mesoderm near the root of the dorsal mesentery. Two substantial masses of cells, one on each side, form in this region and come to lie close to the developing kidney. It seems likely from the studies of Keene and Hewer that as development proceeds, the original mass of cells making up the cortex becomes capped and then surrounded by a second mass of cells derived approximately from the same site as the first. The original or inner mass forms what is called the *provisional* or *fetal cortex of the gland,* and the second or outer mass that subsequently covers it, the *permanent cortex.*

In the meantime, ectodermal cells have migrated from the neural crests (or from the neural tube itself —the source of these cells is somewhat uncertain) to form the celiac ganglia. However, some of the ectodermal-derived cells, instead of developing into ganglion cells at this site, migrate farther afield and into the substance of the cortical tissue to take up a position in its central part. A continuous migration of cells from the developing celiac ganglia proceeds almost until the time of birth (and perhaps later), so that by this time a substantial number of cells have taken up a position in the central part of the adrenal gland to comprise its medulla. Thus the cells of the medulla are cells of the same kind as those that become neurons of the sympathetic nervous system. Their functional relation to the sympathetic system will be described when we later consider the medulla.

The provisional or fetal cortex—derived from the first group of mesodermal cells to separate from the coelomic epithelium—becomes arranged into cords separated by blood vessels, and the structure as a whole reaches a high state of development during fetal life. Not only do the cells of the provisional cortex

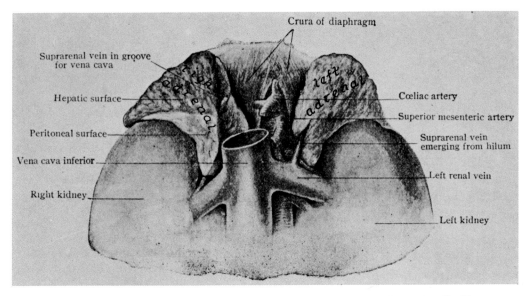

Fig. 25-31. Anterior aspect of adrenal glands hardened in situ. (Huber: Piersol's Human Anatomy. ed. 9. Philadelphia, Lippincott)

comprise the bulk of the cortical tissue that exists at this time, but also they are so numerous as to make the adrenal cortex of the human fetus an organ of impressive size. The cells of the permanent cortex do not develop to any great extent during this time. However, after birth the provisional cortex—so highly developed during fetal life—undergoes a rapid involution. As this occurs, the cells of the permanent cortex begin to differentiate, but for a few years they do not become organized into the 3 zones that characterize the adult cortex.

The fact that the provisional cortex has a somewhat different origin from the permanent cortex and is enormously developed in fetal life but involutes after birth suggests strongly that this provisional cortex should be regarded as an endocrine gland in its own right, having a special function in fetal life. Since it involutes after birth, the thought arises that the trophic hormones that cause its great development during fetal life may perhaps be the gonadotrophic-like hormones (to be described in the next chapter) made by the human placenta during pregnancy, and that they might require the cooperation of the anterior pituitary of the fetus to be effective in the fetus. One difficulty in determining the function of the adrenal cortex in fetal life is that a comparable development of the provisional cortex does not occur in the fetuses of the common experimental animals; hence the experimental study of the provisional cortex of the fetus is correspondingly restricted.

General Microscopic Appearance of the Gland As a Whole

Inspection of a section of the gland with the low-power objective establishes certain prominent landmarks. First, the gland will be seen to have a relatively thick capsule of connective tissue (Fig. 25-32). Next, in the central part of the gland large veins may be seen (Fig. 25-32, *top*). These are the veins of the medulla, and a moderate amount of connective tissue is associated with them. Between this connective tissue and that of the capsule is the parenchyma of the gland. Most of this is cortex, which consists of epithelial secretory cells (despite their origin from mesoderm) that are arranged so as to secrete into wide capillaries. Although the medulla occupies the more central part of the gland and so is surrounded by cortex, the gland is so flattened that the medulla generally appears in a section as a rather thin "filling" in a sandwich of cortex (Fig. 25-32, *top, right*). Moreover, the medulla is not very sharply demarcated from the cortex. However, the cytoplasm of the cells of the medulla is more basophilic than that of the cortical cells; hence, even in a casual low-power inspection of an H and E section, the medulla may generally be identified as a muddy blue layer between two light layers of cortex.

With more detailed study it will be observed that the parenchymal cells of both the cortex and the medulla follow the general plan seen in endocrine glands;

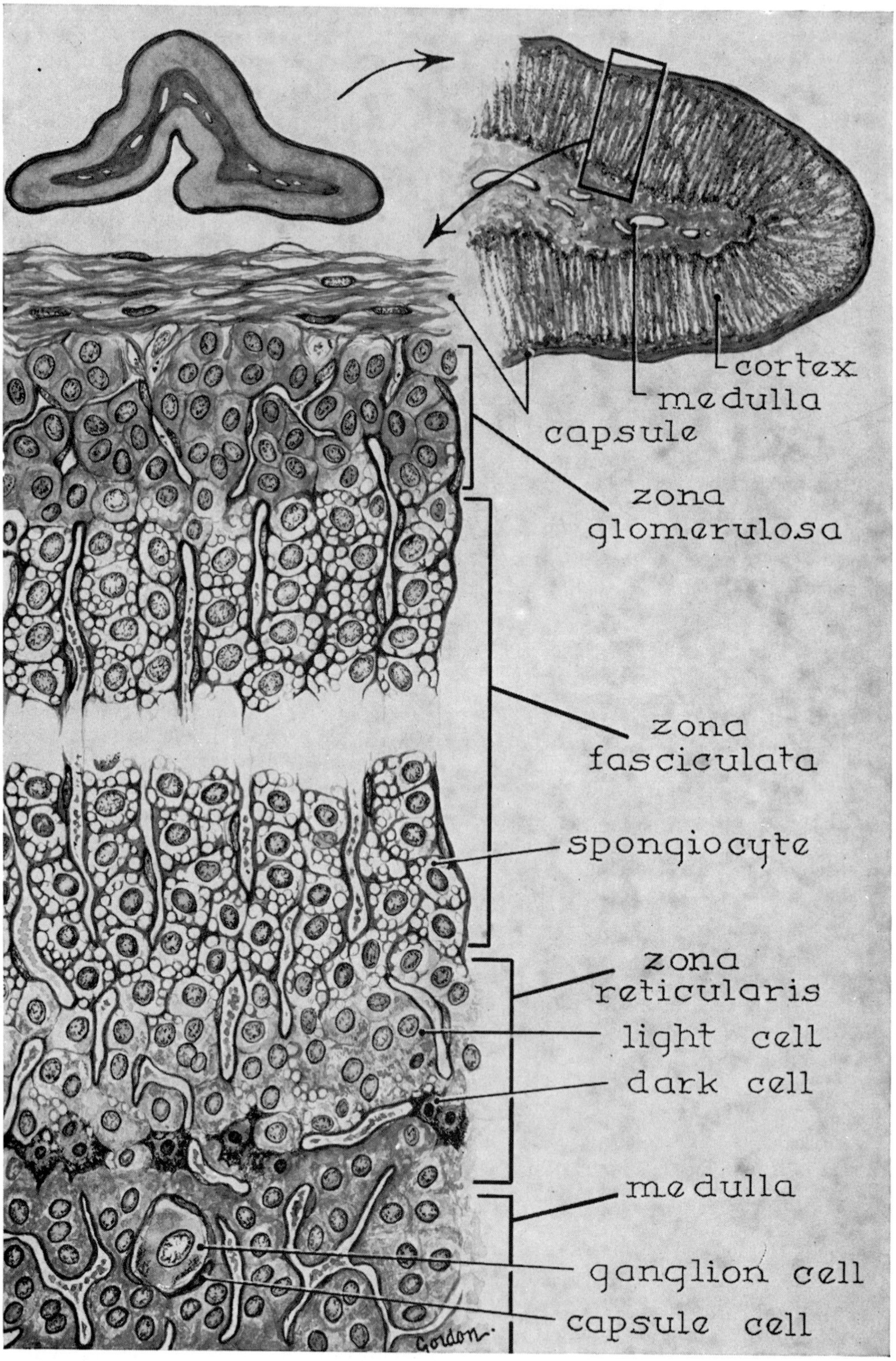

FIG. 25-32. Drawings of various magnifications of an H and E section of an adrenal gland of man.

that is, they are arranged in clumps or cords with vessels between them (Figs. 25-32 and 25-33, *left*). The vessels in the cortex have been described by some authorities as capillaries and by others as sinusoids. In the medulla both narrow capillaries and wider venous channels are found between the clumps and the cords of cells; these drain into the large veins mentioned previously.

THE CORTEX

Microscopic Structure. The parenchymal cells at various levels between the capsule and the medulla reveal 3 different types of arrangement; hence the cortex is said to be composed of 3 different layers or zones. Immediately beneath the capsule the parenchymal cells are groups into little, irregular clusters (the *zona glomerulosa*) with capillaries between the clusters (Fig. 25-32). Beneath this is a thick layer (the *zona fasciculata*), in which the cells are arranged in fairly straight cords that run at right angles to the surface and have straight capillaries between them (Fig. 25-32). Between the zona fasciculata and the medulla is a relatively thin layer (the *zona reticularis*), in which the cells are disposed in cords that run in various directions and anastomose with one another (Fig. 25-32). Wide capillaries occupy the interstices between the cords. The 3 zones described above usually are not sharply defined from one another.

The parenchymal cells of the zona glomerulosa tend to be columnar. Their nuclei are somewhat smaller and darker than those of the next zone; likewise their cytoplasm is of a more even texture, but it contains some lipid droplets.

The cells of the zona fasciculata are roughly polyhedral. Their nuclei are larger and less dense than those of the zona glomerulosa. Their cytoplasm, in H and E sections, appears to be extensively vacuolated, because in life it contains large numbers of lipid droplets (Fig. 25-32). Indeed, this feature of the cells of this zone is so pronounced that the cells here are sometimes termed *spongiocytes*. Cholesterol is said to be more concentrated in these cells than in any other part of the body. The cholesterol esters in these lipid droplets serve as precursors of the steroid hormones made by these cells. With appropriate technics these cells can also be shown to contain considerable quantities of ascorbic acid (vitamin C). The adrenocorticotrophic hormone (ACTH), if given in sufficient amounts, rapidly depletes from these cells much of their cholesterol and ascorbic acid. Both tests—the depletion of these cells of either ascorbic acid or cholesterol—have been used in experimental animals to

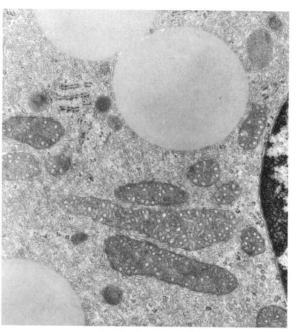

FIG. 25-33. Electron micrograph ($\times$ 28,600) showing a portion of a cell of the zona fasciculata of human adrenal cortex. The large pale circular area and parts of two others represent cuts through lipid droplets. These store cholesterol esters which serve as a precursor of steroid hormones. Near the upper left the section has passed through three flattened vesicles of rER; the dark polyribosomes on their outer surfaces permit them to be easily distinguished. The large objects in the main part of the picture are mitochondria; what appears as little holes in their substance are due to tubular cristae being cut in cross or oblique section. The cytoplasm between the mitochondria is literally packed with tubules of sER. The enzymes of both the mitochondria and the sER are concerned in the synthesis of the steroid hormones. (Illustration courtesy of Prof. John A. Long)

assay the potency of solutions of ACTH. The cells are rich in mitochondria; the EM has shown these to differ from mitochondria in most cells in that in some the cristae tend to be tubular villi (Fig. 25-33) instead of relatively flat shelves.

The cells of both the zona glomerulosa and zona fasciculata contain large amounts of smooth-surfaced endoplasmic reticulum which is concerned in the production of the steroid hormones that they produce. They also contain cisternae of rough-surfaced endoplasmic reticulum as well as a few lysosomes. These can be seen in Figure 25-33.

The cells of the zona reticularis vary in appearance. Some have small dark nuclei and acidophilic cytoplasm and appear to be degenerating. Others have lighter nuclei and cytoplasm. Some cells here contain considerable quantities of pigment (Fig. 25-32).

The Hormones of the Cortex and Their Biological Effects

The adrenal cortex (or substitution therapy, which is now possible) is essential to life. This was ascertained in the last century when Thomas Addison described a disease, subsequently designated by his name, which caused a person afflicted with it to become increasingly weak until he or she suffered complete prostration and died. It was noted that this downhill course was associated with a pigmentation of the skin and anemia. Addison found that patients with this particular clinical picture revealed at autopsy a diseased condition of their adrenal glands. It was, of course, not established until this century that the clinical picture seen in the disease was due to a lack of hormones produced by the adrenal cortex. Now that the hormones are available, people who would otherwise suffer from this disease can be maintained in health.

Unlike the hormones we have considered in the preceding pages which are peptides, polypeptides, proteins or glycoproteins, the hormones produced by the adrenal cortex and which will be described here, together with the hormones produced by sex glands, which will be described in the next two chapters, are what are termed steroids. They are all derived from cholesterol and all have a basic 4-ring structure but differ from one another in certain other respects but not sufficiently to suggest that the differences would account for their having such profoundly different biological effects.

The two major types of hormones produced by the cortex are termed glucocorticoids and mineralocorticoids. In addition, the cortex produces, in a minor way, some hormones of the sex variety. We shall briefly describe in turn these hormones and their biological effects.

The Glucocorticoids

The most important of the active glucocorticoids is cortisol, also called hydrocortisone. Cortisol exerts a great many effects in the body. The precise way it produces these effects is not well understood.

Effects of Cortisol on Protein and Carbohydrate Metabolism. So far as protein is concerned, hydrocortisone is in general a catabolic hormone. In the liver it tends to stimulate the conversion of protein into carbohydrate. However, to do this it must stimulate the synthesis of the protein enzymes that have this effect. This effect is associated with the increased synthesis of RNA so it is believed that cortisol acts at the level of genes, turning on the appropriate ones to bring about its effects.

Since insulin also causes liver cells to accumulate glycogen, it should be explained that the ways in which hydrocortisone and insulin exert this effect are quite different. Insulin acts to cause liver cells to take up glucose from the blood and to store it as glycogen; in other words, the glycogen that appears in liver cells as a result of insulin activity lowers the blood sugar level. On the other hand, hydrocortisone acts to cause the production of carbohydrate in liver cells from protein or protein precursors; hence hydrocortisone can cause glycogen to be laid down in liver cells without taking glucose from the blood and so lowering the blood sugar level; indeed, its action in causing the formation of carbohydrate from protein provides extra sugar for the blood and tends to raise the level of blood sugar. Insulin, therefore, has an antidiabetogenic effect in that it tends to lower the blood sugar level and cortisol has a diabetogenic effect in that it tends to raise the blood sugar level. Normally, of course, these two effects are nicely balanced, but in the absence of either hormone the effects of the other are manifested.

Effect on Lymphatic Tissue. The catabolic effect of hydrocortisone is manifested by its effect on lymphatic tissue also; the administration of the hormone leads to a rapid reduction in the size of the thymus gland, the spleen and other depots of lymphatic tissue. It was believed that in sufficiently large doses it could actually cause a breakdown of lymphocytes, but it is now generally considered that its effect is to inhibit DNA synthesis and so inhibit mitosis. The reduction in size of the lymphocyte depots would therefore have to be explained by the normal rapid turnover of cells in these depots.

Suppression of Growth. In addition to affecting lymphatic tissue, hydrocortisone affects other connective tissues. Its administration while fractured bones are healing leads to the formation of less callus tissue than usual. Hydrocortisone also inhibits the proliferation of fibroblasts in the healing of wounds in ordinary fibrous connective tissue. Given in sufficient amounts, it slows the growth of the epiphyseal disks of young rats; this effect, however, could be explained by cortisol's inhibiting the secretion of growth hormone by the somatotrophs by a negative feedback. Hydrocortisone can also inhibit the production of an immune response, for this requires more cells and also protein synthesis if antibodies are to be produced.

Anti-inflammatory Effect. Cortisone has an ability to suppress allergies and inflammatory responses, probably in ways other than those already described. A possibility here is that it stabilizes the cell membranes and/or the membranes of lysosomes. It could also suppress the formation of histamine.

The effect most easily observed when hydrocortisone is administered is the effect that it has in causing eosinophils to leave the blood vascular system, presumably to enter the substance of the connective tissues; so it produces an *eosinopenia.* In many species it causes lymphocytes to leave the bloodstream in a similar way. Cortisol has other effects, but describing them is beyond the scope of this book.

The Control of the Secretion of Cortisol. The secretion of cortisol is controlled primarily by a negative feedback mechanism that acts between it and the corticotrophs of the anterior pituitary. Thus when the level of cortisol tends to fall in the blood, more ACTH is secreted and this stimulates the adrenal cortex to produce more cortisol. As the blood level of cortisol increases, the secretion of ACTH is slowed and by this means cortisol levels are maintained at normal levels. However, the normal level of cortisol does not seem to be static, for it appears that ACTH secretion is greater in the early morning hours so that in the afternoon the level of cortisol in the blood falls to about half of that attained in the morning. It appears that this normal rhythm is due to the rhythmic secretion of the corticotrophin-releasing factor. It is also believed that the corticotrophin-releasing factor is also the important factor in causing excessive ACTH and hence excessive cortisol secretion in stress situations.

The Mineralocorticoids

These control the sodium and potassium balance in the body by affecting kidney tubules so as to increase their ability to resorb sodium into the blood. The most potent mineralocorticoid is *aldosterone.* Aldosterone thus conserves body sodium. In Addison's disease, a condition already mentioned, or in adrenalectomized animals, sodium is lost from the body into the urine, and potassium accumulates in the blood. Some amelioration of this state of affairs which, if prolonged, leads to death, can be accomplished by the administration of extra sodium chloride; for example, adrenalectomized rats can be kept alive for long periods of time by putting sodium chloride in their drinking water. The giving of mineralocorticoids to such animals will, of course, restore their ability to retain salt.

Control and Site of Their Secretion. There is convincing evidence to the effect that the mineralocorticoids are secreted only by the cells of the zona glomerulosa. Furthermore, the secretory functions of these cells are almost entirely independent of ACTH. The main factor controlling the secretion of aldosterone seems to be the concentration of angiotensin II in the bloodstream and, as was described in the previous chapter, this is formed from angiotension I which in turn is formed from renin which is secreted by the JG cells of the kidney. The secretory activity of the JG cells is, in turn, stimulated by a fall in blood pressure or a lowered sodium content of blood; the latter is shown by increased granulation of JG cells occurring under conditions of adrenalectomy or a low sodium intake.

Sex Hormones

The steroid hormones of the third group made by the adrenal cortex are of the sex variety. The chief kinds are weak androgens. Such sex hormones as are made by the adrenal cortex are probably mostly produced by the cells of the zona reticularis. The ability of the adrenal cortex to produce sex hormones becomes important in understanding how certain disorders of the adrenal gland can be responsible for pseudohermaphrodites—for example, chromosomal females developing masculine sex characteristics.

CELL RENEWAL IN, AND EFFECTS OF ACTH ON, THE CORTEX

There are differences of opinion. One concept is that the cells of the glomerulosa and cells of the fasciculata are relatively independent. First, the glomerulosa cells are thought to secrete the mineralocorticoids, and the cells of the fasciculata, the glucocorticoids. Second, the cells of each of these 2 zones are thought to undergo division and so keep up their cell content indefinitely. Third, the zona glomerulosa and its secretion of mineralocorticoids are thought to be relatively independent of anterior pituitary control and ACTH is thought to act only on the cells of the fasciculata; in support of this concept is the fact that after hypophysectomy, the zona glomerulosa of rats is little affected, but the fasciculata atrophies profoundly.

There are reasons, however, for considering that the zona glomerulosa is the germinative zone. In support of this are the facts that the transplanted autologous capsule of an adrenal gland to which some of the glomerulosa is still attached will regenerate a new cortex, and that rats with these transplants will live. Moreover, it has been shown that transplants of the gland minus its capsule and zona glomerulosa do not grow and survive. Therefore, transplantation experiments in rats suggest that the zona glomerulosa is the regenerative zone of the adrenal cortex.

Another point should be mentioned, namely, that there seems to be some species difference in connection with the zone of the cortex that is affected by ACTH. In our experience (Ham and Haist) in following the day-to-day histologic changes in the adrenal glands of dogs given crude anterior pituitary extracts, we found literally enormous numbers of mitotic figures in the zona glomerulosa but only occasional ones in the zona fasciculata (Fig. 25-34). So, although the zona glomerulosa may be concerned chiefly with secreting mineralocorticoids, there is evidence that it also serves as the chief regenerative zone for cells of the fasciculata that secrete glucocorticoids.

The role and control of the zona reticularis is not clear. If it is assumed that the zona glomerulosa is the germinative zone and acts to maintain the cell population of the cortex, it could be assumed that cells formed in the glomerulosa slowly move down the cords of the fasciculata and finally die in the reticularis. This is the "graveyard" concept of this zone. It has been suggested, however, that it is concerned with producing

sex hormones, although it seems probable that those that are produced in the adrenal are produced also in the zona fasciculata.

The Adrenal Medulla

Microscopic Structure. The cells of the medulla are of the large, ovoid columnar type and are commonly seen in ordinary sections to be grouped together in clumps and irregular cords that are arranged around the blood vessels (Fig. 25-35). Many of them contain fine granules that are colored brown with chrome salts. This is called the *chromaffin reaction,* and it can be observed in the gross by exposing the freshly cut surface of the gland to a weak solution of chrome salts or chromic acid, whereupon the medulla of the gland becomes brown.

The same reaction can be observed in a test tube if the two hormones of the gland are mixed with chrome salts or chromic acid, an indication that the reaction observed in the cells is caused by the presence in the

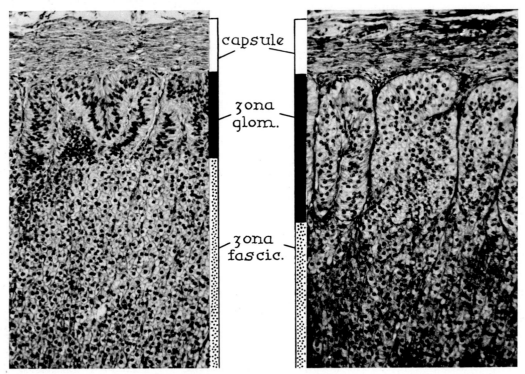

Fig. 25-34. (*Left*) Low-power photomicrograph of a section of the outer part of the cortex of the adrenal gland of a normal dog. (*Right*) Photomicrograph, at the same magnification, of a similar section of the adrenal cortex of a dog that had received several daily injections of an anterior pituitary extract containing adrenocorticotrophin. Observe the great thickening of the zona glomerulosa. High-power inspection shows many mitotic figures in this zone under these conditions.

cells of granules of hormone that are destined for secretion. Although the reaction is called the chromaffin reaction because it was assumed to be due to the granules having a special affinity for chromic acid or chrome salts, it can be produced if other oxidizing agents are used instead of chromic acid.

Development of Knowledge of Function. The medulla is not essential to life. It was the first endocrine gland from which an extract was prepared that was active when it was injected into other animals (Oliver and Schafer, 1894). It was also the first gland from which a pure crystalline hormone was prepared; this was accomplished in 1901. The hormone was named epinephrine. A proprietary name for it is Adrenalin. More than half a century later it was shown that what were believed to be pure extracts of the gland actually contain two substances: epinephrine and norepinephrine (noradrenaline). The two substances have somewhat different effects.

It is not thought that the medulla secretes its two hormones rapidly enough to produce major physiologic effects under ordinary conditions but only under extraordinary conditions. We shall elaborate:

How Secretion by the Medulla Is Affected by Emotional and Physical Stress. As was explained when we dealt with the development of the gland, the parenchymal cells of the adrenal medulla are derived from the same group of cells as those that become the sympathetic ganglion cells of the celiac plexus. However, after migrating into the central part of the adrenal cortex, only a few of them develop into ganglion cells (Figs. 25-32 and 25-35). Most of the young developing cells do not differentiate into ganglion cells proper; instead, they differentiate into secretory cells that are arranged along blood vessels (Fig. 25-35). Nevertheless, they occupy the same position on the 2-neuron sympathetic chains as do the ganglion cells themselves; therefore, they are innervated by *preganglionic* fibers instead of by postganglionic fibers, as are the other types of secretory cells in the body.

From the foregoing it is obvious that, developmentally, the secretory cells of the adrenal medulla and the postganglionic neurons of the sympathetic division of the autonomic nervous system should be very much alike, and it is not surprising that they should function similarly.

Since norepinephrine is secreted at the nerve endings of sympathetic nerve fibers, it seems reasonable to assume that if there were a sudden secretion of medullary hormones, which in man is mostly epinephrine, into the circulation from the secretory cells of the adrenal medulla (which are the counterparts of postganglionic neurons whose nerve endings secrete nor-

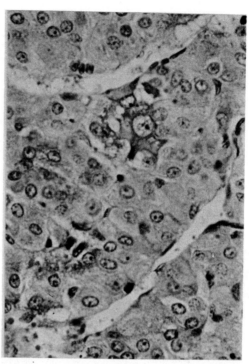

Fig. 25-35. Photomicrograph of H and E section of adrenal medulla. Note the ganglion cell a little above the center. (Photomicrograph by H. Whittaker)

epinephrine), the action of the chemical mediator of the nervous impulse at the sympathetic division released at the terminations of axons of postganglionic fibers of the sympathetic system would be reinforced, and hence it would temporarily dominate the parasympathetic division. When an individual suffers a severe frustration—for example, if he is kept from obtaining something he wants very badly, or prevented from running away from a situation that he considers very dangerous—he may experience an emotional reaction (rage or fear). The development of rage or fear is generally associated with an increase of sympathetic activity over parasympathetic. The increased sympathetic activity results not only in more norepinephrine being produced at sympathetic nerve endings but also in the parenchymal cells of the adrenal medulla, with their very direct sympathetic connections, being stimulated to produce their hormones more rapidly than usual. Enough epinephrine and norepinephrine enter the bloodstream to reinforce the norepinephrine effect at sympathetic nerve endings all over the body.

Both norepinephrine and epinephrine do many things in the body that more or less supercharge it temporarily to help it to fight harder or run away faster. The body becomes geared for "fight or flight."

result of the afferent stimulation involved in severe cold, pain and other stress conditions.

The two hormones of the adrenal medulla, epinephrine (adrenaline) and norepinephrine (noradrenaline) are described chemically as catecholamines or as the catechol hormones because they are amines with a catechol group in their molecular structure. Both act as reducing agents, but norepinephrine forms a darker pigment than epinephrine does when sections are treated with oxidizing agents, and this has led to the finding that the pigment formed in response to oxidizing agents is darker in some cells than in others and hence to the concept that there is specialization in the adrenal medulla, with some cells producing norepinephrine and some, epinephrine.

Chemically, the building block of both hormones is tyrosine. This first becomes converted to dopa (dihydroxyphenylalanine), then to dopamine, and then to norepinephrine. The formation of epinephrine involves the methylation of norepinephrine.

Fine Structure. The most striking feature of the medullary cells is their content of dark granules (Figs. 25-36 and 25-37). Each granule is enclosed by a smooth-surfaced membrane (Fig. 25-38) and is denser in its core than in its periphery. Granules are of an average diameter of about 200 millimicrons. In different cells the number of granules varies somewhat; this is probably due to the fact that cells are in different stages of secretory activity. Another factor accounting for differences in the granules in different cells is that there are two types of cells, one specialized to secrete norepinephrine (Fig. 25-36) and the other specialized to secrete epinephrine (Figs. 25-37 and 25-38). The site of formation of the granules in the cells is complicated because the problem of the formation of these granules is different from that of the synthesis of a protein: granule formation does not involve linking amino acids together in specific sequences, but merely bringing about successive changes in an amino acid. The fact that the granules are enclosed by smooth-surfaced membranes would suggest that a packaging process at least occurs in the Golgi apparatus. Membrane-enclosed granules move to the surface of the cell, where their contents are discharged. Empty membranous shells that are left behind have been seen at the cell membrane. The other features of the cytoplasm are not remarkable. The medullary cells do not have an abundance of rough-surfaced vesicles as would be expected if the cell synthesized protein for secretion. However, they do contain a moderate content of free ribosomes.

Blood Vessels, Lymphatics and Nerves. Usually, each suprarenal gland is supplied by 3 arteries that

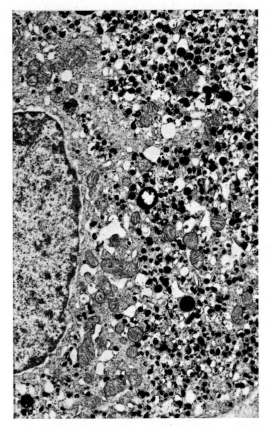

Fig. 25-36. Electron micrograph ($\times$ 9,000) of adrenal medulla of rat, showing part of a cell believed to be of the kind that secretes norepinephrine, which is probably represented by the numerous very dark spherical to oval granules that are loosely enclosed in membranous vesicles in the cytoplasm. Many mitochondria are also present, particularly near the nucleus, which is at the left. (Preparation by Dr. W. R. Lockwood)

The heart beats faster and stronger, the blood pressure becomes increased, and the spleen contracts and adds more blood to the circulatory system. More blood is diverted to striated muscles and less to the viscera. The glycogen of the liver is converted to glucose and liberated into the bloodstream. There are effects on heat production. As will be learned in physiology courses, the effects of the two hormones differ considerably with regard to their affecting the heart rate and increasing the peripheral resistance in the circulatory system, and also in their calorigenic effects and their ability to release sugar into the blood.

An effective secretion of epinephrine and norepinephrine by the cells of the medulla occurs not only in association with emotional states but also reflexly as a

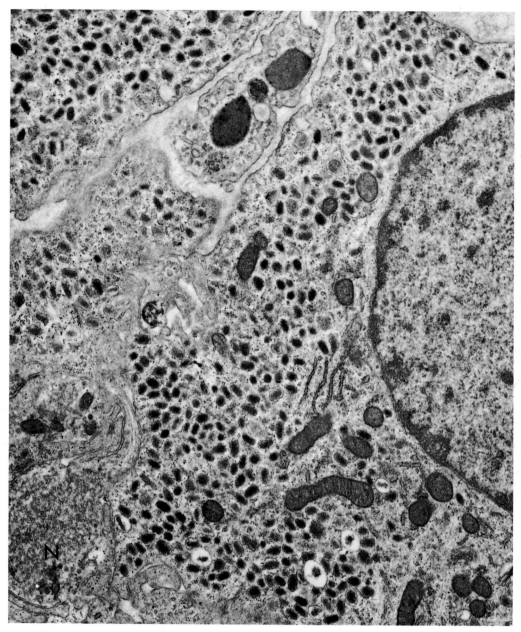

FIG. 25-37. Electron micrograph ($\times$ 18,000) of adrenal medulla of rat, showing cells believed to secrete epinephrine. The granules believed to be epinephrine are less dense than those believed to be norepinephrine and shown in Figure 25-36. Moreover, the epinephrine granules more completely fill the rounded vesicles in which they lie. At the lower left, and labeled N, a nerve ending can be seen.

come from different sources. These break up into many branches as they approach the gland. Some of these supply the capillary beds of the capsule. Others penetrate directly into the medulla to supply the capillary bed of that region with arterial blood. However, the majority empty into the sinusoidal capillaries that run from the zona glomerulosa to the zona reticularis, where they empty into the venous radicles of the medulla. The medullary cells therefore have access to two different types of vessels: the capillaries, which are

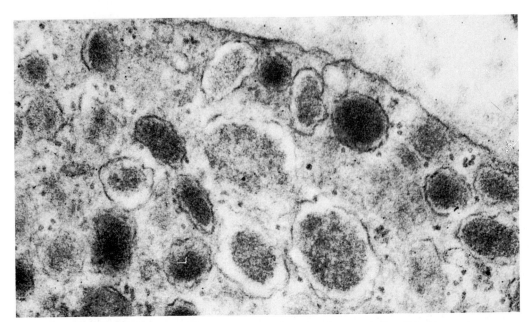

FIG. 25-38. A higher-power electron micrograph showing what are believed to be membrane-enclosed epinephrine granules that are about to be discharged from the cytoplasm. (Preparations by Dr. W. R. Lockwood)

supplied with fresh blood; and the venous radicles that contain blood that has passed along the sinusoidal-like capillaries of the cortex. Both the capillaries and the small venous radicles of the medulla have fenestrated endothelium. It is said that in the zona fasciculata most cells abut on 2 capillaries, one at each of their ends. In ordinary sections, the capillaries of the cortex are often collapsed and hence do not show to advantage.

The capillaries of the medulla also empty into the venous radicles of the part. These unite to form a large central vein which emerges from the hilus of the gland. The central vein has numerous longitudinally disposed smooth muscle fibers in its wall. Veins also arise from the capsule. Lymphatics have been described only where substantial amounts of connective tissue are present in the gland, that is, in association with the larger veins and in the capsule.

Fibers from the parasympathetic system reach the suprarenal gland, but their function, if any, is unknown. Little is known about the functions of the sympathetic fibers that are distributed to the capsule and to the cortex. The significant innervation of the gland is that provided by the preganglionic sympathetic fibers that run directly to the parenchymal cells of the medulla; the chemical mediator here is acetylcholine. True ganglion cells are also present in the medulla (Figs. 25-32 and 25-35).

Paraganglia. The cells of the adrenal medulla, it has been noted, are the result of a migration of developing sympathetic ganglion cells from the site of the developing ganglion to a point some distance from it. This is probably not the only example of the migration of developing sympathetic ganglion cells that occurs, for there are many little clusters of cells that probably originate in the same way to be found behind the peritoneum in various sites. The cells in these little bodies are arranged in clumps and cords and are provided with an extensive blood supply. Since these little bodies are associated with ganglia, they are said to constitute the *paraganglia* of the body. Furthermore, since the cells in these bodies give the chromaffin reactions, the medullary tissue of the adrenal glands and the paraganglia together are often said to constitute the *chromaffin system*.

The Islets of Langerhans

INTRODUCTION

The general features of the islets of Langerhans of the pancreas have already been described (Chapter 22). Here we shall discuss their cells in relation to their internal secretions.

Development of Knowledge. *Diabetes* (*diabetes*, a syphon, or running through) was the name used by the Greeks to designate diseases characterized by a great production of urine (polyuria). In the 18th century it was proved that the urine in most cases of diabetes contained sugar; hence this kind of diabetes was called *diabetes mellitus* (*mellitus,* honeyed) to distinguish it from the other kind (*diabetes insipidus,* described earlier in this chapter) in which polyuria was not associated with glycosuria. It was also realized at this time that it was an ill omen for anyone to begin passing large quantities of sugar-containing urine, for, almost invariably, their health would decline steadily from then on. Many so afflicted literally wasted away, being particularly susceptible while doing so to the development of a great variety of infections and degenerative diseases. Research-minded students may be interested in how progressive steps in the development of knowledge about this condition culminated in replacement therapy that has now saved an incalculable number of lives all over the world.

In 1869 Langerhans discovered the islets in the pancreas that now bear his name. However, he did not suspect that they were little organs of internal secretion. Soon afterward, Kuhne and Lea pointed out that the islets contained extensive capillary networks; this was to help later in making other investigators suspect that they had an endocrine function.

Although Cowley, an English physician, had suggested a full century before that there was some relation between diabetes and the pancreas, it was not until 1889 that this was positively established. At this time, von Mering and Minkowski removed the pancreas from each of a group of experimental animals and found subsequently that the animals upon which they had operated were passing increased amounts of urine, and that it contained sugar. (It has been said that it was noticed that the urine from these dogs attracted large numbers of flies.)

Von Mering's and Minkowski's experiments could be interpreted logically as indicating that a lack of some pancreatic function is responsible for diabetes. But what function? The obvious function of the pancreas known at that time was that of making an external secretion. Nevertheless, the concept of Claude Bernard—that certain bodily functions depend on internal secretions—had by this time made a considerable impression on the scientific world, so further work was done in an attempt to discover whether diabetes results from the pancreas failing to make a proper external or internal secretion. To determine this point, Hedon performed a very ingenious experiment. He showed that a piece of pancreas grafted back into a depancreatized animal would keep the animal free from diabetes even though the graft had no duct connections. In other words, he showed that the anti-

diabetic principle made by the pancreas was absorbed into the blood—it was an internal secretion.

At this time, then, although it was established that diabetes was the result of the lack of an internal secretion, it was not at all clear whether acinous cells or islet cells made the secretion that was secreted into the bloodstream. Indeed, it was not clear whether islet cells were fundamentally different from acinous cells. However, this matter was settled soon afterward by Ssobolew and Schultze. They tied off the pancreatic ducts of experimental animals and found that after a time the acinous tissue of the pancreas all became atrophied, and that only islet tissue was left. Animals that had this operation performed on them, while they suffered from impaired digestion and certain other complaints, did not develop diabetes.

Only one thing more, it appeared, required to be established to lead to the universal acceptance of the islet theory of diabetes: proof that the islets were diseased in those who die of the disease. This was first provided by Opie. At the turn of the century he found that diabetes in most instances was associated with either a lack of islets or with degenerative changes in such islets as were present. It therefore became generally believed that diabetes mellitus was due to the failure of islets to make a hormone, and the as yet theoretical hormone was even given a name—*insulin.*

Two Kinds of Islet Cells Are Discovered. In 1908 Lane, working under the direction of R. R. Bensley, established by histochemical method not only that the granules of islet cells had histochemical properties different from those of zymogen granules (hence, that islet cells were fundamentally different from acinous cells), but also that two kinds of islet cells could be distinguished. He found that certain alcoholic fixatives dissolved the fine cytoplasmic granules from the majority of the cells of the islets but preserved the granules in a minority of the cells. Conversely, fixatives of the same type made up with water instead of alcohol preserved the granules in the majority of the cells but dissolved those from the minority. The numerous cells with the alcohol-soluble granules he termed *beta cells,* and the scarcer ones with alcohol-resistant, water-soluble granules, *alpha cells.* This led to many different staining technics being devised for coloring alpha and beta cells differently (Fig. 25-39).

Although not so common as certain other types of degenerative lesions observed in the islets of diabetics, there was one curious type of islet lesion called hydropic degeneration that was sometimes seen. It was given this name because the cytoplasm of islet cells showing this change appeared to be swollen with a watery fluid and contained little stainable substance

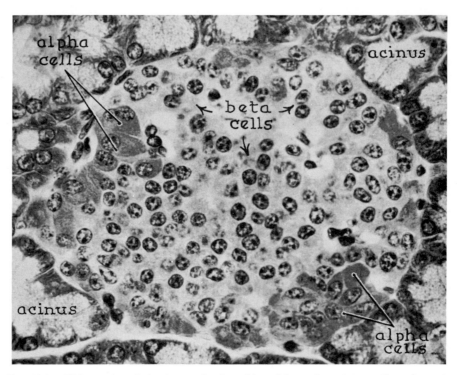

Fɪɢ. 25-39. Oil-immersion photomicrograph of an islet of Langerhans in a section of a guinea pig's pancreas stained by Gomori's method. Alpha cells, with cytoplasm that appears darker than that of the beta cells, may be seen in the periphery of the islet. Most of the interior of the islet is made up of beta cells ranged along capillaries. (Photomicrograph from W. Wilson)

(Fig. 25-40). (More recently, it has been shown that the clear fluid in hydropic beta cells contains a considerable amount of glycogen.) Between 1912 and 1914 both Homans and Allen showed that if most of the pancreas of an animal was removed, and the animal thereafter was fed carbohydrate or protein liberally (1) hydropic degeneration occurred in the islets of the part of the pancreas that had been left intact, and (2) diabetes developed. However, if the animal was given a minimal diet, the islet cells showed no disease, and the animal remained healthy. Using stains based on the findings of Lane and Bensley, both Homans and Allen showed that hydropic degeneration occurred only in the beta cells of the islets, and that this change was preceded by a degranulation of the cells concerned.

These experiments and many others performed by Allen led to the development of what is called the *overwork hypothesis.* Allen showed that if from four fifths to nine tenths of the pancreas were removed from a dog, the remaining portion had enough islets to keep the animal free from diabetes, provided that the dog's diet was restricted. However, he found that if such an animal were fed additional carbohydrate or protein, the beta cells in the fragment of pancreas it possessed would become degranulated and hydropic. He assumed that the extra carbohydrate and protein fed the animals placed increased secretory demands on the beta cells, and that their consequent degranulation and hydropic degeneration were to be interpreted as evidences of exhaustion through overwork. When the increased food intake was continued, he found that the islet lesions became permanent, and that there was no recovery.

The experiments of Allen had, and still have, great implication with regard to the treatment of diabetes. In particular, they have great implication for those who are in danger of developing diabetes, for they show that if any individual overstrains his beta cell capacity by eating too much carbohydrate or protein, beta cells will be destroyed from overwork, and this, of course, will decrease the individual's beta cell capacity and make those that remain more susceptible to overstrain than before.

Although the overwork hypothesis led to better treatment, diabetes remained a widespread and usually fatal disease. It could be expected that many investigators would make attempts to recover the islet hormone from the pancreas of animals so that substitution therapy could be employed in man. Some of these earlier attempts to extract the antidiabetic hormone gave some tantalizingly promising results, but this was as far as they went, and the world remained without substitution therapy for diabetes until the time of Banting and Best.

On the afternoon of October 30, 1920, Banting, then a young medical graduate, read in a medical journal an article about the pancreas in which the findings of Ssobolew and others who had tied off the ducts of the pancreas were described. Banting was very much impressed with the fact that the acinous tissue atrophied after duct ligation, and it is generally believed that he began to suspect that previous attempts to obtain an active extract of islet tissue had failed because the enzymes of the acinous tissue destroyed the islet hormone before it could be extracted. In any event, before going to bed that night he had decided to try making extracts from pancreases after their ducts had been tied off for 6 or 8 weeks so that they presumably would contain only islet and not acinous tissue. The events that occurred between the inception of the idea and the accomplishment of insulin, the collaboration of Best and later of Collip, the inevitable succession of encouraging and discouraging results, the lack of funds and above all the dogged persistence of Banting and finally the emergence of insulin as an effective treatment for diabetes make an inspiring story.

Relation of Other Hormones to Insulin. In 1930, Houssay and Biasotti showed that diabetes produced in animals by removing the pancreas could be ameliorated by removing the pituitary gland as well, and that such animals, instead of declining steadily in health, as do those from which the pancreas only is removed, would live, free from diabetes, for long periods. Some intimation that the pars anterior of the pituitary gland can exert a diabetogenic function had, of course, been given previously by the finding that individuals with certain types of anterior lobe tumors tended to develop diabetes. Furthermore, in 1927, Johns, O'Mulvenny, Potts and Laughton had produced signs of diabetes in dogs by giving them injections of anterior pituitary extract. By 1932 several investigators had also observed this phenomenon. However, one group of investigators, Evans and his collaborators, noted something additional. Whereas all the others had noted signs of diabetes only while injections were continued, Evans and his group observed that two animals continued to have diabetes after the course of injections of anterior pituitary had been finished. One animal recovered after 2 months, but the second was

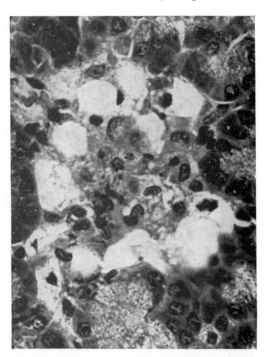

FIG. 25-40. Oil-immersion photomicrograph of an islet of Langerhans in a section of pancreas of a dog that had been given 11 daily injections of anterior pituitary extract that exerted a diabetogenic effect. The beta cells contain large droplets of fluid. This histologic picture is called hydropic degeneration and is an indication of severe overwork on the part of the beta cells. (Ham, A. W., and Haist, R. E.: Am. J. Path., *17*:812)

still diabetic 4 months after the last injection. The importance of this finding was not realized until Young, in 1937, showed that a sufficiently prolonged course of injections of anterior pituitary extract would make dogs permanently diabetic. Richardson and Young made histologic studies of the islets of these dogs. In some islets they found histologic pictures similar to those observed in long-standing cases of diabetes in man; in others they found degranulation and hydropic degeneration of beta cells and, in some, mitotic figures. Subsequently, the author and Haist showed that anterior pituitary injections given daily to dogs caused a progressive degranulation of beta cells, and that this was followed by hydropic degeneration, usually between the 7th and the 11th days (Fig. 25-40). The similarity between the findings with anterior pituitary extracts and those observed by Allen after partial pancreatectomy and liberal feeding was so obvious it was realized that anterior pituitary extracts somehow cause beta cells to overwork to the point of exhaustion and death.

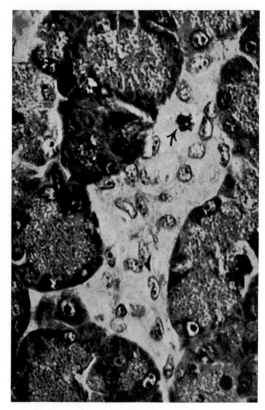

FIG. 25-41. High-power photomicrograph of an islet of Langerhans in a section of pancreas from a dog which had been given 11 daily injections of a diabetogenic anterior pituitary extract and, in addition, enough insulin to protect the beta cells from becoming hydropic from overwork. Observe the mitotic figure in a beta cell.

Crude anterior pituitary hormones contain several trophic hormones as well as growth hormone. Anterior pituitary extracts containing adrenocorticotrophic hormone stimulate the adrenal cortex to make more of the cortical hormone that furthers the conversion of protein and protein precursors to sugar in the body. Long and Lukens and their collaborators demonstrated the effectiveness of the diabetogenic effect of this cortical hormone. In addition, anterior pituitary extracts, by their TSH content, stimulate the thyroid gland; this also increases the need of the animal for insulin. Furthermore, there is evidence that the anterior pituitary extracts act in some manner to render insulin relatively ineffective. Furthermore, in addition to all the other effects they produce, anterior pituitary extracts stimulate cell division in the acini, the small ducts and the islets (Fig. 25-41) in the pancreas. It seems most probable that the chief diabetogenic factor made by the anterior pituitary gland is the growth hormone. One gets the impression that anterior pituitary extracts contain something that activates beta cells in some direct way so that they become exhausted more easily under pituitary stimulation than they would in the absence of anterior pituitary stimulation. In other words, there is some suspicion that some hormone in crude anterior pituitary extracts has a pancreatrophic action.

The foregoing indicates that many diabetogenic influences are normally at work in the body, and that they do not produce diabetes because they are opposed successfully by adequate amounts of the antidiabetogenic hormone, insulin, made by the beta cells of the islets. Diabetes develops when the diabetogenic influences are greater than the beta cell potential of the pancreas.

THE ACTION OF INSULIN

In a normal individual on a normal diet the amount of sugar in the blood remains at a fairly constant level, varying between 0.08 and 0.11 percent. Since it is dissolved in the blood plasma, sugar in this concentration is present in the glomerular filtrate. However, at this concentration, all the sugar in the filtrate can be resorbed as the filtrate passes along the remainder of the nephron. Hence, in a normal individual on a normal diet sugar does not appear in the urine. However, in an untreated diabetic the blood sugar rises above the normal level (*hyperglycemia*) to the point at which the increased amounts in the glomerular filtrate cannot all be resorbed as it courses along the remainder of the nephron; hence sugar appears in the urine (*glycosuria*). The point at which the kidney cannot resorb all the sugar filtered through its glomeruli is said to be its *threshold* for sugar.

The most obvious action of insulin is that it reduces the blood sugar level. It will do this if it is injected either into a diabetic with hyperglycemia or into a normal person. A sufficiently large dose of insulin will reduce the blood sugar level to the point at which convulsions and unconsciousness occur. This is called insulin shock. Enough insulin can lower the blood sugar level to the point at which death ensues. A certain amount of sugar is required in the blood if life is to be supported. Occasionally islet-cell tumors occur; these may cause hyperinsulinism and hypoglycemia.

Insulin acts to lower the blood sugar level by acting at several sites. In a normal individual the sugar absorbed from a hearty meal would raise the blood sugar level substantially were it not for the fact that some of the sugar taken into the blood is stored as glycogen in the parenchymal cells of the liver and in muscle cells. Insulin facilitates this storage phenomenon. Excess sugar that has been absorbed may also be removed from the blood by being converted into fat and stored in the fat depots. Insulin facilitates this change also. Then insulin, in addition, facilitates the metabolism of carbohydrate in muscle cells. In this way it tends to reduce the level of sugar in the blood by speeding up the utilization of carbohydrate. Finally, as has been noted before, insulin opposes the catabolic and antianabolic effects of adrenal cortical hormone.

BETA CELLS

Storage of Insulin. Under normal conditions, only about 1 to 2 days' supply of insulin is stored in the cytoplasm of the beta cells of the pancreas. However, this is an amount sufficient, or almost sufficient, to cause death if it were all discharged into the bloodstream at once. Indeed, a phenomenon much like this actually occurs if an animal is given suitable amounts of alloxan. This chemical exerts a very specific and rapid lethal effect on the beta cells of the islets (Fig. 4-12, *right*). As soon as they are destroyed, their content of stored insulin is almost immediately washed into the bloodstream, and unless sugar is given the animals at this time, they may die of hypoglycemia. If the animal survives this preliminary hypoglycemia, it goes on, of course, to develop hyperglycemia.

Granule Content Seen With the LM. The cytoplasmic granules appear as very fine blue granules in sections stained by Bowie's neutral ethyl violet–Biebrich scarlet stain. Their numbers appear to be representative of the insulin content of the cell. With Haist, we have observed that the number of beta granules revealed by this method become reduced if animals are starved, given insulin or fed a high proportion of fat. Obviously, the reduction in the number of granules under these circumstances is not the result of degranulation from overwork but, instead, to a lack of synthesis due to a lack of work stimulus. Therefore, a reduction in the granule content of beta cells can be caused either by overwork or underwork.

Fine Structure. The mitochondria of both beta and alpha cells are fine in contrast with the coarser ones of acinar cells. Islet cells have Golgi nets in their cytoplasm; these are present between the nuclei of the cells and the surfaces of the cells through which secretion takes place. Well-defined negative Golgi images can be seen with the LM in cells that are actively secreting.

The capillaries of islets are of the fenestrated type. There is a basement membrane around each but there is a minimum of connective tissue to support them; if there were more it would impede their secreting into the capillaries. There is some reason to believe that an increase in pericapillary connective tissue as a result of injury to islets, at least in certain experimental conditions, hinders the delivery of insulin into the capillaries.

The granules of the beta cells differ in different species.

In the rat and the mouse they are round and homogeneous and enclosed in smooth-surfaced membranous vesicles. However, they can be distinguished from alpha granules because they, in contrast with alpha granules, do not, generally, completely fill the membranous vesicles in which they lie; hence, a space can be seen between the edges of beta granules and the membranous vesicles that contain them.

In the dog beta granules often appear as rectangular crystalloid structures. The platelike granules do not fill the rounded membranous vesicles which contain them; hence a comparatively large space can be seen between the long surfaces of the granules and the rounded vesicles in which they lie. In the cat, also, the beta granules have a crystalloid appearance; but in this species the central part of each granule contains a dense rhomboidal or prismatic structure.

In the guinea pig the beta granules have a rounded shape (Fig. 25-42).

In man the beta granules vary from being round to crystalloid in appearance. Here, again, the beta granules, whatever their shape, tend to be withdrawn from the membranous vesicles in which they are contained.

Insulin is a protein which is secreted by the beta cells that produce it. It might therefore be expected that the cells that synthesize and secrete it would have well-developed rough-surfaced vesicles of endoplasmic reticulum and a well-developed Golgi apparatus. However, rough-surfaced vesicles do not appear to advantage in the cytoplasm of beta cells that are well filled with granules. On the other hand, it is easy to find some cells in islets that have cytoplasm that has a great content of rough-surfaced vesicles and few granules (Fig. 25-42). Herman, Sato and Fitzgerald suggest that beta cells pass through two stages, one in which there is much rough-surfaced endoplasmic reticulum, and during which insulin is being synthesized, and then a second stage in which secretion is delivered into the bloodstream.

The material synthesized in the rER is probably proinsulin, which acts more slowly than insulin in reducing blood sugar levels. Normally it is packaged and modified in the Golgi from which it buds off in the form of secretory vesicles which under normal conditions contain insulin. These vesicles are termed granules when seen in sections. The way they are released

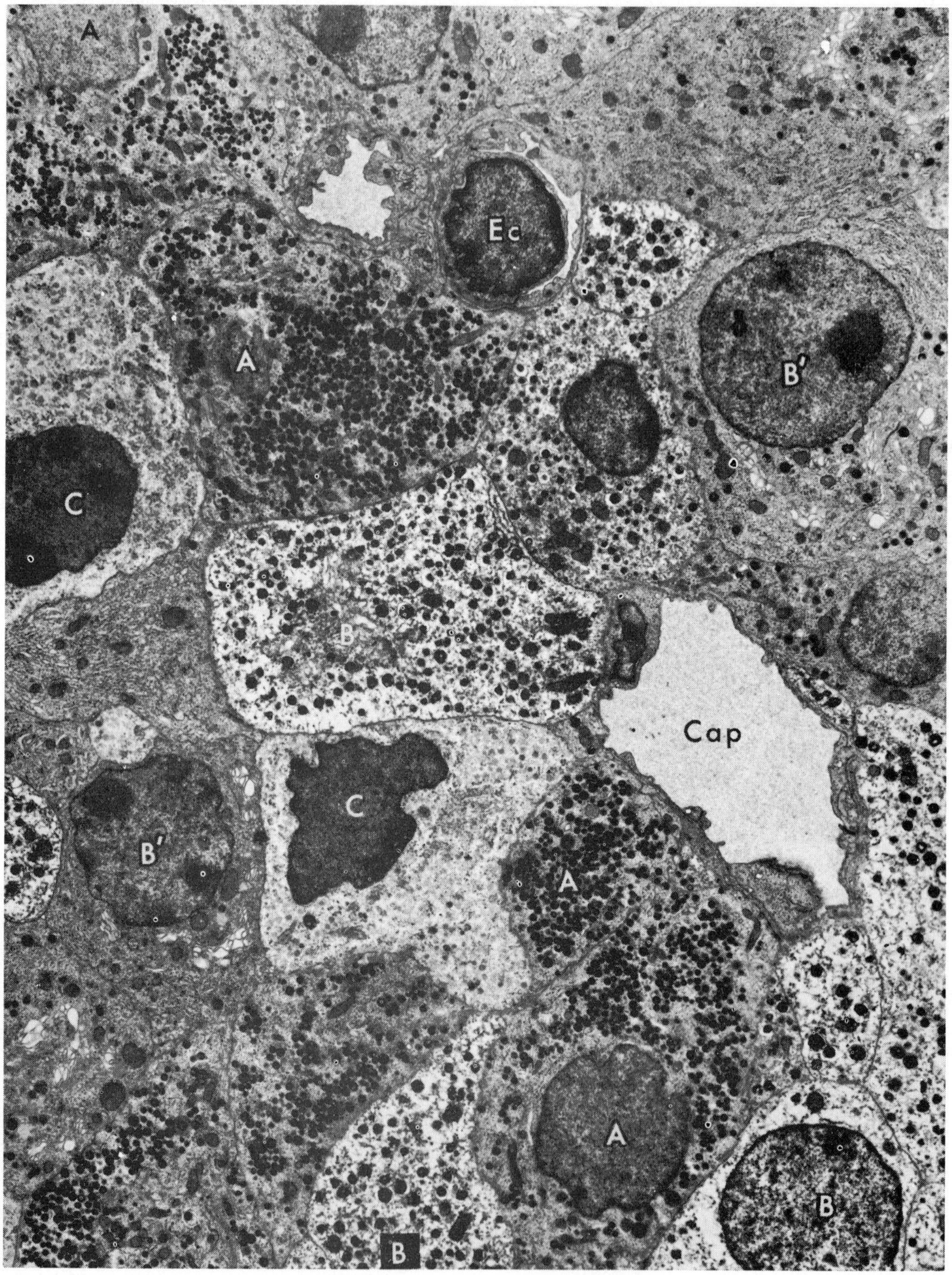

Fig. 25-42. Electron micrograph ($\times$ 3,000) of an islet of Langerhans in a guinea pig, showing alpha cells containing alpha granules (A), beta cells filled with granules (B), beta cells in the stage of synthesizing insulin (B'), a chromophobe (C), a capillary (Cap), and another capillary in which the nucleus of an endothelial cell is present in the section (Ec). (Preparation from L. Herman)

is probably the same as that described for the granules of the secretory cells of the anterior pituitary. Under certain conditions beta cells may secrete proinsulin as such.

Problem of Beta Cell Regeneration. Most diabetics will remain diabetic until someone discovers some way to make their beta cells regenerate. In this sense the cause of persisting diabetes is the inability of the beta cells of the pancreas to regenerate under the stimulus of function. How to induce beta cells to regenerate, or how to induce the ductules of the pancreas to produce beta cells, is a challenging problem for the research worker. The situation is not as hopeless as is the case of neurons, for beta cells can undergo mitosis (see Fig. 25-41).

Control of Insulin Secretion. There is much evidence to show that insulin secretion tends to vary in relation to the blood sugar level and that the blood sugar level controls insulin secretion.

Alpha and Other Islet Cells

Alpha Cells As Seen With the LM. The cytoplasmic granules of alpha cells are larger than those of beta cells. Thus alpha cells can be distinguished from beta cells by several staining methods. Gormori's method is excellent for this purpose (Fig. 25-39). A course of injections of a diabetogenic extract of the anterior pituitary gland, which will cause degranulation of the beta cells, does not commonly cause degranulation of the alpha cells.

In some species—for example, the rat—the alpha cells tend to have a peripheral distribution in islets. In other species, including man and the dog, the alpha cells are scattered throughout the islets but generally show some tendency to form little groups in the more central parts of islets.

The nuclei of alpha and beta cells are different in some species—for example, the guinea pig—but not in most species. Hence alpha and beta cells cannot generally be distinguished in sections by the morphology of their nuclei.

By means of special staining technics, cells that have been termed delta cells and C cells have been demonstrated in the islets of animals of some species. These cells are not numerous, and their functions are unknown.

Fine Structure of Granules of Alpha Cells. The granules of alpha cells are similar in different species, being round, dense and homogeneous, and filling the membranous vesicles in which they lie (Fig. 25-42, *bottom*).

Alpha Cells and Glucagon. It is difficult to know how alpha cells are related to beta cells. They both arise from the same stem cell in fetal development. In some animals (rats) beta cells develop first; in others (rabbits) alpha cells develop first. Alpha cells appear to be unaffected when diabetes is produced by partial pancreatectomy, anterior pituitary extracts or alloxan. Islets composed only of alpha cells may be encountered in the pancreas of diabetics.

It was noticed that sometimes the insulin requirement of an animal in which the beta cells had been destroyed seemed to be greater than that of an animal from which the entire pancreas had been removed. This finding suggested that the pancreas makes some hormone that has an action opposite to that of insulin and raises the blood sugar level. A substance called *glucagon*, which raises blood sugar levels, was then found in certain pancreatic extracts. Much evidence has now been obtained which indicates that the alpha cells produce glucagon; for example, Bencosme has shown that it is not present in extracts of pancreas that have no alpha cells. Glucagon has been shown to cause glucose to be released from the liver into the blood and its secretion is stimulated by low blood sugar levels. It also affects protein and fat metabolism. Its role in the body is not understood as well as that of most hormones.

Nervous Control of Islet Cells. The extent to which islet cell secretion is affected by the autonomic nervous system—and, hence, by severe emotional states—has not been worked out as satisfactorily as might be wished, but there is some indication that the autonomic system may be involved. It has been shown that there are intimate associations between islet cells and ganglion cells in the pancreas. These little aggregates are termed *neuro-insular complexes* (Fig. 25-43). They have been studied by Simard, whose papers should be consulted for further details of their microscopic structure.

The Pineal Body

The pineal body, also called the epiphysis, is a little cone-shaped body about 1 cm. in length. Although it originates from, and remains connected to, the posterior end of the roof of the third ventricle, it projects backward so that it lies dorsal to the midbrain.

Its development begins early in embryonic life. At this time the roof of the diencephalon behind the site of the origin of the chloroid plexus of the third ventricle bulges dorsally as a diverticulum. As development proceeds, the walls of the diverticulum thicken

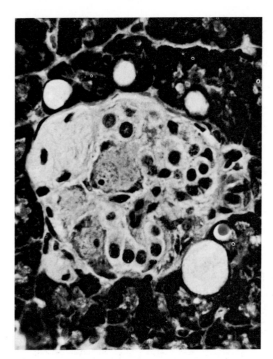

Fig. 25-43. High-power photomicrograph of a section of a rat's pancreas, showing a neuro-insular complex. Note the large ganglion cells in association with islet cells. (Dr. W. S. Hartroft)

a vestigial organ, that is, as the remnant of a structure which in a previous stage of species or individual development served some particular purpose, but which in postnatal life serves no important function. More or less in keeping with this hypothesis is the fact that the pineal body in man reaches its greatest development in childhood, after which it begins and continues to involute. This concept is also supported by the fact that concretions of calcified material called *brain sand* progressively accumulate in it, and the deposition of calcified material in soft tissue is generally regarded as an indication of degenerative change (Fig. 25-44).

In recent years, however, the development of knowledge in other areas—for example, about the chemical mediators of the nervous impulse, neurosecretions and releasing factors—together with the application of the technics of radioautography and electron microscopy to the direct study of the pineal body, have aroused interest in the possibility that the pineal body may serve some function in mammals, and this in turn has generated research activity in this area. One observation in particular has suggested the possibility of function. It has been shown that the pineal takes up radioactive phosphorus faster than any other part of the brain; the high metabolic rate thus indicated suggests that at least it is not a dormant tissue. Before discussing possible functions, we shall first deal with the structure of the two main types of cells that it contains.

Pinealocytes. These are the commonest cells seen in the pineal when a section is viewed with the LM. They are relatively large and are often grouped together in clumps. Their nuclei are large, and have only a moderate amount of condensed chromatin so that their large nucleoli are easily seen (Fig. 25-45). Their cytoplasm contains some clumps of basophilic material which has been shown to dissolve under the influence of RNAase.

The cytoplasm of pinealocytes extends off from their cell bodies in the form of processes; these are very extensive. Furthermore, as we shall see, the cytoplasm of the glial cells also extends off from their cell bodies in the form of processes. Accordingly, the substance of the pineal body in many sites consists of an entanglement of the cell bodies and intertwining processes of pinealocytes and glial cells. The processes stained by iron hematoxylin and seen with the LM in Figure 25-45 cannot be distinguished as belonging to one kind of cell or the other. The point to make here is that the processes of both are extensive, and they intertwine in a remarkable manner.

With the EM the cytoplasm of the pinealocytes reveals the usual organelles, mitochondria, centrioles, a Golgi complex, some dense bodies which are probably

so that the lumen of the outgrowth is gradually obliterated. In postnatal life a lumen is to be seen only at the base of the pineal body, where it is called the pineal recess of the third ventricle.

The outgrowth of the roof of the diencephalon that gives rise to the pineal body contains two types of cells. First, the roof itself contains neuro-ectodermal cells; second, the pia mater, which covers the outgrowth, contains mesenchymal cells. Both types of cell participate in the formation of the pineal body. The neuro-ectodermal cells give rise to parenchymal cells which are termed pinealocytes and also to cells which are generally considered to be glial cells. The mesenchymal cells give rise to the connective tissue of the capsule of the body and to the incomplete partitions of connective tissue that more or less divide the body up into lobules.

On viewing a section of the pineal body, lobules of pinealocytes and glial cells may be seen to be incompletely separated from one another by septa of connective tissue that extend into the body from the capsule and carry blood vessels and nerves into the substance of the gland; some of these irregular partitions can be seen in Figure 25-44. Until relatively recently, the pineal body of the mammal was generally regarded as

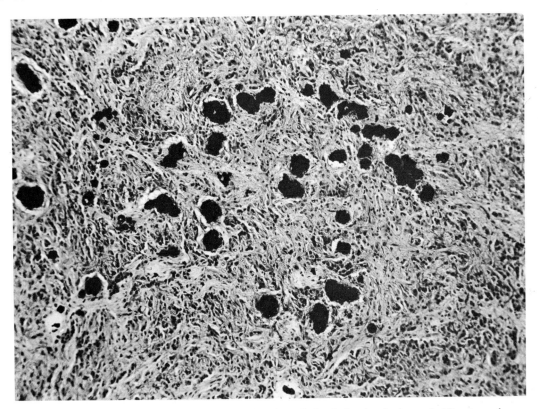

FIG. 25-44. Low-power photomicrograph of section of pineal showing brain sand. (Courtesy of Everett Anderson)

lysosomes, some vesicles of smooth endoplasmic reticulum and some ribosomes arranged as polyribosomes. However, an unusual feature of the cytoplasm is the presence of numerous microtubules (Fig. 25-46). These are from 220 to 300 Å in diameter and of indefinite length. With suitable staining and the best of resolution these can be shown to show a cross striated or beaded appearance. In the cell bodies the microtubules are randomly disposed, but in the processes of the pinealocytes they mostly run parallel to the process. The processes end on the borders of other pinealocytes, on glial cells and at blood vessels.

Glial Cells. With the LM these are recognized fairly readily by their nuclei, which are more flattened and have more of their chromatin condensed than the nuclei of pinealocytes. Some have more or less of a triangular shape (Fig. 25-47). Often 2 or 3 are seen close together. Their cytoplasm is more basophilic than that of pinealocytes.

With the EM the glial cells reveal the usual organelles, including some microtubules, but not so many as are in pinealocytes. The most striking feature of their cytoplasm, however, is its extensive content of fine filaments that are 50 to 60 Å in diameter and commonly arranged in bundles (Fig. 25-47). Filaments such as these are not seen in pinealocytes. The filaments in the processes of the glial cells run parallel to the processes and they insert, as do the tonofibrils of epithelial cells, in attachment plaques at cell membranes. Another way the cytoplasmic organelles of pinealocytes and glial cells differ is that the mitochondria of the glial cells have a much denser matrix than those of pinealocytes. The processes of the glial cells end mostly as bulbous expansions on pinealocytes, other glial cells, or on the cells lining perivascular spaces. Their endings sometimes contain much glycogen.

POSSIBLE FUNCTIONS

The pineal has been investigated by removing the pineal body from young animals, and by grafting a series of pineal transplants into an animal. Various types of extracts made from pineal bodies have been fed or injected into animals. The effects of pineal tumors on men and women have been noted. Biochemi-

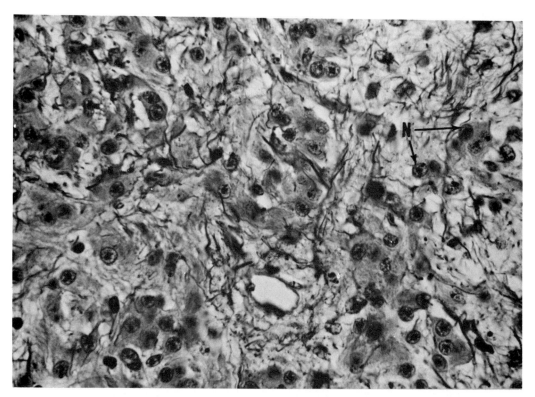

FIG. 25-45. Photomicrograph ($\times$ 500) of section of bovine pineal stained with Heidenhain's iron hematoxylin and showing pinealocytes which have relatively large nuclei (N) and prominent nucleoli. Many densely stained processes can be seen, but it is not possible to tell in this type of preparation whether they belong to the pinealocytes or the glial cells. (Anderson, Everett: J. Ultrastruct. Res.: Supplement 8, May, 1965)

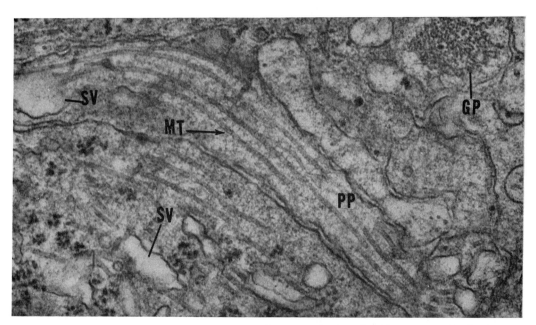

FIG. 25-46. Electron micrograph ($\times$ 76,000) of a longitudinal section of a process of a bovine pinealocyte showing microtubules (MT) and some smooth-surfaced vesicles (SV). Some poly-ribosomes (unlabeled) are evident at the lower left. The process of a glial cell is seen at GP. Material fixed in glutaraldehyde and osmium and stained with uranyl acetate and lead citrate. (Anderson, Everett: J. Ultrastruct. Res: Supplement 8, May, 1965)

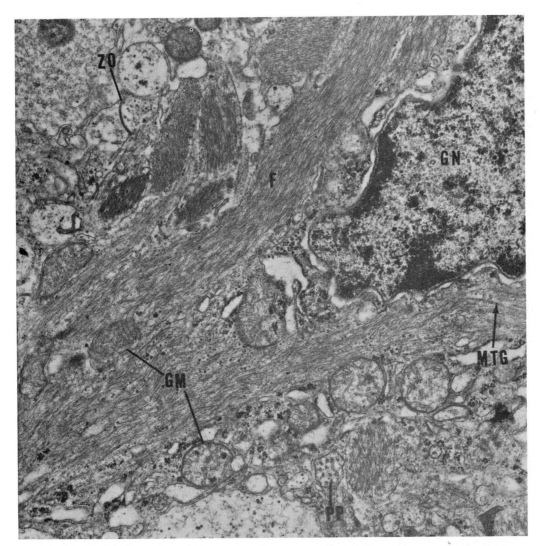

Fig. 25-47. Electron micrograph (× 30,000) of a section of bovine pineal showing part of a glial cell. The somewhat flattened nucleus (GN) is at upper right. Note the bundles of fine filaments (F) in the cytoplasm. A few microtubules are seen (MTG). Mitochondria are labeled GM; note that they possess a very dense matrix. PP indicates the cross section of the process of a pineal-ocyte. ZO indicates a tight junction between the surfaces of the processes of two glial cells. (Anderson, Everett: J. Ultrastruct. Res.: Supplement 8, May, 1965)

cal assays have been made on pineal preparations. The net result of all this study is difficult to assess.

There seems to be some evidence to suggest that there may be some association between the sexual development and the pineal body in the male in that the pineal seem to have some function that inhibits the anterior pituitary gland from secreting gonadotrophic hormone prematurely. However, the nature and significance of this association is still obscure.

Giving pineal extracts to invertebrates affects their ability to react by color changes to light. It might therefore be questioned if some product of the pineal gland in invertebrates has an effect on melanocytes. In this connection a substance called *melatonin* has been extracted from ox pineal glands and has been shown to cause the opposite of the dispersion of pigment in melanocytes that is effected by MSH in frogs. The pineal extract causes the pigment of melanocytes to congregate around their nuclei (MSH causes it to disperse). However, there are other substances (for example, the catechol hormones) that act similarly but not so profoundly, and hence it is difficult to know if these findings are in any way indicative of any normal function of the pineal gland in this respect in mammals.

Nerve Supply. The pineal is well supplied with nerves which enter the gland via the trabeculae. Fibers penetrate into the substance of the gland, and nerve endings have been seen in association with pinealocytes, glial cells and capillaries. Vesicles can be seen in nerve endings, but no cholesterinase activity has as yet been demonstrated in association with the endings. Because of the origin of the pinealocytes and the abundant nerve supply of the pineal, with endings that terminate in association with cells, it might be thought that if the pineal has any function, it would be something of the nature of a neurohormone.

For those who wish details, a most comprehensive account of the microscopic structure of the pineal at the level of both the LM and, in particular, the EM is to be found in the monograph by Everett Anderson.

References and Other Reading

The Hypophysis: The Pituitary Gland as a Whole

Atwell, W. J.: The development of the hypophysis cerebri in man with special reference to the pars tuberalis. Am. J. Anat., *37:*159, 1926.

Daniel, P. M.: The anatomy of the hypothalamus and pituitary gland. *In* Martini, L., and Ganong, W. F. (eds.): Neuroendocrinology. vol. 1, p. 15. New York, Academic Press, 1966.

Ezrin, C.: The pituitary gland. Ciba Clin. Symp. *15:*71, 1963.

————: Chapters 1-4. *In* Ezrin, C., Godden, J. O., Volpé, R., and Wilson, R. (eds.): Systemic Endocrinology. Hagerstown, Maryland, Harper and Row, 1973.

Ganong, W. F., and Martini, L. (eds.): Frontiers in Neuroendocrinology. New York, Oxford University Press, 1969.

Green, J. D.: The histology of the hypophyseal stalk and medium eminence in man, with special reference to blood vessels, nerve fibers and a peculiar neurovascular zone in this region. Anat. Rec., *100:*273, 1948.

————: The comparative anatomy of the hypophysis with special reference to its blood supply and innervation. Am. J. Anat., *88:*225, 1951.

————: The comparative anatomy of the portal vascular system and of the innervation of the hypophysis. *In* Harris, G. W., and Donovan, B. T. (eds.): The Pituitary Gland. vol. 1, p. 127. Berkeley, University of California Press, 1966.

Green, J. D., and Harris, G. W.: Observation of the hypophysioportal vessels of the living rat. J. Physiol., *108:*359, 1949.

Green, J. D., and van Breemen, V. L.: Electron microscopy of the pituitary and observations on neurosecretion. Am. J. Anat., *97:*177, 1955.

von Lawzewitsch, I., and Sarrat, R.: Comparative anatomy and the evolution of the neurosecretory hypothalamic-hypophyseal system. Acta anat., *81:*13, 1972.

Wislocki, G. B.: The meningeal relations of the hypophysis cerebri. II. An embryological study of the meninges and blood vessels of the human hypophysis. Am. J. Anat., *61:*95, 1937.

————: The vascular supply of the hypophysis cerebri of the rhesus monkey and man. Proc. A. Res. Nerv. Ment. Dis., *17:*48, 1938.

The Anterior Lobe and Its Relation to the Hypothalamus

Bain, J., and Ezrin, C.: Immunofluorescent localization of the LH cell of the human adenohypophysis. J. Clin. Endocrinol., *30:*181, 1970.

Burgers, A. C. J.: Melanophore-stimulating hormones in vertebrates. Ann. N.Y. Acad. Sci., *100:*669, 1963.

Ezrin, C.: The Hypophysis, the Pineal Gland. *In* Netter, F. H. (ed.): The Ciba Collection of Medical Illustrations. vol. 4, Endocrine System and Selected Metabolic Diseases. p. 3. Summit, N.J. Ciba, 1965.

Ezrin, C., and Murray, S.: The cells of the human adenohypophysis in pregnancy, thyroid disease and adrenal cortical disorders. Colloques Internationaux du Centre National de la Recherche Scientifique, vol. 15, 1963.

Farquhar, M. G.: Fine structure and function in capillaries of the anterior pituitary gland. Angiology, *12:*270, 1961.

————: Processing of secretory products by cells of the anterior pituitary gland. Mem. Soc. Endocrinol., 19, Subcellular Organization and Function. *In* Heller, H., and Lederis, K. (eds.): Endocrine Tissues. London, Cambridge University Press, 1971.

Fortier, C.: Hypothalamic control of anterior pituitary. Comp. Endocrinol., *1:*1, 1963.

Guillemin, R., and Burgus, R.: The hormones of the hypothalamus. Sci. Am., *227:*24, 1972.

Halmi, N. S.: Two types of basocells in the rat pituitary, thyrotrophs and gonadotrophs vs. beta and delta cells. Endocrinology, *50:*140, 1952.

Halmi, N. S., McCormick, W. F., and Decker, D. A., Jr.: The natural history of hyalinization of ACTH-MSH cells in man. Arch. Path., *91:*318, 1971.

Harris, G. W.: Neural Control of the Pituitary Gland. London, Edward Arnold, 1955.

Herlant, M.: The cells of the adenohypophysis and their functional significance. Int. Rev. Cytol., *17:* 1964.

Hymer, W. C., and McShan, W. H.: Isolation of rat pituitary granules and the study of their biochemical properties and hormonal activities. J. Cell Biol., *17:*67, 1963.

von Lawzewitsch, I., Dickmann, G. H., Amezúa, L., and Pardal, C.: Cytological and ultrastructural characterization of the human pituitary. Acta anat. *81:*286, 1972.

Lee, T. H., and Lerner, A. B.: Isolation of melanocyte-stimulating hormone from hog pituitary gland. J. Biol. Chem., *221:*943, 1956.

Lerner, A. B., and Takahashi, Y.: Hormonal control of melanin pigmentation. Recent Progr. Hormone Res., *12:*203, 1956.

Pearse, A. G. E.: Observations on the localisation, nature and chemical constitution of some components of the anterior hypophysis. J. Path. Bact., *64:*791, 1952.

Purves, H. D.: Cytology of the adenohypophysis. *In* Harris, G. W., and Donovan, B. T. (eds.): The Pituitary Gland, vol. 1, p. 147. Berkeley, University of California Press, 1966.

Purves, H. D., and Griesbach, W. E.: The significance of the Gomori staining of the basophiles of the rat pituitary. Endocrinology, *49:*652, 1951.

Rinehart, J. F., and Farquhar, M. G.: The fine vascular organization of the anterior pituitary gland. Anat. Rec., *121:*207, 1955.

Salazar, H., and Peterson, R. R.: Morphologic observations concerning the release and transport of secretory products in the adenohypophysis. Am. J. Anat., *115:*199, 1964.

Siperstein, E., Nichols, C. W., Jr., Griesbach, W. E., and Chaikoff, I. L.: Cytological changes in the rat anterior pituitary from birth to maturity. Anat. Rec., *118:*593, 1954.

Wilson, W. D., and Ezrin, C.: Three types of chromophil cells of the adenohypophysis. Am. J. Path., *30:*891, 1954.

THE POSTERIOR LOBE—THE NEUROHYPOPHYSIS

Bargmann, W.: Neurosecretion. Int. Rev. Cytol., *19:*183, 1966.

Bargmann, W., and Scharrer, E.: The site of origin of the hormones of the posterior pituitary. Am. Sci., *39:*255, 1951.

Barrington, E. J. W.: An Introduction to General and Comparative Endocrinology. Chapter II. Oxford, Clarendon Press, 1963.

Bodian, D.: Nerve endings, neurosecretory substance and lobular organization of the neurohypophysis. Bull. Johns Hopkins Hosp., *33:*354, 1951.

————: Herring bodies and neuroapocrine secretion in the monkey. An electron microscope study of the fate of the neurosecretory product. Bull. Johns Hopkins Hosp., *118:*282, 1966.

Duncan, D.: An electron microscope study of the neurohypophysis of a bird, Gallus domesticus. Anat. Rec., *125:*457, 1956.

Palay, S. L.: Neurosecretory phenomena in the hypothalamo-hypophyseal system of man and monkey. Am. J. Anat., *93:*107, 1953.

————: An electron microscope study of the neurohypophysis in normal, hydrated and dehydrated rats. Anat. Rec., *121:*348, 1955.

————: The fine structure of the neurohypophysis. *In* Waelsch, H. (ed.): Progress in Neurobiology. II. Ultrastructure and Cellular Chemistry of Neural Tissue. p. 31. New York, Paul B. Hoeber, 1957.

Rennels, E. G., and Drager, G. A.: The relationship of pituicytes to neurosecretion. Anat. Rec., *122:*193, 1955.

Sawyer, W. H.: Neurohypophyseal hormones. Pharmacol. Rev., *13:*225, 1961.

Scharrer, B.: Neurohumors and Neurohormones: Definitions and Terminology. J. Neuro-Visc. Rel. (Suppl. 9):1, 1969.

Scharrer, E., and Scharrer, B.: *In* Handbuch der mikroskopischen Anatomie des Menschen. vol. 6, p. 953. Berlin, Springer-Verlag, 1954.

————: Neurosecretion. Physiol. Rev., *25:*171, 1945.

————: Neurosecretion. Recent Progr. Hormone Res., *10:*183, 1954.

Scharrer, E. A., and Wittenstein, G. J.: The effect of the interruption of the hypothalamo-hypophyseal neurosecretory pathway in the dog. Anat. Rec., *112:*387, 1952.

THE THYROID GLAND: FOLLICULAR CELLS

General

Werner, S. C., and Ingbar, S. (eds.): The Thyroid, A Fundamental and Clinical Text. ed. 3. New York, Harper, 1971.

Special

Axelrad, A. A., Leblond, C. P., and Isler, H.: Role of iodine deficiency in the production of goiter by the Remington diet. Endocrinology, *56:*387, 1955.

Bowers, C. Y., Schally, A. V., Reynolds, G. A., and Hawley, W. D.: Interactions of L-thyroxine of L-triiodothyronine and thyrotrophin-releasing factor on the release and synthesis of thyrotrophin from the anterior pituitary gland of mice. Endocrinology, *81:*741, 1967.

Brookhaven Symposia in Biology No. 7. The Thyroid. Upton, N.Y., Brookhaven National Laboratory, 1955.

Follis, R. H., Jr.: Experimental colloid goiter in the hamster. Proc. Soc. Exp. Biol. Med., *100:*203, 1959.

Gross, J.: Thyroid hormones. Brit. Med. Bull., *10:*218, 1954.

————: The dynamic cytology of the thyroid gland. Int. Rev. Cytol., vol. 6, 1957.

Marine, D., *et al.:* The relation of iodine to the structure of the thyroid gland. Ann. Intern. Med., *1:*349, 1908.

Nadler, N. J.: Synthesis and release of thyroid hormones. Fed. Proc., *21:*628, 1962.

————: Anatomy of the thyroid gland. *In* Werner, S. (ed.): The Thyroid. ed. 3. New York, Harper & Row, 1969.

Nadler, N. J., Young, B. A., Leblond, C. P., and Mitmaker, B.: Elaboration of thyroglobulin in the thyroid follicle. Endocrinology, *74:*333, 1964.

Pitt-Rivers, R., and Tata, J. R.: The Thyroid Hormones. 2 vols. International Series of Monographs on Pure and Applied Biology. London, Permagon Press, 1959.

Podoba, J., and Langer, P. (eds.): Naturally Occurring Goitrogens and Thyroid Function. Symp. Czechoslovak Acad. Sci. Bratislava, Slovak Acad. Sci. Publ., 1964.

Studer, H., and Greer, M. A.: The Regulation of Thyroid Function in Iodine Deficiency. Bern, Huber, 1968.

Wayne, E. J., Koutras, D. A., and Alexander, W. D.: Clinical Aspects of Iodine Metabolism. Oxford, Blackwell, 1964.

THE LIGHT CELLS OF THE THYROID AND CALCITONIN

Bussolati, G., and Pearse, A. G. E.: Immunofluorescent localization of calcitonin in the "C" cells of pig and dog thyroid. J. Endocrinol., *37:*205, 1967.

Copp, D. H., Davidson, A. G. F., and Cheney, B. A.: Evidence for a new parathyroid hormone which lowers blood calcium. Proc. Canad. Fed. Biol. Soc., *4:*17, 1961.

Copp, D. H.: *In* Bourne, G. H. (ed.): The Biochemistry and Physiology of Bone. vol. 2, p. 337. New York. Academic Press, 1972.

Copp, D. H., Cameron, E. C., Cheney, B. A., Davidson, A. G. F., and Henze, K. G.: Evidence for calcitonin—a new hormone from the parathyroid that lowers blood calcium. Endocrinology, *70:*638, 1962.

Copp, D. H., Cockcroft, D. W., and Kyett, Y.: Ultimobranchial origin of calcitonin, hypocalcemic effect of extracts from chicken glands. Canad. J. Physiol. Pharmacol., *45:*1095, 1967.

Copp, D. H.: Historic development of the calcitonin concept. Am. J. Med., *43:*648, 1967.

Foster, G. V., MacIntyre, I., and Pearse, A. G. E.: Calcitonin production and the mitochondrion-rich cells of the dog thyroid. Nature, *203:*1029, 1964.

Godwin, M. C.: Complex iv in the dog with special emphasis on the relation of the ultimobranchial body to interfollicular cells in the postnatal thyroid. Am. J. Anat., *60:*299, 1937.

Hirsch, P. F., and Munson, P. L.: Thyrocalcitonin. Physiol. Rev., *49:*548, 1968.

Hirsch, P. F., Voelkel, E. F., and Munson, P. L.: Thyrocalcitonin: hypocalcemic hypophosphatemic principle of the thyroid gland. Science, *146:*412, 1964.

MacIntyre, I.: Calcitonin: a general review. Calc. Tiss. Res., *1:*173, 1967.

Marks, S. C.: The thyroid parafollicular cell as the source of a potent osteoblast-stimulating factor: evidence from osteopetrotic mice. J. Bone Joint Surg., *51A:*875, 1969.

Nonidez, J. F.: The origin of the "parafollicular" cells, a second epithelial component of the thyroid gland of the dog. Am. J. Anat., *49:*479, 1932.

Pearse, A. G. E.: The cytochemistry of the thyroid "C" cells and their relationship to calcitonin. Proc. Roy. Soc. Biol., *164:*478, 1966.

Pearse, A. G. E., and Carvalheira, A. F.: Cytochemical evidence for an ultimobranchial origin of rodent thyroid C cells. Nature, *214:*929, 1967.

Rasmussen, H., and Pechet, M. A.: Calcitonin. Sci. Am., *223*(3):42, 1970.

Taylor, S. (ed.): Calcitonin. Proc. Symp. Thyrocalcitonin and the C Cells. London, Heinemann, 1968.

Young, B. A., and Leblond, C. P.: The light cells as compared to the follicular cell in the thyroid gland of the rat. Endocrinology, *73:*669, 1963.

See also References to Calcitonin at the end of Chapter 15.

THE PARATHYROID GLANDS

Albright, F., and Reifenstein, E. C.: The Parathyroid Glands and Metabolic Bone Disease. Baltimore, Williams & Wilkins, 1948.

Barnicot, N. A.: The local action of the parathyroid and other tissues on bone in intracerebral grafts. J. Anat., *82:*233, 1948.

Bhaskar, S. N., Schour, I., Greep, R. O., and Weinmann, J. P.: The corrective effect of parathyroid hormone on genetic anomalies in the dentition and the tibia of the *ia* rat. J. Dent. Res., *31:*257, 1952.

Bhaskar, S. N., Weinmann, J. P., Schour, I., and Greep, R. O.: The growth pattern of the tibia in normal and *ia* rats. Am. J. Anat., *86:*439, 1950.

Chang, H.: Grafts of parathyroid and other tissues to bone. Anat. Rec., *111:*23, 1951.

Drake, T. G., Albright, F., and Castleman, B.: Parathyroid hyperplasia in rabbits produced by parenteral phosphate administration. J. Clin. Invest., *16:*203, 1937.

Greep, R. O., and Talmadge, R. V. (eds.): The Parathyroids. Springfield, Ill., Charles C Thomas, 1961.

Grollman, A.: The role of the kidney in the parathyroid control of the blood calcium as determined by studies on the nephrectomized dog. Endocrinology, *55:*166, 1954.

Ham, A. W., Littner, N., Drake, T. G. H., Robertson, E. C., and Tisdall, F. F.: Physiological hypertrophy of the parathyroids, its cause and its relation to rickets. Am. J. Path., *16:*277, 1940.

Howard, J. E.: Present knowledge of parathyroid function, with especial emphasis upon its limitations. *In* Wolstenholme, G. E. W., and O'Connor, C. M. (eds.): Ciba Foundation Symposium on Bone Structure and Metabolism. p. 206. London, J. & A. Churchill, 1956.

Howard, J. E., and Thomas, W. C.: The biological mechanisms of transport and storage of calcium. Canad. Med. Assoc. J., *104:*699, 1971.

McLean, F. C.: The parathyroid glands and bone. *In* Bourne, G. H. (ed.): The Biochemistry and Physiology of Bone. p. 705. New York, Academic Press, 1956.

Munger, B. L., and Roth, S. I.: The cytology of the normal parathyroid glands of man and Virginia deer. A light and electron microscopic study with morphologic evidence of secretory activity. J. Cell Biol., *16:*379, 1963.

Yendt, E. R.: The parathyroids and calcium metabolism. *In* Ezrin, C., Codden, J. O., Volpé, R., and Wilson, R. (eds.): Systemic Endocrinology. p. 95. Hagerstown, Maryland, Harper and Row, 1973.

See also references on bone resorption in Chapter 15.

SOME REFERENCES ON THE ADRENAL GLAND

Bennett, H. S.: Life history and secretion of cells of the adrenal cortex of the cat. Am. J. Anat., *67:*151, 1940.

———: Cytological manifestations of secretion in the adrenal medulla of the cat. Am. J. Anat., *69:*333, 1941.

Bennett, H. S., and Kilham, L.: The blood vessels of the adrenal gland of the adult cat. Anat. Rec., *77:*447, 1940.

Cannon, W. B.: Bodily Changes in Pain, Hunger, Fear and Rage. New York, Appleton, 1920.

Cannon, W. B., and Rosenblueth, A.: Autonomic Neuroeffector Systems. New York, Macmillan, 1937.

Currie, A. R., Symington, T., and Grant, J. K. (eds.): The Human Adrenal Cortex. Baltimore, Williams & Wilkins, 1962.

Deane, H. W., and Greep, R. O.: A morphological and histochemical study of the rat's adrenal cortex after hypophysectomy, with comments on the liver. Am. J. Anat., *79:*117, 1946.

Eisenstein, A. B. (ed.): The Adrenal Cortex. Boston, Little Brown and Co., 1967.

———: Endocrine control of the adrenal gland. Anat. Rec., *109:*41, 1951.

Feldman, J. D.: Histochemical reactions of adrenal cortical cells. Anat. Rec., *107:*347, 1950.

Hagen, P., and Welch, A. D.: The adrenal medulla and the biosynthesis of pressor amines. Recent Prog. Hormones Res., *12:*27, 1956.

Hewer, E. E., and Keene, M. F. L.: Observations on the development of the human suprarenal gland. J. Anat., *61:*302, 1927.

Holmes, W. N.: Histological variations in the adrenal cortex of the golden hamster with special reference to the X zone. Anat. Rec., *122:*271, 1955.

Idelman, S.: Ultrastructure of the mammalian adrenal cortex. Int. Rev. Cytol., *27:*181, 1970.

Jayne, E. P.: Cytology of the adrenal gland of the rat at different ages. Anat. Rec., *115:*459, 1953.

Jones, I. C.: The Adrenal Cortex. London, Cambridge University Press, 1957.

Kitchell, R. L., and Wells, L. J.: Functioning of the hypophysis and adrenals in foetal rats: Effects of hypophysectomy, adrenalectomy, castration, injected ACTH, and implanted sex hormone. Anat. Rec., *112:*561, 1952.

Lever, J. D.: Electron microscopic observations on the adrenal cortex. Am. J. Anat., *97:*409, 1955.

Long, C. N. H.: Pituitary-adrenal relationships. Ann. Rev. Physiol., *18:*409, 1956.

Long, J. A., and Jones, A. L.: Observations on the fine structure of the adrenal cortex of man. Lab. Invest., *17:*355, 1967.

Miale, J. B.: Connective tissue reactions—a critical review: I. The effects of ACTH and cortisone on allergic reactions and the collagen diseases. Ann. Allergy, *9:*530, 1951.

Moon, H. D. (ed.): The Adrenal Cortex. New York, Hoeber, 1961.

Prunty, F. T. G. (ed.): The adrenal cortex. Brit. Med. Bull., *18*:89, 1962.

Ralli, E. P. (ed.): Proceedings of Third Conference on the Adrenal Cortex. New York, Macy, 1952.

Schaberg, A.: Regeneration of the adrenal cortex in vitro. Anat. Rec., *122*:205, 1955.

Selye, H.: Physiology and Pathology of Exposure to Stress. Montreal, Acta, 1950.

Symington, T.: Functional Pathology of the Human Adrenal Gland. Baltimore, Williams & Wilkins, 1969.

Swinyard, C. A.: Growth of human suprarenal glands. Anat. Rec., *87*:141, 1943.

Tepperman, J.: Metabolic and Endocrine Physiology. Chicago, Year Book Medical Publishers, 1962.

Vane, J. R., Wolstenholme, G. E. W., and O'Connor, M.: Andrenergic Mechanisms. Ciba Foundation Symposium. Boston, Little, Brown & Co., 1960.

Williams, R. G.: Studies of adrenal cortex: Regeneration of the transplanted gland and the vital quality of the autogenous grafts. Am. J. Anat., *81*:199, 1947.

Yates, R. D.: A light and electron microscope study correlating the chromaffin reaction and granule ultrastructure in the adrenal medulla of the Syrian hamster. Anat. Rec., *149*:237, 1964.

Some References on the Islets of Langerhans, Including Many of the Historic Contributions That Helped to Elucidate Their Functions

Allen, F. M.: Studies Concerning Glycosuria and Diabetes. Cambridge, Harvard University Press, 1913.

———: Pathology of diabetes: I. Hydropic degeneration of islands of Langerhans after partial pancreatectomy. J. Metabolic Res., *1*:5, 1922.

Banting, F. G., and Best, C. H.: The internal secretion of the pancreas. J. Lab. Clin. Med., *7*:251, 1922.

Bencosme, S. A.: The histogenesis and cytology of the pancreatic islets in the rabbit. Am. J. Anat., *96*:103, 1955.

Bencosme, S. A., and Lazarus, S. S.: Glucagon content of pancreatic tissue devoid of alpha cells. Proc. Soc. Exp. Biol. Med., *90*:387, 1955.

Bencosme, S. A., and Liepa, E.: Regional differences of the pancreatic islet. Endocrinology, *57*:588, 1955.

Bencosme, S. A., Mariz, S., and Frei, J.: Studies on the function of the alpha cells of the pancreas. Am. J. Clin. Path., *28*:594, 1957.

Bensley, R. R.: Structure and relationships of the islets of Langerhans. Harvey Lect., *10*:250, 1915.

Bensley, S. H.: Solubility studies of the secretion granules of the guinea pig pancreas. Anat. Rec., *72*:131, 1938.

Bensley, S. H., and Woerner, C. A.: The effects of continuous intravenous injection of an extract of the alpha cells of the guinea pig pancreas on the intact guinea pig. Anat. Rec., *72*:413, 1938.

Best, C. H., Campbell, J., Haist, R. E., and Ham, A. W.: The effect of insulin and anterior pituitary extract on the insulin content of the pancreas and the histology of the islets. J. Physiol., *101*:17, 1942.

Bowie, D. J.: Cytological studies of the islets of Langerhans in a teleost, Neomaemis griseus. Anat. Rec., *29*:57, 1924.

Campbell, J., Davidson, I. W. F., and Lei, H. P.: The production of permanent diabetes by highly purified growth hormone. Endocrinology, *46*:558, 1950.

Campbell, J., Haist, R. E., Ham, A. W., and Best, C. H.: The insulin content of the pancreas as influenced by anterior pituitary extract and insulin. Am. J. Physiol., *129*:328, 1940.

Dohan, F. C., and Lukens, F. D. W.: Persistent diabetes following the injection of anterior pituitary extract. Am. J. Physiol., *125*:188, 1939.

Evans, H. M., Meyer, K., Simpson, M. E., and Reichert, F. L.: Disturbance of carbohydrate metabolism in normal dogs injected with hypophyseal growth hormone. Proc. Soc. Exp. Biol. Med., *29*:857, 1931-32.

Gomez-Acebo, J., Parrilla, R., and R-Candela, J. L.: Fine struture of the A and D cells of the rabbit endocrine pancreas in vivo and incubated in vitro. I. Mechanism of secretion of the A cells. J. Cell Biol., *36*:33, 1968.

———: Observations with differential stains on human islets of Langerhans. Am. J. Path., *17*:395, 1941.

Gomori, G.: Studies on the cells of the pancreatic islets. Anat. Rec., *74*:439, 1939.

Ham, A. W., and Haist, R. E.: Histological effects of anterior pituitary extracts. Nature, *144*:835, 1939.

———: Histological studies of trophic effects of diabetogenic anterior pituitary extracts and their relation to the pathogenesis of diabetes. Am. J. Path., *17*:787, 1941.

Hédon, E.: Physiologie normale et pathologique du pancréas. Paris, Masson, 1901.

Hellerström, C., Hellman, B., Petersson, B., and Alm, G.: The two types of pancreatic A-cells and their relation to the glucagon secretion. *In* The Structure and Metabolism of the Pancreatic Islets. p. 117. New York, Pergamon Press, 1964.

Homans, J.: The relation of the islets of Langerhans to the pancreatic acini under various conditions of secretory activity. Proc. Roy. Soc. London, s.B., *86*:73, 1912-13.

Houssay, B. A.: Diabetes as a disturbance of endocrine regulation. Am. J. Med. Sci., *193*:581, 1937.

Houssay, B. A., and Biasotti, A.: Le diabète pancréatique des chiens hypophysectomisés. C. R. Soc. biol., *105*:121, 1930.

———: Hypophysectomie et diabète pancréatique chez le crepaud. C. R. Soc. biol., *104*:407, 1930.

———: The hypophysis, carbohydrate metabolism and diabetes. Endocrinology, *15*:511, 1931.

———: Les troubles diabètiques chez les chiens privés d'hypophyse et de pancréas. C. R. Soc. biol., *105*:124, 1930.

Johns, W. S., O'Mulvenny, T. O., Potts, E. B., and Laughton, N. B.: Studies on the anterior lobe of the pituitary body. Am. J. Physiol., *80*:100, 1927.

Lacy, P. E.: Electron microscopic identification of different cell types in the islets of Langerhans of the guinea pig, rat, rabbit and dog. Anat. Rec., *128*:255, 1957.

———: Electron microscopic and fluorescent antibody studies on islets of Langerhans. Exp. Cell Res. (Suppl.), *7*:296, 1959.

———: Electron microscopy of the beta cells of the pancreas. Am. J. Med., *31*:851, 1961.

———: The pancreatic beta cell: structure and function. New Eng. J. Med., *276*:187, 1967.

Lacy, P. E., and Hartroft, W. S.: Electron microscopy of the islets of Langerhans. Ann. N.Y. Acad. Sci., *82*:287, 1959.

Lane, M. A.: The cytological characters of the areas of Langerhans. Am. J. Anat., *7*:409, 1907.

Long, C. N. H., Katzin, B., and Fry, E. G.: The adrenal cortex and carbohydrate metabolism, Endocrinology, *26*:309, 1940.

Long, C. N. H., and Lukens, F. D. W.: The effects of adrenalectomy and hypophysectomy upon experimental diabetes in the cat. J. Exp. Med., *63:*465, 1936.

Long, C. N. H., Lukens, F. D. W., and Dohan, F. C.: Adrenalectomized depancreatized dogs. Proc. Soc. Exp. Biol. Med., *36:*553, 1937.

von Mering, J., and Minkowski, O.: Diabetes mellitus nach Pankreasextirpation. Arch. exp. Path. Pharmakol., *26:*371, 1889.

Munger, B. L.: A phase and electron microscopic study of cellular differentiation in the pancreatic islets of the mouse. Am. J. Anat., *103:*275, 1958.

O'Leary, J. L.: An experimental study on the islet cells of the pancreas in vivo. Anat. Rec., *45:*27, 1930.

Opie, E. L.: Histology of the islands of Langerhans of the pancreas. Bull. Johns Hopkins Hosp., *11:*205, 1900.

————: Pathological changes affecting the islands of Langerhans of the pancreas. J. Exp. Med., *5:*397, 527, 1900-01.

Richardson, K. C.: The influence of diabetogenic anterior pituitary extract on the islets of Langerhans in dogs. Proc. Roy. Soc. London, s.B., *128:*153, 1939-40.

————: Histology of diabetes induced in dogs by injection of anterior-pituitary extracts. Lancet, *1:*1098, 1938.

Richardson, K. C., and Young, F. G.: The "pancreatropic" action of anterior pituitary extracts. J. Physiol., *91:*352, 1937.

Salter, J., and Best, C. H.: Insulin as a growth hormone. Brit. Med. J., *2:*353, 1953.

Schulze, W.: Die Bedeutung der Langerhansschen Inseln in Pankreas. Arch. mikr. Anat., *56:*491, 1900.

Sergeyeva, M. A.: Microscopic changes in the islands of Langerhans produced by sympathetic and parasympathetic stimulation in the cat. Anat. Rec., *77:*297, 1940.

Simard, L. C.: Le complexe neuro-insulaire du pancréas chez les mammifères adultes. Rev. Canad. Biol., *1:*2, 1942.

Ssobolew, L. W.: Zur normalen und pathologischen Morphologie der inneren Secretion der Bauchspeicheldrüse. Virchows Arch. path. Anat., *168:*91, 1902.

Thiéry, J.-P., and Bader, J.-P.: Ultrastructure des îlots de Langerhans du pancréas humain normal et pathologique. Ann. d'Endocrin. (Paris), *27:*625, 1966.

Thomas, T. B.: Cellular components of the mammalian islets of Langerhans. Am. J. Anat., *62:*31, 1937-38.

Woerner, C. A.: Studies of the islands of Langerhans after continuous intravenous injection of dextrose. Anat. Rec., *71:*33, 1938.

Young, F. G.: Experimental investigations on the relationship of the anterior hypophysis to diabetes mellitus. Proc. Soc. Exp. Biol. Med., *31:*1305, 1938.

————: Permanent experimental diabetes produced by pituitary (anterior lobe) injections. Lancet, *2:*372, 1937.

————: The pituitary gland and carbohydrate metabolism. Endocrinology, *26:*349, 1940.

Some References on the Pineal Body

Anderson, E.: The anatomy of bovine and ovine pineals: light and electron microscope studies. J. Ultrastruct. Res., Suppl. 8, May 1965.

Gladstone, R. J., and Wakeley, C. P. G.: The Pineal Organ. London, Ballière, Tindall & Cox, 1940.

Kelly, D. E.: Pineal organs: photoreception, secretion and development. Am. Scientist, *50:*597, 1962.

Kitay, J. I., and Altschule, M. D.: The Pineal Gland. Cambridge, Mass., Harvard University Press, 1954.

Quay, W. B.: Effect of dietary phenylalanine and tryptophan on pineal and hypothalamic serotonin levels. Proc. Soc. Exp. Biol. Med., *114:*718, 1963.

————: Circadian rhythm in rat pineal serotonin and its modifications by estrous cycle and photoperiod. Gen. Comp. Endocrinol., *3:*473, 1963.

————: Cytologic and metabolic parameters of pineal inhibition by continuous light in the rat. Z. Zellforsch., *60:*479, 1963.

Reiter, R. J., and Fraschini, F.: Endocrine aspects of the mammalian pineal gland: a review. Neuroendocrinology, *5:*219, 1969.

Wurtman, R. J., Axelrod, J., and Chu, E. W.: Melatonin, a pineal substance: Effect on the rat ovary. Science, *141:*277, 1963.

26 *The Female Reproductive System*

Introductory Remarks About Sex

Normally, when a female germ cell is fertilized by a male germ cell bearing an X chromosome, the embryo that results develops the form and organs of a female. Correspondingly, when a female germ cell is fertilized by a male germ cell bearing a Y chromosome, the embryo that results develops the form and organs of a male.

However, although an embryo that forms from an ovum that, after fertilization, has an XX complement of chromosomes, can never produce germ cells with Y chromosomes, it is not limited to forming a female reproductive system; for, as we shall see, such an embryo, under certain abnormal environmental circumstances, may develop male rather than female organs. Indeed, it appears that every young embryo, no matter which chromosome complement is present in the ovum from which it arises, has the *potentiality* to develop either type of reproductive system. Nevertheless, since under normal conditions the one of the two potentialities realized in any given embryo is determined by the chromosome complement of the fertilized ovum, it may be concluded that the chromosome constitution, while it does not limit, does exert a profound *directing* influence on the development of the organs and structures that constitute the reproductive system.

The way in which the chromosome complement of the cells of an embryo directs the development of a male or a female reproductive system is not understood. As we shall see, sex hormones probably play some part in the matter, but there are other factors involved.

Indifferent Nature of the Early Gonad. The fundamental organ of either reproductive system is the *gonad* (*gone*, seed) or *sex gland*. There are 2 of either sex in each individual. Those of the female are termed *ovaries;* those of the male, *testes*. The gonads have a dual function in each sex. During the period of sexual maturity the ovaries of females regularly produce mature female germ cells that are capable of being fertilized. They also produce female sex hormones. The testes of males produce male germ cells and male sex hormone.

In the very young embryo the gonads of either sex are said to be indifferent. A histologic examination of one made at this time gives no indication of whether it will later become an ovary or a testis. However, as development proceeds, the organization of cells within the previously indifferent glands becomes indicative of whether they will develop into ovaries or testes. Certain features of the indifferent gonad become suppressed, and others accentuated. As a result of these processes, the embryonic gonads of the 2 sexes soon come to have different microscopic appearances.

On rare occasions both male and female gonads, or parts of gonads, develop and remain in a single individual. For example, the left gonad may develop into a testis, and the right one into an ovary, or both testicular and ovarian elements may develop in the same gonad. The development of both male and female gonadal tissue in the same individual is associated with a disturbed development of the other parts of the reproductive system. Instead of developing only male or female organs and structures, such individuals develop various mixtures of both. Such individuals, then, cannot be classified as either males or females, either by their gonads or by the other organs and structures of their reproductive systems. Therefore, such individuals are called *hermaphrodites* (*Hermēs*, Mercury, *Aphroditē*, Venus). By testing them for Barr bodies, hermaphrodites can be shown to be either chromosomal males or chromosomal females. If a hermaphrodite is a chromosomal female, she will reveal Barr bodies in the cells of such male organs as she possesses.

Effects of Male Sex Hormone on the Development of the Parts of the Reproductive System. One early clue was that it was noticed that when cows gave birth to twins of the opposite sex, the male calf would be born as a normal male, but the female calf often, but not always, would be born with a mixture of female and male organs. Such altered females were termed *freemartins*. Over 50 years ago Lillie showed that this condition was due to the fusion of the membranes that surrounded each of the two developing embryos in the uterus of the cow so that fetal blood could circulate freely between the genetically determined male and the genetically determined female embryos. At this time it was postulated that the reason for the reproductive system of the female embryo being affected, while that of the male was not, was that male hormone from the developing gonads of the male embryo played a dominant role in directing the development of many parts of the reproductive system of an embryo, and if male hormone circulated in a female embryo, it would there suppress the development of the female gonad and also affect the development of other parts of the developing reproductive system, directing its development along male lines. At this time, of course, neither male nor female sex hormones had been isolated.

After male and female sex hormones were isolated and became available for use, many experiments were performed to show that male sex hormone can indeed have a direct and profound effect on stimulating the development of the parts of the reproductive system of an embryo along male lines even though that embryo is a genetically determined female. However, what is even more interesting is the more recent work which indicates that physiological and psychological attributes of maleness may be due to male sex hormones acting on still another organ, namely, some part of the brain (probably the part concerned with the production of releasing factors, as will be described later), and that this effect normally occurs, in male animals in which it has been studied, at an early age, probably shortly before or after birth. Exposure to

male hormone at this time seems to have a more or less permanent effect on behavior patterns, even changing those of females into which male hormone is injected at the right age. Those interested should read S. Levine's article on "Sex Differences in the Brain" in the *Scientific American*, vol. *214*, pages 84 to 90, April 1966.

Pseudohermaphroditism was described in connection with the adrenal gland in the previous chapter.

Introductory Account of the Parts of the Female Reproductive System and Their Functions

The female reproductive system, as may be seen in Figures 26-1 and 26-2, consists of 2 ovaries, 2 oviducts (also called uterine or fallopian tubes), a uterus, a vagina, external genitalia and 2 mammary glands (breasts).

Ovaries. In the sexually mature woman the ovaries are somewhat flattened, solid ovoid bodies, 2.5 to 5.0 cm. long, 1.5 to 3 cm. wide and 0.6 to 1.5 cm. thick (Fig. 26-1). The anterior wall of each is attached to the back of the broad ligament (Fig. 26-1), close to the lateral wall of the true pelvis by means of a short fold of peritoneum called the mesovarium (Fig. 26-9), which conducts vessels and nerves to and from the hilum of the ovary. A rounded ligament, *the ligament of the ovary*, connects the medial end of each ovary with the uterus (Fig. 26-1). The ovary itself is not covered with typical peritoneum but with epithelium (Fig. 26-9) that ranges from columnar to flattened cuboidal. The cut surface of the ovary shows a cortex

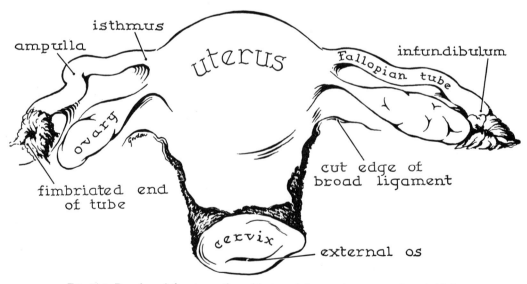

Fig. 26-1. Drawing of the uterus, the oviducts and the ovaries, as seen from behind.

and a medulla; the latter contains many blood vessels and hence sometimes is called the zona vasculosa.

Ovulation and How It Causes Scars on the Surface of the Ovary. The surface of a mature ovary is scarred and pitted; this is due to its having shed many ova (germ cells). As we shall see, these are contained within the cortex in little epithelial bodies called follicles. In a nonpregnant, sexually mature woman a follicle of one ovary matures and ruptures through the ovarian surface (and in doing so liberates an ovum) approximately every 28 days. The phenomenon is known as *ovulation*. Since each time ovulation occurs, an egg cell, surrounded by some epithelial cells, plus some fluid, has to burst through the surface of the ovary, each ovulation results in a break on the ovarian surface which has to heal. Immediately beneath the break the remaining cells of the follicle from which the egg cell was liberated become transformed into a body called a corpus luteum, the endocrine function of which will be described presently. If pregnancy does not occur, the corpus luteum functions for only about 10 to 12 days, after which it degenerates and is replaced by a gradually contracting scar in the ovary immediately beneath the site where the rupture occurred. Scars forming this way from repeated ovulation result in the surface of the ovary becoming increasingly wrinkled and pitted over sites where ovulation has occurred. As we shall see, the fact that the covering (germinal) epithelium of the ovary dips down in the crevices that form in this way is important, for the epithelium at the bottom of a crevice may become pinched off from the surface and form a small inclusion cyst.

If pregnancy occurs after an ovulation, the corpus luteum that forms at the ovulation site continues to develop and function for several months, and by the time it finally degenerates, it has become large enough to leave a relatively large scar in the ovary.

The Path of the Ovum. When a follicle ruptures through the surface of an ovary, an ovum, surrounded by some of the cells of the follicle that still adhere to it, is extruded directly into the peritoneal cavity (Fig. 26-9). As is illustrated in Figure 26-1, the open end of each oviduct is funnel-shaped, and the wide end of the funnel is more or less fitted over the aspect of the ovary from which ova are liberated. Figure 26-1 also shows that the expanded open end of the oviduct is fimbriated (*fimbriae*, fringe); this arrangement permits much of the ovarian surface to be encompassed in such a way that a liberated ovum is led into the lumen of the oviduct.

The oviducts (Fig. 26-1) are the tubes that connect the ovaries to the uterus. Each is covered with peritoneum (the broad ligament is its mesentery). Each oviduct has a muscular wall and is lined with a mucous membrane equipped with ciliated epithelium, which will be described later. Unlike male germ cells (spermatozoa) an ovum cannot move by its own efforts; hence an ovum, delivered into the open end of the oviduct, must be moved to the cavity of the uterus by actions performed by the walls of the oviduct. It is probable that peristaltic contractions that sweep from the open end of the oviduct toward the uterus are chiefly responsible for moving an ovum to the uterus, although the action of the cilia of the epithelial lining of the tubes may assist.

The Usual Site of Fertilization. The mucous membrane of the oviduct is thrown into an extraordinary arrangement of longitudinal folds (Fig. 26-15, *left*). Each fold has a core of lamina propria. These folds probably ensure that an ovum that enters the open end of the tube is kept in close contact on almost all its sides with living cells and compatible fluids as it passes along the tube. These folds probably also provide a similar protection for male germ cells, should these have been introduced into the vagina (Fig. 26-2) of the female, for male germ cells make their way up the cervical canal into the cavity of the body of the uterus (Fig. 26-2), through which they pass to enter the oviducts. It is in the maze created by the folds of mucous membrane in the oviduct that the fertilization of an ovum by a male germ cell occurs (Fig. 26-11). It should therefore not be surprising that fertilization of an ovum can occur in cell cultures because in vivo it actually occurs in fluid that is outside of body substance.

Uterus. The uterus (womb) is a hollow muscular organ with thick walls. It occupies a central position in the pelvis (Fig. 26-2). In shape it resembles an inverted pear that is somewhat flattened. Its narrower part is the body. The uppermost part of the body—that part above the level of the entrance of the oviducts—is the fundus. Since the body of the uterus is somewhat flattened, its central cavity is slitlike, with its anterior and posterior walls in apposition. In its upper part, this slitlike cavity is continuous at each side with the lumen of an oviduct. The cavity of the body narrows below and is continuous with the cervical canal. This, in turn, opens into the vagina (Fig. 26-2).

The Phenomenon of Menstruation. The body of the uterus is lined by a special kind of mucous membrane termed *endometrium* (*metra*, womb) that is pitted with simple tubular glands. It will be described in detail later. In the sexually mature (but not old) nonpregnant woman the innermost (and thicker) part

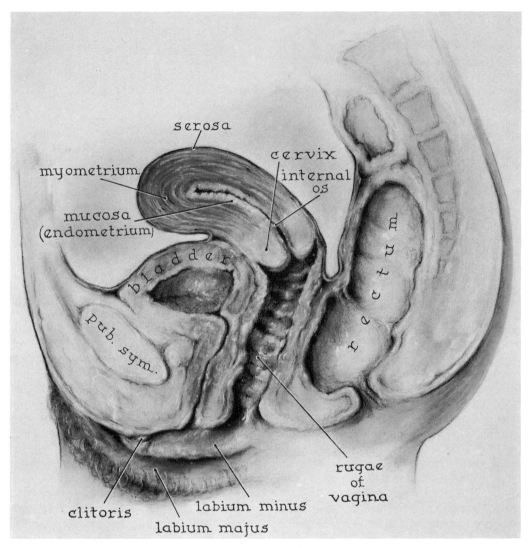

Fig. 26-2. Semidiagrammatic drawing of the parts of the female reproductive system, as seen in a sagittal section.

of this layer breaks down and is exfoliated into the cavity of the uterus approximately every 28 days. The process of exfoliation usually takes about 4 days before its course is run, and during these 4 days the raw surface created by the continuing exfoliation, bleeds. The mixture of blood, glandular secretion and broken-down endometrium delivered into the cavity of the uterus and passed out through the cervical canal and the vagina constitutes the *menstrual (mensis,* monthly*) flow,* and the phenomenon is called *menstruation.* Following menstruation the endometrium regenerates. Ovulation also, it will be recalled, occurs every 28 days. Ovulation, although there is much variation,

does not coincide with menstruation but tends rather to occur about halfway between menstrual periods. Both ovulation and menstruation are the results of the more or less cyclical secretion of hormones as will be described later.

Pregnancy. The liberation of an ovum from an ovary, its fertilization in the oviduct, the changes that occur in it as it passes along the oviduct to the uterus and its implantation into the endometrium—and this marks the beginning of pregnancy—are all illustrated diagrammatically in Figure 26-11.

The further development of the fertilized embedded ovum to form an embryo constitutes the separate subject of *embryology* and hence is dealt with in text-books of embryology. However, the formation of the *placenta,* an organ which permits interchange of dissolved substances between the bloodstreams of mother and embryo, is described later in this chapter.

Menstruation does not occur after a fertilized ovum becomes implanted in the endometrium; hence, a "missed" menstrual period is a time-honored, though by no means invariable, sign of pregnancy. Menstruation does not occur throughout pregnancy.

Parturition. When the fetus has reached full term, parturition (*parturire,* to be in labor) occurs, and a baby is born. The muscle wall of the uterus, which has become very thick during pregnancy, contracts, and the cervix (Fig. 26-2)—the outlet of the uterus— dilates, whereupon the fetus, usually head foremost, slips through the dilated cervix and vagina to reach the outside world. The placenta then separates, and the baby begins its independent existence.

Vagina. The vagina (L. = sheath) is a flattened tube; it serves as a sheath for the male organ in sexual intercourse. Its walls consist chiefly of smooth muscle and of fibroelastic connective tissue; they are a few millimeters thick. It is lined with a mucous membrane that is thrown into transverse folds known as *rugae* (Fig. 26-2). The epithelium is of the stratified squamous nonkeratinizing type. This type of epithelium also covers that part of the cervix that projects into the vagina.

External Genitalia. The external genitalia consist of several structures (Fig. 26-2). A collection of fat deep to the skin that covers the symphysis pubis causes the skin to be raised here in the form of a rounded eminence; this is called the *mons pubis* or *mons veneris.* At puberty this eminence becomes covered with hair. Two folds of skin, the *labia majora* (Fig. 26-2), originate just below the mons pubis. They separate from one another as they pass backward and approach one another again (but do not actually meet) a short distance behind the external opening of the vagina; hence, the vagina opens into the cleft which they enclose. Each of these folds has 2 surfaces covered with skin. The epidermis covering the outer surface of each tends to be pigmented and is equipped with many large hair follicles and sebaceous glands. That of the inner surface also has hair follicles and sebaceous glands, but the hairs are delicate. Sweat glands are also present. The cores of the folds contain fat and some smooth muscle.

Near the anterior end of the cleft between the labia majora is a small body of erectile tissue, the *clitoris* (Fig. 26-2). This is the homologue of the penis of the male. Two delicate folds of skin, the *labia minora,*

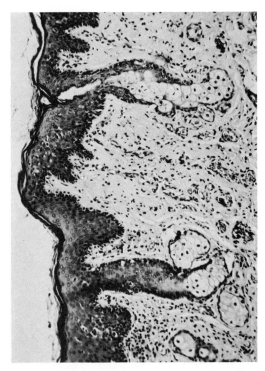

Fig. 26-3. Low-power photomicrograph of a section cut at right angles to the surface of a labium minus. Observe that there are only rudimentary hair follicles; these produce no hairs but are associated with sebaceous glands.

arise just anterior to it. After investing part of the clitoris between them they pass backward, following much the same course as the labia majora to which they lie medial. The labia minora consist of thin folds of skin but possess no hairs (Fig. 26-3). Sebaceous and sweat glands are found on both their surfaces (Fig. 26-3). Although the inner surface of each fold consists of skin, it exhibits the pink color of a mucous membrane.

The Hymen. The labia minora enclose the vestibule of the vagina. In the virgin, an incomplete membranous fold, the *hymen* (Fig. 26-4), projects centrally from the rim of the vestibule and partially occludes the vaginal entrance. Two small glands, the *glands of Bartholin,* which are tubulo-alveolar in type and secrete mucus, are present, one on each side of the vestibule. Each drains into a duct that empties into the groove between the hymen and the labium minus on the side on which the gland is situated. Two elongated masses of erectile tissue, constituting the bulb of the vestibule, are disposed beneath the surface along each side of the vestibule. These two masses approximate

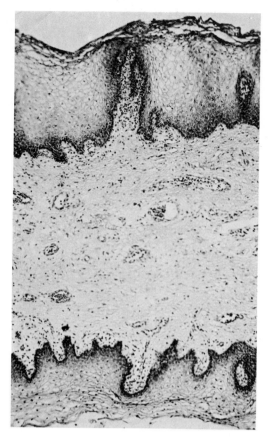

FIG. 26-4. Low-power photomicrograph of a portion of a section cut through the hymen. Observe that both surfaces are covered with stratified squamous nonkeratinizing epithelium and have high papillae.

each other in front. Many mucous glands are present beneath the surface around the vestibule. The urethral orifice is in the midline between the labia minora and between the clitoris and the opening of the vagina (Fig. 26-2).

The external genitalia are richly provided with sensory nerve endings.

Microscopic Structure of the Ovary

Basic Microscopic Features. The ovary consists of a cortex and a medulla. The surface of the cortex is covered with a single layer of epithelium which has, probably incorrectly, been termed germinal epithelium. In young women this is cuboidal (Fig. 26-9), but later in life it becomes flattened over parts of the ovary, though it remains cuboidal in the surface pits and crevices.

The connective tissue substance of the cortex is called its *stroma*. It consists of spindle-shaped cells and intercellular substance. Most of the stroma of the cortex contains a high proportion of cells to intercellular substance; hence in sections it appears heavily nucleated (Fig. 26-5). Moreover, the bundles of cells and fibers that make up most of it run in various directions; hence in sections the stroma of the cortex has a characteristic "swirly" appearance (Fig. 26-5). However, the layer immediately beneath the epithelium differs from the bulk of the stroma in that it has a higher proportion of intercellular substance, and its fiber bundles and cells are both arranged more or less parallel to the surface. This special layer of cortex that is immediately beneath the epithelium is called the *tunica albuginea,* and the white appearance that its name suggests is due to its great content of intercellular substance and lack of vascularity.

The medulla is small as compared to the cortex, and its connective tissue is loosely arranged. It differs further from the cortex in containing more elastic fibers, some smooth muscle cells, spiral arteries and extensive convolutions of veins. The veins may be so large and contain so many blood cells that in a section the student may mistake one for an area of hemorrhage or a hemangioma (a blood vessel tumor). Small blood vessels extend from the medulla into the cortex.

The Development of the Ovary and the Origin of Follicles. The ovaries develop from ridges, termed gonadal or genital ridges, which bulge from the surface of the intraembryonic coelomic cavity. The two ridges are located one on either side of the midline of the embryo between the dorsal mesentery and the mesonephros. Eventually the tissue of these two ridges evolves into the two almond-shaped bodies that are present in later life.

First, the mesodermal cells at the surface of the developing ovary differentiate into a layer of epithelial cells to form a covering for the organ. In other sites in the coelomic cavity surface cells differentiate into the thinner mesothelial cells which line the peritoneal cavity.

Second, beneath the covering epithelium, cords of cells, which have an epithelial appearance similar to that of the covering epithelial cells, appear among the stromal cells. The histologic picture here is reminiscent of that seen in the development of epithelial glands, and as a result a commonly held view has been that the cords of cells that appear in the cortex of the ovary represent downgrowths from the surface epithelium.

Third, about the time when the developing cords of

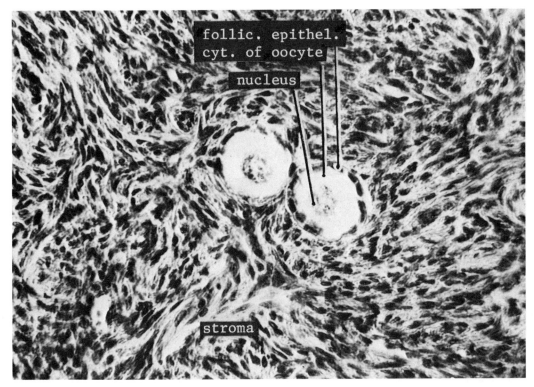

Fig. 26-5. High-power photomicrograph of a section of an ovary of a mature woman, showing "swirly" stroma at 2 primary follicles.

cells are seen, primordial germ cells make their appearance in the cortex of the ovary along with the cells of the cords. It was once assumed that the primordial germ cells develop from cells of the cords by means of cords being broken up into clumps of epithelial cells by stromal cells, after which the central epithelial cell of the clump became a primordial germ cell and the other epithelial cells of the clump formed an epithelial covering for it. A germ cell surrounded by a layer of epithelial cells is called a follicle. However, it was next established that the primordial germ cells do not develop in the ovary but elsewhere, probably in the endoderm of the yolk sac, from which they migrate to the developing ovary and somehow enter its substance at about the time the cords are forming in the cortex. Hence, the epithelium of the ovary is *not* germinal in the sense that it gives rise to the primordial germ cells.

Next, it may be questionable that the covering epithelium is germinal with regard to the cords and/or the epithelial cells that surround the primordial germ cells. If the covering epithelial cell of the ovary is ever germinal in this respect, it subsequently must lose a great deal of its potentiality, for it is now known

that cysts or even tumors that develop from epithelial cells that may become pinched off in crevices on the surface following the repair of a site of rupture of a follicle are of a different character from cysts or tumors that develop from the granulosa (epithelial) cells that surround the germ cells and were supposed to originate from cord cells that in turn were supposed to develop from the germinal epithelium. An alternative source of both the cords and the epithelial cells that surround the germ cells could be stroma cells which, at that time, could be expected to possess a great deal of potentiality.

In the study of histopathology, conceiving of the covering epithelium of the ovary as a germinal epithelium is considered to be a handicap in understanding certain lesions that may develop in the ovary. However, the term *germinal epithelium* is so firmly entrenched in the literature that it has become usual to use it.

The female germ cells that migrate to the ovary and gain entrance to its stroma are called *oogonia*. Early in the development of the ovary they increase greatly in numbers. However, as the prenatal development of the ovary proceeds, most of the germ cells die and, by the time of birth, it has been estimated that there are only around 2,000,000 in the two ovaries and this number is further reduced in postnatal life so that at puberty there are only a few hundred thousand from which only one will develop and be lost from the surface of the ovary every 28 days as a result of ovulation. Ovulation is, of course, interrupted during a pregnancy.

One hopes that the relatively few ova that can be liberated from the ovary of a woman during her life as compared to the vast numbers of oogonia that form in early embryonic development of the ovary results in the survival of the fittest.

Primary (Primordial) Follicles. When in the developing ovary a primordial germ cell becomes enclosed by a single layer of epithelial cells, the little body so-formed is called a *primordial* or *primary follicle* (Fig. 26-5). As noted, vast numbers of oogonia develop but only up to around 400,000 or fewer follicles are in the two ovaries at the time of puberty. Around the end of the third month of embryonic life the oogonia have begun to develop into larger cells; each of these is termed a *primary oocyte*. The cells of the single layer that surrounds each oocyte are termed follicular epithelial cells or, more commonly, *granulosa cells* (why they should be termed granulosa cells is not clear, but this is the common term used for them in pathological and clinical circles).

As was described in Chapter 2 in connection with meiosis and chromosome anomalies, a germ cell has only a haploid number of chromosomes and for this to be achieved a germ cell has to undergo two meiotic divisions. The first of these begins in the germ cells in the ovary in embryonic life.

Soon after primary oocytes develop from oogonia, they enter the prophase of their first meiotic division but they do not complete it at this time. So by the time of birth they are still in the prophase of their first meiotic division, still resting in that stage. They complete their first meiotic division only after puberty and in follicles that are about to rupture at the surface of the ovary (Fig. 26-9), as will be described later.

The Prepuberty Ovary and Its Endocrine Functions. From the time of birth until puberty the ovary grows in size but individual follicles only occasionally begin to grow and develop as follicles do after puberty. It is believed, however, that enough follicles undergo enough development to lead to the formation of some cells that secrete a little estrogen (the generic term for the female sex hormone). It is also believed that up until close to the time of puberty, the hypothalamic center that has the function of secreting the FSH-re-

leasing factor is very sensitive to estrogen and hence the small amounts made by a girl's ovaries up to and around the time of puberty are enough to keep the center from secreting the FSH-releasing factor. However, as puberty nears, the center becomes less sensitive to estrogen so that the small amounts made no longer keep the center suppressed so that it begins to secrete FSH (the follicle stimulating hormone of the anterior pituitary) in a cyclical fashion for reasons that will become apparent as we describe the development and fate of follicles further.

Changes in the Ovary At Puberty; the Beginning of Cyclical Changes. The changes that occur in the human female at the time of puberty are due to the ovaries beginning to come into full function. They do this because they are stimulated to do so by the anterior pituitary gland beginning to secrete gonadotrophic hormones, the follicle-stimulating hormone (FSH) and the luteinizing hormone (LH), also called the interstitial cell secreting hormone (ICSH). To describe how these hormones affect follicles and stroma requires that we first describe primary follicles in somewhat more detail.

Histology of Primary Follicles in the Postpuberty Ovary. Each of the few hundred thousand primary follicles present in the cortical stroma of the ovaries at the time of puberty consists of an oocyte which is around 25 to 30 μ in diameter (Fig. 26-5) enclosed by a single layer of flattened follicular epithelium (Fig. 26-5) which gives the follicle as a whole a diameter of around 40 or so microns. The nucleus of the oocyte is large and pale and with both the LM and the EM its chromatin appears to be fine and dispersed. It contains a nucleolus. Since the nucleus is resting in the prophase of its first meiotic division, it might be thought that it would have the appearance of a mitotic figure, instead of that of an interphase cell in which the chromatin is extended and dispersed. The reason for this appearance seems to be that, after the prophase begins and before it is resumed much later in life, the chromatin threads of the prophase chromosomes become unwound or unfolded sufficiently to lose their appearance of prophase chromosomes and they stay this way until meiosis is resumed years later.

The related subjects of the fine structure of the oocyte and the molecular biology of a cell that may remain in a protracted prophase of meiotic division for several decades are matters more suitably discussed in treatises and textbooks of embryology than here.

At the level of the LM the cytoplasm of an oocyte is pale (Fig. 26-5) and can be shown to possess yolk granules.

The Development of Follicles Under Hormonal Stimulation

Effects of Gonadotrophins on Ovary. First, in the sexually mature nonpregnant female, they cause, once every 28 days or so, several follicles in the substance of an ovary to develop in such a way that they enlarge and approach the surface of the ovary. However, usually only one develops to its full extent (becomes ripe) and ruptures through the surface of the ovary, thus releasing the oocyte it contains into the open end of an oviduct.

The earliest sign of the development of a follicle is given by the follicular epithelial cells. At first these become cuboidal, then columnar, and then, as a result of their proliferation, stratified (Figs. 26-6 and 26-9); the follicle is then known as a secondary follicle. In the meantime, the primary oocyte that it contains increases in size, but its growth is not proportional to that of the follicular epithelium; hence the latter tissue soon comes to constitute the bulk of the follicle. When the primary oocyte has become somewhat more than twice its original diameter, a thick membrane that stains deeply, the *zona pellucida* (Fig. 26-8), develops around it. Probably both the oocyte and the innermost follicular epithelial cells contribute to its formation.

During this period in which the oocyte grows in size it must of course receive nutrients from its exterior. The EM shows that its membrane extends into the zona pellucida in the form of microvilli and, furthermore, the epithelial granulosa cells extend cytoplasmic processes out into and through the zona pellucida to achieve contact with the cell membrane of the oocyte. It is thus via the granulosa cells that the oocyte is provided with food. Furthermore the oocyte evidences the presence of many coated vesicles, which indicates that it absorbs protein as such from its surface.

After the follicular epithelial cells, by their continued division, have become many cells thick, fluid begins to accumulate in little pools between them (Fig. 26-9). These pools of fluid are at first small and are seen roughly halfway between the periphery of the oocyte and the border of the follicle. The precise origin of this fluid which is called *follicular fluid,* is not known; its composition suggests that it is something more than tissue fluid and, hence, that it must be at least modified by the follicular cells among which it accumulates. The follicle continues to enlarge because the follicular epithelial cells continue to proliferate by mitosis, and because fluid continues to accumulate between them. The smaller pools fuse with each other so that larger ones are formed, and the continuance of

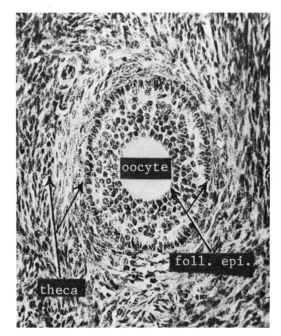

Fig. 26-6. Low-power photomicrograph of a section of an ovary of a mature woman, showing a follicle surrounded by stratified epithelium which has not yet begun to secrete fluid. The plane of section was such that the knife did not pass through the nucleus of the primary oocyte. The theca may be seen indistinctly separated from the ovarian stroma.

this process leads eventually to the bulk of the follicle coming to be composed of a large, more or less central pool of fluid which is not spherical because the oocyte, which is still termed a primary oocyte, together with the follicular cells that cover it, projects into the single large pool of fluid like a little hill from one side (Fig. 26-7). The little hill of follicular cells that contains the ovum is known as the *cumulus oophorus* (*cumulus,* a heap; *oon,* egg; *phorus,* bearer).

While the follicle is developing, as described above, the ovarian stroma that immediately surrounds the follicle becomes organized into a cellular membrane called the *theca* (*theke,* a box).

The cells of this ensheath the epithelial follicle closely and soon become differentiated into 2 layers. The innermost layer, the *theca interna,* is relatively cellular and is provided with many capillaries (Fig. 26-8). The outer layer, the *theca externa,* is more fibrous and not so vascular (Fig. 26-8). However, the line of demarcation between the 2 layers is not usually very distinct.

A fully developed follicle is so large in relation to the thickness of the cortex that it causes a bulge on the

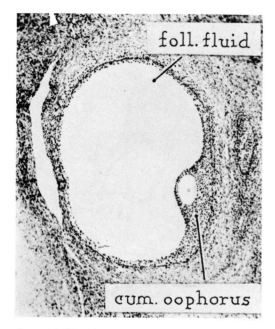

Fig. 26-7. Very low-power photomicrograph of a section of an ovary of a mature woman, showing a developing follicle distended with follicular fluid and the ovum contained in a cumulus oophorus.

surface of the ovary (Fig. 26-9). Moreover, as the follicle develops, the cortex between the outermost part of the follicle and the surface of the ovary becomes very thin.

For the changes, described up to this time, related to the development of a primary follicle into a mature one that bulges from the surface of the ovary to occur, basic levels of FSH and LH must be present in the blood. However, the growth and full development of a follicle is thought to be a primary function of the follicle-stimulating hormone FSH.

In the human female there is at this point a surge in the secretion of LH. This has two effects:

The first is to cause the follicle to undergo some further growth and to burst; how it does this is not known precisely; but its causing increased vascularity in the theca interna with increased tissue fluid production is probably a factor. When the follicle bursts, the secondary oocyte, which is still surrounded by some follicular cells which comprise a *corona radiata* for it, is liberated into, or close to, the open end of the oviduct (Figs. 26-9 and 26-11).

Before considering the second action of LH we shall consider briefly some changes that occur in the oocyte, which at this point is liberated into the oviduct.

At this time the oocyte, which was in late prophase of its first meiotic division, quickly passes through the

other stages of this division. The division of cytoplasm that occurs in this division is very unequal, for one cell, which is now termed the secondary oocyte, retains almost all of the cytoplasm of the primary oocyte, and the other, which is known as a polar body, receives almost none (Fig. 26-11). A second meiotic division then begins in the secondary oocyte but this is not completed unless fertilization occurs, and this does not normally occur until the oocyte is passing along the oviduct (Fig. 26-11). The second meiotic division is also associated with a most uneven distribution of cytoplasm, with another polar body being formed. All polar bodies are discarded. The secondary oocyte, because of the meiotic divisions, has only 23 chromosomes, i.e., the haploid number.

The second action of LH is its triggering the formation of a corpus luteum in the follicle from which the ovum is extruded; this begins to secrete the hormone progesterone.

The Development of a Corpus Luteum. After the ovum and part of the follicular fluid have been extruded at ovulation, the follicle collapses sufficiently to permit the edges of the wound made on the surface of the ovary by the rupture of the follicle to come to-

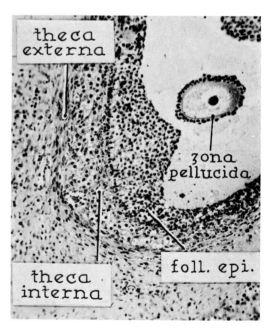

Fig. 26-8. Low-power photomicrograph of a section of an ovary of a mature woman, showing a developing follicle. The secondary oocyte, with some surrounding follicular epithelial cells, appears to be free in the follicle, but this appearance is probably due to the plane of the section. The oocyte shows a well-developed zona pellucida, and the 2 layers of the theca are apparent.

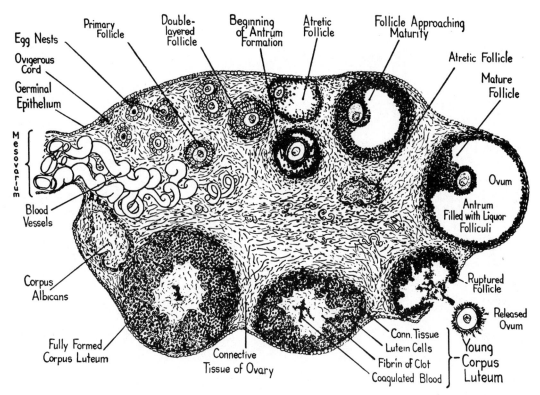

FIG. 26-9. Schematic diagram of an ovary, showing the sequence of events in the origin, the growth and the rupture of an ovarian (graafian) follicle and the formation and the retrogression of corpus luteum. Following clockwise around ovary, starting at the mesovarium. (Patten, B. M.: Human Embryology. New York, Blakiston Division of McGraw-Hill)

gether (Fig. 26-9). Moreover, the reduction in size of the follicle causes the remaining follicular cells and those of the theca interna to be thrown into folds (Fig. 26-9). Only the theca externa retains its original shape. The rupture and subsequent collapse of the follicle usually results in some local bleeding (though in the human female this is not so much as was thought in the past). The escaped plasma and red blood cells become mixed with such follicular fluid as remains in the central part of the follicle. Strands of fibrin then form from the fibrinogen of the escaped plasma.

An early step in the development of the corpus luteum is that the follicular epithelial cells that remain in the follicle enlarge greatly (Fig. 26-10) to become what are called *follicular* or *granulosa lutein* cells. Their cytoplasm becomes abundant as a result of its accumulating lipoid. Lutein pigment also forms in their cytoplasm, but somewhat later. When enough of this accumulates, it imparts a yellow color to the corpus luteum.

The cells of the theca interna, which before ovulation had become enlarged, also become lutein cells and contribute to the size of the corpus luteum. These are called *theca lutein* cells (Fig. 26-10), but, although they are of a connective tissue origin, they develop many of the characteristics of granulosa lutein cells.

Capillaries from the theca interna grow in among the cords and the clumps of lutein cells as the latter develop; hence the corpus luteum comes to have a fairly typical endocrine gland structure (Fig. 26-10). Fibroblasts from the theca interna grow into the more central part of the corpus luteum and there form an undifferentiated type of connective tissue which contains a high proportion of amorphous intercellular substance. This connective tissue tends to surround the remains of the follicular fluid and clotted blood that are still present in the central part of the corpus luteum (Fig. 26-9).

Following ovulation the corpus luteum develops for about 10 to 12 days, attaining a diameter of 1.5 to 2 cm. (Fig. 26-9). The growth that it manifests over this period is probably due to its cells becoming increasingly hypertrophied and not to their undergoing mitosis. Unless the ovum, liberated from the follicle

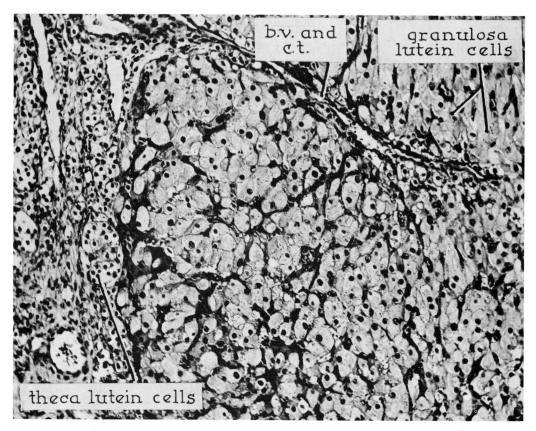

Fig. 26-10. High-power photomicrograph of a portion of a section of a corpus luteum of pregnancy. Observe the large, pale granulosa luteal cells with vacuoles in their cytoplasm. The theca luteal cells are smaller.

before it becomes a corpus luteum, is fertilized, the corpus luteum grows and functions by secreting progesterone only for about 10 to 12 days, after which it begins to involute; this is associated with its vessels collapsing. Moreover, as will be described later, the corpus luteum no longer continues to secrete enough progesterone to maintain the endometrium in a luxuriant condition, so that it begins to show signs of impending disintegration, and is soon mostly cast off (in menstruation).

THE OVARIAN HORMONES: THE FINE STRUCTURE OF THE CELLS THAT PRODUCE THEM AND THE CONTROL OF THEIR SECRETION

The primary hormone made by the ovary is an *estrogen* (estradiol). In the following discussion, we shall use the generic term estrogen for female sex hormone. On being produced in physiological amounts at puberty, estrogen is chiefly responsible for causing the development of the secondary sex characteristics of the female. The other ovarian hormone is progesterone. Both are steroid hormones.

Estrogen Secretion in the Ovarian Cycle. Estrogen is secreted during the 28-day cycle most probably by the cells of the theca interna of the developing follicle. These are fusiform (spindle-shaped) cells well supplied by capillaries. They reveal the usual organelles, rER, sER, Golgi, some free ribosomes and some lysosomes. The cytoplasm, however, contains in addition some lipid droplets. Their mitochondria, moreover, differ from those of most cells in often having some tubular cristae. After ovulation these cells become lutein cells, to be described later.

In most mammals estrogen secretion reaches its peak at the time when the follicle reaches the surface of the ovary and is ready to rupture. In most mammals this is generally the only time that the female will copulate with a male. This, of course, is the very time that coitus is most likely to result in a pregnancy. In the human female estrogen secretion occurs throughout the whole cycle but is somewhat greater at the time of ovulation. As estrogen secretion reaches its peak in the human female it exerts a negative feedback on the hypothalamic centers that secrete the FSH-releasing factor so the further secretion of FSH and hence further follicular growth is inhibited. However, the estrogen peak has the reverse effect on the hypothalamic center controlling LH secretion, for at this time it is stimulated so that there is a surge of secretion of LH, the effects of which have been described in the preceding section.

It should perhaps be mentioned here that the human female differs from most mammalian females in that estrogen secretion by the ovaries does not go through the wide swings that are so common in other mammals, and as a consequence there is no special time induced by hormones which constitutes the only time in their 28-day cycles when women will engage in coitus with a male. In the human, psychological and other factors play important roles.

As already described, a surge secretion of LH by the anterior pituitary at roughly the midpoint of the cycle triggers a corpus luteum to develop from what is left of the ruptured follicle. The cells of the corpus luteum, while continuing to secrete some estrogen, now begin to secrete a hormone called progesterone.

Progesterone Secretion and Its Control. The cells believed to secrete progesterone are the epithelial granulosa cells which become transformed under the influence of LH. During the first phase of the ovarian cycle these cells are of an irregular shape, but, in general, of a cuboidal form. Their nuclei are large and their cytoplasm contains the usual organelles of epithelial cells plus a few lipid droplets. As noted in the growth phase of the follicle, they probably provide nutrients to the oocyte through the zona pellucida by having cellular contacts with the oocyte.

After ovulation the granulosa cells that remain in the follicle change considerably. They enlarge and otherwise develop to become lutein cells. These are characterized particularly by possessing large amounts of sER; in this respect they are like other types of secretory cells involved in synthesizing and secreting steroid hormones. They also have some rER and prominent Golgi stacks and contain a good many lipid droplets.

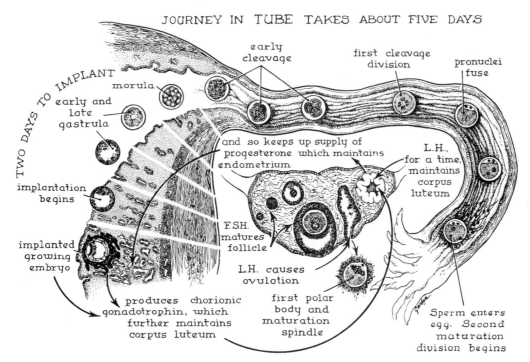

FIG. 26-11. Diagram illustrating the liberation of an ovum from the ovary, its entrance into the oviduct, its fertilization, its passage through the oviduct and its implantation in the endometrium. Study in an anticlockwise direction. The 5 segments of uterine wall that are shown represent from above down the changes that occur in the endometrium from the time of ovulation to the time of implantation. (Redrawn and modified from Dickenson, R. L.: Human Sex Anatomy. Baltimore, Williams & Wilkins)

Fate of the Corpus Luteum. Unless pregnancy occurs, the corpus luteum does not last for more than 10 to 12 days; thus unlike estrogen, progesterone is not made continuously in the nonpregnant female. The chief function of progesterone is to prepare the uterus for the reception of a fertilized ovum. It does this anew each month even in a virgin. The preparation consists of making the endometrium (the lining of the uterus) grow thick and succulent so that a fertilized ovum, on reaching it from the oviduct, may easily become embedded in its lining and be nourished adequately. However, unless this happens the corpus luteum of the ovary regresses after 10 to 12 days and so progesterone production ceases. As a result, the endometrium, brought to a high state of development by this hormone, disintegrates, desquamates and bleeds; this constitutes menstruation. A new 28-day cycle then begins, with a new follicle beginning to develop; this will be discussed presently.

Why the Corpus Luteum Fails. While the formation of the corpus luteum is triggered by a surge of LH secretion at around the midpoint of the cycle, its development for 12 days or so afterward is not dependent on high levels of LH being maintained in the blood. Although some LH may be present, it seems that the life of the corpus luteum is more or less inherently determined in some manner. However, if fertilization of the ovum occurs, the ovum becomes implanted in the lining of the uterus and pregnancy begins. This event interferes with the ovarian cycle. Under these circumstances the corpus luteum that formed does not regress after 12 days or so but continues to develop and secrete progesterone which is required to support the pregnancy (the reason for its persistence will be described presently). It does this for a few months, after which hormones produced by the placenta, to be described in due course, take over its function.

It seems to the author that the hormonal and morphological changes that follow one another throughout the sex cycles of the human female are put in a perspective so that they are much easier to understand— that is, they make more sense, as it were—if one learns also something about the sex cycles of some of the lower animals. After all, it was from the study of these that knowledge developed about what occurred in the human species. So we shall briefly discuss this aspect of the matter.

SEX CYCLES IN LOWER ANIMALS

The Estrous Cycle. In domestic or wild animals the mating impulse is dormant for most of the year in the female and becomes aroused only at certain seasons. At these times the female is said to have come into *heat* or *estrus* (*oistros*, mad desire), and only at these times will a female mate with a male. There is a wide variation among the females of different kinds of animals in the number of times they come into estrus each year. In some kinds that live in the far north, estrus, like Christmas, occurs only once a year, and in still others (rats and mice) it occurs every few days.

It took a long time to find out the cause of estrus. The first step along the way was made when Stockard discovered that the stratified epithelium that lines the vagina of guinea pigs became keratinized at the time of estrus. This change could be regarded as beneficial in that it could provide additional protection for the female from injury by the penis of the male during coitus. Subsequently Allen described the changes that occurred in the epithelium of the mouse during the estrous cycle. The fact that mice from which the ovaries had been removed did not go into estrus and that their vaginal epithelium did not ever become keratinized suggested that both the phenomenon of estrus and the keratinization of the vaginal epithelium were caused by a hormone produced by the ovary at the time of estrus.

Furthermore, the fact that the vaginal epithelium of an ovariectomized mouse never became keratinized provided, for the first time, a way to discover and assay an ovarian hormone, because if an ovarian extract could be shown to keratinize the vaginal epithelium of an ovariectomized mouse, it would prove that it contained the estrus-producing hormone, which, if discovered, would of course be called estrogen. In 1923 Allen (an anatomist) and Doisy (a biochemist), having collected large quantities of follicular fluid from the ovaries of female hogs, succeeded in preparing an extract from the fluid which, when injected into ovariectomized animals, would cause their vaginal epithelium to become keratinized. They were able to assay the strength of their extracts by the same mouse test. Subsequently, the hormone itself was isolated from extracts and its chemical nature determined; in this Doisy played a leading part.

Estrus as such does not occur in the human female. However, its counterpart does occur at about the time of ovulation, because at that time FSH (in the presence of basic amounts of LH) has acted on the ovary both to make it secrete estrogen and to bring a ripe follicle to its surface. But, although the amount of estrogen made by the ovary of the human female is somewhat greater at this time than at other times in the cycle, the proportional increase is not nearly so great as that which occurs in lower animals at the time of estrus.

Progesterone and the Phenomenon of Pseudopregnancy. Estrogen did not explain certain other changes that occurred in women during the menstrual cycle. For example, the histological changes that occur in the lining of the uterus following ovulation were not to be explained by estrogen and, since they were associated with the development of a corpus luteum in the ovary, it was natural that the ovary should be explored to see if it made a second ovarian hormone that caused these changes. Corner and Allen provided evidence for the existence of such a hormone, which was called progesterone. Understanding of its function and the factors that lead to the formation and persistence of corpora lutea was also helped greatly by studying what happens in certain laboratory animals, as follows:

When an isolated female rabbit comes into estrus, ovulation does not occur automatically; instead, the female rabbit remains in estrus until it mates. However, on mating, ovulation occurs. Since, as was discovered, ovulation depends upon the anterior pituitary secreting a surge of LH, it was obvious that in some animals some as yet unknown factor caused the anterior pituitary to secrete enough LH to cause ovulation. Next, if a female rabbit that is in estrus is mated with a *sterile* male, ovulation still occurs; obviously, therefore, ovulation does not depend on male germ cells being introduced into the female but must be caused by such nervous stimulation as is involved in the female's mating with the male.

As was described in the previous chapter in connection with releasing factors, the explanation for this seems to be that afferent impulses set up as a result of coitus are relayed to the hypothalamus, where they cause certain neurons to discharge into the portal circulation the particular releasing factor which controls the secretion of LH. It is to be noted, however, that this mechanism is operative when the rabbit is in estrus and therefore has a relatively high blood level of estrogen. Accordingly, a high blood level of estrogen may be a prerequisite for this releasing factor to be secreted. The females of lower animals mate only when they are in estrus and have a high blood estrogen level.

Human females engage in intercourse at almost any time in the cycle, and there is no evidence to indicate that coitus early in the cycle automatically causes ovulation. It is conceivable that, at about the time when ovulation might occur in any event, coitus might modify the time of ovulation slightly because of afferent impulses causing the secretion of a releasing

factor. But the secretion or effects of a releasing factor that controls LH secretion seem to be dependent on there first being a ripe follicle in the ovary and a relatively high level of estrogen in the blood. The function of the latter may be to wind the biological clock in the hypothalamus so that it is ready to produce the releasing factor that releases LH from the anterior pituitary when it is stimulated to do so, or, in any event, when the proper time arrives.

Pseudopregnancy. In the female rabbit that is mated with a sterile male not only does ovulation occur, but, in addition, corpora lutea develop in the ovary from which the ova are liberated. These for a time grow, develop and secrete, and as a result the animal begins to exhibit all the signs of pregnancy except that its uterus does not contain any embryos. This false pregnancy that develops in the rabbit after it mates with a sterile male, which is due to corpora lutea growing and secreting, is called *pseudopregnancy*. It continues for a considerable time, though not for so long as true pregnancy. Its maintenance is due to the anterior pituitary continuing to secrete LH. However, after a time the corpora lutea in the ovaries involute, and the pseudopregnancy comes to an end. Before discussing why a false pregnancy terminates, we should consider a few other common animals.

The estrus cycle of the rat is different from that of the rabbit, for the isolated female rat remains in estrus for only a few hours and then begins a new estrous cycle. A new cycle is repeated approximately every 4 days. The rat ovulates spontaneously at the time of estrus. Nevertheless, if it does not mate, functional corpora lutea do not develop in its ovaries; hence, no estrogen and progesterone are made by corpora lutea to inhibit the anterior pituitary from secreting FSH, and so after estrus the anterior pituitary immediately begins again to secrete FSH. This brings a new crop of follicles to the surface of one of the ovaries in 4 days' time and stimulates the production of enough estrogen to put the rat into estrus by the time the follicles mature. The rat, therefore, illustrates that the hormones made by the corpora lutea are necessary if the secretion of FSH is to be inhibited immediately after estrus. If a female rat mates with a sterile male at the time of estrus, functional corpora lutea do develop in the ovary, and in the rat enough prolactin (in the rat it is luteotrophin instead of LH) is secreted to maintain the corpora lutea for a while. The latter secrete enough estrogen and progesterone into the bloodstream to cause pseudopregnancy and to prevent the anterior pituitary from secreting FSH, which would cause a new estrous cycle to begin immediately. Therefore the mating of a female rat with a sterile male upsets its estrous cycle. When the pseudopregnancy has run a course of several days, it terminates. When the corpora lutea involute and cease making their hormones, the anterior pituitary thereupon is permitted once again to secrete FSH, and so a new estrous cycle begins.

The estrous cycle of the female of the dog family is different still. An isolated bitch normally comes into estrus twice a year. Ovulation occurs spontaneously at estrus; evidently the high level of estrogen in the blood at the time of estrus winds the biological clock that in this case automatically at the right time sets off the releasing factor that causes the anterior pituitary to secrete LH, which causes ovulation. Moreover, the anterior pituitary, following ovulation, continues to secrete LH and/or prolactin for a considerable time, and, as a result, pseudopregnancy automatically follows estrus in the isolated bitch. This continues approximately half as long as a real pregnancy. Under the influence of the hormones from the corpora lutea, the uterus enlarges, the belly droops, and the mammary glands begin to enlarge. Observing these phenomena, owners of bitches who are not familiar with the phenomena of pseudopregnancy begin to wonder if the isolation they imposed on their pets at the time of estrus was as efficient as they thought. But at about this time the pseudopregnancy terminates. The endometrium, previously built up by the action of progesterone, reverts back to its normal thickness; this is accomplished usually without any external bleeding, although some slight hemorrhages have been observed to occur into the substance of the endometrium at this time.

It should be clear from the foregoing that normal menstruation in the human female is the counterpart of the termination of a pseudopregnancy in lower animals, and that it is precipitated by the failure of a corpus luteum to continue to secrete its hormones, particularly progesterone. The reason for the termination of pseudopregnancy in the human female being associated with such a severe and prolonged event as menstruation, when pseudopregnancy terminates in so many lower animals with almost no disturbance is associated with a special pattern of blood vessels that supply the lining of the uterus in human females; these will be described when we discuss the uterus.

Summary of Hormonal Factors in the Sex Cycle in the Nonpregnant Human Female

Following the failure of the corpus luteum there are not enough steroid sex hormones in the blood to suppress the secretion of the FSH-releasing factor by nerve cells in the hypothalamus. The releasing factor, therefore, flows through the blood of the portal system that supplies the anterior lobe of the pituitary and stimulates specific gonadotrophs to secrete FSH. FSH, together with a basic level of secretion of LH, causes follicles to develop in the ovary and approach its surface. One follicle (usually) becomes fully developed. Meanwhile, the cells of the theca interna of the developing follicles or follicle produce estrogen, and the blood level of estrogen rises. As already mentioned, this may help wind a biological clock in the hypothalamus which automatically at the proper time gives off a signal—the secreting of a releasing factor—which causes the anterior pituitary to secrete a surge of LH. At the time this has occurred, the estrogen level of the blood has risen to a height sufficient to inhibit the further secretion of FSH-releasing factor, and so FSH secretion ceases to be effective. The LH, however, which is secreted by the anterior pituitary at this time causes ovulation and triggers the development of a functional corpus luteum in the ovary in the follicle from which the ovum was extruded. The corpus luteum secretes both estrogen and progesterone; these, over the life of that corpus luteum, probably both—but particularly the estrogen—act to continue the inhibition of the secretion of the releasing factor for FSH, which inhibition began about the time of ovulation. The progesterone builds up the endometrium so that it would be receptive to a fertilized ovum. However, if pregnancy does not occur, the corpus luteum after about 12 days begins to involute. It was thought in the past that the reason for this was that LH secretion failed. It may be that the life of the corpus luteum is predetermined unless pregnancy occurs. However, if pregnancy occurs, as will be described shortly, another hormone (chorionic gonadotrophin) which has many effects like those of LH appears in the blood, and it maintains the corpus luteum. But if pregnancy does not occur, the corpus luteum involutes. Since the endometrium was built up by the progesterone secreted by the corpus luteum, the withdrawal of progesterone that occurs when the corpus luteum involutes causes menstruation. Since the estrogen and, to some extent, the progesterone produced by the corpus luteum have been inhibiting the anterior pituitary (via the hypothalamus and the releasing factor that affects FSH) from secreting FSH, the failure of the corpus luteum (which results in the cessation of estrogen and progesterone secretion from this source) releases the anterior pituitary from this suppressant so that it immediately begins to secrete FSH again, and a new ovarian cycle is on its way.

ANOVULATORY CYCLES

Occasionally, women experience bleeding from the endometrium at the time of menstruation without ovulation having occurred and thus without the development of a corpus luteum in the ovary. These unusual instances of menstrual bleeding without previous ovulation (anovulatory menstruation) are probably due to preceding variations in the level of blood estrogen. We shall elaborate:

If estrogen is withdrawn—for example, by the removal of the ovaries from a sexually mature woman —the endometrium may bleed as a consequence. Furthermore, if estrogen is given to a female at a standard rate for a time and then the dosage is considerably reduced, but not entirely stopped, bleeding from the endometrium will occur not immediately but *only* after an interval of some days. Therefore it is believed that the bleeding that occurs in anovulatory menstruation is to be explained as a delayed response to the reduction in the estrogen output of the ovary that occurs following the maturation of a follicle.

Anovulatory cycles in women are probably not as rare as has been thought; de Allende has shown that a perfectly healthy woman may have 3 or 4 anovulatory cycles a year, with a higher proportion near puberty and the menopause.

THE CORPUS LUTEUM OF PREGNANCY

If pregnancy does not occur, a corpus luteum reaches a diameter of from 1.5 to 2 cm. It then begins to involute. Its capillaries collapse, and the lutein cells disintegrate. As its characteristic cells degenerate further, it shrinks in size, and it finally becomes a small white scar called a *corpus albicans* (Figs. 26-9 and 26-12).

If pregnancy occurs, the corpus luteum continues to grow and function and attains a diameter of about 5 cm. in the third month of pregnancy. At that time, or somewhat later, it begins to involute. However, the involution of a corpus luteum of pregnancy at this late date does not cause menstruation, because by this time the placenta is producing progesterone, and hence the involution of the corpus luteum of pregnancy does not cause a progesterone deficiency. Indeed, it appears that the ovary containing the corpus luteum of pregnancy may be removed earlier than was believed in the past without interrupting the pregnancy because of the placenta's becoming competent in a few months to make enough progesterone to support pregnancy. The involution of a corpus luteum of pregnancy leaves a substantial scar in the ovary.

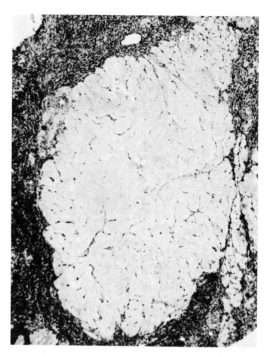

FIG. 26-12. Very low-power photomicrograph of a section of an ovary of a mature woman, showing a corpus albicans that has formed as a result of the degeneration of a corpus luteum of menstruation.

The Cause of the Persistence and Growth of the Corpus Luteum in Pregnancy—Chorionic Gonadotrophin. Why should pregnancy prevent a corpus luteum in an ovary from involuting 12 days or so after ovulation? The reason for the corpus luteum continuing to develop is that a new hormone that acts very much like LH with regard to the corpus luteum is made by the trophoblastic cells of what will become the placenta, soon after the ovum becomes implanted in the endometrium (Fig. 26-11). This hormone is usually called *chorionic* or *placental gonadotrophin*. It differs from LH chiefly in that it cannot do everything that LH can do in an animal from which the anterior pituitary gland has been removed. However, if such an animal is given some anterior pituitary gonadotrophic hormone, chorionic gonadotrophin then exerts an LH effect. In other words, given a little collaboration by the anterior pituitary, the action of chorionic gonadotrophin is similar to that of LH.

Pregnancy Tests. So much chorionic gonadotrophin is made in pregnancy that it is excreted in the urine. Indeed, if the urine of a pregnant woman is injected into an animal it causes profound biologic effects. This is the basis for many of the animal tests for pregnancy.

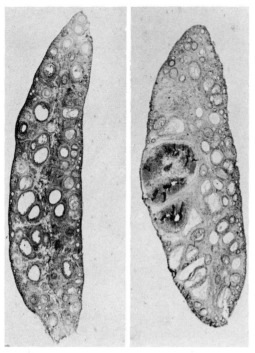

Fig. 26-13. (*Left*) Very low-power photomicrograph of a section of an ovary of a virgin rabbit that was injected with urine from a nonpregnant woman. Mature unruptured follicles may be seen close to the surface. This is the picture seen in a negative test. (*Right*) Very low-power photomicrograph of a section of the ovary of a virgin rabbit that was injected with urine from a pregnant woman. Notice that two of the surface follicles at the left side are very large and are filled with blood as a result of the occurrence of ovulation. On high-power examination, each of these may be seen to have a lining of typical granulosa luteal cells. This is the picture seen in a positive test.

An excellent and instructive one is the Friedman modification of the Aschheim-Zondek test. This will now be described.

It will be recalled that the virgin rabbit, on coming into estrus, remains in estrus, with mature follicles present at the surface of an ovary, until it mates with a male (Fig. 26-13, *left*). In other words, in the rabbit, ovulation awaits the secretion of LH, which occurs normally only as a result of the sexual excitement and the nervous stimulation associated with the act of mating (sometimes the presence of a male in the vicinity is enough to cause enough LH secretion to cause ovulation; hence males should be excluded from the testing laboratory). It is obvious that if some LH were injected into a virgin rabbit in estrus, ovulation would immediately occur, and it would be easy, on

inspecting the ovaries of the rabbit soon afterward, to see that it had occurred, from finding hemorrhagic follicles (Fig. 26-13, *right*) and young corpora lutea. Likewise, if chorionic gonadotrophin were injected into a vein of a rabbit, the same results would be obtained, for this hormone, in an animal with an intact anterior pituitary gland, acts like LH. There is so much chorionic gonadotrophin in the urine of a pregnant woman that a relatively small amount of urine injected into a vein of a virgin rabbit in estrus will cause ovulation and corpus luteum formation (Fig. 26-13, *right*). Since there is no chorionic gonadotrophin in the urine of a nonpregnant woman and not enough LH to have any effect on a rabbit, it is obvious that the injection of urine into a virgin rabbit in estrus permits a decision to be made on whether the urine was obtained from a pregnant or a nonpregnant woman (Fig. 26-13).

Other Tests. The above test was described in some detail because it illustrates some points relevant to the general discussion. Later tests to detect chorionic gonadotrophin in urine have subsequently been devised. One depends on the hormone causing certain female toads to lay eggs, another on chorionic gonadotrophin causing male toads or frogs to liberate spermatozoa in their urine. An esoteric test is the more recent immunological one. This depends on the fact that chorionic gonadotrophin is a glycoprotein, and that it can be adsorbed on red blood cells or even on latex particles. Furthermore, human chorionic gonadotrophin can be purified and used as an antigen which, on being injected into animals, causes them in due course to produce antibodies in their serum which will react with human chorionic gonadotrophin. If red cells (or latex particles) on which human chorionic gonadotrophin has been adsorbed are mixed with antiserum made, say, in rabbits, in response to human chorionic gonadotrophin, the red blood cells (or latex particles) on which the antigen (human chorionic gonadotrophin) has been adsorbed immediately agglutinate. If, however, a test sample of urine or serum from a pregnant woman is mixed with the antiserum before it is mixed with the coated red blood cells or latex particles, agglutination will not occur, because the chorionic gonadotrophin in the sample from the pregnant woman combines with and neutralizes the antibody to chorionic gonadotrophin that was present in the rabbit serum so that it is no longer available to react with the chorionic gonadotrophin adsorbed in the red cells or latex particles. If the sample of urine or serum was taken from a nonpregnant woman, there would be no chorionic gonadotrophin in it to neutralize the antibody in the rabbit serum, and so when the coated red cells or latex particles were mixed with the rabbit serum, the antibody in it would react with the coating and cause the cells or particles to agglutinate. Thus agglutination is a negative test for pregnancy, whereas no agglutination is a positive test.

HORMONAL CONTRACEPTION

One effect of the development of knowledge about sex hormones over the last few decades has had, to say the least, a profound effect on society; this is the application of this knowledge to providing a simple and effective means of contraception for females.

Development of Knowledge. It was known for a long time that a pregnant female did not ovulate during pregnancy. When enough became known about sex and placental hormones it became possible to understand that the reason for ovulation being suppressed in pregnancy was that in pregnancy blood levels of estrogen and progesterone are quickly established that effectively inhibit the mechanisms that would ordinarily lead to the anterior pituitary secreting enough FSH to cause further ovarian follicles to develop and mature in the ovaries. Estrogen has a more potent effect than progesterone in this respect, although in most animals progesterone will prevent ovulation. The source of this estrogen early in pregnancy is the corpus luteum of pregnancy, which, of course, also produces progesterone. Later in pregnancy the placenta (in the human female) also produces estrogen and progesterone.

The next step was to use this knowledge to devise means for preventing ovulation in nonpregnant females. Although there are now various approaches to the problem of hormonal contraception, the first and basic one was and is designed to prevent ovulation by much the same means as occurs naturally during pregnancy.

The oral contraceptives in common use generally contain enough of an estrogenic substance that is effective if taken by mouth, for them, if they are taken regularly following menstruation, to maintain a level of estrogenic activity in the blood that is sufficient to inhibit the secretion of the releasing factor for FSH. Without effective amounts of FSH being secreted, follicles do not ripen in the ovary. Substances with progesterone activity are, in addition, widely used in preparations. These are not as potent as estrogen in inhibiting the secretion of FSH, but they may inhibit to some extent the secretion of LH. The substance having progesterone activity may be taken for only the part of the cycle in which progesterone normally would act on the endometrium to build it up into the premenstrual type. At the proper time in the cycle some days are skipped to cause both estrogen and

progesterone withdrawal, which, of course, brings on menstruation. On the proper day the taking of the preparation is resumed so that estrogen will be available to keep the anterior pituitary from secreting FSH during the next cycle.

It is to be noted that the suppression of ovulation by any of these preparations prevents the regular formation of new corpora lutea in the ovaries of the woman concerned, and hence a nonpregnant woman's production of estrogen and progesterone from this source has to be compensated for, at least in part, by the hormone content of the oral contraceptive being used.

ATRETIC FOLLICLES

It can now be understood that the cortex of the ovary of a sexually mature nonpregnant woman who has borne children may contain a great variety of structures: primary follicles, normal follicles in various stages of development, follicles in various stages of atresia, perhaps a functioning corpus luteum of menstruation and scars of old corpora lutea of menstruation and of pregnancy. We shall now describe some of the features of some of these structures in more detail so that the student may have some general principles for distinguishing between them in sections.

It is to be remembered that, out of several follicles that are stimulated to develop and approach the surface of the ovary of a woman at the time of ovulation, only one usually reaches the final stages of development and maturation and liberates an oocyte. It seems probable, according to Allen, Pratt, Newell and Bland, that the other large ones all undergo atresia. They do not, then, remain in a state of suspended animation, waiting for an opportunity to ovulate in a subsequent month, but die. If ovulation is to occur in another month, a new set of follicles must develop and approach the surface.

In a given section of ovary, there may be, then, many large atretic follicles, and if they are just beginning to undergo atresia, it may be difficult to distinguish them from normal follicles. If atresia has proceeded for any length of time, the student's task is easier, for later on, in atresia, fibroblasts grow into the breaking-down follicle and replace it with connective tissue (Fig. 26-14, *right*). But before this occurs, the detection of atresia requires the use of less obvious criteria. Two early signs of the condition are the pulling away of the follicular epithelium from the theca interna (or a break in the follicular epithelium) and pyknotic nuclei in the follicular epithelial cells. Allen *et al.* note that the cumulus oophorus becomes detached in atresia, but this, of course, cannot be established from the study of a single section. The histologic signs of cell death may, of course, be observed in the ovum in atresia, but the ovum may not be seen in the part of the follicle through which the section under view has been cut.

In distinguishing old atretic follicles from degenerate corpora lutea it is helpful to keep in mind that the term *atresia* is reserved for follicles that degenerate before they mature, and hence that there has been no reason for bleeding to have occurred in them. On the other hand, old corpora lutea, whether of menstruation or pregnancy, usually contain blood pigment that remains behind in them to indicate that they were once the site of a hemorrhage.

The Interstitial Gland

In the ovaries of some species, including man, there may be groups of what appear to be glandular cells scattered about in the stroma. These together are sometimes said to constitute the interstitial gland of an ovary. Individual cells have an appearance that is similar to that of luteal cells, but they are not arranged together to form structures that resemble corpora lutea. It is believed they may originate from follicles that had developed sufficiently for a theca to have begun forming and then the follicles for the most part underwent atresia before the theca developed to a full extent. One reason for this view is that indications of an interstitial gland may be seen in prepuberty ovaries before follicles have begun to mature and rupture. It has been suggested that the cells may at this time in particular produce some female sex hormone but in small quantities which would aid in the prepuberty development of the secondary sex characteristics of the female.

The Ovary After the Menopause

After functioning for 30 odd years, both with respect to liberating ova and secreting hormones, the ovaries appear to become exhausted, and, after a short period during which they function sporadically, they finally cease liberating ova and producing hormones. When they fail to liberate oocytes, there are, of course,

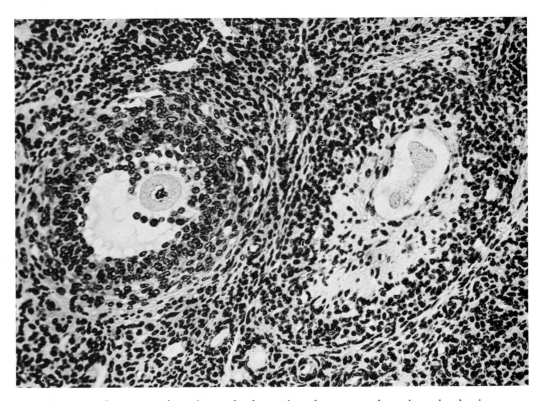

Fig. 26-14. Low-power photomicrograph of a section of an ovary of a guinea pig, showing a normal, developing follicle at the left and an atretic follicle at the right. Observe that the oocyte has degenerated in the atretic follicle, and that fibroblasts have grown into the central part of the follicle.

no new corpora lutea formed, and as a result the endometrium thereafter neither becomes greatly thickened nor collapses each 28 days. The most obvious sign of ovarian failure, then, is that the menses cease; and, indeed, it is for that reason that this time in a woman's life is described as the *menopause* (*mēn,* month, *pausis,* cessation). The menopause usually occurs somewhere between the ages of 45 and 50, and it marks the end of the reproductive life of a woman. Actually, fertility declines rapidly during the 10 years before menopause. An artificial menopause occurs earlier if the ovaries are removed, or if their function is otherwise destroyed as, for example, by irradiation or disease.

The onset of the menopause is usually indicated, though not always, by other signs and symptoms. Commonly, the function of the vasomotor nerves becomes disturbed, and women suffer from what are called "hot flushes." Moreover, they may find it more difficult, for a time, both from physiologic and psychological reasons, to maintain their usual adjustment to life; hence some women exhibit a certain amount of emotional instability at this time. Indeed, in the very badly adjusted, the menopause may precipitate serious mental illness. Other symptoms, such as headache, insomnia and alterations in the rate of the heart beat, are sometimes experienced. Much can now be done to alleviate the more distressing symptoms that occur at this time by the judicious administration of sex hormones.

It should be clearly understood that the hormonal disturbances that occur at the menopause are due to ovarian failure and not to the failure of the anterior pituitary. Indeed, as the estrogen level of the blood falls after the menopause, the negative feedback arrangement between estrogen and FSH leads to FSH being secreted in such increased amounts that fairly large quantities of it appear in the urine. Hence, if the urine of a woman who has passed the menopause is injected into a young animal, it will stimulate follicular development and estrogen production in that young animal and so bring about a precocious puberty in it. There is no point, then, in giving a woman gonadotrophic hormone at this time to stimulate her ovaries. On the other hand, the administration of estrogen to a woman at the time of the menopause could be expected to suppress, to some extent, the increased FSH secretion that ordinarily occurs at this time, as well as to produce other beneficial effects.

The ovary of a woman who has recently passed the menopause is to be distinguished by the relative absence of: (1) primary follicles, (2) follicles in various stages of normal development or showing early atresia,

and (3) recent corpora lutea. As the years pass, the ovary becomes increasingly shrunken, consisting almost altogether of old fibrous tissue.

It seems probable that the falling-off in progesterone production is more abrupt at the menopause than the falling-off in estrogen production. New corpora lutea are necessary if progesterone production is to be carried on for any great length of time. Estrogen production by the ovary, though diminished, may be carried on for some time after the menopause. Estrogens are made by thecal cells. So, as long as theca elements persist in the ovary, as for example in some interstitial gland cells, some estrogen might be produced. Moreover, it is probable that there are some, though not very important, extraovarian sources of estrogen in the body.

The great decrease in estrogen production that occurs at the menopause may be reflected sooner or later in substantial tissue changes in certain parts of the body. Those parts of the female reproductive tract that are dependent on this hormone for the maintenance of their structure tend to become atrophic. For example, the functional capacity of the glands associated with the cervix and external genitalia becomes diminished; the external genitalia themselves tend to atrophy, and the vaginal lining may become very thin and increasingly susceptible to infection. Substitution therapy can do much to relieve these conditions when they occur.

The Oviducts

Each oviduct (Fig. 26-1) is about 12 cm. long and consists of 4 parts: (1) an intramural part—that portion of the tube that extends through the wall of the uterus; (2) an isthmus—the short narrow part of the tube next to the uterus; (3) an ampulla—the longest part of the tube, about the diameter of a pencil and extending from the isthmus to (4) an infundibulum—the flared termination of the tube provided with processes or fimbriae. The wall of the oviduct is made up of 3 layers, a mucous membrane, a muscular coat and an adventitial serous coat (Fig. 26-15).

Mucous Membrane. The epithelium consists of a single layer of columnar cells. There are 2 types of these, ciliated and secretory, and they alternate irregularly with one another (Fig. 26-16, *top*). Their relative and absolute heights vary in relation to different times in the menstrual cycle. Beginning shortly after menstruation, according to Snyder, they both increase in height, and at the time of ovulation they are both about 30 μ high (Fig. 26-16, *top*). Following this, however, the ciliated cells become much shorter, and

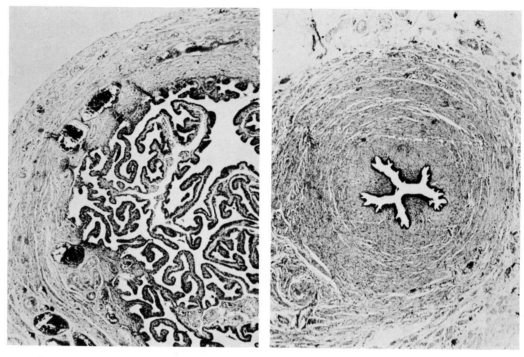

Fig. 26-15. (*Left*) Very low-power photomicrograph of a portion of a cross section of the ampulla of an oviduct of a mature woman. The dark areas in the muscle coat are congested veins. Observe the complex longitudinal folds that are cut in cross section. (*Right*) Very low-power photomicrograph of a cross section of the isthmus of an oviduct.

the nonciliated secretory cells, though they, too, become somewhat shorter, come to project between the ciliated cells into the lumen of the tube, thus making the free epithelial surface somewhat irregular (Fig. 26-16, *bottom*). A few clear cells with dark-staining nuclei may be scattered about in the epithelial membrane close to the basement membrane. They are probably young secretory cells. In addition, occasional lymphocytes are found in this site. It is not believed that the nonciliated cells become ciliated or vice versa. In the past it was generally assumed that the cilia beat toward the uterus and so were an important factor in moving an ovum along the tube to the uterus. However, at least some cilia in some species have been found to beat in the other direction, so other mechanisms involving contractile movements of the muscle of the tube appear to be of primary importance. Ciliated epithelium in this site has been shown to be dependent on the ovary. It is probable that the watery secretions in the tube, whatever they may be, are in some way nutritive or otherwise helpful for the ovum, and that the hormonal stimulation of the cells concerned in making secretions occurs at a time when an ovum would be likely to be passing along the tube. It

is of interest that, for some days, a fertilized ovum lives in this fluid which, in a sense, must act as a culture medium; hence fertilization and the early development of a fertilized ovum actually takes place outside body substance.

The lamina propria of the mucous membrane is of the ordinary connective tissue type except that its cells have potentialities similar to those of the endometrial stroma, for they react similarly if a fertilized ovum inadvertently becomes implanted in the mucosa of the oviduct.

As described in the general account of the parts of the reproductive system, the mucous membrane of the oviduct is thrown into extensive longitudinal folds (Fig. 26-15, *left*). These become reduced in size and extend in the isthmus (Fig. 26-15, *right*) and amount to little more than ridges in the intramural portion of the tube.

Muscle Coat. This consists of 2 layers: an inner one of circularly or somewhat spirally disposed smooth muscle fibers and an outer one of longitudinally disposed fibers. However, the line of demarcation between the 2 layers of muscle is by no means clear-cut, and since some connective tissue extends between the bundles of muscle fibers, the muscle coats may be difficult to identify in anything more than a general way. The inner coat of circular fibers is thickest in the intramural portion of the tube and least prominent in the infundibulum. Peristaltic-like movements of the muscle are believed to be accentuated close to the time of ovulation. The tonus, as well as contractions of the muscle, has been shown to be affected by hormones.

The histologic structure of the serosa is typical.

The Body and the Fundus of the Uterus

The wall of a uterus (Fig. 26-2) varies in thickness from 1.5 cm. to slightly less than 1 cm. It consists of 3 coats which, from without in, are (1) a thin serous coat or *serosa*, (2) a thick muscle coat or *myometrium*, and (3) a mucous membrane or *endometrium*.

The serosa—in reality the peritoneal investment of the organ—consists of a single layer of mesothelial cells supported by a thin connective tissue membrane; it is continuous at each side of the organ with the peritoneum of the broad ligament and is deficient in the lower half of the anterior surface (Fig. 26-2).

The myometrium consists of bundles of smooth muscle fibers separated from one another by connective tissue (Fig. 26-17). The bundles are arranged so as to form 3 rather ill-defined layers. The outermost and innermost layers are thin and consist chiefly of longitudinally and obliquely disposed fibers. The middle layer is much thicker, and in it the smooth muscle fibers tend to be disposed circularly. The larger blood vessels of the wall of the uterus are mostly contained in this middle layer; hence it is sometimes called the *stratum vasculare*. The smooth muscle fibers in this layer, in the uterus of the nonpregnant woman, are about 0.25 mm. in length.

The Growth of the Uterus in Pregnancy. The smooth muscle cells of the myometrium become 10 times as long and many times as thick during pregnancy. The great increase in the thickness of the myometrium in pregnancy is brought about not only by a hypertrophy of previously existing fibers but also by an increase in the number of fibers, the new ones being derived from the division of pre-existing fibers and perhaps also from the transformation of undifferentiated cells in the connective tissue between the bundles into smooth muscle cells.

The Hormonal Basis For the Growth of the Myometrium. Since the placenta (in the human female) produces very large amounts of estrogen during pregnancy, and since estrogens are known to cause a great growth of the myometrium if it is given to ovariectomized animals, as is shown in Figure 26-18, it is as-

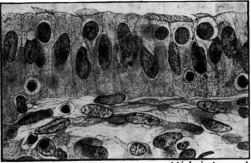
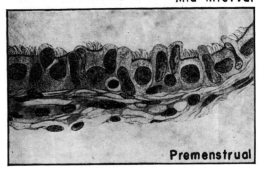

Fig. 26-16. (*Top*) Human oviduct about midinterval stage. (*Bottom*) Tube at premenstrual stage. (Camera lucida drawings; × 700). (Snyder, F. F.: Bull. Johns Hopkins Hosp., *35*:146)

sumed that the great growth of the myometrium in pregnancy is caused primarily by estrogens.

The way in which an estrogen can cause the growth of particular cells in the body must involve the stimulation of protein synthesis in the cells to enable them to enlarge and divide. In the earlier days of hormone research it was assumed that estrogen probably affected protein synthesis and growth by somehow directly affecting certain enzyme-controlled reactions in the cytoplasm. More recent studies, however, have shown that estrogen has a primary effect on the chromatin of the nucleus. It has been shown by radioautography that a labeled estrogen becomes bound to the chromatin of a uterine smooth muscle cell as soon as 2 minutes after it is made available. Other studies indicate that this effect results in the increased production of RNA, and that it accelerates the transport of ribosomal precursor particles which are associated with messenger RNA to the cytoplasm, where polyribosomes appear that have different properties from those present in smooth muscle cells which have not been subjected to estrogen stimulation. The net result is that protein synthesis is increased. Accordingly, the growth effect of estrogen on the smooth muscle cells of

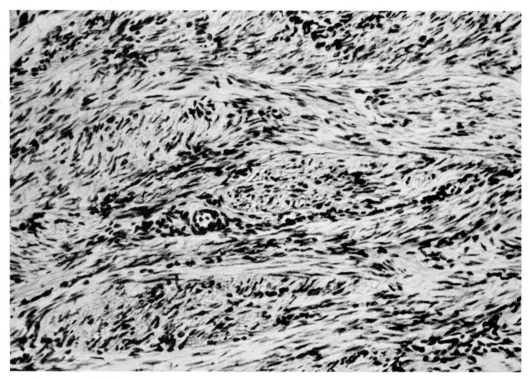

FIG. 26-17. Low-power photomicrograph of a section of the myometrium. Observe the interlacing bundles of smooth muscle fibers.

the uterus seems to be brought about at the level of the genes. The movement of RNA to the cytoplasm, where this primary effect is translated into increased protein synthesis, is also increased.

THE ENDOMETRIUM

This, the mucous membrane that lines the body and the fundus of the uterus, consists of an epithelial lining and a connective tissue lamina propria which is continuous with the myometrium. Customarily, the lamina propria is referred to as the *endometrial stroma*. The stroma is riddled with simple tubular glands whose mouths open through the epithelial surface into the lumen of the uterus, and whose deepest parts almost reach the myometrium (Fig. 26-19, *right*). The glands are composed of columnar epithelium.

It is helpful to describe the endometrium as consisting of 2 chief layers: a thick superficial one, called the *functional* layer, and a thin deep one, called the *basilar* layer. The functional layer is so-called because its character changes greatly during the menstrual cycle; indeed, at menstruation it is mostly shed (Fig. 26-19, *left*). The character of the basilar layer does not change to any great extent during the menstrual cycle,

and it remains through menstruation to regenerate another functional layer after the menstrual flow ceases.

Endometrium During the Menstrual Cycle. As might be supposed, the 28-day menstrual cycle is by no means constant; it may be a few days shorter or several days longer. Furthermore, the length of the cycle may vary in the same individual from time to time. It is usual to number the days in the cycle from the first day of menstruation; this is a concession to medical practice because the first day of menstruation is a date which a patient can set with exactitude. Most commonly, menstruation lasts for 4 days, but periods a day shorter or a day longer are common.

The endometrium passes through several different phases in each cycle. From days 1 to 4 it is said to be in its *menstrual phase* (Fig. 26-19, *left*). From day 4 until a day or two after ovulation the endometrium is said to be in its *estrogenic, proliferative, reparative* or *follicular phase* (Fig. 26-19, *right*). During this time it grows from something less than 1 mm. to 2 or 3 mm. in thickness. Mitosis occurs in both gland and stromal cells. Its growth during this period is encouraged by the estrogen that is being secreted by the ovary as a follicle matures and approaches the surface (hence the terms *estrogenic* and *follicular*). Figure 26-18 illustrates how potently estrogen can affect the growth of a rat uterus.

The last day of the estrogenic phase cannot be set with any exactitude because of the variability of the time of ovulation. Such evidence as exists is somewhat conflicting, but ovulation probably occurs somewhere between days 8 and 20 and rarely before or after this period (see Siegler: *Fertility in Women*). The latter part of the estrogenic phase is often termed the *interval phase*. This term is used to depict that period that ensues after the endometrium has become thoroughly repaired but has not yet begun to be affected by progesterone. The last phase of the menstrual cycle is called either: (1) the *progestational phase*, because the changes that occur in the endometrium during this phase are due to the action of progesterone, or (2) the *progravid* (*gravid*, heavy) *phase*, because pregnancy, when it occurs, begins in this phase, or (3)

the *secretory phase*, because the epithelial cells of the glands actively secrete at this time. This phase begins shortly after ovulation. That the corpus luteum develops and functions for about 10 to 12 days seems to be a much more constant phenomenon in the menstrual cycle than the time of ovulation. The last day or two of the progestational phase is sometimes called the *ischemic* (*ischo*, I keep back, *haima*, blood) *phase* because the vessels that supply the more superficial parts of the functional layer of the endometrium become shut off for variable periods during this time, and the endometrium suffers from a lack of blood supply, as will be described in more detail later.

Microscopic Appearance of Endometrium in Different Phases

The Estrogenic (Interval) Phase. The endometrium in the latter part of the estrogenic (interval)

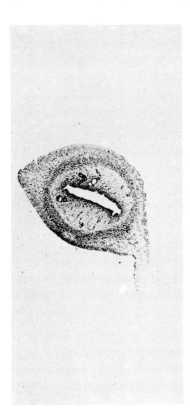 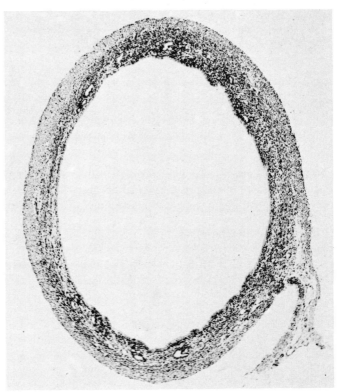

FIG. 26-18. (*Left*) Very low-power photomicrograph of a cross section of one horn of the uterus of a rat a month after its ovaries were removed. The uterus has atrophied as a result of estrogen deficiency. (*Right*) Photomicrograph, at the same magnification, of the same type of preparation made from a rat treated identically, except that the rat from which this specimen was obtained was given large doses of estrogen for a few days before the specimen was recovered. This illustration shows not only that estrogen makes the cells of an atrophied uterus grow but also that estrogen makes its epithelial cells secrete, for this uterus is enormously distended with secretion.

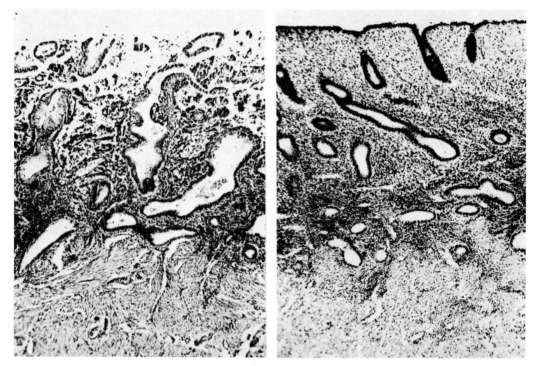

FIG. 26-19. (*Left*) Low-power photomicrograph of a section of the endometrium and the adjacent myometrium near the end of menstruation. Observe the raw inner surface, and notice that all but the most deeply situated parts of the glands and the stroma associated with them are degenerating and being cast away. (*Right*) Low-power photomicrograph of the same region in a section taken from a uterus in which the endometrium was in an early proliferative phase. Observe that the previously raw surface has become epithelized and that the glands are straight.

phase is from 2 to 3 mm. thick. The epithelial cells that line the surface and comprise the glands are columnar and often piled up on one another because of active proliferation. The small amount of mucus they secrete at this time is thin and watery. Patches of ciliated columnar cells are scattered about among the secretory cells. The glands in the functional layer of the endometrium tend to be narrow and straight. The stroma consists of star-shaped mesenchymal cells whose cytoplasmic processes connect with each other. The cells are adherent to a network of reticular fibers. Metachromatically staining amorphous intercellular substance is not so abundant at this time as somewhat earlier. Leukocytes are not common in the stroma in this phase.

The Progestational Phase. In this phase the endometrium becomes more than twice as thick as it was in the interval phase. The increase in thickness is due partly to increased amounts of tissue fluid in the stroma (edema), partly to the glands' accumulating increased amounts of secretion and partly to the increase in the size of stromal cells. Except in the more

superficial part of the functional layer and in the basal layer, the glands become wide, tortuous and sacculated (Figs. 26-20, *left,* and 26-21). Their cells come to contain considerable amounts of glycogen. At first this accumulates between the nuclei and the bases of the cells (Fig. 26-20, *right*), but later it appears between the nuclei and the free borders of the cells; the latter thereupon become ragged in appearance (Fig. 26-21). The secretion in the glands becomes much thicker and more abundant than formerly. The cells of the stroma are enlarged, undergoing what is called a *decidual reaction* (the word *decidua—deciduus,* a falling off—refers to the membrane, into which the functional zone of the endometrium becomes transformed during pregnancy, which is cast off at the time of birth). Stroma cells evidence this reaction by becoming large and pale, and their cytoplasm comes to contain glycogen and lipoid droplets. If pregnancy occurs, the decidual reaction is intensified and persists.

The changes that occur in all but the latter part of the progestational phase are due to the action of progesterone, working in collaboration with such estrogen as is still present in the circulation. It is assumed that, in general, these changes are designed to make the endometrium nutritive for a fertilized ovum; for example, the glycogen that forms may serve as a readily available form of carbohydrate.

The changes that occur toward the end of the progestational phase (provided that pregnancy does not occur) have been described by Markee. This investigator studied them by implanting bits of the endometrium of monkeys into the anterior chambers of their eyes, where they became vascularized and could be observed directly for hours. Markee found that the endometrium, toward the end of what we have termed the progestational phase, begins to regress(shrink). Regression, according to Markee, always precedes menstrual bleeding. In order to explain how the regression of the endometrium, which in all probability occurs because of the decreasing stimulation of both estrogen and progesterone at this time, may act to institute bleeding in and the breakdown of the functional layer of the endometrium, we must first describe the special features of the blood supply of the endometrium. As regression begins, leukocytes invade the endometrium.

Blood Supply of the Endometrium and Its Relation to Menstruation. Daron has studied the arterial supply of the endometrium of the monkey in the various phases of the menstrual cycle by injecting the blood vessels of the animal and then freezing and fixing the uterus *in situ*. Both cleared thick sections and ordinary serial sections were used in his study. Essentially, he found that 2 types of arteries lead from the stratum vascularis of the myometrium to the endometrium. Those of the first type, on approaching the endometrium, assume a coiled form and, without branching to any great extent, maintain their coiled form as they extend through the endometrium to its superficial part; there they terminate in a fountain-like arrangement of precapillary arterioles which supply the capillary beds of the inner part of the endometrium. The second type of artery that Daron describes extends from the stratum vascularis of the myometrium to end, after pursuing a straight course,

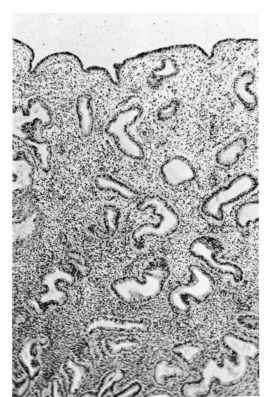
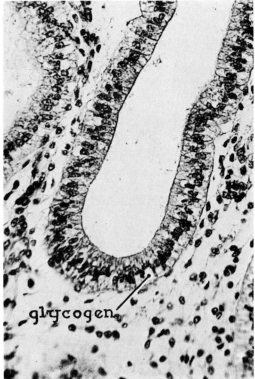

Fig. 26-20. (*Left*) Low-power photomicrograph of the inner portion of the endometrium in the early progestational phase. (*Right*) High-power photomicrograph of one of the glands. At this stage glycogen is present between the nuclei and the bases of their cells.

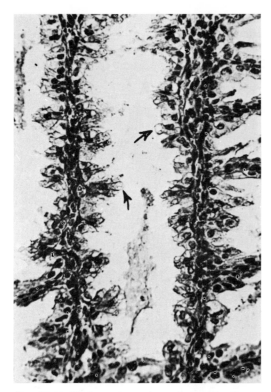

Fig. 26-21. Medium-power photomicrograph of a section of endometrium in the late progestational phase. Observe the ladderlike appearance of the gland photographed, and note that the free borders of the cells of the gland are ragged because there is glycogen at this site (arrows).

have suffered from a lack of blood supply during the period of vasoconstriction), it escapes through their walls into the stroma. By this means little pools of blood accumulate beneath the endometrial surface (Fig. 26-22). These soon rupture through the epithelium into the uterine cavity (Fig. 26-22, *top*). Meanwhile, the coiled artery concerned has become constricted again, and its terminal portions die. The same sequence of events is repeated in other arteries. As small pieces of endometrium become detached, arterioles may bleed directly onto the surface rather than into the stroma. As the deeper parts of the functional layer become involved, veins become opened, and they, too, slowly bleed. Eventually, over a few days, most of the functional layer of the endometrium is lost.

The cause of the progessive disintegration of the endometrium appears to be a lack of blood supply. That the functional layer of the endometrium is supplied by coiled end-arteries facilitates the effectiveness of vasoconstriction in causing an almost complete ischemia of the inner part of the endometrium. That the endometrium regresses and so causes the coiled arteries to become more or less buckled before menstruation, probably further facilitates the effectiveness of the vascoconstriction process in causing the necrosis of the endometrium. The reason for the basal layer's not being lost during menstruation lies in its different blood supply.

The cause of the regression of the endometrium in the latter stages of the progestational phase, and the vasoconstriction of the coiled arteries that follows in its wake, is hormone deficiency. Although both estrogen and progesterone are deficient at this time, progesterone failure is the more important precipitating factor; indeed, menstruation can be delayed by the administration of extra progesterone. Nevertheless, it is to be kept in mind that a reduction in the blood estrogen from the level attained in the midpart of the cycle plays some part in the process, for in anovulatory cycles (which are less common in women but occur commonly in some seasons in monkeys), bleeding occurs at the regular time for menstruation without ovulation having occurred, without a corpus luteum having formed, without progesterone having been secreted and without the endometrium having passed through a proper progestational phase. Hence, estrogen withdrawal, as it is often termed, can by itself cause retraction of the endometrium and bleeding from coiled arteries.

Early Part of Estrogenic Phase. The basal layer of the endometrium, with its separate arterial supply, is left intact throughout the cycle (Fig. 26-19, *left*).

in the deeper layer of the endometrium. The blood supply of at least the more superficial (inner) part of the functional layer of the endometrium, then, is derived from the coiled arteries.

Ischemic and Menstrual Phases. The coiled arteries are of the greatest importance in menstruation; indeed, the phenomenon of menstruation occurs only in those few members of the animal kingdom in which the endometrium of the female has this particular type of blood vessel. Markee found that, as the endometrium regresses, the coiled arteries become increasingly coiled to accommodate themselves to the thinning endometrium. As menstruation approaches, the circulation in them slows, and beginning the day before menstruation, the coiled arteries, one by one, become constricted for prolonged periods of time so that the endometrium that lies over them becomes blanched. After a coiled artery has remained constricted for a time, it dilates, and as blood once more reaches the arterioles and capillaries supplied by the artery (these

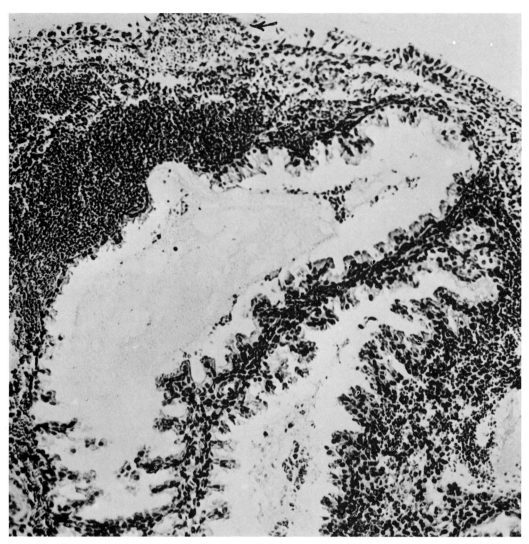

Fɪɢ. 26-22. Medium-power photomicrograph of a section of endometrium at the beginning of menstruation. Observe that a pool of blood has formed in the stroma (*upper left*), that the epithelial lining of the uterus has become discontinuous in the upper middle part of the picture, and that red blood cells are entering the lumen of the uterus at the site indicated by the arrow.

When the menstrual phase has run its course, the epithelium from the glands under the influence of newly secreted estrogen, grows out over the denuded surface and rapidly covers it again (Fig. 26-19, *right*). Mitotic figures become numerous both in the gland and in the stroma cells. Amorphous intercellular substance is formed in noticeable amounts in the stroma; according to both S. H. Bensley and Sylvén, this precedes the substantial formation of reticular fibers, and the amount of it decreases as the fibers develop. Repair is so rapid that an interval type of endometrium is soon produced.

The Placenta

Some General Considerations. The placenta is an organ that develops during pregnancy in the lining of the uterus. When fully developed it has the shape of a flat cake (*placenta*, cake), approximately 15 cm. in diameter and 3 cm. thick. It is fundamentally of fetal origin. Its primary function is to permit substances dissolved in the blood of the mother to diffuse into the blood of the fetus and vice versa. Its design permits this to occur over a vast area. Under normal conditions the blood of the fetus and the blood of the mother

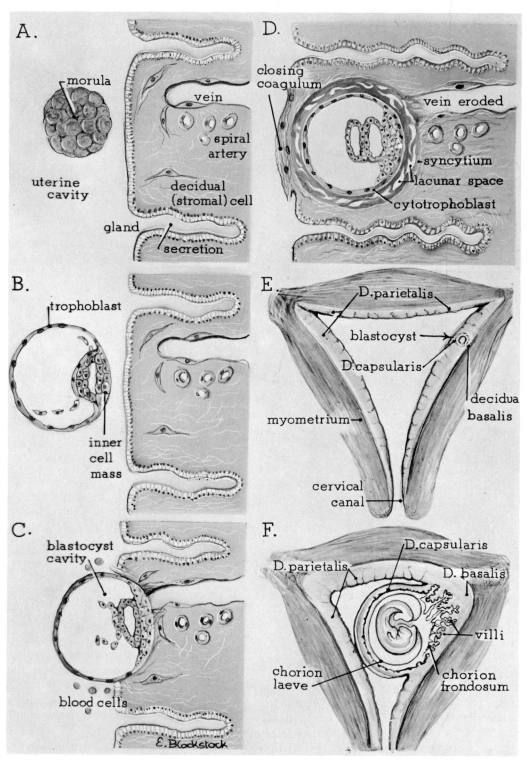

Fig. 26-23. Diagrams A, B, C and D illustrate the stages in the formation of the blastocyst and the embedding of the blastocyst in the uterine wall. The relationships of the growing embryo to the uterus are shown in diagrams E and F.

neither mix nor come into direct contact with one another. They are always separated by what is termed
the placental barrier; this, as we shall see, is a membrane composed of certain tissues. In the placenta,
food and oxygen, dissolved in the mother's blood, diffuse through the placental barrier into the bloodstream
of the fetus, and by this means life and growth are
supported in the fetus until it is born. Likewise, waste
products dissolve through the barrier from the blood
of the fetus to that of the mother and are eliminated
by the mother's excretory organs. Fetal blood passes
to and fro from the fetus to the placenta by means of
blood vessels in the umbilical cord; the latter structure
connects the fetus to the placenta during pregnancy.
At birth the fetus is expressed from the uterus, still
connected by means of the umbilical cord to the placenta. One task of the attending physician is to tie the
umbilical cord, for soon after the delivery of the baby
the placenta becomes detached and is expressed from
the uterus.

THE DEVELOPMENT OF THE PLACENTA

The details are given, more properly than here, in
textbooks of embryology. Here we shall describe only
enough of the process to help make the microscopic
structure of the placenta more readily understandable.

The fertilization of the ovum usually occurs in the
uterine tube (Fig. 26-11). The ovum then passes along
the tube, taking about 4 days to reach the uterus. By
this time several cell divisions have occurred, and it
consists of a clump of cells. Since it now resembles a
mulberry (Fig. 26-23 A), it is called a *morula*. A cavity then appears in this previously solid mass of cells,
after which it is called a *blastocyst* ("cyst" because
it has a cavity, and "blasto" because it will form
something) (Fig. 26-23 B). The blastocyst remains
free in the uterine cavity for only 2 or 3 days (Fig.
26-23 B), after which it becomes *implanted* in the
wall of the uterus (Fig. 26-23 C and D). Usually,
therefore, implantation begins 6 or 7 days after fertilization. At this time the endometrium (Fig. 26-20)
has been under the influence of progesterone for several days; hence it is "receptive" toward the ovum.
The site of implantation may be anywhere on the wall
of the uterus but usually is high up toward the fundus
on the anterior or the posterior wall (Fig. 26-23 E).

The wall of the hollow blastocyst is thin, consisting
of a single layer of cells, the *trophoblast* (Fig. 26-23
B) (*trephein,* to nourish, *blastos,* germ) except where
there is an aggregation of cells called the *inner cell
mass,* which bulges inward from the wall of the blastocyst into its cavity (Fig. 26-23 C and D). The inner

cell mass gives rise to the embryo. Its development is
described in textbooks of embryology. The trophoblast, however, is concerned in the development of the
placenta, so we shall consider it further.

The trophoblast of the blastocyst becomes fixed to
the free surface of the endometrial epithelium. At the
point of contact, the cells of the trophoblast proliferate
to become several cells thick (Fig. 26-23 C). The
uterine epithelium breaks down at this point, probably
because of the enyzmatic activity of the trophoblast.
This leaves a gap in the uterine lining which permits
the blastocyst to sink into the endometrial stroma
(Fig. 26-23 C and D). The defect in the endometrium
is closed temporarily by a plug of fibrin and cellular
debris called the closing coagulum (Fig. 26-23 D).
Later, the endometrial epithelium grows over the embedded blastocyst to restore the uterine lining. The
blastocyst then lies surrounded by stromal cells in the
superficial layer of the endometrium (Fig. 26-23 E).

By the 11th day after fertilization the cells of the
trophoblast have divided and formed 2 layers. The
cells of the inner layer are well defined; this layer is
called the *cytotrophoblast* because it is clearly composed of many individual cells (Figs. 26-23 D and 26-
24). The outer layer is much thicker and does not consist of well-defined cells but of a continuous mass of
cytoplasm containing many nuclei. Since the cells of
this layer are joined together, this layer constitutes a
syncytium (*syn,* together), and the layer itself is
called the *syncytiotrophoblast* (Fig. 26-24, SYN-
CYTIOTROPH). At this stage there are a few small
spaces, called *lacunae* or *lakes* in the syncytium (Figs.
26-23 D and 26-24, LACUNA). By the 15th day these
have increased in size and often become confluent.
Moreover, they are filled with blood from the uterine
veins and the venous sinuses which the trophoblast
has eroded. Only later does the trophoblast erode
maternal (spiral) arteries so that these, too, deliver
blood into these spaces.

As the lacunae enlarge, the strands of trophoblast
left between them are called *primary trophoblastic
villi.* Each villus consists of a core of cytotrophoblast
covered with an outer irregular layer of syncytiotrophoblast. The villi that extend out from the blastocyst around its whole periphery come into contact
with the endometrium in which the blastocyst is
buried, and cells from the villi apply themselves to
the endometrium to form a lining for the cavity in the
endometrium in which the blastocyst lies (Fig. 26-23
D). This lining of the cavity is peripheral to the
blastocyst, and so it is called the peripheral syncytium.
Hence, at this time trophoblast cells form a covering
for the blastocyst and a lining for the cavity in which

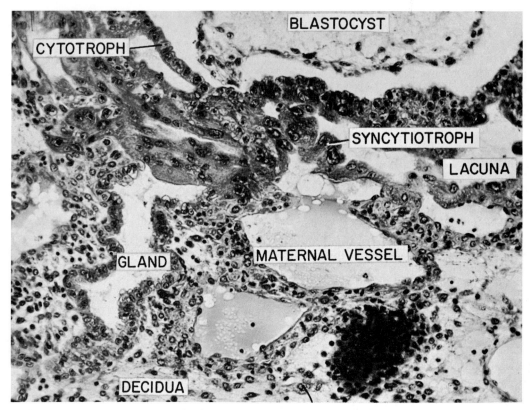

F₁G. 26-24. Part of a 12-day implantation site. Lacunae are lined by syncytium; the latter has
eroded a maternal artery and a uterine gland. The space near the top between embryonic membrane
and trophoblast is an artifact. (Photomicrograph from Professors J. D. Boyd and W. J. Hamilton)

it lies, and between the two are strands of cells, the
villi, which partially separate lacunar spaces (Fig.
26-23 D), which are filled with maternal blood. The
cytotrophoblastic component proliferates rapidly at
the tips of the villous structures that are forming.

The villi at this stage thus consist of cytotrophoblast covered by syncytiotrophoblast. Mitoses are
common in cytotrophoblast but not very common in
the syncytiotrophoblast. It would seem that the latter
grows by cells of the cytotrophoblast fusing to become
syncytiotrophoblast.

The structure of the villi begins to change about
the 15th day. By this time the different germ layers
are forming in the embryo, and mesoderm has grown
out from the developing embryo to form a lining for
the trophoblast that surrounds the blastocyst. When
the trophoblast has gained a lining of mesoderm, it is
called the *chorion* (*chorion,* skin). The mesoderm from
the chorion then extends into the villi to provide them
with mesodermal cores; when this happens, the villi
are called *secondary* or *definitive villi.* These grow and
branch. Fetal blood vessels develop in the mesoderm

in their cores, and later these vessels become connected with the fetal circulation (Fig. 26-27).

So far the changes that have been occurring in the
trophoblast have taken place all around the periphery
of the blastocyst. From here on, developments differ
in various sites around the circumference of the blastocyst. To explain these we must introduce some further
terms.

The endometrium that lies between the blastocyst
and the myometrium is called the *basal plate* (Fig. 26-
23 E, *decidua basalis*), and it is on this side of the
blastocyst that the placenta will develop from the
chorion. This is accomplished by the villi (with their
cores of mesoderm) continuing in this site to grow
and branch. In so doing, they of course continue to
destroy and erode more and more endometrium. As
they do this, the raw surface of the endometrium, as
it becomes exposed, becomes lined with cytotrophoblastic cells from the tips of the villi. Since the lacunae
between villi are filled with maternal blood and the
capillaries of the villi with fetal blood, diffusion of dissolved substances can occur between the maternal

blood in the lacunar spaces and the fetal blood in the capillaries of the villi.

The continuation of the processes described above in the region of the basal plate result in a structural formation of increasing size which in due course is known as the placenta; this will be described in more detail presently.

The Deciduae. All but the deepest layer of the endometrium of the uterus is shed when a baby is born. Since this portion of the endometrium of the pregnant uterus is destined to be shed, much like the leaves of deciduous trees in autumn, all but the deepest layer of the endometrium in a pregnant uterus is referred to as the *decidua* (Fig. 26-23 E). Various areas of the decidua are called by different names which designate their positions relative to the site of the implanted ovum.

The *decidua parietalis* (*parietal* means *forming*, or *situated on, a wall*) lines the entire pregnant uterus except that in the area where the placenta is forming (Fig. 26-23 F).

The *decidua capsularis* is the portion of endometrium that overlies the developing embryo; it forms a *capsule* over it (Fig. 26-23 E and F). As the embryo becomes larger, the decidua capsularis has to cover a larger and larger area, and it becomes very thin and atrophic. After 3 months the size of the chorionic sac that contains the embryo has become so large that the decidua capsularis comes into contact with the decidua parietalis at the opposite surface of the uterus; hence the uterine cavity is obliterated. Thereupon, the decidua capsularis blends with the decidua parietalis, and as it does so, it disappears as a separate layer.

The *decidua basalis* consists of the compact zone of the endometrium that lies between the chorionic sac and its contained embryo and the basal layer of the endometrium (Figs. 26-23 F and 26-25). The decidua basalis becomes the maternal part of the placenta. This is the only part of the placenta that is maternal in origin, and after the placenta is delivered at term, this layer is visible only as poorly defined bits of membrane.

Until about 12 to 16 weeks, the entire surface of the chorionic sac is covered with chorionic villi. As the sac enlarges, those villi associated with the decidua capsularis degenerate and disappear, so that by 16 weeks the greater part of the surface of the sac is smooth. This large area is called the *chorion laeve* (*levis*, smooth) (Figs. 26-23 F and 26-25). The remainder of the surface of the sac, that is, the part adjacent to the decidua basalis, continues to be covered with villi which keep growing and branching. This part, which constitutes the fetal part of the pla-

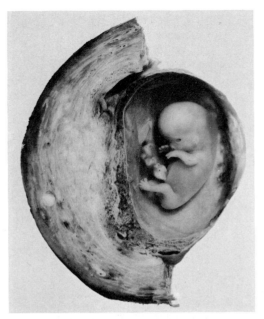

FIG. 26-25. This photograph is of part of the uterine wall with the placenta, fetus and fetal membranes. On the right, the wall of the chorionic sac (in which the fetus lies) is smooth. This is the chorion laeve. On the left, the fetal part of the placenta is formed by the chorion frondosum. This embryo was 36 mm. long. (From Professors J. D. Boyd and W. J. Hamilton)

centa, is called the *chorion frondosum* (Figs. 26-23 F, 26-25 and 26-26). By 16 weeks the placenta is discoid in shape, consisting of the chorion frondosum and the associated decidua basalis. At the time of birth the placenta occupies about 30 percent of the internal surface of the expanded uterus. The progressive increase in its thickness from around the 3rd to the 7th month is due mainly to the villi becoming elongated. The relative weights of placenta and fetus at various stages of pregnancy are: 1 month, 6:1; 4 months, 1:1; birth, 1:7. At birth the placenta weighs about 450 gm., is 15 to 20 cm. in diameter and about 3 cm. thick.

HISTOLOGY OF THE PLACENTA

The Villus. The most important component of the placenta is the chorionic villus. The early villus is a compact, bushlike tuft with its base attached to and arising from the chorion and its tip attached to the decidua. By the 2nd month side branches are formed with free tips, some of which later fuse with similar branches of adjacent villi to create a villous spongework. It is doubtful if such fusion permits anastomosis between fetal blood vessels contained in the respective

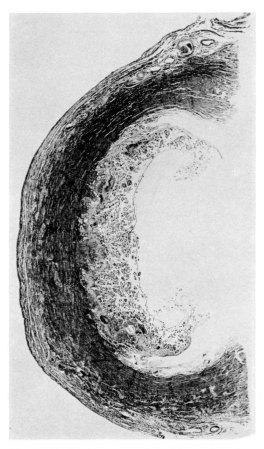

FIG. 26-26. This low-power photomicrograph is of part of the uterus with the placenta in situ, showing numerous villi cut in cross section lying in the intervillous space. The embryo, which was 15 mm. long, has been removed. (From Professors J. D. Boyd and W. J. Hamilton)

cores of fusing villi. However, the cytotrophoblast at the tips of the main villi fuses to form a continuous placental covering for the eroded surface of the decidua basalis. In the fully formed human placenta, there are usually 8 to 15 large villi, each of which, together with its many branches, forms a *fetal cotyledon,* i.e., a fetal lobule.

Villi are alike histologically. A section of placenta cuts villi in all planes, and between them is maternal blood. From any one section of placenta viewed under the microscope, it is difficult for the student to visualize the morphology and the physiology of the respective fetal and maternal circulations, which will be described later, but the student can examine the tissue layers that comprise the *placental barrier* that separates fetal from maternal blood.

In each villus there is a fetal capillary blood vessel lined with typical endothelium (Fig. 26-27). The capillary is contained in the loose connective tissue core of the villus. In the core there are some scattered smooth muscle fibers; these have been described by Arey as spindle-shaped or branching cells containing demonstrable myofibrils. Larger cells with large spherical nuclei (the cells of Hofbauer) also are seen in the cores of villi; possibly these are phagocytic. The trophoblast covering each villus consists of two well-defined layers until approximately the middle of the 3rd month of pregnancy, after which the cytotrophoblast progressively disappears until at term only isolated clumps of its cells are left. Compare *left* and *right* of Figure 26-27 and read caption.

The cytotrophoblast, also called Langhans' layer, consists of large, discrete, pale cells with relatively large nuclei (Figs. 26-24 and 26-27, *left*); the cells rest on a well-defined basement membrane. Their cytoplasm contains vacuoles and some glycogen but no lipid. Wislocki and Bennett considered the vacuoles to be an expression of metabolic exchange instead of a sign of degeneration. Under the EM the cells of the cytotrophoblast, as described by Wislocki and Dempsey, reveal glycogen, mitochondria and ergastoplasm, the last being equivalent to the cytoplasmic basophilia seen with the LM. They found also some material of high electron density located interstitially between cells; this they consider to be iron, which is known to be abundant in the tissue.

The syncytiotrophoblast is a dark, variably thick layer in which numerous small nuclei are irregularly dispersed (Figs. 26-24 and 26-27, *left*). This layer becomes progressively thinner throughout pregnancy (Fig. 26-27, *right*). Its outer surface has an irregular border, which often shows cytoplasmic streamers, an appearance which suggests a considerable plasticity of the cells during life. The EM shows the outer surface to have many microvilli. The cytoplasm ranges from being delicately vacuolated to foamy. It contains mitochondria, Golgi material and lipid droplets. The lipid droplets may be very large and abundant early in pregnancy, but later they become smaller and less numerous. Glycogen is usually absent, or present in very small amounts. After the cytotrophoblast has disappeared, the syncytiotrophoblast rests on a condensed network of reticular fibers.

By the time of birth the layers of tissue that constitute the placental barrier between maternal and fetal blood become very thin (Fig. 26-27, *right*). The outermost layer consists of only a thin layer of syncytium in which a few mitochondria and fat droplets are visible. The cytotrophoblast has mostly disappeared, with only

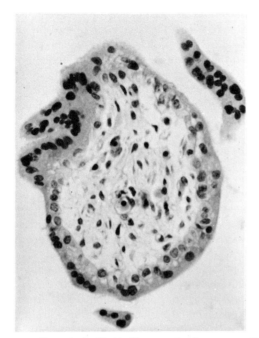 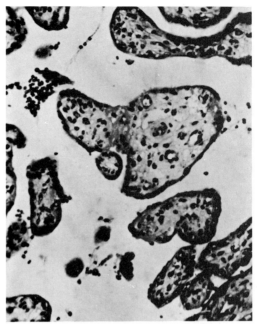

FIG. 26-27. (*Left*) Photograph of a cross section of a villus from a placenta at an early enough stage of pregnancy for the placental villi to show both layers of the trophoblast, the deeper layer being cytotrophoblast and the superficial, syncytiotrophoblast. Note the capillary in the core of the placenta; it contains a nucleated red blood cell. (*Right*) A cross section of a villus from a placenta delivered at full term. The villus is covered only with a thin layer of syncytiotrophoblast. Several capillaries can be seen in the mesenchyme of its core.

occasional cells persisting beneath the layer of syncytium. The middle layer is delicate connective tissue consisting chiefly of reticular fibers. The innermost layer is the endothelium of the fetal capillaries. Wislocki and Dempsey, with the EM, describe the placental barrier as consisting of a layer of syncytium bearing microvilli, a stout basement membrane, a connective-tissue space containing collagenic fibrils, a basement membrane around the capillary and, finally, the endothelium of the fetal capillary.

At intervals along a villus the syncytium is aggregated into protuberances of cytoplasm that contain many nuclei; these protuberances are called *syncytial knots* or *sprouts*. It is known that some of these syncytial sprouts break off to become free in the intervillous space; from here they can pass to the maternal circulation and on to the lungs of the mother.

Present in young placentae and becoming increasingly abundant in older placentae are irregular masses of an eosinophilic, homogeneous substance called *fibrinoid*. Its amount increases progressively during pregnancy; this gives an indication of the age of a placenta. At term aggregations of it many be visible to the naked eye. In sections, fibrinoid is eosinophilic.

As already noted, the maternal part of the placenta consists of the decidua basalis.

The zone where the trophoblastic shell is in contact with the endometrium is variously called the *junctional, composite,* or *penetration zone*. The last term relates to the fact that during the growth of the placenta the maternal tissue undergoes degeneration and necrosis in this zone as it is penetrated by trophoblastic villi. In this zone it is possible to distinguish decidual cells (derived from endometrial stroma) from cytotrophoblastic cells because the former are surrounded with collagenic and reticular fibers, but the latter have no fibrillar material between them. The endometrial stromal cells of the decidua basalis almost all take on the appearance of *decidual* cells; they become large, polygonal, and rich in glycogen and lipid droplets. The epithelial cells lining the endometrial glands during pregnancy are rich in mitochondria, glycogen and lipid droplets. By the 3rd month these glands in the decidua basalis are stretched and appear as horizontal clefts. The decidua basalis as a whole (the basal plate) consists chiefly of a connective tissue stroma, the cells of which are of the decidual type; endometrial glands, fibrinoid, and small clumps of

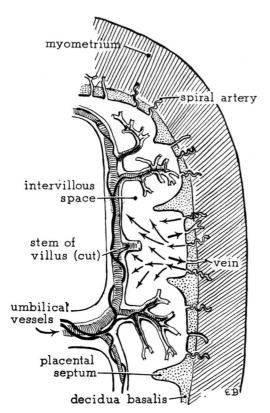

FIG. 26-28. This diagram illustrates the circulation of fetal and maternal blood in the placenta. Blood from the fetus reaches the placenta by the 2 umbilical arteries *(left, dark)*, passes to the villi and is returned to the fetus by the single umbilical vein *(left, cross-hatched)*. Maternal blood enters the intervillous space via numerous spiral arteries and returns to the maternal circulation through many veins. There is no mingling of the two bloods. Placental septae, which subdivide the placenta into cotyledons, are also shown.

projections of decidual tissue between the main villi, extending from the basal plate toward the chorion (Fig. 26-28). Such projections are called *placental septa,* and they divide the placenta into lobules or cotyledons, with each area of placenta between adjacent septa being a *maternal cotyledon* (Fig. 26-28). That the placental septa are mainly of decidual and not trophoblastic origin has been proved recently by Sohval, Gaines and Strauss, who showed that when the fetus was male, the nuclei of the septa are of the female type. Maternal vessels, particularly veins, often make short excursions into the base of a septum; this also suggests that the septa are of decidual and not trophoblastic origin. However, some cells toward the apices of the septa are undoubtedly of fetal origin, being derived from trophoblast and deposited, as it were, on the summits of the septa. From the 4th month, the tissues of the decidua basalis become extraordinarily "loose," being composed chiefly of a very dense venous plexus with dilated and distorted uterine glands. The latter have very thin walls, and secretion persists in them until late in pregnancy. Toward the margins of the placenta, the decidua is more compact.

The Intervillous Space. BLOOD CIRCULATION. The intervillous space develops very rapidly to become an enormous blood sinus bounded on one side by the chorion (chorionic plate) and on the other by the basal plate (Fig. 26-28). The space is labyrinthine in development and in form because the villi in it are variously connected to each other. The space is incompletely divided into compartments by the placental septa. The intervillous space is much expanded toward the embryonic side; this expanded part is the *subchorial lake* or *space.* Here there are only the main stems of the villi, and, just as there is more air space in a dense forest between the trunks of the trees than there is further from the ground between the many branches, there is more space here for blood. The *marginal sinus* is the marginal prolongation of the subchorial lake at the periphery of the placenta, and thus is circular in form when viewed from the surface.

Maternal blood enters the intervillous space through several hundred arterioles that traverse the decidua basalis, there being many such arterioles in each cotyledon or lobule (Fig. 26-28). Blood drains into numerous veins which open over the entire surface of the basal plate. Maternal blood pressure drives the blood entering the intervillous space high up toward the subchorial lake. After bathing the villi, venous blood flows back toward the venous orifices in the basal plate. Contractions of the myometrium and the fetal pulse in the villi possibly assist the circulation.

Attachment of Placenta. One question, not yet

trophoblast cells are also present. As Boyd and Hamilton have described, the fetal syncytium may penetrate through all layers of the maternal endometrium and even into the myometrium. Giant cells may be present in the basal plate, and these are believed to be derived from the fetal syncytium. Passing through the basal plate are spiral arteries which open eventually into the intervillous spaces. They are lined with endothelium, but near their openings they are lined with cells of the syncytiotrophoblast type; these do not institute clotting. This growth of these cells into the maternal spiral arteries probably reduces the pressure at which maternal blood is delivered into the intervillous space.

The maternal decidua is eroded more deeply opposite the main villi than elsewhere, and this leaves

definitely answered, is what mechanism holds the placenta in place. The association of degenerating maternal tissue and fetal trophoblast in the junctional zone, together with the presence of fibrinoid (Nitabuch's membrane), has been noted already, but this does not provide a firm attachment because it is here that separation occurs during labor. Probably the chief mechanism for holding the placenta in place is pressure. The chorionic sac is relatively tense throughout pregnancy, and early in development it fully occupies and obliterates the uterine cavity (Fig. 26-25). The growth of the chorionic sac and its contents requires that the uterus must grow to accommodate it; hence, the uterus hypertrophies, and hyperplasia occurs in the myometrium throughout pregnancy. With the pressure so engendered there would be little tendency for the placenta to move in relation to the uterine wall.

THE TROPHOBLAST AND/OR THE PLACENTA AS A HOMOGRAFT—THEORIES OF WHY REJECTION DOES NOT NORMALLY OCCUR

The fertilized egg and all the cells that develop from it (including those of the trophoblast and placental villi) have 46 chromosomes, half of which are derived from the mother and half from the father. Since the transplantation antigens controlled by paternal genes would be foreign to the female into which the fertilized egg, surrounded by its trophoblast, becomes embedded, it might be expected that a homograft reaction would ensue that would be directed against the paternal antigens and so cause either a rejection of the trophoblast-enclosed embryo or later a rejection of the placenta. Since this does not happen, the question is raised of why the host does not react against the trophoblast and/or the placenta as it would against a homograft of some other kind of tissue, for example, skin.

Perhaps the first matter to discuss is that it is known that there are certain sites (called preferred sites) to which homografts may be transplanted in a body, and in which their cells will survive and even multiply for varying lengths of time. Two such sites are the brain and the anterior chamber of the eye. The cheek pouch of the hamster is another example. The reason they are preferred will be explained shortly.

Next, it will be recalled that cartilage may be transplanted from one person to another with much success. The reason for this seems to be that the cells of cartilage are embedded in semipermeable intercellular substance that is of such a nature that macromolecules do not diffuse through it. Hence, there is no way for antigens on the surface of cartilage cells that are en-

closed in lacunae to come into contact with either circulating lymphocytes or lymphatic tissue or to escape, and so the antigens of the cartilage cells are thought to remain hidden. It is believed that the same reason accounts for the sites mentioned above being preferred sites; namely, there is no lymphatic drainage from them that leads to lymph nodes. For example, the equivalent of lymphatic drainage from the anterior chamber of the eye drains immediately into veins. The substance of the brain contains no lymphatics. The cheek pouch of the hamster is believed to be isolated from lymphatic drainage by a material having the same sort of properties as the intercellular substance of cartilage. The fact that antigens from these sites do not reach regional lymph nodes via lymphatics probably explains why lymphocytes do not readily become sensitized to foreign cells growing in these preferred sites and institute graft-rejection phenomena.

The question therefore arises of whether endometrium under the influence of progesterone is a preferred site. There are, of course, lymphatics in the wall of the uterus, but it seems questionable to the author whether lymphatic capillaries would grow to the surface layer of the endometrium every 28 days when it develops so rapidly under the influence of progesterone. In any event, when the cells of the trophoblast erode the endometrial surface, they, like the cells that cover the placental villi, are mostly exposed to blood rather than to tissue fluid, from which lymph would originate and drain into lymphatics. So there is some reason to think that endometrium that had developed under the influence of progesterone would be, to some extent, a preferred site for the growth of foreign cells.

However, other factors, and probably more important ones, seem to be involved. It has been shown that if fertilized ova are transplanted to any of various sites in the body, from which there is good lymphatic drainage, they will grow and develop. So it might seem as if the cells of the trophoblast did not possess any antigens foreign to their host. But if the host is first immunized against the tissues of the donor of the fertilized egg, the egg transplanted to one of these other sites, say, the kidney, does *not* grow and survive. For the fertilized egg to be rejected in this fashion shows that the cells that are developing from it must have antigens on their surfaces which are foreign to its host. However, it has also been shown that if the fertilized egg is transplanted into the endometrium of a host that has been similarly immunized, the growth and development of the fertilized egg proceeds normally. So the fact that a fertilized egg will grow in any number of locations in a host, locations which would have good lymphatic drainage, shows that a preferred site is not the whole reason for fertilized eggs developing in endometrium; they will develop almost anywhere. However, the fact that in immunized hosts they will grow in the endometrium, when they will not grow elsewhere, shows that the endometrium is a preferred site.

Many theories have been held about why the trophoblast is not quickly rejected when it is transplanted into various body sites and even various species. One concept that has been widely held (see *Embryos and Antigens* by Kirby and Wood) is that cells of the trophoblast (and placental villi) are coated by a material which keeps the cell surfaces of these cells from disclosing their antigens. This material is described as a fibrinoid sort of material, and it is said to be rich in hyaluronic and sialic acids.

At the time of writing there seems to be no doubt about the fact that trophoblast cells do not act as antigenically in any host or in any site as might be expected from their chromosomal complement. It also seems that the endometrium may be a preferred site for their growth. However, although there are interesting and attractive theories to explain both these phenomena, there is a great deal yet to be learned in this fascinating area of research, and when it is learned, the chances are that it will throw further light on how homograft reactions can be suppressed and perhaps also give some leads on how to enhance the immunological defenses of the body against cancer cells.

The Cervix

The cervix is the lowest and relatively narrow segment of the uterus (Fig. 26-22). Since its wall is continuous with the rest of the uterus, it might be thought, with some reason, that its wall would also be composed chiefly of smooth muscle. But a study by Danforth indicated that the amount of smooth muscle and elastic tissue in the wall of the cervix is not as great as has been generally supposed. He found that the wall of the cervix is composed chiefly of dense collagenic connective tissue, and that smooth muscle fibers on the average comprise only about 15 percent of its substance. Furthermore, he found that elastic fibers, except in the walls of its blood vessels, are relatively scarce.

The cervix, it should be remembered, must become widely dilated at parturition in order to permit the passage of the fetus. It is important, for many reasons that will become obvious when clinical work is encountered, to know whether the relaxation of the smooth muscle fibers in its wall is an important factor in permitting the cervix to dilate. Danforth's studies do not suggest that the cervix ordinarily contains

enough smooth muscle to exert a very strong sphincter effect. Hence, it seems that the main factor that permits the cervix to dilate at parturition, in response to the mechanical force exerted upon it, is the softening that occurs in its intercellular substance. This is associated with an increased blood supply and an increased tissue fluid content, which are probably due to the hormones of pregnancy.

Danforth has shown that so little elastic tissue is present in the cervix, except in its blood vessels, that it could scarcely be expected that stretched elastic fibers are a very important factor in bringing about the slow contraction of the cervix that occurs after parturition. What, then, makes the cervix become constricted again? It seems not unlikely that although the cervix does not contain enough smooth muscle to enable it to act as a true sphincter, it does contain enough smooth muscle to help it contract to some extent after birth, particularly since after birth the smooth muscle fibers would be in a stretched state and would have become sensitized to such oxytocin as is secreted by the posterior lobe of the pituitary gland at this time. But its further return probably involves a new organization of its fibrous tissue.

The cervical canal is flattened from before backward. The mucous membrane consists of epithelium and a connective tissue lamina propria. A longitudinal ridge or raphe is present both on the anterior and the posterior surface of the canal, and from these ridges mucosal folds extend at angles toward each side. The ridges do not directly face one another, so that when the lumen is collapsed they fit alongside one another. In addition to the ridges and declivities of the folds there are numerous large, branched, tubular glands. In the vaginal end of the canal these tend to slant from the lumen toward the body of the uterus (Fig. 26-29, *left*).

The epithelium of the mucous membrane (including that of the glands) consists of tall mucus-secreting columnar cells. In H and E sections their cytoplasm is pale, and their deeply stained nuclei are seen to be close to their bases (Fig. 26-29, *right*). Ciliated cells are sometimes seen. The glands extend deep into the lamina propria and even somewhat beyond (Fig. 26-29, *right*). The lamina propria is a cellular type of fibrous connective tissue. The nuclei are of the fibroblast type and are relatively close together. The cytoplasm of the cells cannot be seen clearly in an H and E section; nor can the character of the not overly abundant intercellular substance between the cells be seen to advantage (Fig. 26-29, *right*).

The lamina propria contains no coiled arteries and does not change much during the menstrual cycle.

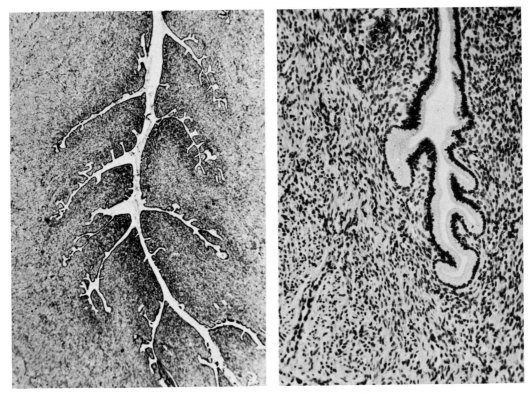

FIG. 26-29. (*Left*) Very low-power photomicrograph of a longitudinal section of the cervix, showing the cervical canal and the glands which extend out from it. The upper end of the photograph represents the end of the section nearest the vagina. (*Right*) Medium-power photomicrograph of the same section, showing the terminal part of one of the glands. The character of the stroma which immediately surrounds the glands and that of the general stroma of the cervix are also shown.

However, the secretion of mucus by the cervical glands becomes increased at the time of ovulation; it is evidently stimulated by estrogen. The glands sometimes become closed off, whereupon they may become converted into cysts. These are called *nabothian follicles.* These may cause elevations on the surface of that part of the cervix that projects into the vagina and so be seen or felt on a vaginal examination.

The portion of the cervix that projects into the vagina is covered by stratified squamous nonkeratinizing epithelium similar to that which lines the vagina (which will be described presently), and with which it becomes continuous. This type of epithelium extends usually for a very short distance into the cervical canal, where it undergoes a transition into the columnar type that lines most of the canal (Fig. 26-30). In some instances the zone of transition between the two types of epithelium is farther in; however, in others the columnar epithelium of the canal may continue out from the canal to cover little areas of the vaginal surface of the cervix close to the beginning of the canal; if so, these areas are termed physiologic erosions. (The stratified squamous nonkeratinizing epithelium which normally covers the cervix is pink-gray in color: columnar epithelium appears red. Hence the term *erosion.*) A factor in producing these is that the lips of the canal may become somewhat everted as a result of childbearing; this tends to expose the columnar epithelium.

The portion of the uterus with which the cervix connects is sometimes termed the isthmus of the uterus. The isthmus is supposed to be the narrowed segment of the organ that begins at its cervical end, where the typical mucous membrane of the cervix begins to change into the endometrial variety. The upper end of the isthmus is supposed to be the site where the lumen becomes constricted (the internal os) before opening out into the wide cavity of the body. However, the landmarks for both the beginning and the end of the isthmus are neither very obvious nor constant in position. The line of transition between the cervical type

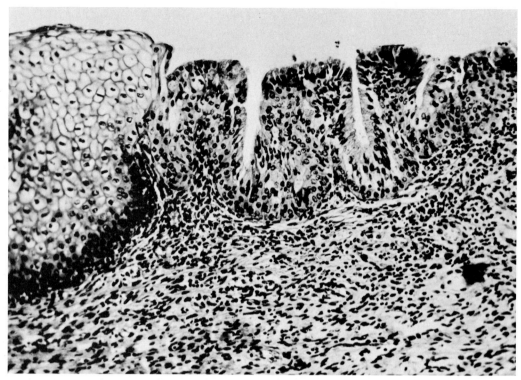

Fɪɢ. 26-30. High-power photomicrograph of a longitudinal section of the cervix near the site where the cervical canal opens into the vagina. The stratified squamous nonkeratinizing epithelium that covers the vaginal portion of the cervix and extends for a very short distance into the canal may be seen at the left, and the columnar epithelium that lines the remainder of the canal, at the right. The zone of transition between the 2 types of epithelium is immediately left of center.

of mucous membrane and the endometrial type may be gradual and the so-called internal sphincter not at all obvious. Danforth has shown that the wall of the so-called isthmus is composed chiefly of smooth muscle, and so he regards the isthmus as part of the body. It does not become dilated in pregnancy as soon as does the body, but when there is a need for more room to accommodate the fetus and the membranes than can be conveniently provided by the body, the isthmus becomes expanded and elongated to provide extra accommodation. Eventually, the more fibrous cervix itself becomes the only segment of the organ that is not expanded during pregnancy. The isthmus, then, is best considered, not as a separate part of the organ, but as the lower end of the body.

The Vagina

The vagina is a musculofibrous tube lined with a mucous membrane (Fig. 26-31). Under ordinary conditions it is collapsed, and the mucous membranes of its anterior and posterior walls are in contact. Except in the upper part of the tube, a longitudinal ridge is present on the mucosal surface of both the anterior and the posterior walls. From these two primary ridges numerous secondary ridges or *rugae* extend toward the sides of the tube (Fig. 26-2). No glands are present in the mucous membrane. The epithelium is of the stratified squamous type, and the way in which its character alters in relation to the level of sex hormones in the bloodstream will be discussed presently. The lamina propria on which the epithelium rests is of a dense connective-tissue type. It may exhibit lymph nodules. Farther out toward the muscle coat, the lamina propria —which in this site is sometimes regarded as a submucosa—becomes loose in texture and contains numerous blood vessels, particularly veins. Elastic fibers are numerous in the lamina propria directly under the epithelial lining, and they extend out through the mucous membrane to the muscular layer. The latter contains both longitudinally and circularly disposed smooth muscle fibers, but these are not gathered into discernible layers (Fig. 26-31). Longitudinally disposed fibers predominate. A fibrous adventitia lies outside the muscular coat and this connects the vagina with adjacent structures. The upper part of the posterior wall of the vagina is covered with peritoneum (Fig. 26-2).

Vaginal Smears. In recent years it has become common to study, particularly by means of films or smears, the cells that are found in the vagina. Such cells as are present in vaginal washings may be derived from: (1) the endometrium of the body of the uterus, (2) the cervical canal, and (3) the vaginal surface of the cervix or the lining of the vagina. Their study may be informative for two reasons. (1) Since the character of cells in these various sites is affected by the particular hormone concentrations that exist in the bloodstream, the cells found in vaginal washings may give some indication about the state of the hormone balance of the individual at the time they are obtained; and (2) cells indicative of having desquamated from an early cancer, growing in the cervix or the body of the uterus, may sometimes be found on an otherwise routine check of a patient and so indicate the need for more detailed examination for cancer. For both these reasons it has become common practice to study, by the film method, cells obtained by gently wiping the lining of the vagina or the covering of the cervix and the cells aspirated or otherwise obtained from the entrance of the cervical canal.

Cyclic Changes in the Vaginal Epithelium. The earlier investigators who attempted to prepare ovarian extracts that contained sex hormones had no ready way to find out if their extracts contained the active hormones they sought. In other words, there were no biologic tests by which the hormone content of any given extract could be assayed conveniently and accurately. Therefore, it was of the greatest importance when Stockard and Papanicolaou discovered, in 1917, that the vaginal epithelium of the guinea pig becomes keratinized at the time of estrus. Hence, whether or not any given guinea pig was in estrus could be ascertained by noting the presence or the absence of keratinized cells in a vaginal smear. A little later, Allen worked out the estrous cycle of the mouse and found that the vagina also became keratinized at the time of estrus. Therefore, it became obvious that the keratinization of the vaginal epithelium was one of the effects of the estrus-producing hormone. Mature mice and rats come into estrus spontaneously every 4 days and in between these periods of estrus the epithelium changes its character as will be described presently.

The changes that occur in the vaginal epithelium throughout the 28-day cycle of the mature human fe-

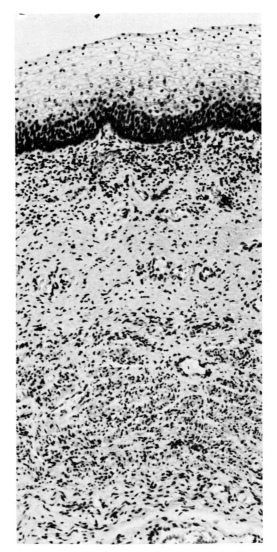

Fig. 26-31. Very low-power photomicrograph of a section of the wall of the vagina. Note that the more superficial epithelial cells are large and pale because of their glycogen content. The smooth muscle coats of the wall may be seen below the middle of the photograph.

male are not nearly so pronounced as those that occur in many lower animals. However, such changes as do occur are more easily interpreted in the light of a knowledge of the pronounced ones that occur in the estrous cycle of the rat or the mouse. Therefore, this will be described briefly.

As noted before, the rat and the mouse have a 4-day estrous cycle. This is divided into 4 periods: *proestrus, estrus, metaestrus* and *diestrus*. In proestrus, follicles approach the surface of the ovary, the uterus

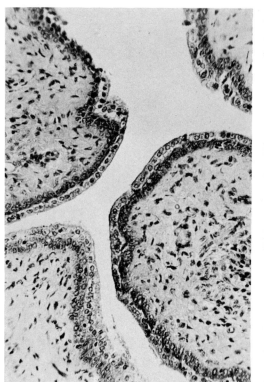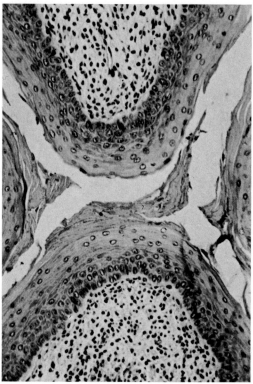

Fɪɢ. 26-32. (*Left*) Low-power photomicrograph of a portion of a cross section of the vagina of a rat from which the ovaries were removed. This shows that, under conditions of estrogen deficiency, the vaginal epithelium becomes thin, and the superficial cells nucleated. (*Right*) A similar praparation from a rat treated identically, except that it was given a large injection of estrogen 2 days before the section was obtained. Observe that the epithelium has become greatly thickened, and that the surface layers are heavily keratinized. This picture is similar to that seen in a normally occurring estrus.

becomes swollen with secretion, and its blood vessels become engorged. The epithelium of the vagina becomes thick as a result of proliferation in its deeper layers, but its most superficial cells are still nucleated. However, cells with kerato-hyalin granules appear beneath the superficial nucleated cells. The epithelial membrane thus comes to have a 2-layered appearance. In estrus or thereabouts, ovulation occurs, and throughout this stage the uterus remains swollen and red. The vaginal epithelium has now become thick and heavily keratinized (Fig. 26-32, *right*), and the mating impulse is aroused. The keratinized epithelium probably plays a protective function in the mating procedure. If mating does not occur, the animal passes into the metaestrus stage. As this progresses, the uterus becomes smaller and the vaginal epithelium much thinner (similar to Fig. 26-32, *left*). The basement membrane disappears, and polymorphonuclear leukocytes invade the epithelium and pass through it to appear

in great numbers among the epithelial cells that are seen in vaginal smears (Fig. 26-33, *left*). In diestrus, the uterus is small and pale, and the vaginal epithelium is still thin. However, polymorphonuclear leukocytes are confined mostly to the superficial layers of the epithelium. As proestrus develops, great mitotic activity occurs in the deeper layers of the epithelium, and it becomes thick again.

Since only the superficial cells desquamate, they are the only type seen in vaginal smears. Hence, in estrus, the vaginal smears contain only keratinized cells (Fig. 26-33, *right*). As metaestrus proceeds, vaginal smears contain, first, keratinized cells and then later nucleated cells and large numbers of the polymorphonuclear leukocytes that are making their way through the epithelium at this stage (Fig. 26-33, *left*). The diestrus stage is characterized by nucleated epithelial cells and leukocytes. In proestrus, the leukocytes have disappeared, so only nucleated epithelial cells are present.

The Epithelium of the Human Vagina. The epithelial lining of the human vagina is stratified and substantial (Fig. 26-31). Its deepest stratum consists of a single layer of cylindrical cells with oval nuclei. The next stratum is several cell layers in thickness. The cells in this stratum are polyhedral in shape, and it is said that they are joined together with intercellular bridges something like those in the stratum spinosum of the epidermis of thick skin; however, the cells in this stratum of the vaginal epithelium do not have a prickly appearance. The next stratum consists of a few layers of more flattened cells; these contain glycogen. Since this dissolves away in the ordinary preparation of sections, the cells of this and the more superficial strata appear swollen and empty. The most superficial stratum consists of several layers of more flattened but somewhat swollen cells, all of which possess nuclei.

The epithelium lining the vagina of the human female differs in two important respects from that lining the vagina of the mouse or the rat. First, since there is no true period of estrus in the human female, there is no time in the menstrual cycle when the epithelium becomes frankly keratinized. At the time of ovulation, which is the counterpart of estrus, the epithelium may show certain tendencies toward keratinization, but, unless the epithelium is unduly exposed to air or some other unusual environmental factor, it does not develop true keratin; hence, the surface cells always contain nuclei. Second, the epithelial cells of the more superficial layers of the vaginal epithelium tend to accumulate considerable quantities of glycogen in their cytoplasm, particularly at the time of ovulation. This has two possible functions: (1) it may serve as nutriment for male germ cells during their passage through this organ, and (2) it is fermented by bacteria in the vagina which convert it to lactic acid, and this may be an important factor in maintaining a suitable type of bacterial flora in the vagina.

The appearance of the cells that desquamate from the lining of the vagina and from the covering of the vaginal surface of the cervix has been studied at great

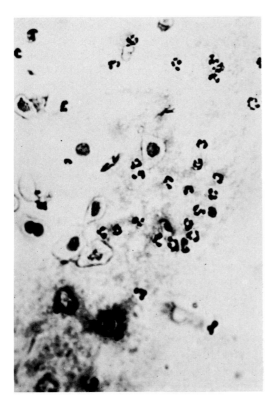 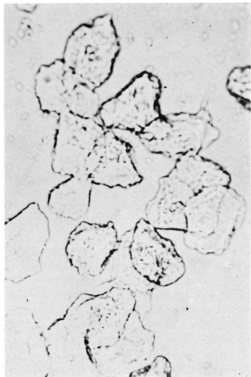

Fig. 26-33. (*Left*) High-power photomicrograph of a stained vaginal smear obtained from a rat in the later stages of metaestrus. Note the nucleated epithelial cells and the characteristic polymorphic nuclei of many granular leukocytes. (*Right*) High-power photomicrograph of a stained vaginal smear obtained from a rat in estrus. Observe that the smear contains nothing but large, very pale-staining, non-nucleated squames of keratin.

length by Papanicolaou by the smear method; his publications should be consulted for full information on this matter. Essentially, such progesterone as is secreted during the menstrual cycle appears to have no effect on the vaginal epithelium. The amount of estrogen secreted at the time of ovulation, while not enough to cause keratinization, does, however, have some effect. Papanicolaou considers that there is a relative increase in acidophilic cells with small dark nuclei in the vaginal smear at this time. The development of acidophilic properties by the surface epithelial cells is evidently preliminary to cells becoming keratinized, but this is as far as the process usually goes. There are also other criteria that may be employed. Evidently, in the hands of an experienced individual, the study of desquamated vaginal cells in smears may be helpful in determining the time of ovulation and the effectiveness of estrogen therapy and in diagnosing atrophic conditions of the vaginal epithelium that are due to estrogen deficiency.

The ability of estrogen to thicken and even keratinize the vaginal epithelium is taken advantage of in the treatment of certain vaginal infections, particularly those that occur in children, for in them the epithelium is thin and vulnerable.

The Mammary Glands (Breasts or Mammae)

Development. The first step in the development of mammary glands in man occurs near the end of the 6th week of embryonic life. At this time, in embryos of either sex, the ectoderm becomes thickened along two lines, each of which runs from the axilla to the groin of the same side. These are called the "milk lines," and their epithelial cells have the potentiality to grow down into the underlying mesenchyme at any point along either line to form mammary glands. Usually, in man, invasion of the underlying mesenchyme by epithelial cells destined to form mammary glands occurs at only one site along each line. However, in many animals mammary glands develop at many sites along each line so that in later life such animals have two rows of mammary glands with which to feed their large families. Occasionally, extra mammary glands develop along the milk line in man (and sometimes elsewhere); if so, they are called *supernumerary nipples* or *breasts*. Among civilized peoples supernumerary breasts are usually removed surgically for cosmetic and other reasons. Aberrant mammary gland tissue in the axilla may not become obvious until pregnancy or lactation causes it to swell.

As the embryo develops, the epithelial cells at the

point along the milk line where a breast is to develop form a little cluster from which up to 20 or more separate cords of epithelial cells push into the underlying mesenchyme in various directions. Each one of these original cords of cells develops into a separate compound exocrine gland; hence, each breast is actually composed of many separate compound glands, each of which empties by a separate duct through the nipple. During fetal life the cords of cells that invade the mesenchyme branch to some extent and tend to become canalized so that at birth a rudimentary duct system has formed. At birth there is no obvious difference between the degree to which the glands of the female and the male infant are developed. During the first few days of life the glands of a baby may become distended for reasons to be described later. The condition soon subsides.

Changes at Puberty. As puberty approaches, the breasts of the female, which up to this time have been flat, become enlarged and more or less hemispheric in shape. The nipple becomes more prominent. The changes in the breasts constitute one of the secondary sex characteristics of the female that appear at this time. Most of the increase in their size is due to fat accumulating in the connective tissue between their lobes and lobules. At puberty the epithelial duct system develops beyond a rudimentary stage, but this change is not so striking as the increased amount of fat in the connective tissue. It is not believed that true secretory units develop at this time; the formation of these awaits pregnancy.

In the male, the mammary glands usually experience no or little change at puberty, remaining flat. Uncommonly, some considerable enlargement closely resembling that which occurs in the female may occur: this condition is called *gynecomastia*.

Estrogen, probably in conjunction with some lactogenic hormone (the secretion of which would be dependent on estrogen appearing in the circulation), brings about the changes in the female breast described above. The progesterone that is periodically secreted from the time of puberty onward may play a contributing role. Estrogen given to males tends to make their rudimentary mammary glands develop into the feminine type.

Histologic Structure of a Resting Breast. The breast of a sexually mature nonpregnant female is termed a *resting breast* to distinguish it from one that is in the process of active growth in pregnancy or one that is functioning in lactation.

The *nipple* is a cylindrico-conical structure of a pink or brownish-pink color. It is covered with stratified squamous keratinized epithelium. Numerous papillae of an irregular shape extend into the epidermis from the dermis to approach the surface closely; hence, over papillae the epidermis may be very thin (Fig. 26-34). The main ducts from each of the many separate glands that make up the breast are called the *lactiferous ducts,* and they ascend through the nipple (Fig. 26-34) to open by separate orifices on its summit; the orifices are so minute that they cannot be seen with the naked eye. The epithelium of the lactiferous ducts, close to their orifices, is similar to that which covers the nipple. Deeper in the nipple the lactiferous ducts are lined with 2 layers of columnar epithelial cells that rest on a basement membrane.

The substance of the nipple consists of dense connective tissue and smooth muscle (Fig. 26-34). The fibers of the latter are arranged both circularly around the lactiferous ducts and parallel with and close beside them as they ascend through the nipple. Many blood vessels and encapsulated nerve endings are also present.

The epidermis of the nipple, like that of the vagina, is sensitive to estrogen. In relation to the problem of "sore nipples"—a condition which develops when some women attempt to nurse their babies—it is perhaps of interest to note that estrogen may be lacking in a woman shortly after she has given birth to a baby. The reason for this is that the function of estrogen production is largely taken over by the placenta during pregnancy; hence, when the placenta is delivered after birth, a woman is deprived of what has been her chief source of this hormone. Eventually, of course, her ovaries will produce a sufficiency, but it is possible that there may be a period of time when the epidermis of the nipple suffers from a lack of stimulation by estrogen. Indeed, Gunther ascribes one type of sore nipple to estrogen deficiency, and, in some experiments in collaboration with Gunther, the author found that feeding human placenta tissue to rats greatly thickened the epidermis of their nipples. However, there are certain complications, too involved to discuss here, in connection with attempting to use estrogen to thicken the epidermis of the nipples of women who have just begun to nurse their babies.

The skin surrounding the nipple, the areola, is of a rosy hue. It becomes pigmented in pregnancy, and after pregnancy never returns to its original shade; it always retains some pigment. Large modified sweat glands, but not so large or so modified as the mammary glands themselves, lie beneath the areola and open onto its surface; these are called the areolar glands (of Montgomery). Sebaceous glands and large sweat glands are present around the periphery of the areola. Smooth muscle fibers are disposed, both circu-

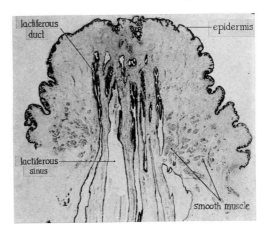

Fig. 26-34. Very low-power photomicrograph, lightly retouched, of a section of a nipple cut perpendicular to the skin surface.

larly and at right angles to the skin surface, beneath the areola.

The lactiferous ducts from the different lobes of the breast converge under the areola to enter the base of the nipple. As they near the point at which they converge, the ducts are believed to become somewhat expanded. These widened segments of the ducts are termed the *lactiferous sinuses* (Fig. 26-34), and in the lactating breast, they are believed to act as little reservoirs for milk. Whether these expanded portions of the ducts may be seen in the gross when a resting breast is dissected is questionable.

The many separate glands that are drained by individual ducts through the nipple constitute the lobes of the breast. Each lobe consists of many lobules; hence, each main lactiferous duct gives rise to many branches that, since they run within lobules, are called *intralobular ducts.* The parenchyma of the lobes and the lobules is generally considered to be disposed in the subcutaneous tissue (the superficial fascia). Nevertheless, the parenchyma of the mammary glands which, it must be remembered, develops from the epidermis of the skin, does not, in a sense, entirely escape the confines of the dermis. It will be recalled that the dermis consists of 2 layers, and that of these the papillary layer that abuts directly on the epidermis is more cellular and of a finer texture than the coarser and noncellular reticular layer that lies deep to it (Fig. 26-35). When cords of epidermis grow down into the mesenchyme to form the duct system of the breast, it seems that they carry, as it were, the developing papillary layer of the dermis along with them to form a soft cellular connective tissue wrapping for each duct (Fig. 26-35) or a common wrapping for small adjacent

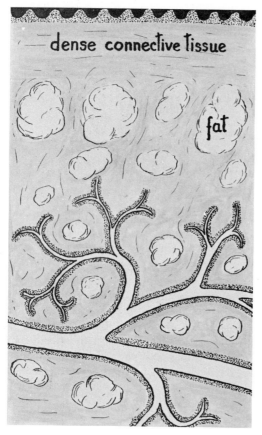

dense connective tissue

fat

FIG. 26-35. Diagram to show the relation of the layers of the dermis to the connective tissue of the breast. The papillary layer of the dermis and the intralobular connective tissue of the breast are comparable and are both stippled in the illustration. The dense connective tissue dermis of the skin is seen to be prolonged deeply, in the form of septa or ligaments, which pass between lobules of fat, to become continuous with the interlobular connective tissue of the breast.

groups of ducts. Then, between these single ducts or groups of epithelial ducts so wrapped, substantial bundles and partitions of coarse noncellular connective tissue extend down from the reticular layer of the dermis that overlies the breast to separate the lobes and the lobules from one another and to hold the whole breast parenchyma tightly to the skin (Fig. 26-35). The larger of these bundles and partitions are termed the *suspensory ligaments of Cooper*. Fat accumulates in them (Fig. 26-35), so that they hold the fat of the breast in place as well as the epithelial parenchyma. Fat also accumulates in the connective tissue between the breast parenchyma and the skin that overlies it and the fascia that lies beneath it.

From the foregoing, the appearance of a section cut from almost any site in a resting breast, and in any plane, may be anticipated. In such a section, epithelial parenchyma will be scanty indeed, and such as is present consists only of single ducts or little clusters of ducts widely separated from one another by connective tissue (Fig. 26-36). Most of the ducts seen in a section are cut obliquely or in cross section; occasionally, a portion of one may be cut in longitudinal section. Occasionally, a large lactiferous duct may be observed in a section that has been cut more or less haphazardly from the breast, but almost all the ducts that are commonly seen are of the different orders of branches that arise from the lactiferous ducts. Since the branches of the main ducts run out into the lobules that dangle, as it were, from the main ducts, most of the ducts seen in a section are inside lobules and hence are termed intralobular ducts. Their walls are generally composed of 2 layers of epithelial cells that have pale cytoplasm and pale oval nuclei. The long diameters of the nuclei in the inner layer of cells are commonly at right angles to the direction of the duct, and those of the outer layer are parallel with the duct. But the arrangement of epithelial cells in these ducts is variable. The epithelial cells of the ducts rest on a basement membrane.

Each duct is surrounded by a tunic of relatively cellular connective tissue that is about as thick as the duct is wide (Fig. 26-36). This cellular connective tissue that abuts on the epithelium of the ducts is the counterpart of the papillary layer of the dermis that abuts on the epidermis (Fig. 26-35). The cellular connective tissue that surrounds the individual ducts in a group of ducts may be confluent. Since this *cellular* connective tissue that invests the ducts is inside lobules, it is termed *intralobular* connective tissue. Fibroblasts are numerous in it and may be easily identified by their large, oval, pale and apparently naked nuclei (Fig. 26-36). Macrophages, lymphocytes and plasma cells are also normal cellular constituents of the intralobular connective tissue.

Single ducts or groups of ducts, invested with intralobular connective tissue, are separated from one another by thick partitions of coarse and *relatively noncellular* dense *interlobular* connective tissue. The connective tissue of these may be regarded, as is indicated in Figure 26-35, as a deep extension of the reticular layer of the dermis (the larger partitions seen are the suspensory ligaments of Cooper). The interlobular connective tissue often contains lobules of fat within its substance; the fat of the breast, then, is tied to the skin by the interlobular connective tissue.

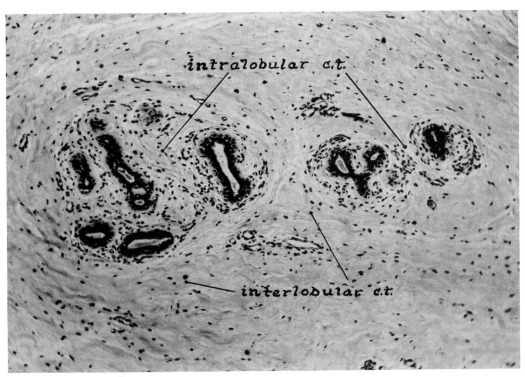

Fɪɢ. 26-36. Low-power photomicrograph of a section of a resting breast. Observe that the ducts are each surrounded by cellular intralobular connective tissue and that the 2 lobules shown are separated and otherwise surrounded by relatively noncellular interlobular connective tissue.

Changes That Occur in the Breast at Pregnancy. The resting breast probably contains no secretory alveoli but consists only of a duct system. As pregnancy proceeds, a great development of the duct system occurs, and, finally, secretory alveoli develop at the ends of the smaller branches of the duct system. By the end of the 5th month of pregnancy the lobules are packed (and greatly expanded) with alveoli (Fig. 26-37). The intralobular connective tissue becomes broken up as alveoli bud from the ducts within lobules, so that the intralobular connective tissue eventually becomes reduced to a series of filmlike partitions between adjacent alveoli; however, these contain extensive capillary networks. The alveoli themselves are composed of a single layer of columnar cells. Curved myoepithelial cells are sometimes seen to be fitted around their periphery. Because of the great expansion of epithelial elements within the lobules, the partitions of interlobular connective tissue become greatly stretched and thinned (Figs. 26-37 and 26-38).

Most of the epithelial growth that occurs in the breast in pregnancy occurs before the end of the 6th month. In the later stages of pregnancy further growth occurs, but very slowly. However, the breasts continue to enlarge; this is due chiefly to the cells of the alveoli beginning to secrete a fluid that expands them (and the breast) from within. This secretion is not milk; milk appears only after parturition, as will be explained presently.

Cause of Growth of Breasts in Pregnancy. Several hormones are involved, and it is difficult to be too precise about any of their actions because all species on which experiments are done do not react the same way, and, furthermore, the fact that the secretion of one hormone affects the secretion of other hormones makes it difficult to determine exactly just which hormone does what.

If intact animals are given enough estrogen, the mammary glands promptly develop. In some species estrogen by itself seems to be enough to prepare the glands for function. However, in some animals it seems that progesterone is also required to bring about the full development of secretory alveoli. In any event, estrogen is certainly involved in bringing about the great development of the epithelial component of the breast in pregnancy.

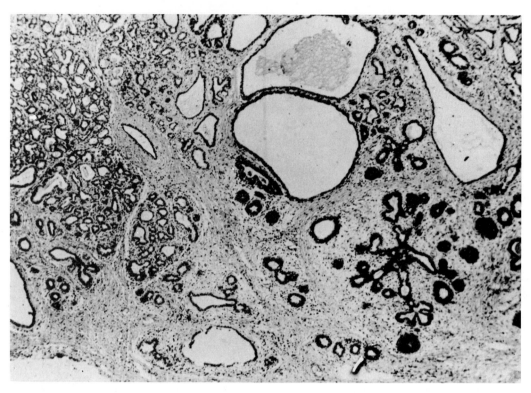

Fɪɢ. 26-37. Low-power photomicrograph of a section of a breast from a woman in the 5th month of pregnancy. The ducts have proliferated and, at the left side, they have given rise to alveoli.

However, estrogen, or a combination of estrogen and progesterone, will not bring about the full development of the mammary glands in a hypophysectomized animal. Accordingly, it seems that pituitary hormones or the hormones of the target glands that they control are also concerned in the phenomenon of the development of the breasts in pregnancy. In particular, evidence indicates that the growth hormone (somatotrophin), the lactogenic hormone and adrenal glucocorticoids all participate with estrogen and progesterone in causing the development of the breasts. However, the anterior pituitary is not essential because experiments are on record which show that the pituitary gland may be removed from a pregnant animal, and, provided that the placenta remains intact and functional, the mammary glands will continue to develop. In this connection it should be mentioned that the placenta makes a lactogenic-like hormone as well as (in the human female) quantities of chorionic gonadotrophin, estrogen and progesterone.

When more is learned about how different hormones affect the growth and secretory functions of cells, it should be possible to be more specific about the roles of the different hormones in this instance. However,

there is no doubt about the fact that estrogen is a key hormone in this connection because it can affect the growth of mammary gland tissue even if it is applied locally.

The Lactating Breast. As noted before, most of the increase in the size of the breasts from the 6th month on is due to secretion accumulating in the alveoli and the ducts. As this secretion is made, some appears and escapes from the nipple (in women who have previously borne children, this may occur relatively early in pregnancy). This secretion is not milk but a somewhat different fluid termed *colostrum*. After parturition, colostrum is secreted more abundantly but only for 2 or 3 days, after which the breasts (in human females) begin to secrete milk.

Colostrum contains a higher concentration of protein than does milk but very little fat. It also contains fragments of cells and even whole cells of a large size. These frequently contain phagocytosed fat and are called *colostrum bodies*. It is probable that these cells are phagocytes that have made their way through the epithelium of the alveoli and so gained entrance to their lumens.

It was once commonly believed that a large proportion of the milk obtained by a baby at a single nursing was secreted during the nursing period. It is now generally accepted that almost no milk is secreted during this time, and that milk is secreted and accumulates during the intervals between nursings.

MICROSCOPIC STRUCTURE. In the lactating breast the lobules are packed with secretory alveoli, among which some intralobular ducts may be seen (Fig. 26-38). In general, the interlobular septa are greatly thinned; those illustrated in Figure 26-38 are wider than most. The appearance of alveoli in different parts of a lactating breast varies in that the alveoli in some parts of the breast have high columnar cells and others low columnar cells. Some alveoli are distended with secretion, and some contain only a little. It is probable that the alveoli of different parts of the same breast may, at the same time, be in different stages of a secretory cycle.

The Fine Structure of the Secretory Cells of the Mammary Gland and the Process of Secretion. Milk contains protein, fat, sugar and mineral salts. It was once believed that the protein of milk was derived from blood protein. However, studies with the EM show that the secretory cells of mammary glands have the same equipment in the more basal parts of their cells for synthesizing protein as other types of cells that produce and secrete protein materials (the latter cells have been described in detail in Chapter 5) namely, abundant cisternae of rough-surfaced endoplasmic reticulum.

The Golgi apparatus is located on the lumen side of the secretory cells, and the indications are that the protein synthesized in the rough-surfaced endoplasmic reticulum is delivered via transfer vesicles to the saccules on the forming face of the Golgi apparatus, and that the protein destined for secretion leaves the mature face of the Golgi apparatus contained in secretory vesicles which move to the lumen side of the cell, where they are discharged into the lumen in much the same manner as occurs in such cells as the zymogenic cells of pancreatic acini.

The fat in the milk is synthesized in the cytoplasm of the secretory cells, probably in the cytoplasmic matrix and probably in much the same manner as fat is synthesized in fat cells, which was described in Chapter 9. Fat droplets move to the free surface of the

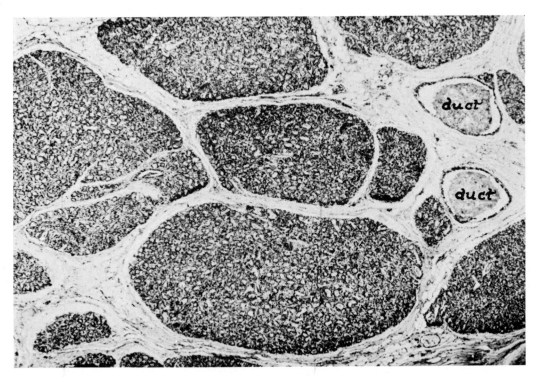

FIG. 26-38. Low-power photomicrograph of a section of a lactating breast. The lobules illustrated, although greatly expanded by a great content of alveoli, are not, in this section, cut through their widest parts. The interlobular septa are thicker in this photomicrograph than they are in most sites in the section.

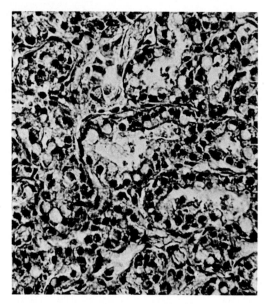

Fig. 26-39. High-power photomicrograph of a small area of a section of a lactating breast. Notice the vacuoles that represent fat droplets in the secretory cells of the alveoli, particularly at their free borders.

cells and are probably extruded by a process best described as reverse pinocytosis, because, in leaving the cell, they become enclosed by cell membrane. In ordinary paraffin sections the fat droplets in the cytoplasm are dissolved, and the spaces they formerly occupied appear as cytoplasmic vacuoles. These are numerous between the free borders of the alveolar cells and their nuclei (Fig. 26-39).

THE CAUSE OF LACTATION AND ITS MAINTENANCE

The lactogenic hormone (prolactin) secreted by mammotrophs of the anterior pituitary is the hormone chiefly responsible for causing the mammary glands to secrete milk. Under ordinary conditions the activity of mammotrophs is suppressed by the secretion of an inhibitory factor by the hypothalamus called PIH (for prolactin inhibiting hormone). Prolactin is secreted in small quantities by the mammotrophs during pregnancy, and a lactogenic-like hormone is also produced by the placenta. These probably collaborate with estrogen in causing the breasts to develop.

The termination of pregnancy, with the expulsion of the placenta, has many effects. The placenta previously has been acting as a hormone factory, making several hormones which could very well inhibit, by negative feedback mechanisms, the production and secretion of similar or other hormones by the glands of

the pregnant woman. When the placenta is delivered at parturition, this suppressive effect on hormone production in the woman's body is removed. One consequence of this may be that the anterior pituitary gland begins to elaborate greatly increased amounts of lactogenic hormone. However, nursing a baby sets up nervous stimuli which act on the hypothalamus *to inhibit* the secretion of PIH—the hypothalamic hormone that ordinarily restrains the secretory activities of mammotrophs. As long as nursing is continued the mammotrophs keep on secreting prolactin.

Ovulation and menstruation may not occur during the time a mother is nursing her baby. However, this is by no means a universal phenomenon, and women can become pregnant again during the nursing period. It is of interest that pregnancy does not interfere with a well-established lactation, and a woman may continue nursing one baby after another has been conceived.

Myoepithelial Cells, Oxytocin and the Milk Ejection Reflex. As occurs in other glands, the secretory alveoli of the mammary gland are each surrounded by cells which have the form of a loose basket, each consisting of a cell body from which many processes extend to clasp more or less the alveolus. These are myoepithelial cells, so-named because they have an epithelial origin and yet contain contractile filaments similar to those of smooth muscle cells. The similiar myoepithelial cells of the secretory alveoli of submaxillary glands are shown in Figure 7-15.

Contrary to what was once thought, the mammary gland continues to secrete in the intervals between nursings, and the milk accumulates in the lumens of alveoli and ducts. Afferent stimuli set up in the mammary gland when a baby begins to nurse reach the paraventricular nuclei of the hypothalamus (Fig. 25-16) to cause neurons to discharge and release oxytocin from the posterior lobe of the pituitary gland. The oxytocin causes the myoepithelial cells of the mammary gland to contract, and this causes the secretion contained in them to be ejected more or less from them to fill the lactiferous sinuses or even spurt through the nipple. In any event, the reflex causes milk to be available at the nipple for the baby to nurse.

A thorough emptying of the breasts at nursing helps maintain and even increase their functional capacities, not only because the nervous stimuli involved restrain the hypothalamus from secreting PIH but also because increased demands for function tend to stimulate the growth of enough further structure to permit the increased functional demands to be met.

Lactation cannot proceed in the absence of the adrenal cortex. The cortical hormone that affects carbohydrate metabolism appears to be the essential factor from this gland. The thyroid hormone also facilitates lactation. Insulin is also necessary.

Regression After Lactation. Since the breasts must be emptied regularly if their structure is to be maintained, and if the secretion of lactogenic hormone is to be continued, the discontinuance of breast feeding, provided that the breasts are not regularly emptied by other means, leads to their gradually regaining almost the same type of microscopic structure as they exhibit before pregnancy begins. They do not return to precisely the same state as before because a few alveoli persist in them. But most of the alveoli are resorbed, and the lobules shrink in size. The partitions of interlobular connective tissue again become thick and strong. It is very important that the breasts be properly supported during the time these partitions are thin, but it is particularly important during the period while the alveoli are being absorbed, the lobules are shrinking in size, and the interlobular partitions are becoming thick again (the 2 to 3 months following the cessation of lactation). If the interlobular septa become "set" in a stretched state, the breasts will subsequently sag unduly.

The Mammary Glands After the Menopause. The changes that occur in the breast after the menopause are various. The general trend that the breast exhibits is toward atrophy, of both its epithelial and its connective tissue components. The intercellular substance of the latter may undergo a hyalin change, but irregular growth and secretory changes may be superimposed upon the general atrophic changes. The epithelium of some ducts may proliferate and that of others secrete and convert the ducts concerned into cysts. Doubtless, estrogen and progesterone deficiency are chiefly responsible for the progressive atrophy that occurs after the menopause.

References and Other Reading

For some General References on sex see next chapter. *See also* textbooks of embryology and endocrinology.

SOME REFERENCES ON THE OVARY, OVIDUCTS, UTERUS AND VAGINA AND ON THE HORMONES PRODUCED BY AND/OR THAT AFFECT ANY OF THESE STRUCTURES

References for the placenta and mammary glands are given separately.

Allen, E.: The menstrual cycle of the monkey, Macacus rhesus. Contrib. Embryol., *19:*1, 1927.

————: The oestrus cycle in the mouse. Am. J. Anat., *30:*297, 1922.

Anderson, E., and Beams, H. W.: Cytological observations on the fine structure of the guinea pig ovary with special reference to the oogonium, primary oocyte and associated follicle cells. J. Ultrastruct. Res., *3:*432, 1960.

Aron, C., Asch, G., and Roos, J.: Triggering of ovulation by coitus in the rat. Int. Rev. Cytol., *20,* 1966.

Aschheim, S.: Pregnanacy tests. J.A.M.A., *104:*1324, 1935.

Austin, C. R.: The Mammalian Egg. Oxford, Blackwell Scientific Publications, 1961.

Bartelmez, G. W.: Histological studies of the menstruating mucous membranes of the human uterus. Contrib. Embryol., *24:*141, 1933.

Bertalanffy, F. D., and Lau, Chosen: Mitotic rates, renewal times, and cytodynamics of the female genital tract epithelia in the rat. Acta Anat., *54:*39, 1963.

Bo, W. J., and Atkinson, W. B.: Histochemical studies on glycogen deposition in the uterus of the rat. Anat. Rec., *113:*91, 1952.

Burrows, H.: Biological Actions of Sex Hormones. ed. 2. London, Cambridge University Press, 1949.

Corner, G. W.: The Hormones in Human Reproduction. Princeton, Princeton University Press, 1942.

Cowell, C. A., and Wilson, R.: The Ovary. *In* Ezrin, C., Godden, J. O., Volpé, R., and Wilson, R. (eds.): Systemic Endocrinology. Hagerstown, Maryland, Harper and Row, 1973.

Crisp, T. M., Dessouky, D. A., and Denys, F. R.: The fine structure of the human corpus luteum of early pregnancy and during the progestational phase of the menstrual cycle. Am. J. Anat., *127:*37, 1970.

Danforth, D. N.: The fibrous nature of the human cervix and its relations to the isthmic segment in gravid and non-gravid uteri. Am. J. Obstet. Gynec., *53:*541, 1947.

Daron, G. H.: The arterial pattern of the tunica mucosa of the uterus in Macacus rhesus. Am. J. Anat., *58:*349, 1936.

de Allende, I. L. C., Shorr, E., and Hartman, C. G.: A comparative study of the vaginal smear cycle of the rhesus monkey and the human. Contrib. Embryol., *31:*1, 1945.

Diczfalusy, E.: Mode of action of contraceptive drugs. Am. J. Obstet. Gynec., *100:*136, 1968.

Enders, A. C.: Observations on the fine structure of lutein cells. J. Cell Biol., *12:*101, 1962.

Guillemin, R.: Hypothalamic factors releasing pituitary hormones. Recent Advances in Hormone Research, *20:*89, 1964.

Hafez, E. S. E., and Blandau, R. J.: The Mammalian Oviduct: Comparative Biology and Methodology. Chicago, University of Chicago Press, 1969.

Hamilton, T. H.: Control by estrogen of genetic transcription and translation. Science, *161:*649, 1968.

Hartman, C. G.: The Time of Ovulation in Women. Baltimore, Williams & Wilkins, 1936.

Hertig, A. T., and Adams, E. C.: Studies on the human oocyte and its follicle. I. Ultrastructural and histochemical observations on the primordial follicle stage. J. Cell Biol., *34:*647, 1967.

Lillie, F. R.: The free-martin; a study of the action of sex hormones in the foetal life of cattle. J. Exp. Zool., *23:*371, 1917.

Markee, J. E.: Menstruation in intraocular endometrial transplants in the rhesus monkey. Contrib. Embryol., *28:*219, 1940.

————: The morphological and endocrine basis for menstrual bleeding. Progr. Gynec., *2:*63, 1950.

McCann, S. M., and Ramirez, V. D.: Neuroendocrine regulation of hypophysio-luteinizing hormone secretion. Recent Advances in Hormone Research, *20:*131, 1964.

Nilsson, O.: Ultrastructure of mouse uterine surface epithelium under different estrogenic influences. pp. 1-387. Uppsala, Almqvist and Wiksells, 1959.

Novak, E., and Everett, H. S.: Cyclical and other variations in the tubal epithelium. Am. J. Obstet. Gynec., *16:*449, 1928.

Ohno, S., Klinger, H. P., and Atkin, N. B.: Human oogenesis. Cytogenetics, *1:*42, 1962.

Papanicolaou, G. N.: The sexual cycle in the human female as revealed by vaginal smears. Am. J. Anat., *52:*519, 1933.

Papanicolaou, G. N., Traut, H. F., and Marchetti, A. A.: The Epithelia of Woman's Reproductive Tract. London, Oxford University Press, 1948.

Parks, A. S. (ed.): Marshall's Physiology of Reproduction. ed. 3. London, Longmans, Green and Co., 1952.

Pederson, E. S.: Histogenesis of lutein tissue of the albino rat. Am. J. Anat., *88:*397, 1951.

Pincus, G.: Control of conception by hormonal steroids. Science, *153:*493, 1966.

Pincus, G., Thimann, K. V., and Astwood, E. B.: The Hormones. vols. 1-5. New York, Academic Press, 1948-64.

Richardson, G. S.: Ovarian physiology. New Eng. J. Med., *294:* May 5, p. 1008; May 12, p. 1064; May 19, p. 1121; and May 26, p. 1183, 1966.

Ryan, K. J., Peters, Z., and Kaiser, J.: Steroid formation by isolated and recombined ovarian granulosa and thecal cells. J. Clin. Endocr. Metab., *28:*355, 1968.

Sharman, A.: Post-partum regeneration of the human endometrium. J. Anat., *87:*1, 1953.

Smith, B. G., and Brunner, E. K.: The structure of the human vaginal mucosa in relation to the menstrual cycle and to pregnancy, Am. J. Anat., *54:*27, 1934.

Smith, P. E., and Engle, E. T.: Differences in the time of onset of uterine bleeding after cessation of estrin and progestin treatments. Anat. Rec., *71:*73, 1938.

Snyder, F. F.: Changes in the human oviduct during the menstrual cycle and pregnancy. Bull. Johns Hopkins Hosp., *35:*141, 1924.

Sotello, J. R., and Porter, K. R.: An electron microscope study of the rat ovum. J. Biophys. Biochem. Cytol., *5:*327, 1959.

Swyer, G. I. M. (ed.): Control of human fertility. Brit. Med. Bull., *26:*1, 1970.

Wislocki, G. B., and Dempsey, E. W.: Histochemical reactions of the endometrium in pregnancy. Am. J. Anat., *77:*365, 1945.

Witschi, E.: Migration of germ cells of human embryos from the yolk sac to the primitive gonadal folds. Carnegie Inst. Contrib. Embryol. *32:*67, 1948.

Yamada, E., Muta, T., Motomura, A., and Koga, H.: The fine structure of the oocyte in the mouse ovary studied with electron microscope. Kurume Med. J., *4:*148, 1957.

Young, A.: Vascular architecture of the rat uterus. Proc. Roy. Soc. Edinburgh, *64:*292, 1952.

Zuckerman, S. (ed.): The Ovary. 2 vols. New York, Academic Press, 1962.

SOME ASPECTS OF PREGNANCY: IMPLANTATION AND THE DEVELOPMENT AND STRUCTURE OF THE PLACENTA

Arey, L. B.: The presence and arrangement of smooth muscle in the human placenta. Anat. Rec., *100:*636, 1948.

Avery, G. B., and Hunt, C. V.: The fetal membranes as a barrier to transplantation immunity. Transplantation, *5:*444, 1967.

Barcroft, J., and Barron, D.: Observations upon form and relations of the maternal and fetal vesels in the placenta of the sheep. Anat. Rec., *94:*569, 1946.

Blandau, R. J. (ed.): The Biology of the Blastocyst. Chicago, University of Chicago Press, 1971.

Boving, B. G.: Implantation. Ann. N.Y. Acad. Sci., *75:*700, 1959.

Boyd, J. D.: Some aspects of the relationship between mother and child. Ulster Med. J., *28:*35, 1959.

Boyd, J. D., and Hamilton, W. J.: The giant cells of the pregnant human uterus. J. Obstet. Gynaec. Brit. Emp., *67:*208, 1960.

————: Development of the human placenta in the first three months of gestation. J. Anat., *94:*297, 1960.

————: The Human Placenta. Cambridge, England, W. Heffer and Sons, 1970.

Boyd, J. D., and Hughes, A. F. W.: Observations on human chorionic villi using the E/M. J. Anat., *88:*356, 1954.

Dempsey, E. W., and Wislocki, G. B.: E/M of human placental villi. Anat. Rec., *117:*609, 1953.

Enders, A. C.: Fine structure of anchoring villi of the human placenta. Am. J. Anat., *122:*419, 1968.

Hamilton, W. J., and Boyd, J. D.: Observations on the human placenta. Proc. Roy. Soc. Med., *44:*489, 1951.

————: Development of the human placenta in the first three months of gestation. J. Anat., *94:*297, 1960.

Kirby, D. R. S., and Wood, C.: Embryos and antigens. Science J., *3:*56, December 1967.

Mossman, H. W.: Comparative morphogenesis of the fetal membranes and accessory uterine structures. Contrib. Embryol., *26*(158):129, 1937.

Paine, C. G.: Observations on placental histology in normal and abnormal pregnancy. J. Obstet. Gynaec. Brit. Emp., *64*(5):668, 1957.

Pierce, G. B., Jr., and Midgley, A. R., Jr.: The origin and function of human syncytiotrophoblastic giant cells. Am. J. Path., *43:*153, 1963.

Ramsey, E. M.: The vascular pattern of the endometrium of the pregnant Rhesus monkey (Macaca mulatta). Contrib. Embryol., *33:*113, 1949.

————: Vascular adaptions of the uterus to pregnancy. Ann. N.Y. Acad. Sci., *75:*726, 1959.

Simmons, R. L., and Russel, P. S.: The histocompatibility antigens of fertilized mouse eggs and trophoblast. Ann. N.Y. Acad. Sci., *129:*35, 1966.

Simmons, R. L., Cruse, V., and McKay, D. G.: The immunologic problem of pregnancy. Am. J. Obstet. Gynec., *97:*218, 1967.

Sohval, A. R., Gaines, J. A., and Strauss, L.: Chromosomal sex detection in the human newborn and fetus from examination of the umbilical cord, placental tissue and fetal membranes. Ann. N.Y. Acad. Sci., *75:*905, 1959.

Terzakis, J. A.: The ultrastructure of normal human first trimester placenta. J. Ultrastruct. Res., *9:*268, 1963.

Villee, C. A.: The Placenta and Fetal Membranes. Baltimore, Williams & Wilkins, 1960.

Villee, D. B.: Development of endocrine function in the human placenta and fetus. New Eng. J. Med., *281:*473, 1969.

Wislocki, G. B., and Bennett, H. S.: Cytology of placental trophoblast. Anat. Rec., *100:*414, 1948.

Mammary Glands

Cowie, A. T., and Folley, S. J.: The mammary gland and lactation. *In* Young, W. C. (ed.): Sex and Internal Secretions. ed. 3, p. 590. Baltimore, Williams & Wilkins, 1961.

Dempsey, E. W., Bunting, H., and Wislocki, G. B.: Observations on the chemical cytology of the mammary gland. Am. J. Anat., *81*:309, 1947.

Gardner, W. U.: The effect of ovarian hormones and ovarian grafts upon the mammary glands of male mice. Endocrinology, *19*:656, 1935.

————: Growth of the mammary glands in hypophysectomized mice. Proc. Soc. Exp. Biol. Med., *45*:835, 1940.

————: Inhibition of mammary growth by large amounts of estrogen. Endocrinology, *28*:53, 1941.

Gardner, W. U., and Chamberlin, T. L.: Local action of estrone on mammary glands of mice. Yale J. Biol. Med., *13*:461, 1941.

Gardner, W. U., and White, A.: Mammary growth in hypophysectomized male mice receiving estrogen and prolactin. Proc. Soc. Exp. Biol. Med., *48*:590, 1941.

Gomez, E. T.: Mammary gland growth in hypophysectomized castrated guinea pigs. Endocrinology, *31*:613, 1942.

Gunther, M.: Sore nipples; causes and prevention. Lancet, *249*:590, 1945.

Jeffers, K. R.: Cytology of the mammary gland of albino rat. Am. J. Anat., *56*:257, 279, 1935.

Linzell, J. L.: The silver staining of myoepithelial cells, particularly in the mammary gland, and their relation to the ejection of milk. J. Anat., *86*:49, 1952.

Nelson, W. O.: Endocrine control of the mammary gland. Physiol. Rev., *16*:488, 1936.

Petersen, W. E.: Lactation. Physiol. Rev., *24*:340, 1944.

Richardson, K. C.: Contractile tissues in the mammary gland with special reference to myoepithelium in the goat. Proc. Roy. Soc. London, Series B, *136*:30, 1949.

Speert, H.: The normal and experimental development of the mammary gland of the Rhesus monkey with some pathological correlations. Carnegie Inst. Contrib. Embryol., *32*:9, 1948.

Trentin, J. J., DeVita, J., and Gardner, W. U.: Effect of moderate doses of estrogen and progesterone on mammary growth and hair growth in dogs. Anat. Rec., *113*:163, 1952.

Turner, C. D.: General Endocrinology. ed. 4. Philadelphia, W. B. Saunders, 1966.

Waugh, D., and van der Hoeven, E.: Fine structure of the human adult female breast. Lab. Invest., *11*:220, 1962.

Wellings, S. R., Grunbaum, B. W., and DeOme, K. B.: Electron microscopy of milk secretion in the mammary gland of the C3H/Crgl mouse. J. Nat. Cancer Inst., *25*:423, 1960.

Wellings, S. R., and Philp, J. R.: The function of the Golgi apparatus in lactating cells of the BALB/cCrgl mouse. An electron microscopic and autoradiographic study. Z. Zellforsch., *61*:871, 1964.

27 The Male Reproductive System

The Parts of the System and Their Functions

The male reproductive system (Fig. 27-1) consists of: (1) two gonads, the *testes,* which produce male germ cells and male sex hormone; (2) a copulatory organ, the *penis,* by which male germ cells may be delivered into the vagina of the female; (3) a long, complicated set of tubes and tubules which lead from the testes to the penis which permits male germs cells made in the testes both to mature and also to be stored before being delivered to the male copulatory organ; and (4) certain glands called the male accessory glands, which have much smooth muscle in their walls. These glands not only provide a fluid vehicle for carrying male germ cells through the copulatory organ in the sexual act, but also, by the reflex contraction of the smooth muscle of their walls during the sexual act (certain voluntary muscles also participate), cause a mixture of their secretions and male germ cells (the mixture is called *semen*) to be expressed vigorously from the penis; this phenomenon, of brief duration, is termed *ejaculation.*

From the foregoing it may be realized that the male reproductive system consists of 4 structures or groups of structures that have somewhat different functions. Before considering the details of the microscopic structure of these and the relation of their microscopic structure to their function, it may be helpful to discuss in a general way some further features that they possess and their relation to one another.

Some General Features of the Testes. Although the testes develop in the abdomen from the indifferent gonads of the embryo, they migrate, in a way to be described in detail later, so that in postnatal life they are contained in the scrotum. This is a pendulous bag that hangs between the curved anteromedial borders of the proximal parts of the thighs (shown, but not labeled, in Fig. 27-1). Its wall is thin, being composed of skin, an incomplete layer of smooth muscle (the dartos) and some subcutaneous tissue. The wall of the scrotum has a considerable surface area, and it is believed that this permits its contents to be maintained at a temperature slightly below that of the body as a whole. This lower temperature is an important requisite in man for the production of male germ cells by the testes. The dartos muscle in the wall of the scrotum contracts in response to cold and certain other types of stimuli; its contraction makes the scrotum smaller and its wall corrugated.

Like the ovaries, the testes perform the two functions of producing germ cells and sex hormone. Male germ cells are called *spermatozoa* (*sperma,* seed; *zōon,* animal). The generic term for substances having male sex hormone activity is *androgen* (*anēr,* man, *gennaō,* I produce).

The structure and the functions of the testes are governed by the gonadotrophic hormone of the anterior pituitary gland. As a boy approaches puberty, the anterior pituitary gland begins to secrete substantial amounts of gonadotrophic hormones. These, in turn, stimulate the testes to begin producing both spermatozoa and androgen. The androgen secreted as a result of the gonadotrophic stimulus brings about the development of the secondary sex characteristics of the male that appear at this time.

The testes have two important functional components. First, tubules, having walls of many cells in thickness and a total length of almost half a mile, are packed into the two testes (Fig. 27-2). These are the *seminiferous* (*semen,* seed, *ferre,* to carry) tubules. Their walls consist of many layers of cells; those cells of the innermost layers are more or less continuously turning into spermatozoa. These become free in the lumens of the tubules. The second important functional component of the testes consists of clumps of endocrine cells, the *interstitial cells.* These are disposed in the connective tissue stroma between the tubules. These produce the androgen that is made by the testes.

Each testis is an ovoid body, 4 to 5 cm. long. It is covered with a thick capsule called the *tunica albuginea* because it contains so much white fibrous tissue (Fig. 27-2). Along the posterior border of each testis, the capsule becomes greatly thickened and extends into the substance of the gland for a short distance to form an incomplete partition. Since it tends to be in the middle of the gland, this abortive partition

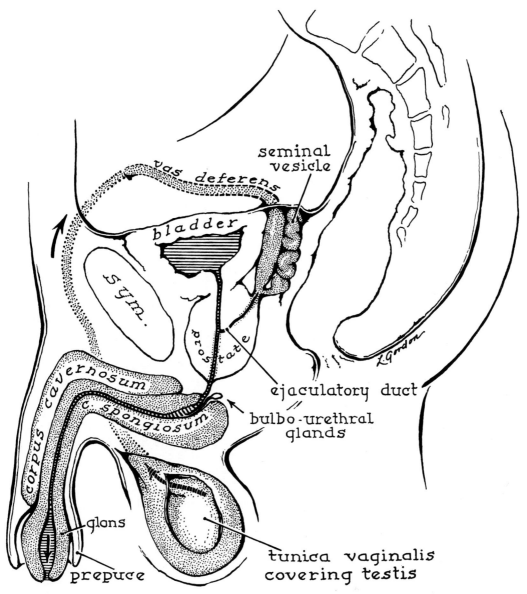

Fig. 27-1. Diagram of the parts of the male reproductive system, showing their connections with one another.

and the thickened part of the capsule from which it arises are said to constitute the *mediastinum* (*mediastinum*, being in the middle) of the testis (Fig. 27-2).

The mediastinum of each testis is riddled with a network of passageways that are lined with epithelium. These constitute the *rete* (*rete*, a net) testis (Fig. 27-2). The seminiferous tubules of the testis all empty into the spaces of the rete.

General Features of the Set of Conducting Tubes and Tubules. The spermatozoa present in the testis or seen in the rete testis are not capable of fertilizing ova. It appears that spermatozoa complete their maturation outside the testis in tubules which are enormously long and convoluted. Some morphologic evidence of this maturation has been observed in the guinea pig in which the spermatozoa were seen to take their definitive shape in the distal part of the tubule only. But the guinea pig is an exception. In most species the changes are more subtle, being mostly biochemical but nevertheless of great importance. The

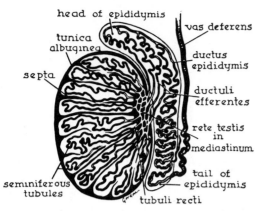

Fig. 27-2. Diagram showing the parts of the testis and the epididymis.

names and the general distribution of the tubules through which the spermatozoa must pass to reach the male copulatory organ will now be given.

The spaces of the rete testis, at the upper part of the mediastinum, drain into 15 to 20 tubules called the *ductuli efferentes* (*effere,* to bring out) that arise in this region (Fig. 27-2). These penetrate the tunica albuginea of the testis and emerge from its upper part. They thereupon pursue an extraordinarily convoluted course as they pass upward. Each tubule is so wound on itself that each forms a little cone-shaped structure. The cones are bound together by loose connective tissue, and together they constitute most of the head of a narrow crescentic structure that caps the upper pole of the testis and extends down along one of its sides. Since the testes are alike (twins), this narrow structure that caps each of them is termed an *epididymis* (*epi,* upon, *didymos,* twin).

Each epididymis has a head, a body and a tail. The head fits over part of the upper pole of the testis and consists essentially of the cones of convoluted ductuli efferentes (Fig. 27-2). The body extends down along the posterolateral border of the testis and consists chiefly of the ductus epididymis. This duct begins in the head where all the ductuli efferentes empty into it. In the body of the epididymis it pursues an extremely convoluted course (Fig. 27-2). This part of it, if unraveled, would be seen to be several yards long. In the tail of the epididymis, which reaches nearly to the lower pole of the testis, the ductus epididymis gradually assumes a less convoluted course and finally emerges from the tail to become the *ductus,* or *vas, deferens* (*deferre,* to carry away) (Fig. 27-2).

The ductus deferens ascends from the tail of the epididymis along the posterior border of the testis, medial to the epididymis. It becomes associated with

blood vessels and nerves and becomes possessed of coverings derived from the anterior abdominal wall, whose lowest medial part it traverses in a region known as the *inguinal canal.* The ductus deferens, together with the blood vessels and the nerves associated with it and the wrappings it obtains from the tissues of the anterior abdominal wall, constitutes a structure known as the *spermatic cord.* The ductus deferens, in the spermatic cord, traverses the inguinal canal, which leads through the muscles and the fascia of the abdominal wall, to enter the abdominal cavity (however, the ductus remains outside the peritoneum). Here the ductus deferens becomes free of its coverings and, after entering and pursuing a course in the pelvis—a course that need not be described here—reaches the back of the urinary bladder (Fig. 27-1). An elongated epithelial-lined sac, the *seminal vesicle* (a blind outpouching of the ductus deferens), lies lateral to it on the back of the bladder (Fig. 27-1). Immediately beyond the point at which the seminal vesicle empties into the ductus deferens, the ductus—which is now the common duct of the testis and the seminal vesicle—is known as the *ejaculatory duct* (Fig. 27-1). This duct pierces the upper surface of the prostate gland, traverses the substance of this gland and empties into the urethra, which structure, in turn, courses through the prostate gland on its way from the bladder to the penis.

General Features of the Glands That Supply the Fluid Vehicle for Spermatozoa. As noted before, the fluid that is delivered through the penis in ejaculation is called semen, and it is a composite of spermatozoa and a fluid vehicle, most of which is supplied by the seminal vesicles and the prostate gland. Moreover, these two structures, as well as containing epithelial secretory cells which provide the fluid vehicle described above, have a considerable amount of smooth muscle in their walls, and the sudden reflex contraction of these muscles at the time of ejaculation provides part of the force required to eject the semen.

The seminal vesicle is lined with secretory cells and its lining is thrown into an enormous number of folds (Fig. 27-19). The secretion produced by its lining cells accumulates in the cavity of the vesicle, and the engorgement of the vesicle that results from this process, together with the filling of the glands of the prostate gland (to be described later), by stimulating the endings of afferent nerves, is probably a very important factor in arousing sex urge in the male.

The prostate gland—about the size and the shape of a horse chestnut—is essentially a rounded mass of smooth muscle and connective tissue, the substance of which is thoroughly riddled by a great many separate compound tubulo-alveolar glands. The prostate gland surrounds the first part of the urethra as the latter emerges from the neck of the bladder (Fig. 27-1). The tubulo-alveolar compound glands that extend throughout its substance all drain, by means of about 2 dozen excretory ducts, into the prostatic portion of the urethra.

The Copulatory Organ. The urethra, which courses through the penis to open through its end, serves, in the act of copulation, as a means whereby semen can be delivered from the body. The penis, under ordinary conditions, is a flaccid structure, and in this state it could not function as a copulatory organ. However, in a male subjected to sufficient erotic influence, the penis becomes greatly increased in size and assumes a more or less erect position. This phenomenon is known as *erection,* and it enables the organ to perform the sexual act. Erection is an involuntary act controlled by the autonomic nervous system. The increased size and the altered position of the organ that occur under these conditions are to be explained by the fact that most of its substance consists of erectile tissue, soon to be described. This is disposed in three long cylindrical bodies arranged, two side by side and known as the *corpora cavernosa,* and one placed medially below the paired ones and known as the *corpus cavernosum urethrae* because in its substance it conducts the urethra from one of its ends to the other (Figs. 27-1 and 27-23). The corpora cavernosa contain a vast number of little cavities, all connected with the vascular system. When the penis is flaccid, the cavities are collapsed and contain only a little blood because the vascular arrangement is such that blood can drain from the cavities more easily than it can enter them. But, under conditions of erotic stimulation, nervous impulses flow to the organ and relax the smooth muscle of the arterial vessels that supply the cavities. This causes greatly increased amounts of blood to enter them, more than can be drained away conveniently. As the cavities of the corpora cavernosa become distended with blood, some of the veins which ordinarily drain blood away from the cavities become compressed. The net result of the great increase of the arterial supply and the impeded venous drainage is that the cavernous bodies become longer, thicker, wider and straighter and, as a consequence, the whole organ becomes enlarged and erect. Subsequently, when the smooth muscle of the arteries that supply the cavities contracts, the rate of drainage of blood from the spaces in the erectile tissue comes to exceed the rate at which it is delivered into the spaces, and, as a result, the organ returns to its flaccid state.

The Testes

Development and Descent. The embryonic development of a testis for the first 5 weeks is the same as that already described for the ovary. The primordial germ cells are derived from the same source as those of the ovary. They migrate to and enter the developing testis during the 5th week and become incorporated into cords of epithelial-like cells that are by this time present in the stroma. The primordial germ cells intermingle with the cells of the cords so that when the cords later develop into tubules, the primordial germ cells of the male, which are called gonocytes, become part of the layer of cells that make up its wall. Eventually the gonocytes become the spermatogonia of the seminiferous tubules that after puberty proliferate as stem cells, with many going through a process of differentiation that results in the formation of male germ cells, spermatozoa. The cells of the sex cords themselves give rise to what are termed the Sertoli (supportive and nutritive) cells of the seminiferous tubules.

Until the end of the 6th week there is little indication of whether a developing gonad will become a testis or an ovary. However, in the 7th week the sex cords become much more clear-cut in the male gonad than in the ovary. Furthermore, the mesenchyme immediately beneath the surface epithelium takes on a distinctive appearance from the deeper stroma, thus indicating that the thick tunica albuginea of the male gonad will form from it later. The interstitial cells, destined to serve an endocrine function in producing male hormone, develop from stroma cells between the epithelial tubules. As development proceeds, the sex cords become continuous with another group of cords that have a different embryologic origin and that become organized somewhat more deeply in the testis; these are the forerunners of the rete. The development of these and the other ducts of the male genital system and the manner in which they become connected with each other involve embryologic considerations too detailed to be dealt with here.

By the 4th month the elongated mass of tissue comprising the embryonic testis has become sufficiently condensed and rounded to have assumed a form suggestive of its adult shape. The cords of epithelium within it, destined to become the seminiferous tubules, have become more sharply defined from the mesoderm-derived stroma that occupies the spaces between them. Some of the cells of the stroma enlarge and become grouped together to constitute clusters of *interstitial cells.* It appears established that these produce androgen (the general term for hormones having male sex hormone activity) during fetal life, and that the testis is much more active an endocrine gland in the fetus than it is after birth until the time of puberty. It seems possible that the development of the interstitial cells of the testis in fetal life is dependent on a trophic-type of hormone made by the placenta.

In the testes of many animals the septa that radiate from the mediastinum out through the testis to the tunica albuginea divide the organ into lobules. However, in the testes of man the septa are incomplete.

Within the imperfectly separated lobules of the testes the cords of cells develop lumens around the seventh year of postnatal life. These seminiferous tubules become arranged in the form of long, convoluted, flattened loops (Fig. 27-2). At the point where each loop closely approaches the mediastinum, the tubule becomes continuous, by means of relatively straight canals (or caniliculi), the *tubuli recti* (*rectus,* straight) (Fig. 27-2), with the rete testis.

The testis originates in the body cavity behind the peritoneum at the medial side of the developing kidney. As development proceeds and the testis migrates downward, the peritoneum bulges out through the anterior abdominal wall, just above the medial end of the inguinal ligament, into the inguinal canal. The elongated tubular pouch of peritoneum so formed is called the *processus vaginalis* (sheathlike extension). The testis, which by this time lies immediately behind the peritoneum, is pulled down into the inguinal canal behind the processus vaginalis. The processus vaginalis traverses the inguinal canal and descends into the scrotum, arriving there at about the 7th month or somewhat later. The testis, pulling the ductus deferens behind it, follows along behind the posterior wall of the processus vaginalis to reach the scrotum shortly before the time of birth. The posterior wall of the processus vaginalis is invaginated by the testis and so covers its lateral and anterior walls as well as its two poles. In this way the testis comes to be provided with visceral peritoneum (the visceral layer of the tunica vaginalis). The remainder of the processus vaginalis lies in its own half of the inner wall of the scrotum and so constitutes the parietal layer of the tunica vaginalis. The canal by which the processus vaginalis communicates with the peritoneal cavity then becomes obliterated (this may occur before birth but usually occurs after).

Hormonal Control of Descent of the Testes and Maldescent. Occasionally, one or both testes fail to descend into the scrotum during fetal life or immediately after birth. Testes that fail to descend may be held up at almost any point along the course that they normally follow. An individual with undescended testes is termed a *cryptorchid* (*kryptos,* concealed; *orchis,*

testis). In some instances undescended testes descend spontaneously during infancy, but in the majority of instances they do not, and measures must be taken to assist them to gain the scrotum. It is important for the testes to descend before age 7, because this is the time when the cords develop lumens to become seminiferous tubules if the testes are in their proper environment. Unless the testes gain the favorable environment of the scrotum, they do not produce spermatozoa; however, the interstitial cells may still produce androgens. As knowledge about sex hormones has increased, it has become apparent that hormones to a considerable degree direct the normal descent of the testes.

As noted before, interstitial cells develop in the testis in significant numbers in the 4th month. This development and the general growth of the organ at this time suggest that it is being stimulated by some trophic hormone. It seems likely that placental gonadotrophin stimulates the growth of the testis of the male early in fetal life; but, as was described in the previous chapter, placental gonadotrophin requires assistance from the anterior pituitary to exert an LH effect, so a pituitary factor would also be involved in making the interstitial cells function as an endocrine gland in fetal life.

The androgens thus secreted would bring about the changes in the inguinal canal that permit the testis to descend through it more readily. It would also facilitate the growth of the scrotum and the ductus deferens. So it seems very probable that the androgen made by the fetal testis is responsible for bringing about these important changes that permit its descent.

Microscopic Appearance of the Testes From Birth to Puberty. The interstitial cells of the testes are not at all prominent during childhood (from birth to 10 years of age). The seminiferous tubules are small and are composed of two types of cells: the gonocytes that are the precursors of the spermatogonia that will later give rise to spermatozoa, and the supporting cells. The latter type of cells, called Sertoli cells, are numerous and show a small irregular nucleus and a poorly delimited cytoplasm. The gonocytes, fewer in number, have a spherical nucleus and a clearly visible cytoplasmic periphery. During adolescence (10 years to 14 years of age), under the stimulation of a pituitary gonadotrophic hormone, the gonocytes, now termed spermatogonia, start to proliferate and eventually produce, in large quantity, the spermatozoa. Simultaneously, the supporting cells increase in volume, and each comes to have a large, pale-staining polymorphous nucleus and much cytoplasm which extends inward from the periphery of the tubule, through the many layers of germ cells that are concerned with

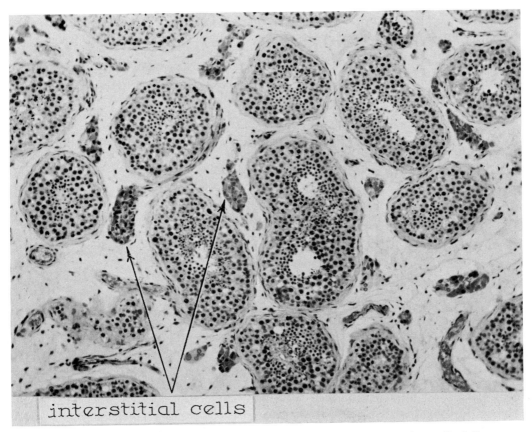

interstitial cells

FIG. 27-3. Low-power photomicrograph of a portion of a section of a testis of man. Seminiferous tubules, cut in cross and oblique section and separated from one another by a slight amount of interstitial connective tissue, may be seen, as well as some groups of interstitial cells.

forming spermatozoa, to the lumen of the tubule. These Sertoli cells (Fig. 27-4, Ser) have several important functions. They nourish the developing germ cells. They also help to provide a barrier (to be described later) between tissue fluid and germ cells in the later stages of formation, and they are involved in the production of a highly specialized tubular fluid. As we shall see, they play an essential role in the process by which spermatozoa are formed. During this period of active growth, the seminiferous tubules develop a lumen while the interstitial cells become distinguishable again in the stroma of the testes. A section of an adult testis showing seminiferous tubules in which spermatogenesis is occurring, and groups of interstitial cells, is illustrated in Figure 27-3.

Spermatogenesis

Terminology. The term spermatogenesis refers to the process by which spermatogonial stem cells give

rise to spermatozoa (male germ cells). The process includes all the changes that occur in a seminiferous tubule as spermatogonia, which lie against the basement membrane of the tubule, give rise to spermatozoa that eventually become free in the lumen of the tubules.

The Tubules in a Section Vary in Appearance. The cellular walls of the tubules are relatively thick because they contain cells in the various steps through which they pass in the process of forming spermatozoa. In an H and E section of a testis in which many seminiferous tubules are cut in cross section, the number of cells (as judged by their nuclei) in the walls of different tubules seems to vary somewhat (Fig. 27-3), which suggests that the process of differentiation that leads to the formation of spermatozoa is more advanced in some sites than in others. Indeed, the final stage of spermatogenesis indicated by the presence of spermatozoa in the innermost layer of cells will be seen only in some of the tubules in a section, so that even a casual glance at a section of testis suggests that the process of spermatogenesis is at different stages in different sites along tubules. The stages will be described in detail shortly.

The Basic Events in Spermatogenesis. The changes that occur in the cells in the walls of the tubules (spermatogenesis) can be thought of as occurring in three zones, from the outer cellular layer of the tubule to its lumen.

First, in the outer zone a spermatogonium undergoes a number of mitotic divisions. Some of each generation of spermatogonia so produced begin to differentiate. The others remain as stem cells. Those that begin to differentiate soon become pushed away from the basement membrane. Here they change slightly and after some further divisions they become cells known as primary spermatocytes. (The morphology of the cells involved here will be described shortly.)

The changes that occur in the next zone of the wall of the tubule depend on primary spermatocytes undergoing a first meiotic division to give rise to secondary spermatocytes which are smaller and which almost immediately undergo a second meiotic division to become what are termed spermatids.

The changes that occur in the innermost zone of the wall of the tubule result in spermatids becoming transformed into spermatozoa. This particular process is called spermiogenesis.

THE CELLS CONCERNED IN SPERMATOGENESIS

Since the cytoplasm of the various cells involved in spermatogenesis does not stain well, such distinctions between cells as are made with the LM are based on the characteristics of their nuclei. Distinguishing different types of closely related cells by nuclear differences can be difficult, because nuclear appearances in sections differ after fixation with different fixatives and, also, in different stages of the cell cycle. They also differ to some extent in different species. Nevertheless, evidence gained from LM studies of stained sections and by additional methods, including radioautography,

indicates that the spermatogonia can be classified into two main types as follows:

Type A spermatogonia in man may present either of two nuclear appearances. In one, called the dark type, although the chromatin granules are fine they stain well so that the nucleus is dark. In the light type the granules are dustlike so the nucleus is relatively pale. Both kinds are seen in Figure 27-4, labeled A. Nucleoli are present in both types, close to the nuclear border (Fig. 27-4). Type A spermatogonia are stem cells. In the rat, when a type A spermatogonium divides it undergoes at least 4 mitotic divisions (the group of cells so formed are shown by the EM to be connected by intercellular bridges as will be described later). The cells resulting from the divisions of A cells, at least in some species, are intermediate cells and these also divide by mitosis to produce B cells. In other species the cells resulting from the division of A cells become B cells. The nuclei of B cells are distinguished by containing deeply stained clumps of chromatin (Fig. 27-4, B) which is in contrast to the fine granules of the nuclei of A cells. The B cells undergo mitosis and the cells they give rise to are called primary spermatocytes (PL in Fig. 27-4).

The Maintenance of the Stem Cell Population. Not all the daughter cells of dividing A type spermatogonia differentiate beyond a point where they lose their potentiality for producing more A cells. Some must always persist as stem cells to maintain the stem cell population. There is, however, some uncertainty about the level at which this result is achieved; prevailing opinion is that it is at the first division of an A cell but there is also some opinion to the effect that cells arising after a few divisions can serve as stem cells.

The Meiotic Divisions of Spermatocytes. Primary spermatocytes are most easily recognized by the appearance of their nuclei when they enter the prophase of the first meiotic division. The prophase of the first meiotic division lasts a relatively long time and is divided into 5 stages. The first stage of the prophase is called the *leptotene stage* (*lepto*, thin; *tainia*, ribbon)

FIG. 27-4. (*On facing page*). Drawings illustrating the various steps of differentiation seen in seminiferous tubules. The illustrations are arranged to demonstrate the 6 typical cellular associations that are found repeatedly in the seminiferous tubules of man. Some of the terms used in this caption are explained in the text a little further on. The 6 associations (stages) are labeled I to VI, respectively. Ser, nucleus of Sertoli cell; A, type A spermatogonia; B, type B spermatogonia; PL, preleptotene primary spermatocytes; L, leptotene primary spermatocytes; Z, zygotene primary spermatocytes; P, pachytene primary spermatocytes; Di, diplotene primary spermatocytes; Sptc-Im, primary spermatocytes in division; Sptc-II, secondary spermatocytes in interphase; S, spermatids at various steps of spermiogenesis; RB, residual bodies. (Clermont, Yves: Am. J. Anat., *112*:35) *See also* Figure 27-5.

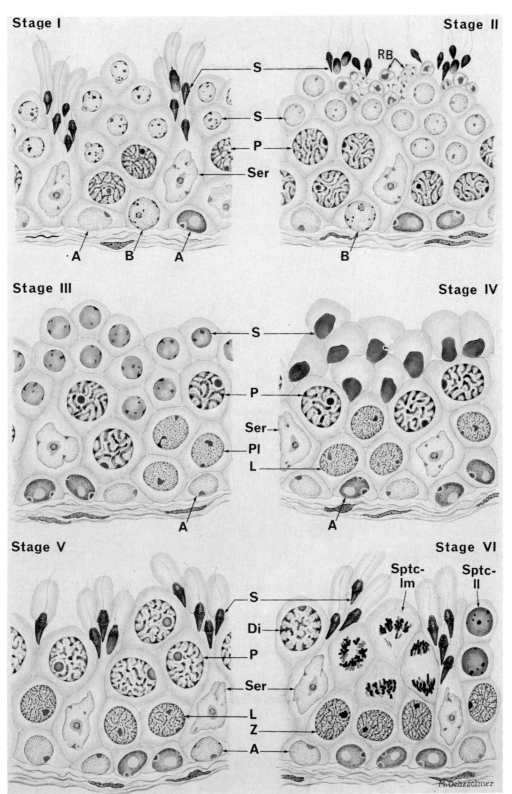

FIGURE 27-4. (*Caption on facing page*)

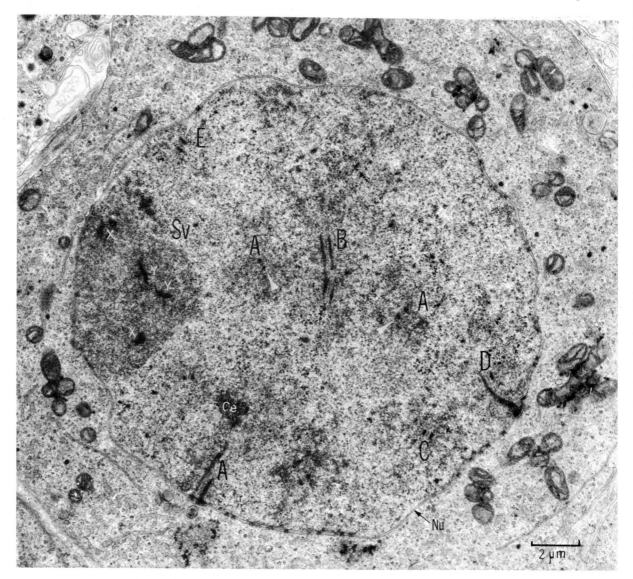

Fig. 27-5. A rat spermatocyte at the pachytene stage of meiotic prophase. In the nucleus there are synaptonemal complexes *A, B, C, D,* and *E,* which are continuous if followed through all sections of this nucleus (see Fig. 27-6). The complexes are attached to the nuclear envelope *Nu.* Inside the sex vesicle *Sv* are the cores on the X-chromosome *X* and the Y-chromosome *Y.* (Preparation by A. Hugenholtz).

because the chromatin threads (chromosomes) that become evident in this stage are very thin and delicate (Fig. 27-4, L). They are dense enough, however, for a section through the nucleus of a primary spermatocyte at this stage to indicate a cell that has entered the prophase (Fig. 27-4, L). It should be mentioned here that the last duplication of DNA to occur in connection with the development of a spermatozoon takes place in the S phase of a primary spermatocyte before

it enters the prophase of the first meiotic division. The primary spermatocyte before it begins prophase is referred to as a *preleptotene spermatocyte* (Fig. 27-4, Pl). DNA duplication is not required as a preliminary to the second meiotic division because in this division the DNA of the cells that divide is halved in forming haploid cells.

The second stage of the prophase of the first meiotic division is called the *zygotene* stage (*zygo,* joined;

tainia, ribbon) because it is in this stage that the homologue of each chromosome seeks out its mate (as was described in the account of meiosis in Chapter 2) to lie beside it (this is known as *synapsis*) and at this stage the chromosomes are said to have formed *bivalents* (*valentia,* strength) because they are now thicker than before (see Z in Fig. 27-4).

The third stage is called the *pachytene stage* (*pachy,* thick) because in this stage the chromosomes become increasingly condensed so they are thicker and shorter (P in Fig. 27-4).

Synaptonemal Complexes. Before describing the next phase of the prophase of the first meiotic division as seen with the LM, we should describe briefly a recent finding that has been made with the EM in connection with synapsis. Studies with the EM have disclosed that when synapsis occurs in both oocytes and spermatocytes, little structures composed of two dark parallel ribbons separated by a narrow space containing less electron dense material are to be seen in the nuclei of the cells at this stage (Figs. 27-5 and 27-6). These structures are called *synaptonemal complexes* (*synapsis,* a coming together; *nema,* thread) to designate that homologue chromosomes have come together to form a structural complex. Several are shown in the nucleus at the pachytene stage in Figures 27-5 and 27-6. It is to be noted that they are attached to the nuclear envelope at both their ends (Fig. 27-6, C and D).

In man there are 23 of these complexes at this stage. The X and Y chromosomes of the male become paired over only a very short distance; they remain almost entirely as single cores in what is termed the sex vesicle (Figs. 27-5 and 27-6). They, too, are attached at both their ends to the nuclear envelope.

As was described in the less detailed account of meiosis in Chapter 2, the synapsis of homologue chromosomes is of vast importance with regard to causing variation in the members of a species. Synapsis provides a means for the exchange of genetic material between each pair of homologous chromosomes involved and so provides for selective forces to act through evolution. The disclosure by the EM of the detailed structure of the arrangements wherein such exchanges are effected opens the door to gaining a better understanding of how they are effected and the factors involved.

The Next Stages of Meiosis. The fourth stage is called the *diplotene* stage (*diplo,* double; *tainia,* ribbon) because at this stage the two chromosomes of each bivalent separate sufficiently to be visible (Fig. 27-4, Di). However, as described in Chapter 2, the chromosome of paternal origin and that of maternal

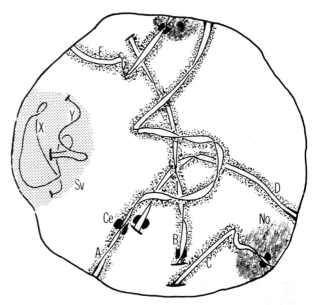

Fig. 27-6. Drawing of a reconstruction of the entire nucleus shown in Figure 27-5. There are 20 synaptonemal complexes in the nucleus but only the five that are visible in Figure 27-5 are shown. These are identified as *A, B, C, D,* and *E.* Each complex represents a set of paired chromosomes, has a centromere (*Ce*) and is attached with both ends to the nuclear envelope. *A* is the longest pair of chromosomes and *C* and *E* are nucleolar (*No*) bearing chromosomes. The sex vesicle *Sv* contains the cores of the *X*- and *Y*-chromosomes which have a small paired region. (Prepared by P. B. Moens)

origin retain contact with one another at some sites along their course; these sites are termed chiasma (which means to cross in the form of an X) because it is at these sites that the crossing over of genes occurs. The fifth and final stage of the prophase meiotic division is termed diakinesis which probably means that the two chromosomes of each bivalent clearly begin to move apart (*dia,* apart; *kinesis,* movement). In this stage the chromosomes are thicker still.

The cell next enters the metaphase with the chromosomes becoming arranged in the equatorial plane. In the anaphase which follows, the 2 chromosomes in each bivalent separate and move toward the two poles of the cell, one chromosome toward each pole (Fig. 27-4, Sptc-Im). Throughout the first meiotic division the two chromatids of each chromosome remain joined at their centromeres; hence the chromatids do not separate as occurs in mitosis. Instead, in the anaphase of the first meiotic division the two chromosomes of each bivalent merely separate from each other. The result is that each of the two daughter cells that form in the telophase in man has only 23 instead of 46 chromosomes—the haploid number instead of the diploid number.

The cells formed as a result of the first meiotic division are called *secondary spermatocytes* (Fig. 27-4, Spct II). They are smaller and closer to the lumen than primary spermatocytes. Since they almost immediately enter the second meiotic division, interphase secondary spermatocytes possess only a haploid num- in the wall of the tubule but they can be seen in various stages of division. Aside from the fact that the secondary spermatocytes possess only a haploid number of chromosomes, the second meiotic division is similar to mitosis, involving the separation of the two chromatids of each chromosome in the anaphase.

Spermatids. The daughter cells formed as a result of the division of secondary spermatocytes are called spermatids (S in Fig. 27-4). At first these are small, roughly rounded cells with round nuclei (S in Fig. 27-4, Stages III and IV). But they soon become elongated cells with ovoid nuclei which take up a position at one end of the cell. The ovoid nucleus of each becomes more or less pointed at the end that faces the wall of the tubule (S in Fig. 27-4, Stages V and VI). They each develop a single flagellum from one of their two centrioles which are present close to the rounded end of the nucleus. The details of their formation will be given in the succeeding text that deals with the study of spermatogenesis with the EM. But first we must deal with the cycle of the seminiferous epithelium and the stages of the cycle that can be identified.

THE CYCLE OF THE SEMINIFEROUS EPITHELIUM

What Is a Cycle? First let us consider cycles in general. With regard to membranes that are many cells in thickness and manifest different cellular compositions at different times, cycles are said to occur if the membrane, which demonstrates a particular structure at a given time, passes through changes in its structure but then returns to the same structure it demonstrated when the cycle began, and does this regularly. In the previous chapter we have had experience with two cycles: first, the menstrual cycle and, second, the cycle that takes place in the epithelium of the vagina of the nonpregnant female mouse and rat. With regard to the latter it was pointed out that the time taken for the cycle was easily determined by taking vaginal smears regularly and then determining the time between appearances of cornified epithelial cells in the smears, which is roughly 4 days.

Differences Between Cycles and Turnovers. In order to avoid possible confusion it should next be explained that the time taken by a cycle in a membrane may or may not be the same as the turnover time of the membrane. In the instance of the menstrual cycle the length of the cycle is approximately the same as its turnover time because almost the whole thickness of the endometrium is lost at menstruation, and so in each menstrual cycle the endometrium must be regenerated from the little that remained. Since almost a whole new membrane is formed in each cycle, the turnover time of the endometrium approximates the time taken by the menstrual cycle. But the time of the cycle of the seminiferous epithelium is not the same as its turnover time because only a small fraction of the cells of the membrane are lost in each cycle—those that have become mature (testicular) spermatozoa.

What is a cycle of the seminiferous epithelium? This is most easily explained if one could observe the same site along the course of a living tubule hour by hour and day by day. If this could be done it would be seen that the cellular constitution seen at this site when the study was begun would soon change and, after passing through many changes in the following period, would return to the same cellular constitution it possessed when the study began. It would thus have passed through a cycle and the time taken for this to happen would be the length of time taken by a cycle of the seminiferous epithelium. However, since it is impracticable to observe the same site in living seminiferous epithelium over a period of days, knowledge of the cycle had to be obtained by more indirect methods as will now be described.

Cell Associations in the Seminiferous Epithelium and How They Change During a Cycle. This subject was at first intensively investigated in small laboratory animals. In many of these it was found that cross sections of seminiferous tubules taken at different sites along the same tubule presented different appearances. For one thing, spermatozoa that had assumed their final form were seen only at some sites, which indicated that the process of spermatogenesis is more advanced at some sites along a tubule than at others. Furthermore, the numbers and state of development of the deeper cells of the wall of the tubule were seen to differ in various sites. Indeed, Clermont described 12 characteristic and different appearances (cell associations) that could be seen in cross sections of the seminiferous tubules of the guinea pig. Other small animals were also shown to demonstrate the same phenomenon. It was concluded that these different cell associations seen at different sites along a tubule represented different *stages* in the process by which spermatozoa were developed.

With this knowledge it was easy to understand that a particular cell association seen at a given site at a given time would change and that sooner or later the same cell association would reappear at this given site. The time taken for it to reappear would be the time taken for a cycle of the seminiferous epithelium.

When the seminiferous epithelium of the tubules of man were studied, the cell associations seen did not seem to be as clear-cut as those of laboratory animals. It was then found that the reason for this was that the cell associations seen in man are not distributed at different sites along the lengths of tubules as they are in laboratory animals but instead they are present with other associations in different sectors of a tubule at the same given cross section. Furthermore, it was found that there are only 6 associations seen in the tubules of man to represent the various stages of spermatogenesis. These are labeled I to VI in Figure 27-4 which shows the various kinds of cells seen in each of these stages with the LM and described in the preceding section. It should be pointed out that the distinction between the different cells involved is made almost entirely by their nuclear morphology and much of it by determining the stage of meiosis the primary spermatocytes are in. The 6 stages are also shown in the low-power pictures in Figure 27-7, in which different stages seen around the circumference of a tubule are marked off from one another by heavy black lines; here too, they are labeled from I to VI. The legend for Figure 27-7 contains a description of the cell types seen in each stage. (For details of the cells in each stage see Figure 27-4.) Both of these figures were taken from the work of Clermont who has provided so much of the information on this subject and whose papers should be read for further information.

The fact that the process of spermatogenesis passes through well-defined stages should not suggest that the cell association seen at one stage is instantaneously transformed into that seen in the next. What may be suggested, however, is that the changes that occur in the seminiferous epithelium do so in more or less of a rhythmic manner.

The Use of Radiography in Determining the Duration of Spermatogenesis and the Length of a Cycle

Only a general concept of how this is done will be given here. In the procedures used to determine either the duration of spermatogenesis or the duration of a cycle of the epithelium advantage is taken of the fact that the only cells that duplicate their DNA in the seminiferous epithelium are spermatogonia and preleptotene primary spermatocytes. This means that if labeled thymidine is made available to the seminiferous epithelium for a very brief period, the only cells that will take up label will be those spermatogonia and preleptotene primary spermatocytes that are at that time in the S phase of the cell cycle. So if label is seen subsequently in any cell concerned in the process of spermatogenesis in the days following the administration of the labeled thymidine, it would have to be label that had been incorporated into a cell when it was either a spermatogonium or a preleptotene primary spermatocyte.

Determining the duration of spermatogenesis is in some ways easier than determining the duration of the cycle. For the former the procedure would be to determine the time after labeling was done when label is seen in mature (testicular) spermatozoa. However, the first labeled spermatozoa that are seen would have originated from labeled preleptotene primary spermatocytes because it takes longer for a labeled spermatogonium to give rise to a labeled spermatozoon than it does for a preleptotene primary spermatocyte to form a spermatozoon. This must be taken into account in calculating the duration of spermatogenesis, which has been estimated in man to be approximately 64 days.

The length of a cycle is somewhat difficult to determine by radioautography. In general it depends on establishing that, immediately after labeling, some primary spermatocytes at the preleptotene stage would be found to be labeled and that they would be in a particular cell association. It could, therefore, be reasoned that, in radioautographs prepared from successively later specimens, the first time some labeled cells are seen in the same cell association in which the first labeled primary spermatocyte was seen, one complete cycle had occurred. However, the different stages of the cycle last for different periods of time and so it might be that one labeled cell was at, say, the first part of that stage when it was seen and the second one at a late part of that stage. In order to take this into account, the times through which different stages persist in the cycle must also be determined. However, the stage of the cycle in which preleptotene primary spermatocytes are duplicating their DNA (Stage III) persists for only a short period and so it can be established that the cycle lasts for 16 days plus or minus one day. It seems furthermore that the process of spermatogenesis extends over 4 cycles. For those who

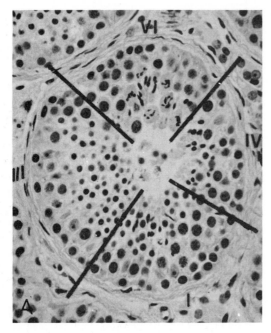

Fɪɢ. 27-7. Low-power photographs of human semi-niferous tubules cut transversely (A) and longitudi-nally (B) to show examples of the distribution of the various cell associations or stages of the cycle in the seminiferous epithelium. In these two photographs the 6 stages of the cycle illustrated in Figure 27-4 can be identified.

Stage I (A) is characterized by spermatogonia (at this magnification the types cannot be identified), pachytene spermatocytes and 2 generations of sper-matids (a young generation with spherical nuclei, an older generation with elongated condensed nu-clei).

Stage II (B) shows, in addition to spermato-gonia and pachytene spermatocytes, generations of young spermatids with spherical nuclei and maturing spermatids lining the lumen and discard-ing their residual cytoplasm.

Stage III (A and B) is characterized by sper-matogonia and preleptotene spermatocytes (not dis-tinguished at this magnification), pachytene sper-matocytes and only 1 generation of spermatids with spherical nuclei.

Stage IV (A and B) is characterized by sper-matogonia, generations of leptotene and pachytene spermatocytes and 1 generation with slightly elongated nuclei.

Stage V (B) is composed of spermatogonia, leptotene or zygotene spermatocytes (not present in this field), pachytene spermatocytes and 1 generation of spermatids with elongated nuclei.

Stage VI (A) shows spermatogonia, 1 generation of early pachytene spermatocytes, maturation divi-sions of primary spermatocytes and 1 generation of spermatids with elongated nuclei. Note that the order in which the stages of the cycle are seen around the tubular lumen is not consecutive but, on the contrary, is variable. (Clermont, Yves: Am. J. Anat., *112:35*)

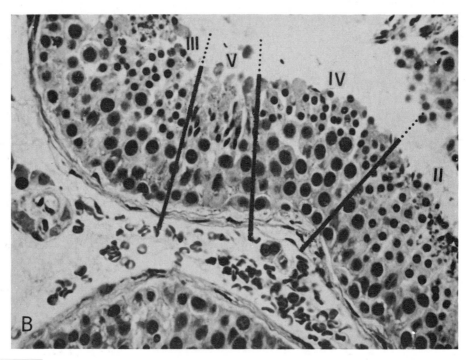

wish more than general information, see references under "Structures and Arrangements in Spermatogenesis."

EM STUDIES ON THE CELLS INVOLVED IN SPERMATOGENESIS

So far, in this account of spermatogenesis as seen with the LM, we have described the various cells involved as if they were distinct, separate entities which of course they seemed to be when examined with the LM. Studies with the EM, however, have now shown that they are not separate entities; instead they are mostly connected to one another by *intercellular bridges* and this may be a factor explaining why they seem to behave in some ways as groups of cells instead of behaving as individual cells would behave.

The cytoplasmic bridges that join the cells together in the process of spermatogenesis result from the two daughter cells that form as a result of each division not becoming completely separated from one another. It will be recalled that in the usual telophase a cleavage furrow appears in the cytoplasm between the two nuclei and deepens until the cytoplasm is completely pinched off at this site so as to separate the two daughter cells. In spermatogenesis, however, the pinching-off process is permanently arrested more or less at the point illustrated in Figure 2-22 and, as a result, the dividing cells remain connected to one another. Subsequent divisions of connected cells results in all the cells that are formed being connected to each other. Figure 27-8 shows 5 cells connected by bridges. The several generations of cells all connected together by cytoplasmic bridges could be said to constitute a *syncytium* (a syncytium is a multinucleated mass of cytoplasm). However, unlike some syncytia, which are formed by the cytoplasm of adjacent cells fusing together, a syncytium that forms in the manner described above develops from a single cell and thus constitutes a clone of a unique type.

Because dividing cells remain connected by bridges it is possible to study the development of spermatogenic cells in relation to the size of groups. A syncytium of 80 cells is more advanced than a group of 40 cells, which in turn is further developed than a group of say, 20 cells. The mapping of cells and their bridges from series of 400 to 600 consecutive sections of rat testicular tubules has been reported by Moens and Go (1971), and the results are summarized in Figure 27-9.

Single cells of the A stem cell type (A_0 in Fig. 27-9) divide to produce a doublet (just to the right of A_0 in Fig. 27-9). If the connecting bridge is broken, two new

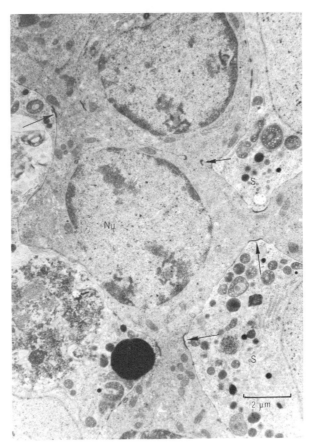

FIG. 27-8. A preleptotene spermatocyte with 4 of its 5 bridges in the plane of section. At this stage of development the morphology is indistinguishable from B spermatogonia. The bridges are marked by arrows. *Nu*, nucleus; *S*, Certoli cell. (Preparation by A Hugenholtz)

A_0 cells would result If it remains intact, the doublet can become committed to spermatogenic development. Successive mitoses yield chains of A spermatogonia which are usually attached to the basement membrane of the testicular tubule. In the diagram (Fig. 27-9) bridges already present in a previous chain are shown as heavy lines, while new bridges are shown as thinner lines. The 5th division gives rise to intermediate spermatogonia, the 6th to B spermatogonia and the 7th to spermatocytes. The entire syncytium moves away from the basement membrane toward the interior of the tubule. The first and second meiotic divisions follow and it appears that the syncytium breaks up into smaller segments as some or all of the Meiosis I bridges fail to persist. The number of divisions that give rise to spermatocytes is usually 7 but varies from 5 to 9.

Division in a given syncytium is synchronous, but a

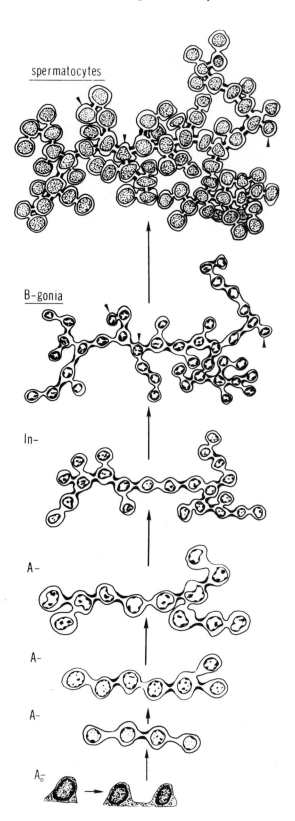

spermatocytes

B-gonia

In-

A-

A-

A-

A-

A₀-

few cells do not divide at all. The spermatocyte syncytium in Figure 27-9 was observed by Moens; the other syncytia in the diagram were deduced from it. The pattern is such that some of the cells—for example, the ones marked by arrowheads—could not have divided.

Spermiogenesis—the Transformation of Spermatids into Spermatozoa. Spermatids are enveloped (encapsulated) by the cytoplasm of Sertoli cells and near the lumen of the tubule (as will be described in connection with Sertoli cells), they undergo a metamorphosis into spermatozoa. In this process they eventually become detached from one another to become free cells.

The newly formed spermatid (Fig. 27-10, *a*) has a central spherical nucleus, a well-delimited Golgi zone close to the nucleus, numerous granular mitochondria and a pair of small centrioles. The formation of the spermatozoon involves elaborate changes in all these cellular structures. The first sign of metamorphosis is seen within the Golgi zone; this is indicated by the formation of a dense granule at the surface of the nuclear membranes (Fig. 27-10, *b*). This granule is called the *acrosomic granule* because it is a little *body* on the extremity (*akron*, extremity) of the nucleus. Its derivatives are PA-Schiff positive, which indicates the presence of carbohydrates. The growing acrosomic granule differentiates into two parts: (1) the *acrosome,* which is a small hemisphere on top of the nucleus (Fig. 27-10, *c*) and (2) the *head cap,* which is a membranelike structure growing around the acrosome on the surface of the nuclear membrane (Fig. 27-10, *c* and *d* and Fig. 27-11). The head cap eventually covers approximately half of the nuclear surface. Once the acrosome and the head cap (the acrosomic system) are well developed, the Golgi zone (Fig. 27-11) becomes detached from the head cap and turns into a "residual Golgi zone" (Fig. 27-10, *d* and *e*). As the acrosomic system develops, one centriole (labeled in Fig. 27-10, *a*) becomes attached to the nuclear membrane in an area opposite the acrosome (Fig. 27-10,

FIG. 27-9. A diagram of syncytial development of rat spermatocytes. The cells remain connected by cytoplasmic bridges following consecutive mitoses. The early division gives rise to type A spermatogonia (*A*) followed by intermediate (*In*) and B spermatogonia. Usually the 7th division produces the spermatocytes which then undergo the two meiotic divisions. Although division is synchronous for the cells of the syncytium as a whole, a few fail to divide (marked by arrowheads). Bridges which persist from previous divisions are outlined heavily. (Prepared by P. B. Moens)

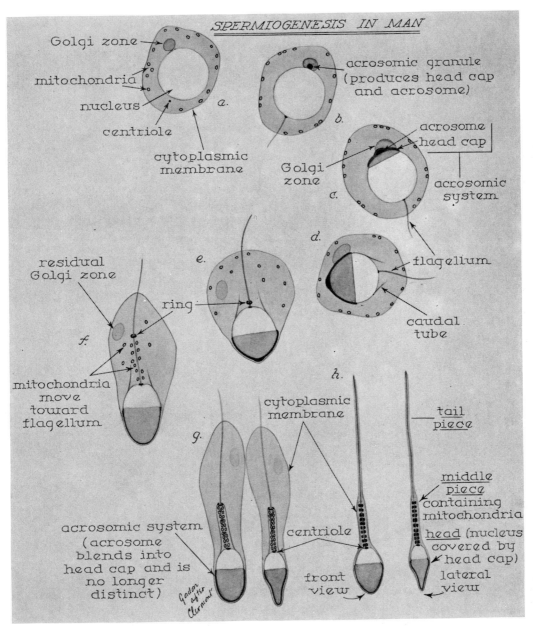

FIG. 27-10. Series of drawings showing the successive steps in the transformation of the spermatid into the spermatozoon. (Modified from Clermont and Leblond: Am. J. Anat., *96:229*)

b and *c*) and gives rise to the vibratile organ of the future spermatozoon, the flagellum (labeled in Fig. 27-10, *c* and *d*). An additional structure appears and surrounds this flagellum; this is the so-called caudal tube, which is made of submicroscopic filaments attached to the nuclear membrane (Fig. 27-10, *d*).

At one step of spermiogenesis, the acrosome and the head cap orient themselves toward the basement membrane of the seminiferous tubule. This is accompanied by a displacement of the nucleus within the cytoplasm of the spermatid toward the cell membrane (Fig. 27-10, *e*). The nucleus then becomes progressively condensed and assumes a slightly flattened and elongated shape. Its anterior end is relatively sharp when it is seen in profile but rounded when it is seen in full face (Fig. 27-10, *g* and *h*). At the surface of the nucleus,

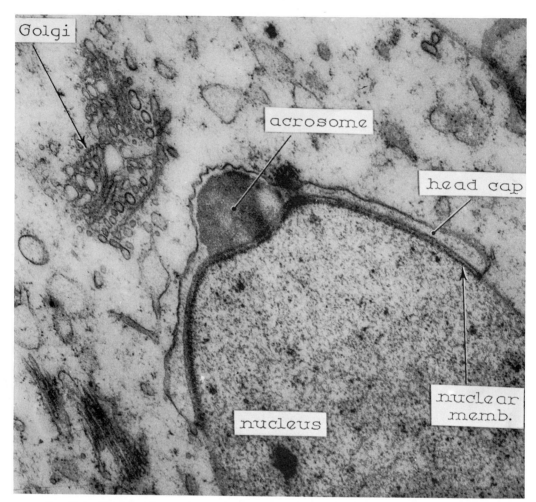

Fɪɢ. 27-11. Electron micrograph (× 39,000) of a section of a human spermatid (corresponding to Fig. 27-10, c), showing, in addition to the nucleus and the Golgi zone, the acrosomic system. The acrosome, a hemispherical dense granule, is inside a vesicular structure, the head cap, which also expands on the nuclear membrane. (Fawcett, D. W., and Burgos, M. H.: Ciba Foundation Colloquia on Ageing. vol. 2, p. 86. London, Churchill)

the acrosome blends into the head cap from which it becomes indistinguishable (Fig. 27-10). Meanwhile, a small ring appears around the flagellum close to the centriole. This ring, once formed, slides along the flagellum for some distance (Fig. 27-10, *e* and *f*). The mitochondria which, up to this stage have been disposed along the cytoplasmic membrane, start to move in the cytoplasm toward the flagellum, and more precisely toward the portion of the flagellum between the centriole and the ring (Fig. 27-10, *f*, *g* and *h*). The mitochondria line up along the flagellum, close to one another, and condense to form a striated collarlike sheath which delimits the middle piece of the future spermatozoon. The fate of the caudal tube is still not

well understood. As the spermatid completes its development, the cytoplasmic surplus, which is not utilized in the formation of the spermatozoon, is cast off and forms a disintegrating *residual body*. However, a thin layer of cytoplasm, delimited by a cytoplasmic membrane, covers the nucleus, the middle piece and the tail piece (except the extremity) of the spermatozoon.

The structure of the tail piece is basically similar to that of cilia (Fig. 27-12), the number and the arrangement of the longitudinal tubules being the same (see Chap. 5). However, along the tubules there are some additional coarse fibers probably of the nature of actin; these coarse fibers make the flagellum of a spermatozoon different from an ordinary cilium.

The net result is that the spermatozoon, though much smaller than the spermatid, retains nuclear elements of the spermatid in its head, some part of its Golgi apparatus in the acrosomic system, most of its mitochondria in the middle piece, and its centrioles: the latter are concerned in the formation of the spindle when cell division occurs in the fertilized ovum. The spermatozoon thus contributes cytoplasmic as well as nuclear components to the ovum. The acrosomic system contains trypsinlike enzymes that play a role in connection with the penetration of the spermatozoon into the ovum.

When fully formed, spermatozoa leave the Sertoli cells and enter the lumens of the seminiferous tubules.

Although their flagella beat, these spermatozoa are probably not very motile and are moved along the system of tubules until they reach the tail end of the epididymis. Then they become fully mature and actively motile and by lashing their tails can move 2 or 3 mm. a minute. In the past it was thought that this enabled them to swim up the female reproductive tract when they are introduced into the vagina. But it now seems that their movement through the reproductive tract is not dependent on the lashing of their flagella although this action may increase Brownian movement and so enhance the possibility of a collision with an ovum.

Spermatozoa were first seen with a microscope by

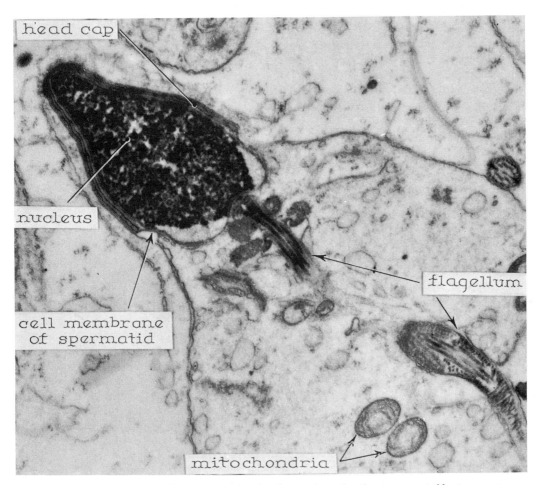

FIG. 27-12. Electron micrograph ($\times$ 25,000) of a section of a human spermatid at a more advanced stage of development (corresponding to Fig. 27-10, g). The nucleus shows a denser osmiophilic material. The head cap is still visible, but the acrosome can no longer be identified. A well-developed flagellum made of numerous filaments is seen extending from the lower end of the nucleus. Mitochondria can also be identified. (Fawcett, D. W., and Burgos, M. H.: Ciba Foundation Colloquia on Ageing. vol. 2, p. 86. London, Churchill)

Ham, a young medical doctor who worked with Leeuwenhoek in the 17th century and whom Leeuwenhoek described as a very modest man.

Spermiogenesis as described above occurs in a special microenvironment different from that in which spermatogonia proliferate and form primary spermatocytes. This matter will be discussed next.

Sertoli Cells and the Blood-Testis Barrier

Dym and Fawcett (1970) have investigated this and should be read for comprehensive information.

The cellular walls of seminiferous tubules are surrounded by a basement membrane of the usual type. But immediately outside the basement membrane there is another membrane which is of the general nature of a wrapping of ordinary connective tissue but is believed to contain a layer of myoid (contractile) cells joined to one another by tight (occludens type) junctions that are generally continuous but sometimes not. The latter type, of course, do not provide a continuous seal between the cells they connect and so permit enough spaces of around 200 Å to exist between the membranes of contiguous cells for tissue fluid and the substances it contains in solution to penetrate to the basement membrane. From there, tissue fluid could bathe the basal part of the cellular wall of the tubule. The tissue fluid is, of course, derived from the capillaries that lie in the interstitial tissue between tubules.

There is, however, not the same free access for tissue fluid or substances dissolved in tissue fluid to reach the cells that evolve in the process later (leptotene spermatocytes, spermatids and spermatogonia), all of which are *not* in contact with the basement membrane that surrounds the tubules. The reason for this is that the spermatogonia that lie between Sertoli cells along the basement membrane become covered by the cytoplasm of the adjacent and much taller Sertoli cells the cytoplasm of which flows over their tops to cover them and preleptotene spermatocytes so thoroughly that the cell membranes of adjacent Sertoli cells in this region can meet and become joined by tight junctions of the occludens type. This has an important effect. First, unlike spermatogonia that abut on the basement membrane and have excellent access to nutrients, the cells nearer the lumen of the tubule, since they do not touch the basement membrane, have no access to tissue fluid because the tight junctions between Sertoli cells prevent tissue fluid from infiltrating between the membranes of contiguous Sertoli cells to reach them. Hence cells such as dividing spermatocytes, spermatids and spermatozoa must obtain their nutrients through

the medium of the cytoplasm of Sertoli cells. Likewise, the fluid in the lumens of the seminiferous tubules must also be derived via Sertoli cell cytoplasm. The Sertoli cells, therefore, form the important component of what is referred to as the blood-testis barrier which is responsible for maintaining a different microenvironment in the inner part of the wall of the seminiferous tubule from that in its outer part.

There is, therefore, a very good reason that observations made long ago with the LM stressed that there was a very close association between Sertoli cells and the differentiating progeny of spermatogonia, and for Sertoli cells being referred to as nurse cells. The EM has disclosed that these cells or parts of cells that with the LM seem to be embedded in the cytoplasm of Sertoli cells retain their own cell membranes and lie in declivities or cavities in the cytoplasm of Sertoli cells that are lined by the cell membrane of the Sertoli cell that is acting as nurse. Hence spermatids, for example, seemingly lying in Sertoli cell cytoplasm, reveal a double cell membrane around them; one belongs to the spermatid and the other to the Sertoli cell. There is an intercellular space between the two membranes.

The irregularly shaped and indented nucleus of a Sertoli cell is easily recognized with the LM. The EM reveals that it contains what is termed a principal nucleolus and two accessory nucleoli. The cytoplasm contains the usual organelles but there is more sER than rER. Golgi stacks are not very prominent. A whorl-like structure situated close to the nucleus and consisting of annulate lamellae of smooth surfaced membranes, arranged around some lipid droplets has been described as being common in Sertoli cells. Lipid droplets and lipofuscin pigment are also common, as are filaments.

Factors Affecting Spermatogenesis. It has already been noted that spermatogenesis does not occur properly unless the testes are maintained at a temperature somewhat lower than that of the body as a whole, and also the cells of the seminiferous tubules are affected by the direct or indirect effect of gonadotrophic hormone. It will be recalled that the capacity of the ovary to produce mature germ cells, under the influence of FSH stimulation, ends more or less suddenly, usually when a woman is between the ages of 45 and 50. An event comparable with this does not occur in the male. In the male, with increasing age, there is usually no more than a slow decline in the ability of the seminiferous tubules to produce mature germ cells, and there are many authentic cases of men having become fathers at a very advanced age.

Spermatogenesis is dependent not only on FSH but also on testosterone, most of which (if not all) is secreted by the interstitial cells soon to be described. Experiments on hypophysectomized rats by Fritz have shown that giving either LH or testosterone allows spermatogonia to develop into primary spermatocytes at the pachytene stage. FSH together with LH or testosterone is necessary for the spermatid stage to be reached, after which LH or testosterone will permit the spermatid to develop further.

The negative feedback mechanism that controls the secretion of FSH is not very well understood. While testosterone can act via the hypothalamus to perhaps inhibit FSH secretion to a slight extent, it has been shown that estrogen has a potent effect in this respect.

Vitamins A and E in particular are required in adequate amounts in the diet if spermatogenesis is to be normal.

Factors Affecting Sperm Morphology. Normal spermatozoa morphologically are a very homogeneous population each with a well defined species-dependent structure. The normal human spermatozoon head, for example, is shaped like a flattened ellipsoid, whereas a mouse sperm head has a marked hooked shape. Packaged into the head of each normal sperm is the haploid chromosome complement of the species. The head is known to be very rigid, of high density and resistant to a large number of physical and chemical agents—an ideal package for such important contents.

In an ejaculate from a healthy donor, most spermatozoa are of normal morphology. Some, however, have a noticeably abnormal morphology—about 20 to 25 percent of spermatozoa in man; in mice, from 1 to 16 percent, depending upon the strain. In the same donor, however, whether he be man or mouse, the percentage of ejaculate spermatozoa with abnormal shape remains constant over long periods. MacLeod describes the causes of what can be temporary variations from a usual pattern.

Certain factors are known to increase the percentage of abnormally shaped sperm that will develop in mice subjected to certain influences. Among these are ionizing radiation, heat and chemical agents. The list of chemicals includes certain pesticides, certain antitumor drugs, and other pharmaceutical agents as well as known carcinogens and mutagens. Moreover in man, x-rays, severe allergic reactions and certain antispermatogenic agents have been reported to show similar effects. Elevated levels of sperm abnormalities have been related to lower fertility in man.

Concentration in Semen. It has been estimated that there are usually more than 100,000,000 spermatozoa in each cubic centimeter of semen in fertile men, and 2 or more cubic centimeters of semen are usually delivered in each ejaculation. Although there is much variation in individual cases, it has also been estimated that men whose semen contains only about 50,000,000 spermatozoa per cubic centimeter are not usually so fertile as those whose semen contains considerably more, and those with 20,000,000 or less per cubic centimeter are generally sterile. Although such an enormous number of spermatozoa is produced by the testis, only 1 spermatozoon actually fertilizes the ovum.

Function of Interstitial Cells. In discussing this matter, it is necessary to understand at once that there is a profound difference between fertility and potency in the male. A fertile male may be defined as one who can produce at ejaculation, at least on some occasions, enough semen containing a sufficient number of healthy spermatozoa suspended in a sufficiently normal fluid vehicle to bring about the fertilization of an ovum in a fertile female. A sterile male cannot accomplish the latter part of this function. Potency refers to another matter—the ability of the male to engage in intercourse. This depends fundamentally on the erection of the penis. A potent but sterile male may be able to ejaculate during intercourse, but the semen expressed will not contain a sufficient number of healthy spermatozoa to cause fertilization of an ovum.

The basis for fertility is spermatogenesis in the seminiferous tubules, which, as noted, is dependent on FSH and LH or testosterone. The basis for establishing potency is testosterone production by the interstitial cells; this is controlled by LH. Sterility need not cause impotence. Indeed, even eunuchs, though necessarily sterile, are not necessarily impotent unless their testes have been removed before puberty. The reason for this is that if there has been enough time for the androgen produced by the testes after puberty to have thoroughly masculinized the individual, to have established a heterosexual drive and to have permitted reflexes dependent on this drive to be formed, then the individual concerned may have remained potent because of the persistence of the reflexes even though his testes have been removed. Androgens, nevertheless, are concerned with the maintenance of the sex drive in the normal male, but it should be realized that psychological factors are also very important in the maintenance of the drive, once the basis for it has been established by androgens.

A male may be sterilized at operation either by removing the testes or by tying off and cutting the ducti deferentes (vasectomy). The latter operation prevents the egress of spermatozoa from the testes, but the interstitial cells continue to produce androgen, which leaves the testes by way of the bloodstream. The testes of the cryptorchid produce androgen, although in less than normal amounts, and usually do not produce

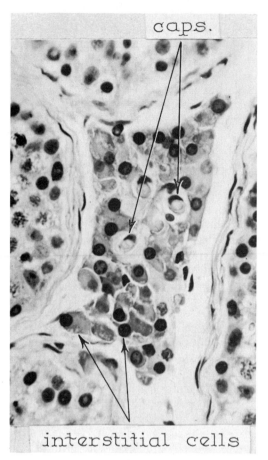

caps.

interstitial cells

Fig. 27-13. High-power photomicrograph of a portion of a section of a human testis. Several blood capillaries (*caps.*) cut in cross section may be seen in an island of interstitial cells. This group of cells lies in the connective tissue between the seminiferous tubules. (Section provided by Y. Clermont)

spermatozoa. As it is possible for a male to be potent but sterile, it is also possible for an otherwise fertile male to be impotent. In such males, impotency is usually due to emotional factors which interfere with the functioning of the autonomic nervous system in such a way that the blood flow into the cavernous tissue of the penis is not sufficient to cause erection.

The secretion of testosterone by the interstitial cells seems to be regulated by the anterior pituitary through a negative feedback mechanism that involves the hypothalamus and a releasing factor and perhaps also the pineal gland which is thought to secrete an anti-gonadotrophic factor in the sustained absence of light. When the amount of androgen in the bloodstream decreases, the anterior pituitary probably secretes addi-

tional LH. Then, when this stimulates androgen production and causes increased amounts to be delivered into the bloodstream, the secretion of LH by the anterior pituitary is temporarily suppressed. It should be anticipated, then, that the administration of androgen to a male will tend to suppress the secretion of LH by his anterior pituitary gland.

Microscopic Appearance of Interstitial Cells. It has been pointed out that in fetal life interstitial cells develop from the mesenchymal cells of the stroma between the developing seminiferous tubules, and that they are much more prominent in the fetal testis from the 4th month on than they are in the postnatal testis between birth and puberty. In the sexually mature male these interstitial cells are distributed either singly or in clumps in the stroma between the tubules, usually in the angular crevices that are created by the round tubules being packed together (Fig. 27-3). They are large cells, measuring up to 20 or more microns in diameter (Fig. 27-13). Their spherical to oval nuclei are pale and contain one or more nucleoli. Some interstitial cells are binucleated. In H and E sections the peripheral cytoplasm may be vacuolated because lipoid droplets have been dissolved from it in the preparation of the section. The cytoplasm immediately surrounding the nucleus may appear to be granular. Some interstitial cells contain a pigment which is probably lipofuscin.

The interstitial cells constitute an unusual type of endocrine gland. They do not develop from an epithelial surface, as do most glands, but from a mesenchymal stroma. Since they are scattered about in the stroma, which is abundantly provided with capillaries, they have access to the vascular system (Fig. 27-13). All in all, they constitute a very diffuse type of endocrine gland.

Fine Structure. The organelle that characterizes the cytoplasm of interstitial cells is sER which, as already noted, is associated with the production of steroid hormones (Fig. 27-14). This is widely distributed mostly in the form of branching tubules. In addition, the cytoplasm contains some mitochondria, some rER, a few Golgi stacks and some inclusions. An interesting type of the latter are crystalloids (Fig. 27-15). Fawcett and Burgos have shown with the EM that the crystalloids have a complex but orderly internal structure; when they are sectioned, they present an appearance not unlike that of a woven fabric (Fig. 27-15, *bottom*).

How the Hormone of the Testis Produces Its Effects on Target Cells. The physiologically important androgen in the male is testosterone. Testosterone affects, and is affected by, body cells to different ex-

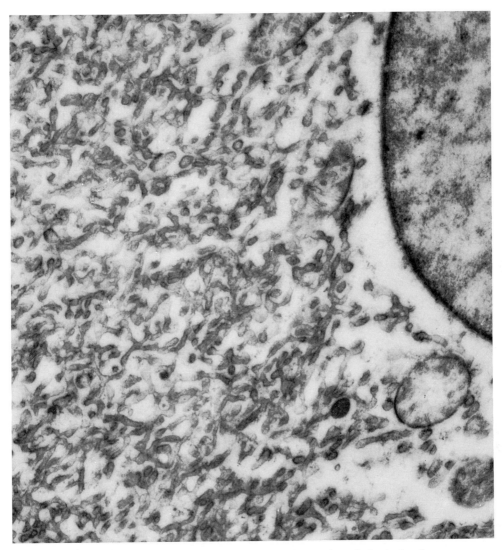

FIG. 27-14. This electron micrograph ($\times$ 33,000) is of a section of the testis of an opossum and shows part of an interstitial cell. Part of a nucleus is seen at top left, with 4 mitochondria adjacent to it. The remainder of the field is filled with a network of interconnected tubules of agranular endoplasmic reticulum. (From Drs. A. K. Christensen and D. W. Fawcett)

tents. Unlike the kinds of hormones that affect only cells that have special receptors on their cell membranes that initiate responses when contacted by the special hormone, testosterone is thought to enter most cells, but it may affect them or be affected by them slightly or not at all. In the liver cells it may undergo extensive metabolic change. In still other cells which can be termed androgen-responsive cells, it is changed, and in a changed form it stimulates both growth and secretion. In rats and mice the androgen-responsive cells, in a decreasing order of responsiveness, have been

found to be in the prostate, seminal vesicles, preputial gland, kidney and skin.

It seems that the reason for certain cells being responsive to its effects is that responsive cells have the ability to convert testosterone to 5-dihydrotestosterone; this conversion occurs in both the cytoplasm and the nuclei of responsive cells that take up testosterone. In the cytoplasm of responsive cells, the dihydrotestosterone is reduced further to other metabolites. In the nuclei of these cells, however, the dihydrotestosterone is not itself altered but becomes bound, by

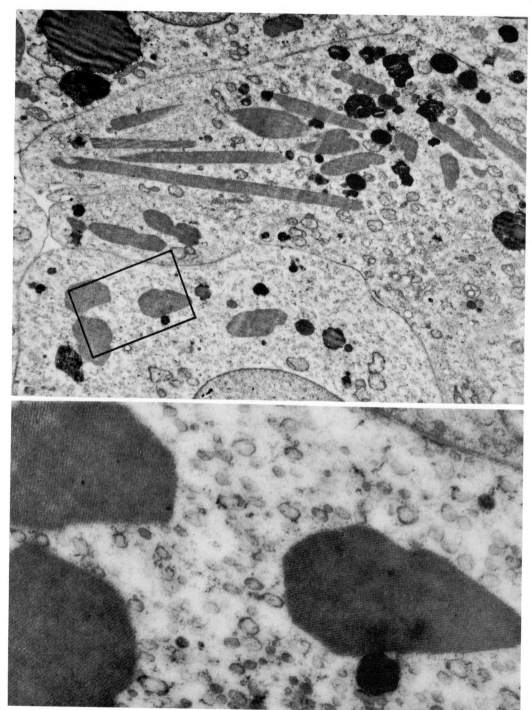

FIG. 27-15. (*Top*) Electron micrograph ($\times$ 8,550) of a section of parts of several interstitial cells. In the cytoplasm, in addition to dark osmiophilic bodies (lipid droplets and pigment granules of a lipoid nature), crystalline structures are visible (the crystalloids of Reinke). (*Bottom*) Electron micrograph ($\times$ 51,750) showing a higher magnification of a section of a crystalloid in which a highly ordered internal structure is apparent. (Fawcett, D. W., and Burgos, M. H.: Ciba Foundation Colloquia on Ageing. vol. 2, p. 86. London, Churchill)

means of a protein, to euchromatin, which, as was described in Chapter 4, is the chromatin that in an interphase nucleus is uncoiled and giving off information. The enzyme that in the nucleus converts testosterone to dihydrotestosterone is tightly bound to the euchromatin-protein complex, though the binding is probably not of the covalent type.

If dihydrotestosterone becomes available in a nucleus and becomes bound to the euchromatin, this would suggest that it acts at the level of the genes by increasing the amount of RNA that is formed, which would result in the affected cells synthesizing more protein and hence increasing in size. Since many of the androgen-sensitive cells of the prostate and seminal vesicles are secretory cells, it seems likely that the metabolic processes concerned in producing all of the components of the secretions of these cells are also stimulated.

As may be recalled from having read Chapter 6, the insect hormone *ecdysone* is a steroid hormone and if it is injected into an immature insect, it causes a puffing on the giant chromosomes that are seen in the salivary glands of insects. The sites where the puffing occurs are sites where transcription is occurring.

Tubuli Recti and Rete Testis. The seminiferous tubules, as they approach the region of the mediastinum testis, become straight and are known as the *tubuli recti;* they empty into the rete testis of the mediastinum (Fig. 27-2). Spermatogenesis does not occur in the tubuli recti, which are lined by tall Sertoli-like cells. The spaces of the rete are lined by cuboidal epithelium.

The Epididymis

The general structure of the epididymis is described in the first part of this chapter. The further details of its microscopic structure follow.

The epididymis is invested in a fibrous covering similar to but somewhat thinner than the tunica albuginea of the testis.

Ductuli Efferentes. The ductuli efferentes, in the cone-shaped bodies in which they are arranged, are held together by a delicate vascular connective tissue. The ductules themselves consist of an epithelial lining, a basement membrane and a thin layer of smooth muscle associated with some elastic fibers. The epithelium exhibits alternating groups of high columnar cells which have typical motile cilia and low columnar cells which usually do not. The latter cells are probably secretory. From a study of the epididymis of the guinea pig, Mason and Shaver suggested that the combined action of the rete testis, the ductuli efferentes

and the proximal portion of the ductus epididymis is to remove from the excretory product of the testes not only excess fluid but also extraneous materials carried with this mass. This reabsorption of fluid at the level of the epididymis would also create a negative pressure which would facilitate the transportation of the spermatozoa from the seminiferous tubule to the epididymis.

Ductus Epididymis. The convoluted ductus epididymis, which together with the connective tissue that holds its coils together (Fig. 27-16) comprises the body and the tail of the epididymis, consists of an epithelial lining, a basement membrane and a thin coat of circularly disposed smooth muscle fibers.

The epithelium, all along the ductus epididymis, is actually pseudostratified columnar epithelium because it contains both small basal cells and tall columnar cells. The tall cells, however, form a continuous even surface. From the tall cells tufts of long branching microvilli project toward the lumen from the free margins of the cells (Fig. 27-17). These cytoplasmic processes were called *stereocilia* (*stereos,* solid), but they do not contain the microtubules characteristic of true cilia. Secretion granules and vacuoles may be seen in the cytoplasm between the free margins of the cells and their nuclei.

The Ductus Deferens

The ductus or vas deferens is a sufficiently substantial structure to be palpated easily through the skin and the subcutaneous tissue. Its firm consistency is due to its very thick muscular wall and relatively narrow lumen (Fig. 27-18).

The mucous membrane consists of an epithelial lining and a lamina propria of connective tissue that contains a high content of elastic fibers. It is thrown into longitudinal folds of only moderate height. As in the ductus epididymis, the epithelium is pseudostratified columnar, and here again the tall columnar cells show stereocilia (Fig. 27-17). At the level of the ampulla the columnar cells lose their stereocilia.

The muscular coat consists of 3 layers (Fig. 27-18, *bottom*). The inner and the outer layers are each thinner than the middle layer and are composed of longitudinally disposed fibers. The thick middle layer is composed of circularly disposed fibers. The adventitia consists of a loose elastic type of connective tissue and blends with the tissues comprising the spermatic cord, which contains arteries, numerous veins, nerves and some longitudinally disposed striated muscle fibers (cremaster muscle). The veins are particularly prominent and form the *pampiniform* (*pampinus,* tendril)

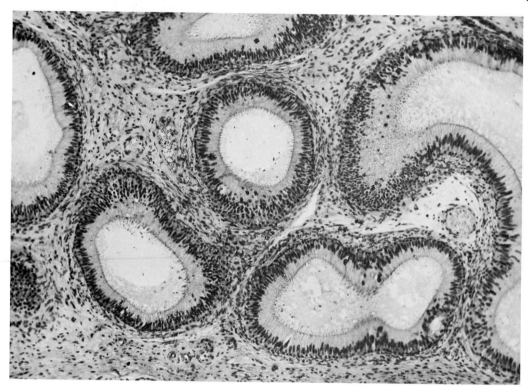

Fɪɢ. 27-16. Low-power photomicrograph of a section of epididymis, showing the ductus epididymis cut in cross and oblique section. For detail see Figure 27-17.

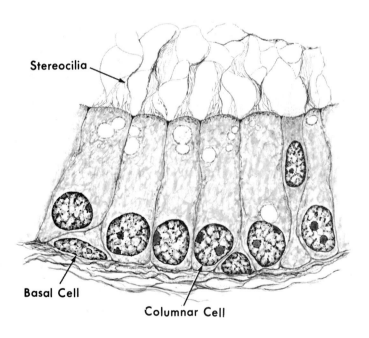

Fɪɢ. 27-17. Drawing of epithelium of ductus epididymis showing the pseudostratified nature of the epithelium and stereocilia. (Illustration courtesy of Y. Clermont)

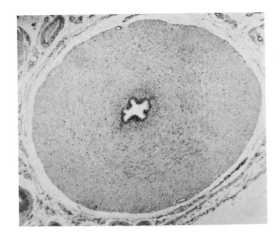

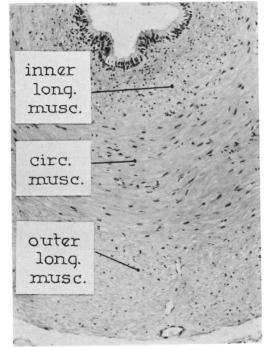

inner long. musc.

circ. musc.

outer long. musc.

Fig. 27-18. Low-power and high-power photomicrographs of an H and E section of the ductus deferens.

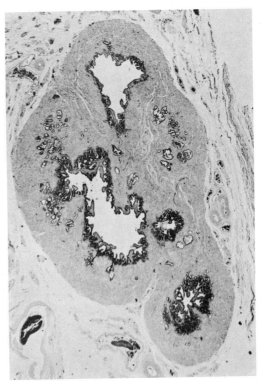

Fig. 27-19. Very low-power photomicrograph of a cross section of a seminal vesicle.

The Seminal Vesicles

The size and the function of the seminal vesicles are controlled to a great degree by hormones; hence, the size and the shape of these structures vary considerably in relation to age. In the sexually mature male they are elongated bodies, 5 to 7 cm. or more long, and somewhat less than half as wide at their widest point. Their form tapers toward the end at which they join the ductus deferens.

To prevent confusion, it should be explained that the structure seen on gross dissection and called the *seminal vesicle* is essentially a tube that is much longer and much narrower than it appears at first sight. The vesicle is coiled and convoluted. The various coils and convolutions, where they touch one another, are adherent through the medium of connective tissue (Fig. 27-19); this is the cause of the form and the organization of the body seen on gross inspection. This connective tissue must be dissected if the seminal vesicle is to be unraveled and seen in its true form; if this is done, it will be found to consist of a tube about 15 cm. long. The coils and the convolutions are such that if a cross section is cut through the undissected body,

plexus; the plexus is so named because the veins wind around the duct similar to the way in which tendrils of plants wind around other bodies for support. This is a common site for veins to become varicosed.

A short distance before the ductus deferens is joined by the seminal vesicle, it becomes dilated to form an ampulla. Here the muscular coat, though still thick, is thinner than in the other parts of the duct, and the lumen is considerably larger. The mucous membrane is thrown into very complicated folds similar to those of the seminal vesicle (Fig. 27-19).

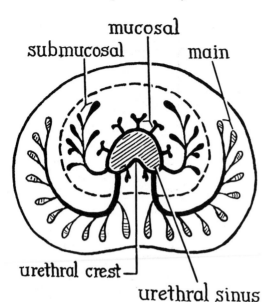

mucosal

submucosal   **main**

urethral crest

urethral sinus

Fig. 27-20. Diagram of a cross section of the prostate gland, showing the distribution of the mucous, the submucous and the main glands and where their ducts open. (Redrawn and slightly modified from Grant, J. C. B: A Method of Anatomy. ed. 4. Baltimore, Williams & Wilkins)

the seminal vesicle will be cut simultaneously at several points along its length (Fig. 27-19).

The wall of the tube exhibits 3 coats: an outermost one of fibrous connective tissue which contain a substantial content of elastic fibers, a middle muscular coat and a lining mucous membrane.

The muscular coat is substantial but not so thick as that of the ductus deferens. It consists of 2 layers: an inner one of circular fibers and an outer one of longitudinal fibers.

The mucous membrane of the seminal vesicle is thrown into an extraordinary series of folds (Fig. 27-19). These permit the vesicle to have an enormous area of secretory epithelium; they also permit the tube to become distended with secretion without the undue stretching of the membrane of secretory cells that line the vesicle. The epithelial lining consists essentially of a layer of tall columnar cells, but, between these and the lamina propria, small cells may be irregularly distributed. The small cells in some instances may form a continuous membrane, deep to the tall cells.

Since the folds of mucous membrane are so very numerous and may branch, the lamina propria of the seminal vesicle, as seen in a section, seems to contain glands. However, the glandular appearance, like that

presented by the mucous membrane of the gallbladder, is due only to the extensive folding of the mucous membrane.

It was once believed that the seminal vesicle served as a storehouse for spermatozoa. The finding of spermatozoa in the seminal vesicle after death does not necessarily provide support for this theory because spermatozoa may migrate into the vesicles after death. The epithelial cells of the vesicles provide an elaborate, thick, yellow, sticky secretion. This is delivered into the ejaculatory duct during ejaculation, and it serves as one of the fluids that constitute a vehicle and also provide nutritive materials for the spermatozoa.

The relation of the structure and the function of the seminal vesicles and the prostate gland to hormones is similar and will be discussed when the microscopic anatomy of the prostate gland has been considered.

The Prostate Gland

The prostate gland is commonly described as being about the size and the shape of a horse chestnut but it is narrower below than above (Fig. 27-1). It surrounds the urethra as the latter emerges from the bladder. It is obvious that in this site enlargements of its substance might obstruct the outlet from the bladder. Unfortunately, enlargements of its substance that exert this effect are relatively common in men who have passed middle life. Their cause is obviously hormonal, for the reverse of enlargement—atrophy—occurs if the testes are removed. The removal of the prostate gland, or some part of it, to free the urethra from obstruction is a relatively common operation in older men.

The prostate gland is of a firm consistency. It is surrounded by a thin capsule that contains both connective tissue and smooth muscle fibers and is to be differentiated from the fascia that lies outside it.

As has already been noted, the substance of the prostate gland is made up of a large number of individual glands; these open by separate ducts into the prostatic urethra and are embedded in a stroma that is a mixture of smooth muscle and fibrous connective tissue.

A cross section of the prostate gland shows that the lumen of the prostatic urethra is V-shaped, with the apex of the V pointing forward (Fig. 27-20). The part of the posterior wall in the urethra that bulges forward to make the cross-section appearance of its lumen V-shaped is termed the *urethral crest* (Fig. 27-20). The two arms of the V that pass laterally and backward constitute the *urethral sinuses* (Fig. 27-20).

The glands that are embedded in the substance of

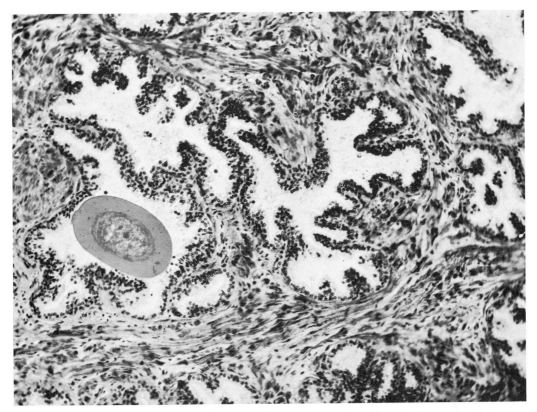

FIG. 27-21. Medium-power photomicrograph of a small area of a section of the prostate gland. Notice the smooth muscle fibers in the stroma of the gland and the concretion in the lumen of a secretory unit on the left.

the prostate are of 3 different orders of size and are distributed in 3 different areas that are arranged more or less concentrically around the urethra. The mucosal glands are the smallest and are disposed in the periurethral tissue (Fig. 27-20). They are of the greatest importance in connection with the enlargements of prostatic substance that occur in older men, for it is these glands that commonly overgrow to form *adenomatous* (*aden,* gland; *oma,* tumor) *nodules*. The submucous glands are disposed in the ring of tissue that surrounds the periurethral tissue (Fig. 27-20). The main, external or proper prostatic glands—and these provide the bulk of the secretion of the gland—are disposed in the outer and largest portion of the gland (Fig. 27-20). The mucosal glands open at various points around the lumen of the urethra, but the ducts of the submucous and main prostatic glands open into the posterior margins of the urethral sinuses (Fig. 27-20).

The prostate gland is imperfectly divided into 3 lobes by the passage through it of the ejaculatory ducts. Each lobe is imperfectly subdivided into lobules.

The ducts that drain the lobules of the bulk of the organ sweep backward to empty into the urethral sinuses (Fig. 27-20). In the lobules, the ducts branch into tubulo-alveolar secretory units. These not only produce secretion but also are adapted to storing secretion. As a consequence they may be greatly dilated. To accommodate large amounts of stored secretion, the epithelial lining of the gland is greatly folded, and papillary projections of mucous membrane extend into their lumens at many sites (Fig. 27-21). This arrangement, together with the fibromuscular stroma that is disposed both between and within the lobules (Fig. 27-21), gives the gland a distinctive microscopic appearance.

In the healthy, sexually mature male the epithelium of the secretory units and ducts (except immediately before they enter the urethra) is of a tall columnar type. Smaller flattened or rounded cells may be distributed irregularly beneath the tall columnar cells. The tall cells have well-developed Golgi networks between their nuclei and their free borders. Blebs of

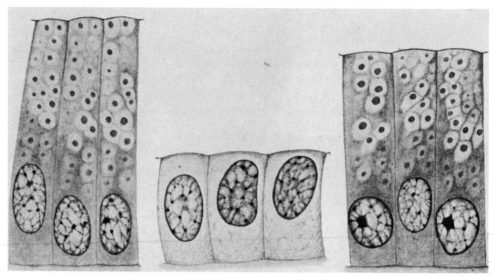

Fɪɢ. 27-22. (*Left*) Cells from the lining of the seminal vesicle of a normal rat. (*Center*) Cells from the same site 20 days after castration. (*Right*) Cells from the same site 20 days after castration; this rat received 29 injections of testis extract, beginning immediately after castration. (Moore, C. R., Hughes, W., and Gallagher, T. F.: Am. J. Anat., *45*:133)

secretion may sometimes be seen, apparently leaving the free surfaces of the cells. Concretions of secretion, which may be calcified to some extent, are not uncommon in the secretory units of the prostate glands of older men (Fig. 27-21, *left*). The epithelium rests on a fibrous connective tissue lamina propria that contains an abundant supply of capillaries.

The secretion of the prostate gland is a thin, somewhat milky fluid. It contains, among other ingredients, quantities of an enzyme known as acid phosphatase; the function of this is not known, but its detection in the bloodstream is of use in the diagnosis of malignant tumors that arise from the secretory cells of the prostate gland.

Effects of Hormones on the Seminal Vesicles and the Prostate Gland. Androgen production by the testes is required to bring about the full development of the seminal vesicles and the prostate gland. Castration, after these structures have fully developed, causes them to atrophy. The most striking microscopic change brought about by castration occurs in the epithelium.

In a sexually mature male the epithelial cells of the seminal vesicles are of the tall columnar type. Their cytoplasm, between their nuclei and free borders, contains abundant secretory granules, each of which tends to be surrounded by a halo (Fig. 27-22, *left*). If the testes are removed, the epithelial cells shrink, becoming more or less cuboidal (Fig. 27-22, *center*). Secre-

tory granules disappear from their cytoplasm. Moore, Hughes and Gallagher have shown that both the height of the epithelial cells of the seminal vesicles and their normal content of secretory granules can be restored by injections of androgen (Fig. 27-22, *right*).

Moore, Price and Gallagher have shown also that the secretory cells of the prostate shrink in height if the testes are removed, and that the prominent Golgi networks of the cells become greatly reduced in size. Both their height and their well-developed Golgi networks can be restored by injections of androgen.

As already noted, testosterone is the physiologically important androgen in the male, and the way in which it probably exerts its effects within androgen-sensitive cells has already been described.

Estrogen injected into male animals causes the epithelium of the seminal vesicles and the prostate gland to change from a tall secretory type into a low nonsecretory type. Moreover, estrogen induces a hypertrophy of the fibromuscular stroma of the prostate and the walls of the seminal vesicles.

The fact that the vigor of the secretory cells of the prostate gland is dependent on androgen is taken advantage of in the treatment of some malignant tumors that arise from these cells. A certain proportion of cancers of the prostate gland are benefited by castration. Being denied androgen, even malignant epithelial cells of the prostate gland may experience diminished function and growth activity. Likewise, in some instances prostatic cancers respond in a similar fashion to treatment with estrogens.

The hormonal basis for the nonmalignant overgrowths of prostatic tissue that so commonly obstruct the urethrae of older men is not thoroughly understood. Both the glandular tissue and the stroma of the prostate gland participate in these overgrowths.

The Penis

Microscopic Structure. The substance of the penis consists essentially of 3 cylindrical bodies of erectile (cavernous) tissue (Fig. 27-23). Two of these, the corpora cavernosa, are arranged side by side in the dorsal half of the organ (Fig. 27-23); this arrangement makes the dorsal surface of the otherwise more or less cylindrical penis somewhat flattened. The third long body of erectile tissue is called the corpus cavernosum urethrae because it conducts the urethra in its substance (Fig. 27-23) from one of its ends to the other (Fig. 27-1). It is also termed the corpus spongiosum. This cavernous body lies ventral to the paired corpora cavernosa. Moreover, it extends somewhat beyond the corpora cavernosa and becomes expanded into a more or less blunt cone-shaped body, the *glans;* this constitutes the free end of the penis (Fig. 27-1).

Each cavernous body is surrounded by a stout sheath of connective tissue called a *tunica albuginea* (Figs. 27-23 and 27-24). In the corpora cavernosa, this sheath consists chiefly of collagenic fibers arranged in an inner circular and an outer longitudinal layer, but it also contains elastic fibers. The tunics covering the paired corpora cavernosa come into contact with one another along the midline of the penis and fuse to form a median septum (Fig. 27-23); this is thickest and most complete near the root of the penis. The sheath surrounding the corpus cavernosum urethrae is more elastic than that covering the other 2 bodies. In the glans, a true tunica albuginea is deficient; here the dermis of the skin that covers the glans serves as a tunica albuginea and is continuous with the cavernous tissue that is deep to it.

The 3 cavernous bodies (except where the paired corpora cavernosa are fused) are bound together by elastic areolar tissue called the *fascia penis* (Fig. 27-23). This also provides a flexible attachment for the skin that covers the penis. The epidermis of the skin of the penis is thin. No coarse hairs are present except near the root of the organ. A circular fold of skin extends forward to cover the glans; this is called the *prepuce* (Fig. 27-1). It is usually sufficiently elastic to permit its being retracted. However, in some instances it is not, and it may fit too tightly over the glans; this

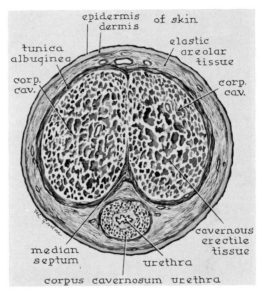

FIG. 27-23. Diagram of a cross section of the midsection of the penis.

condition is called *phimosis.* Modified sebaceous glands are present on the inner surface of the fold; the secretion from these, in a prepuce that cannot be retracted, may accumulate and serve as an irritant. The common operation by which the prepuce is removed is called *circumcision.*

The substance of the cavernous bodies consists of a 3-dimensional network of trabeculae. These are composed of connective tissue and smooth muscle and are covered with endothelium (Fig. 27-24). Between the trabeculae are spaces; since the trabeculae are covered with endothelium, the spaces are lined with endothelium. These spaces tend to be larger in the more central parts of the cavernous bodies and smaller near their periphery (Fig. 27-23). The substance of the glans is made up of convolutes of large veins rather than of spaces separated by trabeculae.

Blood Supply and the Mechanism of Erection. The arterial supply is of two sorts. Branches from the arteria dorsalis end in capillary beds which supply nutriment to the tissues of the organ, including those of the cavernous bodies. From the capillaries of the trabeculae, blood drains into the spaces. The spaces communicate in such a fashion that blood emptied into them can make its way to the more peripheral parts of the bodies, where the spaces communicate with plexuses of veins that are disposed close to the periphery of each cylindrical body. The blood that is instrumental in causing erection is derived chiefly from another and larger set of arteries that enters the sub-

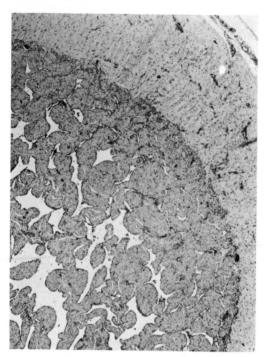

FIG. 27-24. Low-power photomicrograph of a portion of a cross section of a penis, showing the curved tunica albuginea at the upper right, with erectile tissue at the lower left.

stance of the bodies and there gives off branches that are conducted to the spaces by way of the trabeculae. These arteries have thick muscular walls, and, in addition, many possess inner thickenings of longitudinal muscle fibers that bulge into their lumens. Many of these arteries that are disposed along the trabeculae are coiled and twisted when the penis is flaccid; this accounts for their being called *helicine* arteries. Many of the terminal branches of these arteries open directly into the spaces of the cavernous tissue.

The smooth muscle of the arteries and the smooth muscle in the trabeculae are supplied both by sympathetic and parasympathetic fibers. Under conditions of erotic stimulation, the smooth muscle of the trabeculae and the helicine arteries relaxes. The arteries tend to straighten, and as a result blood flows freely from them into the spaces. As blood collects in the spaces and dilates them, the venous plexuses in the peripheral parts of the bodies become compressed. With more blood being delivered into the spaces of the cavernous bodies, and with venous drainage from the bodies being impeded, the bodies become enlarged and turgid. The corpus cavernosum urethrae does not become so turgid as its two companions because its sheath is more elastic.

The phenomenon of the penis returning to its flaccid state after erection is termed *detumescence*. This is brought about by the helicine arteries becoming constricted and by the smooth muscle in the trabeculae contracting; this slowly forces blood from the organ.

The penis is richly provided with a great variety of sensory nerve endings.

The Male Urethra

The male urethra is a tube of mucous membrane. In some sites its lamina propria, which is primarily fibroelastic tissue, contains smooth muscle fibers and, in many sites, glands. Three facts about the urethra that the student will soon be able to verify when he learns, in his clinical years, to pass a catheter, are that it is about 8 inches long, its course is not straight but instead exhibits a reverse curve (Fig. 27-1), and (if the catheter employed is of too fine a caliber) its lining is the seat of many small diverticulae.

The male urethra is commonly described as consisting of 3 parts. On leaving the urinary bladder the urethra enters the base of the prostate gland and courses through it to leave its apex. This portion of the urethra is described as its *prostatic part*. It then pierces the fasciae of the urogenital diaphragm. Accordingly, this portion of it is termed its *membranous part*. It then enters the expanded root (the bulb) of the corpus cavernosum urethrae (Fig. 27-1) and then extends through the entire length of this cavernous body to the apex of the glans (Fig. 27-1), where its *external orifice* is situated. The part of the urethra contained in the corpus cavernosum urethrae is called its *cavernous* or *spongy part*.

The prostatic portion of the urethra is more or less V-shaped in cross section. The apex of the V-shaped posterior wall points forward and is called the urethral crest (Fig. 27-20). A conical elevation on the crest is termed the *colliculus,* and a small diverticulum, the remains of the fetal müllerian ducts, opens through it. The slitlike openings of the ejaculatory ducts may be seen, one on each side of the colliculus, on the urethral crest. The sites of the openings of the prostatic ducts have already been described.

As was noted in Chapter 24, the epithelium of the urinary bladder is of the transitional type (Fig. 27-25 A). The epithelium that lines the first part of the prostatic urethra is of the same type (Fig. 27-25 B). However, in the part of the prostatic urethra nearest the membranous urethra the epithelium changes to the pseudostratified or stratified columnar variety (Fig. 27-25 C).

The lamina propria of the prostatic urethra is com-

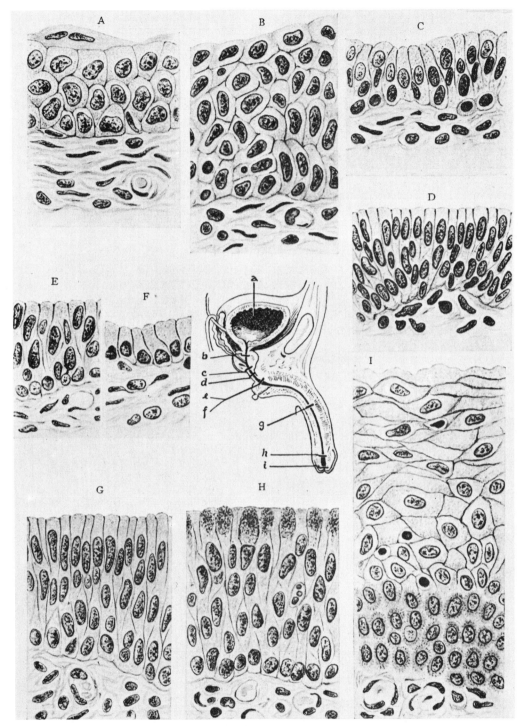

FIG. 27-25. The epithelial lining of the human male urethra at the different regions shown in the central diagram (× 600). (A) Wall of bladder. (B) Inner portion of prostatic urethra. (C) Outer portion of prostatic urethra. (D) Membranous portion of urethra. (E) Ampulla of urethra on sides and bases of folds. (F) Ampulla of urethra on crest of folds. (G) Middle of cavernous urethra. (H) Inner portion of fossa navicularis. (I) Outer portion of fossa navicularis. (Addison: Piersol's Normal Histology. ed. 15. Philadelphia, Lippincott)

posed essentially of fibroelastic connective tissue. It is very vascular, chiefly because of its great content of venules. Indeed, over the urethral crest the lamina propria contains so many venules and veins that it is sometimes described as erectile tissue. Smooth muscle fibers are also present in the mucous membrane of the prostatic urethra. These are disposed in 2 layers; the innermost one consists of longitudinal fibers, and the outer layer, of circular fibers. The latter are highly developed at the internal urethral orifice, where they, reinforced by certain smooth muscle fibers from another source, comprise the *sphincter of the bladder.*

The membranous part of the urethra is the shortest part, being about 1 cm. long. The lining cells here are tall columnar in type and are stratified (Fig. 27-25 D). Some smooth muscle is present in the lamina propria, but the circular fibers in particular are less numerous than they are in the prostatic portion of the urethra. However, in the membranous urethra, striated muscle fibers of the urogenital diaphragm surround the tube; these comprise the *sphincter muscle of the urethra.* This muscle is sometimes called the *external sphincter of the bladder.* Two small bodies, each about as large as a pea, the *bulbo-urethral* or *Cowper's glands,* are disposed on the undersurface of the membranous urethra, close to its midline (Fig. 27-1). Their ducts run forward and medially to open, sometimes by a common opening, on the lower surface of the first part of the cavernous portion of the urethra (Fig. 27-1), next to be described. The glands themselves are of the tubulo-alveolar type, and their secretory cells are mostly of the mucous type. These glands either secrete more copiously, or their secretion is expressed from them because of the contraction of the smooth muscle fibers in their stroma and the voluntary muscle outside them, under conditions of erotic stimulation.

The cavernous or spongy part of the urethra is its longest part. As noted before, the urethra becomes expanded in the bulb of the corpus cavernosum urethrae to form the *bulb* of the urethra (Fig. 27-1). The urethra becomes expanded again in the glans; this expansion of it is termed the *terminal* or *navicular fossa* (Fig. 27-1).

The epithelium in the cavernous part of the urethra is of the stratified columnar type, although simple columnar epithelium may be present on the crests of folds (Fig. 27-25, E, F and G). In the inner part of the terminal fossa some goblet cells may be present (Fig. 27-25 H). In the outer part of the terminal fossa the epithelium becomes stratified squamous in type (Fig. 27-25 I). This in turn becomes continuous with the stratified squamous keratinizing epithelium that covers the glans.

In the cavernous portion of the urethra the smooth muscle of the urethra proper fades out to be replaced, as it were, by the smooth muscle of the septa of the erectile tissue through which the urethra passes.

Two groups of glands are associated with the urethra. These are often termed the *glands of Littre.* One group, the *intramucosal* glands, consists of small simple glands disposed in its lamina propria. Although these are present in all parts of the urethra, they are most numerous in its cavernous part. The second group constitutes the *extramucosal* glands. They are somewhat larger than the intramucosal type. Their ducts commonly pass to the urethra at acute angles. The extramucosal glands are not so widely distributed as the intramucosal glands. Both types secrete mucus. In addition to possessing glands, the lining of the urethra is beset with numerous small outpouchings of its mucous membrane; these are called *lacunae.* The glands described above may open into these.

References and Other Reading

SOME GENERAL REFERENCES ON REPRODUCTION

Beatty, R. A.: The genetics of the mammalian gamete. Biol. Rev., *45:*73, 1970.
Odell, W. D., and Moyer, D. L.: Physiology of Reproduction. St. Louis, C. V. Mosby, 1971.
Parkes, A. S. (ed.): Marshall's Physiology of Reproduction. London, Longmans, Vol. 1, Parts 1 and 2, 1960; Vol. 2, 1962; Vol. 3, 1966.
Young, W. C. (ed.): Sex and Internal Secretions. vols. 1 and 2. Baltimore, Williams and Wilkins, 1961.

SOME GENERAL REFERENCES ON THE TESTIS

Johnson, A. D., Gomes, W. R., and Vandemark, N. L. (eds.): The Testis. vol. 1, Development, Anatomy and Physiology; vol. 2, Biochemistry; vol. 3, Influencing Factors. New York, Academic Press, 1970.
Rosenberg, E., and Paulsen, C. A. (eds.): Advances in Experimental Medicine and Biology. The Human Testis. New York, Plenum Press, 1970.

SOME REFERENCES ON THE DEVELOPMENT OF THE TESTIS

Gier, H. T., and Marion, G. B.: Development of the mammalian testis. *In* The Testis. vol. 1. New York, Academic Press, 1970.
Gondos, B., and Conner, L. A.: Ultrastructure of developing germ cells in fetal rabbit testis. Am. J. Anat., *136:*23, 1973.
Lording, D. W., and de Kretser, D. M.: Comparative ultrastructural and histochemical studies of interstitial cells of rat testis during fetal and postnatal development. J. Reprod. Fertil., *29:*261, 1972.
Sawyer, G. I. M.: Post-natal growth changes in the human prostate. J. Anat., *78:*130, 1944.

Vilar, O.: Histology of the human testis from neonatal period to adolescence. *In* Advances in Experimental Medicine and Biology. The Human Testis. New York, Plenum, 1970.

SOME REFERENCES ON HORMONAL AND STEROID INFLUENCES IN THE TESTIS

General

Allanson, M., and Parkes, A. S.: Cytological and functional reactions of the hypophysis to gonadal hormones. *In* Marshall's Physiology of Reproduction. vol. 3. London, Longmans, Green and Co., 1966.

Donovan, B. T., and Harris, G. W.: Neurohumoral mechanisms in reproduction. *In* Marshall's Physiology of Reproduction. vol. 3. London, Longmans, Green and Co., 1966.

Go, V. L. W., Vernon, R. G., and Fritz, I. B.: Studies on spermatogenesis in rats. III. Effects of hormonal treatment on differentiation kinetics of the spermatogenic cycle in regressed hypophysectomized rats. Can. J. Biochem., *49*:768, 1971.

Gomes, W. R.: Metabolic and regulatory hormones influencing testis function. *In* The Testis. vol. 3. New York, Academic Press, 1970.

Hall, P. F.: Endocrinology of the testis. *In* The Testis. vol. 2. New York, Academic Press, 1970.

Karlson, P., and Sekeris, C. E.: Biochemical mechanisms of hormone action. Acta Endocrinol. (Kobenhaun), *53*:505, 1966.

Kellie, A. E.: Biochemistry of the gonadal hormones and related compounds. *In* Marshall's Physiology of Reproduction. vol. 3. London, Longmans, 1966.

Moore, C. R., Price, D., and Gallagher, T. F.: Rat-prostate cytology as a testis-hormone indicator and the prevention of castration changes by testis-extract injections. Am. J. Anat., *45*:17, 1930.

Morris, C. J. O. R.: The chemistry of gonadotrophins. *In* Marshall's Physiology of Reproduction. vol. 3. London, Longmans, 1966.

Odell, W. D., and Moyer, D. L.: Dynamic relationship of the testis to the whole man. *In* Physiology of Reproduction. St. Louis, C. V. Mosby, 1971.

Parkes, A. S.: The internal secretions of the testis. *In* Marshall's Physiology of Reproduction. vol. 3. London, Longmans, 1966.

Parkes, A. S., and Deanesley, R.: Relation between the gonads and the adrenal glands. *In* Marshall's Physiology of Reproduction. vol. 3. London, Longmans, 1966.

Reiter, R. J., and Fraschini, F.: Endocrine aspects of the mammalian pineal gland: a review. Neuroendocrinology, *5*:219, 1969.

Rosemberg, E., and Paulsen, C. A. (eds.): Regulation of Testicular Function. Role of the hypothalamus. Testicular-pituitary interrelationship. Metabolic effects of gonadotropins. Influence of gonadotropins on testicular function (a collection of 13 papers). *In* Advances in Experimental Medicine and Biology. The Human Testis. New York, Plenum, 1970.

Steinberger, E.: Hormonal control of mammalian spermatogenesis. Physiol. Rev., *51*:1, 1971.

Symposium on Hormonal Control of Protein Biosynthesis. J. Cell. Comp. Physiol., *66*, Suppl. 1, 1965.

Tata, J. R.: Growth and developmental hormones as tools for the study of biosynthetic control mechanisms. J. Sci. Industr. Res., *25*:355, 1966.

Williams-Ashman, H. G.: New facets of the biochemistry of steroid hormone action. Cancer Res., *25*:1096, 1965.

Effects on Cellular Level

Anderson, K. M., and Liao, S.: Selective retention of dihydrotestosterone by prostatic nuclei. Nature, *219*:277, 1968.

Bruchovsky, N., and Wilson, J. D.: The conversion of testosterone to 5α-androstan-17β-ol-3-one by rat prostrate in vivo and in vitro. J. Biol. Chem., *243*:2012, 1968.

Dorrington, J. H., Vernon, R. G., and Fritz, I. B.: The effect of gonadotrophins on the 3′,5′-AMP levels of seminiferous tubules. Biochem. Biophys. Res. Commun., *46*:1523, 1972.

Liao, S., and Lim, A. H.: Prostate nuclear chromatin: An effect of testosterone on the synthesis of ribonucleic acid rich in cytidylyl (3′,5′) guanosine. Proc. Nat. Acad. Sci., *57*:379, 1967.

Lipsett, M. B.: Steroid secretions by the human testis. *In* Advances in Experimental Medicine and Biology. The Human Testis. New York, Plenum, 1970.

——— and Savard, K.: Subcellular structure and synthesis of steroids in the testis. *In* Advances in Experimental Medicine and Biology. The Human Testis. New York, Plenum, 1970.

Sluyser, M.: Effect of testosterone on the binding of prostate histone to DNA in vitro. Biochem. Biophys. Res. Commun., *22*:336, 1966.

Williams-Ashman, H. G., and Shimazaki, J.: Some metabolic and morphogenetic effects of androgens on normal and neoplastic prostate. *In* Weisler, R. W., *et al.* (eds.): Endogenous Factors Influencing Host-Tumor Balance. p. 31. Chicago, University of Chicago Press, 1967.

SOME REFERENCES ON STRUCTURES AND ARRANGEMENTS IN SPERMATOGENESIS

General

Bishop, M. W. H., and Walton, A.: Spermatogenesis and the structure of mammalian spermatozoa. *In* Marshall's Physiology of Reproduction, vol. 1, Part 2. London, Longmans, Green and Co., 1968.

Bruce, W. R., and Meistrich, M. L.: Spermatogenesis in the Mouse. Proc. 1st Internat. Conf. on Cell Differentiation. p. 295. Copenhagen, Munksgaard, 1972.

Courot, M., Hochereau-de Reviers, M., and Ortavant, R.: Spermatogenesis. *In* The Testis. vol. 1. New York, Academic Press, 1970.

Roosen-Runge, E. C.: The process of spermatogenesis in mammals. Biol. Rev., *37*:343, 1962.

Odell, W. D., and Moyer, D. L.: The testis and the male sex accessories. *In* Physiology of Reproduction. St. Louis, C. V. Mosby, 1971.

Structures and Arrangements

Branes, D.: The fine structure of prostatic glands in relation to sex hormones. Int. Rev. Cytol., *20*, 1966.

Bröckelmann, J.: Fine structure of germ cells and Sertoli cells during the cycle of the seminiferous epithelium in the rat. Z. Zellforsch., *59*:820, 1963.

Burgos, M. H., Vitale-Calpe, R., and Aoki, A.: Fine structure of the testis and its functional significance. *In* The Testis. vol. 1. New York, Academic Press, 1970.

Clermont, Y.: The cycle of the seminiferous epithelium in man. Am. J. Anat., *112*:35, 1963.

————: Spermatogenesis in man. A study of the spermatogonial population. Fertil. Steril., *17:*705, 1966.

Clermont, Y., and Trott, M.: Duration of the cycle of the seminiferous epithelium in the mouse and hamster determined by means of radioautography. Fertil. Steril., *20:*805, 1969.

————: Kinetics of spermatogenesis in mammals: seminiferous epithelium cycle and spermatogonial renewal. Physiol. Rev., *52:*198, 1972.

Clermont, Y., and Leblond, C. P.: Spermiogenesis of man, monkey, ram and other mammals as shown by the "periodic acid-Schiff" technique. Am. J. Anat., *96:*229, 1955.

Dym, M., and Fawcett, D. W.: Further observations on the number of spermatogonia, spermatocytes, and spermatids connected by intercellular bridges in the mammalian testis. Biol. Reprod., *4:*195, 1971.

Dym, M., and Fawcett, D. W.: The blood-testis barrier in the rat and the physiological compartmentation of the seminiferous epithelium. Biol. Reprod., *3:*308, 1970.

Fawcett, D. W.: A comparative view of sperm ultrastructure. Biol. Reprod., *2* (Suppl. 2):90, 1970.

Fawcett, D. W., and Burgos, M. H.: Observations on the cytomorphosis of the germinal and interstitial cells of the human testis. *In* Ciba Foundation Colloquia on Ageing. vol. 2, p. 86. London, J. & A. Churchill, 1956.

Fawcett, D. W., and Ito, S.: The fine structure of bat spermatozoa. Am. J. Anat., *116:*567, 1965.

Fawcett, D. W., Eddy, E., and Phillips, D. M.: Observations on the fine structure and relationships of the chromatoid body in mammalian spermatogenesis. Biol. Reprod., *2:*129, 1970.

Fawcett, D. W., and Phillips, D. M.: Observations on the release of spermatozoa and on the changes in the head during passage through the epididymis. J. Reprod. Fertil., *5* (Suppl.):405, 1969.

Firlit, C. F., and Davis, J. R.: Morphogenesis of the residual body of the mouse testis. Quart. J. Microscop. Sci., *106:*93, 1965.

Forer, A., *et al.*: Spermatozoan tails. Nature (New Biol.), *243:*128, 1973.

Hannah-Alava, A.: The premeiotic stages of spermatogenesis. Adv. Genet., *13:*157, 1965.

Heller, C. G., and Clermont, Y.: Kinetics of the germinal epithelium in man. Recent Prog. Hormone Res., *20:*545, 1964.

Koehler, J. K.: Human sperm head ultrastructure: a freeze-etching study. J. Ultrastruct. Res., *39:*520, 1972.

de Kretser, D. M.: Ultrastructural features of human spermiogenesis. Z. Zellforsch., *98:*477, 1969.

Lam, D. M. K., Furrer, R., and Bruce, W. R.: The separation, physical characterization and differential kinetics of spermatogonial cells of the mouse. Proc. Nat. Acad. Sci., *65:*192, 1970.

Loir, M., and Wyrobek, A.: Density separation of mouse spermatid nuclei. Exp. Cell Res., *75:*261, 1972.

Macklin, C. C., and Macklin, M. T.: The seminal vesicles, prostate and bulbo-urethral glands. *In* Cowdry's Special Cytology. ed. 2, p. 1771. New York, Hoeber, 1932.

Percy, B., Clermont, Y., and Leblond, C. P.: The wave of the seminiferous epithelium in the rat. Am. J. Anat., *108:*47, 1961.

Phillips, D. M.: Substructure of the mammalian acrosome. J. Ultrastruct. Res., *38:*591, 1972.

Rattner, J. B.: Observations of centriole formation in male meiosis. J. Cell Biol., *54:*20, 1972.

Rattner, J. B., and Brinkley, B. R.: Ultrastructure of mammalian spermiogenesis. II. Elimination of the nuclear membrane. J. Ultrastruct. Res., *36:*1, 1971.

Rowley, M. J., Berlin, J. D., and Heller, C. G.: The ultrastructure of four types of human spermatogonia. Z. Zellforsch., *112:*139, 1971.

Rowley, M. J., Teshima, F., and Heller, C. G.: Duration of transit of spermatozoa through the human male ductular system. Fertil. Steril., *21:*390, 1970.

Solari, A. J., and Tres, L. L.: Ultrastructure and histochemistry of the nucleus during male meiotic prophase. *In* Advances in Experimental Medicine and Biology. The Human Testis. New York, Plenum, 1970.

Chromosomes and Meiosis

Dronamraju, K. R.: The function of the Y-chromosome in man, animals, and plants. Adv. Genet., *13:*227, 1965.

Esponda, P., and Stockert, J. C.: Localization of RNA in the synaptonemal complex. J. Ultrastruct. Res., *35:*411, 1971.

Fuge, H., and Muller, W.: Murotubuli contact on anaphase chromosomes in first meiotic division. Exp. Cell Res., *71:*241, 1972.

Moens, P. B.: The structure and function of the synaptinemal complex in *Lilium* sporocytes. Chromosoma, *23:*418, 1968.

————: Mechanisms of chromosome synapsis at meiotic prophase. *In* Bourne, G. H., and Danielli, J. F. (eds.): Internat. Rev. Cytol., *35:*117, 1973.

Moses, M. J.: Synaptinemal complex. Ann. Rev. Genet., *2:*363, 1968.

Ohno, S.: Morphological aspects of meiosis and their genetical significance. *In* Advances in Experimental Medicine and Biology. The Human Testis. New York, Plenum, 1970.

Polani, P. E.: Centromere localization at meiosis and position of chiasmata in male and female mouse. Chromosoma, *36:*343, 1972.

Rimpau, J., and Lelley, T.: Attachment of meiotic chromosomes to nuclear membrane. Z. Pflanzenzuchtung, *67:*197, 1972.

Schnedl, W.: End to end association of X and Y chromosomes in mouse meiosis. Nature (New Biol.), *236:*29, 1972.

Interstitial Cells

Christensen, A. K.: Fine structure of testicular interstitial cells in humans. *In* Advances in Experimental Medicine and Biology. The Human Testis. New York, Plenum, 1970.

Hooker, C. W.: The intertubular tissue of the testis. *In* The Testis. vol. 1. New York, Academic Press, 1970.

Murakami, M., and Kitakara, Y.: Cylindrical bodies derived from endoplasmic reticulum in Leydig cells of rat testis. J. Electron Microsc. (Tokyo), *20:*318, 1971.

Reddy, J., and Svobodka, D.: Microbodies (peroxisomes) identification in interstitial cells of testis. J. Histochem. Cytochem., *20:*140, 1972.

Tsang, W. N., Lacy, D., and Collins, P. M.: Leydig cell differentiation, steroid metabolism by interstitium in-vitro and growth of accessory sex organs in rat. J. Reprod. Fertil., *34:*351, 1973.

Some References on the Metabolic Activities of the Testis and Semen

Amann, R. P.: Sperm production rates. *In* The Testis. vol. 1. New York, Academic Press, 1970.

Bishop, D. W.: Sperm Motility. Physiol. Rev., *42:*1, 1962.

Bishop, M. W. H., and Walton, A.: Metabolism and motility of mammalian spermatozoa. *In* Marshall's Physiology of Reproduction. Vol. 1. Part 2. London, Longmans, Green and Co., 1968.

Blackshaw, A. W.: Histochemical localization of testicular enzymes; Free, M. J.: Carbohydrate metabolism in the testis; Johnson, A. D.: Testicular lipids; Davis, J. R., and Langford, G. A.: Testicular proteins; Gledhill, B. L.: Nucleic acids of the testis. All four references *in* The Testis. vol. 2. New York, Academic Press, 1970.

Hotta, Y., Parchman, L. G., and Stern, H.: Protein synthesis during meiosis. Proc. Nat. Acad. Sci., *60:*575, 1968.

Lam, D. M. K., and Bruce, W. R.: The biosynthesis of protamine during spermatogenesis of the mouse: extraction, partial characterization and site of synthesis J. Cell Physiol., *78:*13, 1971.

Mann, T.: The Biochemistry of Semen and of the Male Reproductive Tract. New York, John Wiley and Sons, 1964.

Moresi, V.: Chromosome activities during meiosis and spermatogenesis. J. Reprod. Fertil., *Suppl. 13:*1, 1971.

Nelson, L.: Quantitative evaluation of sperm motility control mechanisms. Biol. Reprod., *6:*319, 1972.

Phillips, D. M.: Comparative analysis of mammalian sperm motility. J. Cell Biol., *53:*561, 1972.

Setchell, B. P.: Testicular blood supply, lymphatic drainage and secretion of fluid. *In* The Testis. vol. 1. New York, Academic Press, 1970.

————: Characteristics of testicular spermatozoa and the fluid which transports them into the epididymis. Biol. Reprod., *1* (Suppl. 1):40, 1969.

Suzuki, H.: Effects of Vitamin E-deficiency and high salt supplementation on changes in kidney and testis of rats. Tohoku J. Exp. Med., *106:*329, 1972.

Some References on the Effects of Chemicals, X-irradiation, and Heat on Spermatogenesis

Bateman, A. J., and Epstein, S. S.: Dominant lethal mutations in mammals. *In* Hollaender, A. (ed.). Chemical Mutagens, Principles and Methods for Their Detection. vol. 2. New York, Plenum Press, 1971.

Bruce, W. R., Furrer, R., and Wyrobek, A. J.: Abnormalities in the shape of murine sperm after acute testicular X-irradiation. Mut. Res. (in press, 1974)

Carlson, W. D., and Gassner, F. X. (eds.): Effects of Ionizing Radiation on the Reproductive System. New York, Macmillan, 1964.

Dym, M., and Clermont, Y.: Role of spermatogonia in the repair of the seminiferous epithelium following x-irradiation of the rat testis. Am. J. Anat., *128:*265, 1970.

MacLeod, J.: The significance of deviations in human sperm morphology. *In* The Human Testis. p. 481. New York, Plenum Press, 1970.

Meistrich, M. L., Eng, V. W. S., and Loir, M.: Temperature effects on the kinetics of spermatogenesis in the mouse. Cell Tissue Kinet., *6:*379, 1973.

Röhrborn, G.: The activity of alkylating agents. I. Sensitive mutable stages in spermatogenesis and oogenesis; ———— and Schleiermacher, E.: II. Histological and cytogenetic findings in spermatogenesis. *In* Vogel, F., and Rohrborn, G. (eds.): Chemical Mutagenesis in Mammals and Man. New York, Springer-Verlag, 1970.

Some Related Readings

Beer, A. E., and Billingham, R. E.: Immunobiology of mammalian reproduction. Adv. Immunol., *14:*1, 1971.

Brackett, B. G.: Mammalian fertilization in vitro. Fed. Proc., *32:*2065, 1973.

Davajan, V., Nakamura, R. M., and Saga, M.: Role of immunology in the infertile human. Biol. Reprod., *6:*443, 1972.

Gould, K. G.: Application of in vitro fertilization. Fed. Proc., *32:*2069, 1973.

Lyon, M., Gleniste, P. H., and Hawker, S. G.: Do H-2 and T-loci of mouse have a function in haploid phase of sperm? Nature, *240:*152, 1972.

Metz, C. B.: Role of specific sperm antigens in fertilization. Fed. Proc., *32:*2057, 1973.

Parkes, A. S.: The biology of spermatozoa and artificial insemination. *In* Marshall's Physiology of Reproduction. Vol. 1, Part 2. London, Longmans, Green and Co., 1968.

Sherman, J. K.: Synopsis of the use of frozen human semen since 1964: State of the art of human semen banking. Fertil. Steril., *24:*397, 1973.

28 *Afferent Nerve Endings and Organs of Special Sense*

Background Material—Some Basic Principles. Man is able to experience many kinds of sensation. A somewhat elementary list of the senses would include touch, pressure, heat, cold, pain, smell, sight, hearing, position and movement.

First, for the normal person to perceive any sensation, a nervous impulse must be set up at the peripheral termination of an afferent neuron chain that leads via the central nervous system (CNS) to the general region of the brain that is concerned with perceiving sensation. Second, the *kind* of sensation that is perceived when nervous impulses arrive from a particular chain of neurons depends on the particular part of this general region of the brain to which this neuron chain is connected. For example, impulses arriving at one part of this region give rise to the sensation of light. Those that arrive at another part give rise to the sensation of touch, and so on. Third, neuron chains that lead to the particular part of this region that is connected with the perception of light, originate in the eye. Likewise, those that arrive at the part of this region of the brain that is concerned with the perception of touch lead from nerve endings all over the body that set off nervous impulses when they are touched. Accordingly, if it were possible to connect up the neuron chains that lead from touch receptors from all over the body to the part of the brain concerned with perceiving light, a person on being touched would perceive light and not touch. In other words, the perception of different sensations depends on nervous impulses arriving at different special parts of the general portion of the brain that is concerned with the perception of sensation.

The next point to make is that the neuron chains that lead to different parts of the region of the brain concerned with sense perception all begin from terminations that are specifically designed to be easily stimulated by the kind of energy that is concerned with producing the sensation this kind of energy invokes.

How different forms of energy could affect various gadgets to complete electrical circuits is illustrated in Figure 17-8. Although setting off nervous impulses is more complex than completing an electrical circuit, the receptors for touch are designed to set off nervous impulses as a result of very delicate contacts. Those concerned with heat must be warmed in order to institute a nervous impulse. Certain cells in the eye set off nervous impulses from the reception of light. Others, such as those concerned with taste and smell react to chemical stimulation by setting off nervous impulses. In other words, different kinds of receptors are designed to be particularly sensitive to different forms of energy and also in some instances (e.g., touch and pressure) to different amounts of the same kind of energy. Furthermore, the right kinds of receptors are connected by neuron chains to the right parts of the region of the brain that is concerned with the perception of different sensations.

The receptors concerned with smell, sight, hearing, taste, and perception of movement and position in relation to gravity are aggregated into what are called *organs of special sense*. These will be described after considering the receptors that give rise to the sensations of touch, pressure, cold, warmth, pain and also certain afferent impulses that are derived from muscles and tendons, which do not necessarily appear in consciousness, and those from joints which are concerned with kinesthetic sensation (to be defined presently).

The Receptors Concerned in Pressure, Touch, Cold, Warmth and Pain

These receptors are morphologically classified into two groups: (1) naked nerve endings, and (2) encapsulated endings. The naked nerve endings seem to be the more primitive—designed, as it were, to initiate reflexes that move an animal away from an environment not conducive to its survival. The encapsulated endings serve what might be termed more sophisticated roles, although the particular functions of some of them are still somewhat obscure. It was thought, for example, that Krause's end bulbs (Fig. 28-1 E) were

936

specialized endings for cold and corpuscles of Ruffini (Fig. 28-1 D) for heat. Now there is a growing tendency to group encapsulated endings of this type (with the exception of Pacinian corpuscles, Fig. 28-1 C) into a single general category of sensory end bulbs which are present in many locations in the body and whose function, as well as structure, is not very well known. However, until more is known about the sensory end bulbs we shall continue to describe what have been called Krause's end bulbs and the corpuscles of Ruffini much as they have been described in the past but recognizing that they probably represent a kind of structure that varies somewhat in appearance in different locations and that their particular roles are probably not as specific about sensitivity to cold and heat as was once believed.

To initiate a nervous impulse at a nerve ending the nerve ending must be depolarized. The way this is accomplished would in general seem to depend on some form of energy making the cell membrane (the axolemma) of the nerve ending more permeable so that sodium ions, normally in excess on the exterior of the membrane, where they create a positive charge, diffuse through the membrane to its inner surface, which causes the positive charge on its exterior to disappear at this site. It is assumed here that the student has read Chapter 17 and knows that this would initiate a nervous impulse that could be relayed to the brain.

Not very much is known about the way in which at least some forms of energy affect receptor nerve endings to set off waves of depolarization. Since there is some clue as to how pressure receptors may function, we shall begin by describing them.

Pressure Receptors—Pacinian Corpuscles. One is illustrated in the center of Figure 28-1. They are known as corpuscles of Vater-Pacini or, more commonly, as pacinian corpuscles, and are regarded as the organs of deep pressure, and possibly also of vibration sense. They are distributed in the deep regions of the subcutaneous tissue, in the connective tissues near tendons and joints, in the interosseous membranes of the leg and the forearm, in the perimysium of muscles, in the pancreas and its mesentery, in serous membranes, under mucous membranes, in the mammary glands and in the external genitalia of both sexes.

Each is made up of a central elongated granular mass covered with many concentric, thin layers. According to Shanthaveerappa and Bourne, the outermost layers are connective tissue, comparable to the connective tissue perineurium of a nerve trunk. Beneath this layer, however, and comprising the bulk of the corpuscle, the concentric layers are believed by these authors to be layers of squamous epithelial cells, which they believe represent a continuation of the epithelial layer that they have described as lining the connective tissue perineurial sheaths of nerve trunks, and which they believe to be of ectodermal origin. A little connective tissue and some capillaries may lie between adjacent sheets of epithelial cells. The structure so obtained has an appearance, when sectioned longitudinally, of a longitudinally sliced onion (Fig. 28-1 C). The peripheral laminae are thicker than those more centrally located. At one pole the nerve fiber enters. It seems probable that the myelin extends far enough into the corpuscle to have one node of Ranvier inside the corpuscle (not shown in Fig. 28-1). The axon terminates in a small swelling in the region of the central granular material. The neurolemma and the endoneurium of the nerve fiber seem to blend with the capsule of the corpuscle.

There is a theory about how the nerve ending within this type of structure could become depolarized on pressure; it is that if a pacinian corpuscle is squeezed by pressure, it elongates. Its elongation in turn would stretch the nerve fiber within it, including the axolemma over its terminal part, and this could make the axolemma more permeable to sodium ions, so that the naked part of the ending within the corpuscle would become depolarized.

Touch. The sensation aroused by touch is subserved by 3 types of receptors: *Meissner's corpuscles, Merkel's disks* and *naked nerve endings,* in particular by basketlike arrangements of naked endings that are disposed around the bases of *hair follicles.*

MEISSNER'S CORPUSCLES are distributed in the connective tissue papillae of the skin just below and perpendicular to the epidermis. These corpuscles are not distributed evenly, being most numerous on the palmar surface of the fingers, the lips, the margins of the eyelids, the nipples and the external genital organs. They are somewhat ovoid structures made up of a central mass of irregular cells penetrated by irregularly curved nerve endings (Fig. 28-1 B), and they possess a many-layered capsule that is continuous with the coverings associated with the afferent nerve fiber.

In the borders of the tongue, and probably in certain other sensitive epithelium, some rudimentary corpuscles of Meissner, called MERKEL'S DISKS, are found. These consist of expanded disks on the terminal twigs of the branches of nerve fibers that penetrate the stratified squamous epithelium. Each terminal disk is attached to a modified epithelial cell.

Many of the hair follicles are surrounded by a BASKETLIKE ARRANGEMENT OF NERVE FIBERS with several types of expanded endings. These are stimu-

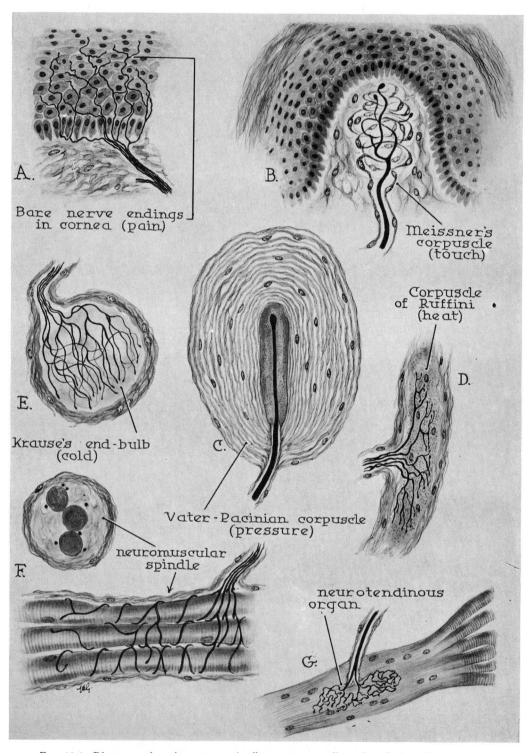

Fig. 28-1. Diagrams of various types of afferent nerve endings described in the text. The drawing of a longitudinal section of a neuromuscular spindle in the lower left corner is no longer adequate; for an up-to-date illustration see Figure 28-2.

lated by the movement of the hairs. Around the hair follicles of rodents this arrangement is still more complicated, and special tactile hairs are present around the nose and the mouth.

The cornea of the eye is sensitive to touch, and it contains only naked nerve fibers.

Why delicate touch should cause any of these terminations of nerve fibers to become depolarized is not understood.

Heat and Cold Receptors. Skin is not everywhere equally sensitive in detecting the presence of a small object that is either colder or warmer than the skin. There are spots where warmth is more easily detected and other spots where cold is more easily detected. These sites, it has been thought, could be correlated with the presence of one or the other, respectively, of two types of encapsulated receptors.

The receptor of warmth has been described as the CORPUSCLE OF RUFFINI, lying deep in the skin or even in the subcutaneous tissue. These are present generally but are particularly numerous in the subcutaneous connective tissue deep to the plantar surface of the foot. This receptor is composed of a loose arborization of nerve fibers ending in flattened expansions and interspersed with a peculiar granular material dotted with nuclei. Elongated connective tissue bundles and fibroblasts give support to the structure (Fig. 28-1 D).

The KRAUSE END-BULB has been thought to be the receptor for cold. These end-bulbs are most prevalent in the dermis of the conjunctiva, the mucosa of the tongue and the external genitalia. Two structurally different types have been described. The simpler is composed of a granular mass enclosed in a connective tissue capsule continuous with the endoneurium of the afferent nerve fiber; the nerve itself penetrates the end-bulb and terminates near the superior pole of the granular mass in a light thickening. The more complex variety is found in the conjunctiva. The afferent nerve, instead of ending bluntly, branches repeatedly in the bulb and ends in several free, enlarged terminations (Fig. 28-1 E). Since it can be shown that extreme heat and cold can be detected in sites, most notably the cornea of the eye, where there are only free nerve endings, it is apparent that free endings also can serve as heat and cold receptors.

Pain Receptors. The element or unit of the receptive mechanism for pain is not a small encapsulated structure innervated by a single nerve fiber but rather an appreciable area over which the naked terminal branches of one neuron are distributed. In the cornea the naked branches of one neuron extend between epithelial cells (Fig. 28-1 A) over as much as one quarter to one half of its surface area. In any area of

normally innervated skin the terminals of many such units overlap intricately.

Pain fibers in the skin arise from a nerve plexus deep in the corium by way of a superficial plexus of unmyelinated and thin myelinated fibers. The fibers leaving this superficial plexus are all unmyelinated, though they may have their origin in myelinated fibers. These naked fibers branch freely and end in fine, beaded terminals beneath and between the cells of the deep layers of the epidermis. Naked endings are also present in many of the connective tissues of the body, but not in all.

The pain endings do not respond selectively to one variety of stimulus but to any type, whether it be mechanical, chemical or thermal, provided that it is sufficiently intense. Therefore, the sensation of pain serves a protective purpose, giving warning of the injurious nature of a stimulus rather than information as to its specific quality.

Afferent Impulses From Muscle and Tendons

Although most of the afferent impulses that arise from afferent nerve endings in muscle and tendons do not appear in consciousness, they are, of course, of the greatest importance in activating reflexes which are concerned in everything from enabling an individual to raise a cup of coffee to his lips, to walk down a street or to type a manuscript such as this. First we shall consider neuromuscular spindles and describe a little about how they can participate in reflexes.

Neuromuscular Spindles, the Stretch Reflex. Figure 17-7 illustrates a common reflex called the knee jerk. This reflex is initiated by striking the patellar tendon just below the patella. The patella, of course, is attached to the tendon of the quadriceps muscle. So when the patellar tendon is tapped and indented, it causes a slight stretching of the quadriceps muscle. This sudden slight stretching is immediately reflected by the contraction of the quadriceps muscle, which by shortening causes the foot to kick briskly forward. This reflex involves only two neurons, an afferent neuron that synapses with a motor (efferent) neuron in the spinal cord, as is shown in Figure 17-7. This reflex is called the *stretch reflex*. The afferent stimulation is generally attributed to structures within the muscle, called neuromuscular spindles, being stretched longitudinally. Neuromuscular spindles, as we shall see, are somewhat complicated structures, and, as will be learned in physiology, they serve somewhat complicated functions. We shall now describe them and explain first the basis for the stretch reflex.

Neuromuscular spindles, according to Cooper and

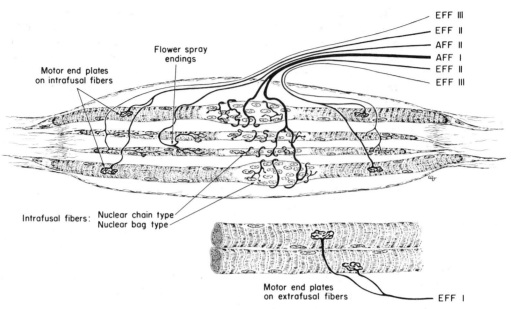

Fig. 28-2. Diagrammatic drawing of a muscle spindle showing the nuclear bag and the nuclear chain types of intrafusal fibers and their afferent and efferent innervation. For details see text. Below some extrafusal fibers and their efferent innervation are shown.

Daniel, in the lumbrical muscles of the hand are about 5.0 mm. long and about 200 μ in diameter. Each is enclosed in a shorter connective tissue capsule which is extensible. Spindles are distributed here and there in striated muscles. They are attached to the muscle in which they are distributed by their ends and in such a way that when the muscle as a whole is stretched, the spindle is stretched. One end of a spindle may be attached to the tendon of a muscle. Within the capsule there are a few to several muscle fibers that are narrower and different in other respects from ordinary striated muscle fibers. Because they are within the spindle, they are termed *intrafusal* (*fusus*, spindle) fibers. The ordinary striated muscle fibers outside the spindles are called *extrafusal* fibers.

According to Cooper and Daniel, the intrafusal fibers of the spindles of man are of two types. One type, the larger, of which there may be from 1 to 4 in a spindle, is known as the *nuclear bag type* of intrafusal fiber. The other type is the more numerous, there being anywhere from 1 to 10 in a spindle, and is termed the *nuclear chain type* of fiber.

The nuclear bag type of fiber is larger and longer than the nuclear chain type (Fig. 28-2). Furthermore, in their midsections, nuclear bag fibers are expanded, and there are no striations, but, as their name indicates, there are many nuclei. The nuclear bag fibers, moreover, may extend through the ends of capsules

into the substance of the striated muscle, where they appear as small groups running for several mm. The region of the nuclear bag is not contractile; hence only the portions of nuclear bag fibers that extend from the nuclear bag region toward each end are contractile.

The nuclear chain type of intrafusal fiber is narrower and shorter than the nuclear bag type. Furthermore, the midsections of the fibers are not expanded, but the myofibrils are here replaced by a chain of large single nuclei (Fig. 28-2).

Most spindles in man contain both types of fibers. A few, near the ends of muscles, may have only nuclear bag fibers.

The Afferent Innervation of the Nuclear Bag Type of Fiber. The nuclear bags lie close together, and each receives a terminal branch from the largest myelinated afferent fiber (labeled AFF I in Fig. 28-2). Each terminal branch of this fiber is wound around a nuclear bag in a spiral fashion; hence this afferent ending is called an annulospiral ending; its annulospiral nature, however, is not so pronounced in man as in certain other species. This ending is essentially a stretch receptor. If the muscle is suddenly stretched, as when the patellar tendon is tapped, as in Figure 17-7, the neuromuscular spindles in the muscle are stretched, and this causes the annulospiral afferent nerve endings that surround each nuclear bag to be stretched. This stretching makes the axolemma of the terminal fibers more permeable, and, as a result, a wave of depolarization is initiated. The nervous impulse thus generated flows to the spinal cord in the afferent neurons, as is shown in Figure 17-7, and each afferent neuron there synapses with a large motor neuron in the same segment of the cord, and the motor (efferent) neuron carries a nervous impulse, via motor end-plates, to some of the ordinary (extrafusal) muscle fibers of this muscle (EFF I in Fig. 28-2), which thereupon contract, and so the stretch reflex is completed.

The afferent neuron in the spinal cord synapses not only with efferent neurons in the same segment but also with other afferent neurons that pass to the cerebellum, which is the part of the brain that is concerned in muscular coordination. The stretch reflex is believed to play an important role in the maintenance of muscle tone.

The Afferent Innervation of Nuclear Chain Fibers. These, as are shown in Figure 28-2, receive afferent fibers from two sources. First, small branches of the large afferent fibers that provide annulospiral endings for the nuclear bags also supply the region of a nuclear chain with similar endings. Second, smaller and separate afferent fibers that enter the spindle (AFF II in Fig. 28-2) end generally in what are termed flower spray or secondary endings on the nuclear chain fiber on either one or both sides beyond the so-called annulospiral endings. The way that afferent impulses arising from the stretching of the flower spray endings are concerned in reflexes involves physiological considerations too complex to discuss here.

Efferent (Motor) Endings in Spindles. The portions of both types of intrafusal fibers that lie between their heavily nucleated regions and the ends of the capsule are supplied by fine motor fibers, the γ (gamma) fibers (EFF II and III in Fig. 28-2) that are much finer than the α (alpha) fibers (labeled EFF I) that innervate the extrafusal fibers. The fibers terminate in small motor end-plates or in multiple (*en grappe*) grapelike endings. The small nerves are numerous and much more difficult to follow than the larger AFF I and AFF II fibers to the afferent endings. The small motor nerves end on portions of the intrafusal muscle fibers, which, unlike the heavily nucleated areas, are clearly striated and contractile. The function of these contractile parts of the intrafusal fibers is not to cause a shortening of the muscle as a whole; instead, their function is probably to stretch the noncontractile nuclear bag or nuclear chain regions of the intrafusal fibers. The contraction of these very small muscle fibers can have little effect on the length of the spindle; its length is much more dependent on the activity of the extrafusal fibers to which it is attached. Hence,

strong efferent stimulation of the contractile parts of intrafusal fibers can, by causing the afferent endings to be stretched, in turn cause a reflex contraction of the muscle (the extrafusal fibers). Another thing that stimulation, probably of the grapelike motor endings, can do is to set up small maintained stretches of the afferent endings.

The system that controls the fine motor fibers to the spindle is regulated by efferent fibers that descend via the spinal cord from various parts of the brain, about which much will be learned in neurophysiology.

Afferent Nerve Endings in Tendons and Joints

Neurotendinous organs are found at the junctions of muscles and tendons and in the aponeuroses of muscles. These consist of small bundles of collagenic fibers with numerous nuclei, enclosed within a capsule of connective tissue (Fig. 28-1 G). A large myelinated nerve fiber enters the structure, usually at its middle, and there subdivides into smaller unmyelinated branches, terminating in leaflike plates. They provide information about tension.

Nerve Endings in Joint Structures. As was noted under nerve supply in Chapter 17, which deals with joints, Gardner has pointed out the presence of numerous corpuscular type endings in the capsules of synovial joints. Since these endings are in sites where they would be compressed by certain types of joint movement, it seems probable that they are also important in connection with kinesthetic sensation, which is the conscious recognition of the orientation of the different parts of the body with respect to each other as well as of rates of movement of the different parts of the body.

The way in which the various types of endings described above—and probably simpler types of endings also—are involved in the complicated but effective ways in which the muscles of man can perform, both reflexly and also at the direction of the conscious mind, is a matter that forms an interesting aspect of courses and texts on the nervous system and neurophysiology.

The Organs of Special Sense— The Olfactory Organ

In the introduction to Chapter 17 it was explained that, as multicellular organisms evolved, the first neurons that developed represented specializations of surface ectodermal cells (Fig. 17-4). As evolution proceeded, the nerve cell bodies of most afferent neurons came to migrate, as it were, along their axons, even-

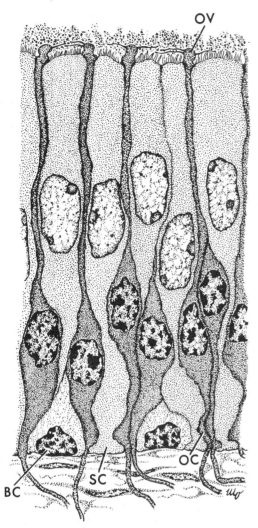

FIG. 28-3. Diagrammatic drawing of a section of olfactory epithelium as seen with the LM. OV, olfactory vesicle; BC, basal cell; SC, sustentacular cell, and OC, olfactory cell.

tually to take up a more central and better-protected position in cerebrospinal ganglia. However, there was one exception to this general rule, because in olfactory areas the cell bodies of afferent neurons are at the surface.

There are 2 olfactory areas, one in each of the 2 nasal cavities. The mucous membrane lining the nasal cavities in the 2 olfactory areas constitutes the *olfactory organ*. The nerve cell bodies present in the epithelium of the mucous membrane at this site are highly sensitive in their ability to be selectively stimulated by odors of different kinds. It should be kept in mind that having nerve cell bodies at the surface is a more hazardous arrangement than having them deeply disposed, with their fibers running to the surface, for if a mucous membrane containing nerve cell bodies is injured by a disease process or by trauma, the nerve cell bodies that are destroyed cannot be regenerated, whereas a surface innervated by fibers alone can be reinnervated after an injury by the regeneration of fibers from the cell bodies of deeply situated nerve cells. So, as might be expected, the sense of smell is often impaired; indeed, Smith from his investigations has estimated that on the average about 1 percent of the fibers of the olfactory nerve (which leads from the receptors to the brain) are lost each year of life. In some individuals all olfactory fibers are lost at a comparatively early age, usually as a result of the destruction of the olfactory cells in the membrane by the infections to which the nasal mucous membrane is so commonly susceptible.

Gross Characteristics. The mucous membrane of the olfactory areas is of a yellow hue. It is disposed so as to line most of the uppermost part of the roof of each nasal cavity, beginning in front of the anterior termination of the superior concha and extending backward for about 1 cm. From the roof it extends down both sides of each nasal cavity: on the lateral side it extends so that it covers most of the superior concha, and on the medial side it extends for about 1 cm. down the nasal septum.

Microscopic Structure. The mucous membrane of the olfactory organ consists of a thick pseudostratified epithelium (Fig. 28-3) and a thick lamina propria.

The *epithelium* consists of 3 kinds of cells: (1) sustentacular, (2) olfactory or sensory, and (3) basal.

The SUSTENTACULAR (*sustentaculum,* a prop) cells are tall cylindrical cells disposed perpendicular to the surface (Fig. 28-3, SC). In their deeper parts they are much narrower than in their superficial parts. Although in the more superficial part of the membrane they are packed closely together, their more or less cylindrical shape precludes their constituting an imperforate layer. The free surfaces of the sustentacular cell are covered with microvilli (Fig. 28-3). The delicate processes of the sensory or olfactory cells, the cell bodies of which lie more deeply (OC in Fig. 28-3), are able to reach the surface by way of the crevices left between the sustentacular cells (Fig. 28-3).

The cytoplasm of the sustentacular cells contains a yellow-to-brown pigment; this accounts for the yellow color of the olfactory area in the gross.

The nuclei of the sustentacular cells are disposed just above the middle of the epithelial membrane. They are oval and lightly stained, and since they lie in approximately the same plane, they appear in a section that is cut at right angles to the surface as a row or two of light oval nuclei that runs parallel to the surface (Fig. 28-3). This row or two of oval nuclei is commonly referred to as the *narrow zone of oval nuclei* to contrast it with the more deeply disposed *wide zone of round nuclei* (of the sensory cells) that lies below it (Fig. 28-3).

Deep to their nuclei the cytoplasm of the sustentacular cells becomes narrower and extends to the basement membrane, except in sites where basal cells (Fig. 28-3) prevent their cytoplasm from reaching the basement membrane.

The basal cells (BC in Fig. 28-3), which are more or less triangular, are disposed irregularly along the deepest layer of the epithelium. Their nuclei are darker than those of the sustentacular cells but a little lighter than those of the sensory cells.

The SENSORY OR OLFACTORY cells are of the nature of bipolar nerve cells; hence each has a cell body and a nerve fiber extending from each of its ends (Fig. 28-3): one, a dendrite; and the other, an axon. The sensory cells, like the sustentacular cells, are arranged perpendicular to the surface. Their cell bodies are fitted between the sustentacular cells in the region where they become greatly narrowed (immediately below the narrow zone of oval nuclei). The nuclei of the sensory cells in this region constitute the broad zone of round nuclei (Fig. 28-2). The dendrites of the bipolar cells ascend toward the surface in the crevices between the sustentacular cells.

Each olfactory cell (Fig. 28-3, OC) has an axon which passes into the lamina propria. Toward the other pole of the cell, the cytoplasm on the superficial side of the nucleus continues toward the surface as a narrow process which terminates in what is generally termed the olfactory vesicle (OV in Fig. 28-3); the vesicle, however, is not hollow, as its name implies; instead, it is a solid bulblike mass of cytoplasm that bulges through the surface. At its point of entry through the surface it is connected to adjacent sustentacular cells by means of a type of junctional complex which would seem to be of the adhaerens type. In the sustentacular cells a terminal web (TW in Fig. 28-4) connects with the complex.

In some sites the terminal superficial parts of the olfactory cells are contiguous with one another. In such sites in the guinea pig, Arstila and Wersäll have described tight junctions.

The olfactory vesicles contain some vesicles of smooth-surfaced endoplasmic reticulum, and some microtubules and mitochondria as well as the bases of the olfactory cilia. The cilia each have a basal body (BB, which can be seen in both longitudinal and cross

section in the olfactory vesicle in Fig. 28-4). The basal bodies have 9 triplets in their walls. The shafts of the cilia, close to the olfactory vesicle, contain both 2 central microtubules and 9 peripheral doublets, as most cilia do. Farther out, however, the cilia narrow considerably (Fig. 28-4), and in their long narrow (and more distal) portions, which follow, only 2 tubules are generally seen. The cilia tend to be roughly parallel to the surface of the olfactory organ over much of their lengths. Because of their large number, they combine to form more or less a layer on top of the microvilli of the sustentacular cells; in this layer they are cut in various ways (Fig. 28-4).

The axon from each olfactory cell passes into the lamina propria. The axons are unmyelinated, and in the lamina propria they become aggregated to form bundles of *olfactory nerve fibers*.

The function of the BASAL cells is unknown; they may be of the nature of reserve cells for forming new sustentacular cells when the need arises.

The *lamina propria* is fibroelastic connective tissue. In its deeper part it contains many veins, and in some of its deeper areas it has almost the character of erectile tissue.

BOWMAN'S GLANDS. The secretory portions of tubuloalveolar glands (the glands of Bowman) are disposed in the lamina propria of the olfactory mucous membrane. Indeed, these glands, according to Smith, are *confined* to the olfactory area; hence, if they are seen in what appears to be adjacent respiratory mucous membrane, it may be inferred that the latter was once olfactory mucous membrane but has suffered so much from injury that it has lost its olfactory character. The ducts of the glands lead through the epithelium to the surface. The fine structure of the cells of the glands of Bowman has received detailed study by Frisch; the principal cell type has abundant smooth-surfaced endoplasmic reticulum (which fact may suggest the presence of lipid in their secretion). The glands make a thin secretion which is often described as having some of the characteristics of mucus, and it presumably constantly freshens the thin layer of fluid which continuously bathes the olfactory cilia on the surface of the organ. The gases responsible for odors are thought to dissolve in this fluid.

OLFACTORY NERVE. Bundles of olfactory nerve fibers are encountered in the lamina propria. As noted before, these are composed of unmyelinated axons of the sensory cells. Collectively, these constitute the *olfactory nerve*, which pierces the skull by way of the cribriform plate of the ethmoid bone to reach the brain.

Relation of Structure to Function. How an individual is able to distinguish different kinds of odors

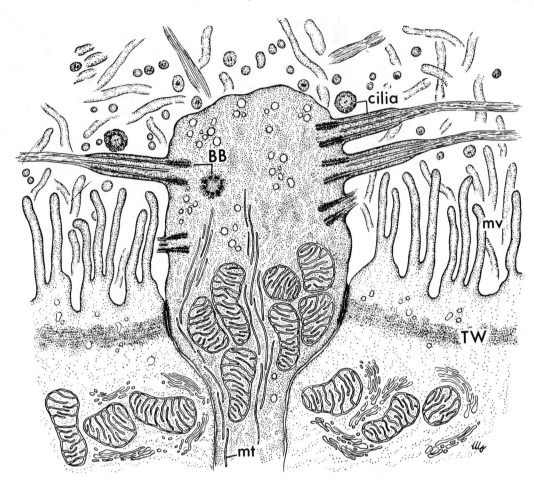

Fɪɢ. 28-4. Diagrammatic drawing to illustrate the fine structure of an olfactory vesicle and adjacent areas. BB, basal body; mv, microvilli; TW, terminal web, and mt, microtubule. (Based on study of D. Frisch: Am. J. Anat., *121*:87, 1967)

and their relative weakness or strength is a matter that is not well understood. Moreover, the problem does not lend itself readily to animal experimentation. Much of the factual basis for speculation on this matter has been obtained from studies made on individuals whose sense of smell has returned, at least in part, after the olfactory organ has been injured by a disease process which was not severe enough to destroy all the sensory cells but only of sufficient severity to render them functionless temporarily, after which most of them recovered.

It might be assumed that the sensory cells of the olfactory area itself would be specialized so that different ones would be sensitive to different odors. However, there are so many different kinds of odors that it is inconceivable that there could be special receptors for each and every kind; this leads, then, to the concept of the existence of olfactory cells specialized for only certain basic odors. The reason for man's being able to discern such a great variety of odors could be due to various combinations of the receptors for the basic odors being stimulated by these different complex odors. Support for this idea has been derived from finding that when the sense of smell is being recovered after having been lost, a few odors may smell as before, others are different than they were before, and still others cannot be smelled at all.

Moreover, there is evidence to suggest that the different receptors for the different kinds of basic odors are not spread evenly throughout the olfactory area; hence damage to one part of the organ may result in certain substances smelling different from before or not at all, whereas other substances under these conditions smell both quantitatively and qualitatively as before.

It would seem, then, that a reasonable working

hypothesis in the light of present knowledge would be: (1) that olfactory cells are of different types, specialized to be easily stimulated by certain basic odors; (2) that the receptors for the basic types of odors are not distributed evenly throughout the whole olfactory area but are segregated to some extent; and (3) that man's ability to recognize such a great variety of different odors is due to these different odors stimulating different combinations of the receptors for the basic odors.

The Eye

The eye, except for being rounded, has most of the structural features of the common and familiar camera. The eyelids comprise its shutter (Fig. 28-5). The eye has an iris diaphragm (Figs. 28-5 and 28-14). This has an advantage over the kind found in cameras, for it contracts and dilates automatically in relation to the amount of light available. The eye has a lens (Fig. 28-5); this, being composed of altered transparent epithelial cells, is more elastic than the glass lens of a camera. Advantage is taken of its elasticity, for the lens of the eye is suspended in such a way that muscle action can alter its shape and so change its focal length. As a consequence, the eye need not be shortened or elongated when objects at different distances are successively brought into focus as is necessary in a camera with a rigid lens. The plastic or metal sides and back of a camera have their counterpart in the eye in a strong connective tissue membrane, the *sclera* (Fig. 28-5). The counterpart in the eye of the light-sensitive film used in a camera is a membrane of living cells of

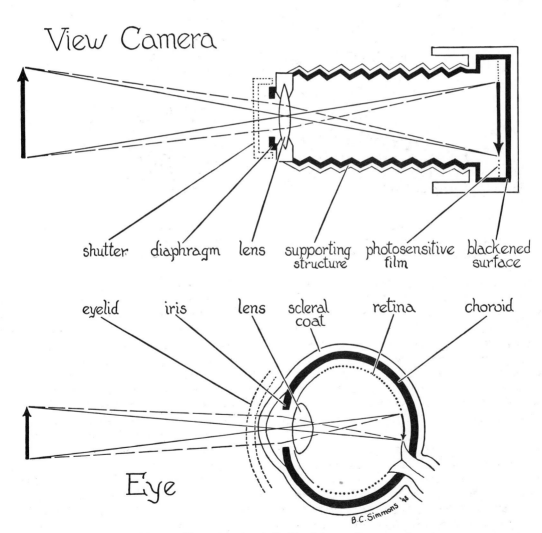

Fig. 28-5. Diagram illustrating the similarities between the eye and a camera.

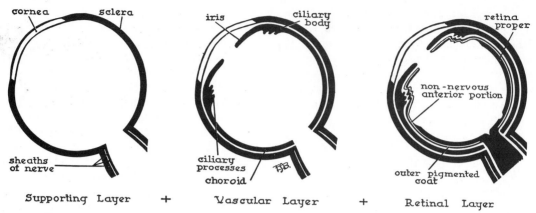

Supporting Layer   +   Vascular Layer   +   Retinal Layer

FIG. 28-6. (*Left*) Diagram of the supporting coat of the eye. (*Center*) Diagram showing the vascular coat of the eye inserted on the inside of the supporting coat. (*Right*) Diagram showing the retinal coat of the eye on the inside of the outer 2 coats.

nervous origin, the *retina,* which lines not only the back but the sides of the eye as well (Fig. 28-5). Then, finally, just as black paint is used to blacken all the interior surfaces of a camera that might leak or reflect light, black pigment is distributed generously between the retina and the sclera and in other sites where it would be useful.

However, unlike many modern cameras, the lens of the eye is not placed at its very front; in this respect the eye is like an old-fashioned camera which has its external aperture covered with a glass window to keep out the dust, and its lens inside, a short distance behind the glass window. The transparent window in the central part of the front of the eye is of a curved form and is called the *cornea* (Fig. 28-7). This is composed chiefly of a tough but transparent type of dense connective tissue that is continuous with the opaque connective tissue of the sclera that surrounds and supports the remainder of the eye.

Windows not only permit householders to see out; they also permit the curious to see in. The cornea is like a window in this respect as well, for, with an instrument called the ophthalmoscope, the physician can direct a beam of light into the eye and at the same time look through the instrument and study the appearance of the various structures within the eye as they are successively illuminated. By this means much useful information not only about the eye but about the health of the body as a whole may be obtained.

GENERAL STRUCTURE

The eye is nearly spherical and about an inch in diameter. It is contained in the anterior part of a bony socket, the *orbit.* Between the eye and the bony wall

of the orbit in which it lies are fat, connective tissue, muscles and the glandular tissue that provides the tears. The eye is suspended by ligaments in such a fashion that voluntary muscles in the orbit (but outside the eye) can move the eye so that one can look up and down and from side to side.

In describing the eye we shall describe first the structure of its *wall,* then its contents (these constitute the *refractive media* of the eye), and finally the *accessory structures* of the eye such as eyelids, tear glands and ducts, and so on.

The Wall of the Eye. The wall of the eyeball consists of 3 layers which, from without in, are designated by the general terms of (1) supporting layer, (2) middle layer and (3) retinal layer (Fig. 28-6). All 3 layers are not present in all parts of the wall of the eye.

The SUPPORTING LAYER consists essentially of a dense connective tissue membrane. Around most of the eye this is called the *sclera* (*scleros,* hard) (Fig. 28-6). The sclera is white in color; the part of the sclera that shows is the "white" of the eye (Fig. 28-14). The part of the supporting layer covering the central part of the anterior portion of the eye bulges forward slightly and is transparent; this is called the *cornea* (Fig. 28-6). The supporting layer completely encloses the other layers of the eye except at one site posteriorly where there is an opening to permit the optic nerve to enter the eyeball.

The MIDDLE LAYER of the wall of the eye is often called the *uveal* (*uva,* grape) *layer* or *tract* because when the sclera is dissected away, the middle layer is exposed and is seen to resemble the skin of a blue grape in that it is pigmented and surrounds the jelly-like contents of the eye. The middle layer of the eye is very vascular; hence it is sometimes called the *vascular layer* of the eye.

The middle illustration in Figure 28-6 shows that the middle layer lies on the inner surface of the supporting layer. In the posterior two thirds of the eye, the middle layer consists of only a thin membrane; this thin posterior segment of the middle layer is called the *choroid*. Moreover, in this illustration it will be seen that toward the anterior part of the eye the middle layer becomes thickened to form what is called the *ciliary body*. This, as a thickened rim of tissue, encircles the anterior part of the eye. From it, what are termed the *ciliary processes* extend inward (Fig. 28-6, *center*). The middle layer of the eye continues anteriorly to constitute the *iris* (diaphragm) of the eye (Fig. 28-6, *center*). The iris is the pigmented part of the eye that may be seen through the cornea (Fig. 28-14); depending on the pigment content of the iris, eyes are said to be blue, brown or some other color. Indeed, pigment is abundant in all parts of the middle coat; this helps to lightproof the wall of the eye and to cut down reflection. The middle coat of the eye conducts blood vessels, and, in addition, in its anterior part it contains smooth muscle. The smooth muscle in the iris causes its aperture, the *pupil* of the eye (Fig. 28-14), to contract or dilate. The smooth muscle of the ciliary body affects the tension of the ligament that suspends the lens, not in the way that might at first be expected, i.e., by its contraction tensing the ligament that suspends the lens, but, instead, by its contraction easing the tension on the ligament. This is how it permits the eye to accommodate its focus for near objects. The muscle of the ciliary body is, then, an important factor in the mechanism of accommodation.

The position of the RETINAL LAYER is illustrated on the right side of Figure 28-6. It consists of 2 layers; the one that lines the middle coat of the eye is pigmented. The layer of the retina that in turn lines the pigmented layer is composed of nervous tissue. The nervous part of the retina, as such, does not extend into the anterior part of the eye (Fig. 28-6, *right*), for there, light could not be focused on it. The nervous part of the retina contains special nerve cells called *rods* and *cones;* these are the *photoreceptors*. In addition, the retina contains the cell bodies of many conductor neurons and many nerve fibers. Most of the latter stream toward the site at which the optic nerve leaves the eye through the scleral layer (*lower right*, Fig. 28-6).

Refractive Media of the Eye. Light passes through the following media before it reaches the retina:

1. The substance of the cornea (Fig. 28-7).
2. A space between the iris and the lens called the *anterior chamber* of the eye (Fig. 28-7); this is filled with a fluid called *aqueous humor.*
3. The lens (Fig. 28-7).
4. The transparent jellylike material of the vitreous body, which fills the interior of the eye behind the lens (Fig. 28-7).

A beam of light is bent when it passes obliquely from a substance of one refractive index into that of another. The cornea is curved, and the difference between the refractive index of cornea and air is greater than the difference between the refractive indices of any of the media through which light subsequently passes to reach the retina. Hence, with regard to refracting light, the curved anterior surface of the cornea is of the greatest importance. The true lens of the eye has a refractive index which is only slightly greater than that of the aqueous humor in front of it and that of the vitreous body behind it; its function, then, of bringing light to a focus on the retina is not of as great a magnitude as that of the cornea. Its unique importance lies in the fact that, being elastic, its focal length can be changed by the pull of muscles on the ligaments which suspend it; hence it permits light from objects at different distances to be focused sharply.

On passing through the vitreous body and on reaching the retina, light does not immediately strike the photoreceptors, for these are in the part of the nervous layer that lies directly against the pigmented layer of the retina (Fig. 28-16). To reach the photoreceptors, light first must pass through the nerve fibers and the nerve cells present in the inner layers of the nervous coat of the retina (the layers adjacent to the vitreous body). Then, when the light reaches and affects the photoreceptors in the outer layers of the nervous coat of the retina, the nervous impulses, set up by the stimulus of light, must pass in the reverse direction through nerve fibers and nerve cell bodies toward the vitreous body. Here, in the innermost layers of the retina (next to the vitreous), the nervous impulses are conducted by nerve fibers that run to the site of exit of the optic nerve, into which nerve they pass to reach the brain (Fig. 28-16).

DEVELOPMENT

The retina of the eye develops as an outgrowth from the forebrain, which early in development is hollow. Its anterior wall bulges forward to form the primary optic vesicle (Fig. 28-8, 1). The bulge then becomes constricted at its point of origin from the forebrain;

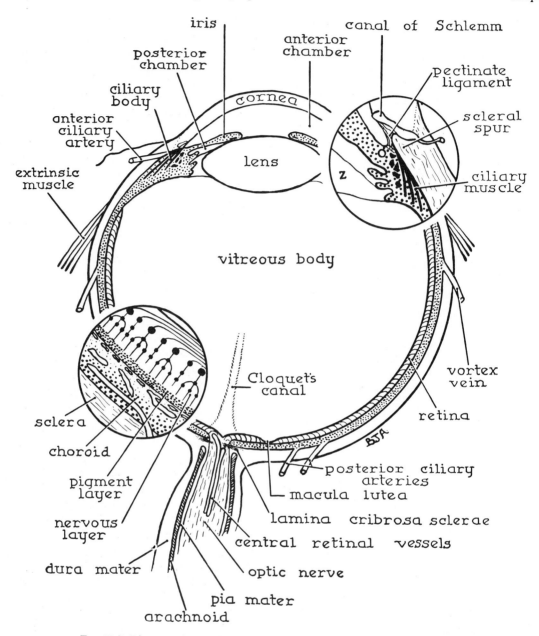

Fig. 28-7. Diagram of a longitudinal section cut through the middle of the eye.

the constricted portion of the bulge is termed the *optic stalk* (Fig. 28-8, 1). While the forebrain is bulging forward to form the optic vesicle, the ectoderm immediately in front of it thickens (Fig. 28-8, 1, lens ectoderm). The anterior wall of the optic vesicle then becomes invaginated so that the optic vesicle becomes cup-shaped, with the wall of the cup having 2 layers (Fig. 28-8, 2 and 3). At the same time the thickened ectoderm in front of the optic vesicle bulges inward to

form the lens vesicle (Fig. 28-8, 2). The lens vesicle then becomes pinched off from the ectoderm from which it arose (Fig. 28-8, 3). The formation of the lens provides an example of induction as was described in Chapter 6. (The further development of the lens will be described shortly along with its microscopic structure.) In the meantime the optic vesicle has become a deep cup, and since its original anterior wall is pressed backward, its original anterior wall constitutes the inner layer of the cup (Fig. 28-8, 3), and this develops into the nervous layer of the retina. The outer wall of the vesicle becomes the outer pigmented layer of the retina, which is black in Figure 28-8, 4.

The actively growing cells in the epithelial elements of the developing eye require a special blood supply, and this is provided, as the eye forms, by an artery that enters by way of the optic stalk. This is called the *hyaloid artery* (Fig. 28-8, 3). This subsequently atrophies as other sources of blood supply are evolved. The origin of the vitreous body is not thoroughly understood; it is a jellylike solution of hyaluronic acid and water.

The mesoderm surrounding the developing eye gives rise to both the middle and the supporting layers of the eye (Fig. 28-8, 4). The eyelids develop as a result of two folds of ectoderm with platelike cores of mesoderm extending over the developing cornea (Fig. 28-8, 4). The substance of the cornea forms from mesoderm,

but ectoderm persists over its anterior surface to form its epithelial covering (Fig. 28-8, 4). The anterior chamber develops as a result of the formation of a space in the mesoderm in this area (Fig. 28-8, 4). Epithelium from the optic vesicle continues forward to form a lining for the back of the ciliary body and the iris, both of which form from mesoderm (Fig. 28-8, 4).

Microscopic Structure of the Parts of the Eye and Their Relation to Function

CORNEA

The cornea is the anterior part of the supporting layer of the eye (Fig. 28-6, *left*). It is a transparent, nonvascular membrane. It has a shorter radius of curvature than the remainder of the wall of the eye. Since it is exposed, it is subject to cuts, abrasions and other kinds of trauma. It is important in treating injuries

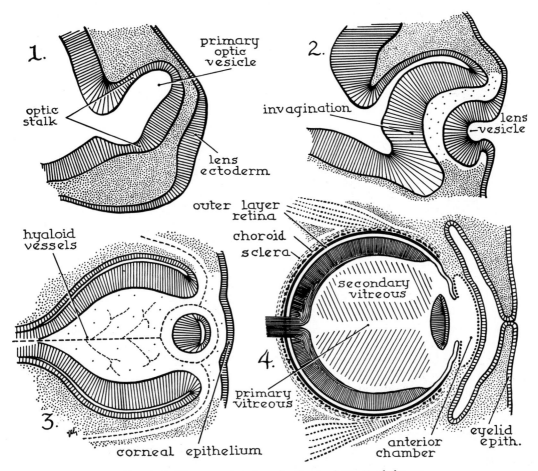

FIG. 28-8. Diagrams of 4 stages in the development of the eye.

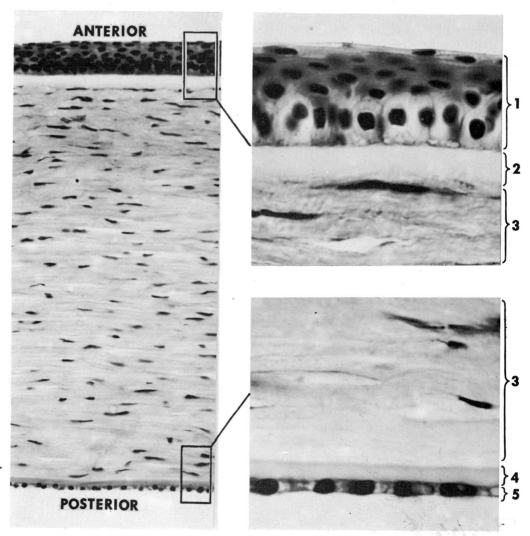

FIG. 28-9. (*Left*) Low-power photomicrograph of a section of the cornea. (*Right*) High-power photomicrographs of parts of the cornea: (1) stratified squamous epithelium; (2) Bowman's membrane; (3) substantia propria; (4) Descemet's membrane; (5) Descemet's endothelium.

of the cornea to know its thickness. Estimates based on measurements made on cadavers are not valid, since the cornea swells after death. In the living it is about 0.5 mm. thick at its central part and somewhat thicker at its periphery.

The cornea (Fig. 28-9) consists chiefly of a special kind of dense connective tissue, containing both cells and intercellular substance, called the *substantia propria* (Fig. 28-9, 3). This is bordered anteriorly and posteriorly by a membrane of homogeneous intercellular substance (Fig. 28-9, 2 and 4). Anteriorly, the cornea is covered with stratified squamous nonkeratinizing epithelium (Fig. 28-9, 1), and posteriorly it is lined

by a single layer of endothelial cells (Fig. 28-9, 5).

The epithelium covering the cornea is several layers in thickness and is replete with nerve endings that are chiefly of the pain type (Fig. 28-1 A). Their stimulation results reflexly in the blinking of the eyelids and in the flow of tears. The surface of the cornea must be kept wet by tears (mucus from the conjunctival glands also helps keep the corneal surface wet); if the nerve pathways concerned in the reflexes described above are destroyed, the corneal surface, on not being frequently wiped by the wet lids, becomes dry and then ulcerated. There are no papillae projecting into the epithelium of the cornea. Furthermore, since the connective tissue beneath it has no capillaries, the epithelium of the cornea is a comparatively long way from a source of nutrition. The diffusion phenomenon on which its cells depend must be very efficient, for corneal epithelium, on being injured, regenerates rapidly. Carbon dioxide is eliminated through the corneal epithelium.

The membrane of intercellular substance on which the basal cells of the corneal epithelium rests is called *Bowman's membrane* (Fig. 28-9, 2). This consists of a transparent homogeneous material. It is generally regarded as a condensation of the intercellular substance of the substantia propria. The EM shows that it contains some collagen. It is regarded as an important protective layer, being resistant to trauma and bacterial invasion. Once destroyed, it does not regenerate. Bowman's membrane does not extend from the cornea into the sclera. The site at which cornea undergoes a transition into sclera (and consequently, where Bowman's membrane ends) is called the *limbus* (*limbus*, a border).

The substantia propria comprises about 90 percent of the thickness of the cornea. It contains flattened connective tissue cells that are disposed between parallel bundles of collagenic fibers called *lamellae* (Fig. 28-9, *left*). While most of the fibers in a lamella are disposed parallel with the surface, those of one lamella run at an angle to those of the next. The fibers of some lamellae join with those of adjacent lamellae to bind the substantia propria together.

In the substantia propria the collagenic fibrils and fibers are embedded in a sulfated mucopolysaccharide. It is assumed that the binding together of collagenic fibrils and fibers in the substantia propria by this substance (as well as their regular arrangement) is responsible for the unique transparency of this membrane.

Deep to the substantia propria is Descemet's membrane (Fig. 28-9, 4). This is composed of a special kind of material that appears to be homogeneous and seems to be chiefly an unusual form of collagen. Applied to the inner side of Decemet's membrane is a single layer of endothelial cells; this layer is called *Descemet's endothelium* (Fig. 28-8, 5).

Fine Structure. The fine structure of the cornea has been investigated with the EM by Sheldon, and that of Descemet's membrane by Jakus. References to their studies are given at the end of this chapter.

Transplantation. Homologous transplants of cornea are made with a considerable amount of success. There were reasons for thinking that cornea, like cartilage, might be different from most other tissues so far as a homograft reaction is concerned because the cornea is normally nonvascular, and it does not contain any

lymphatics. Furthermore, it has a high proportion of intercellular substance to cells. Maumenee says that it has been shown experimentally that the epithelium and the endothelium of a homologous transplant of cornea are lost in a few days. The only cells of the transplant that survive for any length of time are some of the connective tissue cells within the substance of the cornea. It has been shown by Basu and Ormsby, by making corneal grafts from female cats to males, and vice versa, and then determining the chromosomal sex of the cells by the sex chromatin technic, that the connective tissue cells of the graft do live for at least long periods of time. By the same technic it has been shown that the stromal cells of grafts in man live for at least a year, which is as long as they have been followed. The surface epithelium is regenerated from the host, so that it covers the transplant in a few days. The regeneration of the endothelium takes longer. The connective tissue cells within the substance of the cornea are replaced only very slowly from the host.

SCLERA

The sclera is a tough, white, connective tissue membrane that consists of bundles of collagenic fibers with flattened fibroblasts between the bundles (Fig. 28-10). Some elastic fibers are mixed with the collagenic ones. The fibers are not arranged as regularly as those of the substantia propria of the cornea, and the mucopolysaccharide with which they are associated is probably of a somewhat different composition, since the sclera is opaque. The sclera is thick enough to permit its being sutured from the outside without the needle penetrating into the middle layer of the wall of the eye. It is not as thick as the cornea, except at its posterior pole; at the midportion of the globe (the *equator*) it is slightly less than 0.5 mm. thick. However, it is strong enough in adults to withstand very high intraocular pressure, should this condition occur, without stretching.

The relative opacity of the sclera, as compared with the cornea, is due to a very important degree to its greater water content. This can be shown very dramatically by blowing a jet of air on an exposed portion of sclera, for this makes it completely transparent. The reason the cornea remains transparent is that water is lost from its surfaces, so if either of its surfaces becomes damaged, it may become opaque in that area. For example, if some of the vitreous comes and stays in contact with its posterior surface at any point, the cornea becomes opaque at that point.

It is important in connection with testing the intraocular pressure of the eye by means of a tonometer to know that the scleras of different eyes are rigid to different degrees; hence, if the rigidity of the sclera is extreme, it may give an erroneous pressure reading.

At the posterior part of the eye the outermost part of the sclera is continuous with the dural sheath and usually with the arachnoid sheath also of the optic nerve (Fig. 28-7). Its innermost layers are continuous with the pia mater. Moreover, the innermost layer of the sclera, in the form of a perforated disk, bridges what would otherwise be a gap in the sclera, and through this the optic nerve leaves the eye (Fig. 28-22). The fibers of the optic nerve pass through the perforations of the disk. This part of the sclera is called the *lamina cribrosa* (*cribrum,* a sieve).

The sclera as a whole, being composed of dense connective tissue, is poorly supplied with capillaries. However, many larger vessels pierce it obliquely to gain entrance to the middle layer of the eye. The direction of these vessels, in passing through the sclera, is such that on reaching the inner aspect of the sclera they attain a point on the circumference of the eye closer to the anterior pole than the point at which they approached the exterior of the sclera (Fig. 28-7). The anterior ciliary arteries enter beside (or slightly in front of) the ciliary body (Fig. 28-7), and both short and long posterior ciliary arteries pass through the sclera behind the equator (Fig. 28-7). The long posterior ciliary arteries, on entering the middle coat of the eye, take a direct course to the ciliary body; the short ones branch. Four large vortex veins which drain most of the blood from the middle coat pass obliquely backward through the sclera near the equator of the eye (Fig. 28-7). The ciliary arteries have companion veins.

CHOROID

The choroid is that part of the middle layer of the eye behind the ciliary body. It is only 0.1 to 0.2 mm. thick. It consists of 3 layers.

1. **The Epichoroid.** This, its outer layer, consists chiefly of elastic fibers that are attached to the sclera. Many nerve fibers that terminate in *chromatophores* are present in it. The chromatophores are large pigmented cells that may be seen, although they are not labeled, in Figure 28-17. Some have branched irregular cytoplasm like that of an ameba. Whether this pigment is actually produced by these cells or taken up from pigment produced in the retina has been a point of much controversy. During a short phase of early fetal life, before pigment is present, the future pigment cells of the choroid have been found to be dopa-positive. This evidence, along with the fact that fuscin, the pigment of the retina, is slightly different from

melanin, suggests that melanin is produced by the pigment cells of the choroid and thereafter stored *in situ.* It is interesting that melanin pigment recovered from the uveal tract has different antigenic properties from that of other parts of the body. Through the epichoroid run the two unbranching posterior long ciliary arteries. A few smooth muscle fibers are present in this layer in its anterior part; these represent the beginning of the ciliary muscle.

2. **Vessel Layer.** The choroidal vessels that are supplied by the short posterior ciliary arteries and drained by the vortex veins lie in this, the middle layer of the choroid (Fig. 28-17). The stroma is similar to that of the epichoroid.

3. **Choriocapillaris.** This, the inner layer of the choroid network (Fig. 28-17), consists of a single layer of capillaries which, however, are among the largest seen in the body. Some of them, especially those outside the macula (to be described presently), are as wide as sinusoids; these permit a rapid transfer of blood from the arterial to the venous side.

Bruch's Membrane. Separating the choriocapillaris from the outer coat of the retina lies a glassy membrane (*Bruch's membrane*). This has both elastic and basement membrane components, formed by the choroid and the retina, respectively. Bruch's membrane is semipermeable, and through it pass the essential metabolites for the photoreceptors.

CILIARY BODY

The 3 strata of the choroid are continuous anteriorly with the ciliary body. This extends forward to a site where a narrow, short flange of sclera, called the *scleral spur,* projects inward (Figs. 28-7 and 28-10). The ciliary body, as a thickening of the middle coat of the eye, is seen, when an eye is dissected, to form a ring on the inner surface of the sclera behind the scleral spur (Figs. 28-7 and 28-10). When an eye is cut in longitudinal section, the ring is cut in cross section. In cross section it appears as a triangle, with its base facing the anterior chamber and its apex passing into the choroid posteriorly (Fig. 28-7). The elastic epichoroid, in the ciliary body, is replaced by fibers of ciliary muscle. These are of the smooth variety and they comprise the bulk of the ciliary body (Fig. 28-10).

The smooth muscle fibers of the ciliary body are disposed so as to pull in 3 different directions. Accordingly, 3 groups of fibers are distinguished: (1) the *meridional* (a meridian runs from pole to pole, crossing the equator of a globe at right angles) fibers, which arise in the epichoroid near the ciliary body and pass

capsule. As was mentioned in connection with cell membranes in Chapter 8, the present-day evidence suggests that basement membranes are chiefly products of epithelial cells. The capsule of the lens would seem to be a product of the epithelial cells which in due course become transformed into fibers. As the capsule is being formed, the cell membranes of the free surfaces of the epithelial cells seem to become thickened (Fig. 28-13, APM), and at this site adjacent delicate laminae of material appear to be successively added to the forming capsule (Fig. 28-13, C). The capsule, like basement membranes and cell coats in general, is rich in a carbohydrate component that stains brilliantly by the PA-Schiff technic.

The cell membranes of the epithelial cells, as they are forming the capsule, and before they have been transformed into fibers, interdigitate extensively (Fig. 28-13, P). They also contain, close to the cell border where the capsule is forming, many dense bodies (Fig. 28-13, DB); whether or not these are concerned with the formation of the capsule has not yet been ascertained. The lens capsule is constantly under tension and hence constantly "seeks" to make the elastic lens assume a more globular form.

As the lens ages, it loses water and becomes denser and less elastic. Consequently, its range of focus becomes diminished, often sufficiently for individuals to require supplementary lenses (in the form of glasses) for focusing near objectives sharply.

Zonule and the Mechanism of Accommodation. The lens is attached to the ciliary body by means of the *zonule* (Fig. 28-7, *upper right*, Z). The zonule is composed of filaments and fibers. It is sometimes called the *suspensory ligament of the lens.*

The zonule has a broad zone of attachment both to the capsule of the lens around its equator and to the ciliary body (Fig. 28-7). Now it might be thought, as was noted before, that matters would be arranged so that the contraction of the smooth muscle fibers of the ciliary body would pull on the zonule, which would in turn pull on the equator of the lens so that the lens would become flatter and hence accommodated for distant objects. Actually, the contraction of the smooth muscle of the ciliary body produces the opposite effect. Instead of tensing the zonule, the contraction of the smooth muscle of the ciliary body, the fibers of which are firmly attached to the sclera in the region of the scleral spur, pulls the part of the ciliary body to which the zonule is attached, *forward* and *inward*. This effect, since the attachment of the zonule to the ciliary body is posterior to its site of attachment to the lens, relaxes the tension of the zonule and hence permits the lens, which itself is under tension from its capsule, to assume a more globular shape, and hence become accom-

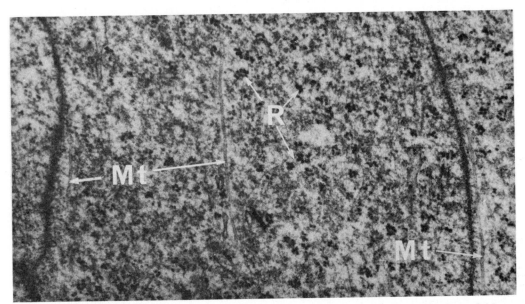

FIG. 28-12. Electron micrograph (× 45,000) of longitudinally sectioned lens fibers from fetal rat at the 18th day of gestation. Microtubules (Mt) are seen, oriented in the long axes of the fibers. Ribosomal aggregates (R) are scattered about in the finely granular substance of the fibers. (Willis, N. R., Hollenberg, M. J., and Braekevelt, C. R.: Canad. J. Ophthalmology, *4*:307, 1969)

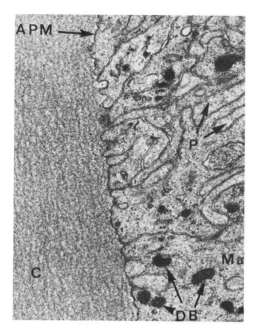

FIG. 28-13. Electron micrograph of the lens capsule and adjacent epithelium of a fetal rat on the 21st day of gestation. C, lens capsule; APM, the thickened and infolded cell membrane of the epithelial cells that are forming the capsule; P, interdigitating lateral processes of contiguous cells; DB, dense bodies, and Ma, cytoplasmic matrix. (Willis, N. R., Hollenberg, M. J., and Braekevelt, C. R.: Canad. J. Ophthalmology, *4*:307, 1969)

modated for close objects. It is to be noted, then, that muscular contraction is required for viewing close objects; this is one reason why reading "tires" the eyes more than viewing distant objects does.

Iris

The iris is a colored disk with a central, variable aperture, the pupil (Fig. 28-14). It is not a flat disk, for the lens pushes against its central part (the *papillary margin*) from behind so that its more central part is more anterior than its periphery (Fig. 28-7).

The space behind the iris, and elsewhere limited by the lens, the vitreous body and the ciliary body, is called the *posterior chamber* of the eye (Fig. 28-7); the space in front of the iris (and at the pupil, in front of the lens), and otherwise limited by the cornea and the most anterior part of the sclera, is called the *anterior chamber* of the eye (Fig. 28-7). Both the anterior and the posterior chambers are filled with a fluid called *aqueous humor*. A certain amount of circulation takes place in this fluid. In all probability the fluid is formed in the posterior chamber and then passes into the ante-

rior chamber, from which it is resorbed by mechanisms to be described presently. Since the posterior border of the pupillary margin of the iris and the anterior surface of the lens press against each other, the iris acts like a valve in that fluid from the posterior chamber can force the pupillary margin of the iris away from the anterior surface of the lens to enter the anterior chamber, but fluid tending to move in the reverse direction presses the pupillary margin of the iris against the lens and so closes the opening between the 2 chambers. Posteriorly, the iris is lined by 2 layers of pigmented epithelial cells continuous with the 2 layers of retinal epithelium that line the ciliary body (Fig. 28-10). Anteriorly, the iris is covered imperfectly with squamous endothelial cells comparable and continuous with those of Descemet's endothelium.

The iris (Fig. 28-10) is well supplied with vessels and networks of nerve fibers. The arteries, branches of the major arterial circle, course spirally through its stroma like a corkscrew, so that their lumens will not be much affected by changes in the radius of the iris. They have a thick collagenous adventitia which prevents kinking when the spirals are compressed and makes the vessels appear as radiating gray lines in pale or blue irises. Throughout the stroma are scattered *chromatophores,* which are concentrated mostly at the anterior border (Fig. 28-10). The vessels do not extend to this border.

Encircling the pupil, about 1.5 mm. from its margin, is a scalloped line formed, in a manner which need not be described here, by the regression of the membrane that extended across the pupil in embryonic life (Fig. 28-14). This line divides the iris into a pupillary and a ciliary portion (Fig. 28-14). Crypts opening ante-

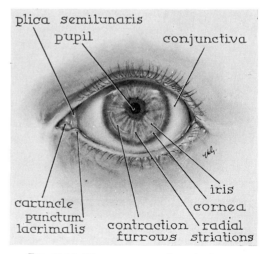

FIG. 28-14. The eye, as seen from in front.

riorly are found in the pupillary portion; they form as a result of the incomplete atrophy of the pupillary membrane. Shorter crypts are also found in the anterior surface of the ciliary portion. The contraction furrows (Fig. 28-14) appear as deeper folds encircling the anterior surface of the iris.

The muscle fibers of the iris are derived from the anterior cells of the pigmented epithelial layer; this is a continuation of the outer retinal layer of the eye. The constrictor of the pupil is the sphincterlike muscle composed of circularly arranged smooth muscle fibers near the pupillary margin. How firmly the iris is held against the anterior surface of the lens depends on the tone of these fibers. The dilator of the pupils is less distinct and consists of a thin sheet of radially disposed fibers near the back of the iris. The fibers are not typical smooth muscle fibers and are called *myoepithelial* cells.

The pupillary size is automatically controlled by a nervous reflex in which the *retina* is the *receptor* organ, and the muscles of the iris the *effectors*. When the eye looks at a bright object, the pupil is reflexly constricted, thereby decreasing the amount of light that can enter the eye, and vice versa. To anyone who has studied photography the pupillary size has a still further significance. A dilated pupil, like a dilated aperture in a camera, results in a diminished "depth" of focus. For this reason, glasses prescribed when the pupil is dilated are likely to be more accurate than those prescribed when the pupil is not.

The color of the iris is due to melanin pigment. As was noted in discussing the color of skin, melanin pigment, seen through a substantial thickness of tissue, appears blue. Hence, if the melanin pigment in the iris is limited to the epithelial cells that line its posterior surface, the iris (provided that the stroma ahead of the pigment is of a usual density) appears blue. If the stroma is somewhat denser than usual, the pigment at the back of the iris gives a gray color to the eye. If sufficient pigment is present in chromatophores in the substance of the stroma as well as in the epithelium at the back of the iris, the iris appears brown. In the white race the final color of the iris is not necessarily developed at the time of birth.

Region of the Angle of the Iris

It has already been observed that the site at which the sclera becomes continuous with the cornea is called the *limbus* (Fig. 28-10) and that immediately behind it the internal surface of the sclera is thrown into a ridge, the *scleral spur*, that extends inward and forward (Fig. 28-10). The scleral spur, of course, encir-

cles the eye. Immediately in front of the scleral spur a furrow dips into the inner layer of the sclera; this is called the *scleral furrow* (in Fig. 28-10 this is not labeled as such but as spaces of Fontana), and it, too, encircles the eye. At the bottom of the furrow a canal (or a group of anastomosing canals) lined by endothelium is situated. This is called the *canal of Schlemm* (Fig. 28-10), and it, too, encircles the eye. In a meridional section, the scleral spur, the scleral furrow and the canal of Schlemm are, of course, all cut in cross section (Fig. 28-10).

The scleral furrow is filled in (over the canal which lies at its bottom) with a loose meshwork of connective tissue; this extends from the cornea, at the anterior side of the furrow, backward to the anterior border of the scleral spur. The spaces in the meshwork were in the past called the *spaces of Fontana* (Fig. 28-10), and they communicate with the anterior chamber. The spaces, which are now commonly referred to as the trabecular spaces, are lined by endothelium; this is continuous with that which lines the cornea and covers the anterior surface of the iris. Hence, aqueous humor is present in the trabecular spaces. The middle (uveal) coat of the eye extends forward to provide a lining for the wall of the eye between the iris and the scleral spur. In the horse this lining is so strong and well developed that it is called the *pecinate ligament*. Sometimes this name is used for its relatively undeveloped counterpart in man (Fig. 28-10).

Ciliary Processes

About 75 little ridges, each about 2.0 mm. long, 0.5 mm. wide and about 1 mm. high, project inward from the ciliary body, immediately behind its point of junction with the iris, into the posterior chamber of the eye. These are termed the *ciliary processes*, and a few are usually to be seen in a single longitudinal section of an eye (Fig. 28-15, *left*).

As is indicated in Figure 28-6 (*center*), the cores of the ciliary processes are the counterparts in this particular region of the choriocapillaris, since they consist chiefly of capillaries that are supported by a delicate connective tissue (Fig. 28-15, *right*). The processes are covered with 2 layers of epithelium; these represent the continuation of the 2 layers of the retina forward (compare the middle and the right drawings in Fig. 28-6). The cells of the deeper of the 2 layers are pigmented (Fig. 28-15, *right*). The superficial layer is called the ciliary epithelium. The epithelial layer, as a whole, rests on a membrane that is continuous with Bruch's membrane and separates the epithelium from the vascular stroma of the processes.

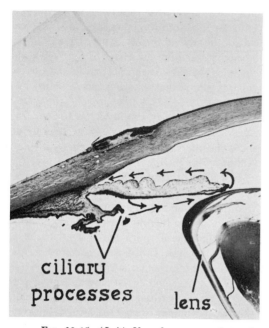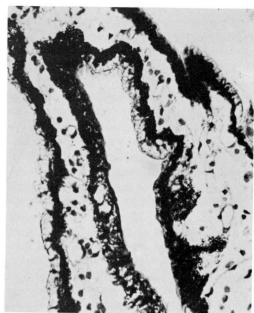

Fig. 28-15. (*Left*) Very low-power photomicrograph of part of a longitudinal section of the eye, showing the ciliary processes. The arrows indicate the course of the circulation of the aqueous humor. (*Right*) High-power photomicrograph of a section of the ciliary processes of a rabbit. Notice the large capillaries in the loose, delicate connective tissue that makes up the stroma of the processes.

With the EM, Pease has shown that the ciliary epithelium (the layer that abuts on the aqueous humor) contains many deep folds of the cell membrane. These begin from the free surface and extend almost through to the deeper sides of the cells. Moreover, Pease has shown that the free surfaces of the cells are covered with a basement membrane. The folds and the basement membrane are both concerned, in all probability, with the transport of fluid required in connection with the secretion of aqueous humor.

Aqueous Humor

Formation, Circulation and Absorption. Aqueous humor is a thin watery fluid containing most of the diffusable substance of blood plasma. Although the albumin-globulin ratio is the same in both aqueous humor and serum, serum has a protein content of 7 percent, whereas aqueous humor contains only 0.02 percent. Like serum, the aqueous humor contains no fibrinogen and therefore cannot clot. It has been a matter of some controversy whether it should be regarded primarily as a dialysate of blood plasma, comparable with tissue fluid, or as a secretion. For one thing it is hypertonic in relation to blood, and in all probability not only the factors concerned in tissue

fluid formation and absorption (hydrostatic and osmotic pressure), but specific cellular activities as well, participate in controlling its quality and its rate of formation and absorption. Friedenwald describes some of the complex cellular activities concerned in the matter, and his paper should be read for further information about this subject.

Although aqueous humor is thin and watery, it has been shown to contain considerable quantities of hyaluronic acid. However, this material, as was explained in Chapter 8, commonly appears in connective tissue as a soft, jellylike, amorphous type of intercellular substance. Its jellylike form in most connective tissues is due to its being present in a highly polymerized state, for its molecular aggregates are of a very large size. It was also observed in Chapter 8 that the enzyme hyaluronidase has the ability to depolymerize hyaluronic acid. It is of interest that it has been determined from studies made on the eyes of cattle that the hyaluronic acid in the aqueous humor is normally about 95 percent depolymerized; this, then, is the reason for the aqueous having such a low viscosity. This suggests that hyaluronidase has a normal function in the eye in keeping the molecular aggregates of hyaluronic acid from becoming large in size. If they did become large in size, they probably could not drain away from the eye by the escape mechanism to be described presently; hence, hyaluronic acid would accumulate in the eye and so change both the physical state and the osmotic pressure of the aqueous humor to the detriment of the eye. It would appear, then, that the action of hyaluronidase in keeping the hyaluronic acid of the eye depolymerized represents a normal physiologic function of the enzyme.

Although the general principles with regard to the formation and the absorption of tissue fluid that have been explained in Chapter 8 are fundamental to the understanding of the formation and the absorption of aqueous humor, there are certain differences in the mechanism that operates in the eye from that which operates in most tissues. These differences are due to the fact that tissue fluid in the eye is under considerably greater pressure than it is in most sites in the body. In most sites the tissues surrounding capillaries are not under very great tension; hence, a relatively low hydrostatic pressure in the capillaries is sufficient to drive tissue fluid out through their walls at their arterial ends. Correspondingly, the tissue substance in which blood vessels are embedded is under so little tension that venules are not compressed, even though the hydrostatic pressure within them is extremely low. However, surrounded by a tough, inelastic, fibrous tunic, the contents of the eye are under constant tension; the usual intraocular pressure ranges from about 20 to 25 mm. of mercury. This requires, then, that the blood within the capillaries of the eye be under a considerably greater hydrostatic pressure than the general intraocular pressure if the osmotic pressure of the colloids of the plasma is to be overcome and tissue fluid (aqueous humor) elaborated. Furthermore, it requires that the blood in intraocular veins also be under considerable hydrostatic pressure; otherwise, the veins within the eye would be collapsed by the intraocular pressure.

Although it is possible that any capillaries close to the anterior or the posterior chambers could contribute to the formation and the absorption of aqueous humor, it is highly probable that the capillaries of the ciliary processes, and to a much lesser extent those at the back of the iris, elaborate most of it. It is not unlikely that the hyaluronic acid of the aqueous is also formed in the delicate connective tissue that forms the cores of the ciliary processes. The most important mechanism for the absorption of aqueous humor is situated in the angle of the iris and will be described presently.

It is to be noted that, since the fibrous tunic of the eye cannot stretch, and since structures within the eye are normally of a constant size and incompressible, a normal intraocular pressure depends on a proper balance between the formation and the absorption of aqueous humor. If conditions should develop in the anterior part of the eye which in another part of the body would cause edema, for example, interference with the absorption of tissue fluid, the eye cannot swell; instead, the intraocular pressure becomes increased. An increase in intraocular pressure sufficient to be incompatible with the continued health of the eye constitutes the condition termed *glaucoma,* and it is obvious that the treatment of the condition would be directed toward increasing the absorption of aqueous humor and/or decreasing its production.

Although under certain conditions aqueous humor can be produced very rapidly and removed very rapidly, it appears that under normal conditions it is formed and absorbed very slowly, probably at about the rate of 2 cu. mm. a minute. After aqueous humor is formed, it passes from the posterior chamber between the lens and the iris to enter the anterior chamber (Fig. 28-15). There it moves toward the angle of the iris, where most of it enters the trabecular spaces (Fontana), from which it is absorbed into the canal of Schlemm.

The canal of Schlemm (Fig. 28-10) probably has no direct communication with the trabecular spaces except perhaps very fine pores that can be seen only with the EM (see Holmberg, Garron, Speakman); hence, aqueous humor, to enter the canal, probably must pass through a delicate membrane, including the endothelium lining the canal. The canal contains aqueous humor during life; this drains outward through *collector trunks* in the sclera. These pass out under the bulbar conjunctiva, where they are known as *aqueous veins* because they contain aqueous humor; in this position they may be seen with a slit lamp during life. The aqueous veins connect with blood-containing veins so that eventually aqueous humor is emptied into the venous system. Interference with the flow of aqueous humor in the collector trunks and the aqueous veins may be a factor in glaucoma. After death, blood may back up into the aqueous and the collecting veins and into the canal of Schlemm so that it may be seen in these sites in sections.

The Vitreous Body

The vitreous body is a mass of transparent gelled amorphous intercellular substance; the cells responsible for its formation are not known with certainty. It is bounded by the internal limiting membrane of the retina, the lens and the posterior zonular membrane

(Fig. 28-7). In addition to transmitting rays of light, its bulk helps, anteriorly, to hold the lens in place and, posteriorly, to keep the inner coat of the retina in apposition with the outer pigmented coat. If vitreous is lost, as occurs unavoidably in some surgical procedures, the 2 latter coats of the retina may become separated.

The vitreous, as has been shown by Adler, also plays a part of the metabolism of the retina, allowing the transfer of metabolites through it.

Through the vitreous body runs Cloquet's canal, the remnant of the primitive hyaloid system or primary vitreous (Fig. 28-8, 4). Cloquet's canal runs from the papilla toward the posterior surface of the lens and is usually inconspicuous in life. In some instances the primitive hyaloid structures persist and may interfere with vision.

The vitreous is denser at its periphery. The dense peripheral vitreous, while it is adherent to the internal limiting membrane of the retina over all its area, is particularly adherent at the papilla. It is also adherent to the posterior surface of the lens near its edge.

Composition of the Vitreous Body. The vitreous body is of the nature of a hydrophilic colloidal system. The dispersed phase of the system probably consists both of a complex protein (vitrein) which has pronounced hygroscopic qualities and *hyaluronic acid*. It contains the crystalloids normally dissolved in aqueous humor. Under normal conditions the vitreous humor is gelled. It is very easily denatured by drying or fixation, and it then exhibits a fibrillar structure that may be seen with the light microscope. However, such fibrillar structure as it possesses during life and imparted to it by its molecular constitution cannot be seen with the ordinary light microscope. It was believed that lost vitreous was not replaced, but Pirie has shown that it re-forms in rabbits.

THE RETINA

In learning the layers of the retina the student should realize that the terms "inner" and "outer" are used (as they are with regard to the layers of the wall of the eye) not with reference to the body as a whole but with regard to the *center* and the *exterior* of the eye. Hence, the inner of any 2 layers of the wall of the eye or of any 2 layers of the retina itself is the layer closer to the center of the eye.

The retina develops from the optic vesicle (an outgrowth from the brain), and at first it is constituted of 2 main layers because the anterior wall of the optic vesicle (Fig. 28-8, 1) becomes invaginated backward into its posterior half to make a 2-layered optic cup

(Fig. 28-8, 2, 3 and 4). It is the inner layer of the optic cup that develops into the nervous portion of the retina. The outer wall of the cup develops into a layer of pigmented epithelium. The cells of this layer are of a somewhat flattened cuboidal shape (Fig. 28-18) when seen in profile and hexagonal when seen in full face. They contain a pigment which is probably an unusual type of melanin called *fuscin* (L., dusky) (Figs. 28-17 and 28-18). It has been reported that these cells in embryonic life before they come to contain pigment are dopa-positive; hence there is reason for assuming that they make the pigment they contain.

The retina is commonly described as consisting of 10 layers. These are labeled from the outside (Figs. 28-17 and 28-18). Therefore, the first layer of the retina is the layer of pigmented epithelium, the layer that develops from the original outer layer of the optic cup. This layer, it should be noted, becomes more firmly attached to the choroid than to the inner and nervous part of the retina from which, it must be remembered, it was originally separated by a cleft. Consequently, when eyes are removed for histologic study, the nervous portion of the retina commonly becomes detached from the layer of pigmented epithelium, which remains adherent to the choroid (Fig. 28-22). The nervous part of the retina is 0.4 mm. thick posteriorly but thins out anteriorly to half this thickness.

The arrangements of the photoreceptor cells are quite different from the usual arrangement seen in afferent neurons. The cell bodies of the photoreceptors are not disposed in ganglia but in the substance of the retina. Furthermore, the cell bodies of the first 2 neurons of the afferent chains that lead from the photoreceptors are also disposed in the retina (Fig. 28-16). If it is remembered that the retina is an outgrowth from the brain, this does not seem so remarkable, for since connector neurons are confined to the tissue of the CNS, and since tissue of the CNS migrates, as it were, into the retina during embryonic development, the presence of connector neurons in the retina might be expected.

In Figure 28-16 the layer of photoreceptors may be seen, apposed to, and projecting slightly into, the layer of pigment epithelium. Each cell in the photoreceptor layer has a dendritic process that extends from the region of the nucleus of the cell outward to the layer of pigmented epithelium. The dendritic processes of the photoreceptors are of 2 general shapes, resembling either *rods* or *cones,* and, accordingly, the photoreceptors are classified as rod or cone cells. The axons of the rod and cone cells pass inward and synapse with the dendrites of the nerve cells in the middle part of the retina. These, of course, are to the inner side of the layer of rod and cone cells and are called *bipolar cells* because they have only 2 processes: a dendrite and an axon (Fig. 28-16). The axons of the bipolar cells pass inward and synapse with the dendrites of the third and innermost layer of nerve cells, the *ganglion cells.* (It should be understood that these cells do not constitute a ganglion; they are called ganglion cells because they are large and otherwise resemble the nerve cells of ganglia.) The axons of the ganglion cells pass inward to the inner border of the retina, where they turn at right angles toward the site of exit of the optic nerve, running in the innermost part of the retina parallel with the surface of the eye (Fig. 28-16).

To affect the rod- and cone-shaped processes of the photoreceptors, light from the vitreous must pass through the inner 2 layers of nerve cells of the retina and through the cell bodies of the photoreceptors themselves. Then, when the light reaches the rod- and cone-shaped dendritic processes of the photoreceptors and nervous impulses are set up, the nervous impulses must pass in the reverse direction, *inward,* through the bipolar and ganglion cells to the innermost part of the retina and from here, along the axons of the ganglion cells, to the site of exit of the optic nerve (Fig. 28-22). Obviously, for this arrangement to be functional, the nerve cells and their processes that are situated to the inner side of the rod- and cone-shaped dendritic processes of the photoreceptors must be readily permeable to light.

Ten Layers. Having gained some knowledge of the arrangement of the nerve cells in the retina, it is easy to learn the 10 classic layers of this structure. These will now be described, and in the following description the photomicrograph of the retina (Fig. 28-17) and the diagram of it (Fig. 28-18), in both of which the layers are numbered, should be consulted with reference to each layer described.

LAYER 1, the *layer of pigment epithelium,* consists of the layer of pigmented epithelial cells (already described) that develops from the outer layer of the optic cup (see also Fig. 28-7).

LAYER 2, the *layer of rods and cones,* consists of the dendritic cytoplasmic processes of the photoreceptors. These are packed closely together, side by side, in this layer, looking like bacilli; hence this layer is sometimes known as the *bacillary layer.*

LAYER 3, was named the *external* or *outer limiting membrane* from studies made on stained sections with the LM. From these studies it was visualized as a sievelike membrane through which the outer parts of the photoreceptor projected and are accordingly supported. With the EM, however, it has become apparent that the dark line seen with the LM, and suggesting a membrane, was probably to be accounted for by very

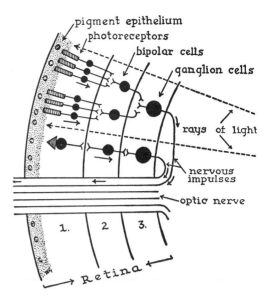

FIG. 28-16. Diagram showing the arrangement of the 3 layers of neurons in the retina. Observe that the light and the nervous impulses travel in opposite directions.

numerous junctional complexes in this area (Fig. 28-19) which connect the ends of the terminal processes of what are termed Müller's cells, and which are a type of glial cell, to the cell membranes of photoreceptors. The cytoplasm of Müller's cells projects through the membrane in the form of microvilli (Fig. 28-19). Müller's cells will be described further in connection with layer 6.

LAYER 4, the *outer nuclear layer,* is the layer formed by the closely packed nuclei of the photoreceptors.

LAYER 5, the *outer plexiform layer,* is the layer in which the axons of the rods and the cones synapse with the dendrites of the bipolar cells. Since several rods may synapse with a single bipolar cell and, except at the fovea (to be described later), more than one cone, the dendrites of bipolar cells must branch into terminal networks; these, suitably stained, give this layer a plexiform appearance.

LAYER 6 is termed the inner nuclear layer. It contains the nuclei of the bipolar cells, Müller's cells and the horizontal cells.

The bipolar cells have already been described.

Müller's cells are a type of neuroglial cell. Although their nuclei are in the inner nuclear layer, their cytoplasm extends all the way from the outer limiting membrane to the inner limiting membrane. The many processes of these cells intrude almost everywhere to provide intimate support in many layers for the nervous elements of the retina. Their inner terminal por-

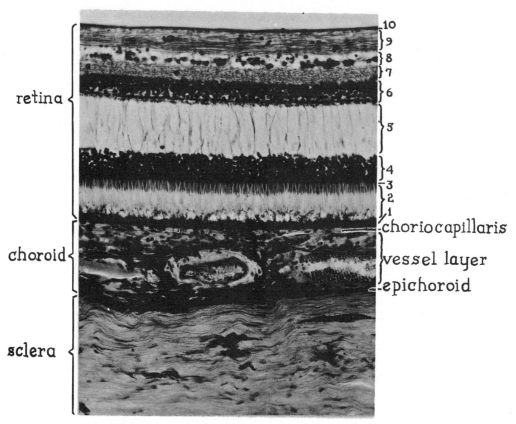

FIG. 28-17. Low-power photomicrograph of a portion of a section cut through the wall of the eye, showing the retina, the choroid and some of the sclera. The numbers refer to the layers of the retina, which are described in the text and shown in diagrammatic form in Figure 28-18.

tions become somewhat expanded to help account for the inner limiting membrane.

The nuclei and the cell bodies of what are termed the *horizontal* cells also lie in the inner nuclear layer. The horizontal cells are neurons, the processes of which connect by means of synapses with cone cells at one site and with cones and rods at other sites.

LAYER 7, the *inner plexiform layer,* is the layer in which the axons of the bipolar cells synapse with the dendrites of the ganglion cells. The latter have fine networks at their terminations; these give the layer a plexiform appearance when sections are suitably stained.

LAYER 8, the *ganglion cell layer,* is the layer in which the large ganglion cells are disposed, together with some neuroglial cells. Retinal blood vessels are also present in this layer.

LAYER 9, the *layer of nerve fibers,* consists of the axons of the ganglion cells; these, after having reached the innermost part of the retina, have turned at right angles to pass thereafter parallel with the inner sur-

face of the retina toward the site of exit of the optic nerve. To aid transparency they possess neither myelin sheaths nor sheaths of Schwann. Spiderlike neuroglial cells, the inner branches of Müller's fibers and blood vessels are also present in this layer.

LAYER 10, the *inner limiting membrane,* is a delicate homogeneous structure composed of the terminations of the processes of Müller's cells.

The Photoreceptors—The Rods and Cones

The two types of photoreceptors (also called visual cells) in the animal kingdom, rods and cones, are both relatively long narrow cells (Fig. 28-20) that resemble each other in many respects. The reason for one kind being called rods and the other cones is that the parts of the cells that project outward, toward and into the pigment layer, and are the parts of these cells that are sensitive to light, are either rod- or cone-shaped.

Since it might be assumed that the parts of the photoreceptors that are sensitive to light would, like the emulsion on a film, face the light, it should be reiterated here that the light-sensitive parts of rods and cones do *not* face the light that enters the eye but face in the opposite direction. Hence, for light to reach these parts of the photoreceptors it must pass not only through all the refractive media of the eye (Fig. 28-7) but also through the other constituents of the retina that are in front of them (refer back to Figures 28-16, and 28-18).

Respective Roles of Rods and Cones. In this connection Young notes that Schultze, a German anatomist, pointed out over a century ago that the retinas of animals whose activities are performed mostly at night or in dim light contained mostly, or entirely, rods. On the other hand, he noted that animals that carry on most of their activities by day had mostly cones in their retinas. He therefore concluded that rods were adapted to functioning in dim light and that cones were specialized for function in bright light. He even surmised that cones were probably responsible for color vision. Both his conclusion and his surmise turned out to be correct. Cats, for example, are equipped only with rods, and although they see well in dim light they see everything in terms of black and white. Birds, however, have cones and color vision which is one reason I gave up attempting to grow my own strawberries.

The Fine Structure of Rods. As can be seen in Figure 28-20, a rod is divided into two main parts by a constriction; these two parts are termed its outer and inner segments respectively. The outer segment is its light-sensitive portion. It is enclosed by a cell membrane and is rod-shaped. The substance of the rod consists of transverse membranous disks that are stacked one above another over its whole length. The disks are of the order of very flattened membranous vesicles. Each disk has a narrow space between its two surfaces and there is a narrow space between each two disks. The disks of rods are shown at high magnification on the right side of Figure 28-21. The disk-containing outer segment of the rod is joined to the remaining part of it, which is called its inner segment, by a constriction which contains a modified cilium (Fig. 28-20). The inner segment consists of two main parts. The first part, adjacent to the constriction, is of about the same diameter as the outer segment and it contains an abundance of mitochondria, many polyribosomes, a Golgi apparatus and a little rER and sER. Microtubules are also present (Fig. 28-20). This part of the inner segment is obviously a site for protein synthesis. The other and innermost part of the inner segment contains the nucleus and, after narrowing considerably, it expands at its termination into a large

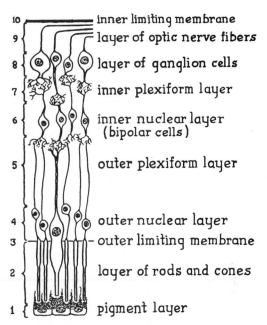

FIG. 28-18. Diagram showing the layers of the retina.

presynaptic structure into which many postsynaptic terminations are inserted. The latter represent the termination of dendrites of the bipolar cells (Fig. 28-16).

The Turnover of the Disks of the Outer Segments of Rods. Throughout this book we have discussed how cell populations are maintained in various parts of the body, and it has been noted that cell turnover is a common way for various parts of the body to be kept in repair. We noted, however, that there is no provision for a turnover of the neurons of the nervous system. The rods and the cones are, of course, types of nerve cells and they are no exception to this general rule. Young, in a most interesting and informative article in *Scientific American,* which anyone interested in the eye would read with both pleasure and profit, has described the sequence of studies which led to an understanding of how the integrity and function of visual cells is maintained throughout life. The turnover required for maintenance is not one of the cells themselves turning over but in the instance of the rods it is a turnover of disks and, in the instance of the cones, a turnover of the important components of the disks. Certain findings led to this conclusion as will now be described.

First, after it became possible to combine the technics of radioautography and electron microscopy it became practicable to follow the synthesis and movement of protein in cells by using labeled amino acids

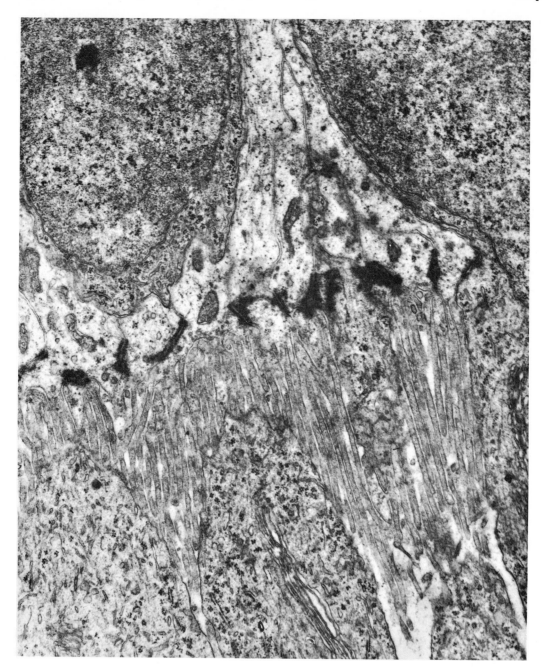

Fig. 28-19. Electron micrograph of section of retina of ground squirrel. Layer 3, the outer limiting membrane, extends across the middle of the picture and is seen to contain many junctional complexes, the fibrillar material of which is electron-dense. These connect the inner segments of photoreceptors to cells of Müller, the cytoplasm of which appears light. Above the middle (layer 3) part of layer 4 is indicated by the presence of two nuclei of cones. Between the parts of the two cone cells light cytoplasm of Müller cells is present. Below the middle numerous microvilli-like processes of Müller cells project between the cytoplasm of the inner segments of photoreceptors (in layer 2). (Hollenberg, M. J., and Bernstein, M. H.: Am. J. Anat., *118*:359, 1966)

as precursors. As was described in the previous edition of this book, Bernard Droz, in 1963, by using this method was able to show that there was a continuous production of protein in the inner segments of rods and also that there was a continuous migration of this protein to the outer segments. Young followed this with further experiments in his laboratory in which it was shown that when the protein reached the outer segment it was at first concentrated at the base of the outer segment. It was then found that this layer of labeled protein that appeared first as the base of the outer segment moved gradually to the end of the segment; in mice and rats this took about 10 days. On reaching the end of the segment the labeled protein disappeared. It was subsequently established that the reason for the labeled protein moving as transverse labeled lines was that the labeled protein had become assembled into a disk and that it was the disk that moved. In other words, there was not only a continuous synthesis of protein but there was also a continuous synthesis of new disks which moved continuously from the base of an outer segment to its end. It was next shown that when disks reached the outer end of a segment they were disposed of by being phagocytosed by the epithelial cells into which the free ends of the outer segments project. It was subsequently shown by Young in radioautographic studies made with Droz that the protein was synthesized in association with the ribosomes in the inner segment,

after which it reached and passed through the Golgi apparatus and from there reached the outer segment by way of the cilium. It was also established that a new disk is produced every 40 minutes.

Some Points About Cones. Young next investigated cone cells and found that new disks are not formed in them after the cone cell has fully developed.

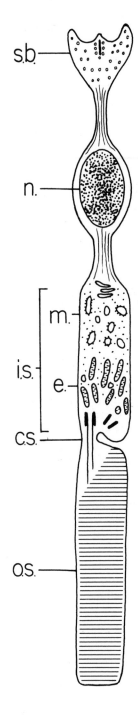

FIG. 28-20. Diagrammatic representation of a photoreceptor of the rod type showing the distribution of the organelles as determined by electron microscopy. Its orientation in this illustration is the same as that of the cells and layers of the retina shown in Figures 28-17 and 28-18 in that the innermost part of this cell is at the top of the illustration and the outermost part at the bottom. The outer segment of the rod (O.S.) contains the disks. The connecting structure between the outer and inner segments is labeled C.S. The inner segment of the rod is labeled i.s. In the outermost part of this a basal body from which a modified cilium extends into the inner part of the outer segment can be seen. The inner segment is commonly described as consisting of two parts, the ellipsoid portion (e) and the myoid portion (m). The former contains abundant mitochondria. The myoid portion contains rER, some free ribosomes and a Golgi apparatus, all of which are shown in the diagram. Farther in, the cell is constricted until it bulges to surround the nucleus (n). It then narrows again and ends in an expansion called the synaptic body (s.b.) because it is here that the photoreceptor is in synaptic association with the terminations of bipolar cells. (Illustration courtesy of Richard W. Young)

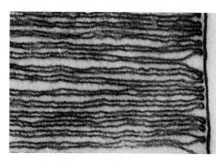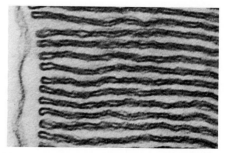

Fig. 28-21. Electron micrographs ($\times$ 100,000). (*Left*) Portion of foveal cone of monkey retina. (*Right*) Portion of outer rod segment of monkey retina. Description given in text. (Dowling, J. E.: Science, *147*:57)

There is, however, a continuous synthesis of protein in them in their inner segments as occurs in rods. Likewise, it moves to the outer segment but, instead of becoming localized to the base of the outer segment, it spreads throughout the outer segment of a cone where it is available to replenish the protein of all the disks and so maintain them in a functioning condition.

Young suggests that the shape of cones is due to the fact that their disks are not replenished. When, during development, disks are first formed, they are smaller than the disks that form later. Since the disks of cones are not replaced, the ones that are formed first are at the outer end of the outer segment while those that are formed later are nearer the bottom of the outer segment and, since the latter are larger, the outer segment would have a cone shape.

The disks of cones are shown on the left side of Figure 28-21. This illustration, however, does not show a feature that is seen at some levels in cones, for at some sites the covering membrane of the cone may turn into the cone as one of the membranes of a disk.

Color vision is to be explained by the fact that there are three types of visual pigment found among cones; these types are specially sensitive to red or blue or green light. Hence, some cones respond to light of one of these wavelengths and others to one of the others. The various other colors we see depend on the relative numbers of the three kinds of cones that are stimulated.

Over much of the retina the nuclei of cones, unlike those of rods, tend to be arranged so that with the LM they are seen in a section as a single row.

The inner end of each cone terminates in a club-shaped expansion; this is sometimes called the *synaptic body* or *cone pedicle*. Hollenberg and Bernstein studied the photoreceptors of the retinas of ground squirrels; these are unique because the photoreceptors are all of the cone type. They found that the pedicles of adjacent cones were often in direct contact with one another, thus providing a basis for interreceptor transmission. Others were separated by processes of Müller cells. The substance of cone pedicles was found to contain numerous synapses with dendrites of cells from the inner nuclear layer. This type of basal process is much more complex than that seen in rods.

Since the layer of rods and cones contains no blood vessels whatsoever, all nourishment comes to this layer from diffusion and largely from the choriocapillaries.

How Light Activates Photoreceptors. This is a very complicated matter of which only superficial description will be attempted here. The pigment in the outer segments of rods and cones that is responsive to light is designated by a general term, *rhodopsin,* and it consists of vitamin A aldehyde, which is called retinal, combined with a protein of the class of opsins. It has been shown that the molecule formed by this combination changes shape under the influence of light and it is thought that this results in some change in the relation of the two components of rhodopsin and that this change, in turn, initiates further changes that cause the membrane of the outer segment to become depolarized and set a nervous impulse on its way.

Sensitivity of the Retina to Light. The sensitivity of the retina to stimulation by light is incredibly great. Hecht *et al.* have estimated that only a single quantum is sufficient to stimulate one rod, and that 6 rods discharging into a common pathway may result in a nervous impulse along the path. There are practically 7 million cones in the human retina and 10 to 20 times that number of rods. Since the number of nerve fibers in the optic nerve has been estimated at from $\frac{1}{2}$ to 1 million, there is, of course, much overlapping of neurons.

MACULA LUTEA AND FOVEA CENTRALIS

Very close to the posterior pole of the eye there is a little depression of the retina; here the retina is more yellow than elsewhere (after death); hence, it is called the *macula lutea* (yellow spot) (Fig. 28-7). The cells and the fibers of the inner layers of the retina diverge from the center of this area so that the photoreceptors in the central and most depressed part of this area, which is called the *fovea centralis,* are not covered to the same extent as the photoreceptors in other parts of the eye. No blood vessels are present in the retina over this area. The receptors here are all cones; moreover, these, though longer than usual, are not so thick as usual; hence, more are packed into this small area than elsewhere. Therefore this area is specialized in several ways for the greatest degree of visual acuity. Only the image formed in this area is interpreted clearly and sharply by the brain. For example, as one reads this page, although he is aware of words arranged in lines from top to bottom, he can see accurately only a very little at a time. In other words, in order that the brain may receive a detailed interpretation of this page, the fovea centralis, like the electron beam originating in the television picture tube, must scan the image of the page, letter by letter, word by word and line by line, from top to bottom. Fortunately, however, most words or groups of words can be recognized from experience merely by their general configuration, thereby saving much time.

Nerve fibers from this specialized area are provided with more room at the papilla (the site of exit of the optic nerve) and consequently are less heaped up and more securely arranged than are the other more converging retinal fibers. Hence, if edema should develop at the papilla, the fibers coming from the macular area are the last to be involved.

OPTIC NERVE

Like the nerve fiber layer of the retina, the optic nerve at the papilla is composed of unmyelinated nerve fibers, containing glial supporting tissue and some capillaries. At the lamina cribrosa, the nerve fibers, arranged in bundles, are interspersed by a fibrous meshwork extending from the sclera (Fig. 28-22). After piercing the lamina cribrosa, the nerve fibers become myelinated, thus swelling the size of the optic nerve (Fig. 28-22). They do not acquire a sheath of Schwann, and, consequently, they resemble the nerve fibers of the white matter of the cord or brain. The sheaths covering the nerve have already been described and are illustrated in Figure 28-7.

INTERNAL APPEARANCE

It has been mentioned above that the eye is the window of the body, and that structures within the eye may be seen from the outside. Indeed, the eye is the only site where structures lying deep to the ectoderm of the body can be seen without artificial exposure or interruption of the integrity of the body surface. Since many of the functional and disease changes which occur in the body are reflected in changes in the structure of the eye, this fact is of great importance.

To look within the eye an instrument called the *ophthalmoscope* is ordinarily used. This provides a bright source of light, the rays of which are projected through the cornea into the patient's eye, thereby providing sufficient light for the operator of the instrument to see the fine structures in the back or fundus of the eye. With another instrument, the slit lamp microscope, the microscopic details of the conjunctiva, the cornea, the iris, the lens, the ciliary body and even the anterior portion of the vitreous can be studied in the living eye.

Figure 28-23 is a black-and-white representation of the fundus of a living right eye as viewed with the ophthalmoscope. The cup-shaped surface of the retina, gray in Figure 28-23, is red (the red reflex) in life because light is reflected back from the red blood cells in the very large capillaries of the choriocapillaris. The whole background has a granular appearance, due in part to the irregular distribution of pigment in the retinal epithelium and in part to the coarse aggregation of pigment cells in the vascular layer of the choroid.

The unmyelinated fibers of the retina (layer 9) converge at the site of exit of the optic nerve. Here, there is much heaping up of the retinal fibers. This constitutes what is known as the *papilla* (Fig. 28-23). In this region the nerve fibers are loosely arranged; consequently, accumulation of tissue fluid in the nervous tissue of the retina results in an obvious swelling of the papilla; this is a valuable early clinical sign of certain pathologic conditions. Since the papilla is of a disklike shape about 1.5 mm. in diameter, it is often called the *optic disk*. It appears much larger when seen through the refracting media of the eye than it does if it is exposed. Because the white lamina cribrosa (white fibrous tissue) is pierced by gray nerve fibers and is supplied by a capillary network, the papilla has a pale pink color in contrast with the redness of the retina elsewhere. Should the capillaries become atrophied, the papilla appears gray, and the little perforations of the lamina cribrosa, now not so obscured, appear more prominent. Should the nerve fibers atrophy, the papilla

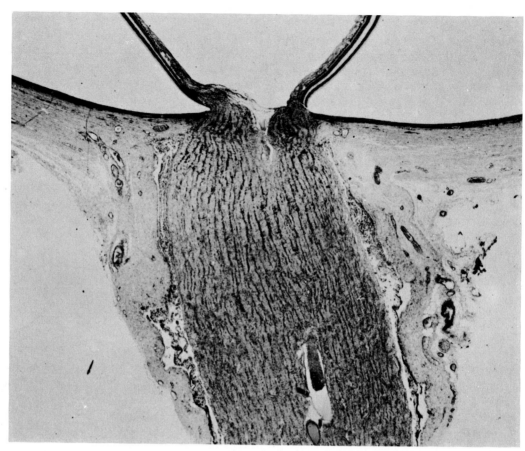

FIG. 28-22. Low-power photomicrograph of a section through the wall of the eye at the site of exit of the optic nerve. Observe that the inner layer of the retina is detached from the outermost layer of pigmented epithelium. Separation commonly occurs along this line when eyes are fixed and sectioned.

becomes chalky white; this appearance may be exaggerated later by the proliferation of glial and fibrous tissue.

The central portion of the papilla, called the *physiologic cup,* is a funnel-like space created by the diverging nerve fibers. An increase in intraocular pressure (and other conditions) may displace the lamina cribrosa and its nerve fibers posteriorly. This results in the whole papilla becoming depressed and cupshaped, a condition referred to as *cupping of the disk.*

The central retinal artery and vein make their appearance at the center of the physiologic cup, and, hugging its medial side (Fig. 28-23), they radiate over the inner surface of the retina, branching as they go (Fig. 28-23).

An area at the posterior pole of the eye, the *macula lutea* (Fig. 28-23), is designed to subserve the highest efficiency for visual acuity. The depressed central part

of this area, the *fovea centralis* (L., central pit), lies about 2.5 papillary diameters laterally from the margin of the papilla and a little below its center. The size of the macula is variable but is usually only slightly larger or smaller than the papilla.

Naturally, large retinal vessels, which would otherwise interfere with vision, do not traverse the macula (Fig. 28-23). Instead, they pass well above and below it in wide curves; this aids the student in locating the macula with the ophthalmoscope. Smaller vessels extend from the curving blood vessels and also from the medial side of the papilla itself into the macular area, but they never quite reach its center, which is left completely nonvascular. Because of yellow pigment in its superficial layers, the macular area appears yellow in the living (in red-free light) or on exposure after death. In ordinary white light it appears darker and redder than the remainder of the retina (Fig. 28-23).

Its darker color is due to an increased amount of pigmentation in the outer pigmented retinal coat, and the increased redness is due to blood contained in the especially large choroidal capillaries disposed behind this area. The fovea centralis, viewed through the pupil, appears to be a minute bright point because light is reflected, as by a mirror, from its concave walls.

Accessory Structures (Adnexa)

Conjunctiva. The conjunctiva is a thin transparent mucous membrane that covers the "white" of the eye as the bulbar conjunctiva (Fig. 28-14) and that lines the eyelid (which is not seen unless the lid is everted)

as the palpebral conjunctiva (Fig. 28-24). The space in the angle formed by the reflection of the palpebral conjunctiva from (and against) the bulbar is called the *fornix.*

The epithelium is characteristically stratified columnar in type with 3 layers of cells: a deep layer of columnar cells, a middle layer of polygonal cells and a superficial layer of flat or low cuboidal cells. The middle layer is absent in most of the palpebral conjunctiva. As the epithelium approaches the lid margin, it changes to stratified squamous in type; this merges with the epidermis of the skin. Scattered through the conjunctival epithelium are mucus-secreting goblet

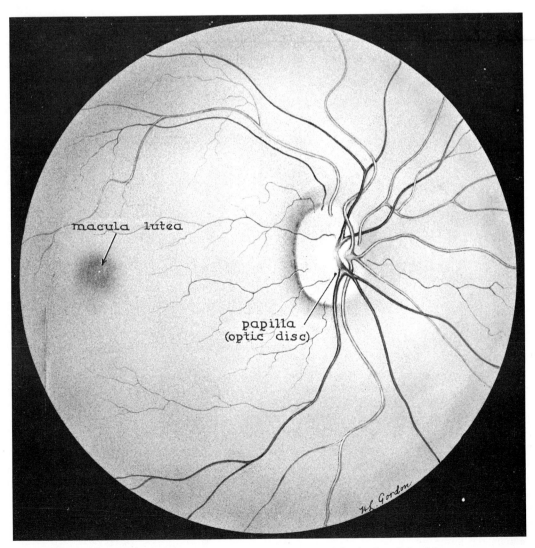

Fig. 28-23. Drawing, in black and white, of the appearance of the fundus of the right eye as seen through the ophthalmoscope.

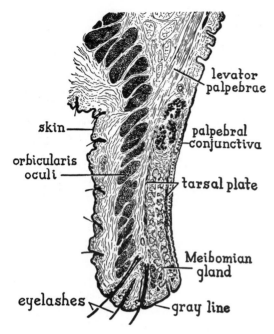

FIG. 28-24. Drawing of a section (low-power) cut perpendicularly through the upper eyelid. (After Duane, A.: Fuch's Textbook of Ophthalmology. ed. 8 revised. Philadelphia, Lippincott)

cells. Near the limbus the epithelium of the bulbar conjunctiva becomes stratified squamous in type and is provided with deep papilla. It is continuous with the epithelium of the cornea.

The substantia (lamina) propria of the conjunctiva consists of delicate fibrous connective tissue; this is particularly loose over the sclera. In it are scattered accumulations of lymphocytes; these form nodules near the fornices. The substantia propria, except in the lid, merges into a more deeply situated and thicker meshwork of collagenous and elastic connective tissue.

The palpebral fissure is the space between the free margins of the 2 lids (Fig. 28-14). At the medial end of the palpebral fissure is a little lake of tears, the lacus lacrimalis. A free fold of conjunctiva, the concave border of which faces the pupil, is present at the medial end of the palpebral fissure; this is called the *plica semilunaris* (Fig. 28-14), and it is probably homologous to the nictitating membrane of birds. In the very angle of the palpebral fissure at its medial end, a little fleshy mass, the *caruncle* (Fig. 28-14), protrudes; developmentally, this is a detached portion of the marginal part of the lower lid; hence it contains a few striated muscle fibers as well as a few hair follicles and sebaceous glands.

Eyelids. Each eyelid is covered on its anterior surface with delicate skin; this contains the follicles of some very fine hairs and some sebaceous and sweat glands (Fig. 28-24). The dermis is of an unusually loose texture, and the subcutaneous tissue, deep to it, in members of the white races, contains almost no fat. The keratin of the epidermis gradually thins out as the skin approaches the free margin of the eyelid, and here the epidermis becomes continuous with the epithelium of the palpebral conjunctiva, which has already been described as lining the inner (posterior) side of the lid (Fig. 28-24).

Each lid is reinforced with a plate of dense connective tissue, the *tarsal plate*. This is placed in the posterior part of the lid so that the palpebral conjunctiva is apposed to its posterior surface (Fig. 28-24). The secretory portions of long, vertically disposed, complex sebaceous glands, called *meibomian glands,* are embedded in the tarsal plate; these open onto the posterior part of the free margin of the lid (Fig. 28-24). Should one of these glands become infected, a painful pealike swelling develops in the lid.

Deep to the skin covering the anterior surface of the lid are bundles of striated muscle fibers of the orbicularis oculi muscle (Fig. 28-24). Some of the collagenic fibers from the aponeurosis of the levator palpebrae muscle pass between these bundles to be inserted into the skin that covers the eyelid. Others connect with the tarsal plate, and still others continue toward the margin of the lid in front of the plate. This latter sheet of connective tissue becomes more areolar as it approaches the margin of the lid, which it reaches to form the gray line, a surgical landmark of some importance. Along this gray line the lid may be split surgically, opening up the submuscular space known to the ophthalmologist as the *intermarginal space.*

The hair follicles of the eyelashes slant anteriorly as they pass to the surface. They are arranged in 3 or 4 rows, just ahead of the gray line. They are provided with sebaceous glands; these are termed the glands of Zeis. Between the follicles, the sweat glands of Moll are disposed. A sty is the result of the infection of either type of gland.

Tear Glands. Tears are produced by the lacrimal gland and several accessory tear glands. The lacrimal gland lies in the superolateral corner of the bony orbit. It is divided by the lateral edge of the levator palpebrae muscle into 2 lobes: a deep orbital lobe and a superficial palpebral lobe. Something less than a dozen ducts run from the gland to empty along the superior fornix. Most of the ducts from the orbital lobe, to reach their termination, pass through the palpebral lobe. Small accessory tear glands, the glands of Krause, are scattered along both fornices, but they are more numerous in the upper one. Still smaller glands are present in the caruncle. It is of interest that the eye may remain healthy in the absence of the lacrimal gland; this suggests that the function of the gland is to some extent that of providing floods of tears on special occasions.

The tear glands develop from the conjunctiva and are of the serous compound tubulo-alveolar type. The secretory cells are of a pyramidal columnar form and contain both fat droplets and secretion granules (Fig. 28-25). The secretory units are surrounded by myoepithelial cells which lie to the inside of the basement membrane.

The secretion of the tear glands is slightly alkaline. In addition to various salts, it contains an enzyme, lysozyme, which is bactericidal. Tears, spread evenly over the cornea and the conjunctiva by the blinking of the lids, keeps the surface of the cornea and the conjunctiva moist; this, as noted before, is an essential function. Floods of tears assist in washing foreign particles from the conjunctival sacs and the cornea.

DRAINAGE OF TEARS. On the free margin of each lid, near its medial end, is a little papilla called the *lacrimal papilla*. A small opening, which, however, can be seen with the naked eye, exists near the summit of the papilla; this opening is termed the *punctum* and it leads into the *lacrimal canaliculus*. This is a small tube that runs first in the lid and then medially so as to meet its fellow from the adjacent lid in a little ampulla that extends outward from the lateral side of a tubular structure called the *lacrimal sac*. The latter decends as the *nasolacrimal duct*, to open through the lateral surface of the inferior meatus of the nose; by means of this mechanism, tears more or less continually drain into the nose. Should any part of this duct system become blocked, tears, produced at only an ordinary rate, run over onto the side of the face.

The puncta and the canaliculi are lined with stratified squamous nonkeratinized epithelium, and the lacrimal sac and nasolacrimal duct with 2 layers of columnar epithelium which contains goblet cells. The lacrimal papilla is rich in elastic fibers.

Taste Buds

The nervous impulses responsible for the sense of taste are set up in little pale-staining bodies which resemble buds or little barrels and are arranged perpendicular to the surface in the epithelium of the mucous membrane of the mouth and the throat (Fig. 28-26). They are most numerous on the upper surface of the tongue, particularly along the sides of the

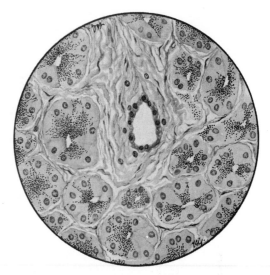

FIG. 28-25. Drawing of a portion of a section (high-power) of the lacrimal gland, showing secretory units and a duct.

grooves that surround vallate papillae. However, they are found on fungiform papillae and even in the epithelium between papillae. A few may be present in other parts of the mouth and in the lining of the throat. It is not unusual to see a taste bud in the epithelium on the laryngeal side of the epiglottis. They have been reported in other parts of the larynx.

A taste bud, like an onion, is constricted at both its ends. Moreover, taste buds, when seen in sections, appear to have a layered structure somewhat similar to that of an onion. This is due to the arrangement of their cells. From the older studies with the LM it was believed that there were two kinds of cells in a taste bud: *sustentacular* cells and *neuroepithelial* taste cells. The sustentacular cells seen in sections had the appearance of slices of cantaloupe; they are narrower at each of their ends than in their midsection, and they pursue a curved course from one end of the bud to the other. At the end of the barrel-shaped structure which reaches almost to the surface, they are arranged so as to surround a little central depression or *pit* which communicates with the surface by means of a fine passageway called the *inner taste pore* which extends through such epithelium as covers the end of the taste bud. The site of this is indicated on Figure 28-26 by an arrow, but the pore itself does not appear in the photomicrograph. (Pores are of such a small caliber that they show only occasionally in sections.) Neuroepithelial taste cells were believed to be intermingled with sustentacular cells in the more central part of the bud as long narrow cells. Their free ends were thought

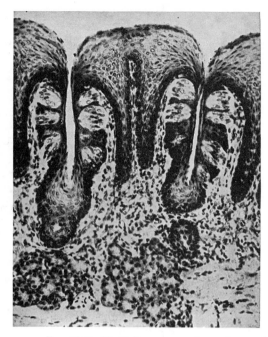 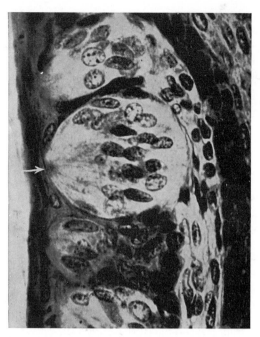

Fig. 28-26. (*Left*) Low-power photomicrograph of a portion of a section cut at right angles to the upper surface of the tongue of a rabbit in the region of the foliate papillae. These papillae, which are well developed only in certain animals, provide an especially good opportunity for seeing taste buds, which are numerous in this illustration. (*Right*) High-power photomicrograph of a taste bud in the epithelium of the side of a foliate papilla of a rabbit. The arrow occupies the approximate site where a pore (not shown) might be expected, and it points to the pit (dark) into which the hairs of the neuroepithelial cells project.

to extend to the pit at the end of the taste bud, where it seemed to give rise to a short hair that extended into the pit. The EM, however has shown that what probably accounted for the hairs of light microscopy are microvilli, a few of which extend into the pore from each taste cell and have stout bundles of filaments in their cores.

The studies of Beidler and Smallman, moreover, strongly suggest that the two kinds of cells described from LM studies merely represent different stages of development of a single cell type. By radioautography they showed that there was a turnover of the cells in a bud, with cells moving from its periphery to its central region. The average life span of a cell was around 250 hours.

In another EM study Murray, Murray and Fujimoto saw and described a third type of cell in taste buds. This cell was characterized by its basal termination showing a density along its cell membrane similar to that seen in presynaptic nerve endings and, furthermore, they observed synaptic type vesicles close to these basal densities. These areas abutted against nerve endings which were not always bulbous in na-

ture, sometimes being merely narrow nerve processes. The arrangements seen suggest that these cells have a polarized function for the transmission of nerve impulses. Whether or not they are the only type of cell having a sensory function seems to remain an open question as does the relation of these cells to the previously described two types.

The sense of taste from the anterior two thirds of the tongue is mediated by way of the chorda tympani division of the facial nerve and from the posterior third by way of the glossopharyngeal nerve. Terminal fibers enter the deep ends of taste buds and end in intimate contact with the neuroepithelial taste cells.

Any substance to be tasted must become dissolved in saliva and pass by means of a pore into the pit at the superficial end of a taste bud; here it affects the ends of the neuroepithelial cells in some fashion so as to cause a nervous impulse to be set up in the fibers associated with the neuroepithelial cells. As is true of smell, there are only certain basic tastes: sweet, sour, salty and bitter, and perhaps alkaline and metallic. Doubtless, there are specialized receptors for each. These are not distributed evenly, so that some tastes are detected more easily in some parts of the tongue than in others. It seems incredible that the great variety of flavors of which we are aware are due to various combinations of these few basic tastes. Actually, it is easy to confuse taste and smell to some degree, and many of the more exotic flavors are probably smelled rather than tasted.

The Ear

INTRODUCTION

Each ear consists of 3 main parts (an external, a middle and an inner part), and each of these 3 parts is in itself termed an ear; hence each (complete) ear is said to consist of an *external ear,* a *middle ear,* and an *inner ear.*

The ear is responsible not only for hearing but also for appreciating (1) how the head is oriented in space in relation to gravitational forces and (2) whether movement of the head takes place (the overcoming of inertia), or, if steady movement of the head is taking place, whether the rate or the direction of the movement is altered. It may seem curious that end-organs concerned in the maintenance of equilibrium are so closely associated with the end-organ for hearing in the body. Actually, however, in the evolutionary scale, the ear was an organ for permitting animals to maintain equilibrium before it was an organ for hearing.

GENERAL STRUCTURE

The *external ear* consists of an appendage, the *auricle,* and a tube, the *external auditory meatus* (*meatus,* a passage or canal), which extends from the auricle into the substance of the skull (Fig. 28-27) to a tiny cavity in the petrous portion of the temporal bone, known as the tympanic cavity or middle ear (Fig. 28-27). The external auditory meatus, although it extends to the middle ear, does not open into it, because a membrane, called the *tympanic membrane* or *eardrum,* extends across the deep end of the external auditory meatus to form a partition between it and the middle ear (Fig. 28-27). This membrane, which thus forms a considerable part of the lateral wall of the middle ear, is of a suitable size and thickness and is maintained under a suitable tension to vibrate in accordance with sound waves that reach it by way of the auricle and the external auditory meatus.

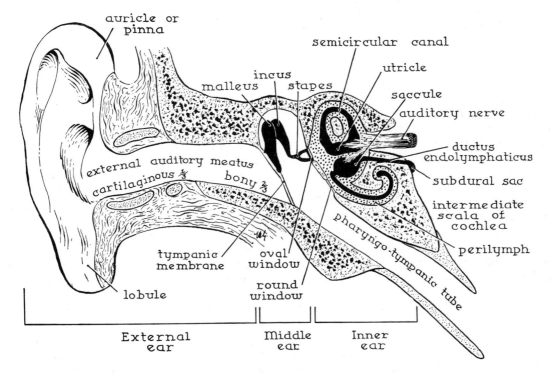

FIG. 28-27. Diagram of an ear, showing the relations of the external, the middle and the inner ear. (Redrawn and modified from Addison: Piersol's Normal Histology. ed. 15. Philadelphia, Lippincott)

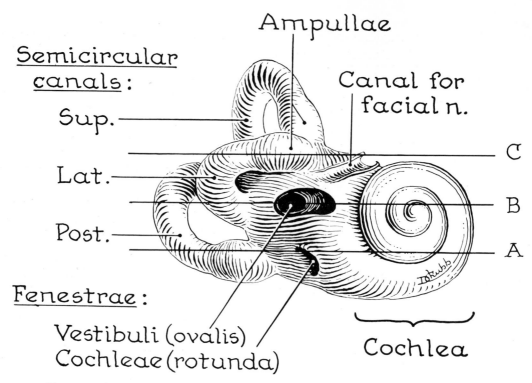

Semicircular canals:
Sup.
Lat.
Post.

Ampullae

Canal for facial n.

C
B
A

Fenestrae:
Vestibuli (ovalis)
Cochleae (rotunda)

Cochlea

FIG. 28-28. An anterolateral view of the bony labyrinth. The oval and round windows (labeled fenestrae) may be seen opening into the vestibule; the cochlea extends from the vestibule to the right, and the semicircular canals, to the left. (Grant, J. C. B.: Method of Anatomy. ed. 4. Baltimore, Williams & Wilkins; lines A, B and C have been added)

Before discussing the general structure and function of the middle ear further, we shall comment briefly on the inner ear, for here are located the special groups of nerve endings which are selectively stimulated by sound, changes in relation to gravity, and alterations in movement.

The inner ear consists of a series of membranous tubes that are disposed in various arrangements and planes, together with 2 membranous sacs with which the membranous tubes communicate (Figs. 28-27, 28-28 and 28-29). This closed system of membranous tubes and sacs is filled with a fluid termed *endolymph*, and at appropriate sites, to be described later, neuroepithelial structures, with special types of nerve endings, are disposed inside these membranous structures. The whole system of membranous tubes and sacs is so like a maze that it is said to constitute the *membranous labyrinth* (*labyrinthos*, a maze). The membranous labyrinth is loosely fitted into a series of spaces and cavities in the bone; these are of a similar pattern to, though somewhat larger than, the membranous labyrinth and are said to constitute the *bony labyrinth*. Although in some sites the membranous labyrinth is attached to the periosteum that lines the wall of the bony labyrinth, the bulk of the membranous labyrinth is suspended in a fluid termed *perilymph* which fills all the space in the bony labyrinth that is not occupied by the membranous labyrinth. To visualize these labyrinths the study of a 3-dimensional model is very helpful.

The most expanded portion of the bony labyrinth lies deep to the bony medial wall of the middle ear; this part of the bony labyrinth is termed its *vestibule* because it is the hallway that would be entered by any microscopic visitor who entered the inner ear from the middle ear. There are no doors opening from the middle ear into the vestibule of the bony labyrinth, so any visitor from the middle ear would have to enter by way of a window. There are two of these in the bony wall that separates the air-filled middle ear from the fluid-filled vestibule of the bony labyrinth; the upper is termed the *oval window* (Fig. 28-28, Vestibuli [ovalis]) and the lower one the *round window* (Fig. 28-28, Cochleae [rotunda]). Both windows normally are closed, but in order to describe how they are closed, we must digress for a moment.

It has already been explained how sound waves set the eardrum into vibration and that the eardrum constitutes a considerable portion of the lateral wall of the middle ear. A chain of 3 tiny bones, with joints between them, extends across the middle ear from its lateral to its medial wall (Fig. 28-27). The free end of the first bone of the chain is attached to the eardrum, and the free end of the last bone in the chain fits into, so as to close effectively, the oval window in the medial wall of the middle ear (Figs. 28-27 and 28-31). Hence, when sound waves set the eardrum in vibration, the chain of bones transmits these vibrations across the middle ear, and since the free end of the last bone of the chain does not fit rigidly into the window (beyond which is the perilymph of the bony labyrinth) but instead, a little like a piston in a cylinder, the vibrations are transmitted to the perilymph in the vestibule. However, fluid is incompressible; hence, every time fluid is pushed in at the oval window, it must push out somewhere else. This occurs at the round window, for this is closed only by a membrane, and this has sufficient elasticity for this purpose. Having described the mechanical arrangements that exist in the ear to permit sound waves eventually to set up vibrations in the perilymph, we shall leave the matter of how these in turn affect nerve endings until certain other details of the bony and membranous labyrinth are considered.

Although the bony labyrinth (Fig. 28-28) has a complex form, it may be helpful to think of it as having 3 main parts. The first of these is the vestibule; this has already been described as its most expanded part, which is disposed immediately medial to the middle ear. The other 2 main parts of the bony labyrinth may be regarded as 2 extensions of the labyrinth from the vestibule, and in these the bony labyrinth is tubular in form. The more anterior of the 2 tubular extensions of the bony labyrinth becomes wound into a spiral, the successive turns of which are of a decreasing radius (Figs. 28-27 and 28-28). Since this coiled part of the bony labyrinth looks something like a snail's shell, it is called the *cochlea* (L., snail shell). The more posterior of the 2 extensions of the bony labyrinth from the vestibule (actually this extension is regarded as a part of the vestibule) takes the form of 3 separate, round, bony tubes, each of which, on leaving the vestibule, follows a semicircular path so that each eventually returns to the vestibule (only one may be seen in Fig. 28-27). Each bony tube communicates at both of

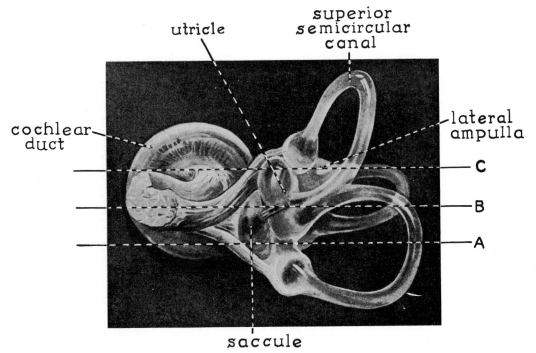

FIG. 28-29. Drawing of the right membranous labyrinth of a human adult (medial and posterior view). It shows the relation between the cochlear duct, the utricle, the saccule, the semicircular canals and the ampullae. (Spalteholtz, W.: Hand Atlas of Human Anatomy. ed. 13. Philadelphia, Lippincott; lines A, B and C have been added)

its ends with the vestibule (Fig. 28-28). These bony tubes are referred to as *semicircular canals,* and it is of great significance that they be disposed in different planes, approximately so that the plane of each is at right angles to the planes of the other two (Fig. 28-28).

As noted before, the membranous labyrinth (Fig. 28-29) is composed of a system of membranous tubes and sacs, and it is fitted loosely into the bony labyrinth. Actually, there are 2 sacs in the membranous labyrinth, and these are both present in the vestibule of the bony labyrinth. The more anterior and smaller of the two is called the *saccule* (*sacculus,* a small sac), part of which is shown in black in Figure 28-27, and the larger and more posterior of the two, the *utricle* (*utriculus,* a little skin bag), part of which is shown in black in Figure 28-27. The 2 sacs are in communication with each other by means of a fine membranous duct.

As was explained before, the membranous labyrinth extends into all parts of the bony labyrinth. The membranous tube that extends into the cochlea is given off from the saccule. On entering the basal turn of the cochlea it becomes known as the *cochlear duct.* It is not, as might at first be imagined, a round tube, but instead it has more of the shape of a ribbon, particularly that of a thick wide ribbon that has been "ironed down" along one of its sides so that one side is much thinner than the other. Such a ribbon would be somewhat triangular in shape when seen in cross section. The cochlear duct, of course, is not solid like a ribbon but is hollow and filled with endolymph. A cross section view of it can be seen in Figure 28-33, where it is labeled *cochlear duct.*

The thicker edge of the ribbonlike cochlear duct is attached to one side of the bony canal of the cochlea by the spiral ligament (Fig. 28-33, *spiral ligament*). The other and thinner edge of the hollow ribbonlike cochlear duct is attached to the other side of the bony canal. Thus the cochlear duct forms a hollow shelf across the bony canal, splitting it into 2 parts along its whole length. In this fashion the cochlear duct ascends the winding turns of the cochlea, always keeping the part of the canal above it—and this is known as the *scala vestibuli* (*scala,* a stairway) (Figs. 28-33 and 28-36)—separated from the part of the canal that lies below it, and which is known as the *scala tympani* (Fig. 28-33). Both the scala vestibuli and the scala tympani are filled with *perilymph.* (This almost is identical with cerebrospinal fluid and is in communication, in a way that need not be described here, with cerebrospinal fluid.) However, the cochlear duct (sometimes termed the *scala media* as in Figure 28-

36) keeps the perilymph in the scala vestibuli separated along the whole course of the cochlea from the perilymph of the scala tympani. (Actually, there is a small opening between the scala vestibuli and the scala tympani at the tip of the cochlea, but this may be disregarded for the time being.)

Since the perilymph in the scala vestibuli and that in the scala tympani are not in free communication with each other, any vibrations in the perilymph in the scala vestibuli, to reach the scala tympani, would have to be transmitted through the thickness of the ribbonlike endolymph-containing cochlear duct. The perilymph in the scala vestibuli connects with the perilymph that bathes the inner aspect of the oval window. This perilymph receives vibrations from the eardrum by way of the chain of bones, the last one of which fits into the oval window. Hence the vibrations of the eardrum are transmitted up into the cochlea by means of the perilymph that extends from the oval window up into the scala vestibuli. However, as was noted before, fluid is incompressible; hence the bone that fits into the oval window cannot push into the window unless the fluid in the bony labyrinth can push out somewhere else. Since the perilymph in the scala tympani is in free communication with that which bathes the inner aspect of the round window, vibrations transmitted into the oval window and through the perilymph of the scala vestibuli can be transmitted through the thickness of the cochlear duct into the perilymph of the scala tympani and from there to the round window, which "gives" sufficiently to permit the above-described mechanism to operate.

The end-organ for hearing consists of a narrow band of special neuroepithelial cells and nerve fibers that is disposed along the floor of the cochlear duct along its whole length. This long end-organ is called the *organ of Corti.* This structure (not labeled) is cut in cross section in Figure 28-33, where it lies above the *basilar membrane* and part of the *osseous spiral lamina.* Most of it is covered by the *tectorial membrane.* Details about its structure will be given later. It is in this organ that the nervous impulses responsible for hearing originate when its special cells are stimulated by vibrations transmitted through the cochlear duct from the perilymph of the scala vestibuli into that of the scala tympani. In all probability, vibrations caused by high notes affect the receptors in the more basal part of the cochlea, and those from low notes, those in the terminal part of the cochlea.

We shall consider next the function of the more posterior extension of the bony labyrinth, the semicircular canals. The semicircular canals (Fig. 28-28), like the cochlea, are filled with perilymph, but each contains, in addition, a membranous tube (part of the membranous labyrinth) which is filled with endolymph (Fig. 28-29). In a special expanded part of each membranous tube, called its *ampulla* (Fig. 28-29), a little mound of neuroepithelial cells called a *crista* (L., a crest) is present in its wall. Another end-organ is located in the utricle. It consists of a little mass of neuroepithelial cells and nerve endings, together with some other features to be described presently, and is called a *macula* (L., a spot). A similar macula is also found in the saccule. Their microscopic structure and functions will be given presently.

MICROSCOPIC STRUCTURE OF THE PARTS OF THE EAR

Auricle. In lower animals the auricle serves 3 purposes. Since it is movable and shaped like a funnel, it can be pointed at the source of a sound, acting as a natural ear trumpet to collect the sound waves and conduct them to the middle ear. Burrowing and aquatic animals can close the auricle over the meatus and in this way keep out dirt and water. In man the auricle can be moved only slightly, but its central area plays an important role in the vertical localization of sound in determining whether a source of sound is above or below the head. It is of little use as a protective structure, and its irregular and flattened shape (Fig. 28-27) would seem to detract from its function as a collector of sound waves.

The shape of the auricle is maintained by its content of yellow elastic fibrocartilage. The auricle is covered with skin on both sides. The subcutaneous tissue on the posteromedial surface is slightly thicker than that on the anterolateral surface and contains some fat cells. Hair follicles with associated sebaceous glands are scattered through the dermis on both sides; these are most prominent near the entrance to the external auditory meatus. At the most dependent part of the auricle lies the *lobule;* this consists of a mass of fat, enclosed in connective tissue septa and covered externally with skin. The relative paucity of nerve endings and the rich capillary bed make the lobule a convenient site for obtaining blood for blood counts.

External Auditory Meatus. This canal leading to the drum is lined with the stratified squamous epithelium of the skin. To prevent the canal from collapsing, its walls have rigid support. In the outer part this support consists of elastic cartilage continuous with the cartilage of the auricle; in the inner part of the meatus the support is provided by bone (Fig. 28-27). In the outer one third of the canal there are many short hairs,

and associated with their follicles are large sebaceous glands. In the submucosa deep to the sebaceous glands there are clusters of tubular *ceruminous* (*cera*, wax) glands; the ducts of these open either directly onto the surface of the canal or into the sebaceous ducts. The ceruminous glands are thought to be modified sweat glands, and their tubules are lined by tall cuboidal or columnar cells. The combined secretion of the sebaceous and the ceruminous glands, called *cerumen*, may accumulate and keep out sound waves. In the inner two thirds of the canal the ceruminous glands are confined to its roof.

Tympanic Membrane. The tympanic membrane is like a sandwich, the filling of which is collagenous connective tissue, and the bread, 2 epithelial coats (Fig. 28-30). The outer epithelial coat is continuous with the stratified squamous epithelium lining the external auditory meatus; it differs from it in having no papillae except short ones near the margin, and also in that over the more central part of the drum it consists of only 2 layers of cells. Furthermore, mitoses are found only in the periphery, but with time the new cells arising from these mitoses migrate toward the center of the drum. Thus the replacement of cells lost from the central region of the drum is accounted for by new cells moving in from the periphery.

The epithelium of the mucous membrane of the middle ear flattens out to exist as a single layer of low cuboidal cells; these form the inner covering of the drum. The middle fibrous filling of the drum consists of 2 layers of collagen fibers; the outer ones are dispersed radially and the inner ones circularly. The upper part of the drum is thin and flaccid because of a lack of collagen filling. Therefore it is known as the *pars flaccida* or *Schrapnell's membrane.*

Middle Ear. The middle ear or tympanic cavity is a tiny epithelial-lined cavity in bone, being roughly the shape of a red blood cell set on edge. The tympanic cavity is described as having 4 walls, a floor and a roof. It is about as high as it is long (about ½ inch), but is very thin. The lateral wall consists largely of the tympanic membrane (Fig. 28-27), and the medial wall is the bone dividing the middle ear from the inner ear. There is a gap between the anterior and the medial walls for a canal, called the *eustachian tube,* which extends forward and communicates with the nasopharynx (Fig. 28-27).

The epithelium lining the cavity consists of simple nonciliated cuboidal cells with no basement membrane. The lamina propria is a thin connective tissue layer, closely adherent to bone. In some areas the cuboidal cells may become several layers thick. When infection

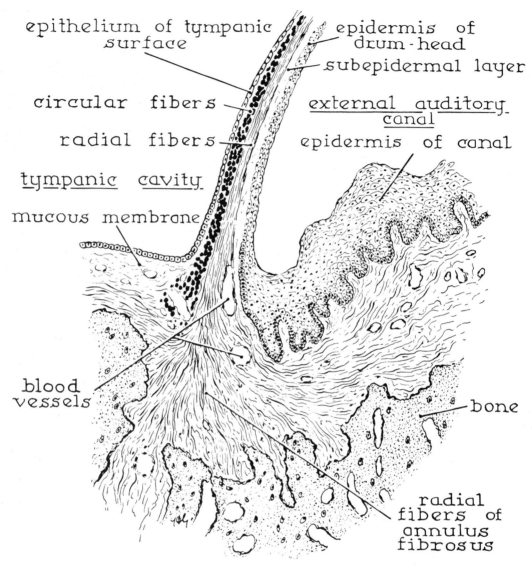

epithelium of tympanic surface

epidermis of drum-head

subepidermal layer

circular fibers

external auditory canal

radial fibers

epidermis of canal

tympanic cavity

mucous membrane

blood vessels

bone

radial fibers of annulus fibrosus

FIG. 28-30. Diagrammatic sketch of a part of the human tympanic membrane (low-power, cut in cross section). It shows the relation of the drum membrane to the external auditory canal and to the tympanic cavity and the attachment of the membrane.

occurs, the epithelium may become ciliated or may change to stratified squamous epithelium.

The middle ear houses 3 small bones or ossicles, 2 muscles and a nerve. The middle ear communicates with the pharynx by means of the *pharyngotympanic* or eustachian tube, and this communication makes the middle ear an air-containing cavity and offers a direct route for infection to reach it from the upper respiratory tract (Fig. 28-27). Indeed, middle ear infections are fairly common complications of head colds, particularly in children. Posteriorly, the tympanic cavity

is continuous with a varying number of alveolar spaces in bone, the *mastoid air cells*. These, too, may become involved in infections that spread up the tube to the middle ear from the nasopharynx.

OSSICLES. The 3 small bones of the middle ear cavity are the *malleus* or *hammer,* the *incus* or *anvil* and the *stapes* or *stirrup* (Fig. 28-27). These bones were doubtless named in the days of the blacksmith shop and have little connotation for the modern student. The malleus is shaped like a crude hammer with a rounded head, a long handle and a spur in the region

of the constricted neck which joins the head to the
handle. The incus is shaped like a molar tooth with a
body or "crown" and a vertical and a horizontal
"root." The stapes, as its name suggests, is shaped
like the stirrup of a riding saddle. It consists of a
head, a neck, 2 limbs and an oval footplate. The head
of the malleus fits into the "crown" of the incus; the
vertical "root" of the incus fits against the head of the
stapes (Fig. 28-27).

The ossicles transmit the vibrations set up in the
tympanic membrane by sound waves to one of the two
windows present in the medial wall of the middle ear.
To do this, the handle of the malleus is firmly attached
to the tympanic membrane (Fig. 28-27) and carries
the vibrations to the incus; the incus transfers the
vibrations to the stapes, causing the footplate of the
stapes, accurately fitted in the oval window, to rock
to and fro. This carries the vibrations to the perilymph
of the vestibule, as has already been explained. During
this transfer, the amplitude of the vibration is decreased, but the force is increased because the ossicles
are so arranged to exert leverage. The ossicles are
atypical long bones, having no epiphyses and reaching
approximately their full size during fetal life. The
malleus and the incus have small central marrow cavities, while the stapes has none in the adult. The "ends"
of these bones are covered with articular cartilage;
they are held together by small ligaments, and the
malleus and the incus are suspended by ligaments from
the roof of the middle ear. The periosteal surfaces of
these bones are covered by the mucous membrane of
the middle ear cavity.

MUSCLES. The 2 muscles of the tympanic cavity
are the *tensor tympani* and the *stapedius*. The tensor
tympani muscle is housed in a bony groove (canal)
above the cartilaginous roof of the eustachian tube;
its tendon crosses the tympanic cavity mediolaterally
to be inserted into the handle of the malleus. The
stapedius muscle is housed in the posterior wall of the
tympanic cavity (Fig. 28-31), and its tendon, issuing
at the summit of a small projection of bone called the
pyramid, is inserted into the neck of the stapes. The
way in which these muscles affect the transmission of
the sound waves by the ossicles is uncertain. The tensor muscle pulls the malleus inward, thus tensing the
tympanic membrane and perhaps accentuating high-
pitched sounds. The stapedius pulls the footplate of
the stapes outward, thus reducing the intralabyrinth
pressure and perhaps making sounds of low frequency
more audible. It has been found that reflex contractions of the stapedius occur during exposure to loud
noise. Therefore it seems that the stapedius plays a

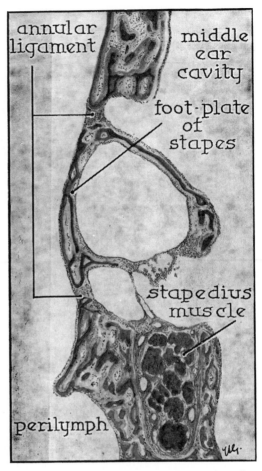

FIG. 28-31. Drawing of a horizontal section (low-
power) of the foot of the stapes and the oval window
of the right ear of a child taken approximately along the
line B in Figure 28-28. It shows the relations of the
stapedius muscle and the annular ligament to the stapes
and the medial wall of the tympanic cavity.

protective role, preventing too violent vibrations from
injuring the special sense organs in the internal ear.

NERVES. The chorda tympani nerve traverses the
middle ear in contact with the inner surface of the
drum. It has no functional concern with the ear. In
addition, branches of many other nerves can be found
in the mucous membrane and the bony walls of the
middle ear. The facial nerve runs in a long canal in the
medial wall of the middle ear. Its only concern with
the ear lies in the fact that it supplies the stapedius
muscle. The tympanic branch of the glossopharyngeal
(Jacobson's nerve) is the great sensory nerve of the
middle ear; the auricular branch of the vagus
(Arnold's nerve) supplies the skin of the external
auditory meatus. An attack of coughing or vomiting

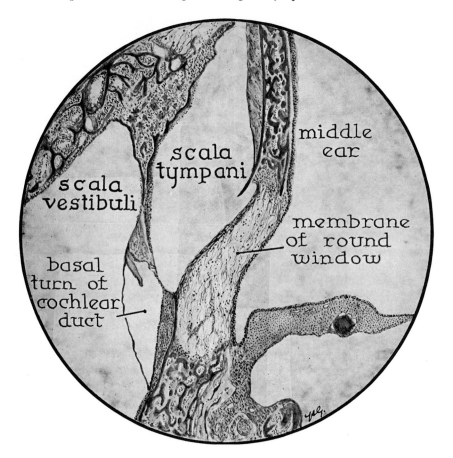

FIG. 28-32. Drawing of a section (low-power) through the round window of the right ear of a child. It shows the relation of the membrane of the round window to the tympanic cavity and the vestibule.

occasionally follows stimulation of the external auditory canal, for example, when a speculum is introduced into it. This is thought to be due to a reflex whose afferent arm is Arnold's nerve.

THE OVAL WINDOW. The footplate of the stapes sits and is fitted accurately in the oval window. Its periphery is attached to the cartilaginous rim of the oval window by the annular ligament composed of strong collagenous and elastic fibers (Fig. 28-31). The mucous membrane lining the middle ear cavity is reflected from this onto the stapes. Through the oval window, vibrations are conducted to the perilymph of the vestibule.

THE ROUND WINDOW. Since fluid is incompressible, there must be some movable object which the perilymph can displace when it is thrust inward at the oval window. This movable object is a moderately elastic membrane which fills in the round window like a flexible windowpane. The membrane has a core of connective tissue and is lined on its middle ear surface by mucous membrane; on its inner side it is lined by the connective tissue of the perilymphatic space of the vestibule (Fig. 28-32).

The Pharyngotympanic Tube. The simple cuboidal epithelium of the middle ear cavity gives way to respiratory epithelium, i.e., pseudostratified ciliated columnar epithelium, in the pharyngotympanic or eustachian tube. There are rugae in the epithelial coat here, and goblet cells can be found in the lining of the cartilaginous part of the tube. Near the pharyngeal end a mixed mucous and serous gland is present in the submucosa. Normally, the mucous surfaces of the tube are in contact, and the tube is open only during swallowing. The pressure in the middle ear can be adjusted rapidly to that of the atmosphere only when this tube is open. Thus, when coming down quickly from heights, one can prevent discomfort by swallowing; this opens the tube and permits the pressure in the middle ear to become equalized with that of the atmosphere.

The Mastoid Air Cells. In early life the mastoid process and all the petrous bone surrounding the inner ear are normally filled with hemopoietic marrow. In the adult, small air pockets continuous with the middle ear cavity have replaced this marrow in the mastoid region. The process whereby the bone is invaded by these air sacs is known as *pneumatization;* it starts as early as the 3rd fetal month, with the greatest extension usually, but not always, occurring between the 3rd year and puberty. The degree of pneumatization of the mastoid area varies greatly from person to person. From a roentgenographic study on pneumatization in a large series of twins, it was concluded that heredity plays a much more important role than middle-ear infection in determining the extent to which the mastoid and the surrounding petrous temporal bone become pneumatized.

The lining of the mastoid air cells is a thin mucoperiosteum; the cuboidal cells of the middle ear cavity here become flattened to a simple squamous type and lie adjacent to the periosteum of the mastoid air cells.

The Cochlea. The bony cochlea, as explained before, is part of the bony labyrinth and consists of a bony tube. In describing the cochlea further it is convenient to speak of it as if it were laid flat on its base; then it can be said that the bony tube of which it is composed winds spirally upward around a central pillar of bone called the *modiolus.* Actually, in position in the body, the apex of the cochlea is directed anterolaterally. However, in describing the microscopic anatomy of this structure, we shall assume that it has been laid flat on its base.

In the account of the general structure of the ear it was explained that the portion of the membranous labyrinth that extends into the bony cochlea was of the shape of a hollow ribbon flattened along one of its edges, and that its 2 edges were in apposition with the 2 sides of the bony canal in which it lies so that it separates the bony canal along its whole length into 2 long spiral chambers, the scala vestibuli and the scala tympani (Figs. 28-33 and 28-36).

A portion of a cross section of the *bony canal* of the cochlea is illustrated in Figures 28-33 and 28-36, and these figures should be referred to frequently as the following description is read. The term *inner,* as used in the following description of the cochlea, refers to the central pillar of the cochlea, the modiolus, a portion of which may be seen housing the spiral ganglion (to be described later) at the bottom of Figure 28-33.

The floor of the cochlear duct, in order to extend from the inner to the outer side of the bony canal of the cochlea, is not so wide as might be thought because both the outer and the inner walls of the bony canal of the cochlea bulge toward the center of the canal of the cochlea to support the floor of the cohlear duct and so make the distance it must bridge narrower. The bulge from the inner wall of the bony canal takes the form of a thin shelf of bone called the *osseous spiral lamina* (Fig. 28-33) because it winds up the modiolus

like the thread on a screw. The bulge from the outer surface of the bony canal is not bone but is of the nature of a thickening of the periosteum that lines the canal; this line of thickened and primarily fibrous periosteum that winds up the turns of the cochlea is called the *spiral ligament* (Fig. 28-33). The floor of the cochlear duct, the *basilar membrane* (Fig. 28-33), bridges the gap between the osseous spiral lamina and the crest of the spiral ligament. The basilar membrane is made up of a dense mat of collagenic and some elastic fibers. The roof of the cochlear duct, in contrast to its floor, is thin, being composed of only 2 layers of squamous epithelial cells; this is called *Reissner's membrane* (Fig. 28-33). The outer wall of the cochlear duct is made up of the spiral ligament already described. The upper and larger part (the part nearer Reissner's membrane) is known as the *stria vascularis* (Fig. 28-33) and is rich in blood vessels which lie directly below a surface layer of deep-staining cuboidal cells. A small part of the outer wall of the cochlear duct, close to the attachment of the basilar membrane to the crest of the spiral ligament, is arranged to form what is known as the *sulcus spiralis externus.* Here, long protoplasmic processes from the surface epithelial cells extend down into the connective tissue of the spiral ligament. Moreover, Shambaugh has found secretory cells, which, though deeply buried in this area, have access to the surface; he suggests that they constitute a secretory mechanism for replenishing endolymph in the cochlear duct.

The Site of the Spiral Organ of Corti. The organ of Corti is the specialized end-organ of hearing. It exists in the form of a long cellular ribbon that runs from one end of the cochlear duct to the other. It lies on the floor of the cochlear duct, and since the cochlear duct is in the form of a spiral, its floor, the basilar membrane, also pursues a spiral course up the duct, and since the ribbonlike organ of Corti lies on the floor of the duct, it, too, pursues a spiral course, and so it is called the *spiral organ of Corti.* This is not labeled in Figure 28-33, but it lies directly above the basilar membrane, which is labeled, and it contains a tunnel which is labeled as such in Figure 28-33. Before giving the details of its structure, we should finish our description of the cochlear duct and its environs.

Except in the area of the organ of Corti, the basilar membrane is lined by low cuboidal cells. To the inner side of the organ of Corti the periosteum of the upper surface of the osseous spiral lamina forms a fleshy elevation, the *limbus spiralis* (Fig. 28-33), which bulges into the duct. The outer margin of this limbus presents a groove known as the *internal spiral sulcus* (Fig. 28-33); the edge of the limbus spiralis that over-

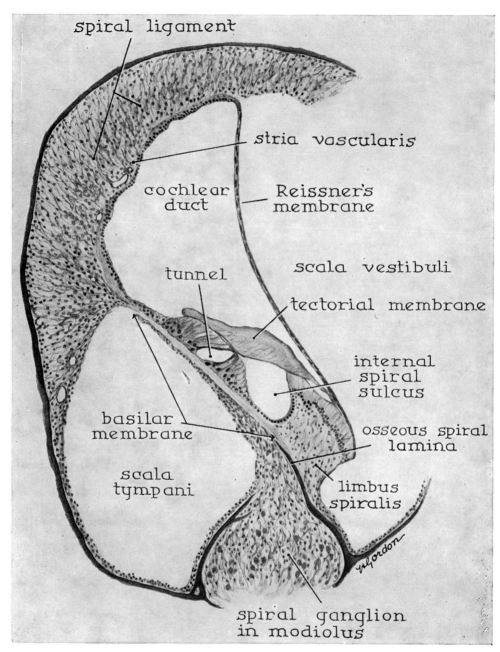

Fig. 28-33. Drawing of a portion of a section (low-power) of the bony cochlea cut parallel to the modiolus and through it along the line B in Figure 28-28. A section cut in this plane cuts the bony tube, as it pursues its spiral course, approximately at right angles at several different sites. Only one cross section of the bony tube is illustrated in this figure; it shows the cochlear duct extending across the bony canal, as well as the features described in the text. The structures in the lower portion of the cochlear duct above the basilar membrane and adjacent part of the osseous spiral lamina are the organ of Corti.

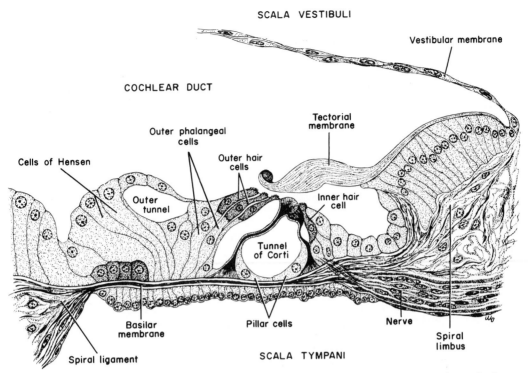

FIG. 28-34. Organ of Corti in the guinea pig (drawn from a light microscope section stained with hematoxylin-eosin). From the base up, the first structure is the epithelium of the scala tympani, which is columnar under the basilar membrane but squamous under the spiral ligament at left and under the spiral limbus at right. The organ of Corti arises from a transformation of the epithelium of the cochlear duct in contact with the basilar membrane, and includes the large epithelial *cells of Hensen* at left, enclosing a space called the outer tunnel; the *outer phalangeal cells,* which are not prominent in this species and support the *outer hair cells;* the *pillar cells* enclosing the tunnel of Corti; the *inner hair cell* supported by the *inner phalangeal cells;* and a row of various epithelial cells from which comes the *tectorial membrane,* which comes quite close to the two types of hair cells. At top, the vestibular membrane separates the cochlear duct from the scala vestibuli. (Illustration provided by C. P. Leblond and Y. Clermont)

hangs this is called the *vestibular lip*. From this lip of the limbus a thin, homogeneous, jellylike membrane extends over and is in contact with the hairs of the hair cells of the organ of Corti (soon to be described). This is the *tectorium* or *tectorial membrane* (Fig. 28-33).

The lining of the scala tympani and of the scala vestibuli (apart from that provided by the basilar membrane, Reissner's membrane and the spiral ligament) is composed of the internal periosteum or endosteum of the bony cochlear canal.

Details of the Structure of the Organ of Corti. The characteristic microscopic structure of the organ of Corti is rigidly maintained along its course in the cochlear duct, particularly in the arrangement of the tunnels and the upright position of the hair cells on the basilar membrane. Two important factors contrib-

uting to this constancy of structure are: first, the basilar membrane, which is continuous with the osseous spiral lamina, offers a rigid base (though capable of vibration). Second, some of the cells of the organ of Corti placed on this base are specially endowed with rigidity (the tunnel pillars, the phalangeal cells and the hair cells themselves) because all of these cells contain thick bundles of fibrillar material that stains with the TPA technic. Because of this internal support, these cells possess the stiffness required to maintain the esoteric shape and arrangement of the components of the organ of Corti along its course.

When the cells of the organ of Corti are listed in a medial direction (from left to right in Fig. 28-34) a group of epithelial cells is first encountered, the tallest of which are the *cells of Hensen* (Fig. 28-34); these have no special characteristics. Next are the *outer pha-*

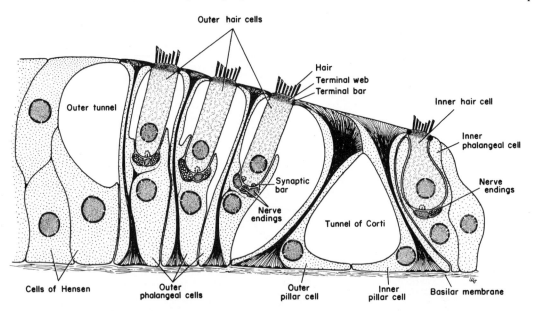

FIG. 28-35. Diagram of the sensory portion of the organ of Corti based on various electron microscopic studies in man and monkey. The cells on the basilar membrane include, from left to right: the cells of Hensen, enclosing the outer tunnel, and then 3 outer phalangeal cells which contain a thin column of rigid material (TPA-stained microtubules) extending from hemidesmosomes at the base to the apical surface (at left of each cell), with a small branch extending to the right below the nerve endings and the base of the outer hair cells. The nerve endings come either from afferent nerves ending in front of synaptic bars of the hair cells (these are sensory nerve endings, finely stippled and labeled in the diagram) or from efferent nerves ending in a swelling containing synaptic vesicles (the vesicles are shown as small circles in some nerve endings of the diagram). Next, the tunnel of Corti is enclosed by the outer and inner pillar cells containing prominent columns of rigid material. At right, the inner hair cell is supported by the inner phalangeal cell. (Illustration provided by C. P. Leblond and Y. Clermont)

langeal cells (Fig. 28-34); these are tall columnar cells which serve as support for the outer hair cells (to be described below), and they also provide support for the nerve endings at the bases of the hair cells. The characteristic feature of an outer phalangeal cell is the presence in its cytoplasm of a TPA-staining column of fibrillar material which starts from half-desmosomes on the membrane at the base of the cell (Fig. 28-34), runs upward through the cytoplasm of the cell, and, just before reaching the bottom of the hair cell which it supports, extends on toward the surface beside the hair cell as a thin process called the phalanx, which is composed of scanty cytoplasm around the TPA-stained column (Fig. 28-35). At the surface of the organ of Corti (that is, on a level with the surface of the hair cells), the phalangeal process, still containing cytoplasm and TPA-stained material, expands into a flat plate connected by junctional complexes to the hair cells. The TPA-stained material of the column and of the plate, when examined in the electron microscope, prove to consist of a thick bundle

of microtubules which end in junctional complexes connecting with hair cells. It may be emphasized that, since the free surface of the phalangeal processes (underlaid by microtubules) is on a level with the free surface of hair cells (which will be shown below to be underlaid by terminal web filaments), they together make up a single plane (which is inadequately named "reticular lamina").

The *outer and inner pillar cells* (Fig. 28-35) are located, one to either side of the tunnel of Corti. They are modified phalangeal cells. Like the previously described phalangeal cells, they extend up to the surface of the organ of Corti. They also each contain a column of TPA-staining material running from base to apex, as indicated in Figure 28-35, but this column is thicker than in phalangeal cells. The EM shows again that the column is composed of packed microtubules.

The hair cells are also classified as outer and inner. There are from 3 to 5 rows of the *outer hair cells* but only 1 row of *inner hair cells*. They demonstrate many interesting features; a notable one is the way in which they are supported. Their bases do not rest on the basilar membrane; instead, as is shown in Figure 28-35, their bases are cradled in cuplike declivities in the cytoplasm of the phalangeal cells. The hair cells themselves are characterized by several features, now to be described.

First, each hair cell has a thick layer of terminal web underlying its free surface and around its edges. This web connects with the junctional complexes, which in turn connect with the TPA-stained material of the phalangeal processes (Fig. 28-35). Second, the free surface of a hair cell has hairlike processes extending from it; these the EM has shown to be large microvilli. They are often referred to as stereocilia. Unlike typical microvilli, they are narrow near their point of origin from the cell, and they widen out in a fanlike way towards their tips. They are arranged on the cell surface in a characteristic pattern, which, when looked at from above, makes up a more or less regular V. At the tip of the V in the young there is a typical cilium. However, in the adult the cilium disappears, although its basal body persists.

A third feature of the hair cells is that their bases have a rounded form, and on this rounded surface there are nerve endings (Fig. 28-35).

As illustrated in Figure 28-35, and described in the legend of that figure, there are two types of nerve endings on the bases of hair cells, afferent and efferent. At the site of contact with an afferent ending there is, in the cytoplasm of the hair cell, a small perpendicular dark rod (the synaptic bar) surrounded by a single row of tiny vesicles (Fig. 28-35).

The sounds received by the external ear and transmitted through the oval window to the perilymph of the scala tympani make the basilar membrane vibrate. This vibration predominates in a given portion of the organ of Corti according to the frequency of the sound. It is further believed that the vibration is transferred to the hair cells, as a result of interaction of their hairs with the tectorial membrane. This somehow causes the hair cells to alter the pattern of action potential activity in the afferent branches of the acoustic nerve which they contact. (It may be added that some large nerve endings, which contain synaptic vesicles, are believed to pass on stimuli to the hair cells. These nerve endings are connected to efferent nerve fibers.)

Nervous impulses from the endings of the nerve fibers at the bases of the hair cells are carried by fibers that run in the basilar membrane (Fig. 28-34) and then between the 2 thin plates of bone that constitute the osseous spiral lamina (Fig. 28-34) to their nerve cell bodies in the *spiral ganglion,* which is housed in the modiolus (Fig. 28-33). These peripheral fibers may

be considered dendrites of the spiral ganglion cells. A single dendrite may have many peripheral branches and so receive stimuli from many hair cells. The bipolar cells of the ganglion send their central processes or axons (as the cochlear division of the auditory nerve) to end synaptically in the cochlear nuclei of the brain stem.

The Vestibule. In the bony vestibule, filled with perilymph, are suspended the sacs of the membranous labyrinth—the utricle and the saccule. These 2 sacs, filled with endolymph, are joined by the short arms of a Y-shaped tube, the *ductus endolymphaticus.* The long arm of the Y extends through the petrous bone to the posterior cranial fossa, where it ends in a blind subdural swelling, the *subdural endolymphatic sac.*

Into the utricle open the ends of the 3 membranous semicircular canals. Each canal has one expanded end or ampulla (Fig. 28-29). The nonexpanded ends of the superior and the posterior ducts have a common opening into the utricle, whereas the others open independently. Hence, for the 3 canals there are 5 openings into the utricle: one opening adjacent to each of the 3 ampullae, one opening from the nonampullated end of the horizontal duct, and one opening common to the nonampullated ends of the superior and posterior ducts. Since each semicircular canal opens at both its ends into the utricle, the semicircle of endolymph in each canal is joined into a circle through the utricular endolymph.

The utricle and the saccule are lined by flattened epithelial cells, usually called *mesothelium,* resting on a connective tissue membrane. The membranous sacs do not fill the bony vestibular space; nor do they lie free in this space, since fine strands of connective tissue connect them to the endosteum lining the bony vestibule. The saccule and the utricle each contains a flat, plaquelike sensory ending, called a *macula* (Fig. 28-36).

Maculae. A macula is somewhat similar cytologically to the organ of Corti. It consists of a thickened epithelium, containing neuroepithelial cells and supporting cells which are separated from a connective tissue layer by a basement membrane.

There are two types of neuroepithelial cells in the maculae: one type is flask-shaped, and the other type is cylindrical. Both kinds are provided at their free ends with a tuft of fine hairs which are similar to those of the organ of Corti (so they also are microvilli and often referred to as stereocilia) except that they may be much longer; some reach at least 100 microns. In addition to 80 or so stereocilia, each of the neuroepithelial cells of the maculae and cristae has also a single kinocilium, which has a more complex structure (9

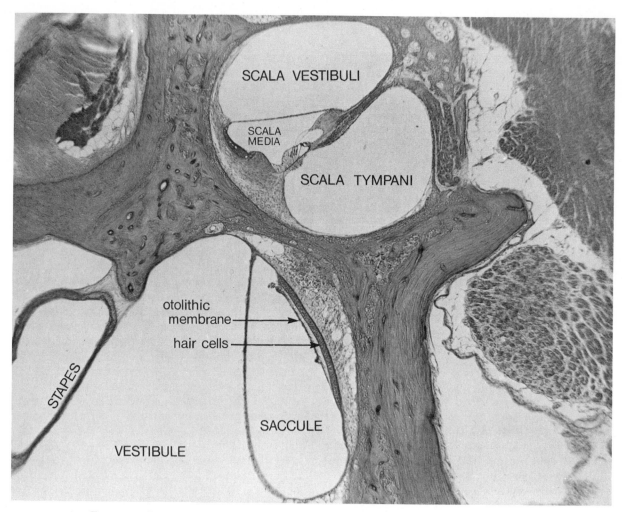

FIG. 28-36. Low-power photomicrograph of a horizontal section cut through the inner ear of a squirrel monkey. It shows the stapes in the oval window, the saccule with the macula adherent to bone and with its surface of hair cells covered by the otolithic membrane, and the organ of Corti (not labeled) in the scala media of the cochlea. (Courtesy of K. E. Money and J. Laufer)

peripheral double tubular filaments and 2 central single tubular filaments) and is longer than the stereocilia. The hairs of the neuroepithelial cells do not float freely in the endolymph but are embedded in a gelatinous membrane called the *otolithic membrane* (*oto,* ear; *lith,* stone) (Fig. 28-36). This membrane includes a surface layer of calcium carbonate crystals that have a specific gravity of approximately 3, much greater than the specific gravity of the surrounding endolymph (see references to Lim and Lane and Lim).

The otolithic membrane lies upon the macula like a flat stone upon a plate. If the head, and therefore the macula (plate), is tilted with respect to gravity, the otolithic membrane (stone) tends to slide down-

hill. This downhill movement pulls on the hairs and alters the activity in the nerve fibers supplying the macula so that the direction and magnitude of the tilt is reported to the brain. Similarly, if the head is given a linear (straight line) acceleration forward, as during the acceleration of an automobile, the otolithic membranes tend to slide on the maculae posteriorly (as a stone on a plate would move during the acceleration of the plate). The utricular otolith organs can therefore be considered to be sensors of gravity and linear acceleration. If the otolithic membranes are removed from the maculae of the guinea pig by centrifuging, the animal loses much of its sense of gravity and fails to show the usual postural responses to tilting and dropping. It is not known whether the saccular otolith organs are part of the organ of balance as the utricular otolith organs are; the saccules may play a role in the sensing of low-frequency vibration. There is, however, opinion to the effect that in man the saccule is probably a sensor of gravity and linear acceleration (*see* Fernandez *et al.*).

The Semicircular Canals. The membranous semicircular canals are lined with a squamous epithelium similar to that lining the saccule and the utricle. This also rests on a framework of connective tissue. The membranous tubes take up only a small part of the bony canal and are eccentrically placed, being in contact with the concave wall of the bony canal. Filaments of connective tissue join the tubes to the more distant parts of the canal, and perilymph fills the interstices.

The outer wall (most distant from the center of the rough circle made by each tube) of each ampulla presents a transverse ridge in its lining, the *crista*. This is composed of neuroepithelial cells (hair cells), connective tissue, nerve fibers and capillaries. The surface epithelium of the crista is similar to that of the macula, possessing both flask-shaped and cylindrical hair cells with large, oval, deep-staining nuclei and supporting cells packed closely, next to the basement membrane (Fig. 28-37). Resting on the surface of the crista is a structure which closely resembles the tectorial membrane; this is called the cupula (L., a cup) (Fig. 28-37). It is a gelatinous noncellular structure which covers the crista and projects up into the endolymph of the ampulla. The cupula differs from the otolithic membrane in that it contains no crystals and has specific gravity equal to that of the surrounding endolymph. In the case of the cupula, the change which causes movement is *angular* acceleration. Angular acceleration, which can be measured in revolutions per minute per second (rpm/sec.), should not be confused with linear acceleration, which can be measured in miles per hour per second (mph/sec.). Angular acceleration is rate of change of rotational velocity, whereas linear acceleration is rate of change of translational (linear) velocity.

It is now known that the cupula is larger than was hitherto believed; it shrinks in the course of histological fixation and dehydration. In life, each cupula extends from the crista completely across the ampulla and closes the lumen of the ampulla like a flap valve or swinging door hinged at the crista. When the head is given an angular acceleration, for example, about the spinal axis, the ring of endolymph in the horizontal semicircular canal (completed in the utricular endolymph) tends to remain stationary because of its in-

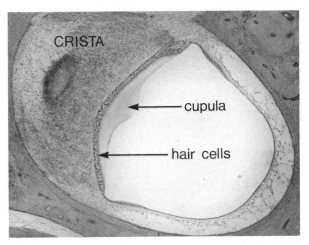

FIG. 28-37. Low-power photomicrograph of a sagittal section cut through the ampulla of a lateral semicircular canal of a squirrel monkey. In life, the crista and cupula together form a complete partition across the ampulla in this plane, but the cupula shrinks greatly with fixation. (Courtesy of Jerry Laufer)

ertia, and the membranous walls move relative to the endolymph. This movement displaces the cupula from its usual position relative to the crista, and the displacement pulls on the hairs and changes the activity in the nerve fibers supplying the crista so that information concerning the angular movement is reported to the brain. The semicircular canals can therefore be considered sensors of angular movement.

If the semicircular canals are discretely inactivated in the cat by experimental surgery, the animal exhibits angular oscillations of the head for several days after the operation, and although it learns to walk normally, it continues to fall down much more frequently than a normal cat. Inactivation of the semicircular canals in dogs produces a similar result and also confers immunity to motion sickness. In man, also, loss of the labyrinths (for example, by meningitis) causes postural instability and immunity to motion sickness.

References and Other Reading

GENERAL

Barr, M. L.: The Human Nervous System. New York, Harper and Row, 1972.

SPECIAL

Afferent Nerve Endings

(References for the olfactory organ, eye, taste buds, and ear are listed under separate headings.)

Boyd, I. A.: The structure and innervation of the nuclear bag muscle fiber system and the nuclear chain muscle fiber system in mammalian muscle spindles. Philos. Trans. Roy. Soc. B., *245:*81, 1962.

Bridgman, C. F.: Comparisons in structure of tendon organs in the rat, cat and man. J. Comp. Neurol., *138:*369, 1970.

Cauna, N.: Structure of digital touch corpuscles. Acta Anat., *32:*1, 1958.

Cauna, N., and Mannan, G.: The structure of human digital Pacinian corpuscles and its functional significance. J. Anat., *92:*1, 1958.

———: Development and postnatal changes in digital Pacinian corpuscles in the human hand. J. Anat., *93:*271, 1959.

Cooper, Sybil, and Daniel, P. M.: Muscle spindles in man; their morphology in the lumbricals and the deep muscles of the neck. Brain, *85:*563, 1963.

Davis, H.: Some principles of sensory receptor action. Physiol. Rev., *41:*391, 1963.

Duthie, H. L., and Gairns, F. W.: Sensory nerve-endings and sensation in the anal region of man. Brit. J. Surg., *47:*585, 1960.

Keller, J. H., and Moffett, B. C., Jr.: Nerve endings in the temporomandibular joint of the Rhesus macaque. Anat. Rec., *160:*587, 1968.

Kennedy, W. R.: Innervation of normal human muscle spindles. Neurology, *20:*463, 1970.

Lewis, T.: Pain. New York, Macmillan, 1942.

Loewenstein, W. R.: Biological transducers. Sci. Am., *203:*98, 1960.

Merrillees, N. C. R., Sunderland, S., and Hayhow, W.: Neuromuscular spindles in the extraocular muscles in man. Anat. Rec., *108:*23, 1950.

Pease, D. C., and Quilliam, T. A.: Electron microscopy of the Pacinian corpuscle. J. Biophys. Biochem. Cytol., *3:*331, 1957.

Sanders, F. K.: Special senses, cutaneous sensation. Ann. Rev. Physiol., *9:*553, 1947.

Shanthaveerappa, T. R., and Bourne, G. H.: New observations on the structure of the Pacinian corpuscle and its relation to the perineural epithelium of peripheral nerves. Am. J. Anat., *112:*97, 1963.

Sinclair, D. C.: Cutaneous Sensation. London, Oxford University Press, 1967.

Straile, W. E.: Encapsulated nerve end-organs in the rabbit, mouse, sheep and man. J. Comp. Neurol., *136:*317, 1969.

Takashi, M., Sakai, I., and Usizima, H.: On the terminal neural apparatus detectible in the retroperitoneum of man—a complex pattern of Pacinian corpuscles. Anat. Rec., *122:*17, 1955.

The Olfactory Organ

Arstila, A., and Wersäll, J.: The ultrastructure of the olfactory epithelium of the guinea pig. Acta Oto-laryng., *64:*187, 1967.

Frisch, D.: Ultrastructure of mouse olfactory mucosa. Am. J. Anat., *121:*87, 1967.

Smith, C. G.: Changes in the olfactory mucosa and the olfactory nerves following intranasal treatment with 1 percent zinc sulphate. Canad. Med. Assoc. J., *39:*138, 1938.

———: Incidence of atrophy of the olfactory nerves in man. Arch. Oto-laryng., *34:*533, 1941.

———: Pathologic changes in olfactory mucosa of albino rats with "stunted" olfactory bulbs. Arch. Oto-laryng., *25:*131, 1937.

———: Regeneration of sensory olfactory epithelium and nerves in adult frogs. Anat. Rec., *109:*661, 1951.

The Eye

Ascher, K. W.: Further observations on aqueous veins. Am. J. Ophthal., *29:*1373, 1946.

Ashton, N.: Anatomical study of Schlemm's canal and aqueous veins by means of neoprene casts; aqueous veins. Brit. J. Ophthal., *35:*291, 1951.

Aurell, G., and Holmgren, H.: Metachromatic substance in cornea with special reference to question of its transparency. Nord. Med., *30:*1277, 1946.

Basu, P. K., Miller, I., and Ormsby, H. L.: Sex chromatin as a biologic cell marker in the study of the fate of corneal transplants. Am. J. Ophthal., *49:*513, 1960.

Basu, P. K., and Ormsby, H. L.: Identification of sex chromatin in corneal stroma cells for the determination of the fate of corneal transplants. Transplant. Bull., *23:*435, 1959.

Cook, C., and Macdonald, R. K.: Effect of cortisone on the permeability of the blood-aqueous barrier to fluorescein. Brit. J. Ophthal., *35:*730, 1951.

Coulombre, A. J.: Cytology of the developing eye. Int. Rev. Cytol., *11,* 1961.

Davson, H.: The Physiology of the Eye. New York, Blakiston Division of McGraw-Hill, 1949.

DeRobertis, E.: Electron microscope observations on the submicroscopic organization of retinal rods. J. Biophys. Biochem. Cytol., *2:*319, 1956.

———: Morphogenesis of the retinal rods; an electron microscope study. J. Biophys. Biochem. Cytol. (Suppl.), *2:*209, 1956.

DeRobertis, E., and Franchi, C. M.: Electron microscope observations on synaptic vesicles in synapses of the retinal rods and cones. J. Biophys. Biochem. Cytol., *2:*307, 1956.

Dowling, J. E.: Foveal receptors of the monkey retina: Fine Structure. Science, *147:*57, 1965.

Droz, B.: Dynamic condition of proteins in the visual cells of rats and mice as shown by radioautography with labeled amino acids. Anat. Rec., *145:*157, 1963.

Duke-Elder, W. S.: Text-book of Ophthalmology. ed. 2. St. Louis, C. V. Mosby, 1938-40.

Duke-Elder, W. S., and Davson, H.: The present position of the problem of the intra-ocular fluid and pressure. Brit. J. Ophthal., *32:*555, 1948.

Duke-Elder, W. S., Davson, H., and Maurice, D. M.: Studies on the intra-ocular fluids. Brit. J. Ophthal., *33:* Part 1, p. 21, January 1949; Part 2, p. 329, June 1949; Part 3, p. 452, July 1949; Part 4, p. 593, October 1949.

Friedenwald, J. S.: The formation of the intraocular fluid. Am. J. Ophthal., *32:*9, 1949.

———: Recent studies on corneal metabolism and growth. Cancer Res., *10:*461, 1950.

Garrow, L. K., and Feeney, M. L.: Electron microscopic studies of the human eye, Part 2. Arch. Ophthal., *62:*966, 1959.

Greaves, D. P., and Perkins, E. S.: Influence of the sympathetic nervous system on the intra-ocular pressure and vascular circulation of the eye. Brit. J. Ophthal., *36:*258, 1952.

Hollenberg, M. J., and Bernstein, M. H.: Fine structure of the photoreceptor cells of the ground squirrel. Am. J. Anat., *118:*359, 1966.

Holmberg, A.: The fine structure of the inner wall of Schlemm's canal. Arch. Ophthal., *62:*956, 1959.

Jakus, M. A.: Studies on the cornea: II. The fine structure of Descemet's membrane. J. Biophys. Biochem. Cytol. (Suppl.), *2:*243, 1956.

Krause, A. C., and Sibley, J. A.: Metabolism of the retina. Arch. Ophthal. (N.S.), *36:*328, 1946.

Langley, D., and Macdonald, R. K.: Clinical method of observing changes in the rate of flow of aqueous humour in the human eye. Brit. J. Ophthal., *36:*432, 1952.

MacMillan, J. A.: Disease of the lacrimal gland and ocular complications. J.A.M.A., *138:*801, 1948.

Mann, I. C.: The Development of the Human Eye. London, Cambridge University Press, 1928.

Meyer, K.: The biological significance of hyaluronic acid and hyaluronidase. Physiol. Rev., *27:*355, 1947.

Meyer, K., and Chaffee, E.: The mucopolysaccharide acid of the cornea and its enzymatic hydrolysis. Am. J. Ophthal., *23:*1320, 1940.

Oppenheimer, D. R., Palmer, E., and Weddell, G.: Nerve endings in the conjunctiva. J. Anat., *92:*321, 1958.

Pease, D. C.: Infolded basal plasma membranes found in epithelia noted for their water transport. J. Biophys. Biochem. Cytol. (Suppl.), *2:*203, 1956.

Pirie, A.: The effect of hyaluronidase on the vitreous humour of the rabbit. Brit. J. Ophthal., *33:*678, 1949.

Polyak, S. L.: The Retina. Chicago, University of Chicago Press, 1941.

Reyer, R. W.: Further studies on lens development from the dorsal iris of Triturus viridescens in the absence of the embryonic lens. J. Exp. Zool., *125:*1, 1954.

————: Regeneration of the lens in the amphibian eye. Quart. Rev. Biol., *29:*1, 1954.

Richardson, K. C.: The fine structure of the albino rabbit iris with special reference to the identification of adrenergic and cholinergic nerves and nerve endings in the intrinsic muscles. Am. J. Anat., *114:*173, 1964.

Sheldon, H.: An electron microscope study of the epithelium in the normal mature and immature mouse cornea. J. Biophys. Biochem. Cytol., *2:*253, 1956.

Sheldon, H., and Zetterqvist, H.: An electron microscope study of the corneal epithelium in the vitamin A deficient mouse. Bull. Johns Hopkins Hosp., *98:*372, 1956.

Sjostrand, F. S.: The electron microscopy of the retina. *In* Smelser, G. K. (ed.): The Structure of the Eye. New York, Academic Press, 1961.

Tokuyasu, K., and Yamada, R.: The fine structure of the retina studied with the electron microscope. J. Biophys. Biochem. Cytol., *6:*225, 1959.

Wanko, T., and Gavin, M. A.: Electron microscope study of lens fibers. J. Biophys. Biochem. Cytol., *6:*97, 1959.

Willis, N. R., Hollenberg, M. J., and Brackevelt, C. R.: The fine structure of the lens of the fetal rat. Canad. J. Ophthal., *4:*307, 1969.

Wolken, J. J.: The photoreceptor structures. Int. Rev. Cytol., *11,* 1961.

Woodin, A. M.: Hyaluronidase as a spreading factor in the cornea. Brit. J. Ophthal., *34:*375, 1950.

Wyburn, G. M., and Bacsich, P.: Survival of retinal elements in subcutaneous homografts. Brit. J. Ophthal., *36:*438, 1952.

Young, R. W.: The renewal of photoreceptor cell outer segments. J. Cell Biol., *33:*61, 1967.

————: The organization of vertebrate photoreceptor cells. *In* Straatsma, B. R., Hall, M. O., Allen, R. A., and Crescitelli, F. (eds.): The Retina: Morphology, Function and Clinical Characteristics. UCLA Forum in Medical Sciences, No. 8. Berkeley and Los Angeles, University of California Press, 1969.

————: A difference between rods and cones in the renewal of outer segment protein. Invest. Ophthalmology, *8:*222, 1969.

————: Visual cells. Sci. Am., *223:*80, 1970.

————: The renewal of rod and cone outer segments in the Rhesus monkey. J. Cell Biol., *49:*303, 1971.

Taste Buds

Beidler, L. N., and Smallman, R. L. S.: Renewal of cells within taste buds. J. Cell Biol., *27:*263, 1965.

Murray, R. G., Murray, A., and Fujimoto, S.: Fine structure of gustatory cells. J. Ultrastruct. Res., *27:*444, 1969.

The Ear

Anson, B. J., and Cauldwell, E. W.: The developmental anatomy of the human stapes. Ann. Otol., *51:*891, 1942.

Bast, T. H.: A historical survey of the structure and function of the cochlea. Ann. Otol., *52:*281, 1943.

Batteau, D. W.: Role of the pinna in localization: theoretical and physiological consequences. *In* Hearing Mechanisms in Vertebrates, A Ciba Foundation Symposium. p. 234-243. London, J. A. Churchill, 1968.

Davies, D. V.: A note on the articulation of the auditory ossicles and related structures. J. Laryng., *62:*533, 1948.

Duvall, A. J., Flock, A., and Wersäll, J.: The ultrastructure of the sensory hairs and associated organelles of the cochlear inner hair cell with reference to directional sensitivity. J. Cell Biol., *29:*497, 1966.

Engström, H., and Wersäll, J.: Structure and innervation of the inner ear sensory epithelia. Int. Rev. Cytol., *7,* 1958.

Fernandez, C., Goldberg, J. M., and Abend, W. R.: Response to static tilts of peripheral neurons innervating otolith organs of the squirrel monkey. J. Neurophysiol., *35:*978, 1972.

Flock, Å.: The structure of the macula utriculi with special reference to directional interplay of sensory response as revealed by morphological polarization. J. Cell Biol., *22:*413, 1964.

————: Electron microscopic and electrophysiological studies on the lateral line canal organ. Acta Oto-laryng. (Suppl.), *199,* 1965.

Flock, Å., and Wersäll, J.: A study of the orientation of the sensory hairs of the receptor cells in the lateral line organ of fish, with special reference to the function of the receptors. J. Cell Biol., *15:*19, 1962.

Hawkins, J. E., Jr.: Cytoarchitectural basis of the cochlear transduct. Sympos. Quant. Biol. (Cold Spring Harbor), *30:*147, 1965.

Hawkins, J. E., and Johnsson, L.-G.: Light microscopic observations of the inner ear in man and monkey. Ann. Otol., *77:*608, 1968.

Johnsson, L.-G., and Hawkins, J. E., Jr.: Otolithic membranes of the saccule and utricle in man. Science, *157:*1454, 1967.

Kimura, R., Lundquist, P. G., and Wersäll, J.: Secretory epithelial linings in the ampullae of the guinea pig labyrinth. Acta Oto-laryng., *57:*517, 1963.

Lim, D. J.: Formation and fate of the otoconia, scanning and transmission electron microscopy. Ann. Otol. Rhinol. Laryngol., *82:*23, 1973.

Lim, J., and Lane, W. C.: Three-dimensional observations of the inner ear with the scanning electron microscope. Trans. Am. Acad. Ophthal. Otolaryngol., 842-872, Sept.-Oct. 1969.

Lundquist, P. G., Kimura, R., and Wersäll, J.: Ultrastructural organization of the epithelial lining in the endolymphatic duct and sac in the guinea pig. Acta Oto-laryng., *57:*65, 1963.

————: Experiments in endolymph circulation. Acta Oto-laryng. (Suppl.), *188:*198, 1964.

Money, K. E., and Friedberg, J.: The role of the semicircular canals in causation of motion sickness and nystagmus in the dog. Canad. J. Physiol. Pharmacol., *42:*793, 1964.

Money, K. E., and Scott, J. W.: Functions of separate sensory receptors of nonauditory labyrinth of the cat. Am. J. Physiol., *202:*1211, 1962.

Montagna, W.: The pigment and fatty substances of the ceruminous glands of man. Anat. Rec., *100:*66, 1948.

Montagna, W., Noback, C. R., and Zak, F. G.: Pigment, lipids and other substances in the glands of the external auditory meatus of man. Am. J. Anat., *83:*409, 1948.

Polyak, S. L., McHugh, G., and Judd, D. K.: The Human Ear. Elmsford, N.Y., Sonotone Corp., 1946.

Potter, A. B.: Function of the stapedius muscle. Ann. Otol., *45:*638, 1936.

Shambaugh, G. E.: Cytology of the Internal Ear. *In* Cowdry's Special Cytology. ed. 2, p. 1333. New York, Hoeber, 1932.

Smith, C. A.: Ultrastructure of the organ of Corti. Advanc. Sci., p. 419, 1968.

————: Electron microscopy of the inner ear. Ann. Otol., *77:*629, 1968.

Wersäll, J.: Studies on the structure and innervation of the sensory epithelium of the cristae ampullares in the guinea pig; a light and electron microscopic investigation. Acta Oto-laryng. (Suppl.), *126:*1, 1956.

————: Efferent innervation of the inner ear. *In* Von Euler, C., *et al.* (eds.): Structure and Function of Inhibitory Neuronal Mechanisms. p. 123. Oxford and New York, Pergamon Press, 1968.

Wersäll, J., and Flock, Å.: Physiological aspects on the structure of vestibular end organs. Oto-laryng. (Suppl.), *192:*85, 1964.

Wersäll, J., Flock, Å., and Lundquist, P. G.: Structural basis for directional sensitivity in cochlear and vestibular sensory receptors. Sympos. Quant. Biol. (Cold Spring Harbor), *30:*115, 1965.

Wiggers, H. C.: The functions of the intra-aural muscles. Am. J. Physiol., *120:*771, 1937.

Index